Mosby's

CANADIAN MANUAL
of DIAGNOSTIC
and LABORATORY TESTS

SECOND CANADIAN EDITION

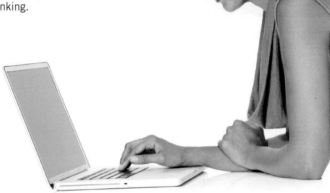

Mosby's

CANADIAN MANUAL of DIAGNOSTIC and LABORATORY TESTS

SECOND CANADIAN EDITION

KATHLEEN DESKA PAGANA, PHD, RN
Professor Emeritus
Department of Nursing
Lycoming College
President, Pagana Keynotes & Presentations
http://www.KathleenPagana.com
Williamsport, Pennsylvania

TIMOTHY J. PAGANA, MD, FACS
Medical Director, Emeritus
The Kathryn Candor Lundy Breast Health Center and The SurgiCenter
Susquehanna Health System
Williamsport, Pennsylvania

CANADIAN EDITOR
SANDRA A. PIKE-MacDONALD, RN, BN, MN, PHD
Professor
School of Nursing
Memorial University of Newfoundland
St. John's, Newfoundland

ELSEVIER

ELSEVIER

MOSBY'S CANADIAN MANUAL OF DIAGNOSTIC AND LABORATORY TESTS,
SECOND CANADIAN EDITION ISBN: 978-0-323-56746-6

Notices

Practitioners and researchers must always rely on their own experience and knowledge in evaluating and using any information, methods, compounds or experiments described herein. Because of rapid advances in the medical sciences, in particular, independent verification of diagnoses and drug dosages should be made. To the fullest extent of the law, no responsibility is assumed by Elsevier, authors, editors or contributors for any injury and/or damage to persons or property as a matter of products liability, negligence or otherwise, or from any use or operation of any methods, products, instructions, or ideas contained in the material herein.

Library of Congress Control Number: 2018944801

VP Medical and Canadian Education: Madelene J. Hyde
Content Strategist (Acquisitions): Roberta A. Spinosa-Millman
Content Development Manager: Luke Held
Content Development Specialist: Kelly Skelton
Publishing Services Manager: Deepthi Unni
Senior Project Manager: Manchu Mohan
Design Direction: Paula Catalano

Last digit is the print number: 9 8 7 6 5 4 3 2

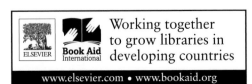

Working together
to grow libraries in
developing countries

www.elsevier.com • www.bookaid.org

Reviewers

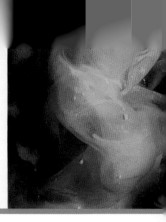

Dana Chorney, RN, BScN, MN
Professor
School of Health and Community
  Services
Durham College
Oshawa, Ontario

Brenda Dafoe Enns, MN, BA
Nursing Instructor
Baccalaureate Nursing Program
Red River College
Winnipeg, Manitoba

Chris Gabourie, CCPf, BHSc
Program Co-ordinator
Academy of Transport Medicine
Ornge Transport Medicine
Toronto, Ontario

Nicole Harder, RN, PhD
Assistant Professor
College of Nursing, Faculty of Health
  Sciences
University of Manitoba
Winnipeg, Manitoba

Joanne Jones, BSN, MSN
Senior Lecturer
School of Nursing
Thompson Rivers University
Kamloops, British Columbia

Nicole L'Italien, RN, BScN, MN
Nursing Faculty
School of Health Sciences
College of New Caledonia
Prince George, British Columbia

Janet MacIntyre, RN, MN, PhD
Faculty of Nursing
University of Prince Edward Island
Charlottetown, Prince Edward Island

Jan Maxwell, MLT, BSc
Professor
Medical Laboratory Science
St. Clair College
Windsor, Ontario

Lisa Purdy, MSc, BSc (MLS), MLT
Director, Medical Laboratory Science Program
Laboratory Medicine & Pathology
University of Alberta
Edmonton, Alberta

Faith Richardson, DNP, RN
Clinician/Educator/Researcher
Kindle Health
Aldergrove, British Columbia

Karla Wolsky, PhD
Chair, NESA BN Programs
Center for Health and Wellness
Lethbridge College
Lethbridge, Alberta

Preface

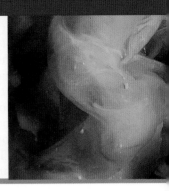

Mosby's Canadian Manual of Diagnostic and Laboratory Tests, Second Canadian Edition, provides the user with an up-to-date, extensive manual that allows rapid access to clinically relevant laboratory and diagnostic tests. The Mosby manual has been adapted to the Canadian health care system by including the following key revisions:

- Canadian coding for diagnostic and laboratory tests
- Canadian (SI) laboratory values
- Canadian legislation
- Canadian statistics
- Canadian standards of practice
- Canadian standard precautions/procedures, practice guidelines, policies
- Canadian specific tests
- Canadian screening protocols
- Canadian recommendations
- Canadian trade and generic drug names
- Canadian test-tube colour-coding classification
- Canadian cultural and racial considerations

A unique feature of the manual is its consistent format, which provides a comprehensive approach to laboratory and diagnostic tests. Tests are categorized according to either the method of testing (e.g., radiography, ultrasonography, nuclear scanning) or the type of specimen (e.g., blood, urine, stool) used for testing. The test results include the range of normal values and units of measure in both the International System of Units (SI) and the conventional units of measure. Every chapter of this book is based on this categorization. Each chapter begins with an alphabetical listing of all tests in the chapter to aid the user in locating discussions quickly. An overview follows the list and contains general information concerning test methods and related patient care.

Chapter 1 includes a discussion of guidelines for proper test preparation and performance. New information on commonly performed laboratory methods includes latex agglutination; agglutination inhibition; hemagglutination; electrophoresis; immunoassay; polymerase chain reaction; and Fluorescence in Situ Hybridization (FISH). Universal precautions or routine practices, such as the use of personal protective equipment and work practice controls, and other clinically important information for the health care provider are included to ensure worker and patient safety during the procedures, as well as accuracy in diagnostic and laboratory testing. This clinical information is essential for health care economics so that tests are performed in a timely manner and do not need to be repeated because of problems in patient preparation, test procedure, or specimen handling.

Communication and collaboration with other health care providers are emphasized. The privacy rules resulting from Canada's *Privacy Act* and the *Personal Information Protection and Electronic*

Documents Act (PIPEDA), as well as the U.S. *Health Insurance Portability and Accountability Act* (HIPAA) and *Standards for Privacy of Individually Identifiable Health Information,* are explained in relation to the health care provider's responsibility to protect access to an individual's personal health information on diagnostic and laboratory test results.

Throughout the book, information is explained in a comprehensive manner to enhance full understanding of each particular test. Every feature of test discussion is geared to provide complete information in a sequence that best simulates priorities in clinical practice. The following information is provided, whenever possible, for a thorough understanding of each diagnostic test:

- *Name of Test.* Tests are listed by their complete name. A complete list of abbreviations and alternative test names follows each main entry.
- *Normal Findings.* Normal laboratory values expressed in SI units are written in boldface purple type; conventional units are presented in parentheses after the SI units. When applicable, values are presented for infants, children, adults, and older adults. Also, where appropriate, values are separated into categories of male and female. We realize that normal ranges for laboratory tests vary significantly, depending on the method of testing and the particular laboratory. For this reason, we strongly encourage the user to check the normal values at the institution where the test is performed. This should be relatively easy because most laboratory reports indicate normal values.
- *Critical Values.* These values reflect results that are well outside the usual range for normal values. Such results generally necessitate immediate intervention. This section is noted with a special icon.
- *Indications.* This section describes the main uses for each test. Emphasis is placed on the type of signs and symptoms that lead to the indications for each test.
- *Test Explanation.* This section provides a comprehensive description of each test. The explanation includes fundamental information about basic pathophysiology in relation to the test methods, what diseases the test results may indicate, and the location where the test is generally performed. Also, in this section, sensations that the patient may experience, test duration, and the type of health care provider involved in the testing are described.
- *Contraindications.* This information alerts the user to situations in which the test should not be performed. As in other segments of the book, each contraindication is fully explained with an in-depth rationale. Situations frequently highlighted in this section include pregnancy, allergies to iodinated or contrast dye, and bleeding disorders.
- *Potential Complications.* This section alerts the user to potential problems that will necessitate astute posttesting assessments and interventions. Not only is each complication fully explained in detail, but also symptoms and appropriate interventions are described. For example, a potential complication of intravenous pyelography is renal failure, especially in older adults. An appropriate intervention may be to hydrate the patient before the test and force fluids afterward.
- *Interfering Factors.* This section includes a thorough discussion of factors that can invalidate or alter the test results. An important feature of this section is the inclusion of drugs that can interfere with test results. Drugs that increase or decrease test values are indicated by a drug icon (■) for quick access.
- *Procedure and Patient Care.* This section emphasizes the role of nurses and other health care providers in diagnostic and laboratory testing by addressing psychosocial and physiologic interventions. Patient teaching priorities are noted with a special icon (✗) to highlight information to be communicated to patients. For quick location of essential information concerning the testing procedure, this section is divided into "before," "during," and "after" time sequences.

Before. This section addresses the need to explain the procedure and to allay the patient's concerns or anxieties. Dietary restrictions, bowel preparations, baseline pretest assessment, and the need for informed consent are discussed.

During. This section provides a complete and thorough description of the testing procedure, alternative procedures, and methods of testing. In most instances, a step-by-step description of testing procedures is provided. This information is important because all health care providers involved in the particular test should have a good understanding of what the procedure entails, to assist more completely in the testing process.

After. This section includes vital information that the nurse or other health care provider should know about postprocedure care of the patient. Specific posttest assessment, medication administration, recognition of posttest complications (with suggestions for nursing interventions), home care, and follow-up are described.

- *Test Results and Clinical Significance.* As the name implies, this section describes the significance of the test findings. A unique feature of this manual, in comparison with other books on diagnostic and laboratory tests, is an extensive discussion of the pathophysiology of the disease process and how it relates to the test result. This enhances the understanding of the diagnostic test and better understanding of many disease processes.

- *Related Tests.* This section, another unique feature of the text, includes a list of tests that are related to the main test under discussion. This list includes tests that provide similar information, tests that provide confirmatory information, and other tests used to evaluate the same organ, disease process, or symptom complex. A short description and page numbers for all related tests make cross-referencing easier. This aids the reader in developing a broader understanding of diagnostic testing and indicates where the reader may obtain more information on the topic of interest.

This logical format emphasizes clinically relevant information. The clarity of the format facilitates a full understanding of content essential to both students and health care providers, and its uniformity allows the user to quickly recognize where information of interest may be found.

Multiple colours have been used to help locate tests, highlight critical information, and generally improve the readability of the text. Another key feature is the use of colour photographs and illustrations throughout the book. Many tables are also included to simplify or summarize complex material regarding clinical care, test categories, or disease processes.

🍁 A new margin icon, a maple leaf, will indicate if the information provides updated Canadian guidelines for easy identification and reference.

Feature boxes are used throughout the book to highlight and summarize important clinical data. They allow the reader to assimilate important information at a glance. There are four types of feature boxes:

 Clinical Priorities,   Age-Related Concerns,

 Cultural Considerations, and   Home Care Responsibilities.

- *Clinical Priorities* boxes emphasize pertinent information specific to understanding and performing a particular test. For example, a patient's coagulation profile must be assessed before invasive studies (e.g., liver biopsy) that may cause bleeding are performed. Chest radiographic examinations should be performed after procedures (e.g., pleural biopsy) that may cause a pneumothorax.

- *Age-Related Concerns* boxes present new research to address primarily pediatric and geriatric priorities. Pediatric priorities include the need for special consideration for different ages.

For example, depending on the child's age, the bowel preparation for the barium enema study is different. Content also includes the normal physiologic changes of aging and how those changes may affect preparation for testing, interpretation of results, and potential complications. For example, an older adult scheduled for intravenous pyelography may be at high risk for dye-induced renal failure that is related to a decrease in renal function, which in turn is associated with aging. A decrease in heart rate, a reduction in myocardial contractility, and a decrease in cardiac output are all age-related physiologic changes that can affect an older adult's response to a stress test.

- *Cultural Considerations* boxes focus on information that can have implications for ordering and interpreting laboratory and diagnostic tests. This is in recognition of the growing body of knowledge related to the cultural implications of laboratory and diagnostic testing. For example, in Canada, members of Indigenous populations are at higher risk than the general population for the development of diabetes; therefore, diabetes screening is critical in these populations in order to intervene early and prevent complications. The percentage of human immunodeficiency virus (HIV)–positive reports is also rising among Canadians of African ancestry, with heterosexual exposure accounting for more than 80% of those positive results; thus, these groups must be recognized as being at high risk, and diagnostic testing may need to be initiated.

- *Home Care Responsibilities* boxes focus on factors that need to be addressed after a test is performed. Because the numbers of procedures being performed on an outpatient basis are increasing, the patient has the responsibility for detecting problems and knowing what to do when they occur. Often, the patient returns home with instructions or guidelines for recognizing problems (such as infection, bleeding, and urinary retention).

The *Bibliography* provides the user with a list of up-to-date, current literature and research on a variety of diagnostic and laboratory tests, including clinical trials, legislative documents, screening guidelines, and recommended protocols. The list provides the user with an opportunity to further explore topics of interest. Related Elsevier texts are also included in the list, as cross-references for understanding laboratory and diagnostic tests.

Appendix A, Alphabetical List of Tests, helps the user locate specific tests at a glance. *Appendix B, List of Tests by Body System,* familiarizes the user with other related studies that the patient may need or that the user may want to review. This information should be especially useful for students and health care providers working in specialized areas. For example, all tests related to infertility are listed in the Reproductive System section. *Appendix C* provides a list of *Common Testing Profiles,* and *Appendix D* provides *Common Abbreviations and Acronyms. Appendix E,* new to this edition, provides a *List of Common Blood Tests and Values.*

A comprehensive index includes the names of all tests and their synonyms and other relevant terms found within the tests.

Common units of measurement are located on the inside front cover.

Many new studies (such as anti-glycan antibodies, cutaneous immunofluorescence antibodies, drug sensitivity genotype testing, galectin-3, serotonin and squamous cell carcinoma antigen) have been added. All other studies have been revised and updated. Outdated tests have been eliminated.

We thank Roberta A. Spinosa-Millman, Kelly Skelton, Wendy Thomas, and Manchu Mohan for their expert guidance and support.

We invite comments from users of this book so that we may improve our goal of providing useful and relevant diagnostic and laboratory test information to users of future editions.

Kathleen D. Pagana
Timothy J. Pagana
Sandra A. Pike-MacDonald

Contents

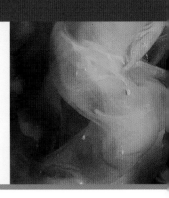

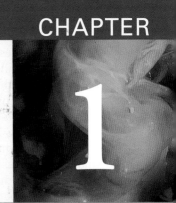
Guidelines for Proper Test Preparation and Performance

OVERVIEW

A complete evaluation of patients with signs or symptoms of disease usually requires a comprehensive history and a thorough physical examination, as well as efficient diagnostic testing. The correct use of diagnostic testing can confirm or rule out the presence of disease and improve the cost efficiency of screening tests in people without signs or symptoms of disease. Finally, appropriate and thoughtfully timed use of diagnostic testing allows monitoring and treatment of diseases.

Furthermore, health care economics necessitates that laboratory and diagnostic testing be performed accurately and in a timely manner. Tests should not have to be repeated because of improper preparation of the patient, incorrect test procedures, or an inappropriate specimen collection technique. The following guidelines describe the responsibilities of health care providers to ensure safety and accuracy in diagnostic testing.

Patient education is the most important factor to ensure accuracy and success of test results. All phases (before, during, and after) of the testing process must be thoroughly explained to the patient. The patient's complete understanding of these phases is essential for the development of nursing processes and standards of care for diagnostic testing.

The interpretation of diagnostic testing is no longer left to the physician alone. In today's complex environment of high-tech testing and economic restrictions, individuals representing many health care professions must be able to interpret diagnostic tests to develop a timely and effective interprofessional plan of care.

CODING FOR DIAGNOSTIC AND LABORATORY TESTS

The International Statistical Classification of Diseases and Related Health Problems, 10th Revision, Canada (ICD-10-CA) and the Canadian Classification of Health Interventions (CCI) provide an alphanumeric designation for diagnoses and inpatient procedures in Canada. The ICD codes are developed, monitored, and copyrighted by the World Health Organization. Using these codes, government health authorities can track diseases and conditions and causes of death and compare health outcomes. All the patient's diseases and conditions can be classified according to an ICD code, which can then be used by health care payers and providers at all points of service. Accurate coding is necessary so that data can be accurately collected, testing accurately interpreted, and medical care properly reimbursed. Complying with this coding requirement is no small task because there are about 140 000 codes in the ICD-10 catalogues. See p. 1186 for a listing of possible diagnostic tests that could be ordered with certain common diseases or conditions. The numbers and letters reflect the ICD-10-CA codes. For additional information about this Canadian coding requirement, see https://www.cihi.ca/en/submit-data-and-view-standards/codes-and-classifications/icd-10-ca.

LABORATORY METHODS

To understand laboratory diagnostic testing, it is helpful to have a basic understanding of commonly performed laboratory methods that can be used on blood, urine, spinal fluid, and other bodily specimens. Most laboratory diagnostic tests use serologic and immunologic reactions between an antibody and an antigen. *Precipitation* is a visible expression of the aggregation of soluble antigens. *Agglutination* is a visible expression of the aggregation of particulate antigens or antibodies. As the specimen is progressively diluted, persistent precipitation or agglutination indicates greater concentrations of the antigen or antibody. Dilution techniques are therefore used to quantify the pathologic antigen or antibody in the specimen. Commonly used laboratory methods and their variations are described below.

Latex Agglutination

Latex agglutination is a common laboratory method in which latex beads (that become visibly obvious when agglutination occurs) are coated with antibody molecules. When mixed with the patient's specimen containing a particular antigen, agglutination will be visibly obvious. C-reactive proteins are identified by this method. In an alternative latex agglutination method (e.g., as needed for pregnancy testing or rubella testing), latex beads are coated with a specific antigen. In the presence of antibodies in the patient's specimen to that specific antigen on the latex particles, visible agglutination occurs.

Agglutination Inhibition

Agglutination inhibition is another laboratory method based on the agglutination process. In this process, if one is trying to identify a particular molecule—for example, hCG (human chorionic gonadotropin)—the patient's specimen is incubated with anti-hCG. Latex particles coated with hCG are then added to the mixture. If the patient's specimen contains hCG, those molecules will attach to the anti-hCG during incubation, leaving no anti-hCG molecules to attach to the hCG-coated latex beads. Therefore, agglutination would not occur because the patient's endogenous hCG "inhibited" the agglutination.

Hemagglutination

Hemagglutination laboratory methods are used to identify antibodies to antigens on the cell surface of red blood cells (RBCs). Like latex, RBC agglutination is visible. Blood typing for transfusions uses this laboratory method. In an alternative method of hemagglutination, different antigens can be bound to the RBC surface. When added to the patient's specimen, specific antibodies can be identified by RBC agglutination.

Electrophoresis

Electrophoresis is an analytic laboratory method in which an electrical charge is applied to a medium on which the patient's specimen has been placed. Migration of charged molecules (particularly proteins) in the specimen can be separated in an electrical field. Proteins can then be identified based on their rate of migration. Serum protein electrophoresis utilizes this method.

Immunoelectrophoresis. Immunoelectrophoresis is a laboratory method that allows the previously electrophoresed proteins to act as antigens to which known specific antibodies are added. This provides specific protein identification. With dilution techniques as described, these particular proteins can be quantified. This method is used to identify gammopathies, hemoglobinopathies, and Bence-Jones proteins.

Immunofixation Electrophoresis. Immunofixation electrophoresis (IFE) is particularly helpful in the identification of certain diseases. In this method, a specific known antibody is added to a previously electrophoresed specimen. The antigen/antibody complexes become fixed (i.e., attached) to the electrophoretic gel medium. When the nonfixed proteins are washed away, the protein immune complexes that remain fixed to the gel are stained with a protein-sensitive stain and can be identified and quantified. IFE is particularly helpful in identifying proteins that exist in very small quantities in the serum, urine, or cerebrospinal fluid.

Immunoassay

Immunoassay is an important laboratory method of diagnosing disease. In the past, *radioimmunoassay (RIA)* was performed using a radioactive label that could identify an antibody/antigen complex at very low concentrations. Unfortunately, there are significant drawbacks of using radioactive isotopes as labels. Radioactive labels have a short half-life and are hard to keep on the shelf. These labels require considerable care to avoid environmental exposure. And finally, the costs associated with disposal of radioactive waste are high.

Enzyme-Linked Immunosorbent Assay. *Enzyme-linked immunosorbent assay (ELISA)* techniques are able to detect immunocomplexes more easily when compared to RIA. This ELISA technique (also known as *enzyme immunoassay [EIA]*) is able to detect antigens or antibodies by producing an enzyme-triggered colour change. In this method, an enzyme-labelled antibody or antigen is used in the immunologic assay to detect either suspected abnormal antibodies or antigens in the patient's specimen. In this method, a plastic bead (or a plastic test plate) is coated with an antigen (e.g., virus). The antigen is incubated with the patient's serum. If the patient's serum contains antibodies to the pathologic viral antigen, an immunocomplex forms on the bead (or plate). When a chromogenic chemical is then added, a colour change is noted and can be spectrophotometrically compared with a control (or reference) serum identification. Quantification of abnormal antibodies in the patient's serum instigated by the viral infection can then be performed. Similarly, EIA can be used for detection of pathologic antigens in the patient's serum. Testing for HIV (human immunodeficiency virus), hepatitis, or cytomegalovirus commonly uses these methods.

Autoimmune Enzyme Immunoassay. *Autoimmune enzyme immunoassay* screening tests are commonly used for the detection of antinuclear antibodies. EIA techniques (similar to what have been described above) are used as the purified nuclear antigens are bound to a series of microwells to which the patient's serum is serially diluted and added. After adding peroxidase conjugated antihuman immunoglobulin G (IgG), a complex antibody/antigen "sandwich" is identified by colour changes.

Chemiluminescent Immunoassays. *Chemiluminescent immunoassays* are extensively used in automated immunoassays. In this technique, chemiluminescent labels can be attached to an antibody or antigen. After appropriate immunoassays are obtained (as described), light emission produced by the immunologic reaction can be measured and quantified. This technique is commonly used to detect proteins, viruses, and nucleic acid sequences associated with disease.

Fluorescent Immunoassays. *Fluorescent immunoassays* consist of labelling an antibody with fluorescein. This fluorescein-labelled antibody is able to bind either directly with a particular antigen or indirectly with anti-immunoglobulins. Under a fluorescent microscope, the fluorescein becomes obvious as yellow-green light. Testing for *Neisseria gonorrhea* or antinuclear antibodies may use these laboratory methods.

With the increasing use of automated analyzers, the use of chemiluminescence and *nephelometry* has become extremely important to allow analyzers to quantify results in great numbers of specimens tested in a short period of time. Nephelometry (in auto analyzers) depends on the light-scattering properties of antigen/antibody complexes as light is passed through the test medium. The quantity of the cloudiness or turbidity in a solution then can be measured photometrically. Automated C-reactive protein, alpha antitrypsin, haptoglobins, and immunoglobulins are often measured using nephelometry.

POLYMERASE CHAIN REACTION

Since the complete human genome sequence became available in 2003, laboratory molecular genetics has become an integral part of diagnostic testing. Molecular genetics depends on an in vitro method of amplifying low levels of specific DNA sequences in a patient's specimen to raise quantities of a potentially present specific DNA sequence to levels that can be quantified by further analysis. This process is called polymerase chain reaction (PCR). This is particularly helpful in the identification of diseases caused by gene mutations (e.g., breast-related cancer in women), in the identification and quantification of infectious agents such as human papillomavirus or HIV, and in the identification of acquired genetic changes that may be present in hematologic malignancies or colon cancer.

In PCR procedures, a known particular target short DNA sequence (ranging from 100 to 1 000 nucleotide pairs) is used. This known DNA sequence "primer" is then placed in a series of reactions with the patient's specimen. These reactions are designed to markedly increase the number of comparable abnormal DNA sequences that potentially exist in the patient's specimen. The increased number of abnormal DNA sequences then can be identified and quantified. In many instances, the nucleic acid of interest is ribonucleic acid (RNA) rather than DNA. In these circumstances, the PCR procedure is modified by reverse transcription (*reverse transcriptase PCR [RT PCR]*). With RT PCR, abnormal RNA can be amplified (increased in number), detected, and quantified.

Real-time PCR uses the same reaction sequence as described. In real-time PCR, fluorescence resonance energy transfer is used to quantify the DNA sequences of interest and identify points of mutation. Real-time PCR provides a product that can be more accurately quantified.

Quantification of PCR-derived DNA/RNA products can be performed in many ways. This can be performed by simple gel electrophoresis, *DNA sequencing*, or using *DNA probes*. DNA probes are presynthesized DNA primers that are used to identify and quantify the amplified DNA produced by the PCR process. Hybridization techniques such as *liquid phase hybridization* interact with a defined DNA probe and the potential targeted DNA in solution. DNA probes have become a very important part of commercial laboratory molecular genetics. Microarray DNA chip technology (*microarray analysis*) places thousands of major DNA probes on one glass chip. After interaction with the patient's specimen, the microarray chip can be scanned with high-speed fluorescent detectors that can quantify each DNA micro sequence. This process is used to identify gene expression of malignancies and has led to a new understanding of the classification, pathophysiology, and treatment of cancer.

FLUORESCENCE IN SITU HYBRIDIZATION (FISH)

Fluorescence in situ hybridization (FISH) uses nucleic probes (short sequences of single-stranded DNA) that are complementary to the DNA sequence to be identified. These nucleic probes are labelled with fluorescent tags that can identify the exact location of the complementary DNA sequence that is being targeted. This method is particularly helpful in the detection of inherited and acquired chromosomal abnormalities common in hematologic and other oncologic conditions, such as lymphomas and breast cancer. Laboratory genetics are also discussed on p. 1139.

ROUTINE PRACTICES

The recent emergence of Ebola hemorrhagic fever and antibiotic-resistant bacteria such as methicillin-resistant *Staphylococcus aureus* (MRSA), along with the continued spread of the hepatitis B virus and HIV, has made all health care organizations aware of the need to protect health care providers. In response to these and other threats, the Public Health Agency of Canada (PHAC), the Canadian Centre for Chronic Disease Prevention and Control, the Canadian Centre for Occupational Health and Safety, and the U.S. Centers for Disease Control and Prevention (CDC) have all endorsed guidelines for routine precautions, also known as routine practices, when caring for patients.

The term *routine practices* has been used by the PHAC since 1999 and refers to a level of care that should be provided to all patients regardless of their infection status. Routine practices are more encompassing than standard or universal precautions because they include strategies to reduce the risk for transmission from patient to health care provider, from patient to patient, and from health care provider to patient. The purpose of using routine practices is to protect health care providers from contracting illnesses from the specimens they handle, the patients they care for, and the environments in which they work (Boxes 1-1 and 1-2). They are based on the assumption that all blood, body fluids, and body tissues contain infectious organisms (bacteria, viruses, and fungi); these materials include serous fluids such as pleural, peritoneal, amniotic, cerebrospinal, and synovial fluids; semen; and vaginal secretions. Routine practices reduce the risk of transmission of these microorganisms to the patient and health care provider.

Routine practices require the use of personal protective equipment (PPE), workplace controls, and engineering controls to protect health care providers from skin and mucous membrane exposure to blood and body fluids. The PHAC and the CDC have developed infection-control guidelines to ensure that health care workers are prepared to meet the global health challenge of caring for a patient with highly infectious diseases and containing the transmission of those diseases (e.g., Ebola). The appropriate level of PPE, comprehensive education on how to put on (i.e., don) and take off (i.e., doff) the PPE, following the proper decontamination protocols, and a commitment to stringent safety precautions can all help to eliminate the risk of transmitting highly infectious diseases from an infected patient. The proper sequence for donning and doffing PPE is presented in Table 1-1.

BOX 1-1 Routine Practices

The following barriers are used in routine practices with all patients to protect against occupational exposure to blood and body fluids:

Personal Protective Equipment (PPE)

PPE includes gowns, gloves, shoe covers, goggles, glasses with side shields, face masks, and protective clothing (including laboratory coat). PPE helps to create a barrier to protect eyes, nose, and mouth and to prevent any blood and body fluids from touching skin, mucous membranes, or personal clothing. Check agency policies for the PPE needed for specific patients.

Work Practice Controls

These techniques reduce the chance of exposure by changing the way a task is performed. Examples are (1) frequent handwashing (see Box 1-2); (2) availability of Ambu bags in strategic locations in the hospital setting; (3) disposal of needles that are "recapped," bent, broken, or removed from syringes; (4) immediate removal of gloves that have a hole or tear; (5) labelling of all disposed patient-related wastes as a "biohazard"; (6) prohibition of eating, drinking, applying cosmetics, or handling contact lenses in patient care areas; and (7) implementation of respiratory hygiene and cough etiquette instructions to contain respiratory secretions in patients and accompanying individuals who have signs and symptoms of a respiratory infection. Routine practices can also include posting signs for visitors with instructions about covering mouths and noses, the use and disposal of tissues, and hand hygiene. Offering masks to coughing patients and encouraging them to keep a distance of at least 1 m from other people can also protect against exposure.

Engineering Controls

These barriers help isolate or remove hazardous materials from the workplace. They can include methods for sharps disposal, such as placing all used needles, contaminated reusable sharps, and other sharps in puncture-resistant containers; the use of laboratory fume hoods to improve ventilation; and the transport of all specimens in leak-proof containers.

If a health care provider has been exposed to blood or other body fluids (e.g., through needlestick injury), testing of the provider and the patient for hepatitis B virus and HIV is necessary.

BOX 1-2 Handwashing

Wash hands with soap and water or alcohol-based hand rub:
- Before and after caring for patients
- Before and after all procedures
- Before handling food
- Before putting on gloves
- After taking off gloves
- After interventions involving blood and body fluids (e.g., venipuncture)

A fundamental principle of routine practices is frequent handwashing, especially between visits with patients and when gloves are changed. Equipment must also be cleaned between visits with patients, and patient rooms must be cleaned daily. All injuries from needles, scalpels, and other sharp devices should be reported and followed up with appropriate testing for infectious disease. Special reusable needles, such as instruments used in the operating room, must be placed in metal containers for transport to a designated area for sterilization or disinfection. Vaccination against hepatitis B virus is another safety precaution recommended by the CDC and the Canadian Centre for Occupational Health and Safety.

TABLE 1-1	Proper Sequence for Donning and Doffing Personal Protective Equipment (PPE)

Donning	Doffing
Remove personal clothing and items and change into scrubs. Inspect PPE prior to donning for defects.	Inspect PPE for any tears, contamination, or cuts. If contamination is visible, disinfect with ABHR or disinfectant wipes.
Perform hand hygiene and put on inner gloves.	Disinfect outer gloves with ABHR or disinfectant wipes.
Put on shoe covers, and gown or coveralls.	Remove apron; roll from inside to outside. Inspect PPE again as above.
Make sure cuffs of inner gloves are tucked under the gown sleeves.	Disinfect outer gloves with ABHR or disinfectant wipes.
Put on an N95 respirator; complete a user seal check.	Remove shoe covers while sitting down and discard. Disinfect and remove outer gloves.
Put on a hood and then outer apron.	Inspect and disinfect inner gloves. Remove inner gloves, perform hand hygiene, and don a clean pair of gloves.
Put on outer gloves; ensure outer glove cuffs are over gown sleeves.	Remove face shield.
	Disinfect inner gloves.
	Remove surgical hood and discard.
	Disinfect inner gloves.
Put on face shield over the surgical hood and N95 respirator.	Unfasten ties of gown and slip hands under the gown at the neck and shoulder and peel gown away from neck and shoulder. Pull gown away from the body, rolling from inside to out and touching only the inside of the gown. Turn contaminated outside toward the inside. Only the clean part of the gown should be visible.
Verify with trained observer and ensure no skin is exposed.	Disinfect and change inner gloves. Don a clean pair of gloves.
Disinfect outer gloves with an alcohol-based hand rub (ABHR) or disinfectant wipe and dry before entering room.	Remove N95 respirator.
	Disinfect inner gloves.
	Disinfect washable shoes.
	Disinfect inner gloves and remove.
	Perform hand hygiene.

Manuel, MacDonald, Alani, et al., 2014

PROPER SEQUENCING AND SCHEDULING OF TESTS

Because of the cost and complexity of laboratory and diagnostic testing, it is important that tests be scheduled in the most efficient sequential manner. Because one type of test can interfere with another, certain guidelines apply when multiple tests must be performed in a limited amount of time. Radiologic examinations that do not necessitate the use of contrast material should precede examinations in which contrast media is required. Radiologic studies involving the use of barium should be scheduled after ultrasonography studies. For example, because contrast agents can obscure visualization of other body areas on subsequent radiologic tests, radiologic studies without contrast should be performed before radiography with iodine contrast dye (such as intravenous pyelography), which in turn should be performed before radiologic studies with barium. Also, stool specimens should be collected before radiologic studies with barium.

Test sequencing affects the ability to perform tests efficiently in a limited time period. An essential component of this process is communication and collaboration with other health care providers in numerous departments.

PROCEDURE AND PATIENT CARE
Before the Test

Patient preparation is vital to the success of any diagnostic test. Patient education is also essential and is discussed later in this chapter. To develop and adhere to patient care guidelines concerning patient preparation for the test, health care providers must understand the procedure. A thorough history to identify contraindications to the specific test is vital. Providers must recognize which patients are at risk for potential complications and counsel them about those complications. The fears and concerns of the patient should be elicited and addressed before testing. To avoid misinterpreting diagnostic test results, providers must document and thoroughly understand ongoing factors (e.g., medications and previous tests) that could interfere with those results.

Pretest preparation procedures must be followed closely. Dietary restriction is often important when patients prepare for tests. Fasting is required for many blood tests and procedures. Studies necessitating fasting should be performed as early in the morning as possible to diminish patient discomfort. Fasting patients can have small amounts of water (no coffee or tea) and take medications with water, unless told not to by their physician. The patient's adherence to dietary restriction is important for accuracy of test results.

Studies such as a barium enema study, colonoscopy, upper gastrointestinal imaging series, and intravenous pyelography are more accurate if the patient has had nothing by mouth (NPO status), which means no food or fluids, not even water, for 8 to 12 hours before the test. Sometimes dietary restrictions are important for safety, especially if a sedative is to be administered during testing; for example, the patient must remain on NPO status for 8 to 12 hours before upper gastrointestinal endoscopy in order to prevent gagging, vomiting, and aspiration. Bowel preparation is necessary for many procedures designed to evaluate the mucosa of the gastrointestinal tract.

Equally important in total patient care is the coordination of ongoing therapy (e.g., physical therapy, administration of medications, other diagnostic testing). The correct timing of testing is key to accurate interpretation of results. For example, blood samples for cortisol, parathyroid hormone, and fasting glucose levels (among others) must be obtained in the early morning hours.

Patient Identification. Proper identification of the patient is critical for safety. The conscious patient should be asked to state his or her full name. The name should be checked against the patient's identification band and requisition slip. The identity of an unconscious patient should be verified by family or friends whenever possible; however, consent for treatment is implied in emergency situations. No specimens should be collected or procedure performed without proper identification of the patient. Costly tests performed on the wrong patient are useless and may be grounds for legal action. Confusion can occur when patients with the same name are on the same nursing unit. Most units have some type of warning or "name alert" to address this concern.

Patient Education. Once the patient is properly identified and the proper test or procedure is scheduled, patient education begins. It is both an ethical and a professional obligation to ensure that patients are informed about the diagnostic tests they are having done and why those tests are needed. An informed patient is also less apprehensive and more cooperative. Patient education helps prepare the patient so that the test will not need to be repeated. Fasting requirements and bowel preparations must be clearly explained to the patient. Written instructions are essential. If such material is used, the patient's literacy and understanding of the material should be validated.

Sometimes medications need to be discontinued for a period of time before certain tests. This information should be determined in consultation with the physician. Medications that are not discontinued may be listed on the requisition or documented in the chart to aid in the interpretation of test results.

Variables Affecting Test Results. Many laboratory tests are affected by individual variables that must be considered when test results are interpreted. Several of these key variables are discussed in the following sections.

Age. Pediatric reference values often differ from adult values. For some tests, values vary according to the age of the infant in weeks. For example, in the first week of life, levels of serum bilirubin, growth hormone, blood urea nitrogen, and fetal hemoglobin are elevated, whereas levels of cholesterol and haptoglobin are decreased. Healthy newborns also have an increase in total white blood cells and decreases in immunoglobulins M and A. For some tests, reference values of children are different from those of adults according to developmental stage. For example, alkaline phosphatase levels in children are much higher than adult values because of rapid bone growth.

Age-related changes are also apparent in the middle and older adult years and can have an effect on adult reference values, including changes to partial pressure of arterial oxygen (Pao_2) in relation to a decrease in respiratory muscle strength. Age-related physiologic changes can also include a decrease in stomach emptying, decreased pH, and altered gastrointestinal motility, thus affecting the absorption of medications and nutrients (e.g., decreased absorption of nutrients can affect albumin and total protein levels). Age-related cardiovascular changes include decreased cardiac output, decreased total body water, and increased adipose tissue, which can cause blood levels of medications to be higher than usual and can affect the storage of lipid-soluble medications and vitamins. Liver and kidney function also decline in older adults, resulting in changes to the metabolism of certain drugs and thus increasing patients' risk for experiencing toxicity and adverse effects. Reference values for cholesterol and triglyceride levels begin to increase in the mid-adult years. Creatinine clearance levels decrease with age in relation to changes in glomerular filtration rate. These age-related physiologic changes and their effect on laboratory values are discussed further in the feature boxes titled Age-Related Concerns.

Gender. Gender is another variable that affects reference values. Differences are usually related to increased muscle mass in men and differences in hormonal secretion. For example, men usually have higher reference values for hemoglobin, blood urea nitrogen, serum creatinine, and uric acid. Men also have higher serum levels of cholesterol and triglycerides than do premenopausal women. Sex-specific hormones also differ: men have higher testosterone levels, and women have higher levels of estrogens, follicle-stimulating hormone, and luteinizing hormones.

Race. In general, race has little effect on laboratory values. It has a greater effect on genetic diseases, such as sickle cell disease in Black people and thalassemia in individuals of Mediterranean descent.

Pregnancy. Many endocrine, hematologic, and biochemical changes occur during pregnancy. Pregnant women have increased levels of cholesterol, triglycerides, lactic dehydrogenase, alkaline phosphatase, and aspartate aminotransferase. They may have lower values of hemoglobin, hematocrit, serum creatinine, urea, glucose, albumin, and total protein.

Cultural Considerations. In general, culture has little effect on laboratory values; however, recognizing the differences in the health status indicators of various cultures is an important step to understanding the effect of culture on interpretation of test results. For example, many of the health status indicators for Indigenous peoples of Canada are different from those of the general population; these indicators include a higher prevalence of diabetes and a higher incidence of tuberculosis. Awareness of the cultural diversity of patients can alert the health care provider to the need for screening and monitoring of specific laboratory values. Interpretation of diagnostic test results in view of cultural considerations is another "way of knowing" that can help to improve the health of culturally diverse populations such as the Indigenous peoples of Canada.

Food Ingestion. Several serum values are markedly affected by food. For example, levels of glucose and triglycerides rise after a meal. To avoid the effects of diet on laboratory tests, many tests are obtained when the patient is in a fasting or NPO state.

Posture. Changes in body position affect the concentration of several components in the peripheral blood. Therefore, it is sometimes important to note whether the patient was supine, sitting, or standing when blood was drawn. Examples of laboratory values affected by posture are levels of norepinephrine, epinephrine, renin, aldosterone, protein, and potassium.

During Testing

Often a number of different health care providers are needed to successfully perform a diagnostic procedure. The health care provider's knowledge of the procedure is a major determinant of the success of the procedure. Furthermore, the presence of a knowledgeable and supportive health care provider during any procedure is invaluable for the patient and for the accuracy of the test.

Specimen Collection. Protocols and guidelines are available for each type of specimen collection. These are essential for appropriate preparation and collection. For example, the selection of the colour-coded tube depends on the type of blood test needed. Guidelines for a 24-hour urine collection must be followed to obtain a representative urine sample. These and other examples are described in detail in the sections on Procedure and Patient Care in different chapters.

Transport and Processing of the Specimen. Preparing the patient and collecting the specimen are essential. Getting the specimen to the laboratory in an acceptable state for examination is just as important. In general, the specimen should be transported to the laboratory as soon as possible after collection. Delays may result in rejection of the specimen. Specimens are usually refrigerated if transportation is delayed.

A Note About Système Internationale d'Unités. The Système Internationale d'Unités (SI units) is a system for reporting laboratory values in terms of standardized international units of measures. This system is currently used in many countries, including Canada. Throughout this book, results are presented in SI units in boldface purple type; conventional units in parentheses follow the SI units when available.

After the Test

Posttest care is an important aspect of total patient care. Attention should be directed to the patient's concerns about possible results or the difficulties of the procedure. Appropriate treatment after testing must be provided. For example, after a barium test, a cathartic is indicated. However, if a bowel obstruction has been identified, catharsis is contraindicated.

Recognition and rapid institution of treatment of complications (e.g., bleeding, shock, bowel perforation) is essential in the care of the patient who has just undergone a diagnostic procedure.

More invasive tests often necessitate heavy sedation or a surgical procedure. In these situations, aftercare is similar to routine postoperative care.

Reporting Test Results. To be clinically useful, results must be reported promptly. In Canada it is mandatory to report critical values that show a marked deviation from reference ranges as soon as they become available (Ontario Association of Medical Laboratories [OAML], 2009). Critical values are results that show a marked deviation from the reference range with no clear indication that the deviations are expected (OAML, 2009). Medical intervention may be needed and these test results must be brought to the attention of the physician. Delays in reporting critical values could be life threatening. Documentation of test results must be included in the appropriate medical records and presented in a manner that is clear and easily interpreted. As in all phases of testing, communication among health care providers is important. Health care providers need to understand the significance of test results. For example, nurses on the evening shift may be the first to see the results of a culture and sensitivity report on a patient with a urinary tract infection. If the results indicate that the infecting organism is not sensitive to the prescribed antibiotic, the physician should be informed and an appropriate antibiotic order obtained.

Guidelines on Disclosing Laboratory Test Results. Ethical and legal standards for the disclosure of test results must strictly follow privacy and confidentiality laws. Canada has two federal privacy laws: the *Privacy Act,* and the *Personal Information Protection and Electronic Documents Act* (PIPEDA). The *Privacy Act* is intended to protect the privacy of an individual's personal information held by government institutions (including information related to race, finances, personal opinions, and medical history) and to provide the patient's right of access to that information. PIPEDA applies to private-sector organizations and does not apply to the not-for-profit organizations such as publicly funded health care institutions. PIPEDA does, however, outline basic disclosure principles that are substantially similar to provincial privacy legislation.

Ontario (*Personal Health Information Protection Act*), New Brunswick (*Personal Health Information Privacy and Access Act*), and Newfoundland and Labrador (NL) (*Personal Health Information Act [PHIA]*) all have privacy legislation that is similar to PIPEDA but the laws apply to health information. The PHIA includes rules for the collection, use, and disclosure of health information about individuals; for the protection of confidentiality of health information; for providing individuals with the right to access their own health information; and for providing a mechanism for complaints. Under the PHIA, a health information custodian (e.g., health care provider) must ensure that all records are retained, transferred, and disposed of in a secure and confidential manner. Consent to collect, use, or disclose personal health information must be obtained from the patient.

The PHIA contains several principles of fair information practices that also govern health care providers' actions when collecting, reporting, and discussing personal information about a patient's diagnosis and health care. One of those principles is the mandate that organizations have a responsibility and accountability to develop policies and processes that are compliant with the PHIA and thus protect access to personal information. Health care providers must inform patients of the purpose for collecting personal information, why it is needed, and how it will be used (e.g., a blood test for electrolytes).

Before any information is collected or any diagnostic tests are conducted, patients must provide informed consent. The collection, use, disclosure, and retention of personal information, such as diagnostic test results, should be limited to the identified purpose, unless there is individual written consent for the release or use of such information. All personal information collected must be accurate and must be safeguarded against loss, theft, unauthorized access, and copying. When requested, personal information such as test results must be accessible to patients, and a simple and easily accessible complaints process must be in place to report any problems. Every province and territory in Canada has a commissioner responsible for overseeing privacy legislation. If patients have a concern about a violation of their rights, they can report it directly to the provincial commissioner or to the Privacy Commissioner of Canada. Compliance with the PIPEDA and provincial privacy laws is an important part of providing diagnostic testing and patient education in Canadian hospitals and communities.

Similar laws exist in the United States, including the *Health Insurance Portability and Accountability Act* (HIPAA) and the *Standards for Privacy of Individually Identifiable Health Information*. The purpose of HIPAA was to improve health care by ensuring the ability of each person to obtain reasonable health care and to allow each individual access to and protection of his or her health care information. As a result of the HIPAA, patients have the right to examine and obtain a copy of their own health records and to request corrections. Information regarding test results can be provided only to the patient and to persons the patient indicates (by signature). Only health care providers may obtain access to a patient's test results. Test results are not given over the phone to patients. Results, whether normal or not, are never left on answering machines or voice mail.

CONCLUSION

Knowledge of the ethical, legal, and professional implications of diagnostic tests and an understanding of the disease process are as important as the communicative skills required to inform the patient and the family of test results. Succinct documentation of test results may be required before the "official" result is included in the patient's chart. Again, a thorough understanding of the test is essential. Adequate follow-up is as important as all previously mentioned factors for successful diagnostic testing. The patient must be educated about home care, the next physician's visit, and treatment options.

Knowledgeable interpretation of diagnostic tests and maintaining privacy are key for effective collaboration among health care providers and patients if the most efficient care is to be provided. The safety and success of diagnostic testing often depend on the nurse and other health care providers. The safety of the patient and health care providers depends on the creation of practice guidelines and standards of care. These can be effectively developed only with a thorough understanding of laboratory and diagnostic testing.

Blood Studies

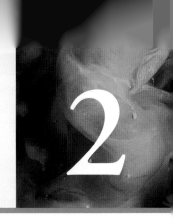

NOTE: *Throughout this chapter, SI units are presented in* boldface colour, *followed by conventional units in parentheses.*

OVERVIEW

TESTS

TESTS

TESTS

2 Blood Studies

TESTS

OVERVIEW

REASONS FOR OBTAINING BLOOD STUDIES

Blood is the body fluid most frequently used for analytic purposes. Blood studies are used to assess a multitude of body processes and disorders. Blood samples can obtain valuable information about the nutritional, hematologic, metabolic, immune, and biochemical status of patients. Common blood studies help assess the quantity of red blood cells (RBCs) and white blood cells (WBCs) and the levels of enzymes, lipids, clotting factors, and hormones. Most blood studies are performed for one of the following reasons:

1. To establish a diagnosis (e.g., high blood urea nitrogen [BUN] and creatinine levels are indicative of renal failure).
2. To rule out a clinical problem (e.g., a normal potassium level rules out hypokalemia).
3. To monitor therapy (e.g., glucose levels are used to monitor treatment of diabetic patients, and partial thromboplastin time [PTT] values are used to regulate heparin therapy).
4. To establish a prognosis (e.g., a declining cluster of differentiation 4 [CD4] counts reflect a poor clinical prognosis for the patient with acquired immune deficiency syndrome [AIDS]).
5. To screen for disease (e.g., prostate-specific antigen levels are used to detect prostate cancer).
6. To determine effective drug dosage and to prevent toxicity. (Peak and trough levels are collected at designated time periods; see p. 229.)

METHODS OF BLOOD COLLECTION

There are three general methods used for obtaining blood samples: venous (venipuncture), arterial, and skin or capillary puncture. Blood collected from these sites differs in several important aspects. For example, arterial blood is oxygenated by the lungs and pumped from the heart to body organs and tissues. Its composition is essentially uniform throughout the body. Venous blood composition varies according to the metabolic activity of the organ or tissue being perfused; it is oxygen deficient in comparison with arterial blood. Variations between arterial and venous blood are often seen in measurements of pH, partial pressure of arterial carbon dioxide ($Paco_2$), and levels of glucose, lactic acid, and ammonia. In contrast, blood obtained by skin or capillary puncture can be a mixture of arterial and venous blood, and levels of analysis (including glucose, bilirubin, and calcium) are markedly different. Capillary puncture blood also includes intracellular and interstitial fluid. By far the most common access for blood withdrawal is venous puncture.

Venous Puncture

Background Information. Because of the ease of obtaining venous blood, this is the primary method of blood collection. It is relatively free of any complications other than injury to veins, as evident from hematomas. Venipuncture is usually obtained in a superficial vein (Figure 2-1). The site most often used is the antecubital fossa of the arm because several large superficial veins are located there. The basilic, cephalic, and median cubital veins are the other most commonly used sites. Veins of the wrist or hand can also be used. When venipuncture cannot be performed on the upper extremities, the femoral vein is the most easily accessible for puncture.

Collection Tubes. Through venipuncture, blood is usually collected into a blood collection tube by means of a Vacutainer Luer adapter and a threaded lock cannula, which is a plastic tube with needle holder attached to a sterile double-ended 20- to 21-gauge needle for adults or 23- to 25-gauge needle for children. Also available are disposable blood collection systems

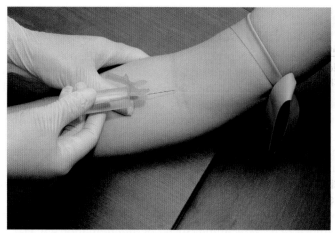

Figure 2-1 Performing venipuncture.

that allow for individual one-time use. Advanced needle technology, which allows for a passive activation of a needle-safety feature as soon as the blood collection is started, is in use in a number of Canadian hospitals. These new needles, which have mechanisms of protection against engineered sharps injury, are replacing the hollow-bore needle, thus reducing the risk for needlestick injury.

A needle and a syringe can also be used to collect the blood sample and then to inject it into the appropriate tube, but this can result in unnecessary trauma to the veins and hemolysis of the blood, which thus affects the values. A 23- to 25-gauge blood collection winged set can also be used to collect blood from the smaller veins in the hand and is often used in older adults when access to veins in the arm is difficult because of poor circulation or dehydration. When a winged blood collection set is used for venipuncture, a nonadditive discard tube must be used to fill the set's tubing space with blood. Anaerobic and aerobic culture bottles can also be used with the winged set or the Vacutainer system to collect blood cultures. Aerobic and anaerobic blood cultures are collected in glass bottles that hold 10 mL of blood.

Collection tubes come in various sizes and hold between 2 and 15 mL of blood. The rubber tops on collection tubes are colour-coded to identify whether the tube is a plain tube (e.g., no preservatives or anticoagulants added); whether the tube contains a specific additive (such as lithium or sodium heparin, oxalate, sodium citrate, or ethylenediamine tetra-acetic acid [EDTA] salts); or whether the tube is chemically clean with no additives. Depending on the tests needed, the analysis is performed on whole blood, serum, or plasma. A centrifuge is used to separate the blood components and to obtain either serum or plasma. Whole blood collected without anticoagulant will clot, and the serum can then be separated out for testing. Whole blood collected with an anticoagulant does not clot, and the plasma can be tested for components such as fibrinogen, which is missing from blood serum.

The selection of the colour-coded tube is based on the requirements of the test. Charts available from the facility should always be followed and checked before selection of the type of tube needed for a particular blood test. Tube top colours and the amount of blood required may vary according to the laboratory and test. A representative chart of the types of blood collection tubes is shown in Table 2-1.

It is recommended to always follow your agency's protocol for the correct blood collection tube and the order for multiple blood collection. Table 2-2 outlines the common order of collection for multiple tube collection as established by the Clinical and Laboratory Standards Institute (2010) and Figure 2-2 demonstrates the correct technique for inverting collection tubes.

TABLE 2-1	Types of Blood Collection Tubes		
Colour of Top	**Additive**	**Purpose**	**Examples**
Red	None (glass) Clot activator (plastic)	To allow blood sample to clot (60 seconds). This enables separation of serum when the serum needs to be tested.	Serum determinations of chemistry profile, bilirubin level, blood urea nitrogen (BUN), and calcium level; routine blood donor screening; and testing for infectious diseases
Red/black	Clot activator and gel for serum separation	Serum separator tube for serum determinations in chemistry and serologic profiles	Chemistry profile, serologic study
Lavender	Liquid- or spray-coated ethylenediamine tetra-acetic acid (EDTA)	To prevent blood from clotting	Whole blood hematologic study, complete blood cell count, platelet count, routine immunohematologic testing, and blood donor screening
Grey	Sodium fluoride/potassium oxalate	To prevent glycolysis	Chemistry profile, glucose and lactose tolerance
Green	Sodium heparin Lithium heparin	To prevent blood from clotting when plasma needs to be tested	Plasma determinations in chemistry, carboxyhemoglobin
Light blue	Buffered sodium citrate; citrate, theophylline, adenosine, and dipyridamole (CTAD)	To prevent blood from clotting when plasma needs to be tested	Hematologic study, prothrombin time (PT), partial thromboplastin time (PTT)
Black	Sodium citrate	Binds calcium to prevent blood clotting	Westergren erythrocyte sedimentation rate (ESR)
Yellow	Sodium polyanethol sulphonate (SPS); acid citrate dextrose (ACD) additives	Preserves red blood cells	SPS for blood cultures specimens in microbiology, ACD for use in blood bank studies, human leukocyte antigen (HLA) phenotyping, and DNA and paternity testing
Gold (serum separator tube [SST])	Spray-coated silica and a polymer gel for serum separation	Collects serum	Chemistry, blood donor screening, and infectious disease testing
Grey/yellow	Thrombin	To ensure clotting within 5 minutes	For stat determinations of chemistry
Red/grey	None	For use as a discard tube or secondary specimen collection tube	
Royal blue	Clot activator (plastic) EDTA salts	To prevent blood from clotting	For measurements of trace elements, toxicology studies, and nutritional-chemistry determinants

2

Blood Studies

TABLE 2-2	Order of Collection for Multiple Tubes	
Tube Stopper Colour	**Type of Collection Tube**	**Mix by Inversion**
Yellow	Blood cultures	8–10 times
Light blue	Sodium citrate tube	3–4 times
Plain red	Serum tube no additive	5 times
Gold or red/black	Serum separator tube with clot activator	5 times
Green, light green, or green/black	Heparin-lithium or sodium	8–10 times
Lavender, tall pink, purple	EDTA	8–10 times
Grey	Sodium fluoride (glucose), potassium oxalate	8–10 times

EDTA, Ethylenediamine tetra-acetic acid.

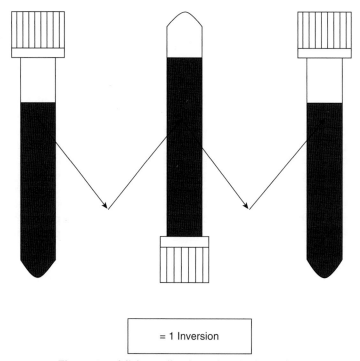

= 1 Inversion

Figure 2-2 Mixing collection tubes by inversion.

Technique

Before

- Identify the patient. Assemble all equipment and supplies (Figure 2-3).
- Explain the procedure and the test to the patient. Explain that mild, brief discomfort may result from the needlestick.
- If fasting is required, verify that this requirement has been followed.

During

- Wash your hands, and bring equipment to the patient's bedside.
- Assist the patient to a supine or a semi-Fowler's position with arm extended and palm up for easy access to the antecubital fossa.

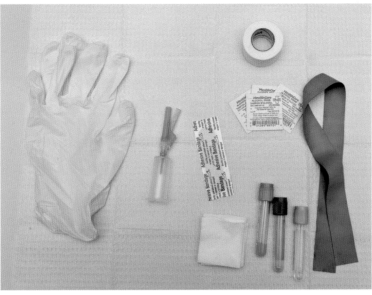

Figure 2-3 Equipment for blood collection.

- Put on gloves.
- Apply a tourniquet several centimetres above the puncture site. Palpate for a firm vein with good rebound.
- Ask the patient to make a fist to distend the veins. If you have difficulty visualizing the veins, ask the patient to open and close the fist several times, ending with it closed.
- Select a vein for venipuncture.
- Cleanse the venipuncture site (usually with 70% isopropyl alcohol or chlorhexidine) moving in a circular motion out 2 inches from the site. Allow the area to dry. If the tourniquet has been on longer than 1 minute, remove it and assess extremity. Wait 1 minute before reapplying tourniquet.
- Perform the venipuncture by entering the skin with the needle bevel up, and the needle at approximately a 15- to 30-degree angle to the skin.
- If you are using a Vacutainer, hold it securely and advance the blood collection tube into the needle of the Vacutainer, as soon as the needle is in the vein. When the tube is filled, remove it. Another blood collection tube can then be inserted into the Vacutainer.
- If you are using a syringe, pull back on the barrel with slow, even tension as blood fills the syringe. Transfer the blood to the appropriate colour tubes.
- Release the tourniquet when the blood begins to flow.

After
- After the blood is collected, place a cotton ball or a 2 × 2 gauze square over the site. Withdraw the needle, and apply pressure to the site until bleeding stops. An adhesive bandage applied over the cotton ball or gauze square usually controls further bleeding.
- Mix blood collection tubes with the additives by gently inverting the tubes as indicated in Table 2-2 and Figure 2-3. Do not vigorously shake the tubes. Specimens collected in the syringe should be transferred to appropriate blood collection tubes and mixed by inversion as indicated.
- Properly dispose of contaminated materials, such as needles and syringes, in a sharps container (Figure 2-4).

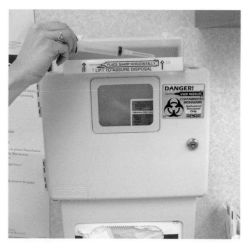

Figure 2-4 Proper disposal of needles and other sharp disposable instruments.

- Remove gloves and wash hands.
- Assess site for bleeding.
- Prepare the blood collection tube label with the patient's name and unique identifier (e.g., medical care plan [MCP] number), specimen collector's name/initials, and date and time of the specimen collection.
- Arrange for prompt delivery of the blood specimen to the laboratory; all samples should be transported to the laboratory preferably within 1 hour or refrigerated. Stat specimens should be transported immediately.
- If the patient fasted before the test, remove diet restrictions.

Potential Complications
Bleeding. After the specimen is collected, apply pressure or a pressure dressing to the venipuncture site. Assess the venipuncture site for bleeding. Instruct patient to apply pressure over the site if necessary.

Hematoma. Hematomas can form under the skin when the vein continues to leak blood. This results in a large bruise. This can usually be prevented by applying pressure to the venipuncture site until clotting occurs. If a hematoma does occur, reabsorption of the blood can be enhanced by the application of warm compresses.

Infection. Instruct the patient to assess the venipuncture site for redness, pain, swelling, or tenderness. These developments are more common in immunocompromised patients and in patients who have undergone lymph node dissection above the venipuncture site.

Dizziness and Fainting. If these occur, prevent injury by helping the patient to a sitting or reclining position. Lowering the patient's head between his or her knees can also help.

Preventing Interfering Factors
- Hemolysis may result from vigorous shaking of a blood specimen. This may invalidate test results. Transferring blood from a syringe to a collection tube can also result in massive hemolysis; therefore, the Vacutainer technique is preferred.

- Collect the blood specimen from the arm without an intravenous (IV) catheter, if possible. IV infusion can influence test results. If it is necessary to collect blood from the arm with an IV catheter, never collect blood above the IV cannula site. Satisfactory samples may be obtained by collecting the blood below the IV cannula; the IV infusion should be turned off for 2 minutes before the venipuncture, and the cannula should be flushed to maintain patency. Select a vein other than the one with the IV device, and collect 5 mL of blood. Discard this sample before collecting blood for analysis.
- Do not use the arm with the dialysis arteriovenous fistula for a venipuncture unless the physician specifically authorizes it.
- Do not perform a venipuncture in the affected arm of a patient who has recently undergone mastectomy; such a patient is at high risk for injury and infection in the affected arm.
- Because of the risk for cellulitis, specimens should not be taken from the side on which an axillary lymph node dissection has been performed.
- To obtain valid results, do not fasten the tourniquet for longer than 1 minute. Prolonged tourniquet application can cause stasis, localized acidemia, and hemoconcentration.

Collecting Blood From an Indwelling Venous Catheter. Follow your unit's guidelines for collecting blood from an indwelling venous catheter, such as a central venous catheter or a peripherally inserted central catheter (PICC). Guidelines specify the amount of blood to be collected from the catheter and discarded before blood is collected for laboratory studies. The guidelines also indicate the amount and type of solution needed to flush the catheter to prevent it from being clogged by blood.

Collecting Multiple Blood Studies. Blood tests are often part of a group of specified tests. This is because patterns of abnormalities may be more useful than single test changes. See Appendix C for suggested blood tests included in multiple blood studies collected for specific diseases and organs.

Arterial Puncture

Background Information. Arterial blood is used primarily to measure the pH, the partial pressure of oxygen (Pao_2), and $Paco_2$. These are often referred to as *arterial blood gas* (ABG) measurements and are described on p. 121. If a patient requires frequent sampling, an indwelling arterial catheter is usually placed in the radial artery. Arterial puncture is used for single or infrequent sampling.

Arterial punctures are more difficult to perform than venipuncture. They also cause a significant amount of discomfort for the patient. The brachial and radial arteries are the arteries most often used for arterial puncture. The femoral artery is linked to higher rates of hematoma and infection and therefore should be reserved for emergency ABG measurements. In patients who have had a cardiac catheter inserted via the brachial artery, the brachial site should also be avoided.

Technique

Before

✗ Explain the procedure to the patient. Inform the patient why this blood test is necessary.
✗ Inform the patient that the test usually causes more discomfort than a venipuncture and that he or she may feel a burning sensation during the procedure.
✗ Stress the importance of staying still during the procedure.
- Gather supplies, including gloves, goggles, a small towel, and an ABG kit with a pre-heparinized syringe.
- Notify the laboratory before you collect arterial blood samples, so that the necessary equipment can be calibrated at the laboratory before the blood sample arrives.

- If the radial site is being used, select the radial artery of the patient's nondominant hand as the first choice.
- Position the patient's palm up with a small towel under the wrist so that the radial artery is closer to the surface.
- Perform the *Allen test* to assess collateral circulation before performing the arterial puncture on the radial artery. To perform the Allen test, make the patient's hand blanch by applying direct pressure to both the radial and ulnar pulses. Then release the pressure over the ulnar artery only. If flow through the ulnar artery is good, flushing will be observed immediately. The Allen test result is then positive, indicating that the ulnar artery is capable of providing blood supply to the hand, and the radial artery can be used for arterial puncture. If the Allen test result is negative (no flushing), repeat it on the other arm. If the results are negative in both arms, choose another artery for puncture. The Allen test is important because it ensures collateral circulation to the hand if thrombosis of the radial artery occurs after the puncture.

During
- Using a circular motion, cleanse the arterial site with 70% isopropyl alcohol, spiralling outward for 30 seconds. Allow the site to dry completely.
- Attach a 20-gauge needle to a syringe containing approximately 0.2 mL of heparin. Individually packaged, disposable ABG sets are available in most hospitals. Prepare the patient for the needlestick. Locate the point where the pulse feels the strongest. Insert the needle at a 30- to 60-degree angle for the radial or brachial artery, and a 60- to 90-degree angle for the femoral artery (Figure 2-5).
- Stop advancing the syringe when blood is seen in the hub of the needle. Arterial pulsations will pump the blood into the syringe, and the pumping will stop when approximately 2 mL of blood has been collected. Remove the needle, and apply pressure to the arterial site for 3 to 5 minutes or 15 minutes if patient has an abnormal clotting time or is receiving anticoagulants. If the femoral artery is used, apply pressure for 30 minutes. A pressure dressing is usually applied. Expel any air bubbles in the syringe.
- Immediately seal the needle and cap the syringe. Gently rotate the syringe to mix the blood and the heparin.

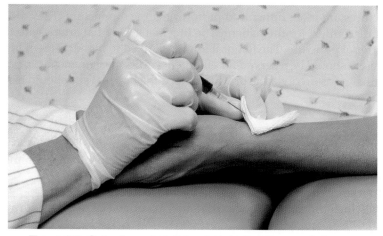

Figure 2-5 Collecting arterial blood. Note that the needle is at a 45-degree angle.

After
- Remove gloves and wash hands.
- Assess site for bleeding.
- On the laboratory slip, indicate whether the patient is receiving any oxygen therapy or is attached to a ventilator; record the patient's temperature and unique identification number (e.g., MCP number).
- Place the arterial blood in a mixture of crushed ice and water, and take it immediately to the chemistry laboratory for analysis. Large cubes or chunks of ice without water do not adequately cool the specimen, and contact of the specimen with solid ice can freeze and therefore hemolyze the blood. For best results, ABG samples should be analyzed within 10 minutes of collection.

Potential Complications

Arterial Thrombosis. Thrombosis can occur after blood is collected and can impair arterial circulation to the hand. This in turn can result in ischemia or necrosis of tissue on the extremity.

Hematoma Formation. Pressure must be applied to the arterial puncture site for at least 3 to 5 minutes to prevent hematoma formation (longer if the patient is receiving anticoagulants and for 30 minutes if the femoral artery is used). If a hematoma results, warm compresses can be used to enhance absorption of the blood.

Bleeding. The site must be carefully assessed for bleeding. An arterial puncture can cause rapid bleeding. This is especially important if the patient has an abnormal clotting time or is taking anticoagulants.

Arterial Occlusion. Check the site frequently for swelling and pulses. Note the colour and temperature, and inquire whether the patient is experiencing any pain, numbness, or tingling, because these are signs of circulatory compromise and must be addressed immediately.

Capillary Blood Collection

Background Information. Capillary blood collection (sometimes called *skin puncture*) allows easy access to capillary blood and carries less risk for complications than do the other methods of blood collection. However, there are distinct differences in the levels of analytes (e.g., glucose) that are measured with venipuncture in comparison with capillary blood collection. Capillary blood collection is the method of choice for obtaining blood from pediatric patients, especially infants, because the collecting of large amounts of blood in repeated venipuncture could result in anemia. However, skin punctures are also commonly used in adult patients for glucose monitoring.

Other puncture sites are the fingertips, earlobes, and heel surfaces. The fingertips are often used in adults and small children. The heel is the site most commonly used in infants. The earlobe can be used to obtain blood in adults and older pediatric patients. The earlobe can also be used to obtain arterialized capillary blood as a possible substitute for arterial blood in determining the pH, $Paco_2$, and Pao_2.

Capillary blood can be collected with finger or heel lancets, which are sterile, disposable instruments often used for glucose monitoring. Microhematocrit tubes are also used to collect capillary specimens. They are disposable narrow-bore plastic or plastic-clad glass capillary tubes that fill by capillary action and hold up to 75 μL of blood.

With changes in health care economics and delivery, the use of capillary blood collection techniques has facilitated blood testing and monitoring in outpatient settings and in the community (e.g., population screening for hyperlipidemia). New painless lancet systems have been developed to help patients monitor their daily capillary blood glucose. Advances in point-of-care capillary blood testing have facilitated the monitoring of laboratory values at home and in the community. ♣ For Diabetes Canada's Clinical Guidelines on Blood Glucose Monitoring, visit http://guidelines.diabetes.ca/fullguidelines.

Technique

Before
- ✗ Identify the patient.
- ✗ Explain the procedure to the patient or family, or both.
- Assemble all supplies. Wash your hands and put on gloves.
- Select an appropriate puncture site. For *newborns,* use a heel lancet; the lateral or medial heel surface is the site most commonly used for blood collection. For *older* infants, children, or adults, use a finger puncture lancet on the lateral aspect of the second, third, or fourth fingertip. Avoid the central tip of the fingers, where the nerve supply is denser.

During
- Warm the puncture site with a warm, moist towel to increase blood flow.
- If you are collecting a capillary blood glucose sample, do not use alcohol to cleanse the site, because this can lead to inaccurate results.
- Wash the patient's hands in warm soapy water, or ask patient to wash hands before procedure.
- Per agency protocol, cleanse the capillary puncture site with the appropriate solution. Allow the site to dry completely.
- Make the puncture with the sterile lancet or other skin puncture device.
- Discard the first drop of blood by wiping it away with a sterile pad.
- Do not milk the site, because this may cause hemolysis of the specimen and introduce excess tissue fluid. Also, avoid using excess pressure on the fingers during blood collection. This, too, may cause hemolysis of the sample.
- Collect the specimen in a microhematocrit tube or on special filter papers.
- If you are using a microhematocrit tube, seal the tube by inserting the dry end into a clay sealant.

After
- Remove gloves and wash hands.
- Assess site for bleeding.
- Initial the blood label, and record the time and date of blood collection. Indicate that the blood was collected by skin or capillary puncture.
- Arrange for prompt transportation of the blood specimen to the laboratory, or complete the blood specimen analysis at the patient's bedside (e.g., glucose monitoring).

Potential Complications

Infection. Assess the skin puncture site for redness, swelling, pain, or tenderness. Although such developments could be indicative of a serious complication, the signs of infection are not usually present immediately following the blood collection procedure. Patients should be educated on how to assess for infection and how to seek advice and treatment.

Hematoma and Bruising. Check the skin puncture site for discoloration, bruising, or swelling. Look for bleeding onto the skin. To prevent this problem, avoid frequent skin punctures or excessive squeezing of the tissue during blood collection.

Artificially High or Artificially Low Blood Glucose Readings. High hematocrit (>50%) may result in an artificially low glucose reading, whereas low hematocrit (<25%) may result in an artificially high glucose reading. Cholesterol levels higher than 13 mmol/L may also result in artificially high glucose readings.

TIMING OF BLOOD COLLECTION

Although many blood specimens can be obtained randomly, some must be collected at specific times. For example, blood for lipoprotein measurement (see p. 355) should be collected after a 12- to 14-hour fast (except for water), because food can alter lipoprotein values. Because glucose levels are related to food intake, an 8-hour fast is required for fasting blood glucose specimens. Glucose tolerance tests (see p. 276) require a measurement of fasting blood glucose level and measurements of glucose levels at 30 minutes, 1 hour, 2 hours, 3 hours, and sometimes 4 hours after glucose administration.

Specimens for therapeutic drug monitoring (see p. 227) must be obtained at specific times that are determined according to the method of drug delivery (e.g., IV or oral), dosage interval, absorption characteristics of the drug, and half-life of the drug. Drug monitoring is especially important for patients taking medications (such as antiarrhythmics, bronchodilators, antibiotics, anticonvulsants, and cardiotonics) because the margin of safety between therapeutic and toxic levels may be narrow. Blood levels can be taken at the drug's peak level (highest concentration) or at the drug's trough level (lowest concentration). Peak levels are useful in tests for toxicity, and trough levels are useful for establishing a satisfactory therapeutic level.

TRANSPORT AND PROCESSING OF BLOOD SPECIMENS

Once blood specimens are obtained, they should be transported promptly to the laboratory. Because the blood cells continue to live in the collection tubes, they will metabolize some of the components in the blood. This can result in alterations in the concentration of some blood components before analysis in the laboratory. Therefore, blood specimens should be delivered to the laboratory for processing within 45 minutes to 1 hour, depending on the test. Stat specimens should be delivered immediately after being collected and analyzed within 10 minutes of collection. Laboratories have written criteria for rejecting a specimen as unsuitable for testing. Box 2-1 lists common reasons for rejecting a blood specimen.

In general, specimens should be tested within 1 hour of collection. If this is not possible, the sample may need to be refrigerated or frozen, depending on the compound being used for testing. Some blood specimens must be sent by mail or special courier from physicians' offices or small hospitals to large reference laboratories. As a result, delays of 24 hours may occur before specimen analysis.

Transport of blood specimens from patients' homes and community settings for analysis at larger hospitals can be a challenge. To avoid errors in specimen transport, all blood collection

BOX 2-1	Criteria for Rejection of Blood Sample

- Improper sample identification, including inaccurate or missing information
- Wrong or outdated collection tube used
- Insufficient blood quantity (quantity not sufficient [QNS])
- Hemolyzed blood sample
- Improper transport of sample (e.g., ABG specimen not on ice)
  - Improper mixing
  - Wrong collection time
- Insufficient filling of anticoagulated tube

tubes should be carried in an upright position and in a locked container to avoid spills. Specimens should be clearly marked "biohazardous materials," and cold packs should be available to cool specimens if necessary. Refer to hospital policies and protocols if blood specimens are being transported for analysis. Each specimen should be in a zip-locked plastic bag with an outside pocket for the laboratory requisition. In this way, specimens can be transported safely and tested accurately.

After testing, the remainder of the blood sample should be saved by the laboratory along with the original sample for 24 hours, to be retested if discrepant results need to be verified. These samples can also be used for additional ("add-on") tests ordered by the physician so as to avoid additional venipunctures. With retesting or "add-on" requests, the stability of the requested serum constituent becomes an important consideration.

Multiphasic screening machines can perform many blood tests quickly and simultaneously with a very small blood sample. An example of this is the sequential multiple analyzer (SMA), which is the name of one instrument used for automatically testing a specific group of tests. An SMA-12 performs 12 tests, whereas an SMA-6 performs 6 tests. Another example is the Astra-7 or Chem-7, which usually includes the following seven studies: sodium, potassium, chloride, CO_2 content, BUN, creatinine, and glucose. See Appendix C for a listing of suggested groups of blood studies that could be used for specific diseases and organ assessment.

REPORTING OF RESULTS

Although accuracy and processing are the prerequisites of good laboratory practice, timeliness in reporting results is essential. To be clinically useful, a test result must be reported promptly. Delays in reporting a result can render the data useless and may adversely affect patient care. The report must also be entered in the appropriate medical record and must be presented in a manner that is clear and easily interpreted. A listing of the patient's medications helps with test result interpretation.

The report of results should include the test results, reporting units, and reference ranges. It is important to note that normal ranges for laboratory tests vary from institution to institution. Serial listing of results is often useful when trends and values make interpretation easier. Comments may be added to help interpret test results; for example, the technologist would indicate whether the sample was hemolyzed.

Because acronyms are used to shorten test names, these code names must be understood for proper interpretation. For example, the acronym *LAP* could stand for *leucine amino peptidase* or for *leukocyte alkaline phosphatase*.

Proper reporting of a "critical" or "panic" value is essential. These values are results well outside the usual range of normal and generally mandate immediate intervention. A good example of this is high or low potassium levels. If these results are phoned to a physician or nurse, verification of this notification must be properly documented.

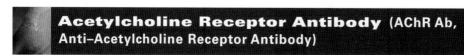

Acetylcholine Receptor Antibody (AChR Ab, Anti–Acetylcholine Receptor Antibody)

NORMAL FINDINGS

≤0.03 nmol/L or negative

INDICATIONS

Antibodies to AChR are used to diagnose acquired myasthenia gravis and also to monitor patients' response to immunosuppressive therapy.

TEST EXPLANATION

Antibodies to AChR occur in more than 85% to 90% of patients with acquired myasthenia gravis, and 63% of patients with only ocular myasthenia gravis have elevated levels. The presence of AChR is virtually diagnostic of this disorder. The measured titre does not correspond well with the severity of myasthenia gravis. In an individual patient with this disorder, however, antibody levels are particularly useful in monitoring response to immunosuppressive therapy. As the patient improves, antibody titre decreases. This test is also used in patients who are suspected of having a thymoma because 59% of such patients also have myasthenia gravis. Because congenital myasthenia gravis is not an autoimmune disease, the AChR test is not helpful in the diagnosis of congenital myasthenia gravis.

AChR blocks neuromuscular transmission by interfering with the binding of acetylcholine to AChR sites on the muscle membrane and preventing muscle contraction. It is this phenomenon that characterizes myasthenia gravis. Three different AChR antibodies are used to test for myasthenia gravis. The AChR-binding antibody is most commonly used. If the result of this test is negative and the diagnosis of myasthenia gravis is highly suspected, the AChR-modulating antibody, which may be more sensitive, is used. Furthermore, a positive result of a modulating antibody test may indicate subclinical myasthenia gravis, which contraindicates the use of curare-like drugs during surgery. The AChR-blocking antibody is the least sensitive test (positive in only 61% of patients with myasthenia gravis), but it can be quantified more accurately. The blocking and modulating antibodies are not often positive for approximately 1 year after onset of symptoms of myasthenia gravis. The method most commonly used for the detection of these AChR antibodies is radioimmunoassay.

INTERFERING FACTORS

- False-positive results may occur in patients with amyotrophic lateral sclerosis who have been treated with cobra venom.
- False-positive results may occur in patients with penicillamine-induced or Lambert-Eaton myasthenic syndromes.
- Patients with autoimmune liver disease may have elevated levels of AChR.
- The use of muscle relaxant drugs (metocurine and succinylcholine) or penicillamine may also cause false-positive results.
- Immunosuppressive drugs may suppress the formation of these antibodies in patients with subclinical myasthenia gravis.

PROCEDURE AND PATIENT CARE

Before

- Explain the procedure to the patient.
- Inform the patient that no fasting is required.
- Inform the patient that the blood sample is usually sent to a reference laboratory. It will take several days before the results are available.

During

- Collect a venous blood sample in a red-top tube.

After

- Apply pressure or a pressure dressing to the venipuncture site.
- Assess the venipuncture site for bleeding.

TEST RESULTS AND CLINICAL SIGNIFICANCE
▲ Increased Levels
Myasthenia gravis,
Ocular myasthenia gravis,
Thymoma: *Fifty-nine percent of patients with thymoma have myasthenia gravis, and 10% of patients with myasthenia gravis have a thymoma.*

RELATED TESTS

Antistriated Muscle Antibody (Antistriational Antibody). This is a serum antibody titre that has been reported to be positive in 95% of patients with myasthenia gravis and thymoma and in 30% of patients with thymoma but without myasthenia gravis.

Cholinesterase (p. 173). Patients with an acquired or congenital deficiency of this enzyme will experience acute myasthenia gravis–like muscle paralysis when a depolarizing agent, such as succinylcholine, is used for anaesthesia induction.

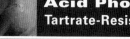

Acid Phosphatase (Prostatic Acid Phosphatase [PAP], Tartrate-Resistant Acid Phosphatase [TRAP])

NORMAL FINDINGS
- Adult/older adult: **<30 ng/mL** (<3.0 *Mcg*/L)

INDICATIONS

Total acid phosphatase—specifically the PAP isoenzyme—is primarily used to document rape or recent sexual intercourse. In the past, it was used in the diagnosis of prostate cancer, but it has been replaced by the use of prostate-specific antigen (p. 434).

TEST EXPLANATION

Acid phosphatase is found in many tissues, including liver, RBCs, bone marrow, and platelets. The highest levels are found in the prostate gland: the PAP isoenzyme. Usually (but not always) levels are elevated in patients with prostatic cancer that has metastasized beyond the capsule to other parts of the body, especially bone. The degree of elevation indicates the extent of disease.

Because acid phosphatase is also found at high concentrations in seminal fluid, this test can be performed on vaginal secretions to investigate alleged rape. This is now the primary use of PAP testing. High levels of acid phosphatase also exist in white blood cells (WBCs; mostly monocytes and lymphocytes). They are helpful in determining the clinical course of lymphoproliferative diseases and hairy cell leukemia. Acid phosphatase is a lysosomal enzyme; therefore, lysosomal storage diseases (such as Gaucher's disease and Niemann-Pick disease) are associated with elevated levels.

In men, half of the total acid phosphatase (nearly all of the PAP) is found in the prostate gland. Lesser amounts are found in the liver, spleen, blood cells, and bone marrow. In women, total acid phosphatase is found in the liver, RBCs, and platelets.

Acid phosphatase can be identified by cellular hydrolysis of naphthol phosphoric acid. The optimal pH for this reaction is acidic. When tartaric acid is added to the solution, hydrolysis of the substance by acid phosphatase is inhibited in prostate cells but not in the cells of hairy cell leukemia. The identification of *tartrate-resistant acid phosphatase* (TRAP) in WBCs is therefore helpful in the diagnosis of hairy cell leukemia (and occasionally other lymphoproliferative diseases). However, the specimens of 5% of patients with hairy cell leukemia are not tartrate resistant. Since 2000, radioimmunoassay and enzyme-linked immunosorbent assay (ELISA) kits have been used to determine acid phosphatase levels (specifically PAP). These methods are more accurate than the biochemical methods previously described and are more easily performed.

INTERFERING FACTORS

- Levels of acid phosphatase (and specifically PAP) may be artificially high in men after a digital rectal examination or after instrumentation of the prostate (e.g., cystoscopy) because of prostatic stimulation. Levels may remain elevated 25% to 50% for up to 48 hours after prostate manipulation. The test should be repeated if elevations occur after a rectal or prostate examination.
- Alkaline and acid phosphatases are very similar enzymes that function at different pH levels. Any condition associated with very high levels of alkaline phosphatase may falsely indicate high acid phosphatase levels.
- Substances that may cause *increases* in levels of acid phosphatase include alglucerase, androgens (in women), and clofibrate (Atromid-S).
- Substances that may cause *decreases* in levels of acid phosphatase include alcohol, fluorides, heparin, oxalates, and phosphates.

PROCEDURE AND PATIENT CARE

Before
- Explain the procedure to the patient.
- Inform the patient that no food or drink restrictions are necessary.
- Note that some laboratories request notification before the blood sample is collected so that immediate attention (<1 hour) can be given to the sample.

During
- Collect a venous blood sample in a red-top tube.
- Handle the tube gently to prevent hemolysis. RBCs contain acid phosphatase.
- On the laboratory slip, note whether the patient has undergone a prostatic or rectal examination or instrumentation of the prostate within the past 24 to 48 hours.

After
- Apply pressure or a pressure dressing to the venipuncture site.
- Assess the venipuncture site for bleeding.
- Deliver the specimen promptly to the laboratory.
- Do not leave the specimen at room temperature for 1 hour or longer; the enzyme is heat and pH sensitive, and acid phosphatase activity will decrease. Once the specimen is received by the laboratory, the use of a preservative and prompt refrigeration are important.

TEST RESULTS AND CLINICAL SIGNIFICANCE

▲ Increased Levels

Prostatic carcinoma,

Benign prostatic hypertrophy,

Prostatitis: *Acid phosphatase and specifically PAP exist in the lysosomes of prostate cells. Diseases affecting prostate tissue destroy those cells, and the lysosomal contents spill into the bloodstream, where they can be detected.*

Multiple myeloma,

Paget's disease,

Hyperparathyroidism,

Metastasis to the bone: *Because acid phosphatase exists in the lysosomes of the bone marrow, diseases affecting the bone are associated with elevations in blood levels.*

Multiple myeloma,

Sickle cell crisis,

Thrombocytosis: *Because acid phosphatase exists in the lysosomes of blood cells, diseases affecting blood cells are associated with elevations in blood levels.*

Lysosomal disorders (e.g., Gaucher's disease): *Because acid phosphatase exists in the lysosomes of many tissues affected by these diseases, elevations in blood levels can be expected.*

Renal diseases,

Liver diseases (such as cirrhosis): *Because acid phosphatase is present in these organs, diseases affecting these organs are associated with elevations in blood levels.*

Rape or sexual intercourse: *PAP levels are elevated in vaginal secretions of a woman who has recently been raped or has recently had sexual intercourse. The PAP assay is a well-documented presumptive assay for the presence of semen.*

RELATED TESTS

Prostate-Specific Antigen (p. 434). This is a more specific test for prostatic cancer.

Alkaline Phosphatase (p. 53). This is a similar enzyme that is more easily identified in an alkaline environment. It is useful in the evaluation of diseases of the liver and bone.

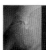

Activated Clotting Time (ACT, Activated Coagulation Time)

NORMAL FINDINGS

70–120 seconds

Therapeutic range for anticoagulation: 150–210 seconds

(Normal ranges and anticoagulation ranges vary according to particular therapy.)

INDICATIONS

The ACT is primarily used to measure the effect of heparin as an anticoagulant during cardiac angioplasty, hemodialysis, and cardiopulmonary bypass surgery.

TEST EXPLANATION

This test measures the time for whole blood to clot after the addition of particulate activators. Like the activated partial thromboplastin time (aPTT, p. 396), it is a measure of the ability of the *intrinsic pathway* (reaction 1) to begin clot formation by activating factor XII (see Figure 2-14, p. 181). The blood clotting status with ACT can help monitor the response to heparin therapy easily and rapidly. Equally important is the use of the ACT in determining the appropriate dose of protamine sulphate required to reverse the effect of heparin on completion of surgical procedures and hemodialysis.

Both the aPTT and the ACT can be used to monitor heparin therapy. However, the ACT has several advantages over the aPTT. First, the ACT is more accurate than the aPTT when high doses of heparin are used for anticoagulation. Thus it is especially useful during clinical situations that necessitate high-dose heparin, such as cardiopulmonary bypass surgery when high-dose anticoagulation is necessary at levels 10 times those used for venous thrombosis. The aPTT is not measurable at these high doses. The accepted goal for the ACT is 400 to 480 seconds during cardiopulmonary bypass surgery.

Second, measurement of the ACT is not only less expensive but also more easily and rapidly performed than that of the aPTT, which is time consuming and requires full laboratory facilities. The ACT can be measured at the patient's bedside. This provides immediate information that can guide further decisions about therapeutic anticoagulation. Because of the capability to measure the ACT at the "point of care," the ACT is particularly useful for patients requiring angioplasty, hemodialysis, and cardiopulmonary bypass.

A nomogram adjusted to the patient's baseline ACT is often used as a guide to reach the desired level of anticoagulation during these procedures. The same nomogram is used in determining the dose of protamine to be administered to neutralize the heparin when a return to normal coagulation is desired on completion of these procedures. The ACT is used in determining when it is safe to remove the vascular access after these procedures. The *modified ACT test* requires a smaller-volume blood specimen, automated blood sampling, standardized blood/reagent mixing, and faster clotting time results than does the conventional ACT test. The modified ACT test is now used more frequently.

INTERFERING FACTORS

- The ACT is affected by several biologic variables, including hypothermia, hemodilution, and platelet number and function.
- Factors affecting the pharmacokinetics of heparin (e.g., kidney or liver disease, heparin resistance) can affect ACT measurements.
- A partially or completely occluded specimen can increase ACT measurements.
- Drugs such as aprotinin (a serine protease inhibitor used during cardiopulmonary bypass surgery) can prolong the ACT when celite is used as the activator.

PROCEDURE AND PATIENT CARE

Before
- Explain the procedure to the patient.

During
- Collect less than 1 mL of blood into a commercial container. Place this container into a whole blood microcoagulation analyzer at the patient's bedside. When a clot is formed, the ACT value is displayed on the machine's screen.
- If the patient is receiving a continuous heparin drip, obtain the blood sample from the arm without the IV catheter.

After

- Apply pressure to the venipuncture site. Remember that the bleeding time will be prolonged because of anticoagulation therapy.
- Assess the patient to detect possible bleeding. Check for blood in the urine and all other excretions and assess the patient for bruises, petechiae, and low back pain.
- For clinical significance, the test results must be evaluated in relation to the timing of heparin administration. A clinical flow sheet should be used to list the test results with the time and route of heparin administration.

TEST RESULTS AND CLINICAL SIGNIFICANCE

▲ Increased Levels

Heparin administration: *Heparin, along with antithrombin III, interrupts the action of several coagulation proteins (except factor VII). As a result, the intrinsic pathway of coagulation is inhibited. This pathway is measured by the ACT and is therefore prolonged.*

Clotting factor deficiencies: *Deficiencies in any clotting factor associated with the intrinsic pathway are associated with prolonged ACT.*

Cirrhosis of the liver: *Coagulation factors are proteins that are synthesized in the liver. Liver disease is therefore associated with a reduction in coagulation factors; this prolongs the time required for the reactions of the intrinsic pathway and prolongs the ACT.*

Coumadin administration: *Deficiencies in the vitamin K clotting factors associated with the intrinsic pathway cause a prolonged ACT.*

Lupus inhibitor: *Lupus inhibitors are autoantibodies against components involved in the activation of the coagulation cascade and thus prolong the ACT.*

▼ Decreased Levels

Thrombosis: *In thrombotic syndromes in which secondary hemostasis is inappropriately stimulated, the ACT may be shortened.*

RELATED TESTS

Partial Thromboplastin Time (p. 396). This test is used to evaluate the intrinsic pathway of secondary hemostasis. It, too, is commonly used to monitor heparin therapy.

Prothrombin Time (p. 446). This test is used to evaluate the extrinsic and common pathways of secondary hemostasis.

Coagulating Factor Concentration (p. 177). This is a quantitative measurement of specific coagulation factors.

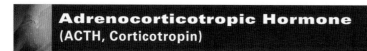

Adrenocorticotropic Hormone
(ACTH, Corticotropin)

NORMAL FINDINGS

Morning: **<18 pmol/L** (<80 pg/mL)
Afternoon/evening: **<11 pmol/L** (<50 pg/mL)

INDICATIONS

The serum adrenocorticotropic hormone (ACTH) study is a test of anterior pituitary gland function that affords the greatest insight into the causes of either Cushing's syndrome (overproduction of cortisol) or Addison's disease (underproduction of cortisol).

TEST EXPLANATION

An elaborate feedback mechanism for cortisol coordinates the function of the hypothalamus, pituitary gland, and adrenal glands. ACTH is an important aspect of this mechanism. Corticotropin-releasing hormone is made in the hypothalamus. This stimulates ACTH production in the anterior pituitary gland, which in turn stimulates the adrenal cortex to produce cortisol. The rising levels of cortisol act as negative feedback and curtail further production of corticotropin-releasing hormone and ACTH.

In patients with Cushing's syndrome, elevations in the ACTH level can be caused by a pituitary ACTH-producing tumour or a nonpituitary (ectopic) ACTH-producing tumour, usually in the lung, pancreas, thymus, or ovary. ACTH levels greater than 44 pmol/L usually indicate ectopic ACTH production. If the ACTH level is below normal in a patient with Cushing's syndrome, an adrenal adenoma or carcinoma is probably the cause of the hyperfunction (Table 2-3).

In patients with Addison's disease, elevation in the ACTH level indicates primary adrenal gland failure, as in adrenal gland destruction caused by infarction, hemorrhage, or autoimmunity; surgical removal of the adrenal gland; congenital enzyme deficiency; or adrenal suppression after prolonged ingestion of exogenous steroids. If the ACTH level is below normal in a patient with adrenal insufficiency, hypopituitarism is most probably the cause of the hypofunction (see Table 2-3).

ACTH can be measured directly by immunoassay. ACTH levels exhibit diurnal variations that correspond to cortisol levels. Levels in the evening (8 PM to 10 PM) are usually half to two-thirds those in the morning (4 AM to 8 AM). This diurnal variation is lost when disease

TABLE 2-3	Cortisol/ACTH Levels in Diagnosis of Adrenal Dysfunction	
Disease	**Cortisol Level**	**ACTH Level**
Cushing's syndrome Adrenal micronodular hyperplasia Adrenal tumour (adenoma, cancer)	High	Low
Cushing's syndrome Cushing's disease (ACTH-producing pituitary tumour) Ectopic ACTH-producing tumour (e.g., lung cancer)	High	High
Addison's disease Adrenal gland failure (e.g., infarction, hemorrhage, congenital adrenal hyperplasia)	Low	High
Hypopituitarism	Low	Low

ACTH, Adrenocorticotropic hormone.

(especially neoplasm) affects the pituitary or adrenal glands. Likewise, stress can blunt or eliminate this normal diurnal variation.

ACTH is measured in amniotic fluid when anencephaly is suspected. Levels are decreased in anencephalic fetuses. (See discussion of amniocentesis on p. 660.)

INTERFERING FACTORS

- Stress (trauma, pyrogen, hypoglycemia), menses, and pregnancy cause levels of cortisol to increase. This is accomplished through elevation of ACTH.
- Recently administered radioisotopes (for scans) can affect levels measured by radioimmunoassay or immunoradiometry.
- Drugs that may cause *increases* in ACTH levels include aminoglutethimide, amphetamines, estrogens, ethanol, insulin, levodopa, metyrapone, spironolactone, and vasopressin.
- Exogenously administered corticosteroids decrease ACTH levels.

✓ Clinical Priorities

- Evaluate the patient for stress factors that could invalidate test results.
- Remember that there is a diurnal variation in ACTH levels that corresponds to variation in cortisol levels. When the sleep pattern is normal, levels are highest in the morning and lowest in the evening.

PROCEDURE AND PATIENT CARE

Before

- Explain the procedure to the patient. Allow plenty of time to answer the patient's questions so as to diminish the patient's stress level as much as possible.
- Keep the patient on NPO status (nothing by mouth) after midnight the day of the test.
- Evaluate the patient for stress factors that would invalidate the test results.
- Evaluate the patient for abnormalities in sleep pattern. When the sleep pattern is normal, the ACTH level is highest between 4 AM and 8 AM and lowest at approximately 9 PM.
- Assess the patient for self-administration of drugs that could affect test results.

During

- Collect the blood specimen in a lavender-top tube or as required by your reference laboratory.
- Chill the blood tube by placing it in a mixture of crushed ice and water, to prevent enzymatic degradation of ACTH.

After

- Apply pressure or a pressure dressing to the venipuncture site.
- Assess the venipuncture site for bleeding.
- Place the specimen tube back in the mixture of crushed ice and water.
- Send it to the chemistry laboratory immediately. ACTH is a very unstable peptide in plasma and should be stored at minus 20°C to prevent artificially low values.

TEST RESULTS AND CLINICAL SIGNIFICANCE

▲ Increased Levels

Addison's disease (primary adrenal insufficiency),

Adrenogenital syndrome (congenital adrenal hyperplasia): *The adrenal glands are not making enough cortisol for the body's needs. The reduced serum cortisol level is a strong stimulus to pituitary production of ACTH.*

Cushing's disease (pituitary-dependent adrenal hyperplasia),

Ectopic ACTH syndrome,

Stress: *ACTH is overproduced as a result of neoplastic overproduction of ACTH in the pituitary gland or elsewhere in the body by an ACTH-producing cancer. Stress is a potent stimulus of ACTH production.*

▼ Decreased Levels

Secondary adrenal insufficiency (pituitary insufficiency),

Hypopituitarism: *The pituitary gland is incapable of producing adequate ACTH.*

Adrenal adenoma or carcinoma,

Cushing's syndrome,

Exogenous steroid administration: *Overproduction or availability of cortisol is a strong inhibitor of pituitary production of ACTH.*

RELATED TESTS

Cortisol, Blood (p. 192) and Cortisol, Urine (p. 953). Cortisol is a hormone produced by the adrenal gland, and abnormal levels are the main determinants of Cushing's syndrome (overproduction) or Addison's disease (underproduction).

Adrenocorticotropic Hormone (ACTH) Stimulation (see following test). This test is used to determine the cause of adrenal insufficiency.

Dexamethasone Suppression (p. 219). This test is used to determine the cause of Cushing's syndrome.

Adrenocorticotropic Hormone Stimulation With Metyrapone (p. 40). This test is used to determine the cause of Cushing's syndrome.

Adrenocorticotropic Hormone Stimulation
(ACTH Stimulation With Cosyntropin, Cortisol Stimulation)

NORMAL FINDINGS

Normal daily cortisol levels:
 8 AM: 110–520 nmol/L (<80 pg/mL)
 4 PM: 50–410 nmol/L (<50 pg/mL)
 Midnight: <140 nmol/L
 Newborn: 55–304 nmol/L
Rapid test: Cortisol levels increase by at least 267 nmol/L (>7 mg/dL) from baseline after cosyntropin administration
 Baseline: >138 nmol/L
 Peak response: >552 nmol/L

INDICATIONS

This test evaluates the ability of the adrenal gland to respond to adrenocorticotropic hormone (ACTH) administration. It is useful in evaluating the cause of adrenal insufficiency and also in evaluating patients with cushingoid symptoms.

TEST EXPLANATION

This test is performed when adrenal insufficiency is detected. An increase in plasma cortisol levels after the infusion of an ACTH-like drug (e.g., cosyntropin) indicates that the adrenal gland is normal and capable of functioning if stimulated. In that case, the cause of adrenal insufficiency would lie within the pituitary gland (hypopituitarism, which is called *secondary adrenal insufficiency*). If little or no rise in cortisol levels occurs after the administration of the ACTH-like drug, the adrenal gland is the source of the problem and cannot secrete cortisol. This is called *primary adrenal insufficiency* (Addison's disease), which may be caused by adrenal hemorrhage, infarction, autoimmunity, metastatic tumour, surgical removal of the adrenal glands, or congenital adrenal enzyme deficiency.

This test can also be used to evaluate patients with Cushing's syndrome. In Cushing's syndrome caused by bilateral adrenal hyperplasia, cortisol elevation is exaggerated in response to the administration of the ACTH-like drug. Patients with Cushing's syndrome caused by hyperfunctioning adrenal tumours (which are usually autonomous and relatively insensitive to ACTH) have little or no increase in cortisol levels over baseline values.

Cosyntropin (Cortrosyn) is a synthetic subunit of ACTH that has the same corticosteroid-stimulating effect as endogenous ACTH in healthy persons. During this test, cosyntropin is administered to the patient, and the ability of the adrenal gland to respond is measured by plasma cortisol levels.

The *rapid stimulation test* is only a screening test. A normal response rules out adrenal insufficiency. An abnormal response, however, requires a 1- to 3-day prolonged ACTH stimulation test to differentiate primary insufficiency from secondary insufficiency. The adrenal gland, however, can also be stimulated by insulin-induced hypoglycemia as a stressing agent. When insulin is the stimulant, cortisol and glucose levels are measured.

INTERFERING FACTORS

▪ Drugs that may cause artificial increases in cortisol levels include prolonged corticosteroid administration, estrogens, and spironolactone.

PROCEDURE AND PATIENT CARE

Before

✗ Have the patient remain on NPO status (nothing by mouth) after midnight the day of the test.

During

Rapid Test

• Determine a baseline plasma cortisol level less than 30 minutes before cosyntropin administration.

- Administer an IV injection of cosyntropin over a 2-minute period. An intramuscular injection may also be used.
- Measure plasma cortisol levels 30 and 60 minutes after drug administration. Measurement with serum or heparinized blood is acceptable.

24-Hour Test
- Determine a baseline plasma cortisol level.
- Start an IV infusion of synthetic cosyntropin for administration over a 24-hour period.
- After 24 hours, measure the plasma cortisol level again.

3-Day Test
- Determine a baseline plasma cortisol level.
- Administer cosyntropin intravenously over an 8-hour period on 2 to 3 consecutive days.
- Measure the plasma cortisol level again 12, 24, 36, 48, 60, and 72 hours after the start of the test.

After
- Apply pressure or a pressure dressing to the venipuncture site.
- Check the venipuncture site for bleeding.

TEST RESULTS AND CLINICAL SIGNIFICANCE

▲ Exaggerated Response

Cushing's syndrome: *Bilateral adrenal hyperplasia.*

Adrenal insufficiency: *Secondary adrenal insufficiency caused by hypopituitarism, exogenous steroid ingestion, or endogenous steroid production from nonendocrine tumour.*

▼ Normal or Below-Normal Response

Cushing's syndrome: *Adrenal adenoma, adrenal carcinoma, ACTH-producing tumour, chronic steroid ingestion.*

Adrenal insufficiency: *Primary adrenal insufficiency (Addison's disease) caused by adrenal infarction, hemorrhage, infection, or metastatic tumour to adrenal gland.*

Congenital enzyme adrenal insufficiency, surgical removal of adrenal gland, and ingestion of drugs, such as mitotane, metyrapone, or aminoglutethimide.

RELATED TESTS

Cortisol, Blood (p. 192). Cortisol is a hormone produced by the adrenal gland and is the main determinant of Cushing's syndrome (overproduction) or Addison's disease (underproduction).

Adrenocorticotropic Hormone (p. 34). This test is used to determine the cause of Cushing's syndrome or Addison's disease.

Dexamethasone Suppression (p. 219). This test is used to determine the cause of Cushing's syndrome.

Adrenocorticotropic Hormone Stimulation With Metyrapone (p. 40). This test is used to determine the cause of Cushing's syndrome.

Adrenocorticotropic Hormone Stimulation With Metyrapone (Metyrapone, ACTH Stimulation With Metyrapone)

NORMAL FINDINGS

Blood

Normal minimal 11-deoxycortisol response: >200 nmol/L (>7 mcg/dL)
Subnormal 11-deoxycortisol response: <200 nmol/L (<7 mcg/dL)
Normal minimal cortisol response: <414 nmol/L (<10 mcg/dL)

24-Hour Urine

Baseline excretion of urinary 17-hydroxycorticosteroid (17-OCHS) is more than doubled.

INDICATIONS

This test is useful in differentiating adrenal hyperplasia from a primary adrenal tumour by determining whether the pituitary-adrenal feedback response mechanism is intact.

TEST EXPLANATION

Metyrapone (Metopirone) is a potent blocker of an enzyme involved in cortisol production. Cortisol production is therefore reduced. When this drug is given, the resulting decrease in cortisol production should stimulate pituitary secretion of adrenocorticotropic hormone (ACTH) by way of a negative-feedback mechanism. Cortisol itself cannot be synthesized because of the metyrapone inhibition at the 11-beta-hydroxylation step, but an abundance of cortisol precursors (11-deoxycortisol and 17-OCHS) will be formed. These cortisol precursors can be detected in the urine or in the blood. This test is similar to the ACTH stimulation test.

In patients with adrenal hyperplasia caused by pituitary overproduction of ACTH, the cortisol precursors are greatly increased. This is because the normal pituitary-adrenal feedback response mechanism is still intact. No response to metyrapone occurs in patients with Cushing's syndrome resulting from adrenal adenoma or carcinoma, because the tumours are autonomous and therefore insensitive to changes in ACTH secretion. This test has no significant advantage over the ACTH stimulation test in the differential diagnosis of Cushing's disease.

This test is also used to evaluate the pituitary reserve capacity to produce ACTH. It can document that adrenal insufficiency exists as a result of pituitary disease (secondary adrenal insufficiency) rather than primary adrenal disease. This test should not be performed if primary adrenal insufficiency is likely because a severe, life-threatening adrenal crisis could be precipitated. A normal response to ACTH should be demonstrated before metyrapone is given.

CONTRAINDICATIONS

- The possible presence of primary adrenal insufficiency, because metyrapone could reduce the production of what little cortisol is produced and thereby precipitate an adrenal crisis.

POTENTIAL COMPLICATIONS

- Addison's disease and addisonian crisis, because metyrapone inhibits cortisol production.

INTERFERING FACTORS

- Recent administration of radioisotopes will interfere with test results performed by radioimmunoassay.
- Chlorpromazine interferes with the response to metyrapone and should not be administered during the testing.

Clinical Priorities

- This test evaluates the intactness of the pituitary-adrenal feedback response mechanism.
- This test should not be performed on patients with adrenal insufficiency. A severe, life-threatening adrenal or addisonian crisis could result.
- Patients should be carefully assessed for impending signs of addisonian crisis, which include glucocorticoid deficiency, drop in extracellular fluid volume, and hyperkalemia. This is a medical emergency and must be treated vigorously.

PROCEDURE AND PATIENT CARE

Before

- Explain the procedure for collecting a 24-hour urine specimen to the patient.
- Obtain a 24-hour urine specimen to measure the baseline 17-OCHS level for the urine test.
- Measure the baseline cortisol level (see p. 192) for the blood test.

During

Blood

- Administer a dose of metyrapone at 11 PM the night before the blood specimen is to be collected.
- Collect a blood specimen to measure cortisol level in the morning (see p. 192).

Urine

- Obtain a 24-hour urine specimen to measure the 17-OCHS baseline level.
- Then collect a 24-hour urine specimen to measure the 17-OCHS level during and again 1 day after the oral administration of a dose of metyrapone, which may be given every 4 hours for 24 hours.

After

- Assess the patient for impending signs of addisonian crisis (muscle weakness, mental and emotional changes, anorexia, nausea, vomiting, hypotension, hyperkalemia, vascular collapse).
- Note that addisonian crisis is a medical emergency that must be treated vigorously. Basically, the immediate treatment includes replenishing steroids, reversing shock, and restoring blood circulation.

TEST RESULTS AND CLINICAL SIGNIFICANCE
▲ Increased Levels

Adrenal hyperplasia: *Cortisol precursors will be significantly increased as a result of accentuating the ACTH effect.*

Adrenal tumour: *Tumours are autonomous and are not affected by inhibitory or stimulatory feedback. There is no apparent change in cortisol precursors.*

Ectopic ACTH syndrome: *This syndrome occurs when neoplasms (usually lung cancer) produce ACTH without regard to regulatory mechanisms. There is no apparent change in cortisol precursors.*

Secondary adrenal insufficiency: *There will be no significant change in cortisol precursors because there is no pituitary function to stimulate the production of ACTH.*

RELATED TESTS

Adrenocorticotropic Hormone (p. 34). This is a direct measurement of ACTH, which is used in the evaluation of Cushing's syndrome and Addison's disease.

Adrenocorticotropic Hormone Stimulation (p. 37). This test is used in a manner similar to the metyrapone test for evaluation of Addison's disease and Cushing's syndrome.

Age-Related Macular Degeneration Risk Analysis (Y402H and A69S)

NORMAL FINDINGS

No mutation noted

INDICATIONS

This test is used for risk assessment and as supportive documentation of macular degeneration.

TEST EXPLANATION

Age-related macular degeneration (ARMD) is recognized as a leading cause of blindness. Blurred or distorted vision and difficulty adjusting to dim light are common symptoms. ARMD, both wet and dry types, is considered a multifactorial disorder, as it is thought to develop because of the interplay among environmental (smoking), genetic (gender, ethnicity) risk, and protective (antioxidants) factors. At least two genetic variants (Y402H and A69S) have been found to be associated with an increased risk for ARMD. The Y402H and A69S genetic variants are common polymorphisms in ARMD. An individual with two copies of the Y402H variant in the gene *CFH* and two copies of the A69S variant in the gene *LOC387715* has an approximate 60-fold increased risk for ARMD. This is significant given how common ARMD is in the general population.

This information can be clinically useful when making medical management decisions (e.g., the use of inflammatory markers) and emphasizing to patients the benefits of smoking cessation and dietary modification. In some cases, genotype information may also assist with clinical diagnosis.

PROCEDURE AND PATIENT CARE
Before

 Explain the procedure to the patient.

During

- Collect a venous sample of blood in a lavender- or a yellow-top tube.

After

- Apply pressure to the venipuncture site.
- Tell the patient that results may not be available for a few weeks.

ABNORMAL FINDINGS

▲ Increased

ARMD: *Patients with abnormal genetics as described are at a marked increased risk for developing macular degeneration.*

Agglutinin, Febrile/Cold

NORMAL FINDINGS

Febrile (warm) agglutinins: no agglutination in titres ≤1:80
Cold agglutinins: no agglutination in titres ≤1:16

INDICATIONS

Febrile agglutinin serologic studies are used to diagnose infectious diseases such as salmonellosis, rickettsial diseases, brucellosis, and tularemia. Neoplastic diseases, such as leukemias and lymphomas, are also associated with febrile agglutinins. Appropriate antibiotic treatment of the infectious agent is associated with a drop in the titre activity of febrile agglutinins. *Cold* agglutinins occur in patients who are infected by other agents, most notably *Mycoplasma pneumoniae.* Other diseases that produce cold agglutinins include influenza, mononucleosis, rheumatoid arthritis, lymphomas, and hemolytic anemia.

TEST EXPLANATION

The febrile and cold agglutinins are antibodies that cause red blood cells (RBCs) to aggregate at high or low temperatures, respectively. They are believed to be a result of infection by organisms with antigenic groups similar to some of those found on the RBCs. Agglutination may occur normally in concentrated serum (<1:32 dilution). Agglutination occurring at titres greater than 1:16 for cold agglutinins and 1:80 for febrile agglutinins is considered abnormal and diagnostic of the infectious agent or disease with which the agglutinins are associated. Agglutinins in high titres can attack RBCs and cause hemolytic anemias. Cold agglutinins are often measured during the suspected acute phase of the disease, and measurement is repeated during the convalescence phase (7 to 10 days later). A fourfold or higher increase in antibody titre is considered diagnostic for the associated infectious diseases. Titre elevation is directly related to severity of infection. High titres of either cold or febrile agglutinins can interfere with blood typing, crossmatching, and transfusion. In older adults, agglutinins can persist for years after an associated illness.

Temperature regulation is critical when these tests are performed. For cold agglutinins, the red-top tube is previously warmed to over 37°C; for febrile agglutinins, the red-top tube is cooled. The specimen is taken to the laboratory immediately so that no hemolysis will occur. Under no circumstances should the cold agglutinin specimen be refrigerated or the febrile agglutinin heated before it reaches the laboratory. At the laboratory, the cold agglutinin specimen is chilled and evaluated for agglutination of RBCs. The febrile agglutinin specimen is heated and also inspected for agglutination of RBCs. Serial dilutions are performed to detect the dilution at which agglutination occurs.

INTERFERING FACTORS

Some antibiotics (cephalosporins and penicillin) can interfere with the development of cold agglutinins.

PROCEDURE AND PATIENT CARE

Before

- Explain the procedure to the patient.
- Inform the patient that no fasting is required.

During

- Collect a venous blood sample in a red-top tube (warmed or cooled; see previous discussion).

After

- Apply pressure or a pressure dressing to the venipuncture site.
- Observe the venipuncture site for bleeding.
- Immediately transport the specimen to the laboratory.

TEST RESULTS AND CLINICAL SIGNIFICANCE

▲ Increased Cold Agglutinins

Viral illness: rapid rise (7 days) peaking at 14 days and falling at 25 days,
Mycoplasma pneumoniae infection,
Infectious mononucleosis,
Influenza,
Nonbacterial infection,
Collagen-vascular diseases (e.g., scleroderma, rheumatoid arthritis),
Cirrhosis,
Systemic lupus erythematosus,
Leukemia, lymphoma, multiple myeloma: *These diseases are associated with very high titres of cold agglutinins.*

▲ Increased Febrile Agglutinins

Salmonella,
Rickettsia,
Brucellosis,
Tularemia,
Leukemia,
Systemic lupus erythematosus,
Lymphoma: *These diseases are associated with high titres of febrile agglutinins.*

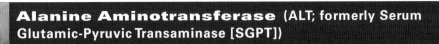

Alanine Aminotransferase (ALT; formerly Serum Glutamic-Pyruvic Transaminase [SGPT])

NORMAL FINDINGS

Older adult: may be slightly higher than adult values
Adult: **5–35 U/L** (5–35 mU/mL)
   Values may be higher in men and in Black patients.

	Male	Female
Infant:		
1–7 days:	6–40 U/L	7–40 U/L
8–30 days:	10–40 U/L	8–32 U/L
1–3 months:	13–39 U/L	12–47 U/L
4–6 months:	12–42 U/L	12–37 U/L
7–12 months:	13–45 U/L	12–41 U/L
Child:		
1–3 years:	19–59 U/L	24–59 U/L
4–6 years:	24–49 U/L	24–49 U/L
14–15 years:	24–54 U/L	19–44 U/L
16–19 years:	24–54 U/L	19–49 U/L

INDICATIONS

This test is used to identify hepatocellular diseases of the liver. It is also an accurate monitor of improvement or worsening of these diseases. In jaundiced patients, an abnormal ALT level indicates that the liver, rather than red blood cell (RBC) hemolysis, is the source of the jaundice.

TEST EXPLANATION

ALT is found predominantly in the liver; lesser quantities are found in the kidneys, heart, and skeletal muscle. Injury or disease affecting the liver parenchyma causes a release of this hepatocellular enzyme into the bloodstream, thus elevating serum ALT levels. Most ALT elevations are caused by liver dysfunction. Therefore, this enzyme is not only sensitive to but also quite specific for hepatocellular disease. In hepatocellular disease other than viral hepatitis, the ratio of ALT to aspartate aminotransferase (DeRitis ratio) is less than 1. In viral hepatitis, the ratio is greater than 1. This is helpful in the diagnosis of viral hepatitis.

INTERFERING FACTORS

- Previous intramuscular injections may cause elevations in ALT levels.
- Drugs that may cause *increases* in ALT levels include acetaminophen, allopurinol, salicylic acid, ampicillin, azathioprine, carbamazepine, cephalosporins, chlordiazepoxide, chlorpropamide, clofibrate, cloxacillin, codeine, dicumarol, indomethacin, isoniazid, methotrexate, methyldopa, nafcillin, nalidixic acid, nitrofurantoin, oral contraceptives, oxacillin, phenothiazines, phenylbutazone, phenytoin, procainamide, propoxyphene, propranolol, quinidine, salicylates, tetracyclines, and verapamil.

Blood Studies

2

PROCEDURE AND PATIENT CARE

Before
☒ Explain the procedure to the patient.
☒ Inform the patient that no fasting is required.

During
• Collect a venous blood sample in a red-top tube.

After
• Apply pressure or a pressure dressing to the venipuncture site.
• Assess the venipuncture site for bleeding. Patients with liver dysfunction often have prolonged clotting times.
• Send the sample to the laboratory for analysis.

TEST RESULTS AND CLINICAL SIGNIFICANCE

▲ Significantly Increased Levels
Hepatitis,
Hepatic necrosis,
Hepatic ischemia

▲ Moderately Increased Levels
Cirrhosis,
Cholestasis,
Hepatic tumour,
Hepatotoxic drugs,
Obstructive jaundice,
Severe burns,
Trauma to striated muscle

▲ Mildly Increased Levels
Myositis,
Pancreatitis,
Myocardial infarction,
Infectious mononucleosis,
Shock: *Injury or disease affecting the liver, heart, or skeletal muscles causes a release of this enzyme into the bloodstream, thus elevating serum ALT levels.*

RELATED TESTS

Aspartate Aminotransferase (p. 130), Gamma-Glutamyl Transpeptidase (p. 261), Alkaline Phosphatase (p. 53), and 5'-Nucleotidase (p. 389). These are other enzymes that exist predominantly in the liver and are measured to provide further information on the function of the liver.

Creatine Kinase (p. 201). This enzyme exists predominantly in heart and skeletal muscle and is measured in a manner similar to that for ALT.

Lactate Dehydrogenase (p. 339). This is an intracellular enzyme; its measurements are used to support the diagnosis of injury or disease involving the heart, liver, RBCs, kidneys, skeletal muscle, brain, and lungs.

Leucine Aminopeptidase (p. 351). This enzyme is specific to the hepatobiliary system. Diseases affecting that system cause elevations in levels of this enzyme.

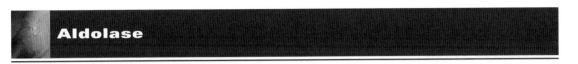

Aldolase

NORMAL FINDINGS

Adult: **<8.0 U/L** (3.0–8.2 Sibley-Lehninger units/dL)
Child (25 months to 16 years): **1.2–8.8 U/L**
Infant (10–24 months): **3.4–11.8 U/L**

INDICATIONS

This test is used to aid in the diagnosis and surveillance of skeletal muscle diseases.

TEST EXPLANATION

Serum aldolase is very similar to the enzymes aspartate aminotransferase (see p. 130) and creatine kinase (see p. 201). Aldolase is an enzyme used in the glycolytic breakdown of glucose. Like aspartate aminotransferase and creatine kinase, aldolase is present in most tissues of the body. This test is most useful for identifying muscular or hepatic cellular injury or destruction. The serum aldolase level is very high in patients with muscular dystrophies, dermatomyositis, and polymyositis. Levels also are increased with injuries such as gangrenous processes and muscular trauma and with such conditions as muscular infectious diseases (e.g., trichinosis), chronic hepatitis, obstructive jaundice, and cirrhosis.

Neurologic diseases causing weakness can be differentiated from muscular causes of weakness with this test. Aldolase values are normal in patients with such neurologic diseases as poliomyelitis, myasthenia gravis, and multiple sclerosis. Aldolase levels are elevated in patients with primary muscular disorders.

INTERFERING FACTORS

- Previous intramuscular injections may cause elevations in aldolase levels.
- Strenuous exercise can cause a transient spike in aldolase level.
- Drugs that may cause *increases* in aldolase levels include hepatotoxic agents.
- Drugs that may cause *decreases* in aldolase levels include phenothiazine.

PROCEDURE AND PATIENT CARE

Before

- Explain the procedure to the patient.
- Inform the patient that a short period of NPO status (4–6 hours) usually enables more accurate results.

During

• Collect a venous blood sample in a red-top tube.

After

• Apply pressure or a pressure dressing to the venipuncture site.
• Observe the venipuncture site for bleeding.

TEST RESULTS AND CLINICAL SIGNIFICANCE

▲ Increased Levels

Muscular Diseases

Muscular dystrophy (highest aldolase levels associated with Duchenne muscular dystrophy),
Dermatomyositis,
Polymyositis

Muscle Injury

Muscular trauma (examples include severe crush injuries, muscular infections [such as trichinosis], delirium tremens, severe burns),
Gangrenous/ischemic processes (such as prolonged shock): *Disease of or injury to muscle causes lysis of the muscle cells. Intracellular enzymes such as aldolase spill into the bloodstream and are detected at elevated levels.*

Hepatocellular Diseases

Hepatitis,
Cirrhosis: *Diseases of the liver cause lysis of the liver cells. Intracellular enzymes such as aldolase spill into the bloodstream and are detected at elevated levels.*

Myocardial Infarction. Infarction of heart muscle causes lysis of the muscle cells. Intracellular enzymes such as aldolase spill into the bloodstream and are detected at elevated levels.

▼ Decreased Levels

Muscle wasting diseases,
Late muscular dystrophy: *As muscle mass decreases, aldolase values decrease.*
Hereditary fructose intolerance: *Without an adequate source of glycogen (i.e., fructose), normal levels of aldolase are not needed.*

RELATED TEST

Creatine Kinase (p. 201). This is another muscular enzyme, and its levels are more frequently used for identifying cardiac and skeletal injury.

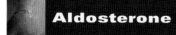

Aldosterone

NORMAL FINDINGS

Blood

Adult: **0.11–0.86 nmol/L**
  Supine: peak, **0.35 nmol/L**; nadir, **0.14 nmol/L** (3–10 ng/dL)

Upright (sitting for at least 2 hours): **<0.03–1.05 nmol/L** (male, 6–22 ng/dL; female, 5–30 ng/dL)
Child/adolescent:
  Newborn: **0.194–5.106 nmol/L** (7–184 ng/dL)
  1 month to 1 year: **0.139 – 2.498 nmol/L** (5–90 ng/dL)
  1–2 years: **0.194–1.499 nmol/L** (7–54 ng/dL)
  2–10 years: **0.083–0.971 nmol/L** (3–35 ng/dL)
  10–15 years: **0.056–0.611 nmol/L** (2–22 ng/dL)

Urine
17–70 nmol/24 hour (2–26 *Mcg*/24 hour)

INDICATIONS

This test is used to diagnose hyperaldosteronism. To differentiate primary aldosteronism (adrenal disease) from secondary aldosteronism (extra-adrenal disease), a plasma renin assay must be performed simultaneously with the aldosterone test.

TEST EXPLANATION

Aldosterone, a hormone produced by the adrenal cortex, is a potent mineralocorticoid. Production of aldosterone is regulated primarily by the renin-angiotensin system. This system works as follows: A decreased effective renal blood flow triggers pressure-sensitive renal glomerular elements to release renin. The renin then stimulates the liver to secrete angiotensin I, which is converted to angiotensin II in the lung and kidney. Angiotensin II is a potent stimulator of aldosterone (see Figure 2-21, p. 461).

Secondarily, aldosterone is stimulated by adrenocorticotropic hormone (ACTH), low serum sodium levels, and high serum potassium levels. Aldosterone, in turn, stimulates the renal tubules to absorb sodium (and then water) and to secrete potassium in the urine. In this way, aldosterone regulates serum sodium and potassium levels. Because water follows sodium transport, aldosterone also partially regulates water absorption (and plasma volume).

Increased aldosterone levels are associated with primary aldosteronism, in which a tumour (usually an adenoma) of the adrenal cortex (Conn syndrome) or bilateral adrenal nodular hyperplasia causes increased production of aldosterone. The typical pattern for primary aldosteronism is an increase in aldosterone level and a decrease in renin level. The renin level is low because the increased aldosterone level disables the renin-angiotensin system. Patients with primary aldosteronism characteristically have hypertension, weakness, polyuria, and hypokalemia.

Increased aldosterone levels also occur with secondary aldosteronism caused by nonadrenal conditions. These include the following:
- Renal vascular stenosis or occlusion
- Hyponatremia (from diuretic or laxative abuse) or low salt intake
- Hypovolemia
- Pregnancy or use of estrogens
- Malignant hypertension
- Potassium loading
- Poor perfusion states (e.g., heart failure)
- Decreased intravascular volume (e.g., cirrhosis, nephrotic syndrome)

In secondary aldosteronism, aldosterone levels and renin levels are high.

The aldosterone assay can be performed on a 24-hour urine specimen or a plasma blood sample. The advantage of the 24-hour urine sample is that short-term fluctuations are eliminated.

Sampling plasma values is more convenient, but they are affected by short-term fluctuations. Factors that can rapidly cause fluctuation in aldosterone levels include the following:
- *Diurnal variation:* Aldosterone levels peak in early morning. In late afternoon, the levels are half those of the morning.
- *Body position:* In the upright position, plasma aldosterone levels are greatly increased.
- *Diet:* Levels of both urine and plasma aldosterone are increased by low-sodium diets and are decreased by high-sodium diets. (Diets high and low in potassium have the opposite effects.)

A 24-hour urine collection is therefore much more reliable because the effect of these interfering factors is dampened.

Primary aldosteronism can be diagnosed by demonstrating little or no increase in renin levels after aldosterone stimulation (in which salt restriction serves as the stimulant). This is because aldosterone is already maximally secreted by the diseased adrenal gland. Also, patients with primary aldosteronism fail to suppress aldosterone after saline infusion (1.5 to 2 L of normal saline solution infused between 8 AM and 10 AM). Aldosterone can be measured in blood obtained from adrenal venous sampling (see p. 1023). In this situation, high levels from the right and left adrenal veins are diagnostic of bilateral adrenal hyperplasia. Unilateral high aldosterone levels are found in patients with aldosterone-producing tumours of the adrenal gland or renal artery stenosis. Renin levels are usually measured at the same time. High unilateral renin levels in combination with unilateral high aldosterone levels indicate renal artery stenosis. Aldosterone-producing tumours of the adrenal gland are characterized by unilateral high levels of adrenal vein aldosterone and low levels of renin.

Clinical Priorities

- Aldosterone levels exhibit a diurnal variation, with levels peaking early in the morning and lowering in the late afternoon.
- Body position affects aldosterone levels. Levels are greatly increased in the upright position. Usually patients should be sitting up for at least 2 hours before blood is collected.
- Levels of both urine and plasma aldosterone are increased by low-sodium diets and are decreased by high-sodium diets. Patients should maintain a normal-sodium diet (~3 g/day) for at least 2 weeks before blood or urine collection.
- A random aldosterone test result is of no significant value unless plasma renin activity is measured at the same time.

INTERFERING FACTORS
- Strenuous exercise and stress can stimulate adrenocortical secretions and increase aldosterone levels.
- Excessive licorice ingestion can cause decreases in aldosterone levels because licorice produces an aldosterone-like effect.
- Values are influenced by posture, diet, pregnancy, and diurnal variations.
- Patient position can significantly affect aldosterone levels.
- Aldosterone levels can be three to five times higher with low-sodium diets.
- If the test is performed by radioimmunoassay, recently administered radioactive medications will affect test results.
- Drugs that may cause *increases* in aldosterone levels include diazoxide (Proglycem), hydralazine (Apresoline), nitroprusside (Nipride), diuretics, laxatives, potassium, and spironolactone.

Drugs that may cause *decreases* in aldosterone levels include angiotensin-converting enzyme inhibitors (e.g., captopril), fludrocortisone (Florinef), licorice, and propranolol (Inderal).

PROCEDURE AND PATIENT CARE

Before

- Explain the procedure for blood collection to the patient. Usually the patient is asked to be in the upright position (at least sitting) for a minimum of 2 hours before blood is collected. On occasion, blood is collected again before the patient gets out of bed. Inform nonhospitalized patients when to arrive at the laboratory and to maintain the upright position for at least 2 hours.
- Inform the patient that no fasting is necessary.
- Explain the procedure for collecting a 24-hour urine sample.
- Give the patient verbal and written instructions regarding dietary and medication restrictions.
- Instruct the patient to maintain a normal-sodium diet (~3 g/day) for at least 2 weeks before blood or urine collection.
- Consult with the patient's physician whether drugs that alter sodium, potassium, and fluid balance (e.g., diuretics, antihypertensives, steroids, oral contraceptives) can be withheld. Test results are more accurate if these drugs are withheld for at least 2 weeks before either the blood or urine test.
- Inform the patient to avoid renin inhibitors (e.g., propranolol) for 1 week before the test, if this is confirmed by the physician.
- Instruct the patient to avoid licorice for at least 2 weeks before the test because of its aldosterone-like effect.

During

Blood Collection

- Collect a venous blood sample in a gold-top (serum separator) tube. For hospitalized patients, the sample is occasionally collected first with the patient in the supine position. A second specimen (upright sample) is collected 4 hours later after the patient has been up and moving.
- Obtain the specimen in the morning.
- On the laboratory slip, indicate whether the patient was supine or standing during the venipuncture.
- Handle the blood specimen gently. Rough handling may cause hemolysis and thereby alter the test results.
- Transport the specimen in a mixture of crushed ice and water to the laboratory.
- Indicate the source of the specimen (i.e., peripheral or adrenal vein).

Urine Collection

- Instruct the patient to discard the first morning specimen and then collect subsequent urine in a pre-acidified container. The first such collection is the start time of the 24-hour collection.
- Collect all urine passed over the next 24 hours in the container.
- Instruct the patient to void before defecating so that the urine is not contaminated by feces.
- Remind the patient not to put toilet paper in the collection container.
- Keep the urine specimen in a mixture of crushed ice and water or keep it refrigerated during the 24 hours.
- Instruct the patient to void as close as possible to the end of the 24 hours and to add this specimen to the collection.

After
Blood Collection
- Apply pressure or a pressure dressing to the venipuncture site.
- Assess the venipuncture site for bleeding.
- Transport the blood specimen promptly to the laboratory.

Urine Collection
- Transport the urine specimen promptly to the laboratory.

TEST RESULTS AND CLINICAL SIGNIFICANCE

▲ Increased Levels

Primary Aldosteronism
Aldosterone-producing adrenal adenoma (Conn disease),
Adrenal cortical nodular hyperplasia,
Bartter syndrome (renal wasting of potassium associated with poor sodium tubule absorption): *Aldosterone is produced in abnormally high quantities by the diseased adrenal gland. Such production is reflected in serum and urine levels.*

Secondary Aldosteronism
Hyponatremia,
Hyperkalemia,
Diuretic ingestion resulting in hypovolemia and hyponatremia,
Laxative abuse: *These are all direct stimulants of aldosterone.*
Stress,
Malignant hypertension,
Poor perfusion states (e.g., heart failure),
Decreased intravascular volume (e.g., cirrhosis, nephrotic syndrome),
Renal arterial stenosis,
Pregnancy and oral contraceptives,
Hypovolemia or hemorrhage: *The renin-angiotensin system is stimulated in these conditions. Renin levels are high, and aldosterone secretion is stimulated.*
Cushing's disease: *Abnormally high ACTH levels secreted by a pituitary adenoma act as a direct stimulant of aldosterone production.*

▼ Decreased Levels

Renin deficiency: *This is very rare and results in aldosterone deficiency.*
Steroid therapy: *ACTH production is suppressed, and therefore aldosterone production is suppressed.*
Addison's disease: *The adrenal cortex is not functional and therefore aldosterone cannot be secreted.*
Patients on a high-sodium diet,
Hypernatremia,
Addison's disease: *These act as potent inhibitors of aldosterone secretion.*
Antihypertensive therapy: *Some antihypertensive medications inhibit aldosterone secretion.*
Aldosterone deficiency,
Toxemia of pregnancy

RELATED TESTS

Sodium, Blood (p. 479); Sodium, Urine (p. 980); Potassium, Blood (p. 420); and Potassium, Urine (p. 976). These are direct measurements of these electrolytes that can help to determine secondary versus primary aldosteronism.

Adrenocorticotropic Hormone (p. 34). This is a test of anterior pituitary gland function.

Renin Assay, Plasma (p. 460). This test is helpful in the differential diagnosis of primary versus secondary aldosteronism.

 Alkaline Phosphatase (ALP)

NORMAL FINDINGS

Older adult: slightly higher than adult values
Adult: **40–160 IU/L** (40-160 U/L)
Child/adolescent:
    1–3 years: **185–383 IU/L**
    4–6 years: **191–450 IU/L**
    7–9 years: **218–499 IU/L**

	Male	Female
10–11 years:	174–624 IU/L	169–657 IU/L
12–13 years:	245–584 IU/L	141–499 IU/L
14–15 years:	169–618 IU/L	103–283 IU/L
16–19 years:	98–317 IU/L	82–169 IU/L

INDICATIONS

ALP is measured in order to detect and monitor diseases of the liver or bone.

TEST EXPLANATION

Although ALP is found in many tissues, the concentrations are highest in the liver, epithelium of the biliary tract, and bone. The intestinal mucosa and placenta also contain ALP. This phosphatase enzyme is called *alkaline* because its function is increased in an alkaline (pH of 9 to 10) environment. This enzyme test is important for detecting liver and bone disorders. Within the liver, ALP is present in Kupffer cells. These cells line the biliary collecting system, and this enzyme is excreted into the bile. Enzyme levels of ALP are greatly increased in both extrahepatic and intrahepatic obstructive biliary disease and cirrhosis. Other liver abnormalities, such as hepatic tumours, hepatotoxic drugs, and hepatitis, cause smaller elevations in ALP levels. Reports have indicated that the most sensitive test to indicate tumour metastasis to the liver is the ALP.

Bone is the most frequent extrahepatic source of ALP; new bone growth is associated with elevated ALP levels. Pathologic new bone growth occurs with osteoblastic metastatic (e.g., breast, prostate) tumours. Paget's disease, healing fractures, rheumatoid arthritis, hyperparathyroidism, and normal-growing bones are causes of elevations in ALP levels as well.

Isoenzymes of ALP are also measured to distinguish between liver and bone diseases. These isoenzymes are most easily differentiated by the heat stability test and electrophoresis. The isoenzyme of liver origin (ALP1) is heat stable; the isoenzyme of bone origin (ALP2) is inactivated by heat. The detection of isoenzymes can help differentiate the source of the pathologic condition associated with the elevated total ALP. ALP1 levels are expected to be high when liver disease is the cause of the elevation in total ALP. ALP2 levels are expected to be high when bone disease is the cause of the elevation in total ALP. Another way to distinguish the cause of elevations in ALP is to simultaneously test for 5'-nucleotidase. This latter enzyme is made predominantly in the liver. If total ALP and 5'-nucleotidase levels are concomitantly elevated, the disease is in the liver. If 5'-nucleotidase is normal, the bone is the most probable source.

Age-Related Concerns

- Young children have increased ALP levels because their bones are growing. This increase is magnified during the adolescent "growth spurt," which occurs at different ages in boys and girls.

INTERFERING FACTORS

- Recent ingestion of a meal can increase the ALP level.
- Young children with rapid bone growth have increased ALP levels. This is most magnified during the adolescent growth spurt. The age at growth spurt differs between girls and boys.
- Drugs that may cause *increases* in ALP levels include albumin made from placental tissue, allopurinol, antibiotics, azathioprine, colchicine, fluorides, indomethacin, isoniazid, methotrexate, methyldopa, nicotinic acid, phenothiazine, probenecid, tetracycline, and verapamil.
- Drugs that may cause *decreases* in ALP levels include arsenicals, cyanides, fluorides, nitrofurantoin, oxalates, and zinc salts.

PROCEDURE AND PATIENT CARE

Before

- Explain the procedure to the patient.
- Inform the patient that fasting is preferred but not required. Overnight fasting may be required for isoenzymes. The ALP level is generally higher after eating.

During

- Collect a venous blood sample in a red-top tube.

After

- Apply pressure or a pressure dressing to the venipuncture site.
- Assess the venipuncture site for bleeding. Patients with liver dysfunction often have prolonged clotting times.

TEST RESULTS AND CLINICAL SIGNIFICANCE

▲ Increased Levels

Primary cirrhosis,

Intrahepatic or extrahepatic biliary obstruction,

Primary or metastatic liver tumour: *ALP is found in the liver and biliary epithelium. It is normally excreted into the bile. Obstruction, no matter how mild, causes elevations in ALP.*

Metastatic tumour to the bone,

Healing fracture,

Hyperparathyroidism,

Osteomalacia,

Paget's disease,

Rheumatoid arthritis,

Rickets: *In these diseases, the ALP comes from the bone.*

Intestinal ischemia or infarction,

Myocardial infarction,

Sarcoidosis

▼ Decreased Levels

Hypophosphatemia: *There is insufficient phosphate to make ALP.*

Hypophosphatasia,

Malnutrition,

Milk-alkali syndrome,

Pernicious anemia,

Scurvy (vitamin C deficiency)

RELATED TESTS

Alanine Aminotransferase (p. 45). This liver enzyme can aid in the differential diagnosis of causes of ALP elevation. If both the alanine aminotransferase and the ALP levels are elevated, hepatocellular disease is suspected.

Aspartate Aminotransferase (p. 130). Measurements of this liver enzyme can aid in the differential diagnosis of causes of ALP elevation. If both the aspartate aminotransferase and the ALP levels are elevated, hepatocellular disease is suspected.

Gamma-Glutamyl Transpeptidase (p. 261). Measurements of this liver enzyme can aid in the differential diagnosis of causes of ALP elevation. If both this and the ALP levels are elevated, diseases affecting the biliary tree are suspected.

5'-Nucleotidase (p. 389). Measurements of this liver enzyme can aid in the differential diagnosis of causes of ALP elevation. If both the 5'-nucleotidase and the ALP levels are elevated, diseases affecting the biliary tree are suspected.

Acid Phosphatase (p. 30). Measurements of this bone enzyme can aid in the differential diagnosis of causes of ALP elevation. If both the acid phosphatase and the ALP levels are elevated, bone disease is suspected.

Creatine Kinase (p. 201). This enzyme exists predominantly in heart and skeletal muscle.

Lactate Dehydrogenase (p. 339). Measurements of this intracellular enzyme are used to support the diagnosis of injury or disease involving the heart, liver, red blood cells, kidneys, skeletal muscle, brain, and lungs. If ALP and lactate dehydrogenase are elevated, liver disease is suspected.

Leucine Aminopeptidase (p. 351). This enzyme is specific to the hepatobiliary system. Diseases affecting that system cause elevations in levels of this enzyme.

Allergy Blood Testing (IgE Antibody Test, Radioallergosorbent Test)

NORMAL FINDINGS

Total immunoglobulin E (IgE) serum levels: >0.35 kIU/L

INDICATIONS

Allergy blood testing is an alternative to allergy skin testing in diagnosing allergy as a cause of a particular symptom complex. It is also useful in identifying the specific allergen affecting a patient. It is particularly helpful when allergy skin testing is contraindicated.

TEST EXPLANATION

Measurement of serum IgE is an effective method to diagnose allergy and specifically identify the allergen (the substance to which the person is allergic). Serum IgE levels increase when allergic individuals are exposed to the allergen. Various classes of allergens can initiate the allergic response. They include animal dandruff, foods, pollens, dusts, moulds, insect venoms, drugs, and agents in the occupational environment.

Although skin testing (see p. 1123) can also identify a specific allergen, measurement of serum levels of IgE is helpful when a skin test result is questionable, when the allergen is not available in a form for dermal injection, or when the allergen may incite an anaphylactic reaction if injected into the patient. IgE is especially helpful in cases in which skin testing is particularly difficult (e.g., in infants or in cases of dermatographism or widespread dermatitis). However, it is important to note that an assay for IgE is expensive and the results are not available immediately. The decision concerning which method to use to diagnose an allergy and to identify the allergen depends on the elapsed time between exposure to an allergen and testing, the class of allergen, the age of the patient, the possibility of anaphylaxis, and the affected target organ (e.g., skin, lungs, intestine).

IgE levels, like provocative skin testing, are used not only to diagnose allergy but also to identify the allergen so that an immunotherapeutic regimen can be developed. Increased levels of total IgE can be diagnostic of allergic disease in general. Specific IgE blood testing, however, is an in vitro test for specific IgE directed to a specific allergen. Since the development of liquid allergen preparations, the use of in vitro blood allergy testing has increased considerably. It is more accurate and safer than skin testing.

Once the allergen has been identified, the treatment for most patients includes avoidance of the allergen and use of bronchodilators, antihistamines, and possibly steroids. If aggressive antiallergy treatment is provided before the test, IgE levels may not rise despite the existence of an allergy.

Allergy to latex-containing products is an increasingly common allergy for which certain industrial and most medical personnel are at risk. It is an allergy that may develop in otherwise nonallergic patients because of overexposure. Furthermore, patients with latex exposure are at risk for allergic reaction if they undergo operative procedures or any procedure for which the health care providers wear latex gloves. In these patients, a latex-specific IgE can be easily identified with the use of an enzyme-labelled immunometric assay. This test is 94% accurate.

Of the many methods of measuring IgE, one of the most commonly used is the radioallergosorbent test. In this method, the serum of a patient suspected of having a specific allergy is mixed with a specific allergen. The antibody-allergen complex is then incubated with one or more radiolabelled monoclonal anti-IgE antibodies. The total amount of IgE can be measured. Enzyme-conjugated, radioimmunometric, colorimetric, fluorometric, or chemiluminometric methods are used for allergen-specific IgE quantification. Accuracy varies between 45% and 95%, depending on the allergen.

CONTRAINDICATIONS

- The presence of multiple allergies, because testing will yield no information regarding identification of the specific allergen.

INTERFERING FACTORS

- Concurrent diseases associated with elevated immunoglobulin G (IgG) levels cause false-negative results.
- Drugs that may cause *increases* in IgE levels include corticosteroids.

PROCEDURE AND PATIENT CARE

Before
- Explain the procedure to the patient.
- Explain to the patient that the suspected allergen will be mixed with the patient's blood specimen in the laboratory. The patient will not be exposed to the allergen.
- Determine whether the patient has recently been treated with a corticosteroid for allergies.

During
- Collect a venous blood sample in a gold-top (serum separator) tube.

After
- Apply pressure or a pressure bandage to the venipuncture site.

TEST RESULTS AND CLINICAL SIGNIFICANCE

Allergy-Related Diseases

Asthma,
Dermatitis,
Food allergy,
Drug allergy,
Latex allergy,
Occupational allergy,
Allergic rhinitis,
Angioedema: *All these diseases are immunoreactive conditions. IgE is the mediator of the "allergic response," and levels of IgE are expected to be elevated in these diseases.*

RELATED TESTS

Allergy Skin Testing (p. 1123). Skin testing is the easiest and least expensive manner of determining specific allergic reactions. However, skin testing is not available for many allergens and may cause an anaphylactic response.

Immunoglobulin Electrophoresis (p. 327). This test is used to assist in the diagnosis of several different disease states. Levels of IgE are occasionally elevated, which indicates that the disease is associated with an allergic response.

Alpha$_1$-Antitrypsin (AAT, A$_1$AT, AAT Phenotyping)

NORMAL FINDINGS

0.85–2.13 g/L (85–213 mg/dL)

INDICATIONS

Serum alpha$_1$-antitrypsin determinations are obtained in patients with a family history of emphysema, because there is a familial tendency for a deficiency of this antienzyme. In serum, deficiencies in or absence of this enzyme can cause the early onset of disabling emphysema. A similar deficiency in alpha$_1$-antitrypsin is observed in children with cirrhosis and other liver diseases.

Alpha$_1$-antitrypsin is also an acute-phase reactant protein that is elevated in the presence of inflammation, infection, or malignancy. It is not specific with regard to the source of the inflammatory process.

TEST EXPLANATION

Alpha$_1$-antitrypsin inactivates endoproteases (protein catabolic enzymes that are released in the body by degenerating and dying cells), such as trypsin and neutrophil elastase, that can break down elastic fibres and collagen, especially in the lung. Deficiencies of alpha$_1$-antitrypsin can be genetic or acquired. Acquired deficiencies can occur in patients with protein-deficiency syndromes (e.g., malnutrition, liver disease, nephrotic syndrome, neonatal respiratory distress syndrome). People with alpha$_1$-antitrypsin deficiency develop severe panacinar (although usually more severe in the lower third of the lungs) emphysema in the third or fourth decade of life. Their major clinical symptoms usually include progressive dyspnea with minimal coughing. Chronic bronchitis is prominent in those patients with deficient alpha$_1$-antitrypsin levels who smoke. Bronchiectasis can also occur in these patients.

Inherited alpha$_1$-antitrypsin deficiency is associated with symptoms earlier in life than acquired alpha$_1$-antitrypsin disease. The inherited condition is also commonly associated with liver and biliary disease. Alpha$_1$-antitrypsin genetic phenotyping has shown that most persons have two alpha$_1$-antitrypsin "M" genes (designated *MM*) and alpha$_1$-antitrypsin levels above 2.50 g/L. "Z" and "S" gene mutations are typically associated with alterations in serum levels of alpha$_1$-antitrypsin. Individuals who are *ZZ* or *SS* homozygous have serum levels below 0.5 g/L and often near zero.

In the *MZ* or *MS* heterozygous state, serum levels of alpha$_1$-antitrypsin are diminished or low normal. Approximately 5% to 14% of the adult population have this heterozygous state, which is considered to be a risk factor for emphysema. Homozygous individuals have severe pulmonary and liver disease very early in life. Alpha$_1$-antitrypsin genetic phenotyping is particularly helpful when blood alpha$_1$-antitrypsin levels are suggestive but not definitive.

Alpha$_1$-antitrypsin is measured qualitatively through immunochemical methods. Quantification is possible but rarely useful with phenotyping. Routine serum protein electrophoresis (p. 440) is a good screening test for alpha$_1$-antitrypsin deficiency because alpha$_1$-antitrypsin accounts for approximately 90% of the protein in the alpha$_1$-globulin region on electrophoresis.

INTERFERING FACTORS

- Serum levels of alpha$_1$-antitrypsin can double during pregnancy.
- Drugs that may cause *increases* in alpha$_1$-antitrypsin levels include oral contraceptives.

PROCEDURE AND PATIENT CARE

Before

- Explain the procedure to the patient.
- Verify with the laboratory performing the study that no fasting is required. Inform the patient accordingly.

During

- Collect a venous blood sample in a red-top tube.

After

- Apply pressure or a pressure dressing to the venipuncture site.
- Observe the venipuncture site for bleeding.
- If the results show the patient is at risk for emphysema, begin patient teaching. Include such factors as avoidance of smoking, infection, and inhaled irritants; proper nutrition; adequate hydration; and education about the disease process of emphysema.
- If the test result is positive, genetic counselling is indicated. Other family members should be tested to determine their and their children's risks.

TEST RESULTS AND CLINICAL SIGNIFICANCE

▲ Increased Levels

Acute and chronic inflammatory disorders,

Stress,

Infection,

Thyroid infections: *Because alpha$_1$-antitrypsin is an acute-phase reactant protein, elevated levels can be expected when the body is subjected to any inflammatory reaction or stress.*

▼ Decreased Levels

Early onset of emphysema (in adults),

Neonatal respiratory distress syndrome,

Cirrhosis (in children): *These diseases result from a lack of inhibition of endoprotease activity (no alpha$_1$-antitrypsin available) within the body. Collagen is broken down, which leads to the destruction of lung and liver structures.*

Low serum proteins: *Diseases such as malnutrition, end-stage cancer, nephrotic syndrome, protein-losing enteropathy, and hepatic failure are associated with lack of protein synthesis. Alpha$_1$-antitrypsin is a protein and is therefore not produced in adequate quantities in these diseases.*

RELATED TESTS

C-Reactive Protein (p. 199). This also is an acute-phase reactant protein that can help to distinguish whether a rise in alpha$_1$-antitrypsin is caused by coronary inflammation.

Erythrocyte Sedimentation Rate (p. 236). This also is an acute-phase reactant protein that can help confirm an inflammatory reaction to an acute illness.

Alpha-Fetoprotein (AFP, Alpha$_1$-Fetoprotein)

NORMAL FINDINGS

Adult: 0–40 *Mcg*/L (<40 ng/mL)
Child (ranges are stratified by weeks of gestation and vary among laboratories):

	Female	Male
1–12 months:	0.6–77.0 *Mcg*/L	0.6–28.3 *Mcg*/L
1–3 years:	0.6–11.1 *Mcg*/L	0.6–7.9 *Mcg*/L
4–6 years:	0.6–4.2 *Mcg*/L	0.6–5.6 *Mcg*/L
7–12 years:	0.6–5.6 *Mcg*/L	0.6–3.7 *Mcg*/L
13–18 years:	0.6–4.2 *Mcg*/L	0.6–3.9 *Mcg*/L

INDICATIONS

This test is used as a screening marker of increased risk for birth defects, such as fetal body wall defects, neural tube defects, and chromosomal abnormalities. It can also be used as a tumour marker to identify cancers.

TEST EXPLANATION

Alpha-fetoprotein is an oncofetal protein normally produced by the fetal liver and yolk sac. It is the dominant fetal serum protein in the first trimester of pregnancy and diminishes to very low levels by the age of 1 year. Normally, it is found in very low levels in the adult.

Alpha-fetoprotein is an effective screening serum marker for fetal body wall defects. The most notable of these are neural tube defects, which can vary from a small myelomeningocele to anencephaly. If a fetus has an open body wall defect, fetal serum alpha-fetoprotein leaks out into the amniotic fluid and is picked up by the maternal serum. Normally, alpha-fetoprotein from fetal sources can be detected in the amniotic fluid or the mother's blood after 10 weeks' gestation. Levels peak between 16 and 18 weeks of gestation. Maternal serum reflects that change in amniotic alpha-fetoprotein levels. When elevated maternal serum alpha-fetoprotein levels are identified, further evaluation—with repeated measurements of serum alpha-fetoprotein levels, amniotic fluid alpha-fetoprotein levels, and ultrasonography—is warranted. Other examples of fetal body wall defects are omphalocele and gastroschisis.

Elevated serum alpha-fetoprotein levels in pregnancy may also indicate multiple-fetus pregnancy, fetal distress, fetal congenital abnormalities, or intrauterine death. After correction for age of gestation, maternal weight, race, and presence of diabetes, low alpha-fetoprotein levels are found in mothers carrying a fetus with trisomy 21 (Down syndrome). Other indicators of trisomy are often measured simultaneously: maternal screen testing (p. 369) and nuchal translucency (see section on pelvic ultrasonography, p. 917).

Alpha-fetoprotein is also a tumour marker. Serum levels of alpha-fetoprotein are increased in as many as 90% of patients with hepatomas. The higher the alpha-fetoprotein level is, the greater the tumour burden is. The alpha-fetoprotein level is decreased if the patient is responding to antineoplastic therapy. Alpha-fetoprotein is not specific for hepatomas, although extremely high levels (>500 Mcg/L) are diagnostic for hepatoma. Other neoplastic conditions—such as nonseminomatous germ cell tumours and teratomas of the testes; yolk sac and germ cell tumours of the ovaries; and, to a lesser extent, Hodgkin disease, lymphoma, and renal cell carcinoma—are also associated with elevated alpha-fetoprotein levels. Testing methods for alpha-fetoprotein quantification include radioimmunoassay or enzyme-linked immunosorbent assay (ELISA) with a commercially available kit. Noncancerous causes of elevations in alpha-fetoprotein levels occur in patients with cirrhosis or chronic active hepatitis.

INTERFERING FACTORS
- Fetal blood contamination, which may occur during amniocentesis, can cause increases in alpha-fetoprotein levels.
- Multiple pregnancies can cause increases in alpha-fetoprotein levels.
- Recent administration of radioisotopes can affect values because results are determined by radioimmunoassay.

PROCEDURE AND PATIENT CARE
If an alpha-fetoprotein test is to be performed on amniotic fluid, follow instructions in the "Procedure and Patient Care" section for amniocentesis, p. 660.

Before
- Explain the procedure to the patient.
- Inform the patient that no food or fluid restriction is required.

During
- Collect a venous blood sample in a red-top tube.

After
- Apply pressure or a pressure dressing to the venipuncture site.
- Assess the venipuncture site for bleeding.
- On the laboratory slip, include the gestational age.

TEST RESULTS AND CLINICAL SIGNIFICANCE
▲ Increased Maternal Serum Levels
Neural tube defects (e.g., anencephaly, encephalocele, spina bifida, myelomeningocele),
Abdominal wall defects (e.g., gastroschisis, omphalocele): *If a fetus has an open body wall defect, fetal serum alpha-fetoprotein leaks out into the amniotic fluid and is picked up by the maternal serum.*
Multiple-fetus pregnancy: *The multiple fetuses produce large quantities of alpha-fetoprotein.*
Threatened abortion,
Fetal distress or congenital anomalies,
Fetal death

▲ Increased Nonmaternal Serum Levels

Primary hepatocellular cancer (hepatoma),
Germ cell or yolk sac cancer of the ovary,
Embryonal cell or germ cell tumour of the testes,
　Other cancers (e.g., stomach, colon, lung, breast, lymphoma): *Cancers contain undifferentiated cells that may carry the surface markers of their fetal predecessors.*
Liver cell necrosis (e.g., cirrhosis, hepatitis)

▼ Decreased Maternal Levels

Trisomy 21 (Down syndrome)
Fetal wastage

RELATED TESTS

Maternal Screen Testing (p. 369). This testing includes alpha-fetoprotein and other serum markers that are accurate indicators of increased risk for birth defects.
　Amniocentesis (p. 660). This is a procedure to obtain amniotic fluid for evaluation of fetal health.
　Pelvic Ultrasonography (p. 917). Nuchal translucency is an accurate indicator of trisomy chromosomal abnormalities.

Aluminum (Chromium and Other Heavy Metals)

NORMAL FINDINGS

0-0.22 *Mc*mol/L (0-6 ng/mL) (all ages)
<2.23 *Mc*mol/L (<60 ng/mL) (dialysis patients all ages)

INDICATIONS

This test is used to evaluate aluminum levels in patients with renal failure. Elevated concentrations of aluminum in a patient with an aluminum-based joint implant suggest significant prosthesis wear.

TEST EXPLANATION

Under normal physiologic conditions, the usual daily dietary intake of aluminum (5–10 mg) is completely excreted by the kidneys. Patients in renal failure (RF) lose the ability to clear aluminum and are at risk for aluminum toxicity. Aluminum-laden dialysis water and aluminum-based phosphate binder gels designed to decrease phosphate accumulation increase the incidence of aluminum toxicity in RF patients. Furthermore, the dialysis process is not highly effective at eliminating aluminum. If a significant load exceeds the body's excretory capacity, the excess is deposited in various tissues, including bone, brain, liver, heart, spleen, and muscle. This accumulation causes morbidity and mortality through various mechanisms. Brain deposition has been implicated as a cause of dialysis dementia. In bone, aluminum replaces calcium and disrupts normal osteoid formation.

Aluminum is absorbed from the gastrointestinal (GI) tract in the form of oral phosphate-binding agents (aluminum hydroxide), parenterally via immunizations, via dialysate on patients on dialysis, via total parenteral nutrition (TPN) contamination, via the urinary mucosa through bladder irrigation, and transdermally in antiperspirants. Lactate, citrate, and ascorbate all facilitate GI absorption.

Serum aluminum concentrations are likely to be increased above the reference range in patients with metallic joint prostheses. Serum concentrations >0.371 *Mc*mol/L (10 ng/mL) in a patient with an aluminum-based implant suggest significant prosthesis wear. *Chromium* and other metals can be determined using similar laboratory techniques.

INTERFERING FACTORS

- Most of the common evacuated blood collection devices have rubber stoppers that are made up of aluminum-silicate. A simple puncture of the rubber stopper for blood collection is sufficient to contaminate the specimen with aluminum; therefore special evacuated blood collection tubes are required for aluminum testing.
- Gadolinium- or iodine-containing contrast media that have been administered within 96 hours can alter the test for heavy metals, including aluminum.

PROCEDURE AND PATIENT CARE

Before
☒ Explain the procedure to the patient.
☒ Tell the patient that no fasting is required.

During
- Collect venous blood in a royal blue–top tube. A tan-top (lead only) Becton-Dickinson tube can be used.
- Have the blood sample sent to a central diagnostic laboratory. The results will be available to the local hospital in 7 to 10 days.

After
- Apply pressure to the venipuncture site.

ABNORMAL FINDINGS

▲ Increased Levels

Aluminum toxicity: *Approximately 95% of aluminum load is eliminated renally. If the load exceeds the ability of the kidney to excrete it, aluminum toxicity may occur.*

Amino Acid Profiles (Amino Acid Screen)

NORMAL FINDINGS

Normal values vary for different amino acids.

INDICATIONS

Certain amino acids are measured to identify diseases associated with specific essential amino acid deficiencies. Metabolic screening of newborns includes amino acid profiles.

TEST EXPLANATION

Amino acids are "building blocks" of proteins, hormones, nucleic acids, and pigments. They can act as neurotransmitters, enzymes, and coenzymes. Eight essential amino acids must be provided to the body by the diet. The body can make the others. The essential amino acids must be transported across the gut and renal tubular lining cells. The metabolism of the essential amino acids is critical in the production of other amino acids, proteins, carbohydrates, and lipids. Amino acid levels can thereby be affected by defects in renal tubule or gastrointestinal transport of amino acids.

When a defect is present in the metabolism or transport of any one of these amino acids, excesses of their precursors or deficiencies of their "end product" amino acid are evident in the blood, urine, or both. More than 90 diseases have been found to be associated with abnormal amino acid function. Common examples of amino acid diseases are phenylketonuria and cystinosis.

Most defects of amino acid metabolism are genetic. Sequelae of these diseases may be minimal or catastrophic (developmental delay, growth retardation, and seizures).

Clinical manifestations of these diseases may be prevented if early diagnosis enables appropriate dietary replacement of missing amino acids. Urine testing for specific amino acids is usually used as screening tests to detect some of these errors in amino acid metabolism and transport. Once a presumptive diagnosis is made, amino acid levels can be determined by chromatographic methods on blood or amniotic fluid. The genetic defects that cause many of these diseases are becoming more defined, which allows for diagnosis to be made even earlier in utero.

INTERFERING FACTORS

- Amino acid levels are affected by the circadian rhythm. Levels are usually lowest in the morning and highest by midday.
- Levels of amino acids are generally higher in infants and children than in adults.
- Pregnancy is associated with reduced levels of some amino acids.
- Normal values vary widely, and without genetic corroboratory evidence, only extremely abnormal results are diagnostic.
- Drugs that may cause *increases* in amino acid levels include bismuth, heparin, steroids, and sulphonamides.
- Drugs that may cause *decreases* in some amino acid levels include estrogens and oral contraceptives.

PROCEDURE AND PATIENT CARE

Before

- Obtain a history of the patient's symptoms.
- Obtain a pedigree highlighting family members with amino acid disorders.
- Inform the patient that a 12-hour fast is generally required before blood collection. On occasion, a particular protein or carbohydrate load is ordered to stimulate production of a particular amino acid metabolite.

During
- Collect a venous blood sample in a red-top tube.
- Usually a 24-hour or random urine specimen is required. Perform screening on a spot urine sample by using the first specimen voided in the morning.

After
- In general, genetic counselling is provided before the test. However, the patient or parents who have acute anxiety often require emotional support immediately after a specimen is obtained.

TEST RESULTS AND CLINICAL SIGNIFICANCE

▲ Increased Blood Levels
Specific aminoacidopathies (e.g., phenylketonuria, maple syrup urine disease): *The parent amino acid is present at increased quantities because of a genetic defect that impairs catabolism of that particular amino acid. The excessive buildup of that amino acid is what causes disease.*

Specific aminoacidemias (e.g., glutaric aciduria): *Products in the catabolic pathway of a particular amino acid accumulate. Which particular product accumulates depends on which enzyme is deficient (usually as a result of a genetic defect).*

▼ Decreased Blood Levels
Hartnup disease,
Nephritis,
Nephrotic syndromes:
These diseases result in amino acid deficiencies secondary to increased renal excretion.

▲ Increased Urine Levels
Specific aminoacidurias (e.g., cystinuria, homocystinuria): *Genetic defects in amino acid metabolism cause buildup of precursor amino acids that are then excreted by the kidney. Several other mechanisms affect the pathophysiologic processes of these diseases.*

RELATED TEST
Phenylketonuria. This blood test is routinely performed on newborns to exclude the diagnosis of phenylketonuria. It is part of a group of tests used in neonatal screening.

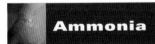

Ammonia

NORMAL FINDINGS
Child and adult: **6–47 Mcmol/L** (10–80 *Mcg/dL*)
Newborn: **<50 Mcmol/L** (90–150 *Mcg/dL*)

INDICATIONS
Ammonia is measured to support the diagnosis of severe liver diseases (fulminant hepatitis or cirrhosis) and for surveillance of these diseases. Ammonia levels are also measured in the diagnosis and follow-up of hepatic encephalopathy.

TEST EXPLANATION

Ammonia is a byproduct of protein catabolism. Bacteria acting on proteins present in the gut make most of the ammonia. By way of the portal vein, it goes to the liver, where it is normally converted into urea and then secreted by the kidneys. Ammonia cannot be catabolized in the presence of severe hepatocellular dysfunction. Furthermore, when portal blood flow to the liver is altered (e.g., as in portal hypertension), ammonia cannot reach the liver to be catabolized. Ammonia blood levels then rise. Congenital enzymatic defects in the urea cycle also can cause a rise in ammonia levels. Finally, impaired renal function diminishes excretion of ammonia, which causes the blood levels to rise. High levels of ammonia result in encephalopathy and coma. Arterial measurement of ammonia levels is more reliable than venous measurement but more difficult to obtain and is therefore not routinely used.

INTERFERING FACTORS

- Hemolysis increases ammonia levels because the red blood cells (RBCs) have approximately three times the ammonia level content of plasma.
- Muscular exertion can increase ammonia levels.
- Cigarette smoking can produce significant increases in ammonia levels within 1 hour of inhalation.
- Ammonia levels may be factitiously increased if the tourniquet is too tight for too long.
- Substances that may cause *increases* in ammonia levels include acetazolamide, alcohol, ammonium chloride, barbiturates, diuretics (loop, thiazide), narcotics, and parenteral nutrition.
- Substances that may cause *decreases* in ammonia levels include broad-spectrum antibiotics (e.g., neomycin), *Lactobacillus* organisms, lactulose, levodopa, and potassium salts.

PROCEDURE AND PATIENT CARE

Before

- Explain the procedure to the patient.
- Inform the patient that no fasting is usually required, but verify this with the patient's physician.

During

- Collect a venous blood sample in a green-top tube. Note that some institutions require the specimen be sent to the laboratory in a container of water and crushed ice.

After

- Apply pressure or a pressure dressing to the venipuncture site.
- Assess the venipuncture site for bleeding. Many patients with liver disease have prolonged clotting times.
- Avoid hemolysis and send the specimen promptly to the laboratory. Out-of-town specimens can be held overnight if frozen.

TEST RESULTS AND CLINICAL SIGNIFICANCE

▲ Increased Levels

Primary hepatocellular disease,
Reye syndrome,
Asparagine intoxication: *The number of functioning liver cells is not sufficient to metabolize the ammonia.*
Portal hypertension,

Severe heart failure with congestive hepatomegaly: *The portal blood flow from the gut to the liver is altered. The ammonia cannot get to the liver to be metabolized for excretion. Furthermore, the ammonia from the gut is rapidly shunted around the liver (by way of gastroesophageal varices) and into the systemic circulation.*

Hemolytic disease of newborn (erythroblastosis fetalis): *RBCs contain high amounts of ammonia. The newborn liver is not mature enough to metabolize all the ammonia presented to it by the hemolysis that occurs in this disease.*

Gastrointestinal bleeding with mild liver disease,

Gastrointestinal obstruction with mild liver disease: *Ammonia production is increased because the bacteria have more protein (blood) to catabolize. An impaired liver may not be able to keep up with the increased load of ammonia that it receives.*

Hepatic encephalopathy and hepatic coma: *These neurologic states are a result of high levels of ammonia acting as false neurotransmitters. The brain cannot function properly.*

Genetic metabolic disorder of urea cycle: *Ammonia is catabolized by the urea cycle. Disruption of that cycle inhibits excretion of ammonia, and levels can therefore rise.*

▼ Decreased Levels

Essential or malignant hypertension,
Hyperornithinemia

RELATED TESTS

Alanine Aminotransferase (p. 45), Aspartate Aminotransferase (p. 130), and Alkaline Phosphatase (p. 53). These tests are all used to evaluate liver function.

Amylase, Blood

NORMAL FINDINGS

Adult: **25–125 IU/L** (25–125 U/L)
Newborn: **<18 IU/L**
Child/adolescent (10–18 years): **<106 U/L**
  Values may be slightly increased during normal pregnancy and in older adults.

Critical Values

More than three times the upper limit of normal (depending on the method)

INDICATIONS

This test is used to detect and monitor the clinical course of pancreatitis. It is frequently ordered when a patient presents with acute abdominal pain.

TEST EXPLANATION

The serum amylase test, which is easy and rapidly performed, is a sensitive indicator for pancreatitis. Amylase is normally secreted from pancreatic acinar cells into the pancreatic duct and then into the duodenum. Once in the intestine, it aids in the catabolism of carbohydrates to their component simple sugars. Damage to pancreatic acinar cells (as in pancreatitis) or obstruction of the pancreatic duct flow (as in pancreatic carcinoma or gallstones in the common bile duct) causes an outpouring of this enzyme into the intrapancreatic lymph system and the free peritoneum. Blood vessels draining the free peritoneum and absorbing the lymph pick up the excess amylase. An abnormal rise in the serum level of amylase occurs within 12 hours of the onset of disease. Amylase is rapidly cleared (in 2 hours) by the kidney; therefore serum levels return to normal 48 to 72 hours after the initial insult. Persistent pancreatitis, duct obstruction, or pancreatic duct leak (e.g., pseudocysts) causes persistent elevation of serum amylase levels.

Although serum amylase is a sensitive test for pancreatic disorders, it is not specific. Other nonpancreatic diseases can cause elevations in amylase levels in the serum. For example, during bowel perforation, intraluminal amylase leaks into the free peritoneum and is picked up by the peritoneal blood vessels. This results in an elevated serum amylase level. A peptic ulcer penetrating into the pancreas also causes elevations in amylase levels. Duodenal obstruction can be associated with less significant elevations in amylase levels. Because salivary glands contain amylase, elevations can be expected in patients with parotiditis (mumps). Amylase is also found in low levels in the ovaries and skeletal muscles. Ectopic pregnancy and severe diabetic ketoacidosis are also associated with hyperamylasemia.

In cases of chronic pancreatic disorders (e.g., chronic pancreatitis) that have resulted in pancreatic cell destruction and cases of massive hemorrhagic pancreatic necrosis, affected patients often do not have high amylase levels because few pancreatic cells may be left to make amylase.

INTERFERING FACTORS

- Serum lipemia factitiously decreases amylase levels with the current laboratory methods.
- IV dextrose solutions can *lower* amylase levels and cause a false-negative result.
- Drugs that may cause *increases* in serum amylase levels include salicylic acid, aspirin, azathioprine, corticosteroids, dexamethasone, ethyl alcohol, glucocorticoids, iodine-containing contrast media, loop diuretics (e.g., furosemide), methyldopa, narcotic analgesics, oral contraceptives, and prednisone.
- Drugs that may cause *decreases* in serum amylase levels include citrates, glucose, and oxalates.

PROCEDURE AND PATIENT CARE

Before

- Explain the procedure to the patient.
- Inform the patient that no fasting is required.

During

- Collect a venous blood sample in a red-top tube.

After

- Apply pressure or a pressure dressing to the venipuncture site.
- Assess the venipuncture site for bleeding.

TEST RESULTS AND CLINICAL SIGNIFICANCE

▲ Increased Levels

Acute pancreatitis,

Chronic relapsing pancreatitis: *Damage to pancreatic acinar cells, as in pancreatitis, causes an outpour-ing of amylase into the intrapancreatic lymph system and the free peritoneum. Blood vessels draining the free peritoneum and absorbing the lymph pick up the excess amylase.*

Peptic ulcer penetrating into the pancreas: *The peptic ulcer penetrates the posterior wall of the duode-num into the pancreas. This causes a localized pancreatitis with elevated amylase levels.*

Gastrointestinal disease: *In patients with perforated peptic ulcer, necrotic bowel, perforated bowel, or duodenal obstruction, amylase leaks out of the gut and into the free peritoneal cavity. The blood and lymphatic vessels of the peritoneum, where levels are demonstrated in excess, pick up the amylase.*

Acute cholecystitis,

Parotiditis (mumps),

Ruptured ectopic pregnancy: *Amylase is also present in the salivary glands, gallbladder, and fallopian tubes. Diseases affecting these organs are associated with elevated levels of amylase.*

Renal failure: *Amylase is cleared by the kidney. Renal diseases reduce excretion of amylase.*

Diabetic ketoacidosis,

Pulmonary infarction,

After endoscopic retrograde pancreatography

RELATED TESTS

Amylase, Urine (p. 941). Amylase can be detected in the urine long after serum amylase levels have returned to normal. If serum amylase levels are normal and pancreatitis is suspected, the period of peak amylase levels may have passed. Amylase levels may still be elevated in the urine.

Lipase (p. 353). Lipase testing is similar to amylase testing except that it is more specific for the pancreas.

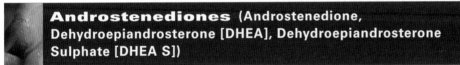

Androstenediones (Androstenedione, Dehydroepiandrosterone [DHEA], Dehydroepiandrosterone Sulphate [DHEA S])

NORMAL FINDINGS

	Male	Female
Androstenedione	1.7–10.5 nmol/L	1.4–15.7 nmol/L
DHEA	2.8–34.6 nmol/L	7.0–52 nmol/L
DHEA S	2.2–9.2 nmol/L	0.3–1.7 nmol/L

INDICATIONS

This test is used for evaluating virilizing syndromes.

TEST EXPLANATION

Androstenediones (androstenedione, DHEA, and its sulphuric ester, DHEA S) are precursors of testosterone and estrone and are made in the gonads and the adrenal gland. Adrenocorticotropic hormone (ACTH) stimulates their adrenal secretion. Androstenedione levels are often elevated in cases of hirsutism and virilization. In the female peripheral tissues and ovaries, androstenedione is converted into testosterone and estrogen. In women, 50% to 60% of testosterone is made in the peripheral tissues, 30% is produced in the adrenal gland, and 20% is produced in the ovary. In women, elevated levels of androstenediones can cause virilizing symptoms such as hirsutism, change in voice, and sterility. Children with congenital adrenal hyperplasia have enzyme defects in the synthesis of cortisol. ACTH secretion is stimulated by the lack of cortisol. As ACTH levels increase, production of androstenediones is stimulated, and levels increase. These hormones are converted into a relatively high level of testosterone by the peripheral tissues. In girls, pseudohermaphroditism results. In boys with similar congenital defects, precocious puberty becomes obvious. This test is also used to assess delayed puberty.

Androstenedione and DHEA secretion is episodic and exhibits a diurnal variation similar to that of cortisol. DHEA S, on the other hand, does not exhibit diurnal variation and is present in the serum at levels much higher than androstenedione or DHEA. Patients with polycystic ovary syndrome (Stein-Leventhal syndrome) have particularly elevated levels of androstenediones. DHEA S levels are particularly high in patients with adrenal carcinoma and, to a lesser extent, in patients with congenital adrenal hyperplasia and Cushing's disease. Normal androstenedione levels are found in patients with Cushing's syndrome caused by benign adrenal tumours.

INTERFERING FACTORS

- A radioactive scan performed 1 week before the test may invalidate the test results, if it is performed by radioimmunoassay.
- Drugs that may cause *increases* in androstenedione levels are clomiphene, corticotropin, and metyrapone.
- Steroids may cause *decreases* in androstenedione levels.

PROCEDURE AND PATIENT CARE

Before

- Explain the procedure to the patient.
- Instruct the patient to have the specimen collected 1 week before or after the menstrual period.
- Inform the patient that fasting before the blood test is preferable, but this should be confirmed with the physician.
- Because peak production of androstenedione is at approximately 7 AM, blood should be collected at approximately that time.

During

- Collect a venous blood sample in a red-top or gold-top tube.
- Indicate the date of the patient's most recent menstrual period on the laboratory form.

After

- Apply pressure or a pressure dressing to the venipuncture site.
- Assess the venipuncture site for bleeding.

TEST RESULTS AND CLINICAL SIGNIFICANCE

▲ Increased Levels

Adrenal tumour: *Some tumours make large amounts of androstenediones, which are then converted by the ovaries and fatty tissue to testosterone and estrogen. The relatively high level of testosterone causes the virilizing signs.*

Congenital adrenal hyperplasia: *This disease is characterized by enzyme defects that prevent conversion of androstenediones to cortisol. Androstenedione levels are increased.*
Ectopic ACTH-producing tumours,
Cushing's disease: *ACTH stimulates the adrenal gland to make large amounts of hormones, including androstenediones.*
Cushing's syndrome: *Large amounts of hormones, including androstenediones, are made in the adrenal gland.*
Stein-Leventhal syndrome,
Ovarian sex cord tumour

▼ Decreased Levels

Primary or secondary adrenal insufficiency,
Ovarian failure,
Oophorectomy: *Production and conversion of androstenediones are decreased.*

RELATED TESTS

Testosterone (p. 489). This test is a direct measurement of testosterone.

Estrogen Fraction (p. 240). This test is a direct measurement of estrogens.

Cortisol, Blood (p. 192). This test is a direct measurement of cortisol, the major adrenal glucocorticosteroid.

Angiotensin

NORMAL FINDINGS

Angiotensin I: **≤25 ng/L** (≤25 pg/mL)
Angiotensin II: **10–60 ng/L** (10–60 pg/mL)

INDICATIONS

This test is performed to identify renovascular hypertension.

TEST EXPLANATION

Renin (p. 460) is an enzyme that is released by the juxtaglomerular apparatus of the kidney. Its release is stimulated by hypokalemia, hyponatremia, decreased renal blood perfusion, or hypovolemia. Renin stimulates the release of angiotensinogen. Angiotensin-converting enzyme (ACE) (p. 73) metabolizes angiotensinogen to angiotensin I and subsequently to angiotensin II and III. Angiotensin then stimulates the release of catecholamines, antidiuretic hormone, ACTH, oxytocin, and aldosterone. Angiotensin is also a vasoconstrictor. Angiotensin is used to identify renovascular sources of hypertension. It can be measured as angiotensin I or angiotensin II. The test is performed by direct radioimmunoassay.

INTERFERING FACTORS

- See Plasma Renin Assay, p. 460.

Blood Studies

2

PROCEDURE AND PATIENT CARE

Before

🖊 Explain the procedure to the patient.

🖊 Instruct the patient to maintain a normal diet with a restricted amount of sodium (approximately 3 g/day) for 3 days before the test.

🖊 Instruct the patient to check with a health care provider about discontinuing any medications that may interrupt renin activity.

During

• Collect a venous blood sample and place it in a chilled lavender-top tube with ethylenediamine tetra-acetic acid (EDTA) as an anticoagulant. Heparin can falsely decrease results.

• Gently invert the blood tube to allow adequate mixing of the blood sample and the anticoagulant.

• Record the patient's position, dietary status, and time of day on the laboratory slip.

• Place the tube of blood on ice, and immediately send it to the laboratory. In the laboratory, the blood will be centrifuged and the serum frozen.

After

• Apply pressure or a pressure dressing to the venipuncture site.

• Observe the venipuncture site for bleeding.

🖊 Tell the patient that usually a normal diet and medications may be resumed.

TEST RESULTS AND CLINICAL SIGNIFICANCE

▲ Increased Levels

Essential hypertension: *A small percentage of these patients have renin hypertension and elevated angiotensin levels.*

Malignant hypertension: *A large percentage of these patients with aggressive hypertensive episodes have elevated angiotensin levels.*

Renovascular hypertension: *Renal artery stenosis or occlusion decreases the renal blood flow, which is a strong stimulant to angiotensin production.*

▼ Decreased Levels

Primary hyperaldosteronism: *This is usually caused by an adrenal adenoma. Aldosterone levels are high and angiotensin levels are low.*

Steroid therapy: *Glucocorticosteroids also have an aldosterone effect, which acts to increase serum sodium levels, decrease potassium levels, and increase blood volume. These responses all tend to diminish angiotensin levels.*

Congenital adrenal hyperplasia: *An enzyme defect in cortisol synthesis causes an accumulation of cortisol precursors, some of which have strong aldosterone-like activity. These act to increase serum sodium levels, decrease potassium levels, and increase blood volume, all of which tend to diminish angiotensin levels.*

RELATED TESTS

Aldosterone (p. 48). This is a direct measurement of aldosterone level. It is used to evaluate hypertension and aldosteronism.

Plasma Renin Assay (p. 460). Plasma renin and angiotensin levels are parallel for each cause of hypertension.

Angiotensin-Converting Enzyme (ACE, Serum Angiotensin-Converting Enzyme [SACE])

NORMAL FINDINGS

8–53 U/L

INDICATIONS

Angiotensin-converting enzyme (ACE) is used to detect and monitor the clinical course of sarcoidosis (a granulomatous disease that affects many organs, especially the lungs). Furthermore, it is used to differentiate between sarcoidosis and other granulomatous diseases and to differentiate active and dormant sarcoid disease.

TEST EXPLANATION

ACE is found in pulmonary epithelial cells and converts angiotensin I to angiotensin II (a potent vasoconstrictor). Angiotensin II is a significant stimulator of aldosterone. ACE is vital in the renin-aldosterone mechanism and therefore important in controlling blood pressure. Despite this, ACE is not very helpful in the evaluation of hypertension. Its value is in the detection of sarcoidosis.

ACE levels are elevated in a high percentage of patients with sarcoidosis. This test is primarily used in patients with sarcoidosis to evaluate the severity of disease and the response to therapy. Levels are especially high with active pulmonary sarcoidosis and can be normal with inactive (dormant) sarcoidosis. Elevated ACE levels also occur in conditions other than sarcoidosis, including Gaucher's disease (a rare familial lysosomal disorder of fat metabolism), leprosy, alcoholic cirrhosis, active histoplasmosis, tuberculosis, Hodgkin disease, myeloma, scleroderma, pulmonary embolism, and idiopathic pulmonary fibrosis. An ACE assay can be performed with spectrophotometry or radioimmunoassay.

INTERFERING FACTORS

- Patients younger than 20 years normally have very high ACE levels.
- Hemolysis or hyperlipidemia may factitiously decrease ACE levels.
- Drugs that may cause *decreases* in ACE levels include ACE inhibitor antihypertensives and steroids.

PROCEDURE AND PATIENT CARE

Before

- Explain the procedure to the patient.
- Inform the patient that no fasting is required.

During

- Collect a venous blood sample in a red-top tube.

After

- Apply pressure or a pressure dressing to the venipuncture site.
- Assess the venipuncture site for bleeding.

TEST RESULTS AND CLINICAL SIGNIFICANCE

▲ Increased Levels

Sarcoidosis: *This is the disease for which this test is primarily performed. The more severe the sarcoidosis is, the greater is the likelihood that ACE levels are increased.*

Other rare diseases that have been found to be associated with ACE elevations include Gaucher's disease, tuberculosis, leprosy, alcoholic cirrhosis, active histoplasmosis, Hodgkin disease, myeloma, idiopathic pulmonary fibrosis, diabetes mellitus, primary biliary cirrhosis, amyloidosis, hyperthyroidism, scleroderma, and pulmonary embolism.

Anion Gap (AG, R factor)

NORMAL FINDINGS

If potassium is used in the calculation: **16 ± 4 mmol/L** (16 ± 4 mEq/L)
If potassium is not used in the calculation: **12 ± 4 mmol/L** (12 ± 4 mEq/L)

INDICATIONS

Calculation of the anion gap assists in the evaluation of patients with acid-base disorders. This calculation is used to attempt to identify the potential cause of the disorder and can also be used to monitor therapy for acid-base abnormalities.

TEST EXPLANATION

The anion gap is the difference between the cations and the anions in the extracellular space and it is calculated in the laboratory as follows: (anion gap = sodium [Na] + potassium [K]) − (chloride [Cl] + bicarbonate [HCO_3^-]). In some laboratories, the potassium is not added into the calculation because the level of potassium in acid-base abnormalities varies. The normal value of the anion gap is adjusted downward if potassium is eliminated from the equation. The anion gap, although not real physiologically, is created by the small amounts of anions in the blood (such as lactate, phosphates, sulphates, organic anions, and proteins) that are not measured. Furthermore, it is important to realize that the HCO_3^- that is measured is actually the venous CO_2, not the arterial HCO_3^-.

This calculation is most often helpful in identifying the cause of metabolic acidosis. As acids such as lactic acid or keto acids accumulate in the bloodstream, bicarbonate neutralizes them to maintain a normal pH within the blood. Mathematically, when HCO_3^- decreases, the anion gap increases. In general, most metabolic acidotic states (except for some types of renal tubular acidosis) are associated with an increased anion gap. The higher the gap is above normal, the more likely it is for a metabolic acidotic state to be present. Proteins can have a significant effect on the anion gap. As albumin (usually negatively charged) increases, the anion gap increases. In the presence of normal albumin levels, a high anion gap is usually a result of an increase in non–chloride-containing acids or organic acids (such as lactic acid or keto acids).

A decrease in the anion gap is very rare but can occur when unmeasured (calcium or magnesium) cations are increased. A reduction in anionic proteins (nephrotic syndrome) also decreases the anion gap. For example, a 1-g/L drop in serum protein is associated with a 2.5-mmol/L drop in the anion gap. Because the anion proteins are lost, the HCO_3^- increases to maintain electrical neutrality. Increase in cationic proteins (some immunoglobulins) also decrease the anion gap. Except for hypoproteinemia, conditions that cause the anion gap to be reduced or negative are relatively rare in comparison with those associated with an elevated anion gap.

Anion gap measurement is also helpful in identifying the presence of a mixed acid-base situation. The ABG measurements are not always fully explanatory, especially if a mixed metabolic acidosis and alkalosis are present concomitantly. An increase in the anion gap despite a normal pH indicates an acidotic component to the metabolic picture. When anion gap measurement is combined with the ABG and electrolyte measurements, complex metabolic clinical pictures can be more clearly elucidated. The anion gap calculation is indicated whenever an acid-base problem exists.

INTERFERING FACTORS

- Hyperlipidemia may cause undermeasurement of sodium and artificially decrease the calculated anion gap.
- Normal values of the anion gap vary according to different normal values for electrolytes, depending on laboratory methods of measurement.
- Drugs that *increase* the anion gap are numerous. Examples are carbenicillin, carbonic anhydrase inhibitors (e.g., acetazolamide), diuretics, ethanol, methanol, penicillin, and salicylate.
- Drugs that *decrease* the anion gap are also numerous. Examples are acetazolamide, lithium, polymyxin B, spironolactone, and sulindac.

PROCEDURE AND PATIENT CARE

Before
- Explain the procedure to the patient.
- Inform the patient that no food or fluid is restricted.

During
- Collect a venous blood sample in a red-top or green-top tube.
- If the patient is receiving an IV infusion, obtain the blood sample from the opposite arm.

After
- Apply pressure to the venipuncture site.
- The sodium, potassium, chloride, and bicarbonate levels are determined by an automated multichannel analyzer. The anion gap is then calculated as indicated in the test explanation section.

TEST RESULTS AND CLINICAL SIGNIFICANCE

▲ Increased Levels

Lactic acidosis,
Diabetic ketoacidosis,
Alcoholic ketoacidosis,
Alcohol intoxication,
Starvation: *These diseases are associated with increased acid ions such as lactate, hydroxybutyrate, or acetoacetate. HCO_3^- neutralizes these acids, HCO_3^- levels fall, and the anion gap mathematically rises.*
Renal failure: *Uremic organic acid anions (e.g., phosphate, sulphates) accumulate in the blood as a result of poor excretion of these acids. The hydrogen combines with the bicarbonate to maintain a homeostatic pH. HCO_3^- levels fall, and the anion gap mathematically rises.*

Increased gastrointestinal losses of bicarbonate (e.g., diarrhea or fistulae): *HCO_3^- and other base losses can occur, thereby mathematically increasing anion gap. Not all gastrointestinal losses result in anion gap differences if mixed electrolyte imbalances occur.*

Hypoaldosteronism: *Aldosterone stimulates acid secretion in the distal renal tubule in exchange for sodium. With deficient quantities of aldosterone, acid builds up and is combined with bicarbonate. HCO_3^- levels fall, and the anion gap rises.*

▼ Decreased Levels

Excess alkali ingestion: *Increase in alkali products (antacids, boiled milk), especially in children, causes increased HCO_3^- products and mathematically decreases the anion gap.*

Multiple myeloma: *The M-chain component of the proteins produced by the neoplastic plasma cells are cationic, causing a compensatory decrease in measured cations and an increase in measured anions to maintain electrical neutrality.*

Chronic vomiting or gastric suction: *The loss of HCl causes a decrease in chloride and an increase in HCO_3^- that mathematically decreases the anion gap.*

Hyperaldosteronism: *Affected patients lose great amounts of potassium and hydrogen ions, which causes a metabolic alkalosis that is associated with a decreased anion gap.*

Hypoproteinemia: *Loss of anionic proteins directly causes a decrease in the anion gap.*

Lithium toxicity: *An increase in inorganic cations decreases the measured cations and thereby decreases the anion gap.*

RELATED TESTS

Sweat Electrolytes (p. 702). Measurement of these electrolytes (sodium, potassium, chloride, and bicarbonate) is necessary to calculate the anion gap.

Arterial Blood Gases (p. 121). This is the method by which acid-base balance is identified and evaluated.

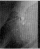

Anticardiolipin Antibody (ACA, aCL Antibodies)

NORMAL FINDINGS

<15.4 immunoglobulin G (IgG) phospholipid units/mL
<21.6 immunoglobulin M (IgM) phospholipid units/mL

INDICATIONS

This test yields positive results in some patients with systemic lupus erythematosus (SLE). The presence of this antibody increases the risk for antiphospholipid syndrome (i.e., venous or arterial thrombosis, thrombocytopenia, recurrent spontaneous abortions). The anticardiolipin antibody test is performed on patients with SLE to determine whether the patients are at risk for developing the complications just described.

TEST EXPLANATION

Antiphospholipid antibodies include anticardiolipin antibodies and the lupus anticoagulant. The lupus anticoagulant, named for its association with SLE, can act as an anticoagulant to prolong the phospholipid-dependent coagulation test (such as partial thromboplastin time). It is present in half of all patients with SLE. Despite its name, it is not associated with bleeding tendencies. Anticardiolipin antibodies (IgG, IgM) are found in approximately 40% of patients with SLE. Patients with SLE who also have anticardiolipin antibodies and the lupus anticoagulant are at higher risk for antiphospholipid antibody syndrome. The clinical features include venous and arterial thrombosis, neuropsychiatric disorders, recurrent spontaneous abortion, and thrombocytopenia. Strokes in young adults have been associated with elevated levels of these antibodies. Both antibodies may be found in patients with drug-induced lupus and nonautoimmune diseases (e.g., syphilis, acute infection) and in normal older adults.

INTERFERING FACTORS

- Patients who have or had syphilis infections can have a cross-reaction to the radiolabelled antibody used for radioimmune assay or the antibody used for enzyme-linked immunosorbent assay (ELISA). In these patients, therefore, the anticardiolipin antibody test yields a false-positive result.
- These antibodies can be present transiently in patients with infections, acquired immune deficiency syndrome (AIDS), inflammation, autoimmune diseases, or cancer.
- *False-positive* results have been observed in patients who take medications such as chlorpromazine, hydralazine, penicillin, phenytoin (Dilantin), procainamide, and quinidine.

PROCEDURE AND PATIENT CARE

Before
- Explain the procedure to the patient.
- Inform the patient that no fasting is required.

During
- Collect a venous blood sample according to the laboratory protocol.

After
- Apply pressure or a pressure dressing to the venipuncture site.
- Assess the venipuncture site for bleeding.

TEST RESULTS AND CLINICAL SIGNIFICANCE

▲ Increased Levels

Systemic lupus erythematosus: *A patient's results are considered positive, and therefore the patient is at risk for antiphospholipid syndrome, if either anticardiolipin antibodies or the lupus anticoagulant is present.*
Antiphospholipid syndrome

RELATED TESTS

Anti-DNA Antibody (p. 88) and Antinuclear Antibody (p. 98). These tests are used to diagnose SLE.

Anticentromere Antibody (Centromere Antibody)

NORMAL FINDINGS

Negative

If test results are positive, the serum will be titrated. Different degrees of positivity are described as follows: "weak positive" means a positive screening titre (1:40 for human epithelial type 2 cells, 1:20 for kidney cells); "moderately positive" means one dilution above screening titre; and "strong positive" means two dilutions above screening titre.

INDICATIONS

This test is used to support the diagnosis of CREST syndrome (calcinosis, Raynaud's phenomenon, esophageal dysfunction, sclerodactyly, and telangiectasia).

TEST EXPLANATION

A centromere is the region of the chromosome referred to as the *primary constriction* that divides the chromosome into arms. During cell division, the centromere exists in the pole of the mitotic spindle.

Anticentromere antibodies are a form of antinuclear antibodies. They are found in a very high percentage of patients with CREST syndrome, a variant of scleroderma. CREST syndrome is characterized by calcinosis, Raynaud's phenomenon, esophageal dysfunction, sclerodactyly (a hand deformity), and telangiectasia (permanent dilation of superficial capillaries and venules). Anticentromere antibodies, on the contrary, are present in only a small minority of patients with scleroderma, a disease that is difficult to differentiate from CREST syndrome. No correlation exists between antibody titre and the severity of CREST syndrome.

PROCEDURE AND PATIENT CARE

Before

- Explain the procedure to the patient.
- Inform the patient that no fasting is usually required, but confirm fasting with physician first.

During

- Collect a venous blood sample in one red-top tube.

After

- Apply pressure or a pressure dressing to the venipuncture site.
- Assess the venipuncture site for bleeding.

TEST RESULTS AND CLINICAL SIGNIFICANCE

Positive

CREST syndrome

RELATED TEST

Antinuclear Antibody (p. 98). This test is used to diagnose autoimmune-related diseases.

Antichromatin Antibody (Antinucleosome Antibodies [Anti-NCS], Antihistone Antibody [Anti-HST, AHA])

NORMAL FINDINGS

Antinucleosome antibodies:
   No antibodies present in <1:20 dilution
Antihistone antibody:
   None detected: <1.0 U
   Inconclusive: 1.0–1.5 U
   Positive: 1.6–2.5 U
   Strong positive: >2.5 U

INDICATIONS

This test is used to diagnose systemic lupus erythematosus (SLE).

TEST EXPLANATION

There are several chromatin antinuclear antibodies associated with autoimmune diseases. Nucleosome represents the main autoantigen-immunogen in SLE, and antinucleosome antibodies are an important marker of the disease activity. Antinucleosome (antichromatin) antibodies play a key role in the pathogenesis of SLE. Nearly all patients with SLE have antinucleosome antibodies. Antinucleosome antibody is one of the many antinuclear antibodies (see p. 98) that indicate autoimmune diseases. Antinucleosome antibody testing has a sensitivity of 100% and a specificity of 97% for SLE diagnosis. Antinucleosome antibodies show the highest correlation with disease activity. Antinucleosome antibodies also show strong association with renal damage (glomerulonephritis and proteinuria) associated with SLE. Antinucleosome autoantibodies are more prevalent than anti-DNA antibodies in patients with SLE.

   Histone antibodies are present in 20% to 55% of cases of idiopathic SLE and 80% to 95% of cases of drug-induced systemic lupus erythematosus. They occur in less than 20% of other types of connective tissue diseases. This antibody is particularly helpful in identifying patients with drug-induced lupus erythematosus caused by drugs such as procainamide, quinidine, penicillamine, hydralazine, methyldopa, isoniazid, and acebutolol. There are several subtypes of antihistone antibody. In drug-induced lupus erythematosus, a specific antihistone—IgG anti-(H2A-H2B)-DNA—is produced. In most of the other associated diseases (rheumatoid arthritis, juvenile rheumatoid arthritis, primary biliary cirrhosis, autoimmune hepatitis, and dermatomyositis/polymyositis), the antihistone antibodies are of other varying specificities. Various immune testing methods are used to identify these antinuclear antibodies, including enzyme-linked immunosorbent assay (ELISA) and indirect immunofluorescence methods.

PROCEDURE AND PATIENT CARE

Before

- Explain the procedure to the patient.
- Inform the patient that no fasting is required.

During

- Collect a venous blood sample in one red-top or gold-top tube.

After

- Apply pressure to the venipuncture site.
- Assess the site for bleeding.

TEST RESULTS AND CLINICAL SIGNIFICANCE

▲ Increased Levels

Systemic lupus erythematosus: *This disease is most commonly associated with antinucleosome antibodies.*

Drug-induced lupus erythematosus: *This disease is most commonly associated with antihistone antibodies.*

Other autoimmune diseases: *Diseases such as lupus hepatitis are occasionally associated with antinucleosome antibodies.*

RELATED TESTS

Antinuclear Antibody (p. 98). This is a type of antibody commonly associated with autoimmune diseases such as SLE.

Anti-DNA Antibody (p. 88). This is useful in the diagnosis and follow-up of SLE.

Anti–Cyclic Citrullinated Peptide Antibody (Cyclic Citrullinated Peptide Antibody, CCP IgG, Anti-CCP)

NORMAL FINDINGS

Cutoff titre: <53 IU/mL

INDICATIONS

Anti–cyclic citrullinated peptide antibody (anti-CCP) is useful in the diagnosis of patients with unexplained joint inflammation, especially when the traditional blood test, for rheumatoid factor (see p. 467), is negative or below 50 IU/mL.

TEST EXPLANATION

Anti-CCP is formed by the intermediary conversion of the amino acid ornithine to arginine. It appears early in the course of rheumatoid arthritis and is present in the blood of most patients with the disease. When this antibody is detected in a patient's blood, there is a high likelihood that the patient has rheumatoid arthritis. Of patients with early-stage rheumatoid arthritis, 30% to 40% may not have elevation of rheumatoid factor levels, which makes the diagnosis difficult in the initial stage. If the anti-CCP level is elevated, the diagnosis of rheumatoid arthritis can be made even if the rheumatoid factor level is negative. This is particularly important because aggressive treatment in the early stages of rheumatoid arthritis prevents progression of joint damage. Anti-CCP levels may rise years before any clinical onset of arthritis or significant elevation of rheumatoid factor. When the anti-CCP and the rheumatoid factor are measured together, the specificity for diagnosing rheumatoid arthritis is 99.1%. Other autoimmune inflammatory diseases are rarely associated with elevated anti-CCP levels. This test may also be useful in differentiating other entities that can resemble rheumatoid arthritis and, at times, cause rheumatoid factor–positive test results (e.g., polymyalgia rheumatica and parvoviral arthropathy).

Anti-CCP is thought to be directly involved in the pathogenesis of rheumatoid arthritis. Citrullinated proteins are found in inflamed synovial tissue of patients with rheumatoid arthritis and may elicit a humoral mechanism for the joint inflammation that highlights rheumatoid arthritis. The presence of anti-CCP in rheumatoid arthritis indicates a more aggressive and destructive form of the disease. It is also a marker for disease progression. Some authorities believe that anti-CCP–positive rheumatoid arthritis and anti-CCP–negative rheumatoid arthritis are clinically different disease entities; the former has a far worse outcome. Patients with anti-CCP–positive rheumatoid arthritis have more swollen joints and show more radiologic destruction than do anti-CCP–negative patients with rheumatoid arthritis.

Among the various commercially available assays, anti-CCP testing with enzyme-linked immunosorbent assay (ELISA) is well correlated with the same antigen specificity, but the numerical normal values for each assay differ widely.

PROCEDURE AND PATIENT CARE

Before
✗ Explain the procedure to the patient.
✗ Inform the patient that no fasting or preparation is required.

During
• Collect a venous blood sample in a red-top tube.

After
• Apply pressure to the venipuncture site.
• Assess the site for bleeding.

TEST RESULTS AND CLINICAL SIGNIFICANCE

▲ Increased Levels
Rheumatoid arthritis: *Testing for rheumatoid factor and anti-CCP is part of a group of tests often performed to diagnose and monitor rheumatoid arthritis.*

RELATED TESTS
Rheumatoid Factor (p. 467). This is the most widely used test to assist in diagnosis and determining prognosis of rheumatoid arthritis.

Erythrocyte Sedimentation Rate (p. 236). This test is used to assess rheumatoid arthritis disease activity.

C-Reactive Protein (p. 199). This test is used to identify and assess treatment for most inflammatory diseases.

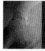

Anti-Deoxyribonuclease-B Titre (Anti–DNase-B [ADB], ADNase-B)

NORMAL FINDINGS

Adult: ≤340 U (≤85 Todd units/mL)
Child:
    Preschool: ≤170 U (≤60 Todd units/mL)
    School age: ≤480 U (≤170 Todd units/mL)

INDICATIONS

This test is performed to indicate previous infection with group A beta-hemolytic streptococci. This is important in patients suspected of having acute rheumatic fever or acute glomerulonephritis.

TEST EXPLANATION

Like the anti–streptolysin O (ASO) titre test, this immunologic test detects antigens produced by group A beta-hemolytic streptococci and yields elevated values in most patients with acute rheumatic fever or poststreptococcal glomerulonephritis. This test is often run concurrently with the ASO test; subsequent testing is usually performed to detect differences in the acute-stage and convalescent blood samples. A rise in the titre of two or more dilution increments between acute-stage and convalescent sera is significant and indicates that a streptococcal infection has occurred. The American Heart Association does not recommend performing this test alone in the evaluation of patients with acute rheumatic fever. It may be more sensitive than ASO testing, but its results are too variable. ASO is the recommended test, but the combination testing kit (Streptozyme), which tests for ASO and anti–deoxyribonuclease-B titre together, is better than either test alone.

INTERFERING FACTORS

▪ Drugs that may cause *decreases* in anti–deoxyribonuclease-B titre include some antibiotics.

PROCEDURE AND PATIENT CARE

Before

☒ Explain the procedure to the patient.
☒ Inform the patient that no fasting is required.

During

• Collect a venous blood sample in a red-top tube.

After

• Apply pressure to the venipuncture site.
• Assess the site for bleeding.

TEST RESULTS AND CLINICAL SIGNIFICANCE

▲ Increased Levels

Acute rheumatic fever,
Poststreptococcal glomerulonephritis

RELATED TEST

Anti–Streptolysin O Titre (p. 109). This is another test to detect previous streptococcal infection.

Antidiuretic Hormone (ADH, Vasopressin, Arginine Vasopressin [AVP])

NORMAL FINDINGS

0.9–4.6 pmol/L (1–5 pg/mL)

INDICATIONS

Antidiuretic hormone (ADH) levels are tested in patients suspected of having diabetes insipidus or the syndrome of inappropriate ADH (SIADH). This test is often performed in patients who complain of polyuria or polydipsia and are found to have marked variations in blood and urine osmolality or sodium levels.

TEST EXPLANATION

ADH, also known as *vasopressin*, is formed by the hypothalamus and stored in the posterior pituitary gland. It controls the amount of water reabsorbed by the kidney. ADH release is stimulated by an increase in serum osmolality or a decrease in intravascular blood volume. Physical stress, surgery, and even high levels of anxiety may also stimulate ADH release. On release of ADH, more water is reabsorbed from the glomerular filtrate at the level of the distal convoluted renal tubule and collecting ducts. This increases the amount of free water within the bloodstream and causes the urine to be highly concentrated.

With low ADH levels, water is excreted, thereby producing hemoconcentration and a more dilute urine. Diabetes insipidus occurs when ADH secretion is inadequate or when the kidneys are unresponsive to ADH stimulation. Inadequate ADH secretion is usually associated with central neurologic abnormalities (neurogenic diabetes insipidus), such as trauma, tumour, or inflammation of the brain (hypothalamus). Surgical ablation of the pituitary gland also results in the neurogenic form of diabetes insipidus; such patients excrete large volumes of free water in the dilute urine. Their blood is hemoconcentrated, which produces a strong thirst.

Primary renal diseases may make the renal collecting system less sensitive to ADH stimulation (nephrogenic diabetes insipidus). Again, in this instance, urine may be diluted by excretion of high volumes of free water. To differentiate ADH deficiency (neurogenic diabetes insipidus) from renal resistance to ADH (nephrogenic diabetes insipidus), a water deprivation test (p. 1012) is performed. During this test, water intake is restricted, urine osmolality is measured, and vasopressin is administered. In neurogenic diabetes insipidus, there is no rise in urine osmolality after water restriction, but there is a rise after vasopressin is given. In nephrogenic diabetes insipidus, there is no rise in urine osmolality after water deprivation or vasopressin administration.

The diagnosis indicated by this test can be corroborated by a serum ADH measurement. Serum ADH levels are low in neurogenic diabetes insipidus but high in nephrogenic diabetes insipidus.

High serum ADH levels are also associated with SIADH. In response to this inappropriately high level of ADH secretion, water is reabsorbed by the kidneys greatly in excess of normal amounts. Thus the patient's blood becomes very diluted, and the urine is concentrated. Blood levels of important serum ions diminish, causing extreme neurologic, cardiac, and metabolic alterations. SIADH can be associated with pulmonary diseases (e.g., tuberculosis, bacterial pneumonia), severe stress (e.g., surgery, trauma), central nervous system tumour, infection, or trauma. Ectopic secretion of ADH from neoplasm (paraneoplastic syndrome) can cause SIADH. The most common tumours associated with SIADH include carcinomas of the lung and thymus; lymphoma; leukemia; and carcinomas of the pancreas, urologic tract, and intestine. Patients with myxedema or Addison's disease also can experience SIADH. Some drugs are known to cause SIADH (see the "Interfering Factors" section).

INTERFERING FACTORS

- Patients with dehydration, hypovolemia, or stress may have increased ADH levels.
- Patients with overhydration, decreased serum osmolality, and hypervolemia may have decreased ADH levels.
- In older patients, the secretion of ADH during the night is decreased in comparison with levels during the day. This lack of secretion is one of the major causes of adult nocturia.
- Use of a glass syringe or collection tube for the sample causes degradation of ADH.
- Drugs that *increase* ADH levels include acetaminophen, barbiturates, cholinergic agents, cyclophosphamide, diuretics (e.g., thiazides), estrogen, narcotics, nicotine, oral hypoglycemic agents (particularly sulphonylureas), and tricyclic or selective serotonin reuptake inhibitor antidepressants.
- Drugs that *decrease* ADH levels include alcohol, beta-adrenergic agents, morphine antagonists, and phenytoin (Dilantin).

PROCEDURE AND PATIENT CARE

Before

- Explain the procedure to the patient.
- Ensure that the patient is adequately hydrated. Instruct the patient to fast for 12 hours.
- Evaluate the patient for high levels of physical or emotional stress.

During

- Collect a venous blood sample in a prechilled plastic anticoagulant tube while the patient is in the sitting or recumbent position.

After

- Apply pressure or a pressure dressing to the venipuncture site.
- Assess the venipuncture site for bleeding.
- The specimen is centrifuged at low temperatures in the laboratory. The serum may be frozen and sent to a reference laboratory on dry ice for testing.

TEST RESULTS AND CLINICAL SIGNIFICANCE

▲ Increased Levels

SIADH,
Central nervous system tumours or infection,

Pneumonia or pulmonary tuberculosis,

Ectopic ADH secretion (usually from lung cancer),

Endocrinopathies, such as myxedema or Addison's disease: *These diseases may be associated with inappropriately high levels of ADH. Patients experience dilutional hyponatremia, hypo-osmolality, and concentrated urine.*

Nephrogenic diabetes insipidus caused by primary renal diseases: *Because of primary renal disease, the kidneys cannot respond to ADH. The patient becomes hemoconcentrated and hyperosmolar. As a result, ADH is maximally stimulated, and yet the kidneys cannot respond.*

Postoperative days 1 to 3,

Severe physical stress (e.g., trauma, pain, prolonged mechanical ventilation): *Stress is a potent stimulator (through the autonomic nervous system) of ADH.*

Hypovolemia,

Dehydration: *Decreased blood volume is a potent direct stimulator of ADH.*

Acute porphyria

▼ Decreased Levels

Neurogenic (or central) diabetes insipidus caused by central nervous system trauma, tumour, or infection,

Surgical ablation of pituitary gland: *The hypothalamus or pituitary ADH-secreting cells are destroyed by these disease processes.*

Hypervolemia: *Increased blood volume is an inhibitor of ADH secretion.*

Decreased serum osmolality caused by overhydration, nephrotic syndrome, psychogenic polydipsia, or IV overinfusion of non–salt-containing fluid: *Decreased serum osmolality is an inhibitor of ADH secretion.*

RELATED TESTS

Water Deprivation (p. 1012). This test is helpful in differentiation of the causes of polyuria (neurogenic diabetes insipidus, nephrogenic diabetes insipidus, psychogenic polydipsia).

Osmolality, Blood (p. 391) and Osmolality, Urine (p. 972). These tests are measurements of solute load in the urine.

Sodium, Blood (p. 479). This is a direct measurement of sodium level in the blood.

Sodium, Urine (p. 980). This is a direct measurement of sodium level in the urine.

Antidiuretic Hormone Suppression (p. 85). This test is used to differentiate SIADH from other causes of hyponatremia or edematous states.

Antidiuretic Hormone Suppression
(ADH Suppression, Water Load)

NORMAL FINDINGS

65% of water load excreted in 4 hours

80% of water load excreted in 5 hours

Urine osmolality (in second hour): ≤**100 mmol/kg**

Urine/serum osmolality ratio: >100

Urine specific gravity: <1.003

INDICATIONS

This test is used to differentiate SIADH from other causes of hyponatremia or edematous states listed in Box 2-2.

TEST EXPLANATION

This test is used to evaluate the possibility of SIADH in patients with electrolyte abnormalities (such as hyponatremia) or edematous states. Usually this test is performed concomitantly with measurements of urine and serum osmolality. Patients with SIADH excrete none or very little of the water load. Furthermore, their urine osmolality is never less than 100, and the urine/serum osmolality ratio is greater than 100. Patients with hyponatremia, other edematous states, or chronic renal diseases excrete up to 80% of the water load and develop midrange osmolality values.

CONTRAINDICATIONS

- The presence of severe pain, nausea, stress, hypovolemia, or hypotension, because antidiuretic hormone is already almost maximally stimulated.

POTENTIAL COMPLICATIONS

- Water intoxication in patients with SIADH, because they are not able to excrete the water load. Symptoms include anorexia, nausea, vomiting, abdominal cramps, confusion, irritability, convulsions, and coma.

INTERFERING FACTORS

- Patients with dehydration, hypovolemia, hypotension, or stress may have increased antidiuretic hormone levels.
- Drugs that *increase* antidiuretic hormone levels include acetaminophen, barbiturates, cholinergic agents, cyclophosphamide, estrogen, narcotics, nicotine, oral hypoglycemic agents, some diuretics (e.g., thiazides), and tricyclic antidepressants.

BOX 2-2	Causes of Hyponatremia or Edema

Hyponatremia
- Syndrome of inappropriate antidiuretic hormone (SIADH)
- Primary (or psychogenic) polydipsia
- Adrenal insufficiency
- Excessive sodium loss (vomiting, diarrhea, diuretics, excessive sweating)
- Pseudohyponatremia associated with excessive nonionic solute load (e.g., hyperglycemia, hyperlipidemia, hyperproteinemia)
- Sickle cell syndrome associated with chronic debilitating diseases

Edematous States
- Heart failure
- Cirrhosis
- Nephrosis
- Myxedema

PROCEDURE AND PATIENT CARE

Before

- Explain the procedure to the patient.
- Instruct the patient to fast after midnight before the test or as ordered by the physician.
- The test is begun early in the morning.
- Inform the patient of the early signs of water intoxication, and instruct the patient to notify you if any occur.
- Place the patient in the recumbent position. The response to water loading in the upright position is reduced because this position is associated with increased antidiuretic hormone.
- One hour before the test, administer 300 mL of water to replace fluids lost overnight. This is not part of the water load.
- Measure the baseline serum sodium or a serum sodium level 24 hours before the test. If the sodium concentration is above a safe level (125 mmol/L), the test can proceed. If not, the test should be cancelled until the sodium is brought to a safe level by water restriction or saline infusion. This precaution minimizes the risk of water intoxication.

During

- Administer water (~20 mL/kg body weight up to 1500 mL) in 10 to 20 minutes.
- Collect urine every hour for 6 hours, and send it to the laboratory for specific gravity and osmolality measurements. (Discard the first morning specimen.)
- Obtain blood for osmolality measurements hourly or at specified times in a red-top (serum) or green-top (heparinized) tube.

After

- Observe the patient for signs of water intoxication.
- If water load clearance does not occur, instruct the patient to restrict water ingestion. Some patients must be admitted for observation.

TEST RESULTS AND CLINICAL SIGNIFICANCE

SIADH

Water excretion: none or very little of the water load
Urine osmolality: >100
Urine specific gravity: >1.020
Urine/serum ratio: >90

Other Hyponatremic or Edematous States (see Box 2-2)

Water excretion: up to 80% of water load
Urine osmolality: <300
Urine specific gravity: >1.020
Urine/serum ratio: <90

RELATED TESTS

Antidiuretic Hormone (p. 83). This is a serum assay for direct measurement of antidiuretic hormone levels. This test is used in the differential diagnosis of neurogenic diabetes insipidus, nephrogenic diabetes insipidus, or psychogenic polydipsia.

Osmolality, Blood (p. 391). This test is a measurement of solute load in the serum.

Osmolality, Urine (p. 972). This test is a measurement of solute load in the urine.

Sodium, Blood (p. 479). This is a direct measurement of sodium level in the blood.

Sodium, Urine (p. 980). This is a direct measurement of sodium level in the urine.

Water Deprivation (p. 1012). This is a test to assist in the differential diagnosis of diabetes insipidus.

Anti-DNA Antibody (Anti–Deoxyribonucleic Acid Antibodies, Antibody to Double-Stranded DNA, Anti–Double-Stranded DNA [Anti–ds-DNA], DNA Antibody, Native Double-Stranded DNA)

NORMAL FINDINGS

Negative: <70 IU/mL
Borderline: 70–200 IU/mL
Positive: >200 IU/mL

INDICATIONS

The anti-DNA antibody test is useful for the diagnosis and follow-up of systemic lupus erythematosus (SLE).

TEST EXPLANATION

This antibody is found in approximately 65% to 80% of patients with active SLE and rarely in patients with other diseases. High titres are characteristic of SLE. Low to intermediate levels of this antibody may be found in patients with other rheumatic diseases and in those with chronic hepatitis, infectious mononucleosis, and biliary cirrhosis. The anti-DNA titre decreases with successful therapy and increases with exacerbation of SLE and especially with the onset of lupus glomerulonephritis. Near-negative values are seen in patients with dormant SLE.

The anti-DNA antibody is a type of *antinuclear antibodies* (ANAs; p. 98). There are two subtypes of anti-DNA antibodies. The first and most commonly found is the antibody against double-stranded DNA (anti–ds-DNA). The second type is the antibody against single-stranded DNA (anti–ss-DNA). The presence of this type is less sensitive and specific for SLE, but it is found in other autoimmune diseases. These antibody-antigen complexes that occur with autoimmune disease are not only diagnostic but are major contributors to the disease process. They induce activity of the complement system, which then may cause local or systemic tissue injury.

Several radioimmunoassay methods are used for measuring anti-DNA antibodies. The Farr method is the oldest and is more sensitive than the lupus erythematosus preparation. It detects anti–ds-DNA and anti–ss-DNA antibodies. As a result, its specificity is not great.

INTERFERING FACTORS

• A radioactive scan performed within 1 week before the test may alter the test results.

• Drugs that may cause *increases* in anti-DNA antibody levels include hydralazine and procainamide.

PROCEDURE AND PATIENT CARE

Before

🖎 Explain the procedure to the patient.
🖎 Inform the patient that no fasting is required.

During

• Collect a venous blood sample in a red-top tube.

After

• Apply pressure or a pressure dressing to the venipuncture site.
• Assess the venipuncture site.

TEST RESULTS AND CLINICAL SIGNIFICANCE

▲ Increased Levels

Collagen-vascular diseases,
Other autoimmune diseases, such as rheumatic fever,
Chronic hepatitis,
Infectious mononucleosis,
Biliary cirrhosis

RELATED TEST

Antinuclear Antibody (p. 98). This is another antibody associated with SLE.

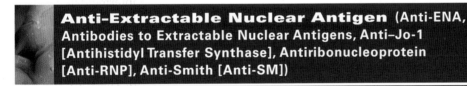

Anti-Extractable Nuclear Antigen (Anti-ENA, Antibodies to Extractable Nuclear Antigens, Anti–Jo-1 [Antihistidyl Transfer Synthase], Antiribonucleoprotein [Anti-RNP], Anti-Smith [Anti-SM])

NORMAL FINDINGS

Negative

INDICATIONS

The anti–extractable nuclear antigens are measured to assist in the diagnosis of systemic lupus erythematosus (SLE) and mixed connective tissue disease (MCTD) and to rule out other rheumatoid diseases.

TEST EXPLANATION

Anti–extractable nuclear antigens are a type of ANAs to certain nuclear antigens that consist of ribonucleic acid (RNA) and protein. The antigen is extracted from the thymus using phosphate-buffered saline solutions and therefore is sometimes referred to as saline-extracted antigen. The most common anti–extractable nuclear antigens are Smith and ribonucleoprotein types.

The anti-Smith antibody is present in approximately 30% of patients with SLE and in approximately 8% of patients with MCTDs. However, it is not present in patients with most other rheumatoid-collagen diseases.

The antiribonucleoprotein antibody is reported in nearly 100% of patients with MCTD and in approximately 25% of patients with SLE, discoid lupus, and progressive systemic sclerosis (scleroderma). In high titres, antiribonucleoprotein is suggestive of MCTD.

The *anti–Jo-1 (antihistidyl transfer synthase)* antibody is present in patients with autoimmune interstitial pulmonary fibrosis and in a minority of patients with aggressive autoimmune myositis. Two other antibodies to anti–extractable nuclear antigens are anti–SS-A and anti–SS-B (see p. 107) and are used mainly in the diagnostic evaluation of Sjögren syndrome.

PROCEDURE AND PATIENT CARE

Before
☒ Explain the procedure to the patient.
☒ Inform the patient that no fasting is required.

During
- Collect a venous blood sample in a red-top tube.

After
- Apply pressure or a pressure dressing to the venipuncture site.
- Assess the venipuncture site for bleeding.
- Check the venipuncture site for infection. Patients with autoimmune disease are immunocompromised.

TEST RESULTS AND CLINICAL SIGNIFICANCE

▲ Increased Anti-Smith Antibodies
SLE

▲ Increased Antiribonucleoprotein Antibodies
MCTD,
SLE,
Discoid lupus scleroderma: *The absence of anti-Smith antibodies and the presence of antiribonucleoprotein antibodies help to differentiate MCTD serologically from SLE and other autoimmune diseases.*

▲ Increased Anti-Jo Antibodies
Pulmonary fibrosis,
Autoimmune myositis

RELATED TESTS

Antinuclear Antibody (p. 98). This is another antibody associated with SLE.
    Anti-DNA Antibody (p. 88). This test is also used to diagnose SLE.

Anti-Glomerular Basement Membrane Antibody (Anti-GBM Antibody, AGBM, Glomerular Basement Antibody, Goodpasture's Antibody)

NORMAL FINDINGS

Tissue
Negative: No immunofluorescence is noted on the basement membrane of the renal or lung tissue.

Blood (by Enzyme Immunoassay)
Negative: <20 units
Borderline: 20–100 units
Positive: >100 units

INDICATIONS

This test is used to detect the presence of circulating glomerular basement membrane antibodies commonly present in autoimmune-induced nephritis (Goodpasture's syndrome).

TEST EXPLANATION

Goodpasture's syndrome is an autoimmune disease characterized by the presence of circulating antibodies against an antigen in the renal glomerular basement membrane and the pulmonary alveolar basement membrane. These immune complexes activate the complement system and thereby cause tissue injury. Patients with this problem usually display a triad of glomerulonephritis (hematuria), pulmonary hemorrhage (hemoptysis), and antibodies to basement membrane antigens. This is a rare form of glomerular nephritis. Approximately 60% to 75% of patients with immune-induced glomerular nephritis have pulmonary complications.

With the use of immunohistochemistry and now with radioimmunoassay, antibodies also can be demonstrated in the glomeruli, the renal tubular basement membrane, and the pulmonary capillary basement membranes. Lung or renal biopsy is necessary to demonstrate these antibodies in tissue. Serum assays are a faster and more reliable method for diagnosing Goodpasture's syndrome, especially in patients in whom renal or lung biopsy may be difficult to perform or contraindicated. Furthermore, serum levels can be used in monitoring response to therapy (plasmapheresis or immunosuppression).

PROCEDURE AND PATIENT CARE

Before
- Explain the procedure to the patient.
- Instruct the patient to fast for 8 hours before the test. Water is permitted during the fast.
- If a lung biopsy or kidney biopsy will be performed to collect the specimen, explain these procedures to the patient.

During
- Collect a venous blood sample in a red-top tube.

After

- Apply pressure or a pressure dressing to the venipuncture site.
- Assess the venipuncture site for bleeding.

TEST RESULTS AND CLINICAL SIGNIFICANCE

Positive

Goodpasture's syndrome
Autoimmune glomerulonephritis
Lupus nephritis

RELATED TESTS

Lung Biopsy (p. 769). This is a test in which lung tissue is obtained for microscopic evaluation.
Renal Biopsy (p. 783). This is a test in which renal tissue is obtained for microscopic evaluation.

 Anti-Glycan Antibodies (Crohn's Disease Prognostic Panel, Multiple Sclerosis Antibody Panel)

NORMAL FINDINGS

Negative

INDICATIONS

This test is used to differentiate multiple sclerosis from other neurologic causes of weakness. It also is used to differentiate Crohn's disease from other forms of inflammatory bowel diseases.

TEST EXPLANATION

Glycans (sugars or carbohydrates) exist on the surface of cells, such as erythrocytes. Anti-glycan antibodies are immunologically directed to these sugar-containing components. Antibodies to glycans can be instigated by bacterial, fungal, and parasitic infections. The use of glycan arrays for systematic screening of patients with multiple sclerosis (MS) and inflammatory bowel disease (particularly Crohn's disease) has been helpful in enabling the diagnosis and prognosis in these patients.

Utilizing enzyme-linked immunosorbent assay (ELISA), these antibodies can be identified and quantified. When used with other antibodies associated with Crohn's disease (such as anti-*Saccharomyces cerevisiae* antibody [ASCA], anti-*laminaribioside carbohydrate* antibody [ALCA], anti-*mannobioside carbohydrate* antibody [AMCA], and anti-*chitobiose carbohydrate* antibody [ACCA]), anti-glycan antibodies are supportive of Crohn's disease over ulcerative colitis or irritable bowel disease. Furthermore, higher levels of these antibodies are associated with a more complicated course of disease.

Other anti-glycan antibodies are specific for MS patients, enabling differentiation between MS patients and patients with other neurologic diseases.

PROCEDURE AND PATIENT CARE

Before

- Explain the procedure to the patient.
- Tell the patient that no fasting is required.

During
- Collect one lavender-, pink-, or green-top tube of venous blood.

After
- Apply pressure to the venipuncture site.

TEST RESULTS AND CLINICAL SIGNIFICANCE
▲ Increased Levels
Crohn's disease,
Multiple sclerosis: *Both of these diseases are associated with elevated levels of anti-glycan antibodies.*

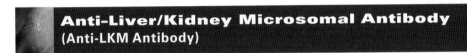

Anti-Liver/Kidney Microsomal Antibody
(Anti-LKM Antibody)

NORMAL FINDINGS
Titres: <1:0

INDICATIONS
This assay is used to diagnose autoimmune hepatitis. This test is performed on patients with suspected autoimmune disorders with liver involvement.

TEST EXPLANATION
There are three different anti–liver/kidney microsomal (anti-LKM) antibodies: anti–LKM-1, anti–LKM-2, and anti–LKM-3. Anti-LKM antibodies are found in patients with autoimmune hepatitis. Anti–LKM-2 is associated with chemical hepatitis, and anti–LKM-3 is elevated in hepatitis D. Anti–LKM-1 is the LKM antibody most commonly measured, and its presence supports the diagnosis of autoimmune hepatitis. The anti-LKM antibodies are directed against the antigens within the hepatocyte. Autoimmune hepatitis is a chronic disorder of the liver characterized by progressive hepatocellular necrosis and inflammation. This disease tends to progress to cirrhosis and liver failure. Autoimmune hepatitis is probably genetic in origin and induced by a viral or chemical hepatitis. Affected patients present with several autoantibodies (antinuclear [p. 98], anti–smooth muscle [p. 104], and anti-LKM). Autoimmune hepatitis may be associated with other rheumatic symptoms such as arthritis, kidney disease, and skin changes.

Anti-LKM antibodies are identified through immunofluorescence assays. Usually all three anti-LKM antibodies are measured in total. However, enzyme immunoassay laboratory methods can separate out each anti-LKM antibody. Elevated levels of anti-LKM antibody are not diagnostic of autoimmune hepatitis but are extremely supportive of the diagnosis.

PROCEDURE AND PATIENT CARE
Before
- Explain the procedure to the patient.
- Explain the importance of performing the test in the morning.

During
- Collect a venous blood sample in a serum separator vacuum tube.

After
- The blood may be sent to a reference laboratory. Results are available in approximately 1 week.

TEST RESULTS AND CLINICAL SIGNIFICANCE

▲ Increased Levels

Autoimmune hepatitis,
Hypergammaglobulinemia: *The pathophysiologic process of these disorders is not known.*

RELATED TESTS

Aspartate Aminotransferase (p. 130) and Alanine Aminotransferase (p. 45). The hepatocellular enzymes are elevated in all forms of hepatitis.

Antinuclear Antibody (p. 98). These antibodies are also elevated in autoimmune hepatitis.

Anti–Smooth Muscle Antibody (p. 104). This test is used to diagnose chronic active hepatitis, which often has an autoimmune origin.

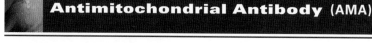

Antimitochondrial Antibody (AMA)

NORMAL FINDINGS

No antimitochondrial antibodies (AMAs) at titres >1:5

INDICATIONS

The AMA test is used primarily to aid in the diagnosis of primary biliary cirrhosis.

TEST EXPLANATION

AMA is an anticytoplasmic antibody directed against a lipoprotein in the mitochondrial membrane. Normally the serum does not contain AMA at a titre greater than 1:5. AMAs are found in 94% of patients with primary biliary cirrhosis. This disease may be an autoimmune disease that occurs predominantly in young or middle-aged women. It has a slow progressive course characterized by elevated levels of liver enzymes, especially alkaline phosphatase and gamma-glutamyl transpeptidase, and by a positive AMA test result. Liver biopsy (see p. 766) is usually necessary to confirm the diagnosis because the AMA test can yield positive results in patients with chronic active hepatitis, drug-induced cholestasis, autoimmune hepatitis (e.g., scleroderma, systemic lupus erythematosus), extrahepatic obstruction, or acute infectious hepatitis. There are several subgroups of AMA. The M-2 subgroup is suspected to be highly specific for primary biliary cirrhosis. For the AMA test, immunofluorescence assay or enzyme-linked immunosorbent assay (ELISA) techniques can be used.

PROCEDURE AND PATIENT CARE

Before

☒ Explain the procedure to the patient.
☒ Inform the patient that no fasting or special preparation is required.

During

• Collect a venous blood sample in a red-top tube.

After

• Apply pressure or a pressure dressing to the venipuncture site.
• Check the venipuncture site for bleeding. Patients with jaundice often have bleeding disorders in association with vitamin K deficiency.

TEST RESULTS AND CLINICAL SIGNIFICANCE

▲ Increased Levels

Primary biliary cirrhosis: *AMA test result is positive in 90% to 100% of affected patients.*
Chronic active hepatitis: *AMA test result is positive in 30% of affected patients.*
Systemic lupus erythematosus,
Syphilis,
Drug-induced cholestasis,
Autoimmune hepatitis (e.g., scleroderma, systemic lupus erythematosus),
Extrahepatic obstruction,
Acute infectious hepatitis: *AMA test result is positive in 2% to 5% of affected patients.*

RELATED TESTS

Anti–Smooth Muscle Antibody (p. 104). This is another anticytoplasmic antibody that usually is present in patients with chronic active hepatitis and in 30% of patients with primary biliary cirrhosis.

Alkaline Phosphatase (p. 53). Although alkaline phosphatase is found in many tissues, the concentrations are highest in the liver, biliary tract epithelium, and bone.

Gamma-Glutamyl Transpeptidase (p. 261). This enzyme is found in the liver and is measured to detect liver cell dysfunction and cholestasis.

Antimyocardial Antibody

NORMAL FINDINGS

Negative (if positive, serum will be titrated)

INDICATIONS

This test is used to detect an autoimmune source of myocardial injury and disease. Antimyocardial antibodies may be detected in rheumatic heart disease, cardiomyopathy, postthoracotomy syndrome, and after myocardial infarction. This test is used not only in the detection of an autoimmune cause for these conditions but also for monitoring response to treatment.

TEST EXPLANATION

A positive antimyocardial antibody test result is associated with several forms of heart disease. Antimyocardial antibodies may be detected before the development of clinical symptoms of heart disease. An immunologic basis has been suspected in rheumatic heart disease for a long time. Research has now documented the presence of serum antibodies against myocardial components and deposition of immunoglobulin and complement in areas around lesions. Antibodies against heart muscle are also found in 20% to 40% of patients after cardiac surgery and in a smaller number of patients after myocardial infarction. These antibodies are usually associated with pericarditis that follows the myocardial injury associated with cardiac surgery or myocardial infarction (Dressler's syndrome). Antimyocardial antibodies have also been detected in patients with cardiomyopathy. Their role in this latter disease is unknown.

The antimyocardial antibody test may be performed by indirect immunofluorescence technique. The patient's serum is added to a rat heart muscle extract. Antigen-antibody immune complexes are identified by immunofluorescent antihuman antibodies. Positive results (increased immunofluorescence) are reported in titres.

PROCEDURE AND PATIENT CARE

Before
- Explain the procedure to the patient.
- Inform the patient that no fasting or special preparation is necessary.

During
- Collect a venous blood sample in a red-top tube.

After
- Apply pressure or a pressure dressing to the venipuncture site.
- Check the venipuncture site for bleeding.

TEST RESULTS AND CLINICAL SIGNIFICANCE

▲ Increased Levels

Rheumatic heart disease,

Streptococcal infection: *The myocardial antigen may be associated with streptococcal organisms because the antibody may occur in patients with other streptococcal diseases.*

Postthoracotomy (cardiac surgery) syndrome,

After myocardial infarction (Dressler's syndrome): *Myocardial injury occurs, and the antibody develops. The antibody-antigen complex may incite the pericarditis that follows the myocardial injury.*

Cardiomyopathy: *The association of cardiomyopathy and antimyocardial antibodies is unknown. Whether the antibodies cause or contribute to the development of cardiomyopathy is being studied.*

Anti-Neutrophil Cytoplasmic Antibody (ANCA)

NORMAL FINDINGS

Negative

INDICATIONS

This blood test is used to assist in the diagnosis of Wegener granulomatosis. It also is used to monitor the course of the disease, to monitor the response to therapy, and to provide early detection of relapse.

TEST EXPLANATION

Wegener granulomatosis is a regional systemic vasculitis in which the small arteries of the kidneys, lungs, and upper respiratory tract (nasopharynx) are damaged by a granulomatous inflammation. Diagnosis can be made through biopsy of clinically affected tissue. Serologic testing plays a key role in the diagnosis of Wegener granulomatosis and other systemic vasculitis syndromes. Most patients with Wegener granulomatosis have circulating autoantibodies against neutrophil cytoplasm, which are useful in the diagnosis.

Anti–neutrophil cytoplasmic antibodies (ANCAs) are antibodies directed against cytoplasmic components of neutrophils. When ANCAs are detected with indirect immunofluorescence microscopy, staining produces two major patterns: cytoplasmic ANCA (c-ANCA) and perinuclear ANCA (p-ANCA). Specific immunochemical assays demonstrate that c-ANCA consists mainly of antibodies to proteinase 3 and p-ANCA consists of antibodies to myeloperoxidase. The antigen-specific immunochemical assay, used to characterize ANCA (rather than the pattern of immunofluorescence microscopy), is more specific and more clinically relevant; therefore, the terms *proteinase 3–ANCA* and *myeloperoxidase-ANCA* are used.

The proteinase 3 autoantigen is highly specific (95% to 99%) for Wegener granulomatosis. When the disease is limited to the respiratory tract, the proteinase 3 autoantigen is present in approximately 65% of patients. When Wegener granulomatosis is inactive, the percentage of positive titres drops to approximately 30%. Most patients with Wegener granulomatosis limited to the kidney do not have positive proteinase 3 levels.

The myeloperoxidase autoantigen is found in 50% of patients with Wegener granulomatosis centred in the kidney. It is also present in patients with non–Wegener granulomatosis glomerulonephritis, such as microscopic polyangiitis.

PROCEDURE AND PATIENT CARE

Before

🖎 Explain the procedure to the patient.
🖎 Inform the patient that no fasting is required.

During

- Collect a venous blood sample in the tube specified by the laboratory performing the test.

After

- Apply pressure or a pressure dressing to the venipuncture site.
- Observe the venipuncture site for bleeding.

TEST RESULTS AND CLINICAL SIGNIFICANCE

▲ Increased Levels

Wegener granulomatosis,
Microscopic polyarteritis,
Idiopathic crescentic glomerulonephritis,
Ulcerative colitis,
Primary sclerosing cholangitis,
Autoimmune hepatitis,
Churg-Strauss vasculitis,
Active viral hepatitis,
Crohn's disease: *The mechanism by which ANCAs are associated with these diseases is unknown.*

Antinuclear Antibody (ANA)

NORMAL FINDINGS

Negative at 1:40 dilution

INDICATIONS

ANAs are measured in order to diagnose systemic lupus erythematosus (SLE) and other autoimmune diseases. These antibodies are used to screen primarily for SLE. Because almost all patients with SLE develop autoantibodies, a negative ANA test result excludes the diagnosis. If the ANA test result is positive, other antibody studies must be performed to corroborate the diagnosis.

TEST EXPLANATION

Autoantibodies are directed to nuclear material (ANAs) or to cytoplasmic material (anticytoplasmic antibodies; Tables 2-4 and 2-5). Many abnormal antibodies are present in patients with autoimmune (which include rheumatic or connective tissue) diseases. ANA is a group of protein antibodies that react against cellular nuclear material. ANA is quite sensitive for detecting SLE. Positive results occur in approximately 95% of patients with this disease; however, many other rheumatic diseases are also associated with ANA (Table 2-6). The ANA test, therefore, is not specific for SLE (Table 2-7). ANA can be tested as a specific antibody or as a group with nonspecific antigens.

ANA tests are performed with different assays (indirect immunofluorescence microscopy or by enzyme-linked immunosorbent assay [ELISA]), and results are reported as titres with a particular type of immunofluorescence pattern (when positive). Low-level titres are considered negative, whereas increased titres are positive and indicate an elevated concentration of ANAs.

ANA appears on indirect immunofluorescence as fluorescent patterns in cells that are fixed to a slide and are evaluated under an ultraviolet-light microscope. Different patterns are associated with a variety of autoimmune disorders. When a more specific subtype of ANA is evaluated (see Table 2-4), the specificity of the pattern is increased for the various autoimmune diseases

TABLE 2-4	Common Antinuclear Antibodies and Diseases They Cause
Common Antinuclear Antibodies	**Disease**
Anti–soluble nucleoprotein	SLE
Anti–extractable nuclear antibody	SLE, MCTD
Anti-Smith	SLE
Antiribonuclear protein	MCTD, SLE, PSS
Anti–Jo-1 antihistidyl	Polymyositis, dermatomyositis
Antinucleolar	PSS, SLE
Anticentromere	CREST syndrome
Anti–SS-A (Ro) and Anti–SS-B (La)	Sjögren syndrome, SLE
Rheumatoid arthritis precipitin	RA, Sjögren syndrome
Anti–scleroderma-70	PSS

CREST, Calcinosis, Raynaud's syndrome, esophageal dysfunction, sclerodactyly, and telangiectasia; *MCTD,* mixed connective tissue disease; *PSS,* progressive systemic sclerosis (scleroderma); *RA,* rheumatoid arthritis; *SLE,* systemic lupus erythematosus.

TABLE 2-5	Common Anticytoplasmic Antibodies and Diseases They Cause
Common Anticytoplasmic Antibody	**Disease**
Antimitochondrial	Primary biliary cirrhosis
Anti–neutrophil cytoplasmic	Wegener granulomatosis
Antimicrosomal	Chronic active hepatitis
Antiribosomal	Systemic lupus erythematosus
Anti-RNA	Scleroderma (systemic sclerosis)

TABLE 2-6	Autoimmune Disease and Positive Antibodies
Autoimmune Disease	**Positive Antibodies**
Systemic lupus erythematosus (SLE)	ANA, SLE prep, dsDNA, ssDNA, anti-DNP, SS-A
Drug-induced SLE	ANA
Sjögren syndrome	RF, ANA, SS-A, SS-B
Scleroderma	ANA, Scl-70, RNA, dsDNA
Raynaud's disease	ACA, Scl-70
Mixed connective tissue disease	ANA, RNP, RF, ssDNA
Rheumatoid arthritis	RF, ANA, RANA, RAP
Primary biliary cirrhosis	AMA
Thyroiditis	Antimicrosomal, antithyroglobulin
Chronic active hepatitis	ASMA

ACA, Anticardiolipin antibody; *AMA,* antimitochondrial antibody; *ANA,* antinuclear antibody; *ASMA,* anti–smooth muscle antibody; *DNP,* dinitrophenol; *ds-DNA,* double-stranded DNA; *RANA,* rheumatoid arthritis nuclear antigen; *RAP,* rheumatoid arthritis precipitin; *RF,* rheumatoid factor; *RNP,* ribonucleoprotein; *Scl-70,* scleroderma antibody; *SS-A* and *SS-B,* antibodies to anti–extractable nuclear antigens; *ss-DNA,* single-stranded DNA.

TABLE 2-7	Disease and Percentage of Patients With ANAs
Disease	**ANA Positive**
Systemic lupus erythematosus	95%
Progressive systemic sclerosis (scleroderma)	70%
Rheumatoid arthritis	30%
Sjögren syndrome	60%
Dermatomyositis	30%
Polyarteritis	1%

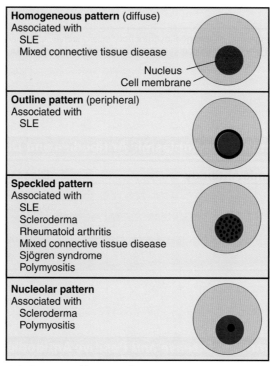

Homogeneous pattern (diffuse)
Associated with
  SLE
  Mixed connective tissue disease
      Nucleus
  Cell membrane

Outline pattern (peripheral)
Associated with
  SLE

Speckled pattern
Associated with
  SLE
  Scleroderma
  Rheumatoid arthritis
  Mixed connective tissue disease
  Sjögren syndrome
  Polymyositis

Nucleolar pattern
Associated with
  Scleroderma
  Polymyositis

Figure 2-6 Patterns of immunofluorescent staining for antinuclear antibodies (ANAs).

(Figure 2-6). An example of a positive result might be as follows: "Positive at 1:320 dilution with a homogenous pattern." This particular test result is considered positive if ANA is found in a titre with a dilution of more than 1:32. In general, the higher the titre of a certain ANA antibody known to be associated with a certain autoimmune disease, the more likely it is that disease exists, and the more active the disease is. As the disease becomes less active because of therapy, the ANA titres can be expected to fall.

The ANA test is often used to screen patients with suspected SLE. If the ANA test result is negative, the patient probably does not have SLE. In approximately 5% of patients with SLE, however, the ANA test yields a negative result. If the result is positive, other corroborative serologic tests are performed (see Table 2-6). In this text, the more commonly clinically used ANA subtypes are discussed separately.

INTERFERING FACTORS

⚖ Drugs that may cause a *false-positive* ANA test result include acetazolamide, salicylic acid, chlorothiazides, chlorprothixene, hydralazine, penicillin, phenylbutazone, phenytoin, procainamide, streptomycin, sulphonamides, and tetracyclines.

⚖ Drugs that may cause a *false-negative* test result include steroids.

PROCEDURE AND PATIENT CARE

Before

✗ Explain the procedure to the patient.

✗ Inform the patient that no fasting or preparation is required.

During

• Collect a venous blood sample in a red-top tube.

After

• Apply pressure or a pressure dressing to the venipuncture site.

• Assess the venipuncture site for bleeding.

✗ Because patients with an autoimmune disease are usually immunocompromised, they should be instructed to check for signs of infection at the venipuncture site. These patients often take steroids, which further compromise their immune system.

TEST RESULTS AND CLINICAL SIGNIFICANCE

▲ Increased Levels

Systemic lupus erythematosus (SLE): *The signs and symptoms of this disease are vague and nonspecific. This disease is associated with a significant production of various autoimmune antibodies. Any organ in the patient's body can be the target of these autoantibodies. The immune complexes incite the complement system and thereby incite tissue damage.*

Rheumatoid arthritis: *The autoimmune response is targeted to the synovial tissues.*

Periarteritis (polyarteritis) nodosa: *The autoimmune response is targeted to the small vessels of various organs.*

Dermatomyositis,

Polymyositis: *The autoimmune response is targeted to the skeletal muscle.*

Scleroderma: *The autoimmune response is targeted to the endothelium of blood vessels. Fibrosis then occurs. This, combined with deposit of collagen-related tissue, incites the organ changes seen in the skin, gastrointestinal tract, and other internal organs.*

Sjögren syndrome: *The autoimmune response is targeted to the exocrine glands (lacrimal and salivary).*

Raynaud's phenomenon: *This phenomenon is characterized by episodic digital ischemia, manifested by blanching and then cyanosis of the fingers in cold temperatures, followed by rubor on rewarming. It is associated with many autoimmune diseases. The term* Raynaud's disease *refers to this phenomenon without an associated autoimmune disease.*

Other immune diseases,

Leukemia,

Infectious mononucleosis,

Myasthenia gravis,

Cirrhosis,

Chronic hepatitis

RELATED TESTS

Anticentromere Antibody (p. 78). This test is used to diagnose CREST syndrome (calcinosis, Raynaud's phenomenon, esophageal dysfunction, sclerodactyly, and telangiectasia).

Anti-DNA Antibody (p. 88). This test is used to diagnose SLE.

Anti–Extractable Nuclear Antigen (p. 89). This test is used to diagnose SLE and mixed connective tissue disease.

Antiscleroderma Antibody (p. 103). This test is used to diagnose scleroderma.

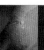

Anti-Parietal Cell Antibody (APCA)

NORMAL FINDINGS

Negative

INDICATIONS

Anti–parietal cell antibody (APCA) testing is used to diagnose an autoimmune cause of pernicious anemia.

TEST EXPLANATION

Parietal cells exist in the proximal stomach and produce hydrochloric acid and intrinsic factor. Intrinsic factor is necessary for the absorption of vitamin B_{12} (see p. 541). APCAs are found in nearly 90% of patients with pernicious anemia. Nearly 60% of those patients also have anti–intrinsic factor antibodies. It is thought that these antibodies contribute to the destruction of the gastric mucosa in pernicious anemia. APCA is also found in patients with atrophic gastritis, gastric ulcers, and gastric cancer.

APCA is present in other autoimmune-mediated diseases such as thyroiditis, myxedema, juvenile diabetes, Addison's disease, and iron-deficiency anemia. Between nearly 10% and 15% of the normal population have APCA. With advancing age, the incidence of APCA increases (especially in relatives of patients with pernicious anemia).

Laboratory testing is usually performed by indirect immunofluorescence with the Fluoro-Kit. With this test system, APCA can cross-react with other antibodies, especially anticellular and antithyroid antibodies. Titre levels greater than 1:240 are considered positive.

PROCEDURE AND PATIENT CARE

Before

☒ Explain the procedure to the patient.
☒ Inform the patient that no fasting or special preparation is necessary.

During

• Collect a venous blood sample in a red-top tube.

After

• Apply pressure or a pressure dressing to the venipuncture site.
• Check the venipuncture site for bleeding.

TEST RESULTS AND CLINICAL SIGNIFICANCE

▲ Increased Levels

Pernicious anemia,

Atrophic gastritis: *APCA and anti–intrinsic factor antibodies may destroy the parietal cell in the gastric antrum through complement fixing antibodies against the parietal cell surface.*

Hashimoto thyroiditis,

Myxedema,

Insulin-dependent diabetes mellitus,

Addison's disease: *These autoimmune diseases may be interrelated in a manner that is not yet clear.*

RELATED TEST

Schilling Test (p. 862). With the use of this test, the ability to absorb vitamin B_{12} is evaluated. This test is also used in the evaluation of patients with pernicious anemia.

Antiscleroderma Antibody (Scl-70 Antibody, Scleroderma Antibody)

NORMAL FINDINGS

Negative

INDICATIONS

This antibody is diagnostic for scleroderma (progressive systemic sclerosis) and is present in 45% of patients with that disease.

TEST EXPLANATION

Scl-70 antibody is an ANA. On the fluorescence ANA test, under the ultraviolet-light microscope, a specific pattern is created for the Scl-70 antibody. The pattern is a speckled group of dots throughout the nucleus (see Figure 2-6, p. 103). The test can be performed by fluorescence testing, enzyme-linked immunosorbent assay (ELISA), and enzyme immunoassay. Progressive serial dilutions are carried out.

Scleroderma is a multisystem disorder characterized by inflammation with subsequent fibrosis of the small blood vessels in skin and visceral organs, including the heart, lungs, kidneys, and gastrointestinal tract. A collagen-like substance is also deposited into the tissue of these organs. In general, the higher the titre of Scl-70 antibody, the more likely it is that scleroderma is present, and the more active the disease is. As the disease becomes less active as a result of therapy, the Scl-70 antibody titres can be expected to fall.

The absence of this antibody does not exclude the diagnosis of scleroderma. The antibody is rather specific for scleroderma but is occasionally seen in other autoimmune diseases, such as systemic lupus erythematosus (SLE), mixed connective tissue disease, Sjögren syndrome, polymyositis, and rheumatoid arthritis.

INTERFERING FACTORS

▎ Drugs that may cause *increases* in Scl-70 levels include salicylic acid, isoniazid, methyldopa, penicillin, propylthiouracil, streptomycin, and tetracycline.

PROCEDURE AND PATIENT CARE

Before

☒ Explain the procedure to the patient.
☒ Inform the patient that no fasting is required.

During

• Collect a venous blood sample in a red-top tube.

After

• Apply pressure or a pressure dressing to the venipuncture site.
• Assess the venipuncture site for bleeding.

TEST RESULTS AND CLINICAL SIGNIFICANCE

Positive

Scleroderma,

CREST syndrome (calcinosis, Raynaud's phenomenon, esophageal dysfunction, sclerodactyly, and telangiectasia): *CREST is a variant of scleroderma. In both diseases, the autoimmune response is targeted to the endothelium of blood vessels. Fibrosis then occurs. This, in combination with deposit of collagen-related tissue, incites the changes seen in the skin, gastrointestinal tract, and other internal organs.*

RELATED TEST

Antinuclear Antibody (p. 98). This group of antibodies is used to diagnose SLE and other autoimmune diseases such as scleroderma.

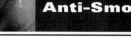

Anti-Smooth Muscle Antibody (ASMA)

NORMAL FINDINGS

No anti–smooth muscle antibody (ASMA) at titres >1:20

INDICATIONS

The ASMA test is used primarily to aid in the diagnosis of autoimmune chronic active hepatitis (CAH), which has also been referred to as "lupoid" CAH.

TEST EXPLANATION

ASMA is an anticytoplasmic antibody directed against actin, a cytoskeletal protein. The serum normally does not contain ASMA at a titre greater than 1:20. ASMA is the most commonly recognized autoantibody in the setting of CAH. It appears in 70% to 80% of patients with CAH. In some types of CAH, tests for ASMA antibodies do not yield positive results.

This disease may be an autoimmune disease, and it occurs predominantly in women. The clinical presentation of CAH is similar to that of viral hepatitis. That clinical picture, along with serologic and pathologic criteria, must exist for more than 6 months to be classified as CAH.

ASMA is not specific for CAH, and the test result can be positive in patients with viral infections, malignancy, multiple sclerosis, primary biliary cirrhosis, and *Mycoplasma* infections. Usually the titre of ASMA is low in these diseases. With CAH, the titre is usually higher than 1:160. The titres are not helpful in predicting prognosis, nor do they indicate response to therapy. ASMA is also used to distinguish autoimmune hepatitis from systemic lupus erythematosus. For the ASMA test, immunofluorescence assay or enzyme-linked immunosorbent assay (ELISA) techniques are used.

PROCEDURE AND PATIENT CARE

Before
- Explain the procedure to the patient.
- Inform the patient that no fasting or special preparation is required.

During
- Collect a venous blood sample in a red-top tube.

After
- Apply pressure or a pressure dressing to the venipuncture site.
- Check the venipuncture site for bleeding. Patients with jaundice often have bleeding disorders in association with vitamin K deficiency.

TEST RESULTS AND CLINICAL SIGNIFICANCE

▲ Increased Levels

CAH,
Mononucleosis hepatitis: *ASMA is positive in 70% to 80% of affected patients.*
Primary biliary cirrhosis,
Viral hepatitis,
Multiple sclerosis,
Malignancy,
Intrinsic asthma: *ASMA is positive in approximately 30% of affected patients.*

RELATED TESTS

Alkaline Phosphatase (p. 53), Aspartate Aminotransferase (p. 130), and other liver enzyme measurements. These enzymes exist within the hepatocytes, and their levels are elevated in patients with hepatitis.

Antimitochondrial Antibody (p. 94). This antibody is most frequently associated with primary biliary cirrhosis. Positive titres of AMA are found in 30% of the patients with CAH.

Anti–Liver/Kidney Microsomal Antibody (p. 93). This antibody is helpful in the diagnosis of autoimmune hepatitis.

Antispermatozoal Antibody (Sperm Agglutination and Inhibition, Sperm Antibodies, Antisperm Antibodies, Infertility Screen)

NORMAL FINDINGS
Negative

INDICATIONS
The antispermatozoal antibody test is an infertility screening test used to detect the presence of sperm antibodies. Antibodies directed toward sperm antigens can diminish fertility.

TEST EXPLANATION
This test is commonly used in the evaluation of a couple experiencing infertility. Antisperm antibodies may be found in the blood of men with blocked efferent ducts of the testes (a common cause of low sperm counts or poor sperm mobility) and in 30% to 70% of men who have had a vasectomy. Reabsorption of sperm from the blocked ducts results in the formation of autoantibodies to sperm as a result of sperm antigens interacting with the immune system. These antibodies can be agglutinins or cytotoxic. The effect of immunoglobulin A antisperm antibodies on the sperm tail is associated with poor motility and poor penetration of cervical mucus. Immunoglobulin G (IgG) antisperm antibodies are associated with blockage of sperm-ovum fusion. High titres of IgG autoantibodies are often associated with postvasectomy degeneration of the testes, which explains why 50% of men remain infertile after successful repair of vasectomy.

In men, high serum titres of antispermatozoal antibody are considered strong evidence of infertility. Low titres are of unknown significance because this is not an uncommon finding in normal fertile men. Serum antispermatozoal antibodies are found in nearly 20% of women. However, many of these women become pregnant. The significance of this antibody in women is therefore unclear.

Antispermatozoal antibodies can also be detected in the sperm of infertile men and in the cervical mucus of infertile women. It is often necessary to identify these antibodies in the serum and other body fluids in the thorough evaluation of infertility.

PROCEDURE AND PATIENT CARE
Before
🖐 Explain the procedure to the patient.

Sperm Specimen
🖐 Inform the man that he should avoid ejaculation for at least 3 days before the semen specimen is collected.
• Give the male patient the proper container for the sperm collection.
🖐 If the specimen is to be collected at home, be certain the patient is instructed to take it to the laboratory for testing within 2 hours of collection.

During
• Collect a venous blood sample from both the male and the female patients in red-top tubes.

Sperm Specimen
• Have the man collect the ejaculate in a plastic container.

Vaginal Mucus Specimen
- Collect 1 mL of cervical mucus and place it in a plastic vial.

After
- Apply pressure or a pressure dressing to the venipuncture sites.
- Check the venipuncture sites for bleeding.
- For a sperm, blood, or cervical specimen, the specimen may be placed in a plastic vial, frozen, and sent to a reference laboratory on dry ice.
- Instruct the couple when and how to obtain the test results.

TEST RESULTS AND CLINICAL SIGNIFICANCE

Infertility: *Antispermatozoal antibodies may be present in the man or the woman and may inhibit the number or motility of sperm or the ability of the sperm to penetrate the ovum.*

Blocked efferent ducts in the testes: *This is considered a common cause of male infertility. Reabsorption of sperm from the blocked ducts results in the formation of autoantibodies to sperm as a result of sperm antigens interacting with the immune system.*

Vasectomy: *Reabsorption of sperm from the occluded vas deferens results in the formation of autoantibodies to sperm as a result of the interaction between sperm antigens and the immune system.*

RELATED TESTS

Sims-Huhner Test (p. 701). This test consists of a postcoital examination of the cervical mucus to measure the ability of the sperm to penetrate the mucus and maintain motility. It is used in the diagnostic workup of infertility. This analysis is also helpful in documenting cases of suspected rape by testing the vaginal and cervical secretions for sperm.

Luteinizing Hormone Assay and Follicle-Stimulating Hormone (p. 361). These hormones are useful for determining the pituitary effect on gonadal function and spermatogenesis.

Semen Analysis (p. 695). This test is used to evaluate the quality of sperm. Semen analysis is used to evaluate infertility and to document the adequacy of operative vasectomy.

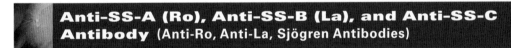

Anti-SS-A (Ro), Anti-SS-B (La), and Anti-SS-C Antibody (Anti-Ro, Anti-La, Sjögren Antibodies)

NORMAL FINDINGS
Negative

INDICATIONS

These three ANAs are used to diagnose Sjögren syndrome.

TEST EXPLANATION

Anti–SS-A, anti–SS-B, and anti–SS-C antibodies are subtypes of ANAs (see Table 2-4, p. 99) and react to nuclear antigens extracted from human B lymphocytes. Anti–SS-A and anti–SS-B produce a speckled immunofluorescent pattern when seen under the ultraviolet-light microscope. They are strongly associated with Sjögren syndrome. This disease is an immunologic abnormality characterized by progressive destruction of the lacrimal and salivary exocrine glands, which leads to mucosal and conjunctival dryness. This disease can occur by itself (primary) or in association with other autoimmune diseases, such as systemic lupus erythematosus (SLE), rheumatoid arthritis, and scleroderma. When it is associated with autoimmune disease, it is referred to as *secondary Sjögren syndrome*.

Anti–SS-A antibodies may be present in approximately 60% to 70% of patients with primary Sjögren syndrome. Anti–SS-B antibodies may be present in approximately 50% to 60% of patients with primary Sjögren syndrome. When anti–SS-A and anti–SS-B antibodies are present, Sjögren syndrome can be diagnosed accurately. These antibodies are rarer when secondary Sjögren syndrome is associated with rheumatoid arthritis. In fact, SS-B is found only in primary Sjögren syndrome. Anti–SS-C is present in approximately 75% of patients with rheumatoid arthritis or patients with secondary Sjögren syndrome associated with rheumatoid arthritis. However, anti–SS-A and anti–SS-B are almost never found in patients with Sjögren syndrome associated with rheumatoid arthritis. Therefore, these antibodies are also useful in differentiating primary from secondary Sjögren syndrome.

Anti–SS-A can also be present in 25% of patients with SLE. This is particularly useful in "ANA-negative" patients with SLE because these antibodies are present in the majority of such patients. Anti–SS-B is rarely found in patients with SLE. In general, the higher the titre of anti–SS antibodies is, the more likely Sjögren syndrome is to be present, and the more active the disease is. As Sjögren syndrome becomes less active as a result of therapy, the anti–SS antibody titres can be expected to fall.

PROCEDURE AND PATIENT CARE

Before
☒ Explain the procedure to the patient.
☒ Inform the patient that no fasting is required.

During
• Collect a venous blood sample in a red-top tube.

After
• Apply pressure or a pressure dressing to the venipuncture site.
• Assess the venipuncture site for bleeding.
☒ Patients with autoimmune disease have a compromised immune system; therefore educate patients on signs and symptoms of infection and the need for follow-up if necessary.

TEST RESULTS AND CLINICAL SIGNIFICANCE

Positive

Sjögren syndrome: *When titres of anti–SS-A or anti–SS-B are high, Sjögren syndrome can be diagnosed with confidence.*

Rheumatoid arthritis: *When titres of anti–SS-C are high, rheumatoid arthritis with or without Sjögren syndrome can be diagnosed with confidence.*

ANA-negative SLE: *Anti–SS-A is present in most affected patients.*

Neonatal lupus: *Anti–SS-A is present in 95% of affected patients.*

RELATED TESTS

Antinuclear Antibody (p. 98). This test is used to diagnose SLE and other autoimmune diseases.

Anticentromere Antibody (p. 78). This test is used to diagnose CREST syndrome (calcinosis, Raynaud's phenomenon, esophageal dysfunction, sclerodactyly, and telangiectasia).

Anti-DNA Antibody (p. 88). This test is used to diagnose SLE.

Anti–Extractable Nuclear Antigen (p. 89). This test is used to diagnose SLE and mixed connective tissue disease.

Antiscleroderma Antibody (p. 103). This test is used to diagnose scleroderma.

Anti-Streptolysin O Titre (ASO Titre)

NORMAL FINDINGS

Adult/older adult: ≤160 Todd units/mL
Child:

- 6 months to 2 years: ≤50 Todd units/mL
- 2–4 years: ≤160 Todd units/mL
- 5–12 years: 170–330 Todd units/mL

Newborn (0–6 months): similar to mother's value

INDICATIONS

This test is used primarily to determine whether a previous streptococcal infection has caused a poststreptococcal disease, such as glomerulonephritis, rheumatic fever, bacterial endocarditis, and scarlet fever. Anti–streptolysin O (ASO) levels are highest in glomerulonephritis and rheumatic fever.

TEST EXPLANATION

The ASO titre is a serologic procedure demonstrating the reaction of the body to infection caused by group A beta-hemolytic streptococci. The *Streptococcus* organism produces streptolysin O, an enzyme that has the ability to destroy (lyse) red blood corpuscles. Because streptolysin O is antigenic, the body reacts by producing ASO, a neutralizing antibody. ASO appears in the serum 1 week to 1 month after the onset of a streptococcal infection; a high titre is not specific for a certain type of poststreptococcal disease (e.g., rheumatic fever vs. glomerulonephritis) but merely indicates that a streptococcal infection is present or has occurred.

When ASO levels are elevated in a patient with glomerulonephritis or endocarditis, it is safe to assume that the disease was caused by streptococcal infection. ASO is of no value for diagnosing acute streptococcal infection; cultures for streptococci are required for diagnosis. However, cultures are useless during the latent period of the poststreptococcal disease (~2 to 3 weeks after initial infection). ASO testing is very helpful at this point. Serial ASO testing may be performed to detect the difference between the acute and convalescent blood samples. Serial measurements of ASO over several weeks, which may demonstrate a rise followed by a slow fall, are much more significant in the diagnosis of a previous streptococcal infection than is a single titre. The highest incidence of positive results is during the third week after the onset of acute symptoms of the streptococcal disease. By 6 months, only approximately 30% of affected patients have abnormal titres.

Another immunologic test, anti–deoxyribonuclease-B (anti–DNase-B; p. 82), also detects antigens produced by group A streptococci. The anti–DNase-B level is elevated in most patients with acute rheumatic fever and poststreptococcal glomerulonephritis.

When ASO and anti–DNase-B are performed concurrently, 95% of previous streptococcal infections are detected. If both repeatedly yield negative results, there is no reason to suspect that the symptoms are caused by a poststreptococcal disease. The Streptozyme test is often used as a screening test to detect any one of multiple *Streptococcus*-induced antibodies.

INTERFERING FACTORS

- Increased beta-lipoprotein levels can neutralize streptolysin O and can result in a false-positive ASO titre.
- Drugs that may cause *decreases* in ASO levels include adrenocorticosteroids and antibiotics. Antibiotics reduce the number of streptococcal organisms and thereby suppress ASO production. Steroids are immunosuppressive and thereby suppress ASO production.

PROCEDURE AND PATIENT CARE

Before

- Explain the procedure to the patient.
- Inform the patient that no fasting is required.

During

- Collect a venous blood sample in a red-top tube.
- Avoid hemolysis of the blood specimen.

After

- Apply pressure or a pressure dressing to the venipuncture site.
- Observe the venipuncture site for bleeding.
- Note that ASO testing may be repeated to determine the highest level of increase.

TEST RESULTS AND CLINICAL SIGNIFICANCE

▲ Increased Levels

Streptococcal infection: *ASO titres do not develop during the early days of the infection. It is only after the second week of an untreated infection that the ASO titre rises.*
Acute rheumatic fever,
Bacterial endocarditis: *ASO titres are highest in these diseases.*
Acute glomerulonephritis: *As many as 50% to 75% of affected patients do not have high ASO titres.*
Scarlet fever,
Streptococcal pyoderma: *ASO titres are often not elevated in these diseases.*

RELATED TEST

Anti–Deoxyribonuclease-B Titre (p. 82). Like the ASO test, this immunologic test also detects antigens produced by group A beta-hemolytic streptococci and yields positive results in most patients with acute rheumatic fever or poststreptococcal glomerulonephritis.

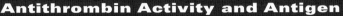

Antithrombin Activity and Antigen Assay (Antithrombin III [AT-III], Functional Antithrombin III Assay, Heparin Cofactor, Immunologic Antithrombin III, Serine Protease Inhibitor)

NORMAL FINDINGS

Antithrombin Activity

Newborn: 35%–40%
>6 months to adult: 80%–130%

Antithrombin Antigen Assay

Plasma: >50% of control value
Serum: 15%–34% lower than plasma value
Immunologic: **170–300 mg/L** (17–30 mg/dL)
Functional: 80%–120%
    Values vary according to laboratory methods.

INDICATIONS

This test is used to evaluate patients suspected of having hypercoagulable states. It is also used to help identify the cause of heparin resistance in patients receiving heparin therapy.

TEST EXPLANATION

Antithrombin III (AT-III) is an alpha$_2$-globulin produced in the liver. It inhibits the serine proteases involved in coagulation (factors II, X, IX, XI, and XII). In normal homeostasis, coagulation results from a balance between AT-III and thrombin. A deficiency of AT-III increases coagulation or the tendency toward thrombosis. A hereditary deficiency of AT-III is characterized by a predisposition toward thrombus formation. This is passed on as an autosomal dominant abnormality. In individuals with hereditary AT-III deficiency, thromboembolic events typically develop in the early twenties. These thromboembolic events are usually venous. Acquired AT-III deficiency may develop in patients with cirrhosis, liver failure, advanced carcinoma, nephrotic syndrome, disseminated intravascular coagulation, and acute thrombosis. AT-III is also decreased as much as 30% in pregnant women and in women who take estrogens.

AT-III provides most of the anticoagulant effect of heparin. AT-III must be present in order for heparin to express its effect. Patients who have AT-III deficiency may be heparin resistant and require unusually high doses for an anticoagulation effect. In general, patients respond to heparin if AT-III levels are at least 60% of normal.

There are two methods of testing for AT-III. The first is a "functional" assay in which AT-III activity is measured. The second is an "immunologic" assay in which the AT-III level is actually quantified. Through both these methods, two types of inherited AT-III syndromes can be identified. In type I, the immunologic assay measurement is reduced (decreased amount of AT-III), but the functional assay measurement is normal (AT-III activity is normal). In type II, the immunologic assay measurement is normal (normal levels of AT-III), but the functional assay measurement is low (AT-III activity is reduced).

Asymptomatic individuals with an AT-III deficiency should receive prophylactic anticoagulation to increase their AT-III levels before any medical or surgical interventions in which inactivity increases the risk of thrombosis. Levels of AT-III may be increased in patients with acute hepatitis, obstructive jaundice, and vitamin K deficiency and in patients who have undergone kidney transplantation.

INTERFERING FACTORS

▌ Drugs that may cause *increases* in AT-III levels include anabolic steroids, androgens, oral contraceptives (containing progesterone), and sodium warfarin.

▌ Drugs that may cause *decreases* in AT-III levels include fibrinolytics, heparin, L-asparaginase, and oral contraceptives (containing estrogen).

PROCEDURE AND PATIENT CARE

Before

✗ Explain the procedure to the patient.

✗ Inform the patient that no fasting is required.

During

• Collect a venous blood sample in a light blue– or red-top tube.

After

• Apply pressure or a pressure dressing to the venipuncture site.

• Assess the venipuncture site for bleeding. Patients receiving heparin therapy may develop a hematoma at the venipuncture site.

• Send the specimen to the laboratory immediately after collection.

TEST RESULTS AND CLINICAL SIGNIFICANCE

▲ Increased Levels

Kidney transplant,

Acute hepatitis,

Obstructive jaundice,

Vitamin K deficiency: *The exact mechanisms for these levels are not known.*

▼ Decreased Levels

Disseminated intravascular coagulation,

Hypercoagulation states (e.g., deep-vein thrombosis): *In these diseases, the AT-III is consumed by the thrombotic process.*

Hepatic disorders (especially cirrhosis): *AT-III is a protein whose synthesis is reduced by liver dysfunction.*

Nephrotic syndrome,

Protein-wasting diseases (malignancy): *Proteins are either lost or otherwise used up, and the amino acid pool is depleted. Therefore, AT-III cannot be made.*

Hereditary familial deficiency of AT-III: *Inadequate amounts of AT-III or adequate amounts of inactive AT-III are made. Anticoagulation is inhibited, and thrombotic events occur.*

RELATED TESTS

Coagulating Factor Concentration (p. 177). This test measures the concentration of specific coagulating factors in the blood.

Protein C, Protein S (p. 437). This is part of the evaluation of patients with coagulation disorders.

Lupus Anticoagulant (p. 76 [anticardiolipin antibodies]). This test is done in many patients with thrombus.

Anti–Thyroglobulin Antibody (Thyroid Autoantibody, Thyroid Anti–Thyroglobulin Antibody, Thyroglobulin Antibody)

NORMAL FINDINGS

<116 IU/mL

INDICATIONS

This test is used as a marker for autoimmune thyroiditis and related diseases.

TEST EXPLANATION

Thyroglobulin autoantibodies bind thyroglobulin (Tg), a major thyroid-specific protein that plays a crucial role in thyroid hormone synthesis, storage, and release. Tg remains in the thyroid follicles until hormone production is required. Tg is not secreted into the systemic circulation under normal circumstances. However, follicular destruction through inflammation (Hashimoto's thyroiditis or chronic lymphocytic thyroiditis and autoimmune hypothyroidism), hemorrhage (nodular goitre), or rapid disordered growth of thyroid tissue (as may be observed in Graves' disease or follicular cell-derived thyroid neoplasms) can result in leakage of Tg into the bloodstream. This results in the formation of autoantibodies to Tg in some individuals. Of individuals with autoimmune hypothyroidism, 30% to 50% will have detectable anti-Tg autoantibodies (Table 2-8).

The antithyroglobulin test is usually performed in conjunction with the antithyroid peroxidase antibody test (p. 115). When this is done, the specificity and sensitivity are greatly increased. Antithyroglobulin assay is a Quantitative Chemiluminescent Immunoassay. Normal results vary based on the methodology used. A small percentage of the normal population has antithyroglobulin antibodies. Normally women tend to have higher levels than men.

TABLE 2-8	Thyroid Diseases and the Incidence of Antithyroid Antibodies	
Condition	**Anti–Thyroglobulin Antibody**	**Anti–Thyroid Peroxidase Antibody**
Hashimoto thyroiditis	70%	95%
Graves' disease	55%	75%
Myxedema	55%	75%
Nontoxic goitre	5%–50%	27%
Thyroid cancer	20%	20%
Normal, male	2%	3%
Normal, female	10%	15%

ANA, Antinuclear antibody.

Tg antibodies are also used when testing Tg as a marker for follicular cell thyroid cancer. If Tg antibodies are present, Tg is then considered an inaccurate marker for recurrent/metastatic cancer.

INTERFERING FACTORS

- Normal individuals, especially older women, may have anti–thyroglobulin antibodies.

PROCEDURE AND PATIENT CARE

Before

☒ Explain the procedure to the patient.
☒ Inform the patient that no fasting is required.

During

- Collect a venous blood sample in a red-top tube.

After

- Apply pressure or a pressure dressing to the venipuncture site.
- Assess the venipuncture site for bleeding.

TEST RESULTS AND CLINICAL SIGNIFICANCE

▲ Increased Levels

Chronic thyroiditis (Hashimoto thyroiditis): *Anti–thyroglobulin antibodies attack the globulin in the thyroid cells. The immune complex creates an inflammatory and destructive process in the gland, which is mediated through the complement system.*

Rheumatoid arthritis,

Rheumatoid-collagen disease: *The association with other autoimmune diseases is well known; however, the mechanism of this association has not been elucidated.*

Pernicious anemia: *APCAs have been associated with the presence of anti–thyroglobulin antibodies.*

Thyrotoxicosis,

Hypothyroidism,

Thyroid carcinoma: *Thyroglobulin, which leaks out of the thyroid as a result of these destructive diseases, stimulates the immune system to produce anti–thyroglobulin antibodies.*

Myxedema: *The antithyroid microsomal antibodies destroy the thyroid cell, which results in hypofunction of the gland.*

RELATED TESTS

Anti–Thyroid Peroxidase Antibody (p. 115). This test is used in conjunction with the anti–thyroglobulin antibody test to support the diagnosis of thyroid diseases.

Thyroid-Stimulating Immunoglobulins (p. 504). Long-acting thyroid stimulator (LATS) and other thyroid-stimulating immunoglobulins are measured to support the diagnosis of Graves' disease, especially when the differential diagnosis is complex.

Thyroid-Stimulating Hormone (p. 500). This test is used to diagnose primary hypothyroidism and to differentiate it from secondary (pituitary) and tertiary (hypothalamus) hypothyroidism.

Thyroxine, Total (p. 516). This is one of the first tests performed to assess thyroid function. It is used to evaluate thyroid function and to monitor replacement and suppressive medical therapy.

Triiodothyronine (p. 525). A T_3 test is used to evaluate thyroid function, primarily in order to diagnose hyperthyroidism. It is also used to monitor thyroid replacement and suppressive medical therapy.

Anti–Thyroid Peroxidase Antibody
(Anti-TPO, TPO-Ab, Antithyroid Microsomal Antibody, Thyroid Autoantibody)

NORMAL FINDINGS
Titre: <9 IU/mL

INDICATIONS
This test is primarily used in the differential diagnosis of thyroid diseases, such as Hashimoto thyroiditis (in adults) and chronic lymphocytic thyroiditis (in children).

TEST EXPLANATION
Thyroid microsomal antibodies are commonly found in patients with various thyroid diseases. They are present in 70% to 90% of patients with Hashimoto thyroiditis. Microsomal antibodies are produced in response to microsomes escaping from the thyroid epithelial cells surrounding the thyroid follicle. These escaped microsomes then act as antigens and stimulate the production of antibodies. These immune complexes initiate inflammatory and cytotoxic effects on the thyroid follicle. This test is often performed in conjunction with the anti–thyroglobulin antibody test, which greatly increases the specificity and sensitivity.

Although many different thyroid diseases are associated with elevated antimicrosomal antibody levels, the most frequent is chronic thyroiditis (Hashimoto thyroiditis in the adult and lymphocytic thyroiditis in children and young adults; see Table 2-8, p. 113). Both these chronic inflammatory diseases have been associated with other autoimmune (collagen-vascular) diseases. Twelve percent of normal girls and women and 1% of normal boys and men have positive antimicrosomal antibodies.

The most sensitive assay for antimicrosomal antibodies is for the anti–thyroid peroxidase (anti-TPO) antibody. This assay involves the use of radioimmunoassay and enzyme immunoassays. Anti-TPO antibody assay is often performed in conjunction with the anti–thyroglobulin antibody test (see p. 113). When both are performed, the specificity and sensitivity are greatly increased.

Anti-TPO antibody is present in almost all patients with Hashimoto thyroiditis, in more than 70% of those with Graves' disease, and, to a variable degree, in patients with nonthyroid autoimmune disease. The amount of anti-TPO antibody is correlated with the degree of lymphocytic infiltrations (inflammation) in the thyroid. Among healthy people, 5% to 10% have elevated anti-TPO antibody levels.

PROCEDURE AND PATIENT CARE

Before

🖊 Explain the procedure to the patient.
🖊 Inform the patient that no fasting is required.

During

- Collect a venous blood sample in a red-top tube.

After

- Apply pressure or a pressure dressing to the venipuncture site.
- Assess the venipuncture site for bleeding.

TEST RESULTS AND CLINICAL SIGNIFICANCE

▲ Increased Levels

Chronic thyroiditis (Hashimoto thyroiditis): *Antimicrosomal antibodies attack the microsome in the thyroid cells. The immune complex creates an inflammatory and destructive process in the gland, which is mediated through the complement system.*

Rheumatoid arthritis,

Rheumatoid-collagen disease: *The association with other autoimmune diseases is well known. The mechanism of this association, however, is not well known.*

Pernicious anemia: *APCAs have been associated with the presence of antimicrosomal antibodies.*

Thyrotoxicosis,

Hypothyroidism,

Thyroid carcinoma: *Microsomes leak out of the thyroid as a result of the presence of these destructive diseases; they stimulate the immune system to produce antimicrosomal antibodies.*

Myxedema: *Antithyroid microsomal antibodies destroy the thyroid cell, which results in hypofunction of the gland.*

RELATED TEST

Anti–Thyroglobulin Antibody (p. 113). This test is used primarily for the differential diagnosis of thyroid diseases, such as Hashimoto thyroiditis and chronic lymphocytic thyroiditis (in children).

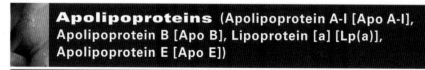

Apolipoproteins (Apolipoprotein A-I [Apo A-I], Apolipoprotein B [Apo B], Lipoprotein [a] [Lp(a)], Apolipoprotein E [Apo E])

NORMAL FINDINGS

Apolipoprotein A-I
Adult/Older Adult
Male: **0.75–1.6 g/L** (75–160 mg/dL)
Female: **0.8–1.75 g/L** (80–175 mg/dL)

Child/Adolescent
6 months–4 years:
    Male: **0.67–1.67 g/L** (67–167 mg/dL)
    Female: **0.60–1.48 g/L** (60–148 mg/dL)
5–17 years: **0.83–1.51 g/L** (83–151 mg/dL)

Newborn–6 Months
Male: **0.41–0.93 g/L** (41–93 mg/dL)
Female: **0.38–1.06 g/L** (38–106 mg/dL)

Apolipoprotein B
Adult/Older Adult
Male: **0.5–1.25 g/L** (50–125 mg/dL)
Female: **0.45–1.2 g/L** (45–120 mg/dL)

Child/Adolescent
Newborn–6 months: **0.11–0.31 g/L** (11–31 mg/dL)
6 months–3 years: **0.23–0.75 g/L** (23–75 mg/dL)
5–17 years:
    Male: **0.47–1.39 g/L** (47–139 mg/dL)
    Female: **0.41–1.32 g/L** (41–132 mg/dL)

Apolipoprotein A-I/Apolipoprotein B Ratio
Male: 0.85–2.24
Female: 0.76–3.23

Lipoprotein (a)
White (fifth to ninety-fifth percentiles):
    Male: **0.22–4.94 g/L** (2.2–49.4 mg/dL)
    Female: **0.21–5.73 g/L** (2.1–57.3 mg/dL)
Black (fifth to ninety-fifth percentiles):
    Male: **0.46–7.18 g/L** (4.6–71.8 mg/dL)
    Female: **0.44–0.75 g/L** (4.4–75 mg/dL)

INDICATIONS

This test is used to evaluate the risk of atherogenic heart and peripheral vascular diseases. These levels may be better indicators of atherogenic risks than are high-density lipoprotein (HDL), low-density lipoprotein (LDL), and very-low-density lipoprotein (VLDL).

TEST EXPLANATION

Apolipoproteins are the protein part of lipoproteins (such as HDL, LDL). In general, apolipoproteins play an important role in lipid transport. They serve as activators to encourage the attachment of lipoproteins to lipoprotein receptors in tissue cells to enable transfer of lipoproteins (carrying fat products) into the cell. Furthermore, apolipoproteins are enzymes related to the lipoprotein synthesis. Apolipoproteins are mostly formed in the liver and intestine. Apolipoprotein synthesis in the intestine is regulated principally by the fat content of the diet.

Apolipoprotein synthesis in the liver is controlled by a host of factors, including dietary composition, hormones (insulin, glucagon, thyroxin, estrogens, androgens), alcohol intake, and various drugs (statins, niacin, and fibric acids). Quantification of apolipoproteins is used as risk factors of atherogenic disease. Still, unsolved methodologic problems within apolipoprotein immunoassays produce significant variability.

There are at least nine types of apolipoprotein, including apolipoproteins A-I, B, and E (Table 2-9). Apolipoprotein A (Apo A) is the major polypeptide component of HDL. Apo A has two major forms: Apo A-I, which constitutes approximately 75% of the Apo A in HDL, and Apo A-II, which constitutes approximately 20% of the total HDL protein. Like the HDL content in the serum, Apo A-I values are also higher in women than in men. Low levels of Apo A are associated with increased risk of coronary artery disease. Therefore, Apo A-I is used as a risk factor for atherogenic vascular disease.

Apo B is the major polypeptide component of LDL and makes up approximately 80% of that protein. Of the protein portion of VLDL, 40% is composed of Apo B. Apo B has been shown to exist in two forms: Apo B-100 and Apo B-48. Apo B-100 is synthesized in the liver and found in lipoproteins of endogenous origin (VLDL and LDL). Apo B-100 has an affinity for the LDL receptor located on cell surfaces in peripheral tissues and is involved with cellular deposition of cholesterol. Because of this, some authorities believe that Apo B-100 is an indicator of atherosclerotic heart disease. Specific apolipoprotein disorders are rare, but knowledge and awareness about the importance of apolipoproteins and their relevance to a variety of clinical disorders are increasing. Familial defective Apo B-100 is an autosomal dominant disorder involving a mutation of Apo B that interferes with binding of LDL. Total cholesterol and LDL-cholesterol levels are raised, and triglyceride levels are normal.

Lipoprotein (a) (Lp[a], referred to as "lipoprotein little a") is another lipoprotein. The two polypeptide components of Lp(a) are Apo(a) and an LDL-like protein. An increased level of Lp(a) may be an independent risk factor for atherosclerosis and is particularly harmful to the endothelium. It has been shown that Apo(a) is a deformed relative of plasminogen, which is responsible for dissolving fibrin clots. This strong resemblance between apolipoprotein and plasminogen may provide a link between lipids, the clotting mechanism, and atherogenesis. Microthrombi containing fibrin on the vessel wall become incorporated into the atherosclerotic plaque. Familial

TABLE 2-9	Summary of Apolipoproteins		
Lipoprotein	**Subcomponents**	**Lipoprotein Component**	**Associated Diseases**
Apolipoprotein A	Apolipoproteins A-I and A-II	HDL	Low levels are a risk factor for atherogenic vascular disease
Apolipoprotein B	Apolipoproteins B-100 and B-48	LDL, VLDL	High levels are a risk factor for atherogenic vascular disease
Lipoprotein (a)	Apolipoprotein (a)	LDL-like proteins	High levels are a risk factor for atherogenic vascular disease
Apolipoprotein C	C1, C2, C3	VLDL	Hyperlipidemia
Apolipoprotein E	E2, E3, E4		Hyperlipidemia, Alzheimer's disease

HDL, High-density lipoprotein; *LDL,* low-density lipoprotein; *VLDL,* very-low-density lipoprotein.

hypercholesterolemia, some forms of renal failure, nephrotic syndrome, and estrogen depletion in women older than 50 years may also be associated with increased levels of Lp(a).

Apolipoprotein C (Apo C) constitutes a large part of VLDL. There are three types of Apo C, called C1, C2, and C3. These are associated with hyperlipidemias. Apo C2 deficiency is a rare autosomal recessive hereditary disorder that leads to an accumulation of chylomicrons and triglycerides. Apo C deficiency is also associated with Tangier disease and nephrotic syndrome.

Apolipoprotein E (Apo E) is also involved in cholesterol transport. Through genotyping, three alleles for Apo E have been identified: E2, E3, and E4. Each person gets an allele from each parent. E3/E3 is the normal genotype. E2/E2 is rare and is associated with type III hyperlipidemia (see Fredrickson's classification, p. 359). E4/E4 or E4/E3 is associated with high LDL levels. The E4 allele has been proposed as a risk factor for Alzheimer's disease, inasmuch as it has a strong association with Alzheimer's disease in the general population. It is not clear how Apo E functions as a risk factor modifying the age at onset in Alzheimer's disease. Apo E is present in the neuritic amyloid plaques (see p. 666) and may also be involved in the neurofibrillary tangle formation, because it binds to tau protein (see p. 666).

INTERFERING FACTORS

All of the apolipoproteins are acute phase reactants, and their levels can be elevated in acutely and chronically ill patients.

Apolipoprotein A-I

- Physical exercise may increase Apo A-I levels.
- Smoking may decrease levels.
- Diets high in carbohydrates or polyunsaturated fats may decrease Apo A-I levels.
- Drugs that may cause *increases* in Apo A-I levels include carbamazepine, estrogens, ethanol, lovastatin, niacin, oral contraceptives, phenobarbital, pravastatin, and simvastatin.
- Drugs that may cause *decreases* in Apo A-I levels include androgens, beta blockers, diuretics, and progestins.

Apolipoprotein B

- Diets high in saturated fats and cholesterol may increase Apo B levels.
- Drugs that may cause *increases* in Apo B levels include androgens, beta blockers, diuretics, ethanol, and progestins.
- Drugs that may cause *decreases* in Apo B levels include cholestyramine, estrogen (in postmenopausal women), lovastatin, neomycin, niacin, simvastatin, and thyroxine.

Lipoprotein (a)

- Drugs that may cause *decreases* in Lp(a) levels include estrogens, neomycin, and niacin.

✓ Clinical Priorities

- Apolipoproteins may be better indicators of atherogenic risks than are HDL, LDL, and VLDL.
- Decreased levels of Apo A-I and increased levels of Apo B-100 are associated with an increased risk of coronary artery disease.
- Research has suggested that increased levels of Lp(a) are associated with a high risk of coronary artery disease.
- A 12- to 14-hour fast is necessary before the test. Only water is permitted during the fast.

PROCEDURE AND PATIENT CARE

Before

✗ Explain the procedure to the patient.

✗ Instruct the patient to fast for 12 to 14 hours before the test. Only water is permitted during the fast.

✗ Inform the patient that smoking is prohibited.

During

- Collect a venous blood sample in a red-top tube.

After

- Apply pressure or a pressure dressing to the venipuncture site.
- Observe the venipuncture site for bleeding.

TEST RESULTS AND CLINICAL SIGNIFICANCE*

▲ Increased Apolipoprotein A-I Levels

Familial hyperalphalipoproteinemia,
Pregnancy,
Weight reduction

▼ Decreased Apolipoprotein A-I Levels

Coronary artery disease,
Ischemic coronary disease,
Myocardial infarction,
Familial hypoalphalipoproteinemia,
Fish eye disease,
Uncontrolled diabetes mellitus,
Tangier disease,
Nephrotic syndrome,
Chronic renal failure,
Cholestasis,
Hemodialysis

▲ Increased Apolipoprotein B Levels

Hyperlipoproteinemia (types IIa, IIb, IV, V),
Nephrotic syndrome,
Pregnancy,
Hemodialysis,
Biliary obstruction,
Coronary artery disease,
Diabetes,
Hypothyroidism,
Anorexia nervosa,
Renal failure

---

*The pathophysiologic processes of these observations have not been well defined.

▼ Decreased Apolipoprotein B Levels

Tangier disease,
Hyperthyroidism,
Inflammatory joint disease,
Malnutrition,
Chronic pulmonary disease,
Weight reduction,
Chronic anemia,
Reye syndrome

▲ Increased Lipoprotein (a) Levels

Premature coronary artery disease,
Stenosis of cerebral arteries,
Uncontrolled diabetes mellitus,
Severe hypothyroidism,
Familial hypercholesterolemia,
Chronic renal failure,
Estrogen depletion,
Apo E-4 allele,
Alzheimer's disease

▼ Decreased Lipoprotein (a) Levels

Alcoholism,
Malnutrition,
Chronic hepatocellular disease

RELATED TEST

Lipoprotein (p. 355). This test is also used to assess the risk of atherogenic vascular disease.

 Arterial Blood Gases (Blood Gases, ABG Measurements)

NORMAL FINDINGS

pH

Adult/child >2 years: 7.35–7.45
Newborn: 7.32–7.49
2 months to 2 years: 7.34–7.46

Partial Pressure of Carbon Dioxide (P_{CO_2})

Adult/child: 35–45 mm Hg
<2 years: 26–41 mm Hg
P_{CO_2} (venous): 40–50 mm Hg

Bicarbonate Ion (HCO_3^-)

Adult/child: **23–29 mmol/L** (23–29 mEq/L)
Newborn/infant: **16–24 mmol/L** (16–24 mEq/L)

Partial Pressure of Oxygen (Po_2)

Adult/child: 80–100 mm Hg
Newborn: 60–70 mm Hg
Po_2 (venous): 40–50 mm Hg

Oxygen Saturation

Adult/child: 95%–100%
Older adult: 95%
Newborn: 40%–90%

Oxygen Content

Arterial: 15–22 volume percent
Venous: 11–16 volume percent

Base Excess/Deficit

0 ± 2 mmol/L (mEq/L)

Alveolar-to-Arterial Oxygen Difference

<10 mm Hg

 Critical Values

pH: <7.25, >7.55
Pco_2: <20 mm Hg, >60 mm Hg
HCO_3^-: **<15 or >40 mmol/L** (mEq/L)
Po_2 (arterial): <40 mm Hg
O_2 saturation: 75% or lower
Base excess/deficit: ±3 mmol/L (mEq/L)

INDICATIONS

Measurement of arterial blood gases (ABGs) provides valuable information in assessing and managing a patient's respiratory (ventilation) and metabolic (renal) acid-base and electrolyte homeostasis. It is also used to assess the adequacy of oxygenation.

TEST EXPLANATION

ABGs are measured to monitor patients on ventilators, monitor critically ill patients who are not on a ventilator, establish preoperative baseline parameters, and regulate electrolyte therapy. Although O_2 saturation monitors can accurately indicate O_2 level, ABG measurements are still used to monitor O_2 flow rates in the hospital and at home. ABG measurement is often performed in conjunction with pulmonary function studies.

Acidity-Alkalinity Measurement

The pH is the negative logarithm of the hydrogen ion concentration in the blood. It is inversely proportional to the actual hydrogen ion concentration. Therefore, as the hydrogen ion concentration decreases, the pH increases, or as the hydrogen ion concentration increases, the pH decreases. Acids found in the blood that are important to pH include carbonic acid (H_2CO_3), dietary acids, lactic acid, and keto acids. The pH is a measure of alkalinity (pH > 7.4) and acidity (pH < 7.35).

In respiratory or metabolic alkalosis, the pH is elevated; in respiratory or metabolic acidosis, the pH is decreased. The pH is usually calculated by a machine that directly measures pH.

Partial Pressure of Carbon Dioxide

The Pco_2 is a measure of the partial pressure of carbon dioxide in the blood. Ten percent of the CO_2 is carried in the plasma and 90% in the red blood cells. Pco_2 is a measurement of ventilation. The faster and more deeply the patient breathes, the more CO_2 is blown off, and Pco_2 levels drop. Pco_2 is therefore referred to as the respiratory component in acid-base determination because this value is controlled primarily by the lungs. As the CO_2 level increases, the pH decreases. The CO_2 level and the pH are inversely proportional. The Pco_2 in the blood and the cerebrospinal fluid is a major stimulant to the breathing centre in the brain. As Pco_2 levels rise, breathing is stimulated. If Pco_2 levels rise too high, breathing cannot keep up with the demand to blow off or ventilate. As Pco_2 levels rise further, the brain is depressed and ventilation decreases further, causing coma.

The Pco_2 level is elevated in primary respiratory acidosis and decreased in primary respiratory alkalosis (Table 2-10). Because the lungs compensate for primary metabolic acid-base derangements, Pco_2 levels are affected by metabolic disturbances as well. In metabolic acidosis, the lungs attempt to compensate by blowing off CO_2 to raise pH. In metabolic alkalosis, the lungs attempt to compensate by retaining CO_2 to lower pH (Table 2-11).

Bicarbonate Ion or Carbon Dioxide Content

Most of the CO_2 content in the blood is HCO_3^-. The bicarbonate ion is a measure of the metabolic (renal) component of the acid-base equilibrium. It is regulated by the kidney. This ion can be measured directly by the bicarbonate value or indirectly by the CO_2 content (see p. 155). It is important not to confuse CO_2 content with Pco_2. CO_2 content is an indirect measurement of HCO_3^-. Pco_2 is a direct measurement of the tension of CO_2 in the blood and is regulated by the lungs.

TABLE 2-10	Normal Values for Arterial Blood Gases and Abnormal Values in Uncompensated Acid-Base Disturbances			
Acid-Base Disturbance	pH	Pco_2 (mm Hg)	HCO_3^- (mmol/L [mEq/L])	Common Cause
None (normal values)	7.35–7.45	35–45	22–26	
Respiratory acidosis	↓	↑	Normal	Respiratory depression (drugs, central nervous system trauma) Pulmonary disease (pneumonia, chronic obstructive pulmonary disease, respiratory underventilation)
Respiratory alkalosis	↑	↓	Normal	Hyperventilation (emotions, pain, respiratory overventilation)
Metabolic acidosis	↓	Normal	↓	Diabetes, shock, renal failure, intestinal fistula
Metabolic alkalosis	↑	Normal	↑	Sodium bicarbonate overdose, prolonged vomiting, nasogastric drainage

TABLE 2-11	Acid-Base Disturbances and Compensatory Mechanisms
Acid-Base Disturbance	**Mode of Compensation**
Respiratory acidosis	Kidneys retain increased amounts of HCO_3^- to increase pH
Respiratory alkalosis	Kidneys excrete increased amounts of HCO_3^- to lower pH
Metabolic acidosis	Lungs "blow off" CO_2 to raise pH
Metabolic alkalosis	Lungs retain CO_2 to lower pH

As the HCO_3^- level increases, the pH also increases; therefore, the relationship of HCO_3^- level to pH is directly proportional. The HCO_3^- level is elevated in metabolic alkalosis and decreased in metabolic acidosis (see Table 2-10). The kidneys also are used to compensate for primary respiratory acid-base derangements. For example, in respiratory acidosis, the kidneys attempt to compensate by reabsorbing increased amounts of HCO_3^-. In respiratory alkalosis, the kidneys excrete HCO_3^- in increased amounts in an attempt to lower pH through compensation (see Table 2-11).

Partial Pressure of Oxygen

This is an indirect measure of the O_2 content of the arterial blood. Po_2 is a measure of the tension (pressure) of O_2 dissolved in the plasma. This pressure determines the force of O_2 to diffuse across the pulmonary alveoli membrane. The Po_2 level is decreased in three situations:
1. Inability to oxygenate the arterial blood because of O_2 diffusion difficulties (e.g., pneumonia, shock lung, congestive failure)
2. When venous blood mixes prematurely with arterial blood (e.g., congenital heart disease)
3. When pulmonary alveoli have been underventilated and overperfused (pickwickian syndrome; e.g., obese patients who cannot breathe properly when in the supine position, or patients with significant atelectasis)

Po_2 is one of the measures used to determine the effectiveness of O_2 therapy.

Oxygen Saturation

O_2 saturation is an indication of the percentage of hemoglobin saturated with O_2. When 92% to 100% of the hemoglobin carries O_2, the tissues are adequately provided with O_2, if O_2 dissociation is normal. As the Po_2 level decreases, the percentage of hemoglobin saturation also decreases. This decrease (see an oxyhemoglobin-dissociation curve) is linear to a certain value. However, when the Po_2 level drops below 60 mm Hg, small decreases in the Po_2 level cause large decreases in the percentage of hemoglobin saturated with O_2. At O_2 saturation levels of 70% or lower, the tissues are unable to extract enough O_2 to carry out their vital functions.

O_2 saturation is calculated by the blood gas machine through the following formula:

$$\text{Percentage of } O_2 \text{ saturation} = \frac{\text{Volume of } O_2 \text{ content Hb}}{\text{Volume of } O_2 \text{ Hb capacity}}$$

Pulse oximetry (see p. 1155) is a noninvasive method of determining O_2 saturation. This can be done easily and continuously. The machine measures O_2 saturation. It actually measures all forms of O_2-saturated hemoglobin, including carboxyhemoglobin (which rises during smoke inhalation or after some inhalants are used). Therefore, in cases of carbon monoxide poisoning when carboxyhemoglobin is high, oximetry inaccurately indicates high O_2 saturation. During oximetry monitoring, a small clip-like sensor is applied to the tip of the patient's finger or earlobe. The oximeter transmits light from one side and records the amount of light on the other side, thus determining O_2 saturation.

Oxygen Content

This is a calculated number that represents the amount of O_2 in the blood. It is calculated as follows:

$$O_2 \text{ content} = O_2 \text{ saturation} \times Hb \times 1.34 + PO_2 \times 0.003$$

Nearly all O_2 in the blood is bound to hemoglobin. O_2 content decreases with the same diseases that diminish Po_2.

Base Excess/Deficit

This number is calculated by the blood gas machine according to the pH, the Pco_2, and the hematocrit. It represents the amount of buffering anions in the blood. HCO_3^- is the largest of these anions. Others include hemoglobin, proteins, and phosphates. Base excess is a way to take all of these anions into account when determining acid-base treatment on the basis of the metabolic component. A negative-base excess (deficit) indicates metabolic acidosis (e.g., lactic acidosis). A positive-base excess indicates metabolic alkalosis or compensation to prolonged respiratory acidosis.

Alveolar-to-Arterial O_2 Difference (A-a Gradient)

This number is calculated as the difference between alveolar O_2 and arterial O_2. The normal value is less than 10 mm Hg. If the A-a gradient is abnormally high, then either diffusion of O_2 across the alveolar membrane is abnormal (thickened edematous alveoli) or unoxygenated blood is mixing with the oxygenated blood. Thickening of alveolar membranes can occur in patients with pulmonary edema, pulmonary fibrosis, and acute respiratory distress syndrome. Mixing of unoxygenated and oxygenated blood occurs in patients with congenital cardiac septal defects, arteriovenous shunts, or underventilated alveoli that are still being perfused (e.g., as with atelectasis or mucus plug).

Interpretation of ABG levels can seem difficult but is really quite easy with a system of evaluation (see Table 2-10). One such system is as follows:

1. Evaluate the pH.
   If the pH is less than 7.35, acidosis is present.
   If the pH is greater than 7.45, alkalosis is present.
2. Next, evaluate the Pco_2.
   If the Pco_2 is high in a patient who has been determined to have acidosis (in step 1), the patient has respiratory acidosis.
   If the Pco_2 is low in a patient who has been determined to have acidosis (in step 1), the patient has metabolic acidosis and is compensating for that situation by blowing off CO_2.
   If the Pco_2 is low in a patient who has been determined to have alkalosis (in step 1), the patient has respiratory alkalosis.
   If the Pco_2 is high in a patient who has been determined to have alkalosis (in step 1), the patient has metabolic alkalosis and is compensating for that situation by retaining CO_2.
3. Next, evaluate the bicarbonate ion (HCO_3^-) level.
   In a patient with respiratory acidosis, HCO_3^- can be expected to be high in an attempt to compensate for this condition.
   In a patient with metabolic acidosis, HCO_3^- can be expected to be low as a reflection of this condition.
   In a patient with respiratory alkalosis, HCO_3^- can be expected to be low to compensate for this condition.
   In a patient with metabolic alkalosis, HCO_3^- can be expected to be high as a reflection of this condition.

Contraindications

Arterial access should not be performed in the following situations:
- The pulse is not palpable.
- Cellulitis or open infection is present in the area considered for access.
- The Allen test result is negative, indicating that there is no ulnar arterial supply to the hand. If, in that case, the radial artery is used for access, thrombosis may occur and jeopardize the viability of the hand.
- There is an arteriovenous fistula proximal to the site of proposed access.
- The patient has a severe coagulopathy.

Potential Complications

- Occlusion of the artery used for access. It is preferable to avoid use of end arteries such as the brachial or femoral artery.
- Penetration of other important structures anatomically juxtaposed to the artery (e.g., a nerve)

INTERFERING FACTORS

- O_2 saturation can be artificially increased by the inhalation of carbon monoxide, which increases the carboxyhemoglobin level.
- In patients with chronic obstructive pulmonary disease (COPD), the stimulus to breathe is not triggered by CO_2 levels (as is normal) but by O_2 levels. If a large amount of O_2 is provided to these patients, they will no longer be stimulated to breathe and will hypoventilate.
- Respiration can be inhibited by the use of sedative-hypnotics or narcotics. Overdosage of these drugs can cause hypoventilation in patients with normal lungs.

Clinical Priorities

- Perform the Allen test to assess collateral circulation before you perform the arterial puncture on the radial artery. A positive Allen test ensures collateral circulation to the hand, if thrombosis of the radial artery should follow the puncture.
- Arterial puncture should not be performed on an arm with an arteriovenous fistula or shunt.
- After the arterial blood is obtained, apply pressure to the puncture site for 3 to 5 minutes to avoid hematoma formation. If the patient has an abnormal clotting time or is taking anticoagulants, apply pressure for approximately 15 minutes.

PROCEDURE AND PATIENT CARE

Before

- Explain the procedure to the patient.
- Notify the laboratory before measuring ABGs so that the necessary equipment can be calibrated before the blood sample arrives.
- Perform the Allen test to assess collateral circulation before you perform the puncture on the radial artery (Figure 2-7). To perform the Allen test, make the patient's hand blanch by obliterating both the radial and the ulnar pulses and then release the pressure over the ulnar artery only. If flow through the ulnar artery is good, flushing can be seen immediately. The Allen test result is then positive, and the radial artery can be used for puncture. If the Allen test is negative (no flushing), repeat it on the other arm. If both arms produce a negative result, choose another artery (femoral) for puncture.
- Note that a positive Allen test result confirms collateral circulation to the hand if thrombosis of the radial artery should follow the puncture.

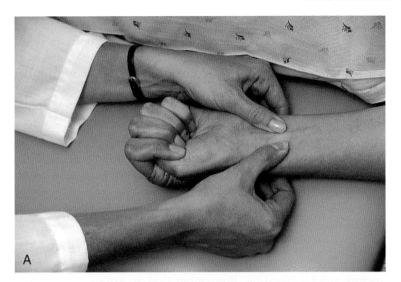

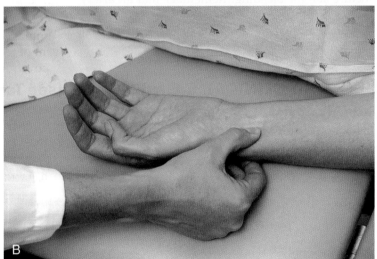

Figure 2-7 The Allen test for evaluating collateral circulation of the radial artery. **A,** Step 1: While the patient's fist is closed tightly, obliterate both the radial and ulnar arteries simultaneously. Instruct the patient to relax the hand, and watch for blanching of the palm and fingers. **B,** Step 2: Release the obstructing pressure from only the ulnar artery. Wait 15 seconds, observing the hand for flushing caused by capillary filling. Flushing indicates a positive Allen test result, which verifies that the ulnar artery alone is capable of supplying the entire hand. If flushing does not occur within 15 seconds, the Allen test result is negative, and the radial artery must not be used for collecting blood.

During

- Note that arterial blood can be obtained from any area of the body in which strong pulses are palpable, usually from the radial, brachial, or femoral artery. The artery chosen for access should have adequate collateral vessels, be easily accessible, and be surrounded by few other vital structures.
- Cleanse the arterial site carefully with an antiseptic (e.g., alcohol or povidoneiodine).
- Use a small-gauge needle to collect the arterial blood in an air-free heparinized syringe.
- After drawing the blood, remove the needle and apply pressure to the arterial site for 3 to 5 minutes.
- Expel any air bubbles in the syringe.

After

- Place the arterial blood on ice and immediately take it to the chemistry or pulmonary laboratory for analysis.
- Hold pressure or apply pressure or a pressure dressing to the arterial puncture site for 3 to 5 minutes to avoid hematoma formation.
- Assess the puncture site for bleeding. Remember that an artery rather than a vein has been accessed.
- If the patient has an abnormal clotting time or is taking anticoagulants, apply pressure for a longer period (approximately 15 minutes).

TEST RESULTS AND CLINICAL SIGNIFICANCE (see Table 2-10)

▲ Increased pH (Alkalosis)

Metabolic Alkalosis

Hypokalemia,

Hypochloremia,

Chronic and high-volume gastric suction,

Chronic vomiting,

Aldosteronism,

Use of mercurial diuretics: *Important acid hydrogen ions are lost. HCO_3^- ions are relatively high.*

Respiratory Alkalosis

Hypoxemic states, such as chronic heart failure (CHF), cystic fibrosis, carbon monoxide poisoning, pulmonary emboli, shock, acute severe pulmonary diseases: *With hypoxemia, breathing is accelerated. CO_2 is blown off.*

Anxiety neuroses,

Pain,

Pregnancy: *These situations are associated with hyperventilation. With hyperventilation, CO_2 is blown off.*

▼ Decreased pH (Acidosis)

Metabolic Acidosis

Ketoacidosis,

Lactic acidosis: *Acid anions build up. Acidosis occurs.*

Severe diarrhea,

Renal failure: *Important base ions are lost. Acid ions are relatively increased and acidosis occurs.*

Respiratory Acidosis
Respiratory failure: *P_{CO_2} builds up, causing acidosis.*

▲ Increased P_{CO_2}

COPD (bronchitis, emphysema),
Oversedation,
Head trauma,
Overoxygenation in a patient with COPD or pickwickian syndrome: *Reduced ventilation causes increased levels of P_{CO_2}.*

▼ Decreased P_{CO_2}

Hypoxemia,
Pulmonary emboli: *Hypoxemia drives the respiratory centre to increase ventilation. With increased ventilation, P_{CO_2} levels decrease.*
Anxiety,
Pain,
Pregnancy: *These situations are associated with rapid ventilation. With increased ventilation, P_{CO_2} levels decrease.*

▲ Increased HCO_3^-

Chronic vomiting or chronic high-volume gastric suction,
Aldosteronism,
Use of mercurial diuretics: *Important acid hydrogen ions are lost. HCO_3^- ions are relatively high. This causes metabolic alkalosis.*
   COPD: *HCO_3^- ions are increased to compensate for chronic hypoventilation (high P_{CO_2}). Compensation occurs for respiratory acidosis.*

▼ Decreased HCO_3^-

Chronic and severe diarrhea,
Chronic use of loop diuretics: *Persistent loss of base ions, including HCO_3^-, occurs. Most of the CO_2 content is HCO_3^-.*
Starvation,
Diabetic ketoacidosis,
Acute renal failure: *Ketoacids are built up. HCO_3^- neutralizes these acids. HCO_3^- levels therefore drop.*

▲ Increased P_{O_2} and O_2 Content

Polycythemia: *The amount of hemoglobin is significantly increased. O_2 content, which saturates the hemoglobin, is also increased.*
Increased inspired O_2,
Hyperventilation: *With increased alveolar O_2 caused by breathing more rapidly or increasing the O_2 in the inspired air, the P_{O_2} and O_2 content can be expected to increase.*

▼ Decreased P_{O_2} and O_2 Content

Anemias: *The amount of hemoglobin is significantly reduced. O_2 content, which saturates the hemoglobin, is also reduced.*
Mucus plug,
Bronchospasm,
Atelectasis,

Pneumothorax,

Pulmonary edema,

Acute Respiratory Distress Syndrome (ARDS),

Restrictive lung disease,

Atrial or ventricular cardiac septal defects,

Emboli: *See rationale below, under increased A-a O$_2$ gradient.*

Inadequate O$_2$ in inspired air (suffocation),

Severe hypoventilation states, such as oversedation or neurologic somnolence: *Without air exchange, Po$_2$ levels fall.*

▲ Increased A-a O$_2$ Gradient

Mucus plug,

Bronchospasm,

Atelectasis,

Pneumothorax,

Pulmonary edema,

ARDS: *Nonventilated lung tissue is still perfused. The perfused blood does not get oxygenated, however, because there is no ventilation in that area of the lung to bring O$_2$ to the blood. The perfused yet unoxygenated blood mixes with the oxygenated blood in the pulmonary veins. By dilution, the O$_2$ content of the mixed blood returning to the heart is lowered. The arterial blood is therefore lowered.*

Atrial or ventricular cardiac septal defects,

Emboli: *The unoxygenated blood gains access to the oxygenated blood by direct shunting. By dilution, the O$_2$ content of the mixed blood returning to the heart is lowered. The arterial blood is therefore lowered.*

RELATED TESTS

Pulmonary Function Tests (p. 1158). This is measurement of lung volume, which aids in the diagnosis and treatment of obstructive and restrictive lung diseases.

Fetal Scalp Blood pH (p. 252). Measurement of fetal scalp blood pH provides valuable information on fetal acid-base status. This screening test is useful clinically for diagnosing fetal distress.

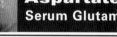

Aspartate Aminotransferase (AST, Formerly Serum Glutamic Oxaloacetic Transaminase [SGOT])

NORMAL FINDINGS

Age	Normal Value (IU/L)
0–5 days	35–140
<3 years	15–60
3–6 years	15–50
6–12 years	10–50
12–18 years	10–40
Adult	7–40
	(Women tend to have slightly lower levels than do men)
Older adult	Slightly higher than adult values

INDICATIONS

This test is used in the evaluation of patients with suspected hepatocellular diseases.

TEST EXPLANATION

This enzyme is found in very high concentrations within highly metabolic tissue, such as the heart muscle, liver cells, skeletal muscle cells, and to a lesser degree in the kidneys, pancreas, and red blood cells (RBCs). When disease or injury affects the cells of these tissues, the cells lyse. The aspartate aminotransferase (AST) is released and picked up by the blood, and the serum level rises. The amount of AST elevation is related directly to the number of cells affected by the disease or injury. Furthermore, the degree of elevation depends on the length of time between the injury and when the blood is collected. AST is cleared from the blood in a few days. Serum AST levels become elevated 8 hours after cell injury, peak at 24 to 36 hours, and return to normal in 3 to 7 days. If the cellular injury is chronic, the elevation in levels will persist.

Because AST exists within the liver cells, diseases that affect the hepatocyte cause elevations in the levels of this enzyme. In acute hepatitis, AST levels can rise to 20 times the normal value. In acute extrahepatic obstruction (e.g., gallstone), AST levels quickly rise to 10 times the norm and then swiftly fall. In patients with cirrhosis, the level of AST depends on the amount of active inflammation.

Serum AST levels are often compared with alanine aminotransferase (ALT) levels. The AST/ALT ratio is usually higher than 1 in patients with alcoholic cirrhosis, liver congestion, and metastatic tumour of the liver. Ratios lower than 1 may be seen in patients with acute hepatitis, viral hepatitis, or infectious mononucleosis. The ratio is less accurate if AST levels exceed 10 times normal.

In acute pancreatitis, acute renal diseases, musculoskeletal diseases, or trauma, serum AST levels may rise transiently. Levels of this enzyme may also be elevated in RBC abnormalities such as acute hemolytic anemia and severe burns. AST levels may be decreased in patients with beriberi or diabetic ketoacidosis and in patients who are pregnant.

INTERFERING FACTORS

- Pregnancy may cause decreases in AST levels.
- Exercise may cause increases in AST levels.
- Levels are artificially decreased in patients with pyridoxine deficiency (such as beriberi, or as in pregnancy), severe long-standing liver disease, uremia, or diabetic ketoacidosis.
- Drugs that may cause *increases* in AST levels include antihypertensives, cholinergic agents, coumarin-type anticoagulants, digitalis preparations, erythromycin, hepatotoxic medications, isoniazid, methyldopa, oral contraceptives, opiates, salicylates, statins, and verapamil.

PROCEDURE AND PATIENT CARE

Before

- Explain the procedure to the patient.
- Avoid giving the patient any intramuscular injection.
- If the patient is taking drugs that could interfere with test results, withhold these drugs, if possible, for 12 hours before the test.

During

- Collect a venous sample of blood in a red-top tube. This is usually done daily for 3 days and then again 1 week later.
- Rotate the venipuncture site.
- Avoid hemolysis.
- On the laboratory slip, indicate whether the patient is taking any drugs that may cause false-positive results.
- Record the time and date of any intramuscular injection given.
- Record the exact time and date when the blood test is performed. This aids in the interpretation of the temporal pattern of enzyme elevations.

After

- Apply pressure or a pressure dressing to the venipuncture site.
- Observe the venipuncture site for bleeding.

TEST RESULTS AND CLINICAL SIGNIFICANCE

▲ Increased Levels

Liver Diseases

Hepatitis,
Hepatic cirrhosis,
Drug-induced liver injury,
Hepatic metastasis,
Hepatic necrosis (initial stages only),
Hepatic surgery,
Infectious mononucleosis with hepatitis,
Hepatic infiltrative process (e.g., tumour): *These diseases cause liver cell injury. The cells die, and lysis of the cells occurs. The contents of the lysed cells (including AST) are spewed out and are picked up by the blood. AST levels thereby become elevated.*

Skeletal Muscle Diseases

Skeletal muscle trauma,
Recent noncardiac surgery,
Multiple traumas,
Severe, deep burns,
Progressive muscular dystrophy,
Recent convulsions,
Heat stroke,
Primary muscle diseases (e.g., myopathy, myositis): *These diseases cause muscle cell injury. The cells die, and lysis of the cells occurs. The contents of the lysed cells (including AST) are spewed out and are picked up by the blood. AST levels thereby become elevated.*

Other Diseases

Acute hemolytic anemia,
Acute pancreatitis: *These diseases cause cell injury in these tissues. The cells die, and lysis of the cells occurs. The contents of the lysed cells (including AST) are spewed out and picked up by the blood. AST levels thereby become elevated.*

▼ Decreased Levels

Acute renal disease,
Beriberi,
Diabetic ketoacidosis,
Pregnancy,
Chronic renal dialysis

RELATED TESTS

Creatine Kinase (p. 201). This enzyme is measured in a manner similar to that of AST and exists predominantly in heart and skeletal muscle.

Alanine Aminotransferase (see p. 45). This enzyme is measured in a manner similar to that of AST and exists predominantly in the liver.

Lactate Dehydrogenase (p. 339). This is an intracellular enzyme measured to support the diagnosis of injury or disease involving the heart, liver, RBCs, kidneys, skeletal muscle, brain, and lungs.

Leucine Aminopeptidase (p. 351). This enzyme is specific to the hepatobiliary system. Diseases affecting that system cause elevations in levels of this enzyme.

Gamma-Glutamyl Transpeptidase (p. 261), Alkaline Phosphatase (p. 53), and 5'-Nucleotidase (p. 389). These enzymes also exist predominantly in the liver.

Beta$_2$-Microglobulin (β_2M)

NORMAL FINDINGS

Blood: **<170 nmol/L** (0.7-1.8 Mcg/mL)
Urine: **<10 mmol/day** (≤300 Mcg/L)
Cerebrospinal fluid: **0.7–1.4 Mcg/mL** (≤2.4 mg/L)

INDICATIONS

This test is used as a tumour marker for blood tumours such as lymphoma or leukemia. Measurements of this protein can also be used in the differential diagnosis of diseases of the kidney.

TEST EXPLANATION

Beta$_2$ microglobulin (β_2M) is a protein that is found on the surface of all nucleated cells and is a major human leukocyte antibody histocompatibility antigen that exists in increased numbers on white blood cells (WBCs) and, in particular, on lymphatic cells. Production of this protein is increased as these cells are produced or destroyed. Therefore, β_2M levels are increased in patients with malignancies (especially lymphoma, leukemia, or multiple myeloma) and in patients with chronic severe inflammatory diseases. Because the degree of elevation can be related to tumour cell load, β_2M is an accurate measurement of tumour disease activity, stage of disease, and prognosis. Therefore, it is an important tumour marker. When central nervous system involvement with these neoplasms is suspected, β_2M can be measured in the cerebrospinal fluid and its levels compared with blood levels. Increased levels are diagnostic of central nervous system involvement.

Blood levels are increased in patients with human immunodeficiency virus (HIV) infection and are a measure of the disease activity. Cytomegalovirus infection is also associated with increased blood levels.

β_2M is excreted by the glomeruli and partially reabsorbed into the blood by the renal tubule. In a patient with renal disease, when blood and urine β_2M levels are obtained simultaneously, glomerular disease can be differentiated from tubular disease: In glomerular disease, blood levels are high and urine levels are low; in tubular disease, the blood levels are low and urine levels are high. Blood levels increase early in kidney transplant rejection.

In patients with aminoglycoside toxicity, β_2M levels become elevated even before creatinine levels. Urine levels are increased in patients with kidney disease caused by high exposure to heavy metals, such as cadmium or mercury. Periodic testing is performed on these workers to detect kidney disease at its earliest stage.

Increased cerebrospinal fluid levels of β_2M indicate central nervous system involvement with leukemia, lymphoma, HIV infection, or multiple sclerosis.

INTERFERING FACTORS

- β_2M is unstable in very acidic urine.
- When this test is performed with radioimmunoassay, results could be affected by recent nuclear imaging.

PROCEDURE AND PATIENT CARE

Before
✕ Explain the procedure to the patient to minimize anxiety.

During

Blood
- Collect a venous blood sample in a red-top tube.

Urine
✕ Instruct the patient to discard the first voided specimen of the day and to begin the 24-hour collection afterwards.
- Have the patient collect all urine passed during the next 24 hours. The patient should post the times of urine collection in a prominent place to prevent accidental disposal of a specimen before the 24-hour period has ended.
- Note that it is not necessary to measure each urine specimen.
✕ Remind the patient to void before defecating so that the urine is not contaminated by feces.
✕ Instruct the patient not to put toilet paper in the collection container.
✕ Encourage the patient to drink fluids during the 24 hours unless this is contraindicated for medical purposes.
✕ Instruct the patient to void as close as possible to the end of the 24-hour period and to add this specimen to the collection.

After
- On the laboratory slip, note the start and end times of the urine collection. Send the specimen to the laboratory promptly.
- Apply pressure to the venipuncture site.

TEST RESULTS AND CLINICAL SIGNIFICANCE

▲ Increased Urine Level

Renal tubule disease,

Drug-induced renal toxicity,

Heavy metal induced renal disease: *These diseases affect the ability of the renal tubule to reabsorb β_2M.*

Lymphomas, leukemia, myeloma,

Acquired immune deficiency syndrome (AIDS): *These diseases are associated with increased production and destruction of lymphocytes or other marrow cells. Increased levels in the blood cause increased renal excretion that overcomes the renal tubule's ability to reabsorb β_2M.*

▲ Increased Serum Level

Lymphomas, leukemia, myeloma,

Glomerular renal disease: *These diseases are associated with increased production and destruction of lymphocytes or other marrow cells.*

Renal transplant rejection: *Because excretion of β_2M is renal, renal transplant rejection reduces excretion, and blood levels of β_2M increase.*

Viral infections (especially HIV and cytomegalovirus),

Chronic inflammatory processes: *The pathophysiologic mechanisms of these processes are not well known. β_2M may act as an acute-phase reactant.*

Bilirubin

NORMAL FINDINGS

Blood

Adult/older adult/child:

    Total bilirubin: **3–22 *Mc*mol/L** (0.2–1.3 mg/dL)

    Indirect bilirubin: **3.4–12.0 *Mc*mol/L** (0.2–0.8 mg/dL)

    Direct bilirubin: **1.7–5.1 *Mc*mol/L** (0.1–0.3 mg/dL)

Newborn total bilirubin: **1.7–180 *Mc*mol/L** (0.1–10.5 mg/dL)

Urine: Negative (**0–0.34 *Mc*mol/L** [0–0.02 mg/dL])

 Critical Values

Adult: **>257 *Mc*mol/L** (>12 mg/dL)

Newborn: **>222 *Mc*mol/L** (>15 mg/dL; immediate treatment required to avoid kernicterus)

INDICATIONS

This test is used to evaluate liver function. It is a part of the evaluation of adult patients with hemolytic anemias and of newborns with jaundice.

TEST EXPLANATION

Bile, which is formed in the liver, has many constituents, including bile salts, phospholipids, cholesterol, bicarbonate, water, and bilirubin. Bilirubin metabolism begins with the breakdown of red

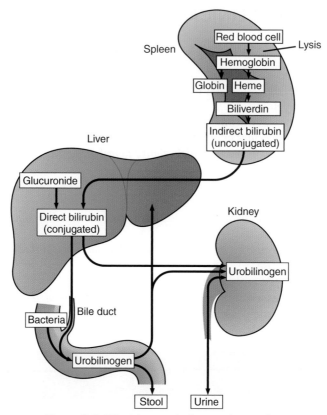

Figure 2-8 Bilirubin metabolism and excretion.

blood cells (RBCs) in the reticuloendothelial system (mostly the spleen; Figure 2-8). Hemoglobin is released from RBCs and broken down to heme and globin molecules. Heme is then catabolized to form biliverdin, which is transformed to bilirubin. This form of bilirubin is called *unconjugated (indirect) bilirubin*. In the liver, indirect bilirubin is conjugated with a glucuronide molecule, which results in conjugated (direct) bilirubin. The conjugated bilirubin is then excreted from the liver cells and into the intrahepatic canaliculi, which eventually lead to the hepatic ducts, the common bile duct, and the bowel.

Jaundice is the discoloration of body tissues caused by abnormally high blood levels of bilirubin. This yellow discoloration is recognized when the total serum bilirubin level exceeds 43 Mcmol/L (2.5 mg/dL). Jaundice results from a defect in the normal metabolism or excretion of bilirubin. This defect can occur at any stage of heme catabolism.

Physiologic jaundice of the newborn occurs if the newborn's liver is immature and does not have enough conjugating enzymes. This results in a high circulating blood level of unconjugated bilirubin, which can pass through the blood-brain barrier and become deposited in the brain cells of the newborn, causing encephalopathy (kernicterus). In newborns, if bilirubin levels are >222 Mcmol/L (15 mg/dL), immediate treatment is necessary to avoid developmental delay. This treatment may include exchange transfusions. High levels of bilirubin in the newborn are often treated with ultraviolet light therapy.

If the defect in bilirubin metabolism occurs after addition of glucuronide, conjugated (direct) hyperbilirubinemia results. Obstruction of the bile duct by a gallstone is the classical example of how obstructed bilirubin excretion causes direct hyperbilirubinemia.

Once the jaundice is recognized either clinically or chemically, it is important in therapy to differentiate whether it is predominantly caused by indirect (unconjugated) or direct (conjugated) bilirubin. This in turn helps elucidate the cause of the defect. In general, jaundice caused by hepatocellular dysfunction (e.g., hepatitis) results in elevated levels of indirect bilirubin. This dysfunction usually cannot be repaired surgically. In contrast, jaundice resulting from extrahepatic dysfunction (e.g., gallstones, tumour blockage of the bile ducts) results in elevated levels of direct bilirubin; this type of jaundice usually can be resolved by open surgery or endoscopic surgery.

The total serum bilirubin level is the sum of the conjugated (direct) and unconjugated (indirect) bilirubin levels. These are separated out when "fractionation" or "differentiation" of the total bilirubin to its direct and indirect parts is requested from the laboratory (Figure 2-9). Normally the indirect (unconjugated) bilirubin makes up 70% to 85% of the total bilirubin. In patients with jaundice, when more than 50% of the bilirubin is direct (conjugated), it is considered hyperbilirubinemia caused directly by gallstones, tumour, inflammation, scarring, or obstruction of the extrahepatic ducts. Indirect hyperbilirubinemia is diagnosed when less than 15% to 20% of the total bilirubin is direct bilirubin. Diseases that typically cause this form of jaundice include accelerated erythrocyte (RBC) hemolysis, hepatitis, and drug reactions.

Delta bilirubin is a form of bilirubin that is covalently bound to albumin. It has a longer half-life than the other forms of bilirubin; therefore, its level remains elevated during the convalescent phases of hepatic disorders, when the conjugated bilirubin has typically returned to normal. It can be derived by the following calculation:

$$\text{Delta bilirubin} = \text{Total bilirubin} - (\text{Direct bilirubin} + \text{Indirect bilirubin})$$

When the defect in bilirubin metabolism occurs after conjugation, elevated levels of direct (conjugated) bilirubin occur. In contrast to the unconjugated form, direct bilirubin is water soluble

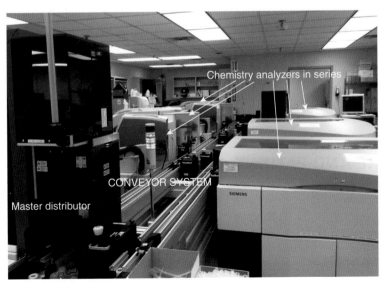

Figure 2-9 Siemens multiple-channel chemistry analyzer. This is one of six chemical analyzer machines that are assembled in series and in which specimens are directed by a computerized master distributor.

and can be excreted into the urine. Therefore, the presence of bilirubin in urine is suggestive of disease affecting bilirubin metabolism after conjugation or defects in excretion (e.g., gallstones). Normally, there may be a small amount of bilirubin in the urine. Testing for bilirubin in the urine is a part of routine urine analysis that can help to distinguish between normal and abnormal amounts of bilirubin in the urine.

Age-Related Concerns

- The physiologic changes of aging can increase a patient's risk for developing hyperbilirubinemia. For example, if hepatic uptake is decreased as a result of an obstruction of the extrahepatic ducts, hyperbilirubinemia can result. Adult patients who experience right-sided heart failure are also at high risk for hyperbilirubinemia caused by decreased perfusion of the kidneys. The nephrotoxicity associated with alcohol hepatitis, infection, use of oral contraceptives, and sepsis can also increase risk for hyperbilirubinemia in older adults.

INTERFERING FACTORS

- Blood hemolysis and lipemia can produce erroneous measurements.
- Drugs that may cause *increases* in blood levels of total bilirubin include allopurinol, anabolic steroids, antibiotics, antimalarials, ascorbic acid, azathioprine, chlorpropamide (Diabinese), cholinergics, codeine, dextran, diuretics, epinephrine, meperidine, methotrexate, methyldopa, monoamine oxidase inhibitors, morphine, nicotinic acid (high doses), oral contraceptives, phenothiazines, quinidine, rifampin, salicylates, steroids, sulphonamides, theophylline, and vitamin A.
- Drugs that may cause *increases* in urine bilirubin levels include allopurinol, antibiotics, barbiturates, chlorpromazine, diuretics, oral contraceptives, phenazopyridine (Pyridium), steroids, and sulphonamides.
- Drugs that may cause *decreases* in blood levels of total bilirubin include barbiturates, caffeine, penicillin, and salicylates (high doses).
- Drugs that may cause *false-negative* results in tests of urine levels include ascorbic acid (vitamin C) and indomethacin (Indocid).
- Substances that may cause *false-positive* results in tests of urine levels include phenazopyridine (Pyridium)–like drugs and urochromes. These substances can colour the urine yellow or orange and foil the colour analysis tests. Bilirubin is not stable in urine, especially when exposed to light.

PROCEDURE AND PATIENT CARE

Before

- Explain the procedure to the patient.
- Note that fasting requirements vary among different laboratories. Some require keeping the patient on NPO status (nothing by mouth), except for water, after midnight the day of the test.

During

Blood

- Collect a venous blood sample in a red-top tube.
- Use a heel puncture for blood collection in infants.
- Prevent hemolysis of blood during phlebotomy.

- Do not shake the tube, because test results may be rendered inaccurate.
- Protect the blood sample from bright light. Prolonged exposure (over 1 hour) to sunlight or artificial light can reduce bilirubin content.

Urine
- Note that this is a spot urine test.
- Collect at least 10 mL of urine for quick, simple testing.
- Use reagent strips (e.g., Multistix) or tablets (e.g., Icotest) for quick, simple testing.

Urine Testing With Multistix Reagent Strips
- Note that this is a firm, plastic strip with seven separate areas for testing pH, protein, glucose, ketones, bilirubin, blood, and urobilinogen.
- For testing bilirubin, obtain a fresh urine specimen and examine it as soon as possible.
- Immerse the dipstick in the well-mixed urine and then remove it immediately to avoid dissolving other reagents.
- Tap the dipstick against the rim of the urine container to remove excess urine.
- Hold the strip horizontally and compare it with the colour chart on the label of the bottle in the designated time period.

Urine Testing With Icotest Tablets
- Place 5 drops of urine on the special test mat.
- Add 2 drops of water. The bilirubin test result is positive if the mat turns blue or purple within the designated time period.
- Note that this test is considered more sensitive than reagent strips for detecting bilirubin.

After
Blood
- Apply pressure or a pressure dressing to the venipuncture site.
- Assess the venipuncture site for bleeding. Patients with jaundice may have prolonged clotting times.

Urine
- Do not reuse reagent strips or Icotest tablets.
- Whether you use strips or tablets or send the urine to the laboratory, note medications that the patient is taking that may affect test results.

TEST RESULTS AND CLINICAL SIGNIFICANCE
▲ Increased Blood Levels of Conjugated (Direct) Bilirubin
Gallstones,

Extrahepatic duct obstruction (tumour, inflammation, gallstone, scarring, surgical trauma): *These diseases cause a blockage of the bile ducts. Bile, which contains bilirubin, cannot be excreted. Blood levels of bilirubin rise.*

Extensive liver metastasis: *The intrahepatic ducts or hepatic ducts become obstructed because of tumour. Bile, which contains bilirubin, cannot be excreted. Blood levels of bilirubin rise.*

Cholestasis from drugs: *Some drugs inhibit the excretion of bile from the hepatocyte into the bile canaliculi. Bile, which contains bilirubin, cannot be excreted. Blood levels of bilirubin rise.*

Dubin-Johnson syndrome,

Rotor syndrome: *Congenital defects in enzyme quantity inhibit metabolism and excretion of bilirubin. Blood levels of bilirubin rise.*

▲ Increased Blood Levels of Unconjugated (Indirect) Bilirubin

Erythroblastosis fetalis,

Transfusion reaction,

Sickle cell anemia,

Hemolytic jaundice,

Hemolytic anemia,

Pernicious anemia,

Large-volume blood transfusion,

Resolution of large hematoma: *RBC destruction occurs. Large amounts of heme are available for catabolism into bilirubin. This quantity exceeds the liver's capability to conjugate bilirubin. Indirect (unconjugated) bilirubin levels rise.*

Hepatitis,

Cirrhosis,

Sepsis,

Neonatal hyperbilirubinemia: *The diseased, injured, or immature liver cannot conjugate the bilirubin presented to it. Indirect (unconjugated) bilirubin levels rise.*

Crigler-Najjar syndrome,

Gilbert syndrome: *Congenital enzyme deficiencies interrupt conjugation of bilirubin. Indirect (unconjugated) bilirubin levels rise.*

▲ Increased Urine Levels of Bilirubin

Gallstones,

Extrahepatic duct obstruction (tumour, inflammation, gallstone, scarring, surgical trauma),

Extensive liver metastasis,

Cholestasis from drugs,

Dubin-Johnson syndrome,

Rotor syndrome: *Defects in bilirubin metabolism and excretion, as discussed earlier, inhibit intestinal excretion of bilirubin. The diseases just listed are associated with direct (conjugated) hyperbilirubinemia. The conjugated bilirubin is water soluble and is excreted, in a small part, in the urine.*

RELATED TESTS

Alkaline Phosphatase (p. 53), Lactate Dehydrogenase (p. 339), Aspartate Aminotransferase (p. 130), Alanine Aminotransferase (p. 45), 5'-Nucleotidase (p. 389), and other liver enzymes. These tests are very helpful in the evaluation of the liver.

Complete Blood Cell Count and Differential Count (p. 187), Haptoglobin (p. 289), and other blood tests. These tests are helpful in the evaluation of hemolytic anemias.

Blood Typing

NORMAL FINDINGS

Compatibility

INDICATIONS

This test is used to determine the blood type of a patient before the patient donates or receives blood and to determine the blood type of expectant mothers in order to assess the risks of Rh incompatibility between mother and fetus.

TEST EXPLANATION

With blood typing, ABO and Rh antigens can be detected in the blood of prospective blood donors and potential blood recipients. This test is also used to determine the blood type of expectant mothers and fetuses. The ABO system, Rh factors, and blood crossmatching are reviewed.

ABO System

Human blood is grouped according to the presence or absence of these antigens. The two major antigens, A and B, form the basis of the ABO system. The surface membranes of group A red blood cells (RBCs) contain A antigens; group B RBCs contain B antigens on their surface; group AB RBCs have both A and B antigens; and group O RBCs have neither A nor B antigens (Table 2-12). In general, a person does not have antibodies to match the surface antigen on his or her own RBCs. That is, individuals with group A antigen (type A) blood do not have anti-A antibodies; however, they do have anti-B antibodies. Similarly, individuals with group B antigens do not have anti-B antibodies but do have anti-A antibodies. People with group O blood have both anti-A and anti-B antibodies (Figure 2-10). These antibodies against A and B blood group antigens are formed in the first 3 months of life as a result of exposure to similar antigens on the surface of naturally occurring bacteria in the intestine.

Blood transfusions are actually transplantations of tissue (blood) from one person to another. It is important that the recipient not have antibodies to the donor's RBCs. If this were to occur, there could be a hypersensitivity reaction, which can vary from mild fever to anaphylaxis with severe intravascular hemolysis. If donor ABO antibodies are present against the recipient's antigens, reactions usually are only minimal unless the recipient is immunocompromised.

TABLE 2-12	Blood Typing		
Blood Type (ABO, Rh)	**Antigens Present**	**Antibodies Possibly Present**	**Percentage of General Population**
O, +	Rh	A, B	35
O, −*	None	A, B, Rh	7
A, +	A, Rh	B	35
A, −	A	B, Rh	7
B, +	B, Rh	A	8
B, −	B	A, Rh	2
AB, +†	A, B, Rh	None	4
AB, −	A, B	Rh	2

*Universal donor.
†Universal recipient.

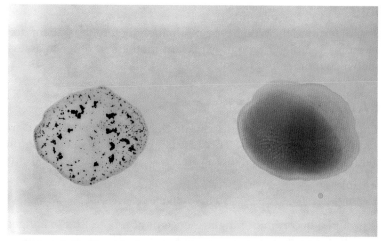

Figure 2-10 Blood typing: agglutination testing on the blood of a person with type A blood. An antigen that is present on the red blood cell combines with anti-A antibody that has been added to a drop of the patient's blood *(left)*. Agglutination (clumping) occurs because of the antigen/antibody complex that is formed. No agglutination is noted when anti-B antibody is added to a drop of the patient's blood *(right)* because patients with type A blood do not have any B antigens.

Individuals with group O blood are considered universal donors because their RBCs do not have antigens. Those with group AB blood are considered universal recipients because they have no antibodies to react to the transfused blood. Group O blood is often transfused in emergency situations in which rapid life-threatening blood loss occurs and immediate transfusion is required. There is no time for crossmatching (~20 minutes). The chance of a transfusion reaction is lowest with type O.

Rh Factors

The presence or absence of Rh antigens on the surface of RBCs determines the classification of Rh positive or Rh negative. Rh factor is the next most important antigen associated with a blood transfusion after ABO compatibility. The major Rh factor is Rho(D). There are several minor Rh factors. If Rho(D) is absent, testing is performed for the minor Rh antigens. If the Rh antigens are not present, the patient is considered Rh negative (Rh−). The incidence of each blood type is noted in Table 2-12.

Rh− individuals may develop antibodies to Rh antigens if exposed to Rh positive (Rh+) blood by prior transfusions or fetal-maternal blood mixing. All women who are pregnant should undergo blood typing and Rh factor determination. If the mother's blood is Rh−, the father's blood should also be typed. If his blood is Rh+, the woman's blood should be examined for the presence of Rh antibodies (by the indirect Coombs test). If the initial screening yields negative results (no antibodies to Rh found), the test is repeated at 28 to 32 weeks and at 36 weeks of pregnancy. If these test results are also negative, the fetus is not at risk. However, if the test result is positive, the fetus is at risk for hemolytic disease of the newborn (erythroblastosis fetalis). This disease results when the mother is Rh− and the fetus is Rh+. Any fetal bleeding that occurs can sensitize the mother to form anti-Rh antibodies. These antibodies cross the placenta and hemolyze the fetal RBCs. Problems ranging from mild fetal anemia to in utero fetal death could occur. The severity of the hemolytic anemia can be evaluated by determining the quantity of bilirubin in the amniotic fluid (Amniocentesis, p. 660).

Rh typing of the mother during pregnancy can prevent hemolytic disease of the newborn. If the mother is Rh−, she should be advised that she is a candidate for Rh immunoglobulin that "neutralizes" the Rh antigen after the delivery. Rh immunoglobulin can reduce the chance of fetal hemolytic problems during subsequent pregnancies.

Blood Crossmatching

Although typing for the major ABO and Rh antigens is no guarantee that a reaction will not occur, it does greatly reduce the possibility of such a reaction. Many potential minor antigens are not routinely detected during blood typing. If allowed to go unrecognized, these minor antigens also can initiate a blood transfusion reaction. Therefore, blood is not only typed but also crossmatched to identify a mismatch of blood caused by minor antigens. In crossmatching, the recipient's serum is mixed with the donor's RBCs in saline solution, and then Coombs serum is added (indirect Coombs test). Only blood products containing RBCs need to be crossmatched. Plasma products do not need to be crossmatched but should be ABO compatible because other cells (white blood cells [WBCs] and platelets) have ABO antigens (Figure 2-11).

Homologous (donor and recipient are different people) and directed (recipient chooses the donor) blood for donation must be rigorously tested before transfusion (Box 2-3). Autologous (recipient and donor are the same person) blood for transfusions, however, is not subject to that same testing. However, autologous blood transfusion is not 100% safe. As a result of the additives used for banking purposes, blood and hypersensitivity reactions can still occur.

An additional complication of blood typing is graft-versus-host disease, in which donor lymphocytes included in the blood transfusion may engraft and multiply in the recipient. These lymphocytes can react against the recipient's tissues. This is most common among immunocompromised patients. Pretransfusion radiation of the unit of blood to be transfused will prevent this problem.

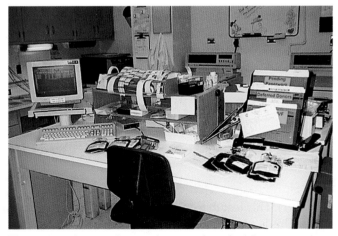

Figure 2-11 Immunohematology section of a laboratory, where units of blood are processed and labelled.

BOX 2-3	Blood Tests Required on Donated Blood

- ABO / Rh typing
- Red Blood Cell Antibody Screen
- Infectious disease testing:
  - HIV serology
  - HTLV
  - Hepatitis virus studies
  - Syphilis
  - West Nile Virus
  - ♣ Chagas Disease (if indicated)

HIV, human immunodeficiency virus; *HTLV,* human T-lymphotropic virus.

INTERFERING FACTORS

- Non-ABO or non-Rh (D) minor antibodies can interfere with obtaining an adequate crossmatch.

PROCEDURE AND PATIENT CARE

Before
🗶 Explain the procedure to the patient.
🗶 Inform the patient that no fasting is required.

During
- Collect a venous blood sample in a red-top tube. (Tube top colour may vary among laboratories.)
- Avoid hemolysis.
- Label the blood tube appropriately before sending it to the laboratory.

After
- Apply pressure or a pressure dressing to the venipuncture site.
- Assess the venipuncture site for bleeding.

TEST RESULTS AND CLINICAL SIGNIFICANCE

ABO type
Rh type
Crossmatch compatibility

RELATED TESTS

Coombs Test, Indirect (p. 191). This test detects circulating antibodies against RBCs.

Amniocentesis (p. 660). This is a test of amniotic fluid, which may demonstrate some evidence of hemolytic disease of the newborn.

CA 19-9 Tumour Marker (Cancer Antigen 19-9)

Blood Studies

2

NORMAL FINDINGS

<37 kU/L (<37 U/mL)

INDICATIONS

CA 19-9 antigen is a tumour marker used for the diagnosis of pancreatic or hepatobiliary cancer, evaluation of response to treatment, and surveillance.

TEST EXPLANATION

CA 19-9 is a carbohydrate cell-surface antigen. It exists on the surface of some cancer cells. Although initially thought to be specific for colorectal cancer, it is now measured primarily in the evaluation of patients with pancreatic or hepatobiliary cancers. In the diagnosis of pancreatic carcinoma, for example, the presence of a pancreatic mass or biliary obstruction and greatly elevated CA 19-9 levels would support the diagnosis of pancreatic cancer over benign pancreatitis. Hepatobiliary cancer is suspected in patients whose presenting symptoms are ascites, jaundice, and elevated CA 19-9 levels. CA 19-9 levels may not be elevated in all patients with pancreatic carcinoma. Approximately 70% of patients with pancreatic carcinoma and 65% of patients with hepatobiliary cancer have elevated levels.

CA 19-9 levels are used in the posttreatment surveillance of patients who have had pancreatic or hepatobiliary cancers. In the few patients with pancreatic or biliary cancer who have a good response to surgery, chemotherapy, or radiation therapy, a decline in serum levels of CA 19-9 confirms this response. A rapid rise in CA 19-9 levels may be associated with recurrent or progressive tumour growth. Mildly elevated levels may exist in patients with gastric cancer, colorectal cancer, hepatoma, and even 6% to 7% of patients with nongastrointestinal malignancies. Levels of CA 19-9 can also be minimally elevated in patients who have pancreatitis, gallstones, cirrhosis, inflammatory bowel disease, or cystic fibrosis.

Because of its lack of sensitivity and specificity, the CA 19-9 test is not effective in screening for pancreatobiliary tumours in the general population.

Clinical Priorities

- CA 19-9 testing is not used as a screening tool for pancreatic or hepatobiliary tumours because of its lack of sensitivity and specificity.
- CA 19-9 testing is used to support the diagnosis of pancreatic or hepatobiliary tumours and to monitor patients' response to treatment.

PROCEDURE AND PATIENT CARE

Before

✗ Explain the procedure to the patient.
✗ Inform the patient that no fasting is required.

During

- Collect a venous blood sample in a red-top tube.
- The blood may be sent to a central diagnostic laboratory for CA 19-9 determinations. The results may not be available for 7 to 10 days.

After

- Apply pressure or a pressure dressing to the venipuncture site.
- Observe the venipuncture site for bleeding.

TEST RESULTS AND CLINICAL SIGNIFICANCE

▲ Increased Levels

Pancreatic carcinoma,
Cholecystitis,
Colorectal cancer,
Hepatobiliary carcinoma,
Cirrhosis,
Gallstones,
Pancreatitis,
Gastric cancer,
Lung cancer,
Inflammatory bowel disease,
Rheumatoid diseases: *CA 19-9 antigen is released from the surface of the cancer cell and leaks into the bloodstream, where it can be detected.*

RELATED TEST

Carcinoembryonic Antigen (p. 159). This is another tumour marker whose levels are elevated in patients with pancreatobiliary cancer.

CA 15-3 and CA 27-29 Tumour Marker
(Cancer Antigen 15-3, Cancer Antigen 27-29)

NORMAL FINDINGS

CA 15-3: <31 kU/L (<31 U/mL)
CA 27-29: <38 kU/L (<38 U/mL)

INDICATIONS

The CA 15-3 and CA 27-29 antigens are tumour-associated serum markers that are measured for breast cancer monitoring.

TEST EXPLANATION

Testing of carcinoembryonic antigen (CEA), the most widely used tumour marker, is limited by poor sensitivity and specificity for patients with breast cancer. Monoclonal antibody technology has enabled the development of tests for CA 15-3 and CA 27-29 antigens. These antigens are not as sensitive for the diagnosis of primary breast cancer as other tumour markers are for their respective tumours; that is, CA 15-3 and CA 27-29 levels are high in only 50% of patients who have a localized breast cancer or a small tumour burden. However, 80% of patients with metastatic breast cancer do have elevated CA 15-3 levels, and 65% have elevated CA 27-29 levels; therefore, the usefulness of these antigen tests as a screening technique in early breast cancers (the most common cancer of women) is quite limited.

Benign breast disease and nonbreast malignancies (e.g., of the lung, pancreas, ovary, or prostate) also can cause elevation of these antigen levels. Measurement of these antigens is useful in monitoring the patient's response to therapy of metastatic breast cancer. A partial or complete response to treatment is confirmed by declining levels. Likewise, a persistent rise in these antigen levels despite therapy is strongly suggestive of progressive disease.

CA 15-3 and CA 27-29 have a high sensitivity but a somewhat lower specificity. Many diseases, both benign and malignant, can cause elevations in these values. Therefore, their measurements cannot be used to diagnose recurrence. However, in the patient who has symptoms, signs, or other test results that indicate recurrence, an elevation in one of these tumour markers would corroborate the diagnosis of recurrent breast cancer. These tumour markers are better suited for indicating response of metastatic disease to treatment (when already elevated). CA 15-3 was the first breast tumour marker available for measurement. The test is usually performed by a reference laboratory with competitive inhibition radioimmune assay. The CA 27-29 marker is tested by immunoradiometric assay.

INTERFERING FACTORS

- Some of the other benign and malignant diseases associated with elevations in levels of these antigens include cancer of the lung, ovary, pancreas, prostate, and colon; fibrocystic disease of the breast; cirrhosis; and hepatitis.

Clinical Priorities

- CA 15-3 and 27-29 tumour markers are not used for screening of early breast cancers.
- These tumour antigens are measured to monitor the patient's response to therapy for metastatic breast cancer. Declining levels suggest that the response to therapy is good; rising levels are suggestive of disease progression.

PROCEDURE AND PATIENT CARE

Before
- Explain the procedure to the patient.
- Inform the patient that no fasting is required.

During
- Collect a venous blood sample in a red-top tube.
- The blood sample may be sent to a central diagnostic laboratory for determinations. The results may not be available for 7 to 10 days.

After
- Apply pressure or a pressure dressing to the venipuncture site.
- Observe the venipuncture site for bleeding.

TEST RESULTS AND CLINICAL SIGNIFICANCE

▲ Increased Levels

Metastatic breast cancer: *Breast cancer antigens on the surface of the breast cancer cell leak into the bloodstream, where they can be detected.*

RELATED TEST

Carcinoembryonic Antigen (p. 159). This is another tumour marker used in the monitoring of breast cancer.

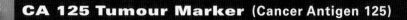

CA 125 Tumour Marker (Cancer Antigen 125)

NORMAL FINDINGS

< 35 kU/L (< 35 U/mL)

INDICATIONS

Measurements of CA 125 are used in the detection of ovarian cancer. They are also used to determine the extent of disease and to monitor the response to treatment.

TEST EXPLANATION

This tumour marker has a high degree of sensitivity and specificity for ovarian cancer. Just as alpha-fetoprotein and human chorionic gonadotropin are accurate tumour markers for germ cell tumours of the ovary, CA 125 is an extremely accurate marker for nonmucinous epithelial tumours of the ovary. CA 125 levels are elevated in more than 80% of women with ovarian cancer.

The CA 125 marker can be used in many ways. By itself, it cannot be used to diagnose ovarian cancer, but it helps support the diagnosis of ovarian cancer. For example, a greatly elevated CA 125 level in women who have abdominal distension, ascites, and a palpable pelvic mass is strong confirmation that the underlying cause is an epithelial ovarian malignancy.

The CA 125 serum tumour marker is also used to determine a patient's response to therapy. In patients responding to treatment comparative serial testing reveals a progressive decline in CA 125 levels. Also, CA 125 tumour markers can help predict whether a second-look (repeat) diagnostic laparotomy will yield positive results. A second-look laparotomy will detect a residual tumour in 97% of patients whose CA 125 level is higher than 3535 kU/L (3535 U/mL), whereas only 56% of patients with ovarian cancer whose CA 125 level is greater than 3535 kU/L (3535 U/mL) will have positive findings on second-look laparotomy. A precipitous fall in CA 125 after two courses of chemotherapy is an accurate predictor of a complete response to chemotherapy and is interpreted as a good prognostic sign.

Finally, CA 125 determinations can be used in posttreatment surveillance of patients with ovarian cancer. Among patients who have had a complete response to radiation therapy, chemotherapy, or surgery, a delayed rise in the CA 125 level is an early predictor of a recurrent tumour in 93%. Abnormal levels can antedate the appearance of obvious recurrent ovarian cancer by 2 to 7 months.

CA 125 is not an effective screening test for the asymptomatic general public because of its lack of specificity. It is used in women at high risk: that is, women who have a strong family history of ovarian cancer or have a breast cancer antigen (*BRCA*) genetic defect (breast cancer genomics, p. 1131). In the general population, elevated levels indicate that either benign or malignant disease is present in 95% of cases.

Elevations in CA 125 levels can be caused by other tumours and benign processes; by diseases that affect the peritoneum, such as cirrhosis, pancreatitis, peritonitis, endometriosis, and pelvic inflammatory disease; and by other malignancies that occur in the female genital tract, pancreas, colon, lung, and breast. In total, 1% to 2% of the normal population have CA 125 levels in excess of 3 535 kU/L (3 535 U/mL).

INTERFERING FACTORS

- The first trimester of pregnancy and normal menstruation may be associated with mild elevations of CA 125 levels.
- Patients with benign peritoneal diseases (e.g., cirrhosis, endometriosis) have mildly increased levels.
- Smoking can artificially increase CA 125 levels.
- Patients who have had recent abdominal surgery may have elevated CA 125 levels for as long as 3 weeks after surgery.

PROCEDURE AND PATIENT CARE

Before

- Explain the procedure to the patient.
- Inform the patient that no fasting or sedation is required.

Clinical Priorities

- CA 125 is measured to detect ovarian cancer and to determine its extent and the patient's response to treatment.
- CA 125 measurement is not an effective screening test for asymptomatic women because of its lack of specificity. It is used in women with a strong history of ovarian cancer.
- CA 125 levels can be assessed to determine the need for a second-look (repeat) diagnostic laparotomy in women being monitored after ovarian cancer therapy.

During

- Collect a venous of blood sample in a red-top tube.
- The blood may be sent to a central diagnostic laboratory for determination of CA 125 level.
- The results are available to the local hospital in 3 to 7 days.

After

- Apply pressure or a pressure dressing to the venipuncture site.
- Observe the venipuncture site for bleeding.
- Provide emotional support to the patient. Cancer testing is very stressful.

TEST RESULTS AND CLINICAL SIGNIFICANCE

▲ Increased Levels

Malignant Disorders
Cancer of the ovary,
Cancer of the pancreas,

Cancer of the colon,

Cancer of the lung,

Peritoneal carcinomatosis,

Cancer of the nonovarian female genital tract,

Cancer of the breast,

Lymphoma: *The CA 125 antigen from the surface ovarian cancer cells leaks into the blood, where it can be detected.*

Benign Disorders

Cirrhosis,

Peritonitis,

Pregnancy,

Endometriosis,

Pancreatitis,

Pelvic inflammatory disease: *The mechanism of elevated CA 125 in these diseases is not known.*

RELATED TESTS

Carcinoembryonic Antigen (p. 159). Levels of this tumour marker can be elevated in ovarian epithelial tumours.

Alpha-Fetoprotein (p. 60). Levels of this tumour marker are elevated in nonepithelial ovarian tumours.

Human Chorionic Gonadotropin (p. 426). Levels of this tumour marker are elevated in nonepithelial ovarian tumours.

Calcitonin (Human Calcitonin, Thyrocalcitonin)

NORMAL FINDINGS

Basal (Plasma)

Male: ≤19 ng/L (≤19 pg/mL)

Female: ≤14 ng/L (≤14 pg/mL)

Calcium Infusion (2.4 mg/kg)

Male: ≤190 ng/L (≤190 pg/mL)

Female: ≤130 ng/L (≤130 pg/mL)

Pentagastrin Injection (0.5 *Mcg*/kg)

Male: ≤110 ng/L (≤110 pg/mL)

Female: ≤30 ng/L (≤30 pg/mL)

INDICATIONS

This test is usually indicated to evaluate individuals with suspected medullary carcinoma of the thyroid. Calcitonin is useful in monitoring response to therapy and predicting recurrences of medullary thyroid cancer. It is also useful as a screening test for patients with a family history of medullary cancer.

TEST EXPLANATION

Calcitonin is a hormone secreted by the parafollicular or C cells of the thyroid gland. Secretion is stimulated by elevated serum calcium levels. Calcitonin contributes to calcium homeostasis. It decreases serum calcium levels by inhibiting bone resorption and increasing calcium excretion by the kidneys.

This test is usually used in the evaluation of patients who have confirmed or suspected medullary carcinoma of the thyroid. Of these patients, 75% have hypersecretion of calcitonin despite normal serum calcium levels. Calcitonin is useful in monitoring response to therapy and predicting recurrences of medullary thyroid cancer. It is also useful as a screening test for patients who have a family history of medullary cancer and are therefore at high risk (20%) for medullary cancer. This is a cancer of the thyroid with a familial tendency, and if it is found late, the prognosis is poor.

This cancer is often associated with multiple endocrine neoplasia syndromes. Routine screening for elevated calcitonin levels can detect medullary cancer early and improve chances for cure. Calcitonin can be used as a tumour marker in monitoring patients with medullary cancer of the thyroid. Increases in calcitonin levels herald progression of the cancer. Declining levels indicate tumour regression. C-cell hyperplasia, a benign calcitonin-producing disease that also has a familial tendency, is also associated with elevated calcitonin levels.

Equivocal elevations in calcitonin levels should be monitored with further provocative testing with the use of pentagastrin or calcium to stimulate calcitonin secretion. *Pentagastrin stimulation* involves an intravenous infusion with blood samples collected before the injection and at 90 seconds, 2 minutes, and 5 minutes after the infusion. The *calcium infusion* test can be performed in a variety of ways, but the most common is to collect blood to establish baseline and then to measure 5- and 10-minute postinfusion blood levels. With medullary cancer of the thyroid, the provocative tests can cause the calcitonin level to rise significantly.

Levels of calcitonin also may be elevated in people with cancer of the lung, breast, and pancreas. This is probably a form of paraneoplastic syndrome in which calcitonin is produced ectopically by the nonthyroid cancer cells.

INTERFERING FACTORS

- Calcitonin levels are often elevated in normal pregnant women and in newborns.
- Drugs that may cause *increases* in calcitonin levels include calcium, cholecystokinin, epinephrine, glucagon, pentagastrin, and oral contraceptives.

PROCEDURE AND PATIENT CARE

Before

- Explain the procedure to the patient.
- Inform the patient that an overnight fast is required. Water is permitted during the fast.

During

- Collect a venous blood sample in a heparinized green-top tube or a chilled red-top tube according to the laboratory's protocol.
- The specimen should be placed immediately in a container of crushed ice and water. The blood may be frozen and sent to a reference laboratory.

After

- Apply pressure or a pressure dressing to the venipuncture site.
- Assess the venipuncture site for bleeding.
- Inform the patient that results may not be available for several days if this specimen is sent to a reference laboratory for analysis.

TEST RESULTS AND CLINICAL SIGNIFICANCE

▲ Increased Levels

Medullary carcinoma of the thyroid,

C-cell hyperplasia: *Calcitonin is secreted by the thyroid in these diseases, despite the calcium blood levels. These abnormalities are not responsive to the normal regulatory feedback mechanisms.*

Oat cell carcinoma of lung,

Breast carcinoma,

Pancreatic cancer: *These cancers can act as autonomous ectopic sites of calcitonin production.*

Primary hyperparathyroidism,

Secondary hyperparathyroidism as a result of chronic renal failure: *These states are associated with high serum calcium levels. High calcitonin levels may be compensatory.*

Pernicious anemia,

Zollinger-Ellison syndrome: *Several familial and nonfamilial multiple endocrinopathies (apudoma) may be associated with high calcitonin levels.*

Alcoholic cirrhosis: *The mechanism is not well defined. The liver may be unable to metabolize hormones well, and high levels of calcitonin result.*

Thyroiditis

RELATED TEST

Calcium, Blood (see following test). This is a direct measurement of the serum calcium level.

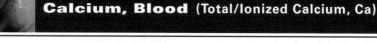

Calcium, Blood (Total/Ionized Calcium, Ca)

NORMAL FINDINGS

Age	mmol/L	(mg/dL)
Total Calcium		
<10 days	1.9–2.60	(7.6–10.4)
Umbilical	2.25–2.88	(9.0–11.5)
10 days to 2 years	2.3–2.65	(9.0–10.6)
Child	2.2–2.7	(8.8–10.8)
Adult*	2.10–2.50	(8.4–10.6)
Ionized Calcium		
Newborn	1.05–1.37	(4.20–5.58)
2 months to 18 years	1.20–1.38	(4.80–5.52)
Adult	1.15–1.35	(4.6–5.1)

*Values tend to decrease in the older adult.

! Critical Values

Total calcium: < 1.65 mmol/L or >3.25 mmol/L (<6 or >13 mg/dL)
Ionized calcium: < 0.80 mmol/L or >1.58 mmol/L (<2.2 or >7 mg/dL)

INDICATIONS

The serum calcium test is used to evaluate parathyroid function and calcium metabolism by directly measuring the total amount of calcium in the blood. Serum calcium levels are used to monitor renal transplant recipients and patients with renal failure, hyperparathyroidism, and various malignancies. They are also used to monitor calcium levels during and after large-volume blood transfusions.

TEST EXPLANATION

Serum calcium is necessary in many metabolic enzymatic pathways. It is vital for muscle contractility, cardiac function, neural transmission, and blood clotting. The serum calcium test is used to evaluate parathyroid function and calcium metabolism by directly measuring the total amount of calcium in the blood. The bones and the teeth act as a reservoir for calcium. When blood levels decrease, parathyroid hormone (PTH) release is stimulated. This hormone acts on the reservoirs to release calcium into the blood. Approximately 50% of the total calcium exists in the blood in its free (ionized) form, and approximately 50% exists in its protein-bound form (mostly with albumin). The serum calcium level is a measure of both. As a result, when the serum albumin level is low (as in malnourished patients), the serum calcium level is also low, and when the serum albumin level is high, the serum calcium level is also high. As a rule, the total serum calcium level decreases by approximately 0.8 mg for every 1-g decrease in the serum albumin level. Serum albumin should be measured with serum calcium.

The ionized form of calcium also can be measured by ion-selective electrode techniques or can be calculated from several available formulas. An advantage of measuring the ionized form is that it is unaffected by changes in serum albumin levels. Many laboratories do not have the equipment to perform the ionized calcium assay. When albumin levels are variable, measurement of ionized calcium can allow more accurate calcium replacement therapy if needed. This is especially true during open heart surgery, major organ transplantation, and renal dialysis.

When the serum calcium level is elevated on at least three separate determinations, the patient is said to have hypercalcemia. Symptoms of hypercalcemia may include anorexia, nausea, vomiting, somnolence, and coma. The most common cause of hypercalcemia is hyperparathyroidism. PTH causes elevations in calcium levels by increasing gastrointestinal absorption, decreasing urinary excretion, and increasing bone resorption. Malignancy, the second most common cause of hypercalcemia, can cause elevations of calcium levels in two main ways. First, tumour metastasis (myeloma, lung, breast, renal cell) to the bone can destroy the bone, causing resorption and pushing calcium into the blood. Second, the cancer (lung, breast, renal cell) can produce a PTH-like substance that drives the serum calcium level up (ectopic PTH). Excess vitamin D ingestion can increase serum calcium by increasing renal and gastrointestinal absorption. Granulomatous infections such as sarcoidosis and tuberculosis are associated with hypercalcemia.

In some instances, a normal serum calcium level does not preclude hypercalcemia. For example, in a patient with a reduced serum albumin level, if the serum calcium level is normal (it, too, should be reduced in this situation), hypercalcemia should be suspected. A similar situation exists in patients with chronic renal failure. These patients have high phosphate levels and other anions that tend to chronically lower serum calcium. As a result, PTH is persistently stimulated to increase calcium levels. The calcium levels return to normal in time, but that "normal" level is actually "high" because it should be low in these patients. This is the classical case of secondary hyperparathyroidism.

Hypocalcemia occurs in patients with hypoalbuminemia. The most common causes of hypo-albuminemia are malnutrition (especially in alcoholic patients) and large-volume intravenous infusions. Half the calcium is bound to albumin; therefore, when the albumin level is low, the calcium level should be low. Large blood transfusions are associated with low serum calcium levels, because the citrate additives used in banked blood for anticoagulation bind the free calcium in the recipient's bloodstream. Intestinal malabsorption, renal failure, rhabdomyolysis, alkalosis, and acute pancreatitis (because of saponification of fat) are also known to be associated with low serum calcium levels. Hypomagnesemia can be associated with refractory hypocalcemia. Symptoms of hypocalcemia include nervousness, excitability, and tetany.

INTERFERING FACTORS

- Vitamin D intoxication may increase serum calcium levels.
- Excessive ingestion of milk may increase levels.
- Serum pH can affect calcium values. A decrease in pH increases calcium levels.
- Prolonged tourniquet application lowers pH and factitiously increases calcium levels.
- There is normally a small diurnal variation in calcium level; levels peak at approximately 9 PM.
- Hypoalbuminemia is associated with decreased levels of total calcium.
- Drugs that may cause *increases* in calcium levels include alkaline antacids, androgens, calcium salts, ergocalciferol, hydralazine, lithium, PTH, thiazide diuretics, thyroid hormone, and vitamin D.
- Drugs that may cause *decreases* in calcium levels include acetazolamide, albuterol, anticonvulsants, asparaginase, aspirin, calcitonin, cisplatin, corticosteroids, estrogens, heparin, laxatives, loop diuretics, magnesium salts, oral contraceptives, and thiazide diuretic.

PROCEDURE AND PATIENT CARE

Before
- Explain the procedure to the patient.
- Inform the patient that no fasting is required; however, the serum calcium measurement may be part of a multichemical analysis in which fasting is required for the other studies.

During
- Collect a venous blood sample in a red-top tube.
- Avoid prolonged tourniquet use.

After
- Apply pressure or a pressure dressing to the venipuncture site.
- Assess the venipuncture site for bleeding.

TEST RESULTS AND CLINICAL SIGNIFICANCE

▲ Increased Levels (Hypercalcemia)
Hyperparathyroidism,
Nonparathyroid PTH-producing tumour (e.g., lung or renal carcinoma): *PTH or a similar hormone mobilizes calcium stores from the bone to the blood.*

Metastatic tumour to bone,

Paget's disease of bone,

Prolonged immobilization: *Bone destruction or thinning causes calcium to leak from the bone and into the blood.*

Milk-alkali syndrome: *With increased ingestion of milk products or antacids (which contain calcium), the serum calcium level can be elevated.*

Vitamin D intoxication: *Vitamin D works synergistically with PTH to increase serum calcium level.*

Lymphoma,

Granulomatous infections such as sarcoidosis and tuberculosis: *These diseases are associated with enhanced levels of vitamin D, which works synergistically with PTH to increase serum calcium level.*

Addison's disease: *Glucocorticosteroids inhibit vitamin D activity. When steroid activity is decreased, vitamin D action is enhanced. Vitamin D works synergistically with PTH to increase serum calcium levels.*

Acromegaly,

Hyperthyroidism

▼ Decreased Levels (Hypocalcemia)

Hypoparathyroidism: *PTH acts to increase serum calcium levels. If PTH levels are reduced, serum calcium levels decline.*

Renal failure,

Hyperphosphatemia secondary to renal failure: *Excess anions, present in patients with renal failure, bind serum calcium.*

Rickets,

Vitamin D deficiency: *Vitamin D acts synergistically with PTH. PTH acts to increase serum calcium levels. Without that synergism, calcium levels decline.*

Osteomalacia,

Hypoalbuminemia,

Malabsorption: *Less calcium is available to the blood.*

Pancreatitis,

Fat embolism: *Pancreatitis is associated with saponification (binding of calcium to fats) of the peripancreatic tissue. This reduces the calcium levels in the blood.*

Alkalosis: *High pH in the blood drives the calcium to intracellular spaces. Blood levels decline.*

RELATED TESTS

Parathyroid Hormone (p. 393). This test is a measurement of PTH, which increases serum calcium levels.

Albumin (p. 440). This test is a direct measurement of serum albumin. Albumin has a major effect on serum calcium metabolism.

Carbon Dioxide Content (CO$_2$ Content, CO$_2$-Combining Power, Bicarbonate [HCO$_3^-$])

NORMAL FINDINGS

Adult/older adult: **21–28 mmol/L** (21–28 mEq/L)

Child: **20–28 mmol/L** (20–28 mEq/L)

Infant: **20–28 mmol/L** (20–28 mEq/L)

Newborn: **13–22 mmol/L** (13–22 mEq/L)

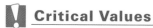 **Critical Values**

<6 mmol/L (mEq/L)

INDICATIONS

The CO_2 content is a measure of CO_2 in the blood. In the peripheral venous blood, this measurement is used to assist in the evaluation of the patient's pH status and electrolyte levels.

TEST EXPLANATION

The serum CO_2 test is usually performed with other electrolyte assessments. It is usually measured by a multiphasic testing machine that also measures sodium, potassium, chloride, blood urea nitrogen, and creatinine. *It is important not to confuse this test with that for partial pressure of carbon dioxide (P_{CO_2}).* This CO_2 content measures H_2CO_3, dissolved CO_2, and the bicarbonate ion (HCO_3^-) that exists in the serum. Because the amounts of H_2CO_3 and dissolved CO_2 in the blood are so small, CO_2 content is an indirect measure of anion. HCO_3^- anion is second in importance to the chloride ion in electrical neutrality (negative charge) of extracellular and intracellular fluid; it plays a major role in acid-base balance.

Levels of HCO_3^- are regulated by the kidneys. Increases occur with alkalosis, and decreases occur with acidosis. This test can be performed on arterial blood, as discussed further on p. 123. When CO_2 content is measured in the laboratory with other serum electrolytes, air affects the specimen, and the P_{CO_2} can be altered. Therefore, venous blood specimens are not ideal for accurate measurements of true CO_2 content or HCO_3^-. They are used primarily as a rough guide for acid-base balance.

INTERFERING FACTORS

- Underfilling the tube with blood allows CO_2 to escape from the serum specimen and may significantly reduce values.
- Drugs that may cause *increases* in serum CO_2 and HCO_3^- levels include aldosterone, barbiturates, bicarbonates, ethacrynic acid, hydrocortisone, loop diuretics, mercurial diuretics, and steroids.
- Drugs that may cause *decreases* in serum CO_2 and HCO_3^- levels include methicillin, nitrofurantoin, paraldehyde, tetracycline, thiazide diuretics, and triamterene.

PROCEDURE AND PATIENT CARE

Before
- Explain the procedure to the patient.
- Inform the patient that no fasting is required.

During
- Collect a venous blood sample in a red-top or green-top tube.

After
- Apply pressure or a pressure dressing to the venipuncture site.
- Assess the venipuncture site for bleeding.

TEST RESULTS AND CLINICAL SIGNIFICANCE

Increased Levels

Severe vomiting,

High-volume gastric suction,

Aldosteronism,

Use of mercurial diuretics: *Important acid hydrogen ions are lost. Levels of HCO_3^- ions are relatively high.*

Chronic obstructive pulmonary disease: *Levels of HCO_3^- ions are increased to compensate for chronic hypoventilation (high P_{CO_2}). This development is also compensation for respiratory acidosis.*

Metabolic alkalosis: *Metabolic alkalosis is defined by an increased amount of HCO_3^- anions in the blood.*

▼ Decreased Levels

Chronic diarrhea,

Chronic use of loop diuretics: *Persistent loss of base ions, including HCO_3^-. Most of the CO_2 content is HCO_3^-.*

Renal failure,

Diabetic ketoacidosis,

Starvation: *Keto acids and other anions are increased. HCO_3^- neutralizes these acids. HCO_3^- levels therefore drop.*

Metabolic acidosis: *Metabolic acidosis is defined by a decreased amount of HCO_3^- anions in the blood.*

Shock: *Lactic acid builds up and is buffered by the HCO_3^-; therefore, HCO_3^- levels diminish.*

RELATED TEST

Arterial Blood Gases (p. 121). This is a battery of arterial blood tests that are used to evaluate acid-base status. Measurements of CO_2 content and HCO_3^- are components of that test.

Carboxyhemoglobin (COHb, Carbon Monoxide)

NORMAL FINDINGS

Nonsmoker: <3% saturation of total hemoglobin

Light smoker: 2%–5%

Heavy smoker: 5%–10%

Newborn: ≥12%

 Critical Values

>20%

INDICATIONS

This test is used to detect carbon monoxide poisoning.

TEST EXPLANATION

This test measures the amount of serum carboxyhemoglobin (COHb), which is formed by the combination of carbon monoxide and hemoglobin (Hb). Carbon monoxide combines with hemoglobin 200 times more readily than oxygen can combine with hemoglobin (oxyhemoglobin). As a result, fewer hemoglobin bonds are available to combine with oxygen. Furthermore, when carbon monoxide occupies the oxygen-binding sites, the hemoglobin molecule is changed so as to bind the remaining oxygen more tightly. This greater affinity of carbon monoxide for hemoglobin and change in oxygen-binding strength does not allow the oxygen to pass readily from the red blood cells (RBCs) to the tissue. Less oxygen is therefore available for tissue cell respiration. This results in hypoxemia. Carbon monoxide poisoning is documented by hemoglobin analysis for COHb. A specimen should be collected as soon as possible after exposure because carbon monoxide is rapidly cleared from the hemoglobin by breathing normal air. Oxygen saturation studies and oximetry yield inaccurate values in carbon monoxide–exposed patients because they measure all forms of oxygen-saturated hemoglobin, including COHb. In these circumstances, the results are normal, even though the patient is hypoxemic.

This test can also be used to evaluate patients with complaints of headache, irritability, nausea, vomiting, and vertigo who may have been unknowingly exposed to carbon monoxide. Its most widespread use, however, is in patients exposed to smoke inhalation, exhaust fumes, and fires. Other sources of carbon monoxide are tobacco smoke, petroleum and natural gas fuel fumes, automobile exhaust, unvented natural gas heaters, and defective gas stoves. Symptoms of carbon monoxide poisoning that are correlated with blood levels are listed in Table 2-13. Carbon monoxide toxicity is treated by administering high concentrations of oxygen to displace the COHb.

Clinical Priorities

- Carbon monoxide combines with hemoglobin 200 times more readily than does oxygen. This results in hypoxemia.
- Carbon monoxide poisoning is documented by the COHb test. Specimens should be collected as soon as possible after exposure because carbon monoxide is rapidly cleared from the hemoglobin by breathing normal air.
- Carbon monoxide toxicity is treated by administration of high concentrations of oxygen to displace the COHb.
- Severe carbon monoxide toxicity may be treated with hyperbaric oxygen.

TABLE 2-13   Symptoms of Carbon Monoxide Poisoning by Level of Hemoglobin Saturation

Level of Carbon Monoxide Saturation of Hemoglobin	Symptoms
10%	Slight dyspnea
20%	Headache
30%	Irritability, disturbed judgement, memory loss
40%	Confusion, weakness, dimness of vision
50%	Fainting, ataxia, collapse
60%	Coma
>60%	Death

PROCEDURE AND PATIENT CARE

Before

🖉 Explain the procedure to the patient or the family.
- Document the patient's history in relation to any possible source of carbon monoxide inhalation.
- Assess the patient for signs and symptoms of mild carbon monoxide toxicity (e.g., headache, weakness, dizziness, malaise, dyspnea) and moderate to severe carbon monoxide toxicity (e.g., severe headache, bright-red mucous membranes, cherry-red blood). Maintain patient safety precautions if the patient appears confused.

During

- Collect a venous blood sample in a lavender-top or green-top tube.

After

- Apply pressure or a pressure dressing to the venipuncture site.
- Assess the venipuncture site for bleeding.
- Treat the patient as indicated by the physician. Usually the patient receives high concentrations of oxygen. Severe carbon monoxide toxicity may be treated with hyperbaric oxygen.
- Encourage respirations to allow the patient to clear carbon monoxide from the hemoglobin.

TEST RESULTS AND CLINICAL SIGNIFICANCE

▲ Increased Levels

Carbon monoxide poisoning

RELATED TESTS

Oximetry (p. 1155). This test is used to easily and continuously monitor oxygen saturation of hemoglobin.

Oxygen Saturation (p. 1155). This test measures the amount of hemoglobin saturated by oxygen.

Carcinoembryonic Antigen (CEA)

NORMAL FINDINGS

<5 Mcg/L (<5 ng/mL)

INDICATIONS

This tumour marker is measured to determine the extent of disease and prognosis in patients with cancer (especially gastrointestinal or breast). It is also used in monitoring the disease and its treatment.

TEST EXPLANATION

Carcinoembryonic antigen (CEA) is a protein that normally is present in fetal gut tissue. By birth, serum levels become undetectable. In the early 1960s, CEA was detected in the bloodstream of adults who had colorectal tumours. It was originally thought to be a specific indicator of the presence of colorectal cancer. Subsequently, however, this tumour marker has been found in patients who have a variety of carcinomas (e.g., breast, pancreatic, gastric, hepatobiliary), sarcomas, and even many benign diseases (e.g., ulcerative colitis, diverticulitis, cirrhosis). Chronic smokers also have detectable CEA levels.

Because the CEA level can be elevated in both benign and malignant diseases, the test is not specific for colorectal cancer. Furthermore, not all colorectal cancers produce CEA. Therefore, CEA testing is not reliable for the detection of colorectal cancer in the general population. Its use is limited to determining the prognosis and monitoring the response of tumour to antineoplastic therapy in a patient with cancer. This is especially helpful in patients with breast and gastrointestinal cancers. The initial pretreatment CEA level is an indicator of tumour burden and therefore of prognosis. Patients with smaller and early-stage tumours are likely to have low, if not undetectable, CEA levels. Patients with more advanced or metastatic tumours are likely to have high CEA levels. A drastic reduction of the preoperative CEA to undetectable levels indicates complete or nearly complete eradication of the tumour. Therefore, this test is used to determine the efficacy of treatment.

This test also is used in the surveillance of patients with cancer. A steadily rising CEA level is occasionally the first sign of tumour recurrence. Therefore, CEA testing is very valuable in the follow-up of patients who have already had potentially curative therapy. However, many (~20%) patients with advanced breast or gastrointestinal tumours may not have elevated CEA levels.

CEA can also be detected in body fluids other than blood. Its presence in those body fluids indicates metastasis. This CEA test is commonly performed on peritoneal fluid or chest effusions. Elevated CEA levels in these fluids indicate metastasis to the peritoneum or pleura, respectively. Likewise, elevated CEA levels in the cerebrospinal fluid indicate metastasis to the central nervous system.

INTERFERING FACTORS

- Smokers tend to have higher CEA levels than do nonsmokers.
- Benign diseases (e.g., cholecystitis, colitis, diverticulitis) and especially liver diseases (e.g., hepatitis, cirrhosis) are also associated with elevated CEA levels.
- Results may vary considerably, depending on the method used for quantification. Because of this, results from different laboratories cannot be compared or interchangeably interpreted.

PROCEDURE AND PATIENT CARE

Before
- Explain the procedure to the patient.
- Inform the patient that no fasting is required.

During
- Collect a peripheral blood specimen. The collecting tube varies according to the commercial laboratory. Diagnostic kits are now available so that CEA can be tested at most local hospitals.
- On the laboratory slip, note whether the patient smokes or has diseases that can affect test results.

After
- Apply pressure or a pressure dressing to the venipuncture site.
- Observe the venipuncture site for bleeding.

TEST RESULTS AND CLINICAL SIGNIFICANCE

▲ Increased Levels

Cancer (gastrointestinal, breast, lung, pancreatic, hepatobiliary): *The cancer cells produce CEA on their cell surface. By a yet unrecognized mechanism, the CEA leaks into the bloodstream. CEA levels then become elevated.*

Inflammation (colitis, cholecystitis, pancreatitis, diverticulitis),

Cirrhosis,

Crohn's disease,

Peptic ulcer: *The mechanism by which benign diseases produce CEA is unknown.*

RELATED TESTS

CA 15-3 and CA 27-29 Tumour Markers (p. 146). These antigens are tumour-associated serum markers for staging breast cancer and monitoring disease treatment.

CA 19-9 Tumour Marker (p. 145). Levels of this tumour marker are elevated in pancreatobiliary tumours and colorectal tumours.

Cell Surface Immunophenotyping (Flow Cytometry Cell Surface Immunophenotyping, Lymphocyte Immunophenotyping, AIDS T Lymphocyte Cell Markers, CD4 Marker, CD4/CD8 Ratio, CD4 Percentage)

NORMAL FINDINGS

Cells	Percentage	Number of Cells/mm^3
T cells	60–95	800–2 500
T helper (CD4) cells	60–75	600–1 500
T suppressor (CD8) cells	25–30	300–1 000
B cells	4–25	100–450
Natural killer cells	4–30	75–500

CD4/CD8 ratio: >1

INDICATIONS

This test is used to detect the progressive depletion of CD4 T lymphocytes, which is associated with an increased likelihood of clinical complications from acquired immune deficiency syndrome (AIDS). Test results can indicate whether a patient with AIDS is at risk for developing opportunistic infections. It is also used to confirm the diagnosis of acute myelocytic leukemia and to differentiate this disease from acute lymphocytic leukemia.

TEST EXPLANATION

All lymphocytes are nurtured by reticulum cells in the bone marrow during development. Normal hematopoietic cells undergo changes in expression of cell surface markers as they mature from stem cells into cells of a committed lineage. Monoclonal antibodies have been developed that react with lymphoid and myeloid glycoprotein antigens on the cell surface of peripheral blood cells.

One kind of lymphocyte, the B lymphocyte, matures in the bone marrow. B lymphocytes provide humoral immunity (produce antibodies). A second type of lymphocyte, the T lymphocyte, matures in the thymus. T lymphocytes are responsible for cellular immunity. A third type of lymphocyte has neither T nor B markers. These lymphocytes are called *natural killer cells* and will chemically attack foreign or cancer cells without prior sensitization. Monoclonal antibodies against cell-surface markers are used to identify the various forms of lymphocytes. The absolute numbers and percentages are then counted by means of flow cytometry. This can be performed on blood or on cell suspensions of tissue.

CD4 helper cells and CD8 cells are examples of T lymphocytes. T lymphocyte counts and especially CD4 cell counts, when combined with results of viral load tests for human immunodeficiency virus (HIV; p. 314), are used to determine when to initiate antiviral therapy. They also can be used to monitor antiviral therapy. Successful antiviral therapy is associated with an increase in CD4 cell counts. Worsening of disease or lack of therapeutic success is associated with decreasing T lymphocyte counts.

There are three related measurements of CD4 T lymphocytes. The first measurement is the total *CD4 cell count.* This is measured in whole blood and is the product of the white blood cell (WBC) count, the lymphocyte differential count, and the percentage of lymphocytes that are CD4 T cells. The second measurement, the *CD4 percentage,* is a more accurate prognostic marker. The percentage of CD4 lymphocytes in the whole blood sample is measured by means of combining immunophenotyping with flow cytometry. This procedure relies on detecting specific antigenic determinants on the surface of the CD4 lymphocyte by antigen-specific monoclonal antibodies labelled with a fluorescent dye. The third prognostic marker, which is also more reliable than the total CD4 cell count, is the *ratio of CD4 (T helper) cells to CD8 (T suppressor) cells.*

Of the three T cell measurements, the total CD4 cell count is the most variable. The diurnal variation in this count is substantial. Because it is a calculated measurement, the combination of possible laboratory error and personal fluctuation can result in wide variations in test results. With the CD4 percentage and CD4/CD8 ratios, very little diurnal variation and laboratory error exist. Results of the Multicenter AIDS Cohort Study, sponsored by a division of the U.S. National Institute of Allergy and Infectious Diseases, suggest that the latter two measurements are more accurate than the total CD4 cell count. However, because the total CD4 cell count was originally thought to be the best marker, this test was used in many of the studies that now form the basis for practice recommendations. It will take time before practice recommendations are based on the more accurate measurements.

The pathogenesis of AIDS is attributed largely to a decrease in the T lymphocyte that bears the CD4 receptor. Progressive depletion of CD4 T lymphocytes is associated with an increased likelihood of clinical complications from AIDS. Therefore, CD4 measurement is a prognostic marker that can indicate whether a patient infected with HIV is at risk for developing opportunistic infections. The measurement of CD4 cell levels is used to decide whether to initiate prophylaxis against *Pneumocystis jiroveci* pneumonia and antiviral therapy and for determining the prognosis of patients with HIV infection.

Both immunodeficiency and the dosage of immunosuppressive medications used after organ transplantation are also monitored with the use of this cell surface immunophenotyping. Lymphomas and other lymphoproliferative diseases are now classified and treated according to the predominant lymphocyte type identified. In some instances, the prognosis of these diseases depends on this lymphocyte phenotyping. The U.S. Department of Health and Human Services (DHHS) Panel on Antiretroviral Guidelines for Adults and Adolescents recommended that CD4 prognostic markers be monitored every 3 to 4 months in all individuals treated with antiretroviral therapy. The CD4 cell count is the major laboratory indicator of immune function in HIV-positive patients and one of the strongest predictors of disease progression and survival. An adequate

CD4 response to treatment is defined as an increase in CD4 cell count in the range of 50 to 150 cells/mm^3 per year. Because the CD4 cell counts gradually fall in virtually all such patients, periodic review of the count can be emotionally stressful for both the patient and the physician: The patient confronts his or her debilitation and mortality, and the health care provider confronts his or her ultimate powerlessness against the relentlessly advancing infections.

As the CD4 cell measurements decrease, the probability of developing AIDS increases. Of patients whose CD4 cell count is less than 100 cells/mm^3, 48% can be expected to develop AIDS within 6 months. It is recommended that antiretroviral therapy be started in patients whose CD4 cell count is less than 350 cells/mm^3 or between 350 and 500 cells/mm^3. Prophylaxis against *P. jiroveci* pneumonia should be started when the CD4 cell count is less than 200 to 300 cells/mm^3.

CD4 prognostic markers also can be useful in guiding the approach to the patient's symptoms. Complaints such as cough and headache are common in the general population; however, in patients infected with HIV, these symptoms often raise concerns about opportunistic infections. If the CD4 cell count exceeded 500 cells/mm^3 in the past 6 months, there is a very low probability that these symptoms result from opportunistic infections. Knowing this, the patient and physician can feel comfortable with routine care.

In *flow cytometry,* thousands of cells can be analyzed in less than 1 minute. The flow cytometer has three components in testing: an optical system, a fluid system, and an electronic system. The *optical* system consists of an argon laser that emits a single wavelength of light at 488 nm (blue region). Cells are labelled with one of several fluorochromes, including fluorescein, phycoerythrin, and peridinin-chlorophyll protein, as a result of the binding of monoclonal antibody–fluorochrome conjugate to a specific blood cell. The fluorochromes are excited by the laser and emit *green* (fluorescein), *orange* (phycoerythrin), and *red* (peridinin-chlorophyll protein) light that is measured through optical filters designed to capture their specific wavelength. The *fluid* system introduces the fluorochrome-bound cells in suspension into a pressurized sheath of fluid that travels through a clear cuvette. The laser light intersects a stream of cells that pass single file through the cuvette. The *electronic* system measures electronic signals from the detectors that provide measures of the magnitude of fluorescence intensity and the extent of light scatter associated with each cell as it passes through the laser. Most clinical flow cytometers measure five parameters on each cell: two nonfluorescence measures (magnitude of forward and side scatter) and three fluorescence measures (green, orange, and red light intensity). Multiple markers can be used simultaneously to identify different cell populations.

Through the use of a combination of monoclonal antibodies that recognize B cell, T cell, and myeloid antigens, it is possible to confirm the diagnosis of acute myelocytic leukemia and to differentiate this disease from acute lymphocytic leukemia if morphologic studies and traditional immunohistochemistry profiles are inconclusive (<15% of cases). It is also helpful in identifying mixed patterns of leukemia that may affect prognosis and treatment. Furthermore, cell surface immunophenotyping through flow cytometry is extremely helpful in differentiating various forms of immunodeficiency diseases.

CONTRAINDICATIONS
- Patients' lack of emotional preparation for the prognosis that the results may indicate.

INTERFERING FACTORS
- Although diurnal variation is usually of no significance, it may have some effect when counts are low. Higher counts can be expected in the late morning hours.
- A recent viral illness can decrease total T lymphocyte counts.

- Nicotine and very strenuous exercise have been shown to decrease lymphocyte counts. However, such data are now being questioned.

 Steroids can *increase* lymphocyte counts.

 Immunosuppressive drugs *decrease* lymphocyte counts.

✓ Clinical Priorities

- Progressive depletion of CD4 T lymphocytes is associated with an increase in complications from AIDS. Examples of such complications are severe immunosuppression, life-threatening opportunistic infections, malignancies, wasting syndrome, and HIV-related encephalopathy.
- The CD4 percentage and CD4/CD8 ratio provide more accurate measurements of CD4 T lymphocytes than does the total CD4 cell count.
- The Public Health Agency of Canada and the U.S. Public Health Service recommend monitoring CD4 cell counts every 3 to 6 months for all persons infected with HIV.

Cultural Considerations

Indigenous people living in Canada make up 3.3% of the total population. Their susceptibility to HIV infection can be affected by many social, economic, and behavioural factors, including high rates of poverty, substance use, and high rates of sexually transmitted infections. In Canada between 1979 and 2003, there were 12 602 positive HIV test results reported to the Centre for Infectious Disease Prevention and Control (CIDPC), of which 851 were Indigenous people. In the same time period, there were 18 934 reported cases of AIDS in Canada, of which 509 were reported to be occurring in Indigenous populations. Indigenous women and youth are at high risk for HIV, with nearly 50% of all of the positive HIV test results occurring in Indigenous women, and positive test results occurring at a younger age in Indigenous people than in non-Indigenous people. Further to HIV susceptibility and culture, the percentage of HIV-positive reports is increasing among Canadians of African ancestry, with heterosexual exposure accounting for more than 80% of those positive test results.

PROCEDURE AND PATIENT CARE

Before

- Explain the procedure to the patient.
- Inform the patient that no fasting or preparation is required.
- Maintain a nonjudgemental attitude toward the patient's sexual practices.
- Allow the patient ample opportunity to express his or her concerns regarding the results.

During

- Record the time of day when the blood specimen is obtained.
- Observe universal body and blood precautions. Wear gloves when you handle blood products from all patients.
- Never recap needles. Used needles and syringes required for obtaining the blood specimen should be disposed of in a puncture-proof container designed for this purpose.
- Collect a venous blood sample in a large green-top tube (containing sodium heparin).
- Collect a venous blood sample in a small lavender-top tube (containing ethylene diamine tetra-acetic acid).

After

- Keep the specimen at room temperature. Do not refrigerate it.
- The specimen must be evaluated within 24 hours.
- Often specimens are sent to a central laboratory.
- Apply pressure or a pressure dressing to the venipuncture site.
- Assess the puncture site for bleeding.
- Instruct the patient to observe the venipuncture site for infection. Patients with AIDS or organ recipients are immunocompromised and susceptible to infection.
- Encourage the patient to discuss his or her concerns regarding the prognostic information that may be provided by these results.

TEST RESULTS AND CLINICAL SIGNIFICANCE

▲ Increased Levels

Chronic lymphocytic leukemia,

B cell lymphoma: *In these conditions, B lymphocyte counts are expected to be increased in tumour tissue or in peripheral blood.*

T cell lymphoma: *In this condition, T lymphocyte counts are expected to be increased in tumour tissue or in peripheral blood (if the bone marrow is heavily involved with tumour).*

▼ Decreased Levels

Organ transplant recipients: *A decreased lymphocyte count is expected and desirable for immunosuppression of organ rejection.*

HIV-positive patients: *When CD4 cell counts are below 200/mm^3, the patient is at increased risk for clinical symptoms from AIDS and the opportunistic infections that accompany this disease.*

Congenital immunodeficiency: *Children with DiGeorge syndrome and thymic hypoplasia have decreased or undetectable levels of B lymphocytes.*

RELATED TESTS

HIV Serology (p. 310). This test is used to detect HIV antibody or antigen in persons at high risk for HIV infection.

HIV Viral Load (p. 314). This test is used to determine the amount of HIV viral load in the blood of an infected patient and is an accurate marker for prognosis and disease progression.

Ceruloplasmin (Cp)

NORMAL FINDINGS

Adults: **230–500 mg/L** (23–50 mg/dL)
Neonates: **20–130 mg/L** (2–13 mg/dL)

INDICATIONS

Ceruloplasmin is an acute-phase reactant protein, and elevated levels can indicate an acute illness. However, the primary use of the ceruloplasmin test is in the diagnosis of preclinical states of Wilson disease.

TEST EXPLANATION

Ceruloplasmin is an alpha$_2$-globulin that binds copper for transport within the bloodstream after it is absorbed from the gastrointestinal tract. Levels are decreased in most cases of Wilson disease, which is an inherited disorder. Patients who are homozygous for the allele for this disease make very little ceruloplasmin. Unbound copper rises to high levels in blood and is toxic to tissues. The copper is deposited in the eyes, brain, liver, and kidneys. Wilson disease is fatal unless early treatment is instituted. If this disease is identified before significant copper deposits affect major organs, the ravages of the disease can be avoided. Ceruloplasmin levels are measured in children at high risk for the disease. Teenagers and young adults with hepatitis, cirrhosis, or recurrent neuromuscular incoordination (signs compatible with Wilson disease) should also undergo this test. Early detection is important because therapy is effective in most cases.

Ceruloplasmin is also an acute-phase reactant protein whose levels become elevated during stress, infection, and pregnancy. However, those levels rise more slowly than do levels of other acute-phase reactants, such as C-reactive protein, and erythrocyte sedimentation rate.

INTERFERING FACTORS

- Values are increased during pregnancy.
- Drugs that may cause *increases* in ceruloplasmin levels include birth control pills, estrogen, methadone, phenytoin, and tamoxifen.

PROCEDURE AND PATIENT CARE

Before
- Explain the procedure to the patient.
- Inform the patient that no fasting is required.

During
- Collect a venous blood sample in a red-top tube.
- Keep the specimen in a container of crushed ice and water.

After
- Apply pressure or a pressure dressing to the venipuncture site.
- Assess the venipuncture site for bleeding.
- Medical follow-up and genetic counselling are indicated when Wilson disease is confirmed.

TEST RESULTS AND CLINICAL SIGNIFICANCE

▲ Increased Levels

Pregnancy,
Thyrotoxicosis,
Cancer,
Acute inflammatory reaction (e.g., infection, rheumatoid arthritis),
Biliary cirrhosis: *These diseases induce the synthesis of ceruloplasmin as an acute-phase reactant.*
Copper intoxication: *Elevation of copper levels stimulates ceruloplasmin production in unaffected individuals.*

▼ Decreased Levels

Wilson disease: *Patients with this disease have a homozygous or heterozygous state and are unable to make ceruloplasmin. Homozygous patients have lower ceruloplasmin levels than do heterozygous patients.*

Normal infants (6 months): *Young infants normally are unable to make adequate amounts of acute-phase reactant proteins (alpha$_2$-globulins) until they are 6 months of age.*

Nephrotic syndrome,

Sprue (celiac disease): *These are protein-losing diseases. Ceruloplasmin is one of the proteins that are lost in these diseases, and blood levels therefore fall.*

Kwashiorkor,

Starvation: *Nutritional deficiencies are associated with low levels of serum proteins, including ceruloplasmin.*

Menkes (kinky-hair) syndrome: *This is an inherited disorder associated with defects in the production of alpha$_2$-globulins such as ceruloplasmin.*

RELATED TESTS

C-Reactive Protein (p. 199) and Erythrocyte Sedimentation Rate (p. 236). These are tests for acute-phase reactant proteins.

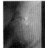

Chloride, Blood (Cl)

NORMAL FINDINGS

Adult/older adult: **98–106 mmol/L** (98–106 mEq/L)
Child: **90–110 mmol/L** (90–110 mEq/L)
Newborn: **96–106 mmol/L** (96–106 mEq/L)
Premature infant: **95–106 mmol/L** (95–106 mEq/L)

Critical Values

<80 mmol/L (<80 mEq/L) or **>115 mmol/L** (>115 mEq/L)

INDICATIONS

This test is performed as a part of multiphasic testing for what are usually called *electrolytes*. By itself, the result of this test does not provide much information. However, with interpretation of the other electrolyte levels, the chloride level can give an indication of acid-base balance and hydration status.

TEST EXPLANATION

Chloride is the major extracellular anion. Its primary purpose is to maintain electrical neutrality, mostly as a salt with sodium. Its production follows sodium (cation) losses and accompanies sodium excesses in an attempt to maintain electrical neutrality. For example, when aldosterone encourages sodium reabsorption, chloride is produced to maintain electrical neutrality. Because water moves with sodium and chloride, chloride also affects water balance. Finally, chloride also serves as a buffer to assist in acid-base balance. As carbon dioxide (and hydrogen cation) increases, bicarbonate must move from the intracellular space to the extracellular space. To maintain electrical neutrality, chloride shifts back into the cell.

Hypochloremia and hyperchloremia rarely occur alone; they usually are part of parallel shifts in sodium or bicarbonate levels. Signs and symptoms of hypochloremia include hyperexcitability of the nervous system and muscles, shallow breathing, hypotension, and tetany. Signs and symptoms of hyperchloremia include lethargy, weakness, and deep breathing.

INTERFERING FACTORS

- Excessive infusions of saline solution can result in increased chloride levels.
- Drugs that may cause *increases* in serum chloride levels include acetazolamide, ammonium chloride, androgens, chlorothiazide, cortisone preparations, estrogens, guanethidine, hydrochlorothiazide, methyldopa, and nonsteroidal anti-inflammatory drugs.
- Drugs that may cause *decreases* in serum chloride levels include aldosterone, bicarbonates, corticosteroids, cortisone, hydrocortisone, loop diuretics, thiazide diuretics, and triamterene.

PROCEDURE AND PATIENT CARE

Before
- Explain the procedure to the patient.
- Inform the patient that no fasting is required.

During
- Collect a venous blood sample in a red-top or green-top tube.

After
- Apply pressure or a pressure dressing to the venipuncture site.
- Assess the venipuncture site for bleeding.

TEST RESULTS AND CLINICAL SIGNIFICANCE

▲ Increased Levels (Hyperchloremia)

Dehydration: *Chloride ions are more concentrated in the blood.*
Excessive infusion of normal saline solution: *Intake of chloride exceeds output, and blood levels rise.*
Metabolic acidosis,
Renal tubular acidosis,
Cushing's syndrome,
Kidney dysfunction,
Hyperparathyroidism,
Eclampsia: *Chloride urinary excretion is decreased.*
Respiratory alkalosis: *Chloride is driven out of the cell in place of bicarbonate ion (HCO_3^-).*

▼ Decreased Levels (Hypochloremia)

Overhydration,
Syndrome of inappropriate secretion of antidiuretic hormone (SIADH): *Chloride is diluted.*
Heart failure: *Chloride is retained with sodium retention but is diluted by excess total body water.*
Vomiting or prolonged gastric suction,

Chronic diarrhea or high-output gastrointestinal fistula: *Chloride cation is high in the stomach and gastrointestinal tract because of hydrochloric acid produced in the stomach.*

Chronic respiratory acidosis,

Metabolic alkalosis: *Chloride is driven into the cell to compensate for the HCO_3^- that leaves the cell to maintain pH neutrality.*

Salt-losing nephritis,

Addison's disease,

Diuretic therapy,

Hypokalemia,

Aldosteronism: *Chloride excretion is increased.*

Burns: *Massive burn can cause severe sodium and chloride losses.*

RELATED TESTS

Sodium, Blood (p. 479), and Potassium, Blood (p. 420). These are other electrolytes commonly measured with chloride.

Arterial Blood Gases (p. 121). This is an arterial blood test used to evaluate acid-base status, including the level of bicarbonate ions.

Chloride, Urine (p. 951). This is a measurement of chloride in the urine.

Cholesterol

NORMAL FINDINGS

Adult/older adult: <5.2 mmol/L (<200 mg/dL)
Child:

Age	Male, mmol/L (mg/dL)	Female, mmol/L (mg/dL)
10–11 years:	3.10–5.90 (120–228)	3.16–6.26 (122–242)
7–12 months (infant):	2.15–5.30 (83–205)	1.76–5.59 (68–216)
0–1 month (newborn):	0.98–4.50 (38–174)	1.45–5.04 (56–195)

INDICATIONS

Cholesterol testing is used to determine the risk for coronary heart disease (CHD). It is also used for evaluation of hyperlipidemias.

TEST EXPLANATION

Cholesterol is the main lipid associated with arteriosclerotic vascular disease. Cholesterol, however, is required for the production of steroids, sex hormones, bile acids, and cellular membranes. Most of the cholesterol that humans eat comes from foods of animal origin. The liver metabolizes the cholesterol to its free form, and cholesterol is transported in the bloodstream by lipoproteins (see p. 355). Nearly 75% of the cholesterol is bound to LDL, and 25% is bound to HDL. Cholesterol is the main component of LDL but only a minimal component of HDL and VLDL. It is the LDL that is most directly associated with increased risk for CHD.

The purpose of cholesterol testing is to identify patients at risk for arteriosclerotic heart disease. Cholesterol testing is usually performed as a part of a lipid profile, in which lipoproteins and triglycerides (see pp. 355 and 523) are evaluated because, by itself, cholesterol is not a totally accurate predictor of heart disease. There is considerable overlap in what are considered "normal" and "high-risk" levels. "Normal" levels have been calculated from a group of patients who have no obvious evidence of CHD. However, this may not be accurate because these patients may have preclinical CHD and may not truly reflect a "no-risk" population.

There is considerable variation in cholesterol levels. Day-to-day cholesterol values in the same individual can vary by 15%. An 8% difference can even be identified within the same day. Positional changes can affect these levels: Levels can decrease by as much as 15% in the recumbent position. As a result, hospitalized patients are expected to have lower levels than outpatients. Because of these significant variations, elevations in cholesterol levels should be corroborated by repeating the study. The two results should be averaged to calculate an accurate cholesterol level for risk assessment.

Because the liver must metabolize ingested cholesterol products, subnormal cholesterol levels are indicative of severe liver diseases. Furthermore, because the main source of cholesterol is diet, malnutrition is also associated with low cholesterol levels. Certain illnesses can affect cholesterol levels. For example, patients with an acute myocardial infarction may have as much as a 50% reduction in cholesterol level for as long as 6 to 8 weeks.

Total cholesterol is used most accurately as a predictor of the risk for CHD, as studied as part of the updated *Framingham Coronary Prediction* algorithm. This prediction model is used to determine a person's risk for developing an ischemic event (angina, myocardial infarction, or myocardial death) over the course of the following decade. Besides cholesterol, other factors used to estimate risk for CHD are age, lipoproteins, blood pressure, cigarette smoking history, diabetes mellitus, and gender.

In this risk model, points are assigned to each factor in the model (Figure 2-12). The total number of points is used to provide the patient's CHD risk. If the CHD risk is divided by age-related data (comparative risk), the patient's risk relative to that of peers can be calculated. The CHD risk can be used to determine whether medicinal cholesterol-lowering intervention is indicated.

Familial hyperlipidemias and hyperlipoproteinemias are often associated with high cholesterol levels.

INTERFERING FACTORS

- Pregnancy is usually associated with elevated cholesterol levels.
- Oophorectomy and postmenopausal status are associated with increased cholesterol levels.
- The recumbent position is associated with decreased cholesterol levels.
- Drugs that may cause *increases* in cholesterol levels include adrenocorticotropic hormone, anabolic steroids, beta-adrenergic blocking agents, corticosteroids, cyclosporine, epinephrine, oral contraceptives, phenytoin (Dilantin), sulphonamides, thiazide diuretics, and vitamin D.
- Drugs that may cause *decreases* in cholesterol levels include allopurinol, androgens, bile salt-binding agents, captopril, chlorpropamide, clofibrate, colchicine, colestipol, erythromycin, isoniazid, liothyronine (Cytomel), monoamine oxidase inhibitors, niacin, nitrates, and statins.

✓ **Clinical Priorities**

- Cholesterol testing is usually performed as part of lipid profile testing, in which lipoproteins and triglycerides are also evaluated.
- Because of considerable variations in cholesterol values, elevated levels should be verified by repeating the test.
- Test preparation usually requires a 12- to 14-hour fast after a low-fat meal. Only water is permitted during the fast.

PROCEDURE AND PATIENT CARE

Before

✗ Instruct the patient to eat a low-fat meal and then fast 12 to 14 hours before the test. Only water is permitted during the fast. Actually, cholesterol levels increase only minimally after a meal. However, early-morning fasting cholesterol levels are more easily compared when measured serially. Furthermore, lipoprotein levels, whose measurements are often ordered simultaneously, are affected by a previous meal. Therefore, fasting is usually requested.

✗ Indicate to the patient that dietary intake for 2 weeks before the test will affect results. Suggest that the patient follow his or her normal diet for at least 1 week before the test.

✗ Instruct the patient to consume no alcohol within 24 hours before the test.

During

- Collect a venous blood sample in a red-top tube.
- The capillary puncture method is also often used for mass screening. There is less than a 5% difference in cholesterol measurements with these two methods.

After

- Apply pressure or a pressure dressing to the venipuncture site.
- Assess the venipuncture site for bleeding.
✗ For patients with high cholesterol levels, provide the following instructions:
  - Low-cholesterol diet
    1. Avoid animal fats.
    2. Replace saturated fats with polyunsaturated fats.
    3. Increase ingestion of fruits and vegetables.
  - Exercise
    - Maintain a healthy body weight.

TEST RESULTS AND CLINICAL SIGNIFICANCE

▲ Increased Levels

Familial hypercholesterolemia,
Familial hyperlipidemia: *Enzymatic deficiencies in lipid metabolism are associated with elevated cholesterol levels.*
Hypothyroidism,
Uncontrolled diabetes mellitus,
Nephrotic syndrome,
Pregnancy,
High-cholesterol diet,

FRAMINGHAM RISK SCORE (FRS)
Estimation of 10-year Cardiovascular Disease (CVD) Risk

Patient's Name: _____

Date: _____

Step 1[1]
In the "points" column enter the appropriate value according to the patient's age, HDL-C, total cholesterol, systolic blood pressure, and if they smoke or have diabetes. Calculate the total points.

Risk Factor	Risk Points		Points
Age	**Men**	**Women**	
30-34	0	0	
35-39	2	2	
40-44	5	4	
45-49	7	5	
50-54	8	7	
55-59	10	8	
60-64	11	9	
65-69	12	10	
70-74	14	11	
75+	15	12	
HDL-C (mmol/L)			
>1.6	-2	-2	
1.3-1.6	-1	-1	
1.2-1.29	0	0	
0.9-1.19	1	1	
<0.9	2	2	
Total Cholesterol			
<4.1	0	0	
4.1-5.19	1	1	
5.2-6.19	2	3	
6.2-7.2	3	4	
>7.2	4	5	

Systolic Blood Pressure (mmHg)	Not Treated	Treated	Not Treated	Treated	
<120	-2	0	-3	-1	
120-129	0	2	0	2	
130-139	1	3	1	3	
140-149	2	4	2	5	
150-159	2	4	4	6	
160+	3	5	5	7	

Smoker	Yes	4	3	
	No	0	0	
Diabetes	Yes	statin-indicated condition		
	No	0	0	

| Total Points | | | | |

Step 2[1]
Using the total points from Step 1, determine the 10-year CVD risk (%).

Total Points	10-Year CVD Risk (%)*	
	Men	Women
-3 or less	<1	<1
-2	1.1	<1
-1	1.4	1.0
0	1.6	1.2
1	1.9	1.5
2	2.3	1.7
3	2.8	2.0
4	3.3	2.4
5	3.9	2.8
6	4.7	3.3
7	5.6	3.9
8	6.7	4.5
9	7.9	5.3
10	9.4	6.3
11	11.2	7.3
12	13.3	8.6
13	15.6	10.0
14	18.4	11.7
15	21.6	13.7
16	25.3	15.9
17	29.4	18.51
18	>30	21.5
19	>30	24.8
20	>30	27.5
21+	>30	>30

* Double cardiovascular disease risk percentage for individuals between the ages of 30 and 59 without diabetes if the presence of a positive history of premature cardiovascular disease is present in a first-degree relative before 55 years of age for men and before 65 years of age for women.
† This is known as the modified Framingham Risk Score.‡

Step 3[1]
Using the total points from Step 1, determine heart age (in years).

Heart Age, y	Men	Women
<30	<0	<1
30	0	1
31	1	2
32	2	3
34	3	
36	4	4
38		
39	5	5
40	6	6
42	7	7
45	8	8
48	9	
51	10	9
54		
55	11	10
57		
59	12	11
60	13	12
64	14	
68	15	13
72		
73	16	14
76		
79		15+
≥80	≥17	

Step 4[2,3]
Using 10-year CVD risk from Step 2, determine (if patient is Low, Moderate or High risk.[1] Indicate Lipid and/or Apo B targets)

Risk Level†	Initiate Treatment If:	Primary Target (LDL-C)	Alternate Target
High FRS ≥20%	• Consider treatment in all (Strong, High)	• ≤2 mmol/L or ≥50% decrease in LDL-C (Strong, Moderate)	• Apo B ≤0.8 g/L or • Non-HDL-C ≤2.6 mmol/L (Strong, High)

Intermediate
FRS 10-19%
	• LDL-C ≥3.5 mmol/L
	  (Strong, Moderate)
	• For LDL-C <3.5 mmol/L consider if:
	  • Apo B ≥1.2 g/L
	  • OR Non-HDL-C ≥4.3 mmol/L
	  (Strong, Moderate)
	• Men ≥50 and women ≥60 with 1 risk factor: low HDL-C, impaired fasting glucose, high waist circumference, smoker, hypertension
		• ≤2 mmol/L or ≥50% decrease in LDL-C
		(Strong, Moderate)
			• Apo B ≤0.8 g/L or
			• Non-HDL-C ≤2.6 mmol/L
			(Strong, Moderate)

Low FRS <10%	• statins generally not indicated	• statins generally not indicated	• statins generally not indicated

Statin-indicated conditions**	• Clinical atherosclerosis*
	• Abdominal aortic aneurysm
	• Diabetes mellitus
	  Age ≥ 40 years
	  15-Year duration for age ≥ 30 years (DM1) Microvascular disease
	• Chronic kidney disease (age ≥ 50 years)
	  eGFR <60 mL/min/1.73 m2 or ACR > 3 mg/mmol
			• statins generally not indicated

Lipid targets LDL-C: _____   or   Apo B: _____

† apoB: apolipoprotein B stat, CVD: cardiovascular disease, FRS: Framingham Risk Score, HDL-C: high-density lipoprotein cholesterol, LDL-C: low-density lipoprotein cholesterol.
* Statins indicated as initial therapy
** Consider LDL-C < 1.8 mmol/L for subjects with acute coronary syndrome (ACS) within past 3 months

1 Adapted from: D'Agostino RB et al.(i). General cardiovascular risk profile for use in primary care. The Framingham Heart Study. Circ 2008;117:743–53.
2 Adapted from: Genest J et al.(i). 2009 Canadian Cardiovascular Society/Canadian Guidelines for the diagnosis and treatment of dyslipidemia and prevention of cardiovascular disease in the adult. Can J Cardiol 2009;25(10):567–579.
3 Adapted from: Anderson T et al.(i). 2012 Update of the Canadian Cardiovascular Society guidelines for the diagnosis and treatment of dyslipidemia for the prevention of cardiovascular disease in the adult. Can J Cardiol. 2013;29(2):151-167.

Provided courtesy of Canadian Cardiovascular Society
Leadership. Knowledge. Community.

Figure 2-12 Estimation of 10-year risk of nonfatal myocardial infarction or coronary death (Framingham Heart Study) in men and women.

Xanthomatosis,

Hypertension,

Myocardial infarction,

Atherosclerosis,

Biliary cirrhosis,

Extrahepatic biliary, stress, and nephrotic syndrome: *The pathophysiologic mechanisms of the association of cholesterol with these diseases are not well known. The association has been noted through observation.*

▼ Decreased Levels

Malabsorption,

Malnutrition,

Advanced cancer: *Most of the cholesterol is synthesized from fat eaten in the diet. When dietary intake is decreased, fat levels and, subsequently, cholesterol levels fall.*

Hyperthyroidism,

Cholesterol-lowering medication,

Pernicious anemia,

Hemolytic anemia,

Sepsis/stress,

Liver disease,

Acute myocardial infarction: *The pathophysiologic mechanisms of the association of cholesterol with these diseases are not well known. The association has been noted through observation.*

RELATED TESTS

Apolipoproteins (p. 116). These polypeptides are associated with lipoproteins and have been used as accurate indicators of risk for CHD.

Lipoprotein (p. 355). HDL and LDL play an important role in the transport of lipids in the bloodstream. Their measurements, too, have been used in the assessment of risk for CHD.

Triglycerides (p. 523). This test is a measure of total triglycerides in the blood. It is a part of the lipid profile.

Cholinesterase (CHS, Pseudocholinesterase, Cholinesterase RBC, Red Blood Cell Cholinesterase, Acetylcholinesterase, Dibucaine Inhibition)

NORMAL FINDINGS

Serum cholinesterase: **8–18 U/mL**

Red blood cell (RBC) cholinesterase: **5–10 U/L**

Dibucaine inhibition: 79%–84%

Values vary with laboratory test methods.

INDICATIONS

This test is performed to detect pseudocholinesterase deficiency before anaesthesia induction or to detect exposure to phosphate poisoning.

TEST EXPLANATION

Cholinesterases hydrolyze acetylcholine and also other choline esters and thereby regulate nerve impulse transmission at the nerve synapse and neuromuscular junction. There are two types of cholinesterases: acetylcholinesterase, also known as "true cholinesterase," and pseudocholinesterase. True cholinesterase exists primarily in the RBCs and nerve tissue. It is not in the serum. Pseudocholinesterase, on the other hand, exists in the serum. Deficiencies in either of these enzymes can be acquired or congenital.

Because succinylcholine (the muscle relaxant most commonly used during anaesthesia induction) is inactivated by pseudocholinesterase, people with an inherited deficiency of pseudocholinesterase enzyme exhibit increased or prolonged effects of succinylcholine. Patients with a genetic variant of pseudocholinesterase may have a nonfunctioning form of pseudocholinesterase and also experience prolonged effects of succinylcholine administration. Muscle paralysis is prolonged and apnea occurs after anaesthesia induction in these patients. This situation can be avoided by measuring serum cholinesterase (pseudocholinesterase) on all patients with a family history of prolonged apnea after surgery. Patients with a nonfunctioning variant of pseudocholinesterase have normal total quantitative pseudocholinesterase levels and yet have prolonged paralytic effects of succinylcholine; therefore, a second test (dibucaine inhibition) is usually also performed. Dibucaine is a local anaesthetic that inhibits the function of normal pseudocholinesterase. The *dibucaine inhibition number* is the percentage of pseudocholinesterase activity that is inhibited when dibucaine is added to the patient's serum sample. If the total pseudocholinesterase level is normal, and dibucaine numbers are low, the presence of a nonfunctioning pseudocholinesterase variant is suspected and the patient will be at risk for succinylcholine-induced prolonged paralysis.

A common form of acquired cholinesterase deficiency, either true cholinesterase or pseudocholinesterase, is caused by overexposure to pesticides or organophosphates. Individuals chronically exposed to these chemicals at work are often monitored by the frequent testing of RBC cholinesterase levels. Other potential causes of reduced cholinesterase levels include chronic liver diseases, malnutrition, and hypoalbuminemia. When found in the amniotic fluid, increased cholinesterase levels represent strong evidence of a neural tube defect.

INTERFERING FACTORS

- Pregnancy decreases test values.
- It is important to recognize that pseudocholinesterase levels cannot be measured in postoperative patients in the recovery room if the patient is not regaining muscular function, because often one or more of the above drugs may be given during the surgery and could invalidate the results.
- Drugs that may cause *decreases* in values include atropine, caffeine, codeine, estrogens, morphine sulphate, neostigmine, oral contraceptives, phenothiazines, quinidine, theophylline, steroids, and vitamin K.

PROCEDURE AND PATIENT CARE

Before

- Explain the procedure to the patient.
- Inform the patient that no fasting is required.
- If the test is performed to whether a presurgical patient is at risk for cholinesterase deficiency, it should be performed several days before the planned surgery.

- If the patient is taking medications that could alter test results, withholding those medications for 12 to 24 hours before the test may be recommended.

During
- Collect a venous blood sample in a red-top tube.

After
- Apply pressure or a pressure dressing to the venipuncture site.
- Assess the venipuncture site for bleeding.

TEST RESULTS AND CLINICAL SIGNIFICANCE

▲ Increased Levels

Reticulocytosis: *Increased RBC precursors are associated with higher levels of true cholinesterase.*
Hyperlipidemia,
Nephrosis,
Diabetes: *Increased levels are observed without any known pathophysiologic condition.*

▼ Decreased Levels

Poisoning from organic phosphate insecticides: *These chemicals inhibit the activity of cholinesterases.*
Hepatocellular disease,
Individuals with congenital enzyme deficiency: *Cholinesterases are not synthesized.*
Malnutrition and other forms of hypoalbuminemia: *Albumin is important in the transport and function of cholinesterases.*

RELATED TEST

Acetylcholine Receptor Antibody (p. 28). This is a measurement of an antibody that blocks the activity of cholinesterases. It is commonly found in patients with myasthenia gravis.

Chromosome Karyotype (Blood Chromosome Analysis, Chromosome Studies, Cytogenetics, Karyotype)

NORMAL FINDINGS

46 chromosomes
Female: 44 autosomes plus two X chromosomes; karyotype: 46,XX
Male: 44 autosomes plus one X chromosome and one Y chromosome; karyotype: 46,XY

INDICATIONS

This test is used to study an individual's chromosome makeup to determine chromosomal defects associated with disease or the risk for developing disease.

TEST EXPLANATION

The term *karyotyping* refers to the arrangement of cell chromosomes from largest to smallest in order to analyze their number and structure. Variations in either can produce numerous developmental abnormalities and diseases. A normal karyotype of chromosomes consists of a pattern of 22 pairs of autosomal chromosomes and a pair of sex chromosomes: XY (male) or XX (female). Chromosomal karyotype abnormalities can be congenital or acquired. These karyotype abnormalities can occur because of duplication, deletion, translocation, reciprocation, or genetic rearrangement.

Chromosome karyotyping is useful in evaluating congenital anomalies, developmental delay, growth retardation, delayed onset of puberty, infertility, hypogonadism, primary amenorrhea, ambiguous genitalia, chronic myelogenous leukemia, neoplasm, recurrent miscarriage, prenatal diagnosis of serious congenital diseases (especially when advanced maternal age is a factor), Turner's syndrome, Klinefelter's syndrome, Down syndrome, and other suspected genetic disorders. To determine the cause of stillbirth or miscarriage, the products of conception also can be studied.

The most common form of karyotyping is performed by banding techniques. This technique provides a method of pairing similar chromosomes on the basis of their size, location of the centromere (constriction that divides the chromosome into long and short arms) and other constrictions, ratio of long to short arms, satellite DNA, and banding patterns. With this method, a characteristic karyotype is determined. An extensive nomenclature system for the types has been developed.

Special chromosome studies can be performed on cells grown in special media to identify certain chromosome abnormalities. DNA testing is now possible through the use of DNA probes and DNA linkage studies.

PROCEDURE AND PATIENT CARE

Before

- Explain the procedure to the patient.
- Determine how the specimen will be collected.
- Obtain preparation guidelines from the laboratory if indicated.
- Be aware that many patients are fearful of the test results and require considerable emotional support.
- Check whether informed consent is required in your province.

During

- Specimens for chromosome analysis can be obtained from numerous sources. Leukocytes from a peripheral venipuncture site are the most easily obtained and most often used for this study.
- Bone marrow biopsy samples and surgical specimens are also sometimes be used as sources for analysis.
- During pregnancy, specimens can be collected by amniocentesis (see p. 660) and chorionic villus sampling (see p. 1134).
- To determine the reason for loss of a fetus, fetal tissue or products of conception can be studied as well.
- Smears and stains of buccal mucosal cells are less costly but do not yield results as accurate as those of other tissue for karyotyping.

After

- Aftercare depends on how the specimen was collected.
- Inform the patient that test results are generally not available for weeks to several months.
- If an abnormality is identified, the entire family line may be tested. This can be exhaustive and expensive.
- If the test results show an abnormality, encourage the patient to verbalize his or her feelings. Provide emotional support.

TABLE 2-14	Common Chromosome Abnormalities
Chromosome Abnormality	**Clinical Manifestation**
Trisomy 21	Down syndrome
Single X	Turner's syndrome
Extra X in male (XXY)	Klinefelter's syndrome
5p deletion	Cri-du-chat syndrome
15q deletion	Prader-Willi syndrome
Partial 3q trisomy	Cornelia de Lange syndrome
Fragile X	Developmental delay
X centromere dislocation	Roberts syndrome
Philadelphia chromosome	Chronic myelogenous leukemia, acute myelogenous leukemia

TEST RESULTS AND CLINICAL SIGNIFICANCE

Abnormal Findings

Chromosome abnormalities can be a cause of congenital anomalies, developmental delay, growth retardation, delayed puberty, infertility, hypogonadism, primary amenorrhea, ambiguous genitalia, chronic myelogenous leukemia, neoplasm, recurrent miscarriage, prenatal diagnosis (e.g., for Down syndrome, Tay-Sachs disease, sickle cell disease) in situations of advanced maternal age, Turner's syndrome, Klinefelter's syndrome, and Down syndrome. Table 2-14 lists a number of the commonly known abnormalities.

RELATED TESTS

Barr Body Analysis. This is an inexpensive test for detecting chromatin material (X chromatin).
    Genetic Testing (p. 1139). This is another method of DNA testing.

Coagulating Factor Concentration (Factor Assay, Coagulating Factors, Blood-Clotting Factors)

NORMAL FINDINGS

Factor	Reference Value (% of "Normal")
II	80–120
V	50–150
VII	65–140
VIII	55–145
IX	60–140
X	45–155
XI	65–135
XII	50–150

INDICATIONS

The coagulating factor concentration test measures the concentration of specific coagulating factors in the blood.

TEST EXPLANATION

These tests measure the quantity of each specific factor suspected to be responsible for putative defects in hemostasis. Testing is available to measure the quantity of the factors listed in Table 2-15. When these factors exist in concentrations below their "minimal hemostatic level," clotting is impaired. These minimal hemostatic levels vary according to the factor involved.

Deficiencies of these factors may be a result of inherited genetic defects, acquired diseases, or drug therapy. Common medical conditions associated with abnormal factor concentrations are listed in Table 2-16. It is important to identify the exact factor or factors involved in the coagulating defect so that replacement of appropriate blood components can be administered (Figure 2-13; see also Table 2-15).

TABLE 2-15	Coagulation Factors*			
Factor	Name	Quantitation of Minimum Hemostatic Normal Values[†]	Abnormal Coagulation Tests Associated With Deficiency	Blood Components to Provide Specific Factor
I	Fibrinogen	2.0–5.0 g/L (60–100 mg/dL)	PT, aPTT	C, FFP, FWB
II	Prothrombin	11–12.5 sec	PT	P, WB, FFP, FWB
III	Tissue factor or thromboplastin	Quantitative sodium (qNa)	PT	
IV	Calcium	See calcium, p. 152		
V	Proaccelerin	50%–100% of control	PT, aPTT	FFP, FWB
VII	Stable factor	50%–100 % of control	PT	P, WB, FFP, FWB
VIII	Antihemophilic factor	50%–150% of control	aPTT	C, FFP, factor VIII concentrate
IX	Christmas factor	50%–150% of control (4 mg/L)	aPTT	FFP, FWB
X	Stuart factor	50%–150% of control (12 mg/L)	PT, aPTT	P, WB, FFP, FWB
XI	Plasma thromboplastin antecedent	65%–135% of control (7 mg/dL)	aPTT	P, WB, FFP, FWB
XII	Hageman factor	50%–150% of control (23–47 mg/mL)	aPTT	
XIII	Fibrin stabilizing factor	Clot is insoluble in a 5-M urea concentration for at least 24 hours		P, C, factor XIII concentrate

aPTT, Activated partial thromboplastin time; *C*, cryoprecipitate; *FFP*, fresh-frozen plasma; *FWB*, fresh whole blood (<24 hours old); *P*, unfrozen banked plasma; *PT*, prothrombin time; *WB*, banked whole blood.
*Recombinant factors are now available for factors VII, VIII, IX, and XIII. Concentrates are also now available for factors II, VII, VIII, IX, and XIII.
[†]Values in purple type are in SI units; values that follow in parentheses are in conventional units.

TABLE 2-16 Conditions Associated With Abnormal Factor Concentrations

Factor	Increased (Excess)	Decreased (Deficiency)
I (Fibrinogen)	Acute inflammatory reactions Trauma Heart disease Cigarette smoking	Liver disease (hepatitis or cirrhosis) DIC Congenital deficiency
II (Prothrombin)	ND	Vitamin K deficiency Liver disease Congenital deficiency Warfarin ingestion
V (Proaccelerin)	ND	Liver disease DIC Fibrinolysis
VII (Proconvertin [stable factor])	ND	Congenital deficiency Vitamin K deficiency Liver disease Warfarin ingestion
VIII (Antihemophilic factor)	Acute inflammatory reactions Trauma/stress Pregnancy Birth control pills	Congenital deficiency (e.g., hemophilia A) DIC
von Willebrand's factor	ND	Congenital deficiency (e.g., von Willebrand's disease) Some acute and chronic leukemias
IX (Christmas factor)	ND	Congenital deficiency (e.g., hemophilia B) Liver disease Nephrotic syndrome Warfarin ingestion DIC Vitamin K deficiency
X (Stuart factor)	ND	Congenital deficiency Liver disease Warfarin ingestion Vitamin K deficiency
XII (Hageman factor)	ND	Congenital deficiency Liver disease DIC

DIC, Disseminated intravascular coagulation; *ND*, not defined (no common diseases states associated with excess of this factor).

The hemostasis and coagulation system is a homeostatic balance between factors encouraging clotting and factors encouraging clot dissolution. The first reaction of the body to active bleeding is blood vessel constriction. In small-vessel injury, this may be enough to stop bleeding. In large-vessel injury, hemostasis is necessary to form a clot that durably plugs the hole until healing can occur. The primary phase of the hemostatic mechanism involves platelet aggregation to the blood vessel (Figure 2-14). Secondary hemostasis then occurs. Secondary hemostasis can be

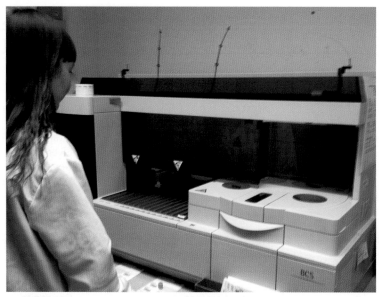

Figure 2-13 Siemens automated hemostasis analyzer. This system can analyze multiple factors involved in hemostasis.

broken down into a series of four reactions that culminate in the production of thrombin and fibrin. These substances act to create a blood clot at the site of vascular injury. In the first reaction, sometimes called the *intrinsic phase of coagulation,* factor XII and other proteins form a complex on the subendothelial collagen in the injured blood vessel. Through a series of reactions, activated factor XI (XIa) is formed and activates factor IX (IXa). In a complex formed by factors VIII, IX, and X, activated factor X (Xa) is formed.

At the same time, the second reaction, the *extrinsic pathway,* is activated and a complex is formed between tissue factor and factor VII. Activated factor VII (VIIa) then is formed. Factor VIIa can directly activate factor X. Alternatively, factor VIIa can activate factors IX and X together. In the third reaction, factor X is activated by the proteases generated in the two previous reactions (factors VIIa and IXa in concert with factor VIII). As an alternative, factor VIIa can activate factors IX and X directly. In the fourth reaction, sometimes referred to as the *common pathway,* factor Xa converts prothrombin in the presence of factor V, calcium, and phospholipid on the platelet surface. Thrombin, in turn, converts fibrinogen to fibrin, which is polymerized into a stable clot. Thrombin also activates factor VIII to stimulate further platelet aggregation and fibrin polymerization.

Almost immediately, three major activators of the fibrinolytic system act on plasminogen, which had previously been absorbed into the clot, to form plasmin. Plasmin causes the fibrin polymer to degenerate into fragments, which are cleared by macrophages.

Roman numerals have been assigned by the order in which the factor had been identified, not by their order in the hemostatic mechanism just described (Table 2-16 lists factor names and routine coagulation test abnormalities associated with factor deficiency).

Fibrinogen, like many other of the coagulation proteins, is considered an acute-phase reactant protein, and its levels are elevated in many severe illnesses. It is also considered a risk factor for coronary heart disease and stroke. Prothrombin is a vitamin K–dependent clotting factor. Its production in the liver requires vitamin K. This vitamin is fat soluble and is dependent on bile for absorption. Bile duct obstruction or malabsorption causes a vitamin K deficiency and results in a reduced quantity of prothrombin and other vitamin K–dependent factors (VII, IX, X). It usually takes approximately 3 weeks before body stores of vitamin K are exhausted.

Hemostasis and Fibrinolysis

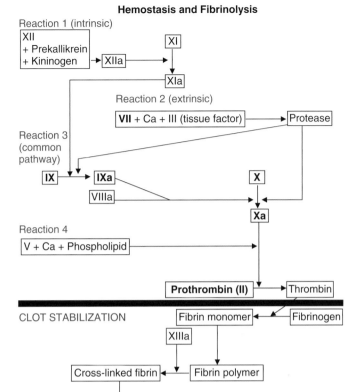

Figure 2-14 Secondary hemostasis (fibrin clot formation) and fibrinolysis (fibrin clot dissolution). Primary hemostasis involves platelet plugging of the injured blood vessel. Secondary hemostasis, as simply described here, takes place most rapidly on the platelet surface after attachment to the fractured endothelium. Four different reactions result in the formation of fibrin. As seen beneath the dark line in the figure, the fibrin clot supports the platelet clump so that the clot does not get swept away by the tremendous "shear forces" of the fast-moving blood cells. Fibrinolysis follows formation of the fibrin clot in order to prevent complete occlusion of the injured blood vessel. Vitamin K–dependent coagulating factors are in boldface type.

Factor VIII is actually a complex molecule with two components. The first component is related to hemophilia A and is involved in the hemostatic mechanism as described previously. The second component is the von Willebrand's factor and is related to von Willebrand's disease. This second component is involved in platelet adhesion and aggregation. Factor XII deficiency is a common cause of prolonged activated partial thromboplastin time in a nonbleeding patient. Patients with factor XII deficiency have been observed to be at increased risk for myocardial infarction and venous thrombosis.

INTERFERING FACTORS

- Many of these proteins are heat sensitive, and their levels decrease the longer the specimen is kept at room temperature.
- Pregnancy or the use of contraceptive medication can increase levels of several of these factors, especially factors VIII and IX. A mild deficiency could be masked.
- Many of these protein coagulation factors are acute-phase reactant proteins. Acute illness, stress, exercise, or inflammation could raise levels.

PROCEDURE AND PATIENT CARE

Before
- ✗ Explain the procedure to the patient.
- ✗ Inform the patient that no fasting is required.

During
- Collect a venous blood sample in a blue-top tube.

After
- Apply pressure or a pressure dressing to the venipuncture site.
- Assess the venipuncture site for bleeding, especially if the patient has had other episodes of clotting deficiency.
- Deliver the blood specimen to the laboratory as soon as possible.
- Freeze the specimen if testing is not going to be performed immediately, because these proteins are very labile.

TEST RESULTS AND CLINICAL SIGNIFICANCE

Fibrinogen
▲ **Increased Levels**
Acute inflammatory reactions,
Trauma: *Fibrinogen is an acute-phase reactant protein.*
Coronary heart disease,
Cigarette smoking: *Elevated fibrinogen levels are merely an observation with no known pathophysiologic process.*

▼ **Decreased Levels**
Liver disease (hepatitis or cirrhosis): *Fibrinogen is not made in adequate volume.*
Consumptive coagulopathy (disseminated intravascular coagulation),
Action of fibrinolysins: *Fibrinolysins act to destroy fibrinogen in the serum.*

Prothrombin
▼ **Decreased Levels**
Vitamin K deficiency,
Liver disease: *Synthesis is diminished.*

Proaccelerin
▼ **Decreased Levels**
Liver disease: *Synthesis is diminished.*

Proconvertin Stable Factor
▼ **Decreased Levels**
Inherited deficiency,
Vitamin K deficiency,
Liver disease,
Warfarin (Coumadin) therapy: *Synthesis is diminished.*

Antihemophilic Factor
▲ **Increased Levels**
Acute inflammatory reactions,
Trauma/stress,
Pregnancy: *Factor VIII is an acute-phase reactant protein.*

▼ **Decreased Levels**
Inherited deficiency (hemophilia A): *Hemophilia A is linked to a sex-linked gene on the X chromosome.*
   Girls and women are rarely affected, because the other X chromosome has a normal gene.
Consumptive coagulation: *This factor is used up, and synthesis cannot match the demand.*

von Willebrand's Factor
▼ **Decreased Levels (von Willebrand's Disease)**
Inherited deficiency,
Autoimmune disease: *Von Willebrand's factor is reduced in quantity.*

Christmas Factor
▼ **Decreased Levels**
Inherited deficiency (hemophilia B),
Liver disease,
Nephrotic syndrome,
Warfarin (Coumadin) therapy: *Synthesis is diminished.*
Consumptive coagulation: *This factor is used up, and synthesis cannot match the demand.*

Stuart Factor
▼ **Decreased Levels**
Inherited deficiency

Hageman Factor
▼ **Decreased Levels**
Inherited deficiency,
Vitamin K deficiency,
Liver disease,
Warfarin (Coumadin) therapy: *Synthesis is diminished.*
Consumptive coagulation: *This factor is used up, and synthesis cannot match the demand.*

RELATED TESTS

Partial Thromboplastin Time, Activated (p. 396). This test is used to evaluate the intrinsic system and the common pathway of clot formation.

Prothrombin Time (p. 446). This test is used to evaluate the adequacy of the extrinsic system and common pathway in the clotting mechanism.

Fibrinogen (p. 254). This coagulating factor is discussed separately.

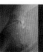

Cold Agglutinins

NORMAL FINDINGS

Screen: negative
Titer: no agglutination ≤1:64

INDICATION

Cold agglutinins are used to identify and investigate cold agglutinin syndrome and unusual infections, such as *Mycoplasma pneumoniae*.

TEST EXPLANATION

Cold agglutinins are antibodies (usually IgM) to erythrocytes. All individuals have circulating antibodies directed against red blood cells, but their concentrations are often too low to trigger disease or symptoms (titers <1:64). In individuals with *cold agglutinin syndrome*, these antibodies are much higher (>1:512). At body temperatures of 28 to 31°C, such as those encountered during winter months, these antibodies can cause a variety of symptoms (from chronic anemia caused by intravascular hemolysis or extravascular sequestration of affected RBCs leading to acrocyanosis of the ears, fingers, or toes because of local blood stasis in the skin capillaries).

There are two forms of cold agglutinin disease, primary and secondary. The primary form has no precipitating cause. Secondary cold agglutinin disease is a result of an underlying condition, notably *Mycoplasma pneumoniae*. The cold agglutinins test is not specific for *Mycoplasma pneumoniae* and is not recommended to diagnose the disease. It does provide supportive information, however. *Mycoplasma pneumoniae* serum antibodies (IgG and IgM) (p. 376) are also supportive of *Mycoplasma* infection.

Other possible conditions associated with cold agglutinins include influenza, mononucleosis, rheumatoid arthritis, lymphomas, HIV, Epstein-Barr virus, and cytomegalovirus. Temperature regulation is important for the performance of this test. Under no circumstances should the cold agglutinin specimen be refrigerated.

The cold agglutinin screen is performed on all specimens first to identify most of those with titer values in the normal range. If the screen is negative, no titration is required. If the screen is positive, a titer with serial saline dilutions is performed.

INTERFERING FACTORS

■ Some antibiotics (penicillin and cephalosporins) can interfere with the development of cold agglutinins.

PROCEDURE AND PATIENT CARE

Before
🖎 Explain the procedure to the patient.
🖎 Tell the patient that no fasting is required.

During
• Collect venous blood in a red-top tube.

After
• Apply pressure to the venipuncture site.
• Transport the specimen immediately to the laboratory.

TEST RESULTS AND CLINICAL SIGNIFICANCE

▲ Increased Levels
Mycoplasma pneumoniae infection,
Viral illness,
Infectious mononucleosis,
Multiple myeloma,
Scleroderma,
Cirrhosis,
Staphylococcemia,
Thymic tumour,
Influenza,
Rheumatoid arthritis,
Lymphoma,
Systemic lupus erythematosus,
Primary cold agglutinin disease: *These diseases are associated with high titers of cold agglutinins of varying concentrations.*

RELATED TESTS

Mycoplasma pneumonia Antibodies (p. 376). The serologic identification of IgG and IgM antibodies to *Mycoplasma* are used to support the clinical diagnosis of the infection.

Complement Assay (C3 and C4 Complement)

NORMAL FINDINGS

Total hemolytic complement: **30–75 kU/L (30–75 U/mL)**
C2: **0.01–0.40 g/L (1–4 mg/dL)**
C3: **0.75–1.75 g/L (75–175 mg/dL)**
C4: **0.22–0.45 g/L (22–45 mg/dL)**

INDICATIONS

Measurements of complement are used primarily to diagnose angioedema and to monitor the activity of disease in patients with systemic lupus erythematosus (SLE), nephritis, membranoproliferative nephritis, or poststreptococcal nephritis.

TEST EXPLANATION

Serum complement is a group of globulin proteins that act as enzymes. These enzymes facilitate the immunologic and inflammatory response. The complement system is important for destroying foreign cells and isolating "foreign" antigens. The total complement, sometimes labelled CH50, is made up of nine major components, C1 through C9. Besides these major components, there are some subcomponents and "inhibitor" components involved in the system. Classic complement activation starts when an immunoglobulin M or G (IgM or IgG) antibody binds with the C1q subcomponent of C1. C1 activates C4, which activates C2 and so on to C9. There are also alternative pathways for the activation of this system.

Once activated, complement acts to increase vascular permeability, allowing antibodies and white blood cells (WBCs) to be delivered to the area of the immune/antigen complex. Complement also acts to increase chemotaxis (attracting WBCs to the area), phagocytosis, and immune adherence of the antibody to antigen. These processes are vital in the normal inflammatory response.

Total complement can be measured by hemolytic tests. For this test, the patient's blood is mixed with antibody-coated red blood cells (RBCs) of sheep. The end point is when 50% of the RBCs are lysed. The patient's blood is serially diluted, and results are reported in complement units per millilitre. Specimens for complement assays may be sent out to reference laboratories. These tests assess the overall function of the entire complement system. The C3 and C4 components can be quantitated by direct immunologic measurement. These subcomponents are measured when total complement has been found to be reduced. C3 makes up the majority of the component of complement. It is made in the liver and, to a lesser degree, in the spleen, skin, and other lymphoid nodules. C4 is made in the bone and lungs.

Reduced complement levels can be congenital, as in hereditary angioedema. Hereditary angioedema is a congenital lack of a C1 "inhibitor" (often called *C1 esterase*). The complement system is overly activated, and the complement components are consumed or used up. As a consequence, serum levels fall.

Acquired complement deficiency occurs with diseases that are associated with increased antibody/antigen complexes. Again, these complexes serve to act as complement activators. If the presence of these complexes is chronic, the complement system is overly activated, and the complement components are consumed or used up. As a consequence, serum levels fall. Diseases associated with immune complexes such as those described include serum sickness, systemic lupus erythematosus, infectious endocarditis, renal transplant rejection, vasculitis, and some forms of glomerulonephritis. When these diseases are treated successfully, complement levels can return to normal.

Complement component levels are increased after the onset of various acute or chronic inflammatory diseases or acute tissue damage. This development is very similar to that of an acute-phase reactant protein.

INTERFERING FACTORS

- C3 is very unstable at room temperature. If the specimen is left standing for more than 1 hour, complement levels could be artificially low. The serum should be separated out and frozen immediately when the specimen is received.

PROCEDURE AND PATIENT CARE

Before
🖉 Explain the procedure to the patient.
🖉 Inform the patient that no fasting or special preparation is required.

During
• Collect a venous blood sample in a red-top tube.

After
• Apply pressure or a pressure dressing to the venipuncture site.
• Observe the venipuncture site for bleeding.

TEST RESULTS AND CLINICAL SIGNIFICANCE

▲ Increased Levels

Rheumatic fever (acute),
Myocardial infarction (acute),
Ulcerative colitis,
Inflammatory illnesses, stress, and trauma: *Complement can develop in a manner very similar to the development of an acute-phase reactant protein. With these illnesses, complement is increased.*
Cancer: *The pathophysiologic mechanism underlying this observation is unknown.*

▼ Decreased Levels

Hereditary angioedema: *Hereditary angioedema is a congenital lack of a C1 "inhibitor" (C1 esterase). The complement system is overly activated, and the complement components are consumed or used up. As a consequence, serum levels fall.*
Severe liver diseases such as hepatitis or cirrhosis: *The liver is the site of synthesis of many of the complement components. Synthesis is decreased in the presence of liver disease. As a consequence, serum levels fall.*
Autoimmune disease (SLE, glomerulonephritis, lupus nephritis, rheumatoid arthritis [severe and active], Sjögren syndrome),
Serum sickness (immune complex disease),
Renal transplant rejection (acute): *These diseases are associated with the increased presence of antibody/antigen complexes, which serve to act as complement activators. The complement system is overly activated, and complement components are consumed or used up. As a consequence, serum levels fall.*
Protein malnutrition,
Anemia,
Malnutrition: *These diseases are associated with protein depletion. Complement is a protein, and its synthesis can be expected to be reduced in these illnesses.*
Infection such as Gram-negative sepsis or bacterial endocarditis,
Glomerulonephritis (specifically poststreptococcal and membranoproliferative): *Alternative pathways of complement activation develop. The complement system is overly activated, and complement components are consumed or used up. As a consequence, serum levels fall.*

COMPLETE BLOOD CELL COUNT AND DIFFERENTIAL COUNT (CBC AND DIFF)

The complete blood cell count (CBC) and differential count are a series of tests of the peripheral blood that provide a tremendous amount of information about the hematologic system and many

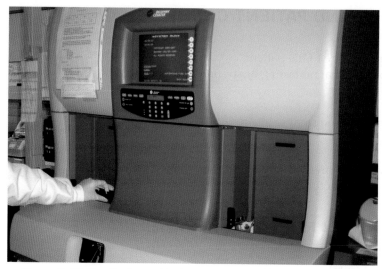

Figure 2-15 The Beckman Coulter automated CBC analyzer can perform many CBC tests in a few minutes. The automated system will notify the technologist if any significant abnormality is noted. Those findings will be corroborated by individual testing.

other organ systems. They are inexpensively, easily, and rapidly performed as screening tests. The CBC and differential count include automated multimeasurement of the following studies (Figure 2-15), which are discussed separately:

Red blood cell (RBC) count (see p. 452)
Hemoglobin (see p. 299)
Hematocrit (see p. 295)
RBC indices (see p. 456)
   Mean corpuscular volume
   Mean corpuscular hemoglobin
   Mean corpuscular hemoglobin concentration
   RBC distribution width (p. 456)
White blood cell (WBC) count and differential count (see p. 549)
   Neutrophils (polynucleated cells, segmented cells, band cells, stab cells)
   Lymphocytes
   Monocytes
   Eosinophils
   Basophils
Blood smear (see p. 738)
Platelet count (see p. 416)
Mean platelet volume (see p. 419)

Coombs Test, Direct (Direct Antiglobulin Test [DAT])

NORMAL FINDINGS

Negative; no agglutination

INDICATIONS

This test is performed to identify immune hemolysis (lysis of red blood cells [RBCs]) or to investigate hemolytic transfusion reactions (Box 2-4).

TEST EXPLANATION

Most of the antibodies to RBCs are directed against the ABO/Rh blood grouping antigens, such as those that occur in hemolytic anemia of the newborn or blood transfusion of incompatible blood. When a transfusion reaction occurs (Box 2-5), the Coombs test can detect the patient's antibodies coating the transfused RBCs. The Coombs test is therefore useful in evaluating suspected transfusion reactions.

Non–blood-grouping antigens can develop on the RBC membrane and stimulate formation of antibodies. Drugs such as levodopa or methyldopa can initial this process. Also, in some diseases, antibodies not originally directed against the patient's RBCs can attach to the RBCs and cause hemolysis, which can be detected by the direct Coombs test. Examples of such antibodies are these:

- Antibodies developed in reaction to drugs such as penicillin
- Autoantibodies formed in various autoimmune diseases
- Antibodies developed in some patients with advanced cancer (e.g., lymphoma)

In many cases, the production of these autoantibodies against RBCs is not associated with any identifiable disease, and the resulting hemolytic anemia is therefore considered idiopathic.

BOX 2-4	Symptoms of Transfusion Reaction

- Fever
- Chills
- Rash
- Flank/back pain
- Bloody urine
- Fainting or dizziness

BOX 2-5	Diagnostic Testing for Suspected Hemolytic Blood Transfusions

- Complete blood cell count (CBC)
- Electrolytes
- Blood urea nitrogen (BUN), creatinine measurements
- Direct Coombs test (recipient blood, before and after transfusion)
- ABO blood typing on donor and recipient blood
- RH typing on donor and recipient blood
- Blood crossmatch
- Prothrombin time
- Partial thromboplastin time (PTT)
- Fibrin split products
- Haptoglobin
- Bilirubin
- Blood cultures on donor and recipient blood
- Urine for free hemoglobin-dipstick testing

The direct Coombs test demonstrates that RBCs have been attacked by antibodies in the patient's bloodstream. The RBCs of patients suspected of having antibodies against RBCs are washed to eliminate any excess free gamma globulins. Coombs serum is added to the RBCs. If the RBCs have antibodies on them, Coombs serum causes agglutination. The greater the quantity of antibodies against RBCs, the more clumping occurs. Such clumping is considered a positive test result, with clumping on a scale of trace amounts to 4. If the RBCs are not coated with auto-antibodies against RBCs (immunoglobulins), agglutination will not occur; this is a negative test result.

INTERFERING FACTORS

- Antiphospholipid antibodies (see p. 76, anticardiolipin antibodies) can cause a false-positive DAT.
- Drugs that may cause *false-positive* results include ampicillin, captopril, cephalosporins, chlor-promazine, chlorpropamide, hydralazine, indomethacin (Indocid), insulin, isoniazid (INH), levodopa, methyldopa, penicillin, phenytoin (Dilantin), procainamide, quinidine, quinine, ri-fampin, streptomycin, sulphonamides, and tetracyclines.

PROCEDURE AND PATIENT CARE

Before

- Explain the procedure to the patient.
- Inform the patient that no fasting is required.

During

- Collect a venous blood sample in a red-top or lavender-top tube.
- Use venous blood from the umbilical cord to detect the presence of antibodies in the newborn.

After

- Apply pressure or a pressure dressing to the venipuncture site.
- Assess the venipuncture site for bleeding.

TEST RESULTS AND CLINICAL SIGNIFICANCE

Hemolytic disease of the newborn,
Incompatible blood transfusion reaction: *Antibodies to the patient's RBCs have been created by mixing of incompatible blood grouping antigens.*
Lymphoma,
Autoimmune hemolytic anemia (rheumatoid/collagen diseases such as systemic lupus erythe-matosus [SLE], rheumatoid arthritis): *Autoantibodies formed in these illnesses attach to RBCs.*
Mycoplasmal infection,
Infectious mononucleosis: *In these illnesses, antibodies develop and, for unknown reasons, attach to the RBCs.*
Hemolytic anemia after heart bypass: *Autoantibodies formed during the use of the heart/lung bypass machine attach to RBCs.*
Adult hemolytic anemia (idiopathic): *Autoantibodies not otherwise associated with any other disease attach to RBCs.*

RELATED TEST

Coombs Test, Indirect (see following test p. 191). This test is used to detect antibodies against RBCs in the serum. It is most commonly used for screening potential blood recipients.

Coombs Test, Indirect (Blood Antibody Screening, Indirect Antiglobulin Test [IAT])

NORMAL FINDINGS

Negative; no agglutination

INDICATIONS

This test is used to detect antibodies against red blood cells (RBCs) in the serum. This laboratory method is used most commonly for screening potential blood recipients.

TEST EXPLANATION

The indirect Coombs test detects circulating antibodies against RBCs. The major purpose of this test is to determine whether the patient has minor serum antibodies (other than the major ABO/Rh system) to RBCs before receiving a blood transfusion. Therefore, this test is the "screening" portion of the "type and screen" routinely performed for blood compatibility testing (crossmatching in the blood bank). This test is also used to detect other agglutinins, such as cold agglutinins that are associated with mycoplasmal infections.

    This test is performed in two stages. In the first stage, a small amount of the recipient's serum is added to donor RBCs containing known antigens on their surfaces. In the second stage, Coombs serum is added after the test RBCs have been cleansed of any free globulins. If antibodies exist in the patient's serum, agglutination occurs. In blood transfusion screening, visible agglutination indicates that the recipient has antibodies to the donor's RBCs. If the recipient has no antibodies against the donor's RBCs, agglutination does not occur; transfusion should then proceed safely without any transfusion reaction. Circulating antibodies against RBCs also may occur in an Rh-negative pregnant woman who is carrying an Rh-positive fetus.

INTERFERING FACTORS

Drugs that may cause *false-positive* results include antiarrhythmics, antituberculins, cephalosporins, chlorpromazine, insulin, levodopa, methyldopa, penicillins, phenytoin (Dilantin), quinidine, sulphonamides, and tetracyclines.

Clinical Priorities

- This test is the "screening" portion of the "type and screen" routinely performed for blood compatibility testing.
- If the recipient of the blood transfusion has antibodies to the donor's RBCs, agglutination occurs. The donor's blood cannot be used for that recipient.
- If the recipient has no antibodies to the donor's RBCs, agglutination does not occur. Transfusion should then proceed safely without any transfusion reaction.

PROCEDURE AND PATIENT CARE

Before

☒ Explain the procedure to the patient.
☒ Inform the patient that no fasting is required.

During

• Collect a venous blood sample in a red-top tube.

After

• Apply pressure or a pressure dressing to the venipuncture site.
• Assess the venipuncture site for bleeding.
• Remember that if the result of this antibody screening test is positive, antibodies are then identified.

TEST RESULTS AND CLINICAL SIGNIFICANCE

Incompatible crossmatched blood: *Anti-ABO/Rh antigens in the donor blood cross-react with the patient's serum.*
Maternal anti-Rh antibodies,
Hemolytic disease of the newborn: *Antibodies result from previous exposure to fetal Rh+ RBCs.*
Acquired immune hemolytic anemia,
Presence of specific cold agglutinin antibody: *Drugs and other illnesses are associated with the development of antibodies detected in the patient's serum.*

RELATED TEST

Coombs Test, Direct (p. 188). This test is performed to identify hemolysis or to investigate hemolytic transfusion reactions.

Cortisol, Blood (Hydrocortisone, Serum Cortisol)

NORMAL FINDINGS

Adult/older adult:
    8 AM: **170–635 nmol/L** (6–23 *Mcg*/dL)
    4 PM: **82–413 nmol/L** (3–15 *Mcg*/dL)
Child (2–11 years):
    8 AM: **28–911 nmol/L** (3–21 *Mcg*/dL)
    4 PM: **28–662 nmol/L** (3–10 *Mcg*/dL)
0–24 months: **28–938 nmol/L** (1–24 *Mcg*/dL)

INDICATIONS

This test is a measure of serum cortisol. It is performed on patients who are suspected to have hyperfunctioning or hypofunctioning adrenal glands.

TEST EXPLANATION

An elaborate feedback mechanism for cortisol coordinates the function of the hypothalamus, pituitary gland, and adrenal glands. Corticotropin-releasing hormone (CRH) is made in the hypothalamus. This stimulates adrenocorticotropic hormone (ACTH) production in the anterior pituitary gland. ACTH stimulates the adrenal cortex to produce cortisol. The rising levels of cortisol act as negative feedback to curtail further production of corticotropin-releasing hormone and ACTH. Cortisol is a potent glucocorticoid released from the adrenal cortex. This hormone affects the metabolism of carbohydrates, proteins, and fats. It has a profound effect on glucose serum levels. Cortisol tends to increase glucose levels by stimulating gluconeogenesis from glucose stores. It also inhibits the effect of insulin and thereby inhibits glucose transport into the cells.

The best method of evaluating adrenal activity is by directly measuring plasma cortisol levels. Normally, cortisol levels rise and fall during the day; this is called the *diurnal variation.* Cortisol levels are highest at approximately 6 AM to 8 AM and gradually fall during the day, reaching their lowest point at approximately midnight. Sometimes the earliest sign of adrenal hyperfunction is only the loss of this diurnal variation, even though the cortisol levels are not yet elevated. For example, individuals with Cushing's syndrome often have upper normal plasma cortisol levels in the morning and do not exhibit a decline as the day proceeds. High levels of cortisol indicate Cushing's syndrome, and low levels of plasma cortisol are suggestive of Addison's disease.

For this test, blood is usually collected at 8 AM and again at approximately 4 PM. The 4 PM value is anticipated to be one to two-thirds of the 8 AM value. Normal values may be transposed in individuals who have worked during the night and slept during the day for long periods of time.

INTERFERING FACTORS

- Pregnancy is associated with increased levels.
- Physical and emotional stress can elevate cortisol levels. Stress stimulates the pituitary-cortical mechanism and thereby stimulates cortisol production.
- Drugs that may cause *increases* in cortisol levels include amphetamines, cortisone, estrogen, oral contraceptives, and spironolactone (Aldactone).
- Drugs that may cause *decreases* in cortisol levels include androgens, aminoglutethimide, betamethasone and other exogenous steroid medications, danazol, lithium, levodopa, metyrapone, and phenytoin (Dilantin).

Clinical Priorities

- Cortisol levels are affected by diurnal variation; levels peak at approximately 6 AM to 8 AM and are lowest at approximately midnight.
- Blood levels are usually measured at 8 AM and again at approximately 4 PM. The 4 PM level is usually one to two-thirds of the morning level.
- Physical and emotional stress can elevate cortisol levels.

PROCEDURE AND PATIENT CARE

Before

🖉 Explain the procedure to the patient to minimize anxiety.

- Assess the patient for signs of physical stress (e.g., infection, acute illness) or emotional stress and report these to the physician.

During

- Collect a venous blood sample in a red-top or green-top tube in the morning after the patient has had a good night's sleep.
- Collect another blood sample at approximately 4 PM.
- On the laboratory slip, indicate the time of the venipuncture.

After

- Apply pressure or a pressure dressing to the venipuncture site.
- Observe the venipuncture site for bleeding.

TEST RESULTS AND CLINICAL SIGNIFICANCE

▲ Increased Levels

Cushing's disease,

Ectopic ACTH-producing tumours,

Stress: *ACTH is overproduced as a result of neoplastic overproduction of ACTH in the pituitary gland or elsewhere in the body by an ACTH-producing cancer. Stress is a potent stimulus for ACTH production. Cortisol rises as a result.*

Cushing's syndrome (adrenal adenoma or carcinoma): *The neoplasm produces cortisol without regard to the normal feedback mechanism.*

Hyperthyroidism: *The metabolic rate is increased and cortisol levels rise accordingly to maintain the elevated glucose needs.*

Obesity: *All sterols are increased in obese persons, perhaps because fatty tissue may act as a depository or site of synthesis.*

▼ Decreased Levels

Adrenal hyperplasia: *The congenital absence of important enzymes in the synthesis of cortisol prevents adequate serum levels.*

Addison's disease: *As a result of hypofunctioning of the adrenal gland, cortisol levels drop.*

Hypopituitarism: *ACTH is not produced by the pituitary gland, which is destroyed by disease, neoplasm, or ischemia. The adrenal gland is not stimulated to produce cortisol.*

Hypothyroidism: *Normal cortisol levels are not required to maintain the reduced metabolic rate of hypothyroid patients.*

RELATED TESTS

Adrenocorticotropic Hormone Stimulation (p. 37). This test is used for the differential diagnosis of Cushing's syndrome or Addison's disease.

Adrenocorticotropic Hormone (p. 34). The serum ACTH study is a test of anterior pituitary gland function that affords the greatest insight into the causes of either Cushing's syndrome (overproduction of cortisol) or Addison's disease (underproduction of cortisol).

Dexamethasone Suppression (p. 219). This test is important for diagnosing Cushing's syndrome and distinguishing its cause.

Cortisol, Urine (p. 953). This test is a measure of urinary cortisol levels. It is performed on patients in whom hyperfunction or hypofunction of the adrenal glands is suspected.

Cotinine

NORMAL FINDINGS

Blood: **0–45 nmol/L** (0–8 Mcg/L)
Urine: **<5 mg/mL**
Saliva: **<0.05 ng/L** (<1.00 μm)

INDICATIONS

Cotinine testing is used as a screening tool to recruit individuals into research studies for smoking cessation, as an outcome marker of treatment efficacy, and for the evaluation of dosage with nicotine replacement therapy. It is also used by insurance companies to determine whether the applicant is a smoker.

TEST EXPLANATION

The word *cotinine* is an anagram of the word *nicotine*. Cotinine is formed when nicotine is metabolized by oxidation. Only 9% of nicotine is excreted intact, whereas 70% is converted to cotinine; therefore, cotinine is an indicator that nicotine has been inhaled or otherwise introduced into the body. Cotinine has an in vivo half-life of approximately 20 hours and is typically detectable for as long as 1 week after the use of tobacco. Because the level of cotinine in the blood is proportionate to the amount of exposure to tobacco smoke, it is a valuable indicator of exposure to tobacco smoke, including secondary (passive) smoke. Cotinine can be measured in the serum, urine, or other biofluids (most commonly the saliva). Cotinine is found in urine from 2 to 4 days after tobacco use.

Although blood study is the most reliable method of testing cotinine, it is also invasive and the most expensive. Blood cotinine levels increase no matter how the tobacco is used (smoked, chew, dip, or snuff products). Cotinine levels are also elevated by the use of any of the nicotine replacement gum, patch, or pill products. Nicotine levels can also be measured, but the half-life of nicotine (~2 hours) is too short to be useful as a marker of smoking status. For smokers, another method of determining tobacco use is expired carbon monoxide. Again, a relatively short half-life (~4 hours) limits the reliability and accuracy of this method. Furthermore, carbon monoxide testing cannot detect the use of smokeless tobacco.

Urine and salivary cotinine levels are less reliable but are more easily obtained and more cheaply performed. Cotinine levels vary by the amount of tobacco used, the use of a filter, the depth of the inhalation, and the size, sex, and weight of the person being tested. Cotinine levels can be elevated when passive smoke inhalation is experienced (Table 2-17). Because hydration status and renal function may affect urinary cotinine results, a spot urine cotinine test is always accompanied by a spot urine creatinine test.

TABLE 2-17   Reference Intervals for Cotinine

	REFERENCE RANGES			
	No Exposure, No Tobacco Use (ng/mL)	Passive Exposure (ng/mL)	Abstinence From Tobacco Use for More Than 2 Weeks (ng/mL)	Active Tobacco Product Use (ng/mL)
Blood	<2	<8	<2	200–800
Urine	<5	<20	<50	1 000–8 000
Biofluid	<2	<8	<2	200–800

Cotinine can be accurately quantified with various laboratory methods, including high-performance liquid chromatography, gas chromatography/mass spectroscopy, enzyme immunoassay, and enzyme-linked immunosorbent assay (ELISA). Qualitative assays (including enzyme immunoassay and ELISA) can be relatively easy to perform on urine and saliva but yield results less accurate than those of blood measurement. Absolute laboratory normal values may vary, depending on the method of testing.

INTERFERING FACTORS

- Menthol cigarettes may increase cotinine levels because the menthol enables the blood to retain cotinine for a longer period of time.

PROCEDURE AND PATIENT CARE

Before

- Explain the procedure to the patient, and indicate the type of specimen needed.
- Obtain an accurate history of recent tobacco use.

During

Blood

- Collect a venous blood sample in a red-top, lavender-top (EDTA), or pink-top (EDTA potassium salts) tube.

Urine

- Obtain a random spot urine specimen of at least 10 mL.
- Immediately transport the specimen to the laboratory.

Saliva

- Ask the patient to spit at least 1 mL into a spit container.
- Alternatively, dental gauze rolls can be placed in the mouth for 15 minutes and then placed in a storage container for transport.

After

- Keep the specimens in a cool place if they cannot be transported to the laboratory immediately.

TEST RESULTS AND CLINICAL SIGNIFICANCE

Tobacco exposure: With even minimal tobacco use, cotinine levels are elevated.

C-Peptide (Connecting Peptide Insulin, Insulin C-Peptide, Proinsulin C-Peptide)

NORMAL FINDINGS

Fasting: **0.26–0.62 nmol/L** (0.78–1.89 ng/mL)
1 hour after glucose load: **1.67–4.0 nmol/L** (5–12 ng/mL)

INDICATIONS

This test is used to evaluate diabetic patients and to identify patients who secretly self-administer insulin. C-peptide is also helpful in monitoring patients with insulinomas (tumours of the insulin-secreting cells of the islets of Langerhans).

TEST EXPLANATION

C-peptide (connecting peptide) is a protein that connects the beta and alpha chains of proinsulin. In the beta cells of the islet of Langerhans in the pancreas, the chains of proinsulin are separated during the conversion of proinsulin to insulin and C-peptide. C-peptide is released into the portal vein in nearly equal amounts. Because it has a longer half-life than insulin, more C-peptide exists in the peripheral circulation. In general, C-peptide levels are correlated with insulin levels in the blood, except possibly in islet cell tumours and in obese patients. The capacity of the pancreatic beta cells to secrete insulin can be evaluated by directly measuring either insulin or C-peptide. In most cases, direct measurement of insulin is more accurate. However, in some instances, direct measurement of insulin does not accurately assess the patient's insulin-generating capability. C-peptide levels more accurately reflect islet cell function in the following situations:

1. In patients with diabetes who are treated with insulin and who have anti-insulin antibodies. This most often occurs in patients treated with old bovine or pork insulin. These antibodies artificially increase insulin levels.
2. In patients who secretly administer insulin to themselves (factitious hypoglycemia). Insulin levels are elevated. Direct insulin measurements in these patients tends to be high, because the insulin measured is self-administered exogenous insulin. However, C-peptide levels in the same specimen are low because exogenously administered insulin suppresses endogenous insulin (and C-peptide) production.
3. In diabetic patients who are taking insulin. The exogenously administered insulin suppresses endogenous insulin production. Insulin levels reflect only the exogenously administered insulin and do not accurately reflect true islet cell function. C-peptide measurements would be a more accurate test of islet cell function. This is performed to determine whether the diabetes is in remission, in which case the patient may not need exogenous insulin.
4. For distinguishing type 1 from type 2 diabetes. This is particularly helpful in patients with newly diagnosed diabetes. A person whose pancreas does not make any insulin (type 1 diabetes) has low levels of insulin and C-peptide. A person with type 2 diabetes has a normal or high level of C-peptide.

The C-peptide test is indicated for the clinical situations just described. Furthermore, C-peptide is used in evaluating suspected insulinoma. It can differentiate insulinoma from factitious hypoglycemia. In the latter condition, C-peptide levels are suppressed by exogenous insulin challenge. With an autonomous secreting insulinoma, C-peptide levels are not suppressed. Furthermore, C-peptide can be used to monitor patients treated for insulinoma. A rise in C-peptide levels indicates a recurrence or progression of the insulinoma. Likewise, some clinicians use C-peptide testing as an indicator of the adequacy of therapeutic surgical pancreatectomy in patients with pancreatic tumours. C-peptide can also be used to diagnose insulin resistance syndrome.

INTERFERING FACTORS

- Because the majority of C-peptide is degraded in the kidneys, renal failure can cause increased levels of C-peptide.
- Drugs that may cause *increases* in levels of C-peptide include oral hypoglycemic agents (e.g., sulphonylureas).

PROCEDURE AND PATIENT CARE

Before

- Explain the procedure to the patient.
- Instruct the patient to fast for 8 to 10 hours before the test. Only water is permitted during the fast.

During

- Collect a venous blood sample in a red-top tube.

After

- Apply pressure or a pressure dressing to the venipuncture site.
- Assess the venipuncture site for bleeding.

TEST RESULTS AND CLINICAL SIGNIFICANCE

▲ Increased Levels

Insulinoma: *Insulin and C-peptide are made concomitantly by the neoplastic cells.*
Pancreas transplant: *Excess C-peptide is produced by the transplanted islet cells.*
Renal failure: *C-peptide is removed from the blood by the kidneys. Diminished kidney function leads to increases in C-peptide levels.*
Administration of oral hypoglycemic agents: *Oral hypoglycemic agents stimulate synthesis of insulin and C-peptide.*

▼ Decreased Levels

Factitious hypoglycemia,
Diabetes mellitus: *The self-administered insulin suppresses endogenous insulin and C-peptide production.*
Total pancreatectomy: *All islet cells have been surgically removed. C-peptide production therefore ceases.*

RELATED TESTS

Glucose, Blood (p. 269). This is a measurement of serum glucose.

Glucagon (p. 267). This is a direct measurement of glucagon, an islet cell hormone that acts to increase serum glucose levels.

Glycosylated Hemoglobin (p. 281). This is a test to measure the amount of glycosylated hemoglobin, which is an indirect measure of the chronic state of glucose levels.

Insulin Assay (p. 330). This is a direct measurement of insulin, an islet cell hormone that acts to decrease serum glucose levels.

 C-Reactive Protein (CRP, High-Sensitivity C-Reactive Protein [hs-CRP])

NORMAL FINDINGS

<10.0 mg/L (<1.0 mg/dL)
Cardiac risk (high-sensitivity C-reactive protein):
   Low: **0.7–1.10 mg/L** (0.07–0.11 mg/dL)
   Moderate: **1.2–1.9 mg/L** (0.12–0.19 mg/dL)
   High: **2.0–3.8 mg/L** (>0.2–0.38 mg/dL)

INDICATIONS

C-reactive protein (CRP) is an acute-phase reactant protein whose elevated levels indicate an inflammatory illness. It is believed to be of value in predicting coronary events.

TEST EXPLANATION

CRP is a nonspecific, acute-phase reactant protein that is measured to diagnose bacterial infectious disease and inflammatory disorders, such as acute rheumatic fever and rheumatoid arthritis. CRP levels are also elevated in the presence of tissue necrosis. CRP levels do not consistently rise with viral infections. CRP is produced primarily by the liver during an acute inflammatory process and other diseases. A positive test result indicates the presence, but not the cause, of the disease. The synthesis of CRP is initiated by antigen-immune complexes, bacteria, fungi, and trauma. CRP is functionally analogous to immunoglobulin G, except that it is not antigen specific. CRP interacts with the complement system.

The CRP test is a more sensitive and rapidly responding indicator than is the erythrocyte sedimentation rate (ESR). In an acute inflammatory change, CRP testing reveals an earlier and more intense increase than does ESR; with recovery, the disappearance of CRP levels precedes the return of ESR to normal. The CRP level also disappears when the inflammatory process is suppressed by anti-inflammatory agents, salicylates, or steroids.

This test is also useful in evaluating patients with an acute myocardial infarction. The level of CRP correlates with peak levels of creatinine kinase-MB (CK-MB) (see p. 201), but CRP levels peak 18 to 72 hours later. Failure of CRP levels to normalize may indicate ongoing damage to the heart tissue. Levels are not elevated in patients with angina.

The development of a *high-sensitivity assay* for CRP (hs-CRP) has enabled accurate measurements at even low levels. Atheromatous plaques in diseased arteries typically contain inflammatory cells. Multiple prospective studies have also demonstrated that baseline CRP level is a good marker of future cardiovascular events. The CRP level may be a stronger predictor of cardiovascular events than is the LDL cholesterol level. When CRP measurement is used together with the lipid profile (see Lipid Tests, Appendix C), it adds prognostic information to that conveyed by the Framingham risk score. Because of the individual variability in hs-CRP, two separate measurements are required to classify a person's risk level. In patients with stable coronary disease or acute coronary syndromes, hs-CRP measurement may be useful as an independent marker for assessing likelihood of recurrent events, including death, myocardial infarction, or restenosis after percutaneous coronary intervention.

Another indicator of inflammation besides CRP that receives considerable attention as a cardiac risk factor is *lipoprotein-associated phospholipase A_2* (Lp-PLA$_2$). Lp-PLA$_2$ promotes vascular inflammation through the hydrolysis of oxidized LDL within the intima, contributing directly to the atherogenic process. When combined with CRP measurement, testing for Lp-PLA$_2$ markedly increases the predictive value in determining risk for a cardiac event, especially in patients whose cholesterol level (see p. 169) is normal. The PLAC test is an enzyme-linked immunosorbent assay (ELISA) in which two highly specific monoclonal antibodies are used to measure the level of Lp-PLA$_2$ in the blood.

The CRP test also may be used postoperatively to detect wound infections. CRP levels increase within 4 to 6 hours after surgery and generally begin to decrease after the third postoperative day. Failure of the levels to fall is an indicator of complications, such as infection or pulmonary infarction.

INTERFERING FACTORS

- CRP levels may be elevated in patients with hypertension, elevated body mass index, metabolic syndrome/diabetes mellitus, chronic infection (gingivitis, bronchitis), chronic inflammation (rheumatoid arthritis), and low HDL/high triglyceride levels.
- Cigarette smoking can cause increases in CRP levels.
- CRP levels can decrease as a result of moderate alcohol consumption, weight loss, and increased activity or endurance exercise.
- Medications that may *increase* CRP levels include estrogens and progesterones.
- Medications that may *decrease* CRP levels include fibrates, niacin, and statins.

PROCEDURE AND PATIENT CARE

Before
- Explain the procedure to the patient.
- Inform the patient that fasting usually is not required; however, some laboratories require a 4- to 12-hour fast. Water is permitted during the fast.

During
- Collect venous blood in one red-top tube.

After
- Apply pressure or a pressure dressing to the venipuncture site.
- Assess the venipuncture site for bleeding.

TEST RESULTS AND CLINICAL SIGNIFICANCE

▲ Increased Levels

Acute, noninfectious inflammatory reaction (e.g., arthritis, acute rheumatic fever, Reiter's syndrome, Crohn's disease),

Collagen-vascular diseases (e.g., vasculitis syndrome, systemic lupus erythematosus),

Tissue infarction or damage (e.g., acute myocardial infarction, pulmonary infarction, kidney or bone marrow transplant rejection, soft-tissue trauma),

Bacterial infections such as postoperative wound infection, urinary tract infection, or tuberculosis,

Malignant disease,

Bacterial infection (e.g., tuberculosis, meningitis): *All these diseases are associated with an inflammatory reaction that instigates the synthesis of CRP.*

Increased risk for cardiovascular ischemic events: *Inflammation of the intimal lining of blood vessels, particularly the coronary vessels, is associated with an increased risk for intimal injury, which leads to plaque occlusions in distal vessel.*

RELATED TESTS

Erythrocyte Sedimentation Rate (p. 236). This is also an acute-phase reactant protein. It is a nonspecific test used to detect inflammatory, infectious, and necrotic processes.

Complement Assay (p. 185). Not only are some of the complement components acute-phase reactant proteins, but CRP interacts with this complex immune system.

Fibrinogen (p. 254). This is an important part of the hemostatic mechanism. It is also an acute-phase reactant protein.

Lipoproteins (p. 355) and Homocysteine (p. 318). These are important risk factors for heart disease.

Creatine Kinase (CK, Creatine Phosphokinase [CPK])

NORMAL FINDINGS

Total Creatine Kinase

Adult/older adult (values are higher after exercise):
  Male: **20–215 IU/L (20–215 U/L)**
  Female: **20–160 IU/L (20–160 U/L)**
Newborn: **68–580 IU/L (68–580 U/L)**

Isoenzymes

CK-MM: 96%–100%
CK-MB: 0%–6%
CK-BB: 0%

INDICATIONS

This test is used to support the diagnosis of myocardial muscle injury (infarction). It can also indicate neurologic or skeletal muscle diseases.

TEST EXPLANATION

Creatine kinase (CK) is found predominantly in the heart muscle, skeletal muscle, and brain. Serum CK levels are elevated when these muscle or nerve cells are injured. CK levels can rise

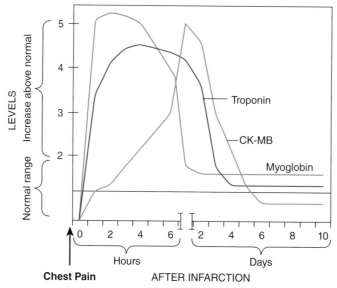

Figure 2-16 Blood studies useful in the diagnosis of myocardial infarction.

within 6 hours after damage. If damage is not persistent, the levels peak 18 hours after injury and return to normal in 2 to 3 days (Figure 2-16).

To test specifically for myocardial muscle injury, electrophoresis is performed to detect the three CK isoenzymes: CK-BB, CK-MB, and CK-MM. The CK-MB isoenzyme portion appears to be specific for myocardial cells. CK-MB levels rise 3 to 6 hours after infarction occurs. If there is no further myocardial damage, the level peaks at 12 to 24 hours and returns to normal 12 to 48 hours after infarction. CK-MB levels do not usually rise with transient chest pain caused by angina, pulmonary embolism, or heart failure. CK-MB levels also rise in patients with shock, malignant hyperthermia, myopathies, or myocarditis. CK-MB levels can become mildly elevated (below the threshold of positive) in patients with unstable angina, and this development signifies an increased risk for an occlusive event. Very small amounts of CK-MB also exist in skeletal muscle. Severe injury to or diseases of the skeletal muscle can also raise CK-MB levels above normal.

The CK-MB isoenzyme level is helpful in both quantifying the degree of myocardial infarction and determining the time of infarction onset. CK-MB measurements are often used to determine appropriateness of thrombolytic therapy, which is used for myocardial infarction. High CK-MB levels suggest that significant infarction has already occurred, thereby precluding the benefit of thrombolytic therapy.

Because the CK-BB isoenzyme is found predominantly in the brain and lung, injury to either of these organs (e.g., cerebrovascular accident, pulmonary infarction) is associated with elevated levels of this isoenzyme.

The CK-MM isoenzyme normally makes up almost all of the circulatory total CK enzymes in healthy people. When the total CK level is elevated as a result of increases in CK-MM, injury to or disease of the skeletal muscle is present. Examples of such disease or injury include myopathies, vigorous exercise, multiple intramuscular injections, electroconvulsive therapy, cardioversion, chronic alcoholism, and surgery. Because CK is made only in the skeletal muscle, the normal value of total CK (and therefore CK-MM) varies according to a person's muscle mass. In large muscular people, a CK level that is higher than average may be a normal condition. Likewise, people of small stature or those with low muscle mass are expected to have low CK levels.

TABLE 2-18	Timing of Appearance and Disappearance of Commonly Measured Cardiac Enzymes After Cardiac Event		
Enzyme	**Level Starts to Rise**	**Level Peaks**	**Level Returns to Normal**
Total CK	4–6 hours	24 hours	3–4 days
CK-MB	4 hours	18 hours	2 days
AST	8 hours	24–48 hours	4 days
LDH	24 hours	72 hours	8–9 days
Troponin T	4–6 hours	10–24 hours	10 days
Troponin I	4–6 hours	10–24 hours	4 days

AST, Aspartate aminotransferase; *CK,* creatine kinase; *CK-MB,* myocardial CK isoenzyme; *LDH,* lactate dehydrogenase.

This is important because high normal CK levels in patients with high muscle mass can mask a myocardial infarction.

Each isoenzyme has been found to have isoforms. The CK-MM isoforms MM1 and MM3 are most useful for cardiac disease. Either an MM3/MM1 ratio or an MB2/MB1 ratio higher than 1 suggests acute myocardial injury.

CK is the main cardiac enzyme studied in patients with heart disease. Because its blood clearance and metabolism are well known, its frequent determination (on admission and at 12 hours and 24 hours) can accurately reflect timing, quantity, and resolution of a myocardial infarction (see Figure 2-16). Lactate dehydrogenase and aspartate aminotransferase are also enzymes that were at one time used to confirm a myocardial infarction. The clearance characteristics of each enzyme are listed in Table 2-18.

Newer blood assays for cardiac markers can rapidly and accurately detect acute myocardial infarction in the emergency room. One of these assays is troponin (see p. 531). Another assay is ischemia-induced albumin (see p. 338).

Clinical Priorities

- Avoid intramuscular injections in patients with cardiac disease. Intramuscular injections can cause elevations in CK levels.
- The CK-MB isoenzyme is helpful in both quantifying the degree of myocardial infarction and timing the onset of the infarction.
- The CK-MB isoenzyme is often used to determine the appropriateness of thrombolytic therapy. High levels may indicate that significant infarction has already occurred, thus precluding a benefit from thrombolytic therapy.

INTERFERING FACTORS

- Intramuscular injections can cause elevations in CK levels.
- Strenuous exercise and recent surgery may cause increases in CK levels.
- Early pregnancy may produce decreases in CK levels.
- Muscle mass is directly related to a patient's normal CK level.

 Drugs that may cause *increases* in CK levels include alcohol, amphotericin B, ampicillin, some anaesthetics, anticoagulants, aspirin, captopril, clofibrate, colchicine, dexamethasone (Dexasone), furosemide (Lasix), lithium, lidocaine, morphine, propranolol, statins, and succinylcholine.

PROCEDURE AND PATIENT CARE

Before

☒ Explain the procedure to the patient.

☒ Discuss with the patient the need and reason for frequent venipuncture in diagnosing myocardial infarction.

• Avoid intramuscular injections in patients with cardiac disease. These injections may artificially elevate the total CK level.

☒ Inform the patient that no food or fluid restrictions are necessary.

During

• Collect a venous blood sample in a red-top tube. This is usually done when the patient first arrives in the emergency department and again 12 hours later, followed by daily testing for 3 days and then at 1 week.

• Rotate the venipuncture sites.

• Avoid hemolysis.

• Record the time and date of any intramuscular injection.

• On each laboratory slip, record the exact time and date of venipuncture. This aids in the interpretation of the temporal pattern of enzyme elevations.

After

• Apply pressure or a pressure dressing to the venipuncture site.

• Observe the venipuncture site for bleeding.

TEST RESULTS AND CLINICAL SIGNIFICANCE

▲ Increased Levels of Total Creatine Kinase

Diseases or injury affecting the heart muscle, skeletal muscle, and brain

▲ Increased Levels of CK-BB Isoenzyme

Electroconvulsive therapy,

Adenocarcinoma (especially breast and lung): *The pathophysiologic mechanism underlying this observation is not known.*

Pulmonary infarction: *The lung tissue has small amounts of CK-BB. With cellular injury of this organ, the contents of the cell, including CK, spill out into the bloodstream, causing elevations in CK-BB isoenzyme levels.*

Diseases that affect the central nervous system (e.g., brain injury, brain cancer, cerebrovascular accident [stroke], subarachnoid hemorrhage, seizures, shock, Reye syndrome)

▲ Increased Levels of CK-MB Isoenzyme

Acute myocardial infarction,

Cardiac aneurysm surgery,

Cardiac defibrillation,

Myocarditis,

Ventricular arrhythmias,

Cardiac ischemia: *Any disease or injury to the myocardium causes CK-MB to spill out of the damaged cells and into the bloodstream, producing elevations in CK-MB levels.*

▲ Increased Levels of CK-MM Isoenzyme

Rhabdomyolysis,

Muscular dystrophy,

Myositis: *Diseases affecting skeletal muscle cause CK-MM to spill out of the damaged cells and into the bloodstream, producing elevations in CK-MM levels.*

Recent surgery,

Electromyography,

Intramuscular injections,

Trauma,

Crush injuries: *Injury affecting skeletal muscle causes CK-MM to spill out of the damaged cells and into the bloodstream, producing elevations in CK-MM levels.*

Delirium tremens,

Malignant hyperthermia,

Recent convulsions,

Electroconvulsive therapy,

Shock: *Anoxic injury from lack of blood supply or repetitive muscular motion can cause injury to skeletal muscle. This causes CK-MM to spill out of the damaged cells and into the bloodstream, producing elevations in CK-MM levels.*

Hypokalemia,

Hypothyroidism: *These diseases have a metabolic effect on skeletal muscle. Muscle injury results. This causes CK-MM to spill out of the damaged cells and into the bloodstream, producing elevations in CK-MM levels.*

RELATED TESTS

Aspartate Aminotransferase (p. 130). Elevated levels of this enzyme may indicate cardiac injury. This finding is not specific to the heart, however.

Lactate Dehydrogenase (p. 339). This intracellular enzyme is measured to support the diagnosis of injury or disease involving the heart, liver, red blood cells (RBCs), kidneys, skeletal muscle, brain, and lungs.

Alanine Aminotransferase (p. 45). This test is used similarly to the test for aspartate aminotransferase and exists predominantly in the liver.

Leucine Aminopeptidase (p. 351). This enzyme is specific to the hepatobiliary system. Diseases affecting that system cause elevation in levels of this enzyme.

Gamma-Glutamyl Transpeptidase (p. 261), Alkaline Phosphatase (p. 53), and 5'-Nucleotidase (p. 389). These enzymes exist predominantly in the liver.

Troponins (p. 531). This is a biochemical marker used to assist in the evaluation of patients with chest pain.

Creatinine, Blood (Serum Creatinine)

NORMAL FINDINGS

Older adult: Decrease in muscle mass may cause decreases in values.

Adult:

Female: **44–97 Mcmol/L** (0.5–1.1 mg/dL)

Male: **53–106 Mcmol/L** (0.6–1.2 mg/dL)

Child/adolescent (1–18 years): **18–62 Mcmol/L** (0.2–0.7 mg/dL)

Infant (7 days to 12 months): **18–35 Mcmol/L** (0.2–0.4 mg/dL)

Newborn (0–1 week): **53–97 Mcmol/L** (0.6–1.1 mg/dL)

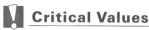

Critical Values

>247 Mcmol/L (>4 mg/dL) (indicates serious impairment in renal function)

INDICATIONS

Creatinine is used to diagnose impaired renal function.

TEST EXPLANATION

This test measures the amount of creatinine in the blood. Creatinine is a catabolic product of creatine phosphate, which is used in skeletal muscle contraction. The daily production of creatine, and subsequently creatinine, depends on muscle mass, which fluctuates very little. Creatinine, like blood urea nitrogen (BUN), is excreted entirely by the kidneys and therefore is directly proportional to renal excretory function. Thus, with normal renal excretory function, the serum creatinine level should remain constant and normal. Besides dehydration, only renal disorders—such as glomerulonephritis, pyelonephritis, acute tubular necrosis, and urinary obstruction—cause an abnormal elevation in creatinine. There are slight increases in creatinine levels after meals, especially after ingestion of large quantities of meat. Furthermore, there may be some diurnal variation in creatinine (nadir at 7 AM and peak at 7 PM).

The serum creatinine test, like the BUN test, is used to diagnose impaired renal function. Unlike BUN level, however, the creatinine level is affected minimally by hepatic function. The creatinine level reflects an approximation of glomerular filtration rate (GFR). The serum creatinine level has much the same significance as the BUN level but tends to rise later. Therefore, elevations in creatinine level suggest chronicity of the disease process. In general, a doubling of creatinine suggests a 50% reduction in the glomerular filtration rate. The creatinine level is interpreted in conjunction with the BUN level. These tests are referred to as *renal function studies:* The BUN/creatinine ratio is a good measurement of kidney and liver function. The normal range is 6 to 25; 15.5 is the optimal adult value for this ratio.

Although serum creatinine level is the biochemical parameter most commonly used to estimate GFR in routine practice, there are some shortcomings to the use of this parameter. Factors such as muscle mass and protein intake can influence serum creatinine level, leading to an inaccurate estimation of GFR. Moreover, in unstable, critically ill patients, acute changes in renal function can make real-time evaluation of GFR with serum creatinine difficult. On the other hand, cystatin C, a protein that is produced at a constant rate by all nucleated cells, is probably a better indicator of GFR. Because of its constant rate of production, its serum concentration is determined only by glomerular filtration. Its level is not influenced by the factors that affect creatinine and BUN levels.

Cystatin C might predict the risk for developing chronic kidney disease, thereby signalling a state of "preclinical" kidney dysfunction. Several studies have found that increased levels of cystatin C are associated with the risk for death, several types of cardiovascular disease (including myocardial infarction, stroke, heart failure, peripheral arterial disease, and metabolic syndrome). For young adults, the average reference interval is higher than **2.9 Mcmol/L** (<0.70 mg/L), and for older adults, the average reference interval is higher than **3.5 Mcmol/L** (0.56 to 0.98 mg/L).

Age-Related Concerns

- Older adults and young children normally have lower creatinine levels as a result of reduced muscle mass. This may potentially mask renal disease in patients at these ages.

INTERFERING FACTORS

- A diet high in meat content can cause transient elevations of serum creatinine levels.
- Drugs that may cause *increases* in creatinine values include angiotensin-converting enzyme (ACE) inhibitors, aminoglycosides (e.g., gentamicin), cimetidine, heavy-metal chemotherapeutic agents (e.g., cisplatin), and other nephrotoxic drugs such as cephalosporins (e.g., cefoxitin).

PROCEDURE AND PATIENT CARE

Before

- Explain the procedure to the patient.
- Inform the patient that no fasting is required.

During

- Collect venous blood in a red-top tube.
- For newborns and infants, blood is usually collected from a heelstick.

After

- Apply pressure or a pressure dressing to the venipuncture site.
- Observe the venipuncture site for bleeding.

TEST RESULTS AND CLINICAL SIGNIFICANCE

▲ Increased Levels

Diseases affecting renal function, such as glomerulonephritis, pyelonephritis, acute tubular necrosis, urinary tract obstruction, reduced renal blood flow (e.g., shock, dehydration, congestive heart failure, atherosclerosis), diabetic nephropathy, nephritis: *In these illnesses, renal function is impaired, and creatinine levels rise.*

Rhabdomyolysis: *Injury of the skeletal muscle causes myoglobin to be released in the bloodstream. Large amounts are nephrotoxic. Creatinine levels rise.*

Acromegaly,

Gigantism: *These diseases are associated with increased muscle mass, which causes the "normal" creatinine level to be high.*

▼ Decreased Levels

Debilitation,

Decreased muscle mass (e.g., muscular dystrophy, myasthenia gravis): *These diseases are associated with decreased muscle mass, which causes the "normal" creatinine level to be low.*

RELATED TESTS

Blood Urea Nitrogen (p. 534). This is a test of renal function. In contrast to the creatinine test, there are many nonrenal factors that can alter the BUN test result.

Creatinine Clearance (see following test). This is a more accurate measurement of renal function. It is a direct measurement of glomerular filtration rate.

Creatinine Clearance (CrCl)

NORMAL FINDINGS

Newborn: **1.2 mL/sec** (72 mL/min)
Adult (<40 years):
   Male: **1.78–2.32 mL/sec** (107–139 mL/min)
   Female: **1.45–1.78 mL/sec** (87–107 mL/min)

Age-Related Concerns

- Adult values decrease **0.06 mL/sec** (6.5 mL/min) with each decade of life after 20 years of age because of a decrease in glomerular filtration rate (GFR).

INDICATIONS

The creatinine clearance is measured to calculate the GFR of the kidneys.

TEST EXPLANATION

Creatinine is a catabolic product of creatine phosphate, which is used in skeletal muscle contraction. The daily production of creatine, and subsequently creatinine, depends on muscle mass, which fluctuates very little. Creatinine is excreted entirely by the kidneys and therefore is directly proportional to the GFR (i.e., the number of millilitres of filtrate made by the kidneys per minute). Creatinine clearance (CrCl) is a measure of the GFR. Urine and serum creatinine levels are assessed, and the clearance rate is calculated.

The amount of filtrate made in the kidney depends on the amount of blood to be filtered and on the ability of the glomeruli to act as a filter. The amount of blood present for filtration is decreased in renal artery atherosclerosis, dehydration, and shock. The ability of the glomeruli to act as a filter is decreased by diseases such as glomerulonephritis, acute tubular necrosis, and most other primary renal diseases. Significant bilateral obstruction to urinary outflow affects glomerular filtration (CrCl) only after it is long-standing.

When one kidney alone becomes diseased, the opposite kidney, if normal, has the ability to compensate by increasing its GFR. Therefore, with unilateral kidney disease or nephrectomy, a decrease in CrCl is not expected if the other kidney is normal.

Several nonrenal factors may influence CrCl. With each decade of age, the CrCl decreases because of a decrease in the GFR. Because urine collections are timed, incomplete collections artificially decrease CrCl. Muscle mass varies among people. With decreased muscle mass, CrCl values are lower. Likewise, ingestion of large amounts of meat temporarily increases CrCl.

The CrCl test requires a 24-hour urine collection and a measurement of the serum creatinine level. CrCl is then computed according to the following formula:

$$CrCl = UV/P,$$

where

U = creatinine concentration in collected 24-hour urine sample
V = volume of urine over 24 hours
P = plasma creatinine concentration

Creatinine values are often used to assess the completeness of a 24-hour urine collection. In patients with normal creatinine levels, the CrCl should indicate whether all the urine has been collected for the full 24 hours.

The 24-hour urine collections used to measure CrCl are too time-consuming and expensive for routine clinical use. However, a new measure to determine the GFR is the *estimated GFR*. In this equation, the serum creatinine level, age, and numbers that vary depending upon sex and ethnicity are used to calculate the GFR with very good accuracy. The prediction equation for GFR is as follows, with

$$GFR\left(mL/min/1.73m^{2210}\right) = 186 \times \left(Pcr\right)^{-1.154} \times \left(age\right)^{-0.203} \times \left(0.742 \text{ if female}\right) \times \left(1.210 \text{ if Black}\right)$$

where Pcr is serum or plasma creatinine level in micromoles per litre (milligrams per decilitre). The GFR is expressed in millilitres per minute per $1.73\,m^2$.

An increasing number of institutions across the country are beginning to report a GFR on patients who are 18 years and older with every serum creatinine measurement ordered. The GFR calculation can be programmed into most laboratory information systems. As a result, chronic renal disease is being recognized more frequently in its early stages. Chronic renal disease can be treated and progression to renal failure slowed or prevented. For example, if a patient with diabetes is found to have a reduced GFR of 49 at an annual examination, that patient's primary care physician can and should take steps to treat the early chronic renal disease. This may include the use of ACE inhibitors, more aggressive treatment of high blood pressure, glycemic dietary control, and treatment of high cardiac risk factors.

Table 2-19 shows population estimates for mean (average) estimated glomerular filtration rate by age. There is no difference between races or sexes when estimated GFRs are expressed per square metre of body surface area. For diagnostic purposes, most laboratories report estimated GFR values above 60 as ">60 mL/min/1.73 m²," not as an exact number.

TABLE 2-19 Mean Estimated GFR by Age	
Age (Years)	**Mean Estimated GFR**
20–29	116 mL/min/1.73 m²
30–39	107 mL/min/1.73 m²
40–49	99 mL/min/1.73 m²
50–59	93 mL/min/1.73 m²
60–69	85 mL/min/1.73 m²
70+	75 mL/min/1.73 m²

GFR, Glomerular filtration rate.

INTERFERING FACTORS

- Exercise may cause increased creatinine values.
- Incomplete urine collection may yield an artificially low value.
- Pregnancy increases CrCl. This is due in part to the increased load placed on the kidneys by the growing fetus.
- A diet high in meat content can cause transient elevation of the serum creatinine and CrCl. When the creatinine is high, its clearance is increased. Therefore, the CrCl overestimates the GFR.
- The estimated GFR may be inaccurate in extremes of age and in patients with severe malnutrition or obesity, paraplegia or quadriplegia, and in pregnant women.
- Drugs that may cause *increases* in CrCl rate include aminoglycosides (e.g., gentamicin), cimetidine, heavy-metal chemotherapeutic agents (e.g., cisplatin), and nephrotoxic drugs such as cephalosporins (e.g., cefoxitin).
- Drugs that may cause a *decrease* in estimated GFR interfere with creatinine secretion (e.g., cimetidine or trimethoprim) or creatinine assay (cephalosporins). In these cases, a 24-hour creatinine clearance may be necessary to accurately estimate kidney function.

PROCEDURE AND PATIENT CARE

Before

- Explain the procedure to the patient.
- Inform the patient that no special diet is usually required.
- Note that some laboratories instruct the patient to avoid cooked meat, tea, coffee, or drugs on the day of the test. Check with the laboratory.

During

- Instruct the patient to discard the initial urine specimen and start the 24-hour collection with the next specimen.
- Instruct the patient to collect all the urine passed during the next 24 hours.
- Show the patient where to store the urine specimen.
- Keep the specimen in a container of water and crushed ice or refrigerated during the 24 hours.
- On the urine container and laboratory slip, indicate the starting time. The patient should post the times of urine collection in a prominent place to prevent accidental discharge of a specimen.
- Instruct the patient to void before defecating so that urine is not contaminated by feces.
- Remind the patient not to put toilet paper in the collection container.
- Encourage the patient to drink fluids during the 24-hour collection unless this is contraindicated for medical purposes.
- Instruct the patient to avoid vigorous exercise during the 24 hours, because exercise may cause an increase in CrCl.
- Instruct the patient to void as close as possible to the end of the 24-hour period and to add this specimen to the collection.
- Make sure that a venous blood sample is collected in a red-top tube during the 24-hour collection.
- Note the patient's age, weight, and height on the requisition sheet.

After

- Apply pressure or a pressure dressing to the venipuncture site.
- Observe the venipuncture site for bleeding.
- Transport the urine specimen promptly to the laboratory.

TEST RESULTS AND CLINICAL SIGNIFICANCE

▲ Increased Levels

Exercise,

Pregnancy,

High cardiac output syndromes: *As blood flow increases to the kidney, GFR and CrCl increase.*

▼ Decreased Levels

Impaired kidney function (e.g., renal artery atherosclerosis, glomerulonephritis, acute tubular necrosis),

Conditions causing decreases in GFR (e.g., heart failure, cirrhosis with ascites, shock, dehydration): *Conditions that are associated with decreases in blood flow to the kidneys will decrease GFR.*

RELATED TESTS

Blood Urea Nitrogen (p. 534). This is a test of renal function. In contrast to the creatinine test, there are many nonrenal factors that can alter the BUN test result.

Creatinine, Blood (p. 205). The creatinine measurement is used to diagnose impaired renal function.

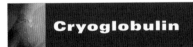

Cryoglobulin

NORMAL FINDINGS

No cryoglobulins detected

INDICATIONS

This test is performed to identify cryoglobulins in patients with symptoms of purpura, arthralgia, or Raynaud's phenomenon. Cryoglobulin testing is used to support the diagnosis of the diseases that are known to be associated with cryoglobulins.

TEST EXPLANATION

Cryoglobulins are abnormal immunoglobulin protein complexes that exist within the blood of patients with various diseases. These proteins precipitate reversibly at low temperatures and redissolve with rewarming. Cryoglobulins can precipitate within the blood vessels of the fingers when exposed to cold temperatures. This precipitation then causes clogging of the blood flow within those blood vessels. Affected patients may have thus symptoms of purpura, arthralgia, or Raynaud's phenomenon (pain, cyanosis, coldness of the fingers).

There are three types of cryoglobulinemia: monoclonal cryoglobulinemia, or type I, which is associated with hematologic disorders and malignancies (e.g., multiple myeloma and Waldenström macroglobulinemia); and mixed cryoglobulinemia, or type II and type III, which are associated with infectious and systemic disorders (e.g., hepatitis C, rheumatoid arthritis, hepatitis B, SLE, endocarditis, and biliary cirrhosis). Approximately 92% of patients with mixed cryoglobulinemia have hepatitis C infection. Testing of cryoglobulins is complicated by the facts that no reference range for cryoglobulins has been widely accepted and that temperature must be strictly controlled during collection of blood samples.

For this test, the blood sample is taken to the chemistry laboratory, where it is allowed to clot at 37°C for 1 hour. It is important that the sample temperature not drop below 37°C until serum separation is complete, to prevent early precipitation. The collection tube is then kept at 4°C and analyzed at 72 hours. Some laboratories wait 7 days if no precipitate forms initially. The specimen is then refrigerated for 24 to 72 hours. After that time, the specimen is evaluated for precipitation. If precipitation is identified, it is measured and recorded, and the cryoglobulins are identified by immunoelectrophoresis. The tube is then rewarmed, and the specimen is reexamined for dissolution of that precipitation. If precipitation of the refrigerated specimen is identified and dissolved on rewarming, the presence of cryoglobulins is verified.

PROCEDURE AND PATIENT CARE

Before
- Explain the procedure to the patient.
- Inform the patient that an 8-hour fast may be ordered by the physician. This will minimize turbidity of the serum caused by ingestion of a recent (especially fatty) meal. Turbidity may make the detection of precipitation rather difficult.

During
- Collect a venous blood sample in a red-top tube that has been prewarmed to 37°C. This can be achieved by submerging the tube in warm water during the transport to the laboratory.

After
- Apply pressure or a pressure dressing to the venipuncture site.
- Observe the venipuncture site for bleeding.
- If cryoglobulins are present, warn the patient to avoid cold temperatures and contact with cold objects in order to minimize Raynaud's symptoms. Instruct the patient to wear gloves in cold weather.

TEST RESULTS AND CLINICAL SIGNIFICANCE

The following is a list of diseases associated with the presence of cryoglobulins:

Connective tissue disease (e.g., systemic lupus erythematosus, Sjögren syndrome, rheumatoid arthritis)

Lymphoid malignancies (e.g., multiple myeloma, leukemia, Waldenström macroglobulinemia, lymphoma)

Acute and chronic infections (e.g., infectious mononucleosis, endocarditis, poststreptococcal glomerulonephritis)

Liver disease (e.g., hepatitis, cirrhosis)

RELATED TESTS

Agglutinin, Febrile/Cold (p. 43). These agglutinins are antibodies that cause red blood cells (RBCs) to aggregate at high or low temperatures, respectively.

Rheumatoid Factor (p. 467). This test is useful in the diagnosis of rheumatoid arthritis. Other diseases, such as systemic lupus erythematosus (SLE), may cause a positive result.

Cutaneous Immunofluorescence Antibodies
(Indirect IFA Antibodies, Anti–Basement Zone Antibodies, Anti–Cell Surface Antibodies)

NORMAL FINDINGS

No evidence of antibodies

INDICATIONS

This test is used to diagnose and monitor autoimmune-mediated dermatitis and paraneoplastic dermatitis.

TEST EXPLANATION

Autoimmune-mediated skin lesions are often associated with the presence of elevated levels of antibodies in the serum (see Antiscleroderma Antibody, p. 103) and in the skin. IgG anti-basement zone (BMZ) antibodies are produced by patients with pemphigoid, epidermolysis bullosa acquisita (EBA), and bullous eruption of lupus erythematosus (LE). The titer of anti-CS antibodies generally correlates with disease activity of pemphigus. This test is useful for confirming a diagnosis of these diseases and monitoring therapeutic response. Indirect immunofluorescence (IF) testing may be diagnostic when histologic or direct IF studies are only suggestive, nonspecific, or negative.

Anti-CS antibodies correlate with a diagnosis of pemphigus.

Anti-BMZ antibodies correlate with a diagnosis of bullous pemphigoid, cicatricial pemphigoid, EBA, or bullous eruption of LE.

Results should be interpreted in conjunction with clinical information, histologic pattern, and results of direct IF study.

PROCEDURE AND PATIENT CARE

Before

- Explain the procedure to the patient.
- Tell the patient that no fasting is required.

During

- Collect a venous blood sample in a red-top tube.

After

- Apply pressure or a pressure dressing to the venipuncture site.
- Assess the venipuncture site for bleeding.

TEST RESULTS AND CLINICAL SIGNIFICANCE

Positive

Pemphigoid,
Pemphigus,
Bullosa acquisita,
Bullous lupus erythematosus,

Paraneoplastic dermatitis: *In these diseases an autoimmune reaction is instigated and directed to the skin and other organs. As a result, IgG, IgA, and IgM antibody levels will increase.*

RELATED TEST

Skin Biopsy. Cutaneous immunofluorescence antibodies can also be detected directly on skin biopsy. This test is confirmatory for autoimmune dermatitis.

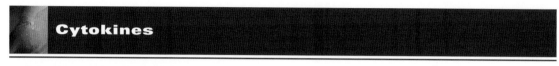

NORMAL FINDINGS

Findings vary by laboratory and technique

INDICATIONS

Cytokine assays are used predominantly for clinical research. Clinically, they may have the following uses:

- Measurement of progression of acquired immune deficiency syndrome (AIDS)
- Measurement of progression of inflammatory diseases, such as rheumatoid arthritis and other autoimmune diseases
- Tumour markers (e.g., for breast cancer, lymphoma, and leukemia)
- Determination of risk for disease (e.g., risk for developing Kaposi sarcoma in patients with AIDS)
- Determination of treatment of disease (e.g., which patients with rheumatoid arthritis may benefit from cytokine therapy)
- Determination of immune function and response
- Monitoring of patients receiving cytokine therapy or anticytokine therapy

TEST EXPLANATION

Cytokines are a group of proteins that have multiple functions but, in general, are produced by immune cells to communicate and orchestrate the immune response. The immune system has many different cells that must act together to effectively protect the body from infection, inflammation, or tumour. The cytokines are made by many different types of cells, including lymphocytes (T cells, B cells), monocytes, and eosinophils. Some cytokines stimulate each other, and some inhibit other cytokines to maintain balance. Originally, cytokines were named by their function (e.g., T cell growth factor, colony-stimulating factor). As more was learned about this complex group of proteins, it became apparent that a single cytokine might act differently on different cells. Therefore, naming the cytokine by function was confusing and misleading. As more cytokines were identified, they were named *interleukins* and numbered by the sequence of discovery. Interleukins, in general, are made by leukocytes. Lymphokines and monokines are made by lymphocytes and monocytes, respectively. Other cytokines include interferon and growth factors.

Cytokines have receptors in other cells to which they attach and instigate a series of intracellular activity that may be associated with secretion, motion, or cell division. In general, cytokines act very close to their cells of origin or even on the cell that generated them. Because their effect is so significant over a small area, cytokines exist in only small quantities. That makes quantitative assays very difficult. Radioimmunoassay, immunoradiometric assays, enzyme-linked immunosorbent assays (ELISAs), and radioreceptor assays are some of the latest laboratory techniques used to accurately measure these proteins.

Cytokines are used therapeutically in stimulating bone marrow production of blood cells in patients with suppression (by chemotherapy) or disease of the bone marrow. They are used as potent anti-inflammatory or antineoplastic agents. Some cytokines are produced at increased levels in particular disease states and are thereby markers for disease extent, progression, and response to therapy. For cancers that are associated with elevated cytokines, they act as tumour markers.

Any list of all of the cytokines and their function quickly becomes inaccurate and imperfect. The discovery of new cytokines and new functions changes so frequently that any such list is outdated by the delay in publication. Likewise, any listing of normal values is just as quickly antiquated because methods of testing change so frequently. It is suggested that "normal values" be cited in reference to the laboratory performing the assay. At present, cytokine quantitative and qualitative assays are used predominantly for research. Cytokine testing, including measurement of cytokine receptor proteins, is often performed as part of multiple blood studies.

Usually, cytokine testing is performed on serum. However, joint fluid is often tested in the evaluation of patients with arthritis. Likewise, if inflammatory encephalitis or meningitis is suspected, cerebrospinal fluid may be the specimen.

INTERFERING FACTORS

- Cells can still produce cytokines after specimen collection. It is best to freeze the specimen.
- Cytokines can become degraded in the specimen container.
- Cytokines can stimulate or inhibit other cytokines while in the specimen container.

PROCEDURE AND PATIENT CARE

Before

- Explain the procedure to the patient.
- Inform the patient that no fasting or preparation is required.

During

- Collect a venous blood sample in a red-top tube.
- Usually such specimens are sent to a reference laboratory.

After

- Apply pressure to the venipuncture site.

TEST RESULTS AND CLINICAL SIGNIFICANCE

Abnormal Findings

AIDS: *The cytokine profile associated with the developing stages of AIDS or the susceptibility to AIDS-related tumours has yet to be determined.*

Various malignancies (breast cancer, lymphoma, and leukemia): *Progression of these tumours may be the result or the instigator of elevated cytokines.*

Impaired immune function: *Cytokines are integral in the function of both cellular and humoral immune response. The exact cytokine profile for immune dysfunction has yet to be determined.*

Rheumatoid arthritis: *Rheumatoid arthritis and other autoimmune diseases may be associated with increases in cytokine levels that are compatible with a strong immune reaction. Measurement of certain cytokines may be important in monitoring more advanced anticytokine treatments for autoimmune diseases.*

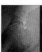

Cytomegalovirus (CMV)

NORMAL FINDINGS

No virus isolated

INDICATIONS

This test is used to identify cytomegalovirus (CMV) in patients in whom the infection is suspected.

TEST EXPLANATION

CMV belongs to the viral family that includes herpes simplex, Epstein-Barr, and varicella-zoster viruses. CMV infection is widespread. Infections usually occur in utero, during early childhood, and in early adulthood. Certain populations are at increased risk. Homosexual men, transplant recipients, and patients with acquired immune deficiency syndrome (AIDS) are particularly susceptible. Infections are acquired by contact with body secretions or urine. Blood transfusions are commonly implicated in the spread of CMV. As much as 35% of patients receiving multiple transfusions become infected with CMV. After infection, there is an asymptomatic incubation period of approximately 60 days. Acute symptoms may then develop. Most patients with acute disease have no or very few (mononucleosis-like) symptoms. Others may have mononucleosis-like symptoms of fever, lethargy, and anorexia. This period is followed by a latent phase. The acute phase can be reactivated at any time.

CMV is the most common congenital infection. Pregnant women can acquire the disease during their pregnancy, or a previous CMV infection can become reactivated at that time. Approximately 10% of infected newborns exhibit permanent damage, usually developmental delay and auditory damage. Fetal infection can cause microcephaly, hydrocephaly, cerebral palsy, developmental delay, or death.

TORCH (toxoplasmosis, other, rubella, CMV, herpes) infections have recognized detrimental effects on the fetus. The effects on the fetus may be direct or indirect (e.g., precipitating abortion or premature labour). Included in the category of "other" are infections (e.g., syphilis). All of these tests are discussed separately.

Virus culture is the most definitive method of diagnosis. However, a culture cannot differentiate an acute infection from a chronic, inactive infection. Immunofluorescence, enzyme-linked immunosorbent assay (ELISA), and latex agglutination methods of identifying anti-CMV antibodies reveal much more information about the activity of the infection. CMV immunoglobulin G (IgG) antibody levels persist for years after infection. The presence of immunoglobulin M (IgM) antibodies, however, indicates a relatively recent infection. Three different CMV antigens can be detected immunologically. They are called *early, intermediate-early,* and *late antigens,* and they indicate onset of infection. CMV inclusion bodies can be identified in the renal cells sloughed into the urine and are detected during a routine urinalysis.

No specific therapy is known for this infection. If the diagnosis is established early by viral culture or serologic study, abortion may be an option. A fourfold increase in CMV titre in paired sera collected 10 to 14 days apart is usually indicative of an acute infection.

PROCEDURE AND PATIENT CARE

Before
✍ Explain the procedure to the patient.

During
- For culture, urine, sputum, or mouth swab is the specimen of choice. Fresh specimens are essential.
- For an antibody or antigen titre, collect blood in a gold-top or red-top tube.
- Collect a specimen from the pregnant woman with suspected acute infection as early as possible.
- Collect the convalescent specimen 2 to 4 weeks later.

After
- Apply pressure or a pressure dressing to the venipuncture site.
- Assess the venipuncture site for bleeding.
- The specimens are cultured in a virus laboratory, which takes approximately 3 to 7 days.

TEST RESULTS AND CLINICAL SIGNIFICANCE
CMV infection

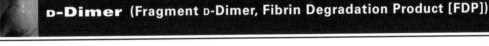

D-Dimer (Fragment D-Dimer, Fibrin Degradation Product [FDP])

NORMAL FINDINGS
<3.0 nmol/L (<0.4 *Mcg*/mL)

INDICATIONS
The D-dimer test is used to identify intravascular clotting.

TEST EXPLANATION
The fragment D-dimer test assesses both thrombin and plasmin activity. D-Dimer is a fibrin degradation fragment that is made through lysis of crosslinked (D-dimerized) fibrin. As plasmin acts on the fibrin polymer clot, fibrin degradation products (FDPs) and D-dimer are produced. The D-dimer assay provides a highly specific measurement of the amount of fibrin degradation that occurs. Normal plasma does not have detectable amounts of fragment D-dimer.

This test provides a simple and confirmatory test for disseminated intravascular coagulation (DIC). Positive results of the D-dimer assay correlate with positive results of FDPs. The D-dimer assay may be more specific than the FDP assay, but it is less sensitive. Therefore, combining the FDP and the D-dimer tests may provide high sensitivity and specificity for recognizing DIC.

Levels of ᴅ-dimer can also increase when a fibrin clot is lysed through thrombolytic therapy. Thrombotic problems such as deep-vein thrombosis (DVT), pulmonary embolism, sickle cell disease, and thrombosis of malignancy are also associated with high ᴅ-dimer levels. Recently, ᴅ-dimer has been used as an effective screening test for DVT. It is able to accurately identify patients with DVT, who then undergo venous duplex scanning (see p. 930). If the ᴅ-dimer test result is negative, its high predictability indicates that the patient does not have DVT, and further duplex scanning may not be necessary.

Finally, the ᴅ-dimer test can be used to determine the duration of anticoagulation therapy in patients with DVT. Among patients with an abnormal ᴅ-dimer level 1 month after the discontinuation of anticoagulant therapy, incidence of recurrent DVT is significant. This incidence can be reduced with reinstitution of anticoagulation therapy.

The ᴅ-dimer can be tested by enzyme-linked fluorescent immunoassay (ELFA), multiple enzyme-linked immunosorbent assay (ELISA) methods, or latex quantitative/qualitative assay. The general consensus is that ELFA is the fastest, most reliable, and least labour-intensive assay (for a single test).

PROCEDURE AND PATIENT CARE

Before
🗶 Explain the procedure to the patient.
🗶 Inform the patient that no fasting is required.

During
• Collect a venous blood sample in a blue-top tube.

After
• Apply pressure or a pressure dressing to the venipuncture site.
• Assess the venipuncture site for bleeding. If the patient is receiving anticoagulants or has coagulopathies, remember that the bleeding time will be increased.

TEST RESULTS AND CLINICAL SIGNIFICANCE

▲ Increased Levels

DIC: *This is a phenomenon of rapid intramicrovascular coagulation and synchronous fibrinolysis. ᴅ-Dimer is produced by the action of plasmin on the fibrin polymer clot.*
Primary fibrinolysis,
During thrombolytic or defibrination therapy: *ᴅ-Dimer is produced by the action of plasmin on the fibrin polymer clot.*
Deep vein thrombosis,
Pulmonary embolism,
Arterial thromboembolism,
Sickle cell anemia with or without vaso-occlusive crisis: *The body's natural reaction to clot development is fibrinolysis. ᴅ-Dimer is produced by the action of plasmin on the fibrin polymer clot.*
Pregnancy,
Malignancy,
Surgery: *These clinical situations are associated with varying degrees of clotting and fibrinolysis. ᴅ-Dimer is produced by the action of plasmin on the fibrin polymer clot.*

RELATED TESTS

The following are tests used to assist in the diagnosis of DIC:

Prothrombin Time (p. 446). This is used to evaluate the adequacy of the extrinsic system and common pathway in the clotting mechanism.

Coagulating Factor Concentration (p. 177). This is a quantitative measurement of specific coagulation factors.

Partial Thromboplastin Time, Activated (p. 396). This test is used to evaluate the intrinsic system and the common pathway of clot formation. It is most commonly used to monitor heparin therapy.

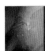 **Dexamethasone Suppression** (DS, Prolonged/Rapid DS, Cortisol Suppression, Adrenocorticotropic Hormone [ACTH] Suppression)

NORMAL FINDINGS

Prolonged Method

Expected values (normal)

Low dose: >50% reduction of plasma cortisol and 17-hydroxycorticosteroid (17-OCHS) levels

High dose: >50% reduction of plasma cortisol and 17-OCHS levels

Rapid Method

Normal: nearly zero cortisol levels

INDICATIONS

The dexamethasone suppression test is important for diagnosing adrenal hyperfunction (Cushing's syndrome) and distinguishing its cause.

TEST EXPLANATION

An elaborate feedback mechanism for cortisol exists to coordinate the function of the hypothalamus, pituitary gland, and the adrenal glands. Corticotropin-releasing hormone is made in the hypothalamus. This stimulates adrenocorticotropic hormone (ACTH) production in the anterior pituitary gland. ACTH stimulates the adrenal cortex to produce cortisol. The rising levels of cortisol act as negative feedback and curtail further production of corticotropin-releasing hormone and ACTH. Cortisol is a potent glucocorticoid released from the adrenal cortex. This hormone affects the metabolism of carbohydrates, proteins, and fats. It has an especially profound effect on glucose serum levels.

The dexamethasone suppression test is based on the dependence of pituitary ACTH secretion on the plasma cortisol feedback mechanism. As plasma cortisol levels increase, ACTH secretion is suppressed; as cortisol levels decrease, ACTH secretion is stimulated. Dexamethasone is a synthetic steroid (similar to cortisol) that suppresses ACTH secretion. Under normal circumstances, this results in reduced stimulation to the adrenal glands and ultimately a drop of 50% or more in plasma cortisol and 17-OCHS levels. This important feedback system does not function properly in patients with Cushing's syndrome.

In Cushing's syndrome caused by bilateral adrenal hyperplasia (Cushing's disease), the pituitary gland is reset upward and responds only to high plasma levels of cortisone and steroids. In Cushing's syndrome caused by adrenal adenoma or cancer (which acts autonomously), cortisol secretion continues despite a decrease in ACTH. When Cushing's syndrome is caused by an ectopic ACTH-producing tumour (as in lung cancer), that tumour is also considered autonomous and continues to secrete ACTH despite high cortisol levels. Again, no decrease occurs in plasma cortisol. Knowledge of the following defects in the normal cortisol-ACTH feedback system is the basis for understanding the dexamethasone suppression test:

Cushing's Syndrome Caused by Bilateral Adrenal Hyperplasia

Low dose: no change
High dose: >50% reduction of plasma cortisol and 17-OCHS levels

Cushing's Syndrome Caused by Adrenal Adenoma or Carcinoma

Low dose: no change
High dose: no change

Cushing's Syndrome Caused by Ectopic ACTH-Producing Tumour

Low dose: no change
High dose: no change

The dexamethasone suppression test also may identify depressed individuals likely to respond to electroconvulsive therapy or antidepressants rather than to psychologic or social interventions. ACTH production is not suppressed after administration of low-dose dexamethasone in these patients.

The *prolonged* dexamethasone suppression test can be performed over a 6-day period on an outpatient basis. The rapid dexamethasone suppression test is easily and quickly performed and is used primarily as a screening test to diagnose Cushing's syndrome. It is less accurate and less informative than the prolonged dexamethasone suppression test, but when its results are normal, the diagnosis of Cushing's syndrome can safely be ruled out. Because of the ease with which the rapid dexamethasone suppression test can be performed, it is useful in clinical medicine.

INTERFERING FACTORS

- Physical and emotional stress can elevate ACTH release and obscure interpretation of test results. Stress is a stimulant of the pituitary gland, which thereby secretes ACTH.
- Drugs that can affect test results include barbiturates, estrogens, oral contraceptives, phenytoin (Dilantin), spironolactone (Aldactone), steroids, and tetracyclines.

PROCEDURE AND PATIENT CARE

Before

- Explain the procedure (prolonged or rapid test) to the patient.
- Obtain the patient's weight as a baseline for evaluating side effects of steroids.

During

Prolonged Test

- Obtain a baseline 24-hour urine collection for corticosteroids (urine 17-OCHS [see p. 959] or urinary cortisol).

- Collect blood for determination of baseline plasma cortisol levels if indicated. Collect 24-hour urine specimens daily over a 6-day period. Because 6 continuous days of urine collections are needed, no urine specimens are discarded except for the first voided specimen on day 1, after which the collection begins.
- On day 3, administer a low dose of dexamethasone by mouth as ordered by the physician.
- On day 5, administer a high dose of dexamethasone by mouth as ordered by the physician.
- Administer the dexamethasone with milk or an antacid to prevent gastric irritation.
- The urine samples for cortisol and 17-OCHS do not need a preservative.
- Note that the creatinine content is measured in all the 24-hour urine collections to demonstrate their accuracy and adequacy.
- Keep the urine specimens refrigerated or in a container of water and crushed ice during the collection period.

Rapid Test
- Give the patient a dose of dexamethasone by mouth at 11 PM as ordered by physician.
- Administer the dexamethasone with milk or an antacid to prevent gastric irritation.
- Attempt to ensure a good night's sleep. The patient may take a sedative or a hypnotic only if absolutely necessary.
- At 8 AM the next morning, collect blood for determination of the plasma cortisol level before the patient arises.
- If no cortisol suppression occurs after administration of the dose of dexamethasone, administer a higher dose to suppress ACTH production. This is referred to as the *overnight 8-mg dexamethasone suppression test*. Patients with adrenal hyperplasia exhibit ACTH suppression. Patients with adrenal or ectopic tumours do not exhibit ACTH suppression.

After
- Evaluate the patient for evidence of gastric irritation.
- Assess the patient for steroid-induced side effects by monitoring weight, glucose levels, and potassium levels.
- Send specimens to the laboratory promptly.

TEST RESULTS AND CLINICAL SIGNIFICANCE
Adrenal Hyperfunction (Cushing's Syndrome)
Cushing's disease,

Ectopic ACTH-producing tumours: *In these illnesses, ACTH is produced without regard to the inhibitory feedback mechanism that normally exists. This is a result of neoplastic overproduction of ACTH in the pituitary gland or elsewhere in the body by an ACTH-producing cancer. ACTH is not suppressed. As a result, cortisol is not suppressed.*

Adrenal adenoma or carcinoma: *Neoplasms of the adrenal glands are not sensitive to the inhibitory feedback mechanism that normally exists. Therefore, ACTH is suppressed by the dexamethasone, but cortisol production (the end point of the test) is not.*

Bilateral adrenal hyperplasia: *The inhibitory feedback mechanism that normally exists in the pituitary-adrenal system is blunted. Therefore, at low dexamethasone doses, no change in cortisol production is observed. At high dexamethasone doses, however, the ACTH and subsequently cortisol are suppressed.*

Mental depression: *ACTH is not suppressed in individuals likely to require electroconvulsive or medicinal therapy for depression.*

RELATED TESTS

Adrenocorticotropic Hormone Stimulation with Cosyntropin (p. 37). This test is used to evaluate the differential diagnosis of Cushing's syndrome or Addison's disease.

Adrenocorticotropic Hormone (p. 34). The serum ACTH study is a test of anterior pituitary gland function that affords the greatest insight into the causes of either Cushing's syndrome (overproduction of cortisol) or Addison's disease (underproduction of cortisol).

Cortisol, Blood (p. 192). This is a direct measurement of the cortisol blood level.

Cortisol, Urine (p. 953). This test is a measure of urinary cortisol. It is performed on patients who are suspected to have hyperfunctioning or hypofunctioning of the adrenal gland.

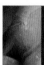
Diabetes Mellitus Autoantibody (Insulin Autoantibody [IAA], Islet Cell Antibody [ICA], Glutamic Acid Decarboxylase Antibody [GAD Ab])

NORMAL FINDINGS

<1:4 titre; no antibody detected

INDICATIONS

This test is used in the evaluation of insulin resistance. It is also used to identify type 1 diabetes and to evaluate suspected allergy to insulin. This antibody test is furthermore used in surveillance of patients who have received pancreatic islet cell transplantation.

TEST EXPLANATION

Type 1 diabetes mellitus is insulin-dependent diabetes (IDDM). This condition is now increasingly recognized as an "organ specific" form of autoimmune disease that results in destruction of the pancreatic islet cells and their products. These antibodies are used in testing to differentiate type 1 diabetes mellitus from type 2 (non–insulin-dependent) diabetes mellitus. Nearly 90% of young patients with type 1 diabetes have one or more of these autoantibodies at the time of their diagnosis. Patients with type 2 diabetes have low or negative titres.

These antibodies often appear years before the onset of symptoms. For screening relatives of patients with IDDM, the test is useful because these relatives are at risk for developing the disease. Of first-degree relatives with both islet cell antibody and insulin autoantibody, 60% to 80% develop IDDM within 10 years. The presence of glutamic acid decarboxylase antibody provides confirmatory evidence. The presence of these antibodies identifies which patient with gestational diabetes will eventually require insulin permanently. Once recognized, diabetes-preventive treatment is instituted. This may include counselling in addition to antibody and glucose monitoring.

Because insulin antibodies appear in nearly all patients with diabetes treated with exogenous (human, bovine, or porcine) insulin, testing for the presence of these antibodies must precede insulin administration. Insulin antibodies develop from impurities in animal insulin or from antigenic stimulation of the insulin molecule. With the increased use of human insulin, the frequency of anti-insulin antibodies has significantly decreased.

The most common type of anti-insulin antibody is immunoglobulin G (IgG), but immunoglobulins A, M, D, and E (IgA, IgM, IgD, and IgE) also have been reported. Most of these insulin antibodies do not cause clinical problems, but their presence may complicate most insulin assays. Anti-insulin antibodies act as insulin-transporting proteins and bind the free insulin. This can reduce the amount of insulin available for glucose metabolism. They may also contribute to insulin resistance (daily insulin requirements exceeding 200 U/day for 2 days). IgM, in particular, may cause insulin resistance. Insulin allergy (most common with animal insulin) may result from IgE antibodies to insulin.

These insulin antibodies are diagnostic of factitious hypoglycemia from surreptitious administration of insulin. In these cases, C-peptide studies may also determine whether hypoglycemia is caused by insulin abuse, because C-peptide is not produced when exogenous insulin is administered.

INTERFERING FACTORS

- When anti-insulin antibodies are measured by radiobinding assay, radioactive scans within 7 days before the assay may interfere with the assay result.

PROCEDURE AND PATIENT CARE

Before

𝄤 Explain the procedure to the patient.
𝄤 Inform the patient that no fasting is required.

During

- Collect a venous blood sample in a plain red-top or a gold-top (blood/serum separator) tube.

After

- Apply pressure to the venipuncture site.

TEST RESULTS AND CLINICAL SIGNIFICANCE

▲ Increased Levels

Insulin resistance: *The anti-insulin antibodies bind insulin and thereby diminish the amount of free insulin available for glucose metabolism.*

Allergies to insulin: *Although allergies occur most frequently with the use of animal-generated insulin, they can also occur with human insulin. A rash or lymphadenopathy may be the manifestation of such an allergy.*

Factitious hypoglycemia: *Because most patients develop anti-insulin antibodies to exogenous insulin, the identification of these antibodies is evidence of the secretive self-administration of insulin in a patient who denies the use of insulin.*

RELATED TESTS

C-Peptide (p. 197). This test is used to evaluate diabetic patients. It is also used to identify patients who secretly self-administer insulin.

Insulin Assay (p. 330). This test is used to diagnose insulinoma (tumour of the islets of Langerhans) and to evaluate abnormal lipid and carbohydrate metabolism. It is used in the evaluation of patients with fasting hypoglycemia.

2,3-Diphosphoglycerate (2,3-DPG in Erythrocytes)

NORMAL FINDINGS

0.79 ± 0.12 mmol/L hemoglobin (12.3 ± 1.87 Mcmol/g of hemoglobin)
4.2 ± 0.64 mmol/L red blood cells (RBCs) (4.2 ± 0.64 Mcmol/mL of RBCs)
  Levels are lower in newborns and even lower in premature infants.

INDICATIONS

This test is used in the evaluation of nonspherocytic anemia.

TEST EXPLANATION

2,3-Diphosphoglycerate (2,3-DPG) is a byproduct of the glycolytic respiratory pathway of the red blood cell (RBC). A congenital enzyme deficiency in this vital pathway alters the RBC shape and survival significantly. Nonspherocytic anemia is the result. Another result of the enzyme deficiency is reduced synthesis of 2,3-DPG. 2,3-DPG controls oxygen transport from the RBCs to the tissues. Deficiencies of this enzyme result in alterations of the oxygen-hemoglobin dissociation curve, which controls release of oxygen to the tissues. Many anemias that are not a result of 2,3-DPG deficiency are associated with increased levels of 2,3-DPG as a compensatory mechanism.

  Usually, 2,3-DPG levels increase in response to anemia or hypoxic conditions (e.g., obstructive lung disease, congenital cyanotic heart disease, after vigorous exercise). Increases in 2,3-DPG decrease the amount of oxygen binding to hemoglobin so that oxygen is more easily released to the tissues when needed (lower arterial partial pressure of oxygen [Pao_2]). Levels of 2,3-DPG are decreased as a result of inherited genetic defects. This genetic defect parallels sickle cell disease and hemoglobin C diseases.

INTERFERING FACTORS

- Levels may be increased after vigorous exercise.
- High altitudes may increase 2,3-DPG levels.
- Banked blood has decreased amounts of 2,3-DPG.
- Acidosis decreases 2,3-DPG levels.

PROCEDURE AND PATIENT CARE

Before

- Explain the procedure to the patient.
- Inform the patient that no fasting is required.

During

- Collect a venous blood sample in a red-top tube.

After

- Apply pressure or a pressure dressing to the venipuncture site.
- Assess the venipuncture site for bleeding.

TEST RESULTS AND CLINICAL SIGNIFICANCE

▲ Increased Levels

Anemia: *In compensation, 2,3-DPG levels increase to provide adequate oxygen to the tissues.*

Hypoxic heart and lung diseases (e.g., obstructive lung disease, cystic fibrosis, congenital cyanotic heart disease): *Hypoxemia stimulates the production of 2,3-DPG.*

Hyperthyroidism: *Increased metabolic processes increase oxygen requirements. This need is met by increased 2,3-DPG.*

Chronic renal failure: *Erythropoietin deficiency as a result of chronic renal failure causes anemia. In compensation, 2,3-DPG levels increase to provide adequate oxygen to the tissues.*

Pyruvate kinase deficiency: *This enzyme is important in the glycolytic respiratory pathway of the RBC. Its function is to metabolize 2,3-DPG byproducts. In the absence of this enzyme, 2,3-DPG is not metabolized, and levels increase.*

Compensation for higher altitudes: *In compensation for the reduced oxygen availability, 2,3-DPG is increased in order to make more oxygen available to the tissues.*

▼ Decreased Levels

Polycythemia: *2,3-DPG is made in the RBC as a result of its glycolytic respiratory process. Increased numbers of RBCs cause a compensatory decrease in 2,3-DPG levels.*

Acidosis: *Decreases in 2,3-DPG levels are associated with metabolic or respiratory acidosis.*

After massive blood transfusion: *Banked RBCs lose 2,3-DPG during storage.*

2,3-DPG disease: *The enzymes required for synthesis of 2,3-DPG are reduced. As a result, 2,3-DPG levels are reduced.*

Respiratory distress syndrome: *The pathophysiologic mechanism underlying this observation is unknown.*

2,3-DPG mutase deficiency,

2,3-DPG phosphatase deficiency: *These enzymes are critical in the synthesis of 2,3-DPG. Reduced levels of the enzymes cause reduction in synthesis of 2,3-DPG.*

RELATED TESTS

Complete Blood Cell Count (p. 187). This is a series of tests that provide information about the hematologic system and many other organ systems.

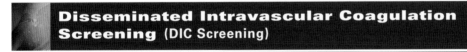

Disseminated Intravascular Coagulation Screening (DIC Screening)

NORMAL FINDINGS

No evidence of disseminated intravascular coagulation (DIC)

INDICATIONS

This group of tests is indicated for patients who are suspected of having acute DIC (demonstrate a coagulopathy), for patients who have chronic DIC (have chronic microembolic processes), and for patients who are at high risk for DIC (have sepsis or advanced cancer).

TEST EXPLANATION

This is a group of tests used to detect DIC. Many pathologic conditions can instigate or are associated with DIC. The more common ones are bacterial septicemia, amniotic fluid embolism, retention of a dead fetus, malignant neoplasia, liver cirrhosis, extensive surgery (especially on the prostate or liver), extracorporeal heart bypass, extensive trauma, severe burns, and transfusion reactions.

In DIC, the entire clotting mechanism is triggered inappropriately. This results in significant systemic or localized intravascular formation of fibrin clots. Consequences of this futile clotting are intravascular clogging of blood flow and excessive bleeding, which result from consumption of the platelets and clotting factors that have been used in intravascular clotting. The fibrinolytic system is also activated to break down the clot formation and the fibrin involved in the intravascular coagulation. This fibrinolysis results in the formation of fibrin degradation products (FDPs; see Thrombosis Indicators, p. 495) which, by themselves, act as anticoagulants; these FDPs only serve to enhance the bleeding tendency.

Organ injury can occur as a result of intravascular clots, which cause microvascular occlusion in various organs. This may cause serious anoxic injury in affected organs. Also, red blood cells (RBCs) passing through partly plugged vessels are injured and subsequently hemolyzed. The result may be ongoing hemolytic anemia. Figure 2-17 summarizes the pathophysiologic mechanisms and effects of DIC. Heparin is sometimes used to treat DIC because it inhibits the ongoing futile thrombin formation. This decreases the use of clotting factors and platelets, and bleeding ceases.

When DIC is suspected in a patient with a bleeding tendency, a series of routinely performed laboratory tests are done (prothrombin time, partial thromboplastin time, bleeding time, and platelet count). If results are abnormal, further testing should be performed (Table 2-20). With these tests, the hematologist can make the appropriate diagnosis with confidence. All these tests are discussed separately in this book.

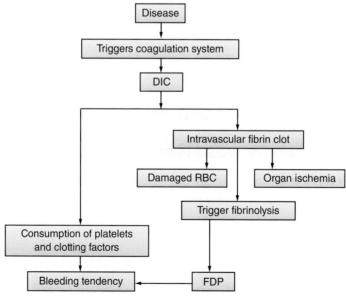

Figure 2-17 Pathophysiologic development of disseminated intravascular coagulation (DIC), which may result in bleeding tendency, organ ischemia, and hemolytic anemia. FDP, fibrin degradation products; RBCs, red blood cells.

TABLE 2-20	Screening Tests for Disseminated Intravascular Coagulation

Test	Result
Platelet count (p. 416)	Decreased
Prothrombin time (p. 446)	Prolonged
Partial thromboplastin time (p. 396)	Prolonged
Coagulating factors (p. 177)	Decreased levels of factors I, II, V, VIII, X, and XIII; more commonly used for diagnosis than for screening
Fibrin degradation products (p. 217)	Increased amounts
Fibrinogen (p. 254)	Decreased level
D-Dimer (p. 217)	Increased level
Fibrinopeptide A (p. 217)	Increased level
Prothrombin fragment (p. 217)	Increased level

Blood Studies

2

RELATED TEST

Protein C, Protein S (p. 437). This test identifies deficiencies in either protein C or protein S, or both. This is part of an evaluation of hypercoagulation.

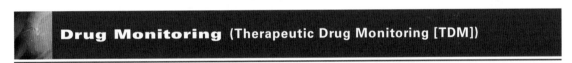

Drug Monitoring (Therapeutic Drug Monitoring [TDM])

NORMAL FINDINGS

Table 2-21 lists the therapeutic ranges for the average patient.

INDICATIONS

This test is performed to monitor drug levels.

TEST EXPLANATION

Therapeutic drug monitoring (TDM) entails measuring blood drug levels to determine effective drug dosages and to prevent toxicity. It is also used to identify patients who are not compliant with their medication regimens. The patient's age and size, extent and rate of drug absorption or excretion, and metabolic rate can all affect drug levels. Measurement of drug levels is very important in patients for whom these variables are outside the normal ranges or who have other diseases that can affect drug levels. Drug monitoring is helpful in patients who take other medicines that may affect drug levels or act in a synergistic or antagonistic manner with the drug to be tested. Some medicines—for example, antiarrhythmics, bronchodilators, antibiotics, anticonvulsants, and cardiotonics—have a very narrow therapeutic margin (i.e., the difference between therapeutic and toxic drug levels is small).

TDM is helpful if the desired therapeutic effect of the drug is not observed as expected. Dosages beyond normal may have to be prescribed. Likewise, if toxic symptoms appear with standard doses, TDM can be used to adjust dosing.

TABLE 2-21   Drug Monitoring Data

		THERAPEUTIC LEVEL*	
Drug	**Use**	**SI Units**	**Conventional Units**
Acetaminophen	Analgesic, antipyretic	66–200 *Mc*mol/L	10–30 *Mc*g/L
Amikacin	Antibiotic	20–30 mg/L	15–25 *Mc*g/mL
Aminophylline	Bronchodilator	55–110 *Mc*mol/L	10–20 *Mc*g/mL
Amitriptyline	Antidepressant	430–900 nmol	120–150 ng/mL
Carbamazepine	Anticonvulsant	17–50 *Mc*mol/L	5–12 *Mc*g/mL
Chloramphenicol	Anti-infective	30–77 *Mc*mol/L	10–20 *Mc*g/mL
Desipramine	Antidepressant	430–675 nmol/L	150–300 ng/mL
Digoxin	Cardiac glycoside	0.6–1.3 nmol/L	0.8–2 ng/mL
Disopyramide	Antiarrhythmic	8.3–22.0 *Mc*mol/L	2–5 *Mc*g/mL
Ethosuximide	Anticonvulsant	280–710 *Mc*mol/L	40–100 *Mc*g/mL
Gentamicin	Antibiotic	5–10 mg/L	5–10 *Mc*g/mL
Imipramine	Antidepressant	550–1015 nmol/L	150–300 ng/mL
Lidocaine	Antiarrhythmic	17–43 *Mc*mol/L	1.5–5 *Mc*g/mL
Lithium	Manic episodes of manic depression psychosis	0.8–1.2 mmol/L	0.8–1.2 mEq/L
Methotrexate	Antitumour agent	90–790 nmol/L	>0.01 *Mc*mol/24 hr
Nortriptyline	Antidepressant	170–495 nmol/L	50–150 ng/mL
Phenobarbital	Anticonvulsant	65–170 *Mc*mol/L	10–30 *Mc*g/mL
Phenytoin	Anticonvulsant	40–80 *Mc*mol/L	10–20 *Mc*g/mL
Primidone	Anticonvulsant	23–55 *Mc*mol/L	5–12 *Mc*g/mL
Procainamide	Antiarrhythmic	17–43 *Mc*mol/L	4–10 *Mc*g/mL
Propranolol	Antiarrhythmic	193–386 nmol/L	50–100 ng/mL
Quinidine	Antiarrhythmic	6–15 *Mc*mol/L	2–5 *Mc*g/mL
Salicylate	Antipyretic, anti-inflammatory, analgesic	1.1–2.2 mmol/L	100–250 *Mc*g/mL
Theophylline	Bronchodilator	55–110 *Mc*mol/L	10–20 *Mc*g/mL
Tobramycin	Antibiotic	5–10 mg/L	5–10 *Mc*g/mL
Valproic acid	Anticonvulsant	350–700 *Mc*mol/L	50–100 *Mc*g/mL

*Levels vary according to the laboratory performing the test.

The ranges listed in Table 2-21 may not apply to all patients because clinical response is influenced by many factors (Box 2-6). Also, different laboratories use different measurement units for reporting test results and normal ranges. It is important that sufficient time pass between the administration of the medication and the collection of the blood sample to allow for adequate absorption and achievement of therapeutic levels.

Blood is routinely used for TDM because results indicate the activity of the drug at any one particular time. Urine drug levels reflect the presence of the drug over the previous several days. Therefore, if data concerning drug levels at a particular time are necessary, blood testing is required. Gas chromatography, thin-layer chromatography, radioimmunoassay, fluorescent immunoassay, and other laboratory methods are used to determine drug levels.

Blood samples can be taken at the drug's peak level (highest concentration) or at the trough level (lowest concentration). Peak levels are useful in tests for toxicity, and trough levels are useful for demonstrating a satisfactory therapeutic level. Trough levels are often referred to as *residual levels*. The time when the sample should be collected after the last dose of the medication varies according to whether a peak or trough level is requested and according to the half-life

BOX 2-6   Factors Influencing Blood Drug Levels

Route of administration
Drug metabolism
Age
Other disease
Drug absorption
Drug excretion
Weight
Laboratory methods
Drug delivery (cardiovascular function)
Dosage
Other medications
Patient compliance with medication regimen

TABLE 2-22   Peak Concentration Times for Some Common Drugs

Drug (Given by Routine Route)	Peak (Hours)
Phenytoin	4–8
Phenobarbital	12
Lithium	1–3
Tricyclic antidepressants	2–6
Procainamide	1–2
Procainamide SR	4
Lidocaine	2
Quinidine	2
Digoxin	$\frac{1}{2}$–$1\frac{1}{2}$
Theophylline	2–3
Gentamicin	$\frac{1}{2}$
Vancomycin	$\frac{1}{2}$–2

of the drug (the time required for the drug blood level to decrease by 50%). Table 2-22 lists the peak concentration times for some commonly used drugs. Both peak and trough levels should be within the therapeutic range. If peak levels are higher than the therapeutic range, the patient may experience toxic effects. It trough levels are below the therapeutic range, drug therapy is inadequate.

TDM is used to alter the dosage of medications that can be analyzed in the laboratory. There are many aspects that can affect proper drug dosing. The most recent evidence known to affect drug dosing has come from improved methods of evaluating a patient's ability to metabolize the drug. The cytochrome P450 (CYP450) system is a major family of all drug-metabolizing enzymes. These metabolic enzymes are found primarily in the human liver.

Several CYP450 enzymes are involved in the metabolism of a significant proportion of drugs such as tricyclic antidepressants, serotonin reuptake inhibitors, neuroleptics, beta blockers, antiarrhythmics, and tamoxifen. CYP2D6 is one of CYP450 enzymes that play an instrumental role in the breakdown and clearance of prescribed drugs. CYP2D6 is a hydroxylase that, along with CYP2C9 and CYP2C19, is responsible for 40% of first-pass hepatic metabolism and is thought to be active in the enzymatic breakdown of 20% to 25% of all medicines now prescribed.

CYP450 genotype testing is a method of evaluating the metabolic effectiveness of the CYP450 system. With cytochrome genotyping, four categories of drug metabolizers can be identified: poor metabolizers, intermediate metabolizers, extensive metabolizers, and ultrametabolizers. Overall, poor metabolizers and, to a lesser extent, intermediate metabolizers are prone to exaggerated adverse effect from drugs metabolized by CYP2D6, whereas normal doses of the same drugs tend to be ineffectual for ultrametabolizers. If a drug (e.g., tamoxifen) must be hydrolyzed to its active form, poor metabolizers do not benefit from normal doses, whereas ultrametabolizers experience drug benefit from even small doses.

Humans inherit two alleles for the *CYP2D6* gene, one from each parent. Each allele may be normal, or "wild-type" (designated *wt*), or variant type (designated *vt*). Thus, genotypically, an individual's alleles may be homozygous wild-type (*wt/wt*), heterozygous (*wt/vt*), or homozygous variant (*vt/vt*). Those with two wild-type alleles have effective metabolic ability, whereas those with one or two variant type alleles may have diminished metabolism. In addition, other drugs that are metabolized by the CYP2D6 enzyme may compete for the enzyme function and diminish the metabolism of another concomitantly administered medication.

This test allows physicians to consider genetic information from patients in selecting medications and dosages of medications for a wide variety of common conditions such as cardiac disease, psychiatric disease, and cancer. This assay is performed predominantly on a buccal smear and subjected to reverse-transcriptase polymerase chain reaction and more specialized techniques such as gene amplification/sequencing.

PROCEDURE AND PATIENT CARE

Before

- Explain the procedure to the patient.
- Inform the patient that no food or fluid restrictions are needed.
- For patients in whom symptoms of drug toxicity are suspected, the best time to collect the blood specimen is when the symptoms are occurring.
- If there is a concern regarding whether an adequate dose of the drug is achieved, it is best to obtain trough levels.

During

- Collect a venous blood sample in a tube designated by the laboratory. *Peak* levels are usually obtained 1 to 2 hours after oral intake, approximately 1 hour after intramuscular administration, and approximately 30 minutes after intravenous administration. *Residual (trough)* levels are usually obtained shortly (0 to 15 minutes) before the next scheduled dose. Consult with the pharmacy for specific times.

After

- Apply pressure or a pressure dressing to the venipuncture site.
- Assess the venipuncture site for bleeding.
- Clearly mark all blood samples with the following information: patient's name, diagnosis, name of drug, time of last drug ingestion, time of sample, and any other medications the patient is currently taking.
- Promptly send the specimen to the laboratory.

TEST RESULTS AND CLINICAL SIGNIFICANCE

Nontherapeutic levels of drugs,

Toxic levels of drugs: *TDM is only a guide to treatment. Therapy may be successful at drug levels below therapeutic range. Levels above therapeutic range may be necessary in some patients to obtain adequate therapy.*

RELATED TEST

Toxicology (p. 986). This is generally a urine test to determine the toxic effect of prescribed and nonprescribed drugs that are often used and abused in criminal behaviour.

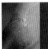

Drug Sensitivity Genotype Testing (AccuType)

NORMAL FINDINGS

No abnormal genetic abnormalities

INDICATIONS

This test is indicated if a patient is taking a medication with no therapeutic effect or is experiencing signs of toxicity at normal therapeutic doses.

TEST EXPLANATION

The efficacy of therapeutic drugs can vary considerably among different patients. Factors that influence these variations include genetic aberrations, patient age, race, body weight or surface area, sex, tobacco use, concomitant medications, and comorbid medical conditions. It is extremely important to identify differences in drug metabolism to preclude the possibility of overdosing or underdosing.

Drug sensitivity genotype testing identifies genetic aberrations that encode various proteins required for drug metabolism. If the gene is abnormal, the protein may be deficient in quantity or character to properly metabolize the medication given to the patient. Various laboratories have "trademarked" their testing methods. A common test is called *AccuType Testing*.

Drug sensitivity genotype testing is available for predicting a patient's response to warfarin, clopidogrel, interferon-ribavirin (and other retroviral medications), metformin, and anti-TB drugs (rifampin/isoniazid).

PROCEDURE AND PATIENT CARE

Before

- Explain the procedure to the patient.
- Tell the patient that no food or fluid restrictions are needed.

During

- Collect a venous blood sample in a whole blood (EDTA, lavender-top tube) or a collection tube designated by the laboratory.
- Alternatively, 1 mL of saliva in an Oragene DNA self-collection kit can be submitted. The specimen should be maintained at room temperature.

After

- Apply pressure or a pressure dressing to the venipuncture site.
- Promptly send the specimen to the laboratory.

TEST RESULTS AND CLINICAL SIGNIFICANCE

Genetic aberrations that may alter drug metabolism: *As a result of knowing genetic aberrations in drug metabolism, drug dosages can be modified to provide the therapeutic dose without risks of toxicity.*

RELATED TEST

Drug Monitoring (p. 227). This test includes a more general discussion of pharmacogenetics.

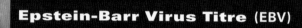

Epstein-Barr Virus Titre (EBV)

NORMAL FINDINGS

Titres ≤1:10: nondiagnostic
Titres 1:10–1:60: indicative of infection at some undetermined time
Titres ≥1:320: active infection

A fourfold increase in titre in paired sera collected 10 to 14 days apart is usually indicative of an acute infection.

INDICATIONS

This test is used to diagnose a suspected Epstein-Barr virus (EBV) infection (infectious mononucleosis).

TEST EXPLANATION

EBV affects more than 90% of individuals during the first two decades of life worldwide. Once infection occurs, the virus becomes dormant but can be reactivated later. EBV infection can produce infectious mononucleosis. Mononucleosis is seen most often in children, adolescents, and young adults. Clinical features include acute fatigue, fever, sore throat, lymphadenopathy, and splenomegaly. Laboratory findings of lymphocytosis, atypical lymphocytes, and transient serum heterophil antibodies are seen in patients with acute EBV infection. Most patients with infectious mononucleosis recover uneventfully and return to normal activity within 4 to 6 weeks. In Africa, EBV has been associated with Burkitt lymphoma. In China, EBV infection has been associated with nasopharyngeal carcinoma.

After recovery from primary EBV infection, patients are lifelong, latent EBV carriers. Since 2005, specific immunologic tests to identify EBV activity indicate that latent EBV infection can reactivate and become associated with a constellation of chronic signs and symptoms resembling infectious mononucleosis. Clinical manifestations of chronic EBV are variable and include nonspecific symptoms, such as profound fatigue (chronic fatigue syndrome), pharyngitis, myalgia, arthralgia, low-grade fever, headache, paraesthesia, and loss of abstract thinking ability.

TABLE 2-23	Serologic Studies and the Timing of Infections		
Serologic Study	**Time From Infection to Appearance of Symptoms**	**Duration of Infection**	**Clinical Significance**
Mononucleosis spot heterophil	5 days	2 weeks	Acute or convalescent infection
VCA-IgM	7 days	3 months	Acute or convalescent infection
VCA-IgG	7 days	Present for life	Acute, convalescent, or old infection
EBNA-IgG	3 weeks	Present for life	Old infection
EA-D	7 days	2 weeks	Acute or convalescent infection

EA-D, Early antigen D (diffuse); *EBNA*, Epstein-Barr virus nuclear antigen; *IgG*, immunoglobulin G; *IgM*, immunoglobulin M; *VCA*, viral capsid antigen-antibody.

Serologic tests are the only method of diagnosing EBV infection. The heterophil agglutination slide test (mononucleosis ["mono"] spot test) helps support the diagnosis. Other, more specific immunologic tests indicate more precisely the timing of the infection (Table 2-23). The viral capsid antigen-antibodies (VCAs) can be immunoglobulin G or M (IgG or IgM). The EBV nuclear antigen (EBNA) is located in the nuclei of the infected lymphocyte. Another EBV antigen is the early antigen (EA). There are two EA antigens. One is spread diffusely about the cytoplasm of the lymphocyte (EA-D), and the other is restricted to only one area of the cytoplasm (EA-R). EA-D is commonly found in nasopharyngeal cancer. EA-R is commonly found in Burkitt lymphoma.

The interpretation of EBV antibody tests is based on the following assumptions:

1. Once the person becomes infected with EBV, the anti-VCA antibodies appear first.
2. Anti-EA (EA-D or EA-R) antibodies appear next or are present with anti-VCA antibodies early in the course of illness. An anti-EA antibody titre greater than 80 in a patient 2 years after acute infectious mononucleosis indicates chronic EBV syndrome.
3. As the patient recovers, anti-VCA and anti-EA antibodies decrease and anti-EBNA antibodies appear. Anti-EBNA antibody persists for life and reflects a past infection.
4. After the patient is recovered, anti-VCA and anti-EBNA antibodies are always present but at lower ranges. On occasion, anti-EA antibody also may be present after the patient recovers.

If an acute infection is suspected to have occurred more than a few weeks before the test, the mononucleosis spot test may be negative. Detecting anti-VCA IgG or EBNA is not helpful because their presence indicates that an EBV infection has occurred sometime in the patient's life but not necessarily recently. Detecting anti-VCA IgM, however, indicates that the syndrome of complaints the patient experienced a few weeks earlier was because of EBV infection.

PROCEDURE AND PATIENT CARE

Before

☒ Explain the procedure to the patient.
☒ Inform the patient that no fasting or special preparation is required.

During

- Collect a venous blood sample in a red-top tube.
- On the laboratory slip, record the date of onset of illness.
- Obtain serum samples as soon as possible after the onset of illness.
- Obtain a second blood specimen 14 to 21 days later.

After

- Apply pressure or a pressure dressing to the venipuncture site.
- Observe the venipuncture site for bleeding.

TEST RESULTS AND CLINICAL SIGNIFICANCE

▲ Increased Levels

Infectious mononucleosis,

Chronic EBV carrier state: *To establish this diagnosis, one of the antibodies should be found in abnormal titres.*

Chronic fatigue syndrome: *EBV antibodies are not found in all cases.*

Burkitt lymphoma,

Nasopharyngeal cancer: *These cancers are frequently associated with EBV carrier states. However, a cause-and-effect relationship has not been determined.*

RELATED TEST

Mononucleosis Spot (p. 375). This test is used to detect heterophil antibodies that can support the diagnosis of EBV infection (infectious mononucleosis).

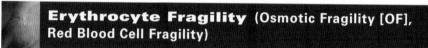

Erythrocyte Fragility (Osmotic Fragility [OF], Red Blood Cell Fragility)

NORMAL FINDINGS

Hemolysis begins at 0.5% NaCl
Hemolysis is complete at 0.3% NaCl

INDICATIONS

This test is performed to detect hereditary spherocytosis and thalassemia when intravascular hemolysis is identified.

TEST EXPLANATION

Red blood cells (RBCs) are bound by a membrane that allows water to pass through while generally restricting the solutes. This process, called *osmosis*, causes RBCs to absorb water when in a hypotonic medium. This results in swelling and, ultimately, hemolysis as the cell bursts. In the osmotic fragility test, used to determine the concentration of solute inside the cell, the cell is subjected to salt solutions of different concentrations. The ability of the normal RBC to withstand hypotonicity results from its biconcave shape, which allows the cell to increase its volume by 70% before the surface membrane is stretched. Once this limit is reached, lysis occurs. When intravascular hemolysis is identified, osmotic fragility testing is used to determine whether the RBCs have increased fragility (tend to burst open when exposed to a highly concentrated NaCl solution) or decreased fragility (tend to burst open in less concentrated, and thus more hypotonic, NaCl solution).

An osmotic fragility test indicates primarily the ratio of surface area to volume of RBCs. The lower the ratio, the more fragile the RBC is. Osmotic fragility of RBCs is defined as the ease with which the cells burst in hypotonic solutions. This is expressed in terms of the concentration of the saline solution in which the cells are hemolyzed. The numbers of cells that burst in varying concentrations of NaCl are plotted on a curve. That curve is compared with a normal curve. If the curve is shaped or shifted to the right, osmotic fragility is abnormally increased (i.e., more cells lyse in more highly concentrated NaCl solutions). If the curve is abnormally shaped or shifted to the left, osmotic fragility is decreased (i.e., fewer cells lyse at comparable NaCl concentrations). It is useful to record the concentration of sodium chloride solution at which 50% lysis (i.e., the median corpuscular fragility) occurs. This value is normally 0.40% to 0.45% of NaCl concentration. Other useful values include the concentration at which lysis begins (minimum resistance) and that at which lysis appears to be complete (maximum resistance). This test is performed by means of automated spectrophotometry.

Round RBCs (spherocytes) have increased osmotic fragility in comparison with normal indented RBCs. In hereditary spherocytosis, the RBC structure is abnormal as a result of a lack of spectrin, a key RBC cytoskeletal membrane protein. The cell membrane becomes unstable, which forces the cell to the smallest volume: that of a sphere. This common disorder is associated with intravascular hemolysis, manifested by increased osmotic fragility, which causes the entire curve to "shift to the right" or causes most of it to be within the normal range with a "tail" of fragile cells.

Thalassemia, on the other hand, is associated with thinner leptocytes whose osmotic fragility is decreased. A single-tube osmotic fragility test has been proposed for thalassemia screening with a range of different saline concentrations. The sensitivity and specificity of a 0.36% buffered saline provide a positive or at least equivocal result in nearly all patients with a thalassemia trait.

INTERFERING FACTORS

- Acute hemolysis because the osmotically labile cells are already hemolyzed and, therefore, not found in the blood specimen. Testing is recommended during a state of prolonged homeostasis with stable hematocrit.
- Dapsone can *increase* osmotic fragility.

PROCEDURE AND PATIENT CARE

Before
- Explain the procedure to the patient or the child's parents.
- Inform the patient that no fasting is required.

During
- Collect a venous blood sample in a green-top (sodium or lithium heparin) tube.
- Avoid hemolysis.

After

- Apply pressure or pressure dressing to the venipuncture site.
- Assess the venipuncture site for bleeding.

TEST RESULTS AND CLINICAL SIGNIFICANCE

▲ Increased Erythrocyte Fragility

Acquired hemolytic anemia,

Hereditary spherocytosis,

Hemolytic disease of the newborn,

Pyruvate kinase deficiency: *These diseases are associated with the presence of abnormal spherocytic RBCs.*

Malaria: *The* Plasmodium *organism causes intravascular hemolysis and creation of rounded RBCs.*

▼ Decreased Erythrocyte Fragility

Thalassemia,

Hemoglobinopathies (proteins C and S disease): *Decreased RBC fragility may result in part from changes in membrane porosity or strength.*

Iron deficiency anemia,

Reticulocytosis: *The shape and relative volume of the cell area affects osmotic fragility.*

RELATED TESTS

Haptoglobin (p. 289). This is an accurate marker of intravascular hemolysis.

Blood Smear (p. 738). RBC shape is identified and quantified.

Erythrocyte Sedimentation Rate (ESR, Sed Rate Test)

NORMAL FINDINGS

Westergren Method

Male: up to 15 mm/hour

Female: up to 20 mm/hour

Child: up to 10 mm/hour

Newborn: 0–2 mm/hour

INDICATIONS

The erythrocyte sedimentation rate (ESR) is a nonspecific test used to detect illnesses associated with acute and chronic infection, inflammation (collagen-vascular diseases), advanced neoplasm, and tissue necrosis or infarction.

TEST EXPLANATION

ESR is a measurement of the rate at which the red blood cells (RBCs) settle in saline solution or plasma over a specified time period. It is nonspecific and therefore not diagnostic for any particular organ disease or injury. Because inflammatory, neoplastic, infectious, and necrotic diseases increase the protein (mainly fibrinogen) content of plasma, RBCs have a tendency to stack up on one another, increasing their weight and causing them to descend faster. Therefore, in these diseases the ESR is increased. The ESR provides the same information as does an acute-phase reactant protein: It occurs as a reaction to acute illnesses as described previously.

The ESR can be measured to detect occult disease. Many physicians use the ESR test in this way for routine evaluation of vague symptoms. Other physicians regard this test as so nonspecific that it is useless as a routine study. The ESR test is occasionally helpful in differentiating disease entities or complaints. For example, in a patient with chest pain, the ESR is increased with myocardial infarction but is normal with angina.

The ESR is a fairly reliable indicator of the course of disease and therefore can be used to monitor disease therapy, especially for inflammatory autoimmune diseases (e.g., temporal arteritis, polymyalgia rheumatica). In general, as the disease worsens, the ESR increases; as the disease improves, the ESR decreases. If the results of the ESR are equivocal or inconsistent with clinical impressions, the C-reactive protein test is often performed.

The ESR has several limitations:
1. As mentioned previously, it is nonspecific.
2. It is sometimes not elevated in the presence of active disease.
3. A number of other factors may influence the results (see "Interfering Factors" section).

ESR elevation may lag behind other indicators early in an infection. Likewise, in the convalescent stage of a disease or infection, the ESR may remain elevated longer than other disease indicators. ESR cannot be used as an indicator of tumour burden in association with neoplastic diseases, such as myeloma or breast cancer.

INTERFERING FACTORS

- The ESR can be artificially low when the collected specimen is allowed to stand longer than 3 hours before the test.
- Pregnancy (second and third trimester) can cause elevations in ESR.
- Menstruation can cause elevated ESR.
- The sedimentation tube must be perfectly vertical. Any tilt can distort results.
- Some anemias can artificially increase the ESR. Correction nomograms for variations in RBC count are available.
- Polycythemia is associated with decreased ESR.
- Diseases associated with increased proteins (e.g., macroglobulinemia) can artificially increase the ESR.
- Drugs that may cause *increases* in ESR include dextran, methyldopa, oral contraceptives, penicillamine, procainamide, theophylline, and vitamin A.
- Drugs that may cause *decreases* in ESR include aspirin, cortisone, and quinine.

PROCEDURE AND PATIENT CARE

Before
- Explain the procedure to the patient.
- Withhold medications that may affect test results, if indicated.

During
- Collect a venous blood sample in a lavender-top tube.

After

- Apply pressure or a pressure dressing to the venipuncture site.
- Assess the venipuncture site for bleeding.
- In the laboratory, the blood is aspirated into a calibrated sedimentation tube and allowed to settle, usually for 60 minutes. The remaining clear area (plasma) is measured as the sedimentation rate.
- An alternative method is performed by measuring the distance (in millimetres) that RBCs descend (or settle) in normal saline solution in 1 hour.
- Transport the specimen immediately to the laboratory.

TEST RESULTS AND CLINICAL SIGNIFICANCE

▲ Increased Levels

Chronic renal failure (e.g., nephritis, nephrosis): *The pathophysiologic mechanism underlying this observation is not well defined.*

Malignant diseases (e.g., multiple myeloma, Hodgkin disease, advanced carcinomas): *Malignant diseases are often associated with increases in abnormal serum protein levels. Diseases associated with increased levels of serum proteins are also associated with increased ESR.*

Bacterial infection (e.g., abdominal infections, acute pelvic inflammatory disease, syphilis, pneumonia),

Inflammatory diseases (e.g., temporal arteritis, polymyalgia rheumatica, rheumatoid arthritis, rheumatic fever, systemic lupus erythematosus [SLE]),

Necrotic diseases (e.g., acute myocardial infarction, necrotic tumour, gangrene of an extremity): *ESR, like levels of acute-phase reactant proteins, is elevated in these acute illnesses.*

Diseases associated with increased protein levels (e.g., hyperfibrinogenemia, macroglobulinemia): *These diseases are associated with increased ESR.*

Severe anemias (e.g., iron deficiency or vitamin B_{12} deficiency): *With lower RBC volumes, the RBCs settle faster than in blood containing normal RBC volume.*

▼ Artificially Decreased Levels

Sickle cell disease,

Spherocytosis: *Diseases that distort the RBC are associated with decreased ESR.*

Hypofibrinogenemia: *Disease associated with decreased protein levels inhibit the sedimentation of RBCs.*

Polycythemia vera: *Increased numbers of RBCs in the blood inhibit the sedimentation of RBCs.*

RELATED TESTS

Complement Assay (p. 185). Some of the complement components are also acute-phase reactant proteins.

Fibrinogen (p. 254). This is an important protein involved in the hemostatic mechanism. It is also an acute-phase reactant protein.

C-Reactive Protein (p. 199). This is also an acute-phase reactant protein.

Erythropoietin (EPO)

NORMAL FINDINGS

5–35 IU/L

INDICATIONS

Erythropoietin is used to assist in differentiating the cause of anemia or polycythemia.

TEST EXPLANATION

Erythropoietin is a glycoprotein hormone produced in the peritubular interstitial cells located in the inner cortex of the kidney. In response to decreased oxygen sensed by these renal cells and perhaps the carotid body cells, the production of erythropoietin is increased. Erythropoietin stimulates the bone marrow to increase red blood cell (RBC) production. As a result, oxygenation in the kidneys is improved, and the stimulus for erythropoietin production is reduced. This feedback mechanism is very sensitive to minimal persistent changes in oxygen levels. In patients with normal renal function, erythropoietin levels are inversely proportional to the hemoglobin concentration.

As a hormone, erythropoietin is often administered to patients who experience anemia as a result of chemotherapy. On occasion, athletes abuse this hormone to improve oxygen-carrying capacity and thereby improve performance.

Erythropoietin testing is performed to assist in the differential diagnosis of patients with anemia and polycythemia. The erythropoietin level is elevated in patients who have low hemoglobin levels because of failure of marrow production or RBC destruction (iron-deficiency or hemolytic anemia, respectively). The anemia results in reduced availability of oxygen to the kidneys, and erythropoietin production is stimulated. However, although patients with renal diseases (or bilateral nephrectomy) are anemic, they do not have elevated erythropoietin levels. The peritubular renal cells are damaged by renal disease. Erythropoietin levels fall, and these patients experience anemia.

Patients who have polycythemia vera as an appropriate response to hypoxemia have elevated erythropoietin levels; patients who have malignant polycythemia vera, however, may have reduced erythropoietin levels. Some renal cell or adrenal carcinomas can produce elevations in erythropoietin levels that are unresponsive to the normal feedback inhibitory mechanisms.

INTERFERING FACTORS

- Pregnancy is associated with elevated erythropoietin levels.
- The use of transfused blood decreases erythropoietin levels.
- Drugs that *increase* erythropoietin levels include adrenocorticotropic hormone (ACTH), birth control pills, and steroids.

PROCEDURE AND PATIENT CARE

Before
- Explain the procedure to the patient.

During
- Collect a venous blood sample in a red-top or red/black-top (gel separator) tube.

After
- Apply pressure or a pressure dressing to the venipuncture site.
- Observe the venipuncture site for bleeding.

TEST RESULTS AND CLINICAL SIGNIFICANCE

▲ Increased Levels

Iron-deficiency anemia,

Megaloblastic anemia,

Hemolytic anemia,

Myelodysplasia,

Chemotherapy,

Acquired immune deficiency syndrome (AIDS): *Decreased RBC production is associated with reduced oxygen-carrying capacity. The specialized renal cells stimulate erythropoietin production as a result.*

Pheochromocytoma,

Renal cell carcinoma,

Adrenal carcinoma: *These and other tumours can be associated with an ectopic site of erythropoietin production.*

▼ Decreased Levels

Polycythemia vera: *Marrow erythroid production is maximal. Oxygen-carrying capacity is maximized. The specialized renal cells reduce erythropoietin production.*

Renal diseases and renal failure: *When the peritubular cells in the kidney are damaged, they cannot produce erythropoietin. Blood levels drop.*

RELATED TESTS

Hemoglobin (p. 299). Erythropoietin is inversely proportional to hemoglobin levels.

Reticulocyte Count (p. 465). This is an important blood test that also is used in differentiating the causes of anemia and polycythemia.

 Estrogen Fraction (Estradiol, Estriol, and Total Estrogen)

NORMAL FINDINGS

	Serum	URINE	
		Mcg/24 hr	nmol/L
Estradiol			
Child <10 years	55 pmol/L	0–6	0–22
Male adult	183.5 pmol/L	0–6	0–22
Female adult			
Follicular phase	73.4–1 284.9 pmol/L	0–13	0–11
Midcycle peak	550–2 753 pmol/L	4–14	15–51
Luteal phase	110–1 652 pmol/L	4–10	15–37
Postmenopausal	≤73.4 pmol/L	0–4	0–15
Estriol*			
Male adult	N/A	1–11	18–67
Female adult			
Follicular phase	N/A	0–14	0–51
Ovulatory phase	N/A	13–54	104–370

Continued

	Serum	URINE	
		Mcg/24 hr	nmol/L
Luteal phase	N/A	8–60	81–296
Menopausal	N/A	1.4–19.6	5.2–72.5
Female, pregnant			
First trimester	132 nmol/L	0–800	0–2 900
Second trimester	132–485 nmol/L	800–12 000	2 900–44 000
Third trimester	108–1 596 nmol/L	5 000–12 000	18 000–180 000
Total Estrogen			
Male adult or child <10 years	N/A	4–25	55–147
Female, not pregnant	20–80 ng/L	4–60	55–294
Female, pregnant	60–400 ng/L		
First trimester	N/A	0–800	0–2 900
Second trimester	N/A	800–5 000	2 900–18 350
Third trimester	N/A	5 000–50 000	18 350–183 000

*Rising estriol levels indicate normal fetal growth.

 Critical Values

Estriol levels 40% below average of two previous values necessitate immediate evaluation of fetal well-being during pregnancy.

INDICATIONS

Estrogen measurements are used to evaluate sexual maturity, menstrual problems, and fertility problems in women. The test of estrogen fraction is also used in the evaluation of boys and men with gynecomastia or feminization syndromes. In pregnant women, it is used to indicate fetal-placental health. In patients with estrogen-producing tumours, it can be used as a tumour marker.

TEST EXPLANATION

There are three major estrogens (estradiol, estrone, and estriol). Estradiol is produced predominantly in the ovary. Women have a feedback mechanism for the secretion of estradiol. Low levels of estradiol stimulate the hypothalamus to produce gonadotropin-releasing factors. These hormone factors stimulate the pituitary to produce follicle-stimulating hormone (FSH) and luteinizing hormone (LH). These two hormones stimulate the ovary to produce estradiol, which peaks during the ovulatory phase of the menstrual cycle. This hormone is measured most often to evaluate menstrual and fertility problems, menopausal status, sexual maturity, gynecomastia, and feminization syndromes or as a tumour marker for patients with certain ovarian tumours.

Estrone is also secreted by the ovary, but most of it is converted from androstenedione in peripheral tissues. Estrone is a more potent estrogen than estriol but is less potent than estradiol. Estrone is the major circulating estrogen after menopause.

Estriol is the major estrogen in pregnant women. Serial urine and blood studies of estriol excretion provide an objective assessment of placental function and fetal normality in high-risk gestations. Excretion of estriol increases at approximately the eighth week of gestation and continues to rise until shortly before delivery. Estriol is produced in the placenta from estrogen precursors, which are made by the fetal adrenal gland and liver. The measurement of excreted estriol is an important index of fetal well-being. Rising values indicate that the fetoplacental unit is functioning adequately. Decreasing values suggest fetoplacental deterioration (failing pregnancy, dysmaturity, pre-eclampsia/eclampsia, complicated diabetes mellitus, anencephaly, fetal death), and the pregnancy must be reassessed promptly. If the estriol level falls, early delivery of the fetus may be indicated.

Serial studies usually begin at approximately 28 to 30 weeks of gestation and are then repeated weekly. The frequency of these estriol determinations can be increased as needed to evaluate a high-risk gestation. Collection may be done daily. Although the first collection is the baseline value, all collection results are compared with previous ones because decreasing values suggest fetal deterioration. Some physicians use an average of three previous values as a control value.

Estriol excretion studies can be performed with blood studies, or a 24-hour urine test. Because urinary creatinine excretion is relatively constant, creatinine clearance is often tested simultaneously to assess the adequacy of the 24-hour urine collection for estriol. A serially increasing estriol/creatinine ratio is a favourable sign in pregnancy. Plasma estriol determinations also can be used to evaluate the fetoplacental unit. These studies can conveniently and rapidly assess the quantity of free estriol in the plasma by radioimmunoassay. The plasma collected by venipuncture is an accurate reflection of the current status of the placenta and fetus. The advantage of the plasma estriol determination is that it is obtained more easily than a 24-hour urine specimen, and the plasma specimen is less affected by medications. All the estrogens can be measured by gas chromatography, but radioimmunoassay techniques are more accurate, and their results are less affected by drugs or birth control pills.

Unfortunately, only severe placental distress decreases urinary estriol sufficiently to be a reliable predictor of fetoplacental stress. Furthermore, plasma and urinary estriol levels have significant daily variation, which may confound serial results. Maternal illnesses, such as hypertension, pre-eclampsia, anemia, and impaired renal function, can also factitiously decrease urinary estriol levels. Because these problems create a high number of false-positive and false-negative findings, most clinicians now use nonstress fetal monitoring (p. 597) to indicate fetal-placental health.

INTERFERING FACTORS

- Recent administration of radioisotopes may alter test results if radioimmunoassay methods are used.
- Glycosuria and urinary tract infections can increase urine estriol levels.
- Drugs that may *increase* estriol levels include adrenocorticosteroids, ampicillin, estrogen-containing drugs, phenothiazines, and tetracyclines.
- Drugs that may *decrease* estriol levels include clomiphene.

PROCEDURE AND PATIENT CARE

Before

- Explain the procedure to the patient.
- If the patient is going to collect the 24-hour urine specimen at home, give her the collection bottle (with a preservative, usually boric acid) and instruct her to keep the urine refrigerated.
- Inform the patient that no food or fluid restrictions are needed.

During

Blood
- Collect a venous blood sample in a red-top tube.

24-Hour Urine
🖉 Instruct the patient to discard the initial urine specimen and start the 24-hour collection with the next specimen.

🖉 Instruct the patient to collect all urine passed during the next 24 hours. Make sure the patient knows where to store the urine container.

- Ask the patient to keep the specimen in a container of water and crushed ice or refrigerated during the 24-hour collection period.

🖉 Instruct the patient to indicate the starting time on the urine container and laboratory slip.

- Further instruct the patient to post the hours for the urine collection in a prominent place to prevent accidentally discarding a specimen.

🖉 Instruct the patient to void before defecating so that the urine is not contaminated by feces.

🖉 Remind the patient not to put toilet paper in the collection container.

🖉 Encourage the patient to drink fluids during the 24 hours.

🖉 Instruct the patient to void as close as possible to the end of the 24-hour period and to add this specimen to the collection.

After
- Apply pressure or a pressure dressing to the venipuncture site.
- Observe the venipuncture site for bleeding.
- Transport the 24-hour urine specimen promptly to the laboratory.

🖉 Inform the patient how and when to obtain the results of this study.

TEST RESULTS AND CLINICAL SIGNIFICANCE

▲ Increased Levels

Feminization syndromes: *Estrogens are increased in these syndromes for a variety of reasons. Male patients begin to develop female secondary sex characteristics.*

Precocious puberty: *Children who develop secondary sexual characteristics at an abnormally early age often have a genetic defect in adrenal cortisol metabolism. As a result, large amounts of sex steroid precursors accumulate and are converted to estrogens by the ovary. This causes precocious secondary sexual changes.*

Ovarian tumour,

Testicular tumour,

Adrenal tumour: *Gonadal tumours (e.g., granulosa thecal cell tumours) secrete estrogens. The higher the levels, the greater the tumour burden. In these instances, estrogen can act as a tumour marker that can be used to monitor the disease.*

Normal pregnancy: *Estriol is the main estrogen whose levels are elevated during pregnancy, although estrone and estradiol levels are also elevated. Multiple pregnancies are associated with particularly high levels of estriol.*

Hepatic cirrhosis,

Liver necrosis: *Estrogens are catabolized, in part, by the liver. If liver function is deficient, estrogens and their precursors accumulate. Adult feminization in male patients can result.*

Hyperthyroidism: *An estrogen-related increase in the production of thyroid-binding globulin produces an elevation of serum total thyroxine (T_4).*

▼ Decreased Levels

A failing pregnancy is associated with reduced placental production of estriol: *Dysmaturity, Rh isoimmunization, pre-eclampsia/eclampsia, anencephaly, fetal death, or any disease that causes fetal distress will be associated with reduced estriol levels.*

Turner's syndrome: *This syndrome is seen in female patients who are missing one X chromosome. They have gonadal dysgenesis to varying degrees.*

Hypopituitarism,

Primary and secondary hypogonadism,

Stein-Leventhal syndrome: *Diseases affecting the organs involved in the synthesis of sex hormones anywhere in the hypothalamus/pituitary/gonadal axis are associated with reduced estrogen levels.*

Menopause: *With normal age-related ovarian failure, estrogen (especially estrone) levels decline.*

Anorexia nervosa: *Reduction in fat intake reduces sterol precursors available for estrogen synthesis.*

RELATED TESTS

Luteinizing Hormone and Follicle-Stimulating Hormone Assay (p. 361). These are measurements of gonadal stimulatory hormones.

Fetal Nonstress Test (p. 597). This is a more accurate test of placental/fetal viability.

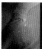

Ethanol (Ethyl Alcohol, Blood Alcohol, Blood EtOH)

NORMAL FINDINGS

None

 Critical Values

>64.8 mmol/L (>300 mg/dL)

INDICATIONS

This test is a measurement of alcohol in the blood. It is used to diagnose alcohol intoxication and overdose.

TEST EXPLANATION

Ethanol depresses the central nervous system and may lead to coma and death. This test is usually performed to evaluate alcohol-impaired driving or overdose. Proper collection, handling, and storage of the blood sample are important for medical/legal cases involving sobriety. The blood test is the specimen of choice. Blood is taken from a peripheral vein in living patients and from the aorta in cadavers. Ethanol also can be detected in the urine, in gastric contents, or by breath analyzer. Conversion tables are available to calculate blood levels on the basis of alcohol levels identified in the various nonblood specimens.

Blood alcohol levels higher than **17.4 mmol/L** (>80 mg/dL) may cause flushing, slowing of reflexes, and visual impairment. Most courts do not consider this level definite proof of intoxication. Individuals with alcohol levels lower than 0.05% weight/volume are not considered to be under the influence of alcohol. Levels higher than 0.08% are considered in Canada to be illegal and definite evidence of intoxication. Depression of the central nervous system occurs with levels higher than **21.7 mmol/L** (>100 mg/dL), and fatalities are reported with levels higher than **86.4 mmol/L** (>400 mg/dL). Levels of blood alcohol higher than **21.7 mmol/L** (>100 mg/dL) can cause hypotension. This is especially important to recognize in trauma patients who are in shock.

INTERFERING FACTORS

- Elevated levels of blood ketones (as in diabetic ketoacidosis) can cause artificial elevation of results of blood and breath tests.
- Alcohols other than ethanol, such as isopropyl (rubbing) alcohol or methanol (grain), are also detected by this test.
- Use of large amounts of isopropyl alcohol in cleansing skin for a needlestick can artificially elevate the test results.

 Clinical Priorities

- This test is used to diagnose alcohol intoxication and overdose.
- To cleanse the venipuncture site, use povidone-iodine or peroxide instead of an alcohol wipe.
- Proper collection, handling, and storage of the blood sample are important for medical/legal cases involving sobriety.
- Patients undergoing these tests should be advised of their legal rights.

PROCEDURE AND PATIENT CARE

Before
- Explain the procedure to the patient.
- Follow the institution's protocol if the specimen will be used for legal purposes.
- Patients should be advised of their legal rights. Sometimes it is most appropriate for a law enforcement officer to advise the patient. The alcohol level may be used as evidence for later court proceedings.

During
- To cleanse the venipuncture site, use povidone-iodine or peroxide instead of an alcohol wipe.
- Collect a venous blood sample in a grey-top or red-top tube according to the agency's protocol.
- If a gastric or urine specimen is indicated, approximately 20 to 50 mL of fluid is necessary.
- Breath samples for analysis are taken at the end of expiration after a deep inspiration.

After
- Apply pressure or a pressure dressing to the venipuncture site.
- Assess the venipuncture site for bleeding.
- Follow the agency's protocol regarding specimen delivery.
- The exact time of specimen collection should be indicated. Also, signatures of the collector and a witness may be needed in some instances for legal evidence.

TEST RESULTS AND CLINICAL SIGNIFICANCE

▲ Increased Levels

Alcohol intoxication or overdose: *Alcohol is rapidly absorbed from the stomach in approximately 1 hour. If the stomach is empty, absorption is faster. Alcohol is metabolized in the liver. A 70-kg person with normal liver function can metabolize approximately 15 mg of alcohol per hour.*

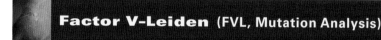

Factor V-Leiden (FVL, Mutation Analysis)

NORMAL FINDINGS

Negative

INDICATIONS

This test is used to diagnose factor V–Leiden thrombophilia.

TEST EXPLANATION

Factor V is an important factor in reaction 4 (common pathway) of normal hemostasis. The term *factor V–Leiden* refers to an abnormal form of factor V in which there is a specific glutamine-to-arginine substitution at nucleotide 1691 in the gene for factor V. That genetic mutation causes a single amino acid replacement (Arg506Gln) at one of three cleavage sites in the factor V molecule. The endogenous anticoagulant protein C (see p. 437) is normally able to break down factor V at one of these cleavage sites. However, protein C cannot inactivate this same cleavage site on factor V–Leiden. Factor V–Leiden is therefore inactivated at a rate approximately ten times slower than normal factor V is inactivated, and this inactivation persists longer in the circulation. This results in increased thrombin generation and a mild hypercoagulable state reflected by elevated levels of prothrombin fragment 1+2 and other activated coagulation markers.

Individuals heterozygous for the factor V–Leiden mutation have a slightly increased risk for venous thrombosis. Homozygous individuals have a much greater risk for devastating thrombosis (e.g., deep-vein thrombosis, arterial thrombosis, or pulmonary embolism).

Individuals who are candidates for factor V–Leiden testing include patients with the following backgrounds:
- A thrombotic event without any predisposing factors
- A strong family history of thrombotic events
- A thrombotic event before 30 years of age
- Deep-vein thrombosis during pregnancy or while taking birth control pills
- Venous thrombosis at unusual sites (e.g., cerebral, mesenteric, portal, or hepatic veins)
- An arterial clot

Factor V–Leiden is a common hereditary blood coagulation disorder present in 3% of the general population. It is the most common genetic cause of venous thrombosis and is associated with 20% to 40% of cases of venous thrombosis. Approximately 10% of patients who have factor V–Leiden eventually experience a thrombotic event.

Testing for factor V–Leiden is sometimes preceded by a screening coagulation test called the *activated protein C (APC) resistance test*. This is a test to identify resistance of factor V to APC. Protein C (see p. 437), in the presence of its cofactors thrombomodulin and thrombin, is enzymatically cleaved to its active form, APC. APC is an important natural anticoagulant (to balance coagulation) that functions by inactivating the critical coagulation factors Va and VIIIa. In patients with thrombosis (many of whom have factor V–Leiden), those factors are resistant to deactivation when exposed to APC. Pregnancy and reactive causes of increased factor VIII can also be associated with APC resistance.

APC resistance testing is performed on citrated plasma (collected in blue-top tubes) from patients with thrombosis in whom activated partial thromboplastin time (aPTT) is normal before anticoagulant therapy. Briefly, a standard aPTT test (see p. 396) is performed in the absence and then in the presence of commercially available APC. In the normal response, the aPTT is prolonged in the presence of APC as a result of the anticoagulant action of this protein. Failure to prolong the aPTT is considered an abnormality caused by "resistance to APC." The results are reported as a ratio of (APC − aPTT)/aPTT; normal results are higher than 2.0. Patients with the lowest APC ratios appear to be homozygous for the abnormal factor V molecule, whereas heterozygous patients appear to have ratios intermediate between the normal range and homozygote levels.

If APC resistance is identified, the patient then may choose to undergo mutation testing by DNA analysis of the F5 gene, which encodes the factor V protein. This testing should be accompanied by professional genetic counselling for the patient and family members.

PROCEDURE AND PATIENT CARE

Before
✍ Explain the procedure to the patient.
- If the patient is receiving heparin by intermittent injection, plan to collect the blood specimen for the aPTT 30 minutes to 1 hour before the next dose of heparin.
- If the patient is receiving a continuous heparin infusion, collect the blood at any time.

During
- Collect a venous blood sample in one or two blue-top tubes.
- If the APC resistance testing reveals APC resistance, genetic counselling is indicated. Then, blood is collected in a lavender-top (ethylenediamine tetra-acetic acid) tube.
- As an alternative, genetic testing can be performed on the patient's cells obtained by a smear of the oral surface of the cheek.

After
- Apply pressure or a pressure dressing to the venipuncture site.
- Assess the venipuncture site for bleeding. Remember that if the patient is receiving anticoagulants, the bleeding time will be increased.
- Results are provided to the patient by a physician and a genetic counsellor.

TEST RESULTS AND CLINICAL SIGNIFICANCE

APC resistance: *This result most probably indicates the presence of factor V–Leiden, but other forms of thrombophilia (predisposition to thrombotic events) can cause APC resistance.*

Factor V–Leiden genetic mutation, homozygous: *Affected patients have received a factor V–Leiden gene from each parent. In these individuals, the risk for thrombotic events exceeds 80 times that of the normal population.*

Factor V–Leiden genetic mutation, heterozygous: *Affected patients have received a factor V–Leiden gene from one parent and a normal factor V gene from the other. In these individuals, the risk for thrombotic events is approximately 10 times that of the normal population.*

RELATED TESTS

Protein C, Protein S (p. 437). This test identifies deficiency in either protein C or protein S, or in both.

Partial Thromboplastin Time, Activated (p. 396). This test is used to confirm or rule out APC resistance and is a preliminary test for identifying individuals with factor V–Leiden.

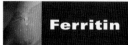
Ferritin

NORMAL FINDINGS

Male: **20–200** *Mcg*/L (20–200 ng/mL)
Female: **20–150** *Mcg*/L (20–150 ng/mL)
Child/adolescent:
  Newborn: **25–200** *Mcg*/L (25–200 ng/mL)
  ≤1 month: **200–600** *Mcg*/L (200–600 ng/mL)
  2–5 months: **50–200** *Mcg*/L (50–200 ng/mL)
  6 months to 15 years: **7–142** *Mcg*/L (7–142 ng/mL)

INDICATIONS

This is the most sensitive test to determine iron-deficiency anemia.

TEST EXPLANATION

The serum ferritin study is a good indicator of available iron stores in the body. Ferritin, the major iron-storage protein, is normally present in the serum in concentrations directly related to iron storage. In normal patients, **1** *Mcg*/L (1 ng/mL) of serum ferritin corresponds to approximately 8 mg of stored iron. Ferritin levels rise persistently in men and postmenopausal women. In premenopausal women, levels stay approximately the same. Decreases in ferritin levels indicate a decrease in iron storage in association with iron-deficiency anemia. A ferritin level lower than 10 mg/100 mL is diagnostic of iron-deficiency anemia. A decrease in serum ferritin level often precedes other signs of iron deficiency, such as decreased iron levels or changes in red blood cell (RBC) size, colour, and number. Only when protein depletion is severe can ferritin be decreased by malnutrition. Increased levels are a sign of iron excess, as seen in hemochromatosis, hemosiderosis, iron poisoning, or recent blood transfusions. Increases in ferritin are also noted in patients with megaloblastic anemia, hemolytic anemia, and chronic hepatitis. Furthermore, ferritin is factitiously elevated in patients with chronic disease states such as neoplasm, alcoholism, uremia, collagen diseases, or chronic liver diseases. The ferritin test is also used in patients with chronic renal failure to monitor iron stores.

A limitation of this study is that ferritin also can act as an acute-phase reactant protein, and ferritin levels may be elevated in conditions that do not reflect iron stores (e.g., acute inflammatory diseases, infections, metastatic cancer, lymphomas). The ferritin level becomes elevated 1 to 2 days after onset of the acute illness, and the level peaks at 3 to 5 days. If iron deficiency coexists in patients with these diseases, it may not be recognized because the levels of ferritin would be factitiously elevated by the concurrent disease.

TABLE 2-24	Results of Iron Studies in Various Clinical States			
Clinical State	**Ferritin**	**Iron**	**Total Iron-Binding Capacity**	**Transferrin Saturation**
Chronic blood loss	↓	↓	↑	↓
Acute blood loss	Normal	↓	Normal	↓
Iron deficiency	↓	↓	↑	↓
Hemolytic anemia	↑	↑	↓	↑
Chronic disease	↑	↓	↓	↓
Hemochromatosis	↑	↑	↓	↑
Pregnancy	↓	↓	↑	↓
Estrogen therapy	Normal	↑	↑	↓
Acute inflammation	↑	Normal	↓	↑

When combined with measurements of the serum iron level and total iron-binding capacity (TIBC), this test is useful in differentiating and classifying anemias. For example, in patients with iron-deficiency anemia, the ferritin, iron, and transferrin saturation levels are low, whereas the TIBC and transferrin levels are high (Table 2-24). Ferritin is measured by either radioimmunoassay or enzyme immunoassay.

INTERFERING FACTORS

- Recent transfusions or recent ingestion of a meal with a high iron content (red meats) may cause elevations in ferritin levels. The iron that is ingested stimulates ferritin production to store the increased serum iron.
- Recent administration of a radionuclide can cause abnormal levels if testing is performed by means of radioimmunoassay.
- Hemolytic diseases may be associated with an artificially high iron content. Iron is freed from the hemoglobin that is released from the hemolyzed RBCs. Ferritin synthesis is increased to store the increased serum iron.
- Acute and chronic inflammatory conditions and Gaucher's disease can artificially increase ferritin levels.
- Disorders of excessive iron storage (e.g., hemochromatosis, hemosiderosis) are associated with high ferritin levels. Ferritin synthesis is increased to store the increased serum iron.
- Iron-deficient menstruating women may have decreased ferritin levels, because their iron stores are generally low as a result of monthly menses.
- Drugs that may *increase* ferritin levels include iron preparations. Ferritin synthesis is increased to store the increased serum iron.

PROCEDURE AND PATIENT CARE

Before
- Explain the procedure to the patient.
- Inform the patient that no fasting is required.

During
- Collect a venous blood sample in a red-top tube.

After

- Apply pressure or a pressure dressing to the venipuncture site.
- Assess the venipuncture site for bleeding.

TEST RESULTS AND CLINICAL SIGNIFICANCE

▲ Increased Levels

Hemochromatosis,

Hemosiderosis: *Increased iron stores in the tissues stimulate ferritin production for storage.*

Megaloblastic anemia,

Hemolytic anemia: *RBCs in with anemias lyse and release iron into the bloodstream. Ferritin production is stimulated to store the excess free iron.*

Alcoholic/inflammatory hepatocellular disease,

Inflammatory disease,

Advanced cancers: *Because ferritin is an acute-phase reactant protein, its production is increased with acute diseases.*

Chronic illnesses such as leukemias, cirrhosis, chronic hepatitis, or collagen-vascular diseases: *The pathophysiologic mechanism underlying this observation is not known.*

▼ Decreased Levels

Iron-deficiency anemia: *When iron stores are decreased, less ferritin is required. Levels diminish accordingly.*

Severe protein deficiency: *Ferritin is a protein. In severely depleted persons, ferritin synthesis is reduced.*

Hemodialysis: *Iron stores can be reduced by dialysis. Decreased iron stores require less ferritin. Levels diminish accordingly.*

RELATED TESTS

Iron Level, Total Iron-Binding Capacity, and Transferrin Saturation (p. 334). These tests include a direct measurement of bound iron in the blood. TIBC is a measurement of all proteins available for binding mobile iron. Transferrin represents the largest quantity of iron-binding proteins.

Transferrin Receptor Assay (p. 521). Transferrin represents the largest quantity of iron-binding proteins.

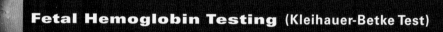

Fetal Hemoglobin Testing (Kleihauer-Betke Test)

NORMAL FINDINGS

<1% of red blood cells (RBCs)

INDICATIONS

This test is performed on pregnant women to determine the presence of fetal-maternal hemorrhage (FMH) and, if it is present, quantify the amount of hemorrhage.

TEST EXPLANATION

Fetal hemoglobin may be present in the mother's blood because of FMH, which causes leakage of fetal cells into the maternal circulation. When large volumes of fetal blood are lost in this way, serious and potentially fetal or neonatal outcomes can result. Massive FMH may be the cause of approximately 1 per 50 stillbirths. No historical or clinical features allow antecedent identification of those in whom FMH may be the cause of an intrauterine death. Therefore, FMH will continue to remain undetected in a large proportion of affected patients.

Leakage of fetal RBCs can begin anytime after the middle of the first trimester. It presumably results from a breach in the integrity of the placental circulation. As pregnancy continues, fetal RBCs become more evident in affected mothers' circulation, so that by term, fetal cells are detectable in the circulation of approximately 50% of affected mothers. Most of these cells, however, are present in the mother's circulation as a result of very small leaks. Small leaks are not implicated in intrauterine death.

Risk factors correlated with the increasing risk for massive FMH include maternal trauma, placental abruption, placental tumours, third-trimester amniocentesis, fetal hydrops, poorly perfused fetal organs, antecedent sinusoidal fetal heart tracing, and twinning. The presence of one or more of these features is an indication for fetal hemoglobin testing.

The standard method of detecting FMH is the Kleihauer-Betke test. This method takes advantage of the differential resistance of fetal hemoglobin to acid. A standard blood smear is prepared from the mother's blood. An acid bath is then used to remove all adult hemoglobin, but it does not remove fetal hemoglobin. Subsequent staining turns fetal cells (containing fetal hemoglobin) rose pink, although the mother's cells are only seen as "ghosts." A large number of cells (e.g., 5 000) are counted under the microscope, and the ratio of fetal to maternal cells is generated.

The flow-cytometric method for fetal hemoglobin determination offers several advantages over the traditional Kleihauer-Betke method. This more objective method has been shown to have improved sensitivity, precision, and linearity in comparison with traditional methods.

FMH becomes of even greater significance when the mother's blood is Rh negative, inasmuch as this is the mechanism through which Rh sensitization could develop if the fetus has paternal Rh-positive blood cells. If this is known to exist, Rh immune globulin (RhoGAM) antibodies directed to Rh-positive fetal cells are given to the pregnant mother (at approximately 28 weeks of pregnancy, and within 72 hours after a birth, miscarriage, abortion, or amniocentesis). RhoGAM is often administered if the Rh-negative mother undergoes any invasive procedure in which she may be exposed to the Rh-positive fetal blood. The RhoGAM antibodies kill the fetal RBCs in the maternal bloodstream before the mother has an opportunity to develop any antibodies to fetal Rh-positive RBCs. This precludes more aggressive anti–fetal RBC activity in the near or remote future. By determination of the amount and volume of fetal blood loss, a dose of RhoGAM can be calculated according to the following formula:

$$\text{Vials of Rh immune globulin} = \frac{\text{Millilitres of fetal blood}}{30}$$

This test is often performed on women who have delivered a stillborn baby to determine whether FMH was a potential cause of fetal death.

INTERFERING FACTORS

- Any maternal condition (such as sickle cell disease) that involves persistence of fetal hemoglobin in the mother will cause a false-positive result.
- If the blood is collected after Caesarean section, a false-positive result could be obtained. Vaginal delivery does result in higher frequency of detection of FMH.

PROCEDURE AND PATIENT CARE

Before

 Explain the procedure to the patient.

During

- Collect a venous blood sample in a red-top tube for serum testing.
- Avoid hemolysis.

After

- Apply pressure to the venipuncture site.
- Emphasize to the patient the importance of antepartum health care.
- Provide emotional support in the event that this test is performed after a stillborn delivery.

TEST RESULTS AND CLINICAL SIGNIFICANCE

▲ Increased Levels

FMH: *Fetal, placental, or maternal pathologic processes can result in leakage of fetal cells into the maternal bloodstream.*

Hereditary persistence of fetal hemoglobin: *With any hemoglobinopathy, fetal hemoglobin is often continually made in RBCs as a compensatory mechanism to ensure adequate tissue oxygenation. This situation is identified through fetal hemoglobin testing and may be a false indicator of FMH.*

Intrachorionic thrombi: *Placental thrombosis causes a breakdown in the maternal-fetal membrane barrier. Fetal cells can cross over into the maternal circulation.*

Fetal Scalp Blood pH (Fetal Oxygen Saturation Monitoring)

NORMAL FINDINGS

pH: 7.25–7.35
Oxygen saturation: 30%–50%
Partial pressure of oxygen (Po_2): 18–22 mm Hg
Partial pressure of carbon dioxide (Pco_2): 40–50 mm Hg
Base excess: 0–10 mmol/L (mEq/L)

INDICATIONS

This test indicates fetal well-being or fetal distress.

TEST EXPLANATION

Measurement of fetal scalp blood pH provides valuable information on fetal acid-base status. This screening test is useful for diagnosing fetal distress.

Although the Po_2, Pco_2, and bicarbonate ion (HCO_3^-) concentration can be measured with the fetal scalp blood sample, the pH is the most useful clinically. The pH normally ranges from 7.25

to 7.35 during labour; a mild decline within the normal range is noted during contractions and as labour progresses.

Fetal hypoxia causes anaerobic glycolysis, which results in excess production of lactic acid. This causes an increase in HCO_3^- concentration (acidosis) and a decrease in pH. Acidosis reflects the effect of hypoxia on cellular metabolism. Low pH levels are strongly correlated with low Apgar scores.

CONTRAINDICATIONS

- Premature membrane rupture, because infection can be instilled into the uterus
- Active cervical infection (e.g., gonorrhea, herpes, human immunodeficiency virus [HIV] infection), because the active infection can be spread to the fetus

POTENTIAL COMPLICATIONS

- Continued bleeding from the puncture site
- Hematoma
- Ecchymosis
- Infection

Clinical Priorities

- The fetal scalp pH indicates fetal well-being or fetal distress.
- Fetal hypoxia causes anaerobic glycolysis, which results in excess production of lactic acid. This causes a decrease in pH.
- Low pH is strongly correlated with low Apgar scores.

PROCEDURE AND PATIENT CARE

Before

- Explain the procedure to the patient.
- Obtain an informed consent from the patient for this procedure.
- Inform the patient that no fasting or sedation is required.
- Also inform the patient that she may be uncomfortable during the cervical dilation and that after the procedure, she may have vaginal discomfort and menstrual-type cramping.

During

- Note the following procedural steps:
  1. Amnioscopy is performed with the mother in the lithotomy position.
  2. The cervix is dilated, and the endoscope (amnioscope) is introduced into the cervical canal.
  3. The fetal scalp is cleansed with an antiseptic and dried with a sterile cotton ball.
  4. A small amount of petroleum jelly is applied to the fetal scalp to cause droplets of fetal blood to bead.
  5. After the skin on the scalp is pierced with a small metal blade, beaded droplets of blood are collected in long, heparinized capillary tubes.

6. The tube is sealed with wax and placed on ice to retard cellular respiration, which can alter the pH.
7. The physician performing the procedure applies firm pressure to the puncture site to retard bleeding.
8. Scalp blood sampling can be repeated as necessary.

• Note that this study is performed by a physician in approximately 10 to 15 minutes.

After
• After delivery, assess the newborn and identify and document the puncture site or sites.
• Cleanse the site of the scalp puncture with an antiseptic solution and apply an antibiotic ointment.

TEST RESULTS AND CLINICAL SIGNIFICANCE
▲ Increased Levels
Fetal distress: *Fetal hypoxia causes anaerobic glycolysis, which results in excess production of lactic acid. This causes an increase in HCO_3^- concentration (acidosis) and a decrease in pH.*

RELATED TEST
Arterial Blood Gases (p. 121). This test provides valuable information in assessing and managing a patient's respiratory (ventilation) and metabolic (renal) acid-base and electrolyte homeostasis. It is also used to assess adequacy of oxygenation.

Fibrinogen (Factor I, Quantitative Fibrinogen)

NORMAL FINDINGS
Adult: **5.8–11.8** *Mc*mol/L (200–400 mg/dL)
Newborn: **3.68–8.82** *Mc*mol/L (125–300 mg/dL)

 Critical Values

Values lower than **2.94** *Mc*mol/L (100 mg/dL) can be associated with spontaneous bleeding.

INDICATIONS
The fibrinogen test is used primarily to aid in the diagnosis of suspected bleeding disorders.

TEST EXPLANATION
Fibrinogen is essential for blood clotting. It is part of the "common pathway" (fourth reaction) in the coagulation system. Fibrinogen is converted to fibrin by the action of thrombin during the coagulation process. Fibrinogen, which is produced by the liver, is also an acute-phase reactant protein. It rises sharply during tissue inflammation or tissue necrosis.

   High levels of fibrinogen have been associated with an increased risk for coronary heart disease, stroke, myocardial infarction, and peripheral arterial disease. Levels may be reduced in patients with liver disease, malnourished states, and consumptive coagulopathies (e.g., disseminated intravascular coagulation). Large-volume blood transfusions are also associated with low levels because banked blood does not contain fibrinogen. Reduced levels of fibrinogen cause prolongation of prothrombin time and partial thromboplastin time.

INTERFERING FACTORS

- Blood transfusions within the previous month may affect test results.
- Diets rich in omega-3 and omega-6 fatty acids reduce fibrinogen levels.
- Drugs that may cause *increases* in fibrinogen levels include estrogens and oral contraceptives.
- Drugs that may cause *decreases* in fibrinogen levels include anabolic steroids, androgens, asparaginase, phenobarbital, streptokinase, urokinase, and valproic acid.

PROCEDURE AND PATIENT CARE

Before
- Explain the procedure to the patient.
- Inform the patient that no fasting is required.

During
- Collect venous blood in a blue-top tube.

After
- Apply pressure or a pressure dressing to the venipuncture site.
- Assess the venipuncture site for bleeding.

TEST RESULTS AND CLINICAL SIGNIFICANCE

▲ Increased Levels
Acute inflammatory reactions (e.g., rheumatoid arthritis, glomerulonephritis),
Trauma,
Acute infection such as pneumonia: *Fibrinogen is an acute-phase reactant protein.*
Coronary heart disease,
Stroke,
Peripheral vascular disease,
Cigarette smoking: *Elevated fibrinogen levels are merely an observation with no known pathophysiologic cause.*
Pregnancy: *Pregnancy is associated with increases in levels of serum proteins (including fibrinogen).*

▼ Decreased Levels
Liver disease (hepatitis, cirrhosis): *Fibrinogen is not made in adequate volume.*
Disseminated intravascular coagulopathy,
Fibrinolysins: *Primary and secondary fibrinolysins act to destroy fibrinogen within the serum.*
Congenital afibrinogenemia: *A genetic defect precludes the synthesis of fibrinogen.*
Advanced carcinoma,

Malnutrition: *Severe protein depletion is associated with reduced levels of fibrinogen (a protein).*
Large-volume blood transfusion: *Fibrinogen does not exist in normal levels in banked blood. The more that is transfused, the more the native fibrinogen is diluted.*

RELATED TESTS

Prothrombin Time (p. 446). This measurement is used to evaluate the adequacy of the extrinsic system and common pathway in the clotting mechanism.

Partial Thromboplastin Time (p. 396). This measurement is used to evaluate the intrinsic system and the common pathway of clot formation. It is most commonly used to monitor heparin therapy.

Coagulating Factor Concentration (p. 177). This is a quantitative measurement of specific coagulation factors.

Thrombosis Indicators (p. 495). These tests are most commonly used to support the diagnosis of disseminated intravascular coagulation.

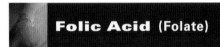

Folic Acid (Folate)

NORMAL FINDINGS

11–57 nmol/L (5–25 ng/mL)

INDICATIONS

This test quantifies the folate level in the blood. It is used in patients who have megaloblastic anemia. It is also used to assess nutritional status, especially in alcoholic patients.

TEST EXPLANATION

Folic acid, one of the B vitamins, is necessary for the normal function of red blood cells (RBCs) and white blood cells (WBCs). It is needed for the adequate synthesis of certain purines and pyrimidines, which are precursors of DNA. It is also used in the synthesis of several amino acids. Vitamin B_{12} is necessary for conversion of inactive 5-methyltetrahydrofolate to tetrahydrofolate, the active form of folate. As with vitamin B_{12}, the folate level depends on adequate dietary ingestion and normal intestinal absorption of this vitamin.

The finding of a low serum folate level means that the patient's recent diet has been subnormal in folate content or that recent absorption of folate has been subnormal. In time, folate levels also drop in the tissues. Tissue folate is best tested by determining the content of folate in RBCs. A low RBC folate level can mean either the presence of tissue folate depletion as a result of folate deficiency, which necessitates folate therapy, or that the patient has primary vitamin B_{12} (see p. 541) deficiency, which blocks the ability of cells to take up folate. In the latter case, the proper therapy is supplementation with vitamin B_{12} rather than with folic acid. For these reasons, it is advisable to determine RBC folate levels in addition to serum folate levels.

Folic acid blood levels are performed to assess folate availability in pregnancy, to evaluate hemolytic disorders, and to detect anemia caused by folic acid deficiency (in which the RBCs are abnormally large, causing a megaloblastic anemia). These RBCs have a shortened life span and impaired oxygen-carrying capacity. If this capacity is low, RBC folate level is measured.

The main causes of folic acid deficiency include dietary deficiency (usually in alcoholic patients), malabsorption syndrome, pregnancy, and certain anticonvulsant drugs. Decreased folic acid levels are seen in patients with folic acid–deficiency anemia (megaloblastic anemia), hemolytic anemia, malnutrition, malabsorption syndrome, malignancy, liver disease, and celiac disease. Some drugs (e.g., anticonvulsants, antimalarials, alcohol, aminopterin, methotrexate) are folic acid antagonists and interfere with nucleic acid synthesis.

Levels of folic acid may be elevated in patients with pernicious anemia. Because such patients do not have an adequate amount of vitamin B_{12} to metabolize folic acid, levels of folate rise in pernicious anemia. The folic acid test should be performed in conjunction with tests for vitamin B_{12} levels.

The folate test is often part of the workup in alcoholic patients to assess nutritional status. Folate must be depleted for at least 5 months before megaloblastic anemia occurs.

Radioimmunoassay or enzyme immunoassay techniques are now the most common methods of folic acid measurement.

INTERFERING FACTORS

- A folate-deficient patient who has received a blood transfusion may have an artificially normal result.
- Because radioimmunoassay is the method of choice for folic acid determination, radionuclide administration should be avoided for at least 24 hours before the radioimmunoassay test.
- Drugs that may cause *decreases* in folic acid levels include alcohol, aminopterin, salicylic acid, ampicillin, antimalarials, chloramphenicol, erythromycin, estrogens, methotrexate, oral contraceptives, penicillin derivatives, phenobarbital, phenytoin, and tetracyclines.

PROCEDURE AND PATIENT CARE

Before

- Explain the procedure to the patient.
- Inform the patient that no fasting is usually required unless ordered by physician.
- Instruct the patient not to consume alcoholic beverages before the test.
- Collect the specimen before starting folate therapy.

During

- Collect a venous blood sample in a red-top tube.
- Avoid hemolysis. Folate in the RBCs can artificially raise serum folate levels when hemolysis of the RBC occurs.
- On the laboratory slip, indicate whether the patient is taking any medications that may affect test results.

After

- Apply pressure or a pressure dressing to the venipuncture site.
- Assess the venipuncture site for bleeding.
- Transport the blood to the laboratory immediately after collection.

TEST RESULTS AND CLINICAL SIGNIFICANCE

▲ Increased Levels

Pernicious anemia: *When the amount of vitamin B$_{12}$ is inadequate for metabolizing folic acid, levels of folate rise.*

Vegetarianism: *Increased ingestion of folate-containing vegetables can lead to increased levels of folic acid.*

Recent massive blood transfusion: *Folate in the hemolyzed RBCs of banked blood can artificially raise serum folate levels.*

▼ Decreased Levels

Malnutrition: *Inadequate intake of folic acid is the most common cause of folate deficiency. This is most common in alcoholic patients. Alcohol also reduces folic acid absorption.*

Malabsorption syndrome (e.g., celiac disease): *Folic acid, like vitamin B$_{12}$, is absorbed in the small intestine. In malabsorption, folic acid is not absorbed. Serum and tissue levels then decline.*

Pregnancy: *Folic acid deficiency in pregnancy probably results from a combination of inadequate intake and increased demand placed by the fetus on the maternal source of folic acid.*

Folic acid deficiency (megaloblastic) anemia,

Hemolytic anemia: *These anemias are the result of folic acid deficiency. The large megaloblastic RBCs cannot flow through small capillaries. Instead, they fracture and hemolyze. The shortened life span ultimately leads to anemia.*

Malignancy,

Liver disease,

Chronic renal disease: *The pathophysiologic mechanism underlying these observations is not known.*

RELATED TESTS

Vitamin B$_{12}$ (p. 541). This is a measurement of the level of vitamin B$_{12}$ in the serum. This test should be performed along with a folic acid test.

Schilling Test (p. 862). This is a test to determine the cause of vitamin B$_{12}$ deficiency.

Complete Blood Cell Count and Differential Count (p. 187). This test is performed routinely and can identify megaloblastic anemia.

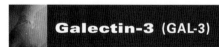

Galectin-3 (GAL-3)

NORMAL FINDINGS

≤22.1 ng/mL

INDICATIONS

This test is helpful in determining the prognosis of heart failure.

TEST EXPLANATION

Heart failure progresses primarily by dilatation of the ventricular cardiac chamber through remodelling in fibrosis as a response to cardiac injury and/or overload. Galectin-3 (GAL-3) is a biomarker that appears to be actively involved in both the inflammatory and fibrotic pathways involved in remodelling. GAL-3 is a carbohydrate-binding lectin whose expression is associated with inflammatory cells, including macrophages, neutrophils, and mast cells. GAL-3 has been linked to cardiovascular physiologic processes, including myofibroblast proliferation, tissue repair, and cardiac remodelling in the setting of heart failure. Concentrations of GAL-3 have been used to predict adverse remodelling after a variety of cardiac insults.

Elevated GAL-3 results indicate an increased risk for adverse outcomes. Elevated levels are associated with increased risk of mortality and prolongation of the symptoms associated with heart failure. Unlike natriuretic peptides, such as beta natriuretic peptides (BNP) (p. 379), GAL-3 is not useful in the diagnosis of heart failure. Testing was performed by quantitative 2-site manual enzyme-linked immunosorbent assay (ELISA).

INTERFERING FACTORS

- Hemolysis increases GAL-3 levels.
- Heterophil antibodies (p. 375) increase GAL-3 levels.

PROCEDURE AND PATIENT CARE

Before

✗ Explain the procedure to the patient.
✗ Tell the patient that no fasting is required.

During

- Collect a venous blood sample in an EDTA (usually lavender) containing tube.

After

- Apply pressure to the venipuncture site.
- Assess the venipuncture site for bleeding.
- Continue with aggressive medical care for suspected CHF.

TEST RESULTS AND CLINICAL SIGNIFICANCE

▲ Increased Levels

Heart failure: *Heart failure is associated with cardiac remodelling. As a result, GAL-3 is secreted into the bloodstream.*

RELATED TESTS

Chest X-Ray (p. 1053). This test may demonstrate an enlarged heart, commonly associated with heart failure. Pulmonary edema can also be noted.

Echocardiography (p. 906). This test is accurate in determining cardiac remodelling and enlarged cardiac ventricles.

Beta Natriuretic Peptides (p. 379). Natriuretic peptides are used to identify and stratify patients with heart failure (HF).

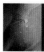 **Fungal Antibody Tests** (Antifungal Antibodies)

NORMAL FINDINGS
No antibodies detected

INDICATIONS
Serologic tests for antibodies are used to support the diagnosis of a recent fungal infection.

TEST EXPLANATION
Fungal infections can be superficial, subcutaneous, or systemic (deep). Serologic antibody testing is performed for the systemic fungal infections (mycoses), which are the most destructive. In general, mycoses are caused by the inhalation of airborne fungal spores. Some of the most serious fungal infections are coccidiomycosis, blastomycosis, histoplasmosis, and paracoccidioidomycosis. These infections start as primary pulmonary infections and can become more diffuse (Table 2-25). They can affect anyone. Systemic infections with *Aspergillus, Candida,* and *Cryptococcus* organisms usually affect only patients with compromised immunity.

The laboratory diagnosis of fungal infections includes direct microscopic visualization, culture, and serologic testing for antibodies. Fungal antibody testing is not highly reliable. Antibodies are present in approximately 70% to 80% of infected patients. When test results are positive, they merely indicate that the person has an active or has had a recent fungal infection. In general, complement fixation or immunodiffusion is the method to detect immunoglobulin G antibodies in the blood. Antibodies to immunoglobulins A and M can also be identified by enzyme immunoassay. In addition, these antibodies can be identified in the cerebrospinal fluid. Tests for these antibodies can be conducted singularly or as a group of blood tests. Cross-reactions can occur (e.g., antibodies to blastomycosis can cross-react with histoplasmosis antigens).

PROCEDURE AND PATIENT CARE
Before
☒ Explain the procedure to the patient.
☒ Inform the patient that no fasting or preparation is required.

TABLE 2-25	Diseases Resulting From Fungal Infections	
Fungus	**Systemic Disease**	**Endemic Area**
Candida albicans	Candidiasis, thrush, yeast of mouth/esophagus	Ubiquitous
Cryptococcus neoformans	Infection of the lung, bloodstream; meningitis	Ubiquitous
Histoplasma capsulatum	Pulmonary infection	Caribbean, Central and South America
Coccidioides immitis	Pulmonary infection	Southwestern United States, Mexico, Central America
Aspergillus	Pulmonary infection	Ubiquitous

During

- Collect a venous blood sample in a red-top or any serum separator (red/black- or gold-top) tube.
- On the laboratory slip, specify the particular antibody or group of antibodies that are to be tested.

After

- Apply pressure or a pressure dressing to the venipuncture site.
- Assess the venipuncture site for bleeding.

 Because some patients with fungal infection may be immunocompromised, instruct the patient to check for signs of infection at the venipuncture site (e.g. warmth, inflammation, drainage from site, swelling).

TEST RESULTS AND CLINICAL SIGNIFICANCE

▲ Increased Levels

Acute fungal infection: *Fungal antibodies develop only with systemic or deep infections. Negative results do not rule out a fungal disease.*

RELATED TEST

Sputum Culture and Sensitivity (p. 791). This is the most common method of laboratory confirmation of a fungal infection. Antifungal therapy sensitivity can be assessed through culture techniques.

Gamma-Glutamyl Transpeptidase (GGTP, g-GTP, Gamma-Glutamyl Transferase [GGT])

NORMAL FINDINGS

Adult male: 8–38 U/L
Adult female: 5–27 U/L
Older adult: slightly higher than adult
Child: similar to adult
Newborn: five times higher than adult

INDICATIONS

This is a sensitive indicator of hepatobiliary disease. It is also used as an indicator of heavy and chronic alcohol use.

TEST EXPLANATION

The enzyme gamma-glutamyl transpeptidase (GGTP) participates in the transfer of amino acids and peptides across the cellular membrane and possibly participates in glutathione metabolism. The highest concentrations of this enzyme are found in the liver and biliary tract. Lesser concentrations are found in the kidneys, spleen, heart, intestines, brain, and prostate gland. Men may have higher GGTP levels than do women because of the additional levels in the prostate. Very small amounts have been detected in endothelial cells of capillaries. This test is used to detect liver cell dysfunction, and it is highly accurate in indicating even the slightest degree of cholestasis. This is the most sensitive liver enzyme for detecting biliary obstruction, cholangitis, or cholecystitis. As with leucine aminopeptidase and 5'-nucleotidase, the elevation of GGTP levels generally parallels that of alkaline phosphatase (ALP) levels; however, GGTP testing is more sensitive. Also, as with 5'-nucleotidase and leucine aminopeptidase levels, GGTP level is not increased in bone diseases as is ALP level. The combination of a normal GGTP level with an elevated ALP level implies skeletal disease. That of an elevated GGTP level and elevated ALP level implies hepatobiliary disease. GGTP level is also not elevated in childhood or pregnancy, as ALP usually is.

Another important clinical value of GGTP testing is that it can detect chronic alcohol ingestion. It is therefore very useful in the screening and evaluation of alcoholic patients. GGTP levels are elevated in approximately 75% of patients with chronic alcoholism.

Why levels of this enzyme are elevated after an acute myocardial infarction is not clear. The elevation may represent the associated hepatic insult (if elevation occurs in the first 7 days) or the proliferation of capillary endothelial cells in the granulation tissue that replaces the infarcted myocardium. The elevation usually occurs 1 to 2 weeks after infarction.

INTERFERING FACTORS

- Values may be decreased in late pregnancy.
- Drugs that may cause *increases* in GGTP levels include alcohol, phenobarbital, and phenytoin (Dilantin).
- Drugs that may cause *decreases* in GGTP levels include clofibrate and oral contraceptives.

PROCEDURE AND PATIENT CARE

Before
- Explain the procedure to the patient.
- Inform the patient that an 8-hour fast is recommended. Only water is permitted during the fast.

During
- Collect a venous blood sample in a red-top tube.

After
- Apply pressure or a pressure dressing to the venipuncture site.
- Assess the venipuncture site for bleeding. Patients with liver dysfunction often have prolonged clotting times.

TEST RESULTS AND CLINICAL SIGNIFICANCE

▲ Increased Levels

Liver diseases (e.g., hepatitis, cirrhosis, hepatic necrosis, hepatic tumour or metastasis, hepato-toxic drugs, cholestasis, jaundice): *Liver and biliary cells contain GGTP. When injured or diseased, these cells lyse, and the GGTP leaks into the bloodstream.*

Myocardial infarction: *The pathophysiologic mechanism is not clear. It may be associated with hepatic insult or the proliferation of capillary endothelial cells in the granulation tissue that replaces the infarcted myocardium.*

Alcohol ingestion: *The pathophysiologic mechanism is not clear. It may be associated with hepatic insult.*

Pancreatic diseases (e.g., pancreatitis, cancer of the pancreas): *Pancreatic cells contain GGTP. When injured or diseased, these cells lyse, and the GGTP leaks into the bloodstream.*

Epstein-Barr virus (infectious mononucleosis), cytomegalovirus infections, and Reye syndrome: *The pathophysiologic mechanism is not clear. It may be associated with subclinical hepatitis that can occur with these infections.*

RELATED TESTS

Alanine Aminotransferase (p. 45) and Aspartate Aminotransferase (p. 130). Levels of these liver enzymes are elevated in hepatocellular disease.

Alkaline Phosphatase (p. 53). This test is used to detect and monitor diseases of the liver or bone.

5′-Nucleotidase (p. 389). Levels of this liver enzyme are elevated in diseases affecting the biliary tree.

Creatine Phosphokinase (p. 201). This enzyme is similar to AST and exists predominantly in the heart and the skeletal muscle.

Lactate Dehydrogenase (p. 339). This intracellular enzyme is used to support the diagnosis of injury or disease involving the heart, liver, red blood cells, kidneys, skeletal muscle, brain, and lungs.

Leucine Aminopeptidase (p. 351). This enzyme is specific to the hepatobiliary system. Diseases affecting that system cause elevation in levels of this enzyme.

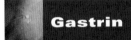

Gastrin

NORMAL FINDINGS

Adult: **0–180 ng/L** (0–180 pg/mL)
Child: **0–125 ng/L** (0–125 pg/mL)
Levels are higher in older adults.

INDICATIONS

This test is used in the evaluation of patients with peptic ulcers to diagnose Zollinger-Ellison syndrome or G-cell hyperplasia.

TEST EXPLANATION

Gastrin is a hormone produced by the G cells located in the distal part of the stomach (antrum). Gastrin is a potent stimulator of gastric acid. When gastric physiologic processes are normal, an alkaline environment (created by food or antacids) stimulates the release of gastrin. Gastrin then stimulates the parietal cells of the stomach to secrete gastric acid. The pH environment in the stomach is thereby reduced. By negative feedback, this low-pH environment suppresses further gastrin secretion.

Zollinger-Ellison syndrome (gastrin-producing pancreatic tumour) and G-cell hyperplasia (overfunctioning of G cells in the distal stomach) are associated with high levels of serum gastrin. Patients with Zollinger-Ellison tumours have aggressive peptic ulcer disease. Unlike routine peptic ulcers, Zollinger-Ellison syndrome and G-cell hyperplasia have a high incidence of complicated and recurrent peptic ulcers. It is important to identify these latter conditions in order to institute more appropriate, aggressive medical and surgical therapy. The serum gastrin level is normal in patients with routine peptic ulcers but greatly elevated in patients with Zollinger-Ellison syndrome or G-cell hyperplasia.

Of importance, however, is that patients who are taking antacid peptic ulcer medicines, have undergone peptic ulcer surgery, or have atrophic gastritis have a high serum gastrin level (in response to alkalinity in the stomach). However, levels usually are not as high as in patients with Zollinger-Ellison syndrome or G-cell hyperplasia.

Not all patients with Zollinger-Ellison syndrome exhibit increased levels of serum gastrin. In some patients, gastrin levels may be at the top of the normal range, which makes it difficult to differentiate the syndrome from routine peptic ulcer disease. Zollinger-Ellison syndrome or G-cell hyperplasia can be diagnosed in such patients by gastrin stimulation tests with calcium or secretin. Patients with these diseases have greatly increased serum gastrin levels in association with the infusion of these drugs.

INTERFERING FACTORS

- Peptic ulcer surgery creates a persistent alkaline environment, which is the strongest stimulant of gastrin production.
- Ingestion of high-protein food can result in an increase in serum gastrin levels to two to five times the normal level.
- Diabetic patients taking insulin may have artificially elevated levels in response to hypoglycemia.
- Drugs that may *increase* serum gastrin levels include antacids and H_2-blocking agents (e.g., esomeprazole, lansoprazole, omeprazole, pantoprazole, rabeprazole). These medications create an alkaline environment, which is the strongest stimulant of gastrin production.
- Calcium or insulin can *increase* gastrin levels by acting as a gastrin stimulant.
- Other drugs that may *increase* gastrin levels include catecholamines and caffeine.
- Drugs that may *decrease* gastrin levels include anticholinergics and tricyclic antidepressants.

PROCEDURE AND PATIENT CARE

Before

- Explain the procedure to the patient.
- Instruct the patient to fast for 12 hours before the test. Water is permitted during the fast.
- Instruct the patient to avoid alcohol for at least 24 hours before the test.

During

- Collect a venous blood sample in a red-top tube.
- For the *calcium infusion test*, administer calcium gluconate intravenously. A pre-infusion serum gastrin level is then compared with specimens taken every 30 minutes for 4 hours.
- For the *secretin test*, administer secretin intravenously. Pre-injection and postinjection serum gastrin levels are measured at 15-minute intervals for 1 hour after injection.
- On the laboratory slip, indicate whether the patient is taking any drugs that may affect test results.

After

- Apply pressure or a pressure dressing to the venipuncture site.
- Observe the venipuncture site for bleeding.

TEST RESULTS AND CLINICAL SIGNIFICANCE

▲ Increased Levels

Zollinger-Ellison syndrome: *This syndrome is associated with high levels of gastrin that is produced by a pancreatic islet cell gastrin-producing tumour.*

G-cell hyperplasia: *The G cells in the antrum of the stomach are hyperplastic and produce increased amounts of gastrin.*

Pernicious anemia,

Atrophic gastritis: *An achlorhydric alkaline environment exists in these illnesses. This is a strong stimulant of gastrin secretion.*

Gastric carcinoma: *Cancer of the stomach usually exists in an achlorhydric alkaline environment. This is a strong stimulant of gastrin secretion.*

Chronic renal failure: *Gastrin is metabolized by the kidneys. Without adequate kidney function, gastrin levels increase.*

Pyloric obstruction or gastric outlet obstruction: *The stomach becomes distended. Gastric distension is a potent stimulant of gastrin production.*

Retained antrum after gastric surgery: *Antral tissue mistakenly left on the duodenal stump after gastric resection is constantly bathed in duodenal alkaline juices. This is a strong stimulant of gastrin secretion.*

RELATED TEST

Gastric Analysis. This is an older test of gastric juices that is used to diagnose Zollinger-Ellison syndrome and to determine the adequacy of antipeptic medical and surgical therapy.

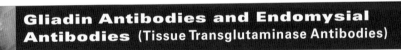

Gliadin Antibodies and Endomysial Antibodies (Tissue Transglutaminase Antibodies)

NORMAL FINDINGS

	Age	Normal
Gliadin immunoglobulin A (IgA)/ immunoglobulin G (IgG)	0–2 years ≥3 years	<20 U <25 U
Endomysial IgA	All ages	Negative
Tissue transglutaminase IgA	All ages	<20 U

INDICATIONS

This test is used to diagnose celiac disease by identifying antibodies to gliadin and gluten in affected patients.

TEST EXPLANATION

Gliadin and gluten are proteins found in wheat and wheat products. Patients with celiac disease cannot tolerate ingestion of these proteins or any products containing wheat. In affected patients, these proteins are toxic to the mucosa of the small intestine and cause characteristic pathologic lesions. Affected patients experience severe intestinal malabsorption symptoms (e.g. nausea, diarrhea, cramping, and vomiting). The only treatment is for the patient to abstain from wheat and wheat-containing products.

When an affected patient ingests wheat-containing foods, gluten and gliadin build up in the intestinal mucosa. These gliadin and gluten proteins (and their metabolites) cause direct mucosal damage. Furthermore, immunoglobulins (antigliadin, anti-endomysial, and anti–tissue transglutaminase antibodies) are made, appearing in the gut mucosa and in the serum of severely affected patients. The identification of these antibodies in the blood of patients with malabsorption is helpful in supporting the diagnosis of celiac disease. However, a definitive diagnosis of celiac disease can be made only when a patient with malabsorption is found to have the pathologic intestinal lesions characteristic of celiac disease. Also, the patient's symptoms must be improved with a gluten-free diet. Both the lesions and the response to diet must be present to confirm the diagnosis.

In patients with known celiac disease, these antibodies can be used to monitor disease status and dietary compliance. Furthermore, these antibodies can be measured to determine whether treatment is successful, inasmuch as the test results become negative in patients on a gluten-free diet.

INTERFERING FACTORS

- Other gastrointestinal diseases such as Crohn's disease, colitis, and severe lactose intolerance can be associated with *elevated* levels of gliadin antibodies.

PROCEDURE AND PATIENT CARE

Before
- Explain the procedure to the patient.
- Inform the patient that no fasting is required.
- Obtain a list of foods that have been ingested in the last 48 hours.
- Assess how many malabsorption symptoms the patient has been experiencing in the previous few weeks.

During
- Collect a venous blood sample in a red-top tube.

After
- Apply pressure to the venipuncture site.
- Assess the venipuncture site for bleeding.

TEST RESULTS AND CLINICAL SIGNIFICANCE

Celiac disease,

Dermatitis herpetiformis: *This is a chronic, extremely itchy rash consisting of papules and vesicles. It is associated with sensitivity of the intestine to gluten in the diet (celiac disease).*

Glucagon

NORMAL FINDINGS
50–100 ng/L (50–100 pg/mL)

INDICATIONS
This test is a direct measurement of glucagon in the blood. It is used to diagnose a glucagonoma. It is also useful in the evaluation of some diabetic patients. In addition, pancreatic function can be investigated with the use of this test.

TEST EXPLANATION
Glucagon is a hormone secreted by the alpha cells of the pancreatic islets of Langerhans. Glucagon is secreted in response to hypoglycemia and increases the blood glucose level by breaking down glycogen to glucose in the liver. It also increases glucose levels in other tissues by inhibiting passage of glucose into cells and by encouraging efflux of glucose from the cell. Glucagon also oxidizes fatty acids to their basic glycerol components to form glucose. As serum glucose levels rise in the blood, glucagon secretion is inhibited by a negative feedback mechanism.

Elevated glucagon levels may indicate the diagnosis of a glucagonoma (i.e., an alpha islet cell neoplasm). Glucagon deficiency occurs with extensive pancreatic resection or with burned-out pancreatitis. Arginine is a potent stimulator of glucagon. If the glucagon levels fail to rise even with arginine infusion, the diagnosis of glucagon deficiency as a result of pancreatic insufficiency is confirmed.

After ingestion of a carbohydrate-loaded meal, the glucagon level normally decreases through an elaborate negative feedback mechanism. This does not occur in patients with diabetes. Furthermore, in patients with insulin-dependent diabetes, glucagon stimulation caused by hypoglycemia does not occur. Arginine stimulation is performed to differentiate pancreatic insufficiency from diabetes. In diabetes, glucagon levels demonstrate an exaggerated elevation in response to arginine administration. In pancreatic insufficiency, glucagon secretion is not stimulated with arginine. In diabetic patients, hypoglycemia fails to stimulate glucagon release, as occurs in a nondiabetic person.

Because glucagon is thought to be metabolized by the kidneys, renal failure is presumably associated with high glucagon levels and, as a result, high glucose levels. When rejection of a transplanted kidney occurs, one of the first signs of rejection may be increased serum glucose levels.

INTERFERING FACTORS
- Test results may be invalidated if a patient has undergone a radioactive scan within the previous 48 hours and glucagon is measured by radioimmunoassay. Administration of radionuclides can affect results.
- Glucagon levels may be elevated after prolonged fasting, stress, or moderate to intense exercise.
- Drugs that may cause *increases* in glucagon levels include some amino acids (e.g., arginine), cholecystokinin, danazol, gastrin, glucocorticoids, insulin, nifedipine, and sympathomimetic amines.
- Drugs that may cause *decreases* in glucagon levels include atenolol, propranolol, and secretin.

PROCEDURE AND PATIENT CARE

Before

- ☒ Explain the procedure to the patient.
- ☒ Inform the patient that fasting is necessary for 10 to 12 hours before the test. Only water is permitted during the fast.

During

- Collect a venous blood sample in a lavender-top tube.

After

- Apply pressure or a pressure dressing to the venipuncture site.
- Assess the venipuncture site for bleeding.
- Place the specimen in a container of water and crushed ice and send it to the laboratory immediately.

TEST RESULTS AND CLINICAL SIGNIFICANCE

▲ Increased Levels

Familial hyperglucagonemia: *A genetic defect causes a predominance of a glucagon precursor.*

Glucagonoma: *Several syndromes, including the more common multiple endocrine neoplasia, are associated with glucagonomas.*

Diabetes mellitus: *The pathophysiologic mechanism underlying this observation is not known.*

Chronic renal failure: *Glucagon is metabolized by the kidney. With loss of that function, glucagon and glucose levels rise.*

Severe stress, including infection, burns, surgery, and acute hypoglycemia: *Stress stimulates catecholamine release. This in turn stimulates glucagon secretion.*

Acromegaly: *Growth hormone is a stimulator of glucagon.*

Hyperlipidemia: *The pathophysiologic mechanism underlying this observation is not well established.*

Acute pancreatitis: *When pancreatic cells are injured during the inflammation, the cells' contents (including glucagon) are spilled into the bloodstream.*

Pheochromocytoma: *Catecholamines are potent stimulators of glucagon secretion.*

▼ Decreased Levels

Idiopathic glucagon deficiency: *The pathophysiologic mechanism underlying this process is not well understood. An autoantibody process may be the cause.*

Cystic fibrosis,

Chronic pancreatitis: *The chronically diseased pancreas cannot produce glucagon.*

Postpancreatectomy status: *In the absence of pancreatic tissue, glucagon secretion does not occur.*

Cancer of the pancreas: *When pancreatic tissue is destroyed by tumour, glucagon secretion does not occur.*

RELATED TEST

Glucose, Blood (see following test). This test is commonly used to diagnose diabetes. Glucose levels are affected by glucagon secretion.

Glucose, Blood (Blood Sugar, Fasting Blood Sugar [FBS])

NORMAL FINDINGS

Adult: **3.9–6.1 mmol/L** (70–110 mg/dL)
Umbilical cord: **2.5–5.3 mmol/L** (45–96 mg/dL)
Premature infant: **1.1–3.3 mmol/L** (20–60 mg/dL)
Neonate (0–28 days): **1.7–3.3 mmol/L** (30–60 mg/dL)
Infant (1 month to 2 years): **2.2–5.0 mmol/L** (40–90 mg/dL)
Child <2 years: **3.3–5.5 mmol/L** (60–100 mg/dL)
Child >2 years to adult:
   Fasting: **<6.1 mmol/L** (70–110 mg/dL) ("fasting" is defined as no caloric intake for at least 8 hours)
   Casual: **11.1 mmol/L** (≥200 mg/dL) ("casual" is defined as any time of day)
Older adult: increase in normal range after 50 years of age

Critical Values

Adult:
   >16.6 mmol/L (>299 mg/dL) may cause disorientation
   >22.2 mmol/L (>400 mg/dL) may cause coma
Fasting adult male: **<2.77 mmol/L** (<50 mg/dL) may cause brain damage
Fasting adult female and child: **<2.22 mmol/L** (<40mg/dL) may cause brain damage

INDICATIONS

This test is a direct measurement of the blood glucose level. It is most commonly used in the evaluation of diabetic patients.

TEST EXPLANATION

Through an elaborate feedback mechanism, glucose levels are controlled by insulin and glucagon. Glucose levels are low in the fasting state. In response, glucagon, which is made in the alpha cells of the pancreatic islets of Langerhans, is secreted. Glucagon breaks glycogen down to glucose in the liver, and glucose levels rise. If the fasting persists, protein and fatty acids are broken down under glucagon stimulation. Glucose levels continue to rise.

   Glucose levels are elevated after eating. Insulin, which is made in the beta cells of the pancreatic islets of Langerhans, is secreted. Insulin attaches to insulin receptors in muscle, liver, and fatty cells, in which it drives glucose into these target cells to be metabolized to glycogen, amino acids, and fatty acids. Blood glucose levels diminish. Many other hormones (e.g., adrenocorticosteroids, adrenocorticotropic hormone [ACTH], epinephrine, growth, thyroxine) can also affect glucose metabolism.

   The serum glucose test is helpful in diagnosing many metabolic diseases. Serum glucose levels must be evaluated according to the time of day they are performed. For example, a glucose level of **7.5 mmol/L** (135 mg/dL) may be abnormal if the patient is in the fasting state, but this level would be within normal limits if the patient had eaten a meal within the previous hour.

   In general, true glucose elevations indicate diabetes mellitus; however, there are many other possible causes of hyperglycemia. Similarly, hypoglycemia has many causes. The most common cause is inadvertent insulin overdose in patients with brittle diabetes. If diabetes is suspected on the basis of elevated fasting blood levels, a glycosylated hemoglobin or glucose tolerance test can be performed.

Glucose determinations must be performed frequently in patients with newly diagnosed diabetes in order to monitor closely the insulin dosage to be administered. Fingerstick blood glucose determinations are often performed before meals and at bedtime. Results are compared with a sliding-scale insulin chart ordered by the physician to provide coverage with subcutaneous regular insulin.

INTERFERING FACTORS

- Many forms of stress (e.g., trauma, general anaesthesia, infection, burns, myocardial infarction) can cause increases in serum glucose levels.
- Caffeine may cause increases in serum glucose levels.
- Many pregnant women experience some degree of glucose intolerance. If this condition is significant, it is called *gestational diabetes.*
- Most intravenous fluids contain dextrose, which is quickly converted to glucose. Most patients receiving intravenous fluids have increased glucose levels.
- Drugs that may cause *increases* in glucose levels include antidepressants (tricyclics), beta-adrenergic blocking agents, corticosteroids, intravenous dextrose infusion, dextrothyroxine, diazoxide, diuretics, epinephrine, estrogens, glucagon, isoniazid, lithium, phenothiazines, phenytoin, salicylates (acute toxicity), and triamterene.
- Drugs that may cause *decreases* in glucose levels include acetaminophen, alcohol, alpha-glucosidase inhibitors, anabolic steroids, biguanides, clofibrate, disopyramide, gemfibrozil, insulin, monoamine oxidase inhibitors, meglitinides, pentamidine, propranolol, sulphonylureas, and thiazolidinediones.

Clinical Priorities

- Serum glucose levels must be evaluated according to the time of day they are obtained. Levels are increased after a recent meal.
- Glucose determinations must be performed frequently in patients with newly diagnosed diabetes in order to determine appropriate insulin therapy. Fingerstick blood glucose determinations are usually performed before meals and at bedtime.
- Many forms of stress can cause increases in serum glucose levels.
- Many drugs affect glucose levels.

PROCEDURE AND PATIENT CARE

Before
- Explain the procedure to the patient.
- For fasting blood glucose determination, the patient must fast for 8 hours before the test. Water is permitted during the fast.
- To prevent starvation, which may artificially raise the glucose levels, the patient should fast no longer than 8 hours.
- Withhold insulin or oral hypoglycemic drugs until after blood is obtained, as per physician's orders.

During
- Collect a venous blood sample in a red-top or grey-top tube.
- Glucose levels can also be evaluated by a fingerstick blood test, with the use of either a visually read test or a reflectance meter. The advantage of the visually read test is that it does not require

an expensive machine. However, the patient must be able to visually interpret the colour of the reagent strip. Using reflectance meters (e.g., Glucometer, Accu Check bG, Stat Tek) improves the accuracy of the blood glucose determination. However, this method is more complex because it requires machine calibration and control testing.

After

- Apply pressure or a pressure dressing to the venipuncture site.
- Observe the venipuncture site for bleeding.
- Be certain that the patient receives a meal immediately after the fasting blood test.

TEST RESULTS AND CLINICAL SIGNIFICANCE

▲ Increased Levels (Hyperglycemia)

Diabetes mellitus: *This disease is defined by glucose intolerance and hyperglycemia. A discussion of the many possible causes is beyond the scope of this book.*

Acute stress response: *Severe stress—including infection, burns, and surgery—stimulates catecholamine release. This in turn stimulates glucagon secretion, which causes hyperglycemia.*

Cushing's syndrome: *Blood cortisol levels are high. This in turn causes hyperglycemia.*

Pheochromocytoma: *Catecholamine stimulates glucagon secretion, which causes hyperglycemia.*

Chronic renal failure: *Glucagon is metabolized by the kidneys. With loss of that function, glucagon and glucose levels rise.*

Glucagonoma: *Glucagon is autonomously secreted, which causes hyperglycemia.*

Acute pancreatitis: *When pancreatic cells are injured during the inflammation, the cells' contents (including glucagon) are spilled into the bloodstream. The glucagon causes hyperglycemia.*

Diuretic therapy: *Certain diuretics cause hyperglycemia.*

Corticosteroid therapy: *High cortisol levels cause hyperglycemia.*

Acromegaly: *Growth hormone stimulates glucagon, which causes hyperglycemia.*

▼ Decreased Levels (Hypoglycemia)

Insulinoma: *Insulin is autonomously produced without regard to biofeedback mechanisms.*

Hypothyroidism: *Thyroid hormones affect glucose metabolism. With diminished levels of this hormone, glucose levels fall.*

Hypopituitarism: *Many pituitary hormones (ACTH, growth hormone) affect glucose metabolism. With diminished levels of these hormones, glucose levels fall.*

Addison's disease: *Cortisol affects glucose metabolism. With diminished levels of this hormone, glucose levels fall.*

Extensive liver disease: *Most glucose metabolism occurs in the liver. When liver function is decreased, glucose levels decrease.*

Insulin overdose: *This is the most common cause of hypoglycemia. When insulin is administered at too high a dose (especially in brittle diabetes), glucose levels fall.*

Starvation: *With decreased carbohydrate ingestion, glucose levels diminish.*

RELATED TESTS

Diabetes Mellitus Autoantibody (p. 222). This test is used in the evaluation of insulin resistance, to identify type 1 diabetes, to evaluate patients with a suspected allergy to insulin, and in surveillance of patients who have received pancreatic islet cell transplants.

Glucose, Urine (p. 957). Testing for glucose in the urine is a part of routine urinalysis. The presence of glucose in the urine reflects the degree of glucose elevation in the blood. Urine glucose tests are also used to monitor the effectiveness of therapy for diabetes mellitus.

Glycosylated Hemoglobin (p. 281). This is an accurate method of indicating average glucose levels over the 100 to 120 days before the test.

Glucose Tolerance (p. 276). This is a test of a patient's capability to handle a glucose load.

Glucose, Postprandial (p. 272). This is a timed glucose measurement after a carbohydrate meal.

Glucagon (p. 267). This is a direct measurement of glucagon, which acts to increase glucose in the blood.

Insulin Assay (p. 330). This is a direct measurement of insulin, which acts to decrease glucose in the blood.

 Glucose, Postprandial (2-Hour Postprandial Glucose [2-Hour PPG], 2-Hour Postprandial Blood Sugar, 1-Hour Glucose Screen for Gestational Diabetes Mellitus, O'Sullivan Test)

NORMAL FINDINGS

2-Hour Postprandial Glucose Measurement

Adult: <7.7 mmol/L (<140 mg/dL)
Child: <7.8 mmol/L (<140mg/dL)

1-Hour Glucose Screen for Gestational Diabetes

<7.9 mmol/L (<140 mg/dL)

INDICATIONS

The 2-hour postprandial glucose test is a measurement of the amount of glucose in the patient's blood 2 hours after a meal is ingested (postprandial). This test is used to diagnose diabetes mellitus.

TEST EXPLANATION

For this study, a meal acts as a glucose challenge to the body's metabolism. Insulin is normally secreted immediately after a meal in response to the elevated blood glucose level and causes the glucose level to return to the preprandial range within 2 hours. In patients with diabetes, the glucose level usually is still elevated 2 hours after the meal. The postprandial glucose test is a screening test for diabetes mellitus that is easily performed. If the readings are higher than **7.8 mmol/L** (140mg/dL) and lower than **11.1 mmol/L** (200 mg/dL), a glucose tolerance test may be performed to confirm the diagnosis. If the 2-hour postprandial glucose level is higher than **11.1 mmol/L** (200 mg/dL), the diagnosis of diabetes mellitus is confirmed. Also, a glucose tolerance or glycosylated hemoglobin test can be performed to corroborate and better evaluate the disease.

The 1-hour glucose screen is used to detect gestational diabetes mellitus, which is the most common medical complication of pregnancy. Gestational diabetes is a carbohydrate intolerance first manifested during pregnancy and affects 3% to 8% of pregnant women; up to 50% of these women develop overt diabetes later in life. The detection and treatment of gestational diabetes may reduce the risk for several adverse perinatal outcomes (e.g., excessive fetal growth and birth trauma, fetal death, neonatal morbidity).

Screening for gestational diabetes is performed with a 50-g oral glucose load, followed by a glucose level determination 1 hour later. This sequence is called the *O'Sullivan test*. Screening is performed between 24 and 28 weeks of pregnancy. However, patients with risk factors such as a previous history of gestational diabetes may benefit from earlier screening. Patients whose serum glucose level equals or exceeds **7.78 mmol/L** (140mg/dL) should be evaluated with a 3-hour glucose tolerance test.

INTERFERING FACTORS

- Smoking during the testing period may increase the blood glucose level.
- Stress, through the catecholamine effect, can increase glucose levels.
- If the patient eats a small snack or eats candy during the 2-hour interval, glucose levels are artificially elevated.
- If the patient is not able to eat the entire test meal or vomits some or all of the meal, levels are artificially decreased.

PROCEDURE AND PATIENT CARE

Before

- Explain the procedure to the patient.
- Usually a fasting blood glucose level is measured before the meal is given. This measurement serves as a baseline glucose level (see p. 269).
- For the 2-hour postprandial glucose test, instruct the patient to fast for 12 hours before the test, as per physician's orders. At the time of testing, instruct the patient to eat the entire meal (with at least 75 g of carbohydrates) and then not to eat anything else until the blood is collected 2 hours later.
- For the 1-hour glucose screen for gestational diabetes, give the fasting or nonfasting patient a 50-g oral glucose load.
- Instruct the patient not to smoke during the test.
- Inform the patient that he or she should rest during the 1- or 2-hour interval, because exercise can increase glucose levels.

During

- Collect a venous blood sample in a red-top or grey-top tube 1 or 2 hours after the patient has eaten the test meal.

After

- Apply pressure or a pressure dressing to the venipuncture site.
- Observe the venipuncture site for bleeding.

TEST RESULTS AND CLINICAL SIGNIFICANCE

▲ Increased Levels

Diabetes mellitus: *This disease is defined by glucose intolerance and hyperglycemia. A discussion of the many possible causes is beyond the scope of this book.*

Gestational diabetes mellitus: *This disease is defined by glucose intolerance and hyperglycemia during pregnancy.*

Malnutrition: *Malnourished patients have very poor glucose tolerance when they start to eat. The pathophysiologic processes underlying this observation and theories about it are not well defined and are multiple.*

Hyperthyroidism: *Thyroid hormone is an ancillary hormone that affects glucose metabolism and acts to increase glucose levels.*

Acute stress response: *Severe stress—including infection, burns, and surgery—stimulates catecholamine release. This in turn stimulates glucagon secretion, which causes hyperglycemia.*

Cushing's syndrome: *Blood cortisol levels are high. This in turn causes hyperglycemia.*

Pheochromocytoma: *Catecholamine stimulates glucagon secretion, which causes hyperglycemia.*

Chronic renal failure: *Glucagon is metabolized by the kidney. With loss of kidney function, glucagon and glucose levels rise.*

Glucagonoma: *Glucagon is autonomously secreted, which causes hyperglycemia.*

Diuretic therapy: *Certain diuretics cause hyperglycemia.*

Corticosteroid therapy: *High cortisol levels cause hyperglycemia.*

Acromegaly: *Growth hormone stimulates glucagon secretion, which causes hyperglycemia.*

Extensive liver disease: *Most glucose metabolism occurs in the liver. With decreased function of the liver, glucose levels decrease.*

▼ Decreased Levels

Insulinoma: *Insulin is autonomously produced without regard to biofeedback mechanisms.*

Hypothyroidism: *Thyroid hormone affects glucose metabolism. With diminished levels of this hormone, glucose levels fall.*

Hypopituitarism: *Many pituitary hormones (adrenocorticotropic hormone [ACTH], growth hormone) affect glucose metabolism. When levels of these hormones are diminished, glucose levels fall.*

Addison's disease: *Cortisol affects glucose metabolism. When levels of this hormone are diminished, glucose levels fall.*

Insulin overdose: *This is the most common cause of hypoglycemia. When insulin is administered at too high a dose (especially in brittle diabetes), glucose levels fall.*

Malabsorption or maldigestion: *The test meal is not absorbed, and glucose levels do not increase.*

RELATED TESTS

Glucose, Blood (p. 269). This test is a direct measurement of the blood glucose level. It is most commonly the initial test in the evaluation of diabetic patients.

Glycosylated Hemoglobin (p. 281). This is an accurate method of indicating glucose tolerance in the recent past.

Glucose Tolerance (p. 276). This is a test of a patient's capability to handle a glucose load.

Glucose-6-Phosphate Dehydrogenase (G6PD Screen)

NORMAL FINDINGS

Negative (screening test) **0.17–0.24 nKat/g hemoglobin** or 12.1 ± 2 U/g hemoglobin

INDICATIONS

This test is used to identify deficiency of glucose-6-phosphate dehydrogenase (G6PD) in patients who have developed hemolysis after taking certain oxidizing drugs. It is especially useful in male patients of certain ethnic populations that are susceptible to this genetic defect.

TEST EXPLANATION

G6PD is an enzyme used in glucose metabolism. G6PD deficiency causes precipitation of oxidized hemoglobin (forms Heinz bodies). This may result in hemolysis of variable severity. This disease is a sex-linked, recessive trait carried on the X chromosome. The full effect of this genetic defect is not seen if the normal gene is present on a second X chromosome to oppose the genetic defect. Because boys and men have no second X gene, the genetic defect is unopposed. Affected boys inherit this abnormal gene from their mothers, who are usually asymptomatic. In these boys, the disease is most severe.

In rare cases when girls have the defective gene on both X chromosomes, the disease is equally severe. Most commonly, however, women act as carriers of the gene in that one X chromosome has the defective gene and the other has the normal gene for G6PD. Carrier women have variable expressions of the disease from no symptoms to moderate symptoms if under a significant degree of stimulation.

G6PD is the most common human enzyme defect, being present in more than 400 million people worldwide. In the United States, G6PD is found mainly in Black people. Approximately 10% to 15% of that population is affected by the disease. Individuals of Mediterranean descent (Italians, Greeks, Sephardic Jews) are also at risk for the genetic defect.

G6PD is an important enzyme involved in the pentose pathway of glucose metabolism that produces the reduced form of nicotinamide adenine dinucleotide phosphate (NADPH) in the red blood cell (RBC). Most of the glucose in a young RBC is metabolized to produce the reduced form of nicotinamide adenine dinucleotide (NADH) by the Embden-Meyerhof pathway. As the RBC ages, the pentose pathway becomes the dominant pathway of glucose metabolism. The NADPH in turn maintains the supply of reduced glutathione, which is used to neutralize free oxidative radicals that damage the RBC. Glutathione protects the RBC against potentially destructive oxidizing states such as infection, pharmacologic agents, or certain foods (such as fava beans). If NADPH is present through the action of G6PD, the RBC is not susceptible to oxidizing agents. When the oxidative effects of glutathione are deficient, as in patients with G6PD deficiency, proteins precipitate on the RBC membrane, which leads to RBC destruction and hemolysis. Patients with severe G6PD deficiency can have chronic or intermittent hemolysis. Individuals with mild deficiency do not have hemolysis without exposure to the oxidizing drugs or oxidizing events. With the administration of an oxidizing drug, hemolysis can start as early as the first day and is usually present by the fourth day. The most common oxidizing drugs known to precipitate hemolysis and anemia in G6PD deficiency are antimalarials, sulpha drugs, nitrofurantoins, aspirin, and phenacetin (Box 2-7). Infections or acidosis can also precipitate a hemolytic process in these patients.

BOX 2-7	Drugs That Precipitate Hemolysis in Patients With G6PD Deficiency

- Acetanilid
- Antimalarials
- Antipyretics
- Ascorbic acid
- Aspirin
- Dapsone
- Methylene blue
- Nalidixic acid
- Nitrofurantoin
- Phenacetin
- Phenazopyridine
- Primaquine
- Quinidine
- Sulpha
- Sulphonamides
- Thiazide diuretics
- Tolbutamide
- Vitamin K (water soluble)

G6PD, Glucose-6-phosphate dehydrogenase.

This test is used to diagnose G6PD deficiency when this condition is suspected. Several different testing methods are available for G6PD screening and testing. G6PD enzyme assay direct quantitation yields the most definitive results.

INTERFERING FACTORS

- With the dye reduction and glutathione screening testing, reticulocytosis caused by a hemolytic episode may be associated with artificially high levels of G6PD.

PROCEDURE AND PATIENT CARE

Before

⬚ Explain the procedure to the patient.
⬚ Inform the patient that no fasting is required.

During

- Collect a venous blood sample in a lavender-top or green-top tube.
- Avoid hemolysis.

After

- Apply pressure or a pressure dressing to the venipuncture site.
- Assess the venipuncture site for bleeding.
⬚ If the test result indicates G6PD deficiency, give the patient a list of drugs that may precipitate hemolysis. Instruct patients with the Mediterranean type of this disease not to eat fava beans. Teach patients to read labels on any over-the-counter drugs for the presence of agents (e.g., aspirin, phenacetin) that may cause hemolytic anemia.

TEST RESULTS AND CLINICAL SIGNIFICANCE

▲ Increased Levels

Reticulocytosis (e.g., pernicious anemia or chronic blood loss): *With the dye reduction and glutathione screening testing, reticulocytosis caused by a hemolytic episode may be associated with artificially high levels of G6PD.*

▼ Decreased Levels

G6PD deficiency

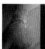

Glucose Tolerance (GT, Oral Glucose Tolerance [OGT])

NORMAL FINDINGS

Serum

Fasting: **4–6 mmol/L** (70–110 mg/dL)
30 minutes after glucose administration: **<11.1 mmol/L** (<200 mg/dL)
1 hour after glucose administration: **<11.1 mmol/L** (<200 mg/dL)
2 hours after glucose administration: **<7.8 mmol/L** (<140 mg/dL)

3 hours after glucose administration: **<6.4 mmol/L** (70–115 mg/dL)
4 hours after glucose administration: **<6.4 mmol/L** (70–115 mg/dL)

Urine
Negative

INDICATIONS
This test is used to assist in the diagnosis of diabetes mellitus. It is also used in the evaluation of patients with hypoglycemia.

TEST EXPLANATION
✤ The Canadian Diabetes Association (2008) defined the criteria for the diagnosis of diabetes. These criteria include sufficient clinical symptoms (polydipsia, polyuria, ketonuria, weight loss) plus either a casual blood glucose level of **11.1 mmol/L** or higher or impaired fasting blood glucose level of 7 mmol/L or higher. The classification of type 1 diabetes, type 2 diabetes, and gestational diabetes mellitus is summarized in Table 2-26.

✤ The Canadian Diabetes Association recommends that individuals older than 40 years be screened for diabetes every 3 years with a fasting blood glucose test. People with additional risk factors, such as Indigenous peoples, or those with a family history should be screened more often as determined by their physician. When the fasting blood glucose level is **6.1 to 6.9 mmol/L**, a 2-hour glucose tolerance test is indicated.

The presence of these criteria for the diagnosis of diabetes should be reconfirmed by repeated testing on a different day in the absence of unequivocal hyperglycemia and metabolic decompensation.

The glucose tolerance test is thus used when diabetes is suspected (in patients with retinopathy, neuropathy, diabetic-type renal diseases), but the criteria for the diagnosis cannot be met without the data obtained by the glucose tolerance test. This test is not part of routine screening for diabetes. The glucose tolerance test may be used for the following:
- Patients with a family history of diabetes
- Patients who are massively obese
- Patients with a history of recurrent infections
- Patients with delayed healing of wounds (especially on the lower legs or feet)
- Women who have a history of stillbirths or delivering large babies
- Patients who have transient glycosuria or hyperglycemia during pregnancy or after myocardial infarction, surgery, or stress

TABLE 2-26	Canadian Diabetes Association Classification of Diabetes
Classification	**Descriptors**
Type 1	Primarily a result of pancreatic beta cell destruction
Type 2	Ranges from primarily insulin resistant with relative insulin deficiency to a main secretory defect with insulin resistance
Gestational diabetes mellitus	Glucose intolerance with onset or first recognition during pregnancy
Other types	Include a wide variety of conditions, mainly genetic forms of diabetes or diabetes associated with other diseases or drug use

Information from Canadian Diabetes Association. (2013). *Canadian Diabetes Association 2013 Clinical Practice Guidelines for the Prevention and Management of Diabetes in Canada.* Toronto: Canadian Diabetes Association.

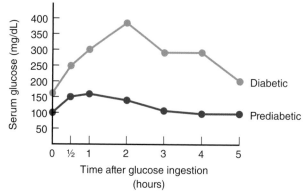

Figure 2-18 Glucose tolerance test curves for a diabetic patient and a prediabetic patient.

In the glucose tolerance test, the patient's ability to tolerate a standard oral glucose load (75 g) is evaluated by obtaining serum and urine specimens for glucose level determinations before glucose administration and then 30 minutes, 1 hour, 2 hours, 3 hours, and sometimes 4 hours after the administration. Normally there is a rapid insulin response to the ingestion of a large oral glucose load. This response peaks in 30 to 60 minutes and returns to normal in approximately 3 hours. Patients with an appropriate insulin response are able to tolerate the dose quite easily, with only a minimal and transient rise in serum glucose levels within 1 to 2 hours after ingestion. Glucose does not spill over into the urine in normal patients.

Patients with diabetes are not able to tolerate this load. As a result, their serum glucose levels become greatly elevated from 1 to 5 hours (Figure 2-18). Also, glucose can be detected in their urine.

Gestational diabetes also can be diagnosed by the glucose tolerance test. In general, the diagnosis of diabetes can be made if two or more of the results exceed the following:
- Fasting: **5.8 mmol/L** (105 mg/dL)
- 1 hour: **10.5 mmol/L** (190 mg/dL)
- 2 hours: **9.1 mmol/L** (165 mg/dL)
- 3 hours: **8.0 mmol/L** (145 mg/dL)

♣ The Canadian Diabetes Association recommends that pregnant women who have not previously had an abnormal glucose tolerance test result should undergo screening between 24 and 28 weeks of pregnancy with a 50-g dose of glucose. This is called the *O'Sullivan test*. A glucose level higher than **7.8 mmol/L** (140 mg/dL) warrants the glucose tolerance test.

Gastrointestinal absorption can vary among individuals. For that reason, some centres prefer to administer an intravenous glucose load rather than depend on gastrointestinal absorption. Also, an occasional patient is unable to tolerate the oral glucose load (e.g., patients with prior gastrectomy, short-bowel syndrome, malabsorption). In these instances, a glucose tolerance test can be performed by administering the glucose load intravenously. The values for the intravenous glucose tolerance test differ slightly from those of the oral glucose tolerance test because intravenous glucose is absorbed faster.

Glucose intolerance also may exist in patients with oversecretion of hormones that have an ancillary effect on glucose level, such as patients with Cushing's syndrome, pheochromocytoma, acromegaly, aldosteronism, or hyperthyroidism. Patients with chronic renal failure, acute pancreatitis, myxedema, type IV lipoproteinemia, infection, or cirrhosis can also have an abnormal result of the glucose tolerance test. Certain drugs, as mentioned in the "Interfering Factors" section, can cause abnormal glucose tolerance test results.

The glucose tolerance test is also used to evaluate patients with hypoglycemia. Hypoglycemia may occur as late as 5 hours after the initial glucose load.

CONTRAINDICATIONS

- Serious concurrent infections or endocrine disorders, because glucose intolerance will be observed even though affected patients may not be diabetic.
- Vomiting part or all of the glucose meal, which invalidates the test.

POTENTIAL COMPLICATIONS

- Dizziness, tremors, anxiety, sweating, euphoria, or fainting may occur during testing. If these symptoms occur, a blood specimen is obtained. If the glucose level is too high, the test may need to be stopped and insulin administered.

INTERFERING FACTORS

- Smoking during the testing period stimulates glucose production; this is an effect of the nicotine.
- Stress (e.g., from surgery, infection) can increase glucose levels.
- Exercise during the test can affect glucose levels.
- Fasting or reduced caloric intake before the glucose tolerance test can cause glucose intolerance.
- Drugs that may cause glucose intolerance include antihypertensives, anti-inflammatory drugs, aspirin, beta blockers, furosemide, nicotine, oral contraceptives, phenothiazines, psychiatric drugs, steroids, and thiazide diuretics.

PROCEDURE AND PATIENT CARE

Before
- Explain the procedure to the patient.
- Educate the patient about the importance of having adequate food intake with adequate carbohydrates (150 g) for at least 3 days before the test.
- Instruct the patient to fast for 12 hours before the test, unless otherwise ordered by the physician.
- Instruct the patient to discontinue drugs (including tobacco) that could interfere with test results.
- Give the patient written instructions explaining the pretest dietary requirements.
- Obtain the patient's weight to determine the appropriate glucose loading dose (especially in children).

During
- Obtain fasting blood and urine specimens.
- Administer the prescribed oral glucose solution: usually 75 g of glucose or dextrose for non-pregnant patients and 100 g for pregnant patients. Several commercial preparations are available. The glucose load may be diluted in as much as 300 mL of a lemon juice/water mixture.
- Give pediatric patients a carbohydrate load that is based on their body weight.
- Instruct the patient to ingest the entire glucose load.
- Inform the patient that he or she cannot eat anything until the test is completed. However, encourage the patient to drink water. No other liquids should be taken during the testing period.
- Inform the patient that tobacco, coffee, and tea are not allowed because they cause physiologic stimulation.

- Collect a venous blood sample in a grey-top tube 30 and 60 minutes after the glucose load and at hourly periods.
- Collect urine specimens at hourly periods.
- During the testing period, assess the patient for reactions such as dizziness, sweating, weakness, and giddiness. (These are usually transient.) If the symptoms are persistent, measure the serum glucose level.
- For the intravenous glucose tolerance test, administer the glucose load intravenously over 3 to 4 minutes.

After

- Apply pressure or a pressure dressing to the venipuncture sites.
- Mark on the tubes the time that the specimens are collected.
- Send all specimens promptly to the laboratory.
- Allow the patient to eat and drink normally.
- Administer insulin or oral hypoglycemics if ordered.
- Assess the venipuncture sites for bleeding.

TEST RESULTS AND CLINICAL SIGNIFICANCE

▲ Increased Levels

Diabetes mellitus: *This disease is defined by glucose intolerance and hyperglycemia. A discussion of the many possible causes is beyond the scope of this book.*

Acute stress response: *Severe stress—including infection, burns, and surgery—stimulates catecholamine release. This in turn stimulates glucagon secretion, which causes hyperglycemia and glucose intolerance.*

Cushing's syndrome: *Blood cortisol levels are high. This in turn causes hyperglycemia and glucose intolerance.*

Pheochromocytoma: *Catecholamines stimulate glucagon secretion, which causes hyperglycemia and glucose intolerance.*

Chronic renal failure: *Glucagon is metabolized by the kidneys. With loss of that function, glucagon and glucose levels rise.*

Glucagonoma: *Glucagon is autonomously secreted, which causes hyperglycemia.*

Acute pancreatitis: *When pancreatic cells are injured during the inflammation, the cells' contents (including glucagon) are spilled into the bloodstream. The glucagon causes hyperglycemia.*

Diuretic therapy: *Certain diuretics cause hyperglycemia.*

Corticosteroid therapy: *High cortisol levels cause hyperglycemia and glucose intolerance.*

Acromegaly: *Growth hormone stimulates glucagon, which causes hyperglycemia and glucose intolerance.*

Myxedema: *Usually these patients have a flat glucose tolerance curve, but they may have a "diabetic curve."*

Somogyi response to hypoglycemia: *This is a reactive hyperglycemia after hypoglycemia that may result from an exaggerated insulin response to the glucose load.*

After gastrectomy: *Patients who have undergone gastrectomy can dump most of the glucose load into the small intestines in just minutes because the normal pylorus is absent. This can cause rapid absorption of glucose into the bloodstream and cause an artificial elevation in glucose level during the early part of the test.*

RELATED TESTS

Diabetes Mellitus Autoantibody (p. 222). This test is used in the evaluation of insulin resistance. It is also used to identify type 1 diabetes and to confirm a suspected allergy to insulin. This antibody test is also used in surveillance of patients who have received pancreatic islet cell transplants.

Glucose, Blood (p. 269). This is the primary screening test to diagnose diabetes.

Glucose, Urine (p. 957). Testing for glucose in the urine is a part of routine urinalysis. The presence of glucose in urine reflects the degree of glucose level elevation in the blood. Urine glucose tests are also used to monitor the effectiveness of therapy for diabetes mellitus.

Glycosylated Hemoglobin (see following test p. 281). This is an accurate method of indicating glucose tolerance in the recent past.

Glucagon (p. 267). This is a direct measurement of glucagon, which acts to increase glucose level in the blood.

Insulin Assay (p. 330). This is a direct measurement of insulin, which acts to decrease glucose level in the blood.

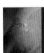

Glycosylated Hemoglobin (GHb, GHB, Glycohemoglobin, Hemoglobin A$_{1c}$ [HbA$_{1c}$], Diabetic Control Index, Glycated Protein)

NORMAL FINDINGS

Nondiabetic adult/child: 4%–5.9%
Good diabetic control: <7%
Fair diabetic control: 8%–9%
Poor diabetic control: >9%
   Values vary according to laboratory methods.

INDICATIONS

This test is used to monitor diabetes treatment. It measures the amount of hemoglobin A$_{1c}$ (HbA$_{1c}$) in the blood. This test provides an accurate long-term index of the patient's average blood glucose level.

TEST EXPLANATION

In adults, approximately 98% of the hemoglobin in the red blood cell (RBC) is hemoglobin A. Approximately 7% of hemoglobin A consists of a type of hemoglobin (HbA$_1$) that can combine strongly with glucose in a process called *glycosylation*. Once glycosylation occurs, it is not easily reversible. HbA$_1$ is actually made up of three components (hemoglobins A$_{1a}$, A$_{1b}$, and A$_{1c}$). HbA$_{1c}$ is the component that most strongly combines glucose. HbA$_{1c}$ makes up the majority of the HbA$_1$. Approximately 70% of HbA$_{1c}$ is glycosylated. Only 20% of hemoglobins A$_{1a}$ and A$_{1b}$ are glycosylated. HbA$_{1c}$ provides the most accurate measurement because it constitutes the majority of glycosylated hemoglobin.

As the RBC circulates, it combines its HbA$_1$ with some of the glucose in the bloodstream to form glycohemoglobin (GHb). The amount of GHb depends on the amount of glucose available in the bloodstream over the RBC's 120-day life span. Therefore, the GHb value reflects the average blood glucose level for the 100- to 120-day period before the test. The more glucose the RBC is exposed to, the greater the GHb percentage is. One important advantage of this test is that the sample can be collected at any time because it is not affected by short-term variations (e.g., food intake, exercise, stress, hypoglycemic agents, patient cooperation). It is also possible for very high short-term blood glucose levels to cause an elevation of GHb levels. Usually, however, the degree of glucose elevation results not from a transient high level but from a persistent, moderate elevation over the entire life of the RBC.

Like GHb, the glucose can nonenzymatically bind to proteins in proportion to the mean blood glucose level. The *glycated protein* is stable until the degradation of the protein. Recall that the average life span of an RBC (and the GHb within) is 120 days. The GHb, therefore, may not reflect more recent changes in glucose levels. Because the turnover rate of proteins is much faster than that of hemoglobin, the measurement of serum glycated proteins (such as *glycated albumin* or *fructosamine*) provides more recent information about glucose levels. Glycated proteins reflect an average blood glucose level of the previous 15 to 20 days. Although an initial single glycated protein result may not distinguish good glucose control from poor control, serial testing provides a much better indication of glucose control.

The GHb or glycated proteins tests are particularly beneficial for the following:
1. Evaluating the success of diabetic treatment and patient compliance.
2. Comparing and contrasting the success of past and new forms of diabetic therapy.
3. Determining the duration of hyperglycemia in patients with newly diagnosed diabetes.
4. Providing a sensitive estimate of glucose imbalance in patients with mild diabetes.
5. Individualizing diabetic control regimens.
6. Providing a sense of reward for many patients when the test shows achievement of good diabetic control.
7. Evaluating diabetic patients whose glucose levels change significantly from day to day (brittle diabetes).
8. Differentiating short-term hyperglycemia in nondiabetic patients (e.g., recent stress or myocardial infarction) and diabetic patients (in whom the glucose level has been persistently elevated).

By a relatively simple calculation, GHb can be correlated accurately with the daily mean plasma glucose (MPG) level, the average glucose level throughout the day. This has been very helpful for diabetic patients and their health care providers in determining and evaluating daily glucose goals. There is a linear relationship between levels of HbA_{1c} (GHb) and plasma glucose level:

$$MPG = (35.6 \times GHb) - 77.3,$$

with a Pearson correlation coefficient (r) of 0.82. Each 1% change in GHb represents a change of approximately $2\,mmol/L$ ($35\,mg/dL$) of MPG level (Table 2-27).

TABLE 2-27	Correlation Between Glycohemoglobin and Mean Plasma Glucose Level	
Glycohemoglobin (Hemoglobin A$_{1c}$)	**Approximate Mean Plasma Glucose Level (mmol/L [mg/dL])**	**Interpretation**
4%	3.61 mmol/L (65 mg/dL)	Nondiabetic range
5%	5.55 mmol/L (100 mg/dL)	Nondiabetic range
6%	7.5 mmol/L (135 mg/dL)	Nondiabetic range
7%	9.44 mmol/L (170 mg/dL)	CDA target
8%	11.38 mmol/L (205 mg/dL)	Action suggested

CDA, Canadian Diabetes Association.

American Diabetes Association (2012). Diagnosis and classification of diabetes mellitus. *Diabetes Care 35* (Supplement 1) 564–571.

INTERFERING FACTORS

- Hemoglobinopathies can affect results because the quantity of hemoglobin A (and, as a result, HbA_1) varies considerably in these diseases.
- Values are artificially elevated when the RBC life span is lengthened because the HbA_1 has a longer period available for glycosylation.
- Abnormally low levels of proteins may falsely indicate normal glycated fructosamine levels despite the fact that glucose levels are high.
- Ascorbic acid may cause artificially low levels of glycated fructosamine.

PROCEDURE AND PATIENT CARE

Before

- Explain the procedure to the patient.
- Inform the patient that no fasting is required.

During

- Collect a venous blood sample in a grey-top or lavender-top tube.

After

- Apply pressure or a pressure dressing to the venipuncture site.
- Assess the venipuncture site for bleeding.

TEST RESULTS AND CLINICAL SIGNIFICANCE

▲ Increased Levels

Newly diagnosed diabetes: *This test is not used to diagnose diabetes because the range of "normal" is so broad; it is best used to assess glycemic control during treatment.*

Poorly controlled diabetes,

Nondiabetic hyperglycemia (e.g., acute stress response, Cushing's syndrome, pheochromocytoma, glucagonoma, corticosteroid therapy, acromegaly): *Patients with these illnesses tend to have persistently elevated glucose levels that cause elevations in GHb and glycated protein levels.*

Patients with splenectomy: *In these patients, RBC survival is prolonged. More time for hemoglobin glycosylation is available. GHb and glycated protein levels increase.*

Pregnancy: *In some women with gestational diabetes or prediabetes, levels of glucose are persistently high, which causes elevations in GHb and glycated protein levels.*

▼ Decreased Levels

Hemolytic anemia,

Chronic blood loss: *RBC survival is shortened. Therefore, there is less time for glycosylation, and GHb and glycated protein levels decrease.*

Chronic renal failure: *These patients have reduced hemoglobin levels as a result of lack of erythropoietin, which is produced in the kidneys. HbA_1 levels are also decreased.*

RELATED TESTS

Glucose, Blood (p. 269). This is the primary screening test for diabetes.

Glucose, Urine (p. 957). Testing for glucose in the urine is a part of routine urinalysis. The presence of glucose in the urine reflects the degree of glucose elevation in the blood. Urine glucose tests are also used to monitor the effectiveness of therapy for diabetes mellitus.

Glucose Tolerance (p. 276). This is a test of a patient's capability to handle a glucose load.

Glucose, Postprandial (p. 272). This is a timed glucose measurement after a carbohydrate meal.

Glucagon (p. 267). This is a direct measurement of glucagon, which acts to increase glucose levels in the blood.

Insulin Assay (p. 330). This is a direct measurement of insulin, which acts to decrease glucose levels in the blood.

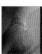

Growth Hormone (GH, Human Growth Hormone [HGH], Somatotropin Hormone [SH])

NORMAL FINDINGS

Male: **<5** *Mcg*/L (<5 ng/mL)
Female: **<10** *Mcg*/L (<10 ng/mL)
Child/adolescent:
  0 to <7 years: **<1–13.6** *Mcg*/L (<1–13.6 ng/mL)
  7 to <11 years: **<1–16.4** *Mcg*/L (<1–16.4 ng/mL)
  11 to <15 years: **<1–14.4** *Mcg*/L (<1–14.4 ng/mL)
  15 to <19 years: **<1–13.4** *Mcg*/L (<1–13.4 ng/mL)

INDICATIONS

This test is used to identify growth hormone deficiency in adolescents with short stature, delayed sexual maturity, or other growth deficiencies. It is also used to document the diagnosis of growth hormone excess in patients with gigantism or acromegaly. In addition, it is often used as a screening test for pituitary hypofunction.

TEST EXPLANATION

Growth hormone, or somatotropin, is secreted by the acidophil cells in the anterior pituitary gland and plays a central role in modulating growth from birth until the end of puberty. An elaborate feedback mechanism is associated with the secretion of growth hormone. The hypothalamus secretes growth hormone–releasing hormone, which stimulates growth hormone release from the pituitary. Growth hormone exerts its effects on many tissues through a group of peptides called *somatomedins*. The most commonly tested somatomedin is somatomedin C (p. 482), which is produced by the liver and has a major effect on cartilage. High levels of somatomedins stimulate the production of somatostatin from the hypothalamus. Somatostatin inhibits further secretion of growth hormone from the pituitary gland. Growth hormone is secreted during sleep, exercise, and ingestion of protein and in response to hypoglycemia.

In the total absence of growth hormone, linear growth occurs at one-half to one-third the normal rate. Growth hormone also plays a role in the control of body anabolism throughout life by increasing protein synthesis, increasing the breakdown of fatty acids in adipose tissue, and increasing the blood glucose level.

If growth hormone secretion is insufficient during childhood, limited growth and dwarfism may result. Also, a delay in sexual maturity may occur in adolescents with reduced growth hormone levels. Conversely, overproduction of growth hormone during childhood results in gigantism; affected persons may reach a height between nearly 7 and 8 feet (213 and 244 cm). An excess of growth hormone during childhood (after closure of long bone end plates) results in acromegaly, which is characterized by an increase in bone thickness and width but no increase in height.

Growth hormone tests are also used to confirm hypopituitarism or hyperpituitarism. Growth hormone assay is the most widely used test for growth hormone deficiency or excess. Because growth hormone secretion is episodic, random assays for growth hormone are not adequate determinants of growth hormone deficiency. Normal growth hormone levels overlap significantly with deficient levels. Low levels may indicate deficiency or may be normal for certain individuals at certain times of the day. To negate time variables in testing, growth hormone samples should be collected 60 to 90 minutes after deep sleep because levels increase during sleep. Also, strenuous exercise can be performed for 30 minutes in an effort to stimulate growth hormone production. Growth hormone levels measured at the end of the exercise period are expected to be maximal. These two methods are helpful in evaluating growth hormone deficiency.

To negate the common variations in growth hormone secretion, screening for insulin-like growth factor 1 (IGF-1) or somatomedin C provides a more accurate reflection of the mean plasma concentration of growth hormone. Virtually no patient with normal IGF-1 levels has acromegaly. IGF-1 is not helpful in evaluating patients with growth hormone deficiency because levels are affected by nutritional status, liver and thyroid function, and age. These proteins are not affected by the time of day or food intake as is growth hormone because they circulate bound to proteins that are durable and long lasting.

A growth hormone stimulation test (p. 287) can be performed to evaluate the body's ability to produce growth hormone in cases of suspected growth hormone deficiency. The growth hormone suppression test is used to identify gigantism in children or acromegaly in the adult. If growth hormone can be suppressed to less than 2 to 4 µ/L, the patient has neither of these conditions. The most commonly used suppression test is the oral glucose tolerance test (p. 276). Through a rise in glucose level, growth hormone normally is suppressed. In acromegalic patients, only a slight or no decrease in growth hormone level occurs.

INTERFERING FACTORS

- Random measurements of growth hormone are not adequate determinants of growth hormone deficiency, because hormone secretion is episodic.
- A radioactive scan performed within the week before the test may affect test results if levels are determined by radioimmunoassay.
- Growth hormone secretion is affected by diet and increased by stress, exercise, and low blood glucose levels.
- Drugs that may cause *increases* in growth hormone levels include amphetamines, arginine, dopamine, estrogens, glucagon, histamine, insulin, levodopa, methyldopa, and nicotinic acid.
- Drugs that may cause *decreases* in growth hormone levels include corticosteroids and phenothiazines.

PROCEDURE AND PATIENT CARE

Before

- Explain the procedure to the patient.
- Ensure that the patient is not emotionally or physically stressed, because this can increase growth hormone levels.
- It is preferred that patients be well rested and are kept on NPO status (nothing by mouth), except for water, after midnight the morning of the test.

During

Growth Hormone
- Collect a venous blood sample in a red-top tube.
- Because approximately two-thirds of the total production of growth hormone occurs during sleep, its secretion also can be measured during hospitalization by obtaining blood samples while the patient is sleeping.

Growth Hormone Suppression Test
- Obtain peripheral venous access with normal saline solution.
- Obtain baseline growth hormone and glucose readings as described previously.
- Administer the prescribed glucose dose.
- Measure growth hormone and glucose levels 30, 60, 90, and 120 minutes after glucose ingestion.

After
- Apply pressure or a pressure dressing to the venipuncture site.
- Assess the venipuncture site for bleeding.
- On the laboratory slip, indicate the patient's fasting status and the times when the blood is collected. Also document the patient's recent activity (e.g., sleeping, walking, eating).
- Because the half-life of growth hormone is only 20 to 25 minutes, send the blood to the laboratory immediately after collection.

TEST RESULTS AND CLINICAL SIGNIFICANCE

▲ Increased Levels

Gigantism,
Acromegaly: *These two syndromes are caused by excess growth hormone.*
Anorexia nervosa: *Starvation stimulates growth hormone secretion.*
Stress,
Major surgery,
Hypoglycemia,
Starvation,
Deep-sleep state,
Exercise: *These situations stimulate growth hormone secretion.*

▼ Decreased Levels

Growth hormone deficiency,
Pituitary insufficiency: *Growth hormone is produced in the pituitary gland. Diseases, tumours, ischemia, and trauma to the pituitary gland or hypothalamus cause growth hormone deficiency.*
Dwarfism: *This is a result of growth hormone deficiency in children.*
Hyperglycemia: *Elevated glucose levels inhibit growth hormone secretion.*
Failure to thrive: *This is a result of growth hormone deficiency in infants and children.*
Delayed sexual maturity: *This is a result of growth hormone deficiency in adolescents.*

RELATED TESTS

Growth Hormone Stimulation (p. 287). This is a test designed to stimulate the secretion of growth hormone. It is required to accurately diagnose growth hormone deficiency.

Somatomedin C (p. 482). Somatomedin C levels parallel growth hormone levels. However, they are not affected by the many factors that cause significant variations in growth hormone results.

Growth Hormone Stimulation (GH Provocation, Insulin Tolerance [IT], Arginine)

NORMAL FINDINGS

Growth hormone levels: >10 *Mc*g/L (>10 ng/mL)

INDICATIONS

The growth hormone stimulation test is used to identify patients who are suspected of having growth hormone deficiency. A normal patient can have low growth hormone levels, but if those levels remain low after growth hormone stimulation, the diagnosis is more accurate.

TEST EXPLANATION

Because growth hormone secretion is episodic, random measurement of plasma growth hormone levels is not adequate support for the diagnosis of growth hormone deficiency. To diagnose this deficiency, growth hormone stimulation tests are indicated. One of the most reliable growth hormone stimulators is insulin-induced hypoglycemia, in which the blood glucose level declines to less than **2.2 mmol/L** (40 mg/dL). Other growth hormone stimulants include vigorous exercise and drugs (e.g., arginine, glucagon, levodopa, clonidine).

Pituitary growth hormone deficiency cannot be diagnosed by identifying a deficiency of growth hormone to just one stimulant, because as many as 20% of normal patients do not respond to the stimulant. Therefore, a double-stimulant test is usually performed: Arginine infusion is followed by insulin-induced hypoglycemia. Arginine is an amino acid that stimulates growth hormone secretion; hypoglycemia also stimulates growth hormone secretion. A growth hormone concentration over 10 mg/L after stimulation effectively rules out growth hormone deficiencies.

Growth hormone also can be stimulated by vigorous exercise. This may entail running or stair-climbing for 20 minutes. Blood samples of growth hormone are obtained immediately, 20 minutes, and 40 minutes afterward. Growth hormone–releasing factor can also be used to stimulate growth hormone. At present, the best method of diagnosing growth hormone deficiency consists of a positive result of a stimulation test followed by a positive response to a therapeutic growth hormone trial. Growth hormone deficiency is also suspected when bone age, as determined by radiographs of the long bones (see p. 1045), indicates that growth is retarded in comparison to chronologic age.

Only minor discomfort is associated with this test, results from the insertion of the intravenous line, and the hypoglycemic response induced by the insulin injection. This discomfort may include postural hypotension, somnolence, diaphoresis, and nervousness. The procedure is usually performed by a nurse under a physician's supervision. It takes approximately 2 hours to perform.

CONTRAINDICATIONS

- Epilepsy, because seizures can be induced by the hypoglycemia
- Cerebrovascular disease, because hypoglycemia may induce stroke
- Myocardial infarction, because the stress associated with the hypoglycemia may cause angina or a myocardial infarction
- Low basal plasma cortisol levels, because affected patients cannot respond to or compensate for the hypoglycemia

POTENTIAL COMPLICATIONS

- Hypoglycemia may be so significant and severe as to cause ketosis, acidosis, and shock. If the patient is under close observation, such developments are unlikely to occur.

INTERFERING FACTORS

- A radioactive scan performed within 1 week before the test may affect test results because radioimmunoassay of growth hormone would be confounded by the previously administered radioisotope.

PROCEDURE AND PATIENT CARE

Before

- Explain the procedure very carefully to the patient and, if appropriate, to the parents.
- Instruct the patient to remain on NPO status (nothing by mouth), except for water, after midnight on the morning of the test.

During

- Note the following procedural steps:
    1. A saline-lock intravenous line is inserted for the administration of medications and the withdrawal of frequent blood samples.
    2. Baseline measurements of blood levels for growth hormone, glucose, and cortisol are obtained.
    3. Venous samples for growth hormone are obtained immediately, 60 minutes, and 90 minutes after injection of arginine, insulin, or both.
    4. Blood glucose levels are monitored at 15- to 30-minute intervals with the glucometer. The blood glucose level should drop to less than **2.2 mmol/L** (40 mg/dL) for effective measurement of growth hormone reserve.
- Monitor the patient for signs of hypoglycemia, postural hypotension, somnolence, diaphoresis, and nervousness.
- The patient may be given ice chips for comfort during the test.

After

- Observe the venipuncture site for bleeding.
- Inform the patient and family that results may not be available for approximately 7 days. Many laboratories run growth hormone tests only once a week.
- After the test, give the patient a sweet snack such as cookies or fruit, and a drink such as apple juice or fruit punch, or an intravenous glucose infusion as per physician's orders.
- Send the blood to the laboratory immediately after collection, because the half-life of growth hormone is only 20 to 25 minutes.

TEST RESULTS AND CLINICAL SIGNIFICANCE

▼ Decreased Levels

Pituitary deficiency,

Growth hormone deficiency: *Diseases (e.g., tumour, infarction, trauma) of the pituitary gland can result in failure of the pituitary gland to secrete either growth hormone or all the pituitary hormones. Growth hormone stimulation tests will fail to stimulate growth hormone secretion.*

RELATED TESTS

Somatomedin C (p. 482). Somatomedin C levels parallel growth hormone levels. However, they are not affected by the many factors that cause significant variations in growth hormone results.

Growth Hormone (p. 284). This test is a direct quantitative assay for growth hormone.

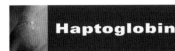

Haptoglobin

NORMAL FINDINGS

Adult: **0.5–2.2 g/L** (50–220 mg/dL)
Newborn: **0–0.1 g/L** (0–10 mg/dL)

 Critical Values

<0.4 g/L (<40 mg/dL)

INDICATIONS

This test is used to identify the presence of intravascular hemolysis. Haptoglobin levels are decreased when significant hemolysis occurs. The test is nonspecific for indicating the type of hemolytic anemia.

TEST EXPLANATION

The serum haptoglobin test is used to detect intravascular destruction (lysis) of red blood cells (RBCs). This process is called *hemolysis*. Haptoglobins are glycoproteins produced by the liver. Haptoglobins are powerful proteins that bind to free hemoglobin. In hemolytic anemias associated with the hemolysis of RBCs, the released hemoglobin is quickly bound to haptoglobin, and the new complex is rapidly catabolized. This results in a diminished amount of free haptoglobin in the serum; this decrease cannot be readily compensated for by normal liver production. As a result, the level of haptoglobin in the serum is transiently reduced.

Haptoglobin levels are also decreased in patients with primary liver disease not associated with hemolytic anemias. This occurs because the diseased liver is unable to produce these glycoproteins. Hematoma can reduce haptoglobin levels by the absorption of hemoglobin into the blood and by binding hemoglobin with haptoglobin.

Haptoglobin concentrations are elevated in many inflammatory diseases, and therefore haptoglobin can be analyzed as a nonspecific acute-phase reactant protein in much the same way as the erythrocyte sedimentation rate (see p. 236). That is, levels of haptoglobin increase with severe infection, inflammation, tissue destruction, acute myocardial infarction, burns, and some cancers.

INTERFERING FACTORS

- Ongoing infection can cause artificial elevations of test results.
- Drugs that may cause *increases* in haptoglobin levels include androgens and steroids.
- Drugs that may cause *decreases* in haptoglobin levels include chlorpromazine, diphenhydramine, indomethacin, isoniazid, nitrofurantoin, oral contraceptives, quinidine, and streptomycin.

PROCEDURE AND PATIENT CARE

Before

🖊 Explain the procedure to the patient.
🖊 Inform the patient that no fasting is required.

During

- Collect a venous blood sample in a red-top tube.
- Avoid hemolysis, which may alter test results.

After

- Apply pressure or a pressure dressing to the venipuncture site.
- Assess the venipuncture site for bleeding.

TEST RESULTS AND CLINICAL SIGNIFICANCE

▲ Increased Levels

Collagen-rheumatic diseases,
Infection (e.g., pyelonephritis, urinary tract infection, pneumonia),
Tissue destruction (e.g., myocardial infarction),
Nephritis,
Ulcerative colitis,
Neoplasia: *These and many other diseases can cause an elevation in levels of haptoglobin, an acute-phase reactant protein.*
Biliary obstruction: *Haptoglobin, after attaching to hemoglobin, is excreted by the liver in the bile. Biliary obstruction diminishes that excretion.*

▼ Decreased Levels

Hemolytic anemia (e.g., erythroblastosis fetalis, autoimmune hemolytic anemias, hemoglobinopathies [sickle cell disease], paroxysmal nocturnal hemoglobinuria, drug-induced hemolytic anemia, or uremia): *Hemolysis occurs, freeing hemoglobin in the plasma. The free hemoglobin is tightly bound to haptoglobin. The complex is catabolized and excreted. Haptoglobin cannot be replaced fast enough, and levels in the blood fall.*
Transfusion reactions: *ABO antibodies bind to ABO antigens on the RBC membrane and cause hemolysis. Hemoglobin is liberated from the RBC. The free hemoglobin is tightly bound to haptoglobin. The complex is catabolized and excreted. Haptoglobin cannot be replaced fast enough, and levels in the blood fall.*
Prosthetic heart valves: *The mechanical trauma of the valve on the RBC causes hemolysis, and hemoglobin is liberated from the RBC. The free hemoglobin is tightly bound to haptoglobin. The complex is catabolized and excreted. Haptoglobin cannot be replaced fast enough, and levels in the blood fall.*
Primary liver disease: *The diseased liver cannot make adequate amounts of haptoglobin. The liver is the sole source of haptoglobin.*
Hematoma,
Tissue hemorrhage: *The free hemoglobin in the hematoma binds the haptoglobin. The complex is catabolized and excreted. Haptoglobin cannot be replaced fast enough, and levels in the blood fall.*

Heinz Body Preparation

NORMAL FINDINGS
No Heinz bodies detected

INDICATIONS
This test is used to detect Heinz bodies, which appear as a result of oxidative denaturation of the hemoglobin molecule.

TEST EXPLANATION
Heinz bodies are water-insoluble precipitates of oxidated-denatured proteins or hemoglobin that form within red blood cells (RBCs). They occur as a result of exposure to oxidative chemicals and drugs. Mutations of hemoglobin (specifically Hb Koln), thalassemias, and defects in the hemoglobin-reductive defence system against oxidation (glucose-6-phosphate dehydrogenase [G6PD] deficiency or pyruvate kinase deficiency) lead to an enhanced tendency toward oxidative hemolysis. The diagnosis of these problems can be established by the detection of Heinz bodies in RBCs through a Heinz body preparation.

Heinz bodies are often associated with hemolytic anemias and the presence of spherocytosis. The pathophysiologic process of these anemias starts with oxidative injury to hemoglobin. As a result, RBC inclusions (Heinz bodies) of variable size and usually eccentric location adhere to the RBC membrane. Smooth movement of the membrane over the cytosol is reduced. These RBCs are selectively blocked from leaving the splenic cords and entering the sinuses. Splenic macrophages attack these RBCs and cause hemolysis. This process can be severe enough to cause intravascular destruction as well, producing hemoglobinemia and hemoglobinuria. Most often the clinical picture includes normocytic anemia in association with splenomegaly.

Agents that commonly induce oxidation of hemoglobin include nitrofurantoin, salicylic acid, acetaminophen, phenazopyridine, phenacetin, dapsone, and other sulphones. Diets high in pickled or smoked foods, consumption of nitrates, recreational drugs, mothballs, and industrial chemicals can also oxidize hemoglobin.

For Heinz body detection, fresh blood is incubated with a supravital stain (such as methyl violet or Nile blue) and examined by microscopy for presence of stained inclusions close to the RBC membrane (Heinz bodies). These RBC granules can be quantified by several different methods but are most commonly counted on microscopy. It is important not to confuse Heinz bodies with other RBC granules, such as Howell Jolly bodies.

PROCEDURE AND PATIENT CARE

Before
- Explain the procedure to the patient.
- Inform the patient that no fasting is required.

During
- Collect a venous blood sample in a lavender-top tube (ethylenediamine tetra-acetic acid [EDTA]), pink-top tube (EDTA salts), or green-top tube (sodium or lithium heparin).

After

- Apply pressure or a pressure dressing to the venipuncture site.
- Assess the venipuncture site for bleeding.

TEST RESULTS AND CLINICAL SIGNIFICANCE

▲ Increased Titre Levels

Unstable hemoglobinopathies (e.g., Hb Gun Hill),
Red cell enzymopathies (e.g., G6PD),
Thalassemia,
Heinz body hemolytic anemia: *These hemolytic anemias are highlighted by the presence of Heinz bodies in RBCs.*

RELATED TESTS

Red Blood Cell Count (p. 452). RBC count is used to identify hemolytic anemia that may be highlighted by Heinz bodies.

Haptoglobin (p. 289). The serum haptoglobin test is used to detect intravascular hemolysis of RBCs.

Helicobacter pylori Antibodies Test (*Campylobacter pylori*, Anti–*Helicobacter pylori* IgG Antibody, *Campylobacter*-Like Organism [CLO] Test, Rapid Urease Test, *H. pylori* Stool Test)

NORMAL FINDINGS

No antibodies present

INDICATIONS

This test is used to detect *Helicobacter pylori* infections. It is indicated in patients who have recurrent or chronic gastric or duodenal ulceration or inflammation. When the *H. pylori* infection is successfully eradicated, the ulcer or inflammation usually heals.

TEST EXPLANATION

H. pylori, a bacterium that can be found in the mucus overlying the gastric mucosa and in the mucosa itself (cells that line the stomach), is a risk factor for gastric and duodenal ulcers, chronic gastritis, or even ulcerative esophagitis. This Gram-negative bacillus is also a class I gastric carcinogen. Gastric colonization by this organism has been reported in approximately 90% to 95% of patients with a duodenal ulcer, in 60% to 70% of patients with a gastric ulcer, and in approximately 20% to 25% of patients with gastric cancer.

Approximately 10% of healthy persons younger than 30 years have gastric colonization with *H. pylori*. The incidence of gastric colonization increases with age; among people older than 60 years, the rates are percentages similar to their ages. Most patients with gastric colonization by *H. pylori* remain asymptomatic and never develop ulceration.

TABLE 2-28   Tests Commonly Used to Detect *Helicobacter pylori* Infection

Test	Advantages
Invasive (Specimen Obtained by Endoscopy)	
Culture	Can determine antibody sensitivity
Urease	Quick and simple
Noninvasive	
Serology	Convenient and inexpensive
Carbon-13 urea breath	Safer and less expensive than endoscopy

Several methods are used to detect the presence of this organism (Table 2-28). The organism can be cultured from a specimen of mucus obtained through a gastroscope (see p. 636). The specimen is plated on an enriched medium such as chocolate or Skirrow medium and incubated for 5 to 7 days at 37°C. The organism can also be detected in a gastric mucosal biopsy sample (from the antrum and greater curvature of the corpus). The organisms can be identified when the tissue is specially stained (e.g., Giemsa or Warthin-Starry). This method yields slightly more accurate results than does the culture technique and is therefore considered the criterion standard for detecting *H. pylori*.

It often takes several weeks before the results are available from cultures. For a patient with symptomatic or active ulcer disease, it is preferable to start treatment before that time. For that reason, rapid urease testing for *H. pylori* has been developed. *H. pylori* is capable of breaking down high quantities of urea because of its capability to produce great amounts of urease, an enzyme that can be found in the lining of the stomach of infected patients. In one such test (the *Campylobacter*-like organism [CLO] test), a small piece of gastric mucosa (obtained through gastroscopy) is inserted into testing gel. Within a few hours, if *H. pylori* organisms are present in the gastric mucosa, the urease (made by the *H. pylori*) turns the gel orange or red. If the colour change does not occur, *H. pylori* is not present. Another rapid urease test involves the use of specially prepared paper on which the gastric mucosa specimen is laid. If *H. pylori* organisms are present, the paper changes colour. A third rapid urease test entails the use of a specially prepared tablet that is dissolved in a small test tube. When the gastric mucosa of an infected patient is added, the solution changes colour. These tests are nearly 95% accurate.

Although *H. pylori* does not survive in the stool, an enzyme-linked immunosorbent assay (ELISA) with a polyclonal anti–*H. pylori* capture antibody can detect the presence of *H. pylori* antigen in a fresh stool specimen. A breath test is also available for the detection of *H. pylori*.

Serologic testing is the most common noninvasive method of diagnosing *H. pylori* infection. It is the easiest test to perform, and no preparation or abstinence from antacids is required. Immunoassays of antibodies to *H. pylori* have been developed and are very accurate in detecting the presence of the organism. The immunoglobulin G (IgG) anti–*H. pylori* antibody test is most commonly used immunoassay. IgG levels become elevated 2 months after infection and stay elevated for more than a year after treatment. Levels of the immunoglobulin A (IgA) anti–*H. pylori* antibody, like the IgG antibody, become elevated 2 months after infection but decrease 3 to 4 weeks after treatment. Levels of the immunoglobulin M (IgM) anti–*H. pylori* antibody are the first to become elevated (~3 to 4 weeks after infection), but this antibody is not detected 2 to 3 months after treatment. Such antibody titres are fast becoming the standard criterion for *H. pylori* detection.

The laboratory methods most commonly performed for immunotesting include ELISA and immunochromatography. Accuracy exceeds 85% with these methods. The antibodies can be detected with a small amount of blood obtained by fingerstick. Serologic testing is often used several months after treatment to document cure of *H. pylori* infection. Serologic testing is also used to corroborate the findings of other *H. pylori* testing methods.

INTERFERING FACTORS

- *H. pylori* can be transmitted by contaminated endoscopic equipment during endoscopic procedures.
- Rapid urease tests can yield false-negative results if the patient uses antacid therapy within the week before the test.

PROCEDURE AND PATIENT CARE

Before

- Explain the procedure to the patient.
- Inform the patient that no fasting is required for the blood test.
- If a biopsy or culture specimen is to be obtained by endoscopy, see discussion of esophagogastroduodenoscopy on p. 636.
- If culture is to be performed, ensure the patient has not had any antibiotic, antacid, or bismuth treatment for 5 to 14 days before the endoscopy.

During

- Collect a venous blood sample according to the protocol of the laboratory performing the test.
- A gastric or duodenal biopsy or specimen of mucus can be obtained by endoscopy. Keep the specimen moist by the addition of 2 to 5 mL of sterile saline solution or other wetting agent as required by the laboratory. Place in a sterile container.
- Transport time for culture specimens must be minimized.

After

- Apply pressure or a pressure dressing to the venipuncture site.
- Assess the venipuncture site for bleeding.
- If endoscopy was used to obtain a culture, see procedure for esophagogastroduodenoscopy (p. 636). The specimen should be transported to the laboratory within 30 minutes after collection.

TEST RESULTS AND CLINICAL SIGNIFICANCE

▲ Increased Levels

Acute and chronic gastritis,
Recurrent duodenal ulcer,
Gastric ulcer,
Gastric carcinoma: *These illnesses are associated with the presence of* H. pylori *infection. Whether the infection is causative or contributive is not well known.*

RELATED TESTS

Gastrin (p. 263). This test is a measure of serum gastrin. This hormone stimulates gastric acid secretion. Oversecretion can cause recurrent peptic ulcers. The initial symptoms may be similar to those of chronic *H. pylori* infection.

Urea Breath Test (p. 1172). This is a breath test used to diagnose *H. pylori* infection.

Esophagogastroduodenoscopy (p. 636). This endoscopic procedure is used to directly biopsy the gastric mucosa for definitive *H. pylori* identification.

Hematocrit (Hct, Packed Red Blood Cell Volume, Packed Cell Volume [PCV])

NORMAL FINDINGS

Adult male: 0.42–0.54 volume fraction (42%–54%)
Adult female: 0.37–0.47 volume fraction (37%–47%)
Pregnant female: >0.33 volume fraction (>33%)
Older adult: values may be slightly decreased.
Child/adolescent:

	Volume Fraction (%)	
	Male	Female
Newborn:	**0.37–0.47** (37%–47%)	**0.38–0.48** (38%–48%)
15–30 days:	**0.41–0.43** (41%–43%)	**0.34–0.42** (34%–42%)
61–180 days:	**0.31–0.38** (31%–38%)	**0.31–0.39** (31%–39%)
6 months to 2 years:	**0.31–0.36** (31%–36%)	**0.31–0.36** (31%–36%)
6–12 years:	**0.31–0.38** (31%–38%)	**0.32–0.39** (32%–39%)
12–18 years:	**0.31–0.41** (31%–41%)	**0.32–0.39** (32%–39%)

 Critical Values

<0.20 volume fraction (<20%) or **>0.60 volume fraction** (>60%)

 Age-Related Concerns

- Values in children are age specific; normal values vary throughout the first 18 years.
- Values are slightly decreased in older adults.

INDICATIONS

The hematocrit (Hct) is an indirect measurement of red blood cell (RBC) number and volume. It is used as a rapid measurement of RBC count. This measurement is repeated serially in patients with ongoing bleeding or as a routine part of the complete blood cell count. It is an integral part of the evaluation of anemic patients.

TEST EXPLANATION

The Hct is the percentage of the total blood volume that is represented by RBCs. The height of the RBC column is measured after centrifugation. It is compared with the height of the column of the total whole blood. The ratio of the height of the RBC column to that of the original total blood column is multiplied by 100%. This is the Hct value. It is routinely measured as part of a complete

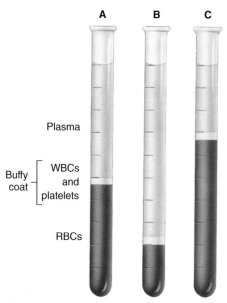

A B C

Plasma

Buffy coat — WBCs and platelets

RBCs

Figure 2-19 Drawing of tubes showing hematocrit levels of normal blood, blood with evidence of anemia, and blood with evidence of polycythemia. Note the buffy coat, located between the packed red blood cells (RBCs) and the plasma. **A,** A normal percentage of RBCs. **B,** Anemia (low percentage of RBCs). **C,** Polycythemia (high percentage of RBCs).

blood cell count. The Hct closely reflects the hemoglobin and RBC values. The Hct in percentage points usually is approximately three times the hemoglobin concentration in grams per decilitre when RBCs are of normal size and contain normal amounts of hemoglobin.

Normal values vary according to gender and age. Women tend to have lower values than men, and Hct values tend to decrease with age. Abnormal values indicate the same pathologic states as do abnormal RBC counts and abnormal hemoglobin concentrations. Decreased levels indicate anemia (reduced number of RBCs). Increased levels can indicate erythrocytosis (Figure 2-19).

Like other RBC values, the Hct can be altered by many factors other than RBC production. For instance, in dehydrated patients, the total blood volume is contracted. The RBCs make up a greater proportion of the total blood volume, and the Hct measurement is therefore artificially high. Likewise, if the RBC is morphologically increased in size, the RBCs constitute a greater proportion of the total blood volume, and Hct is, again, artificially high.

The Hct can be measured in a capillary tube (by skin puncture) by placing the blood in the tube, which is then spun in a microcentrifuge. The percentage of the RBC portion of the column to the whole column is the Hct. This value is most often calculated by automated cell counting machines.

Decisions concerning the need for blood transfusion are usually based on the hemoglobin or the Hct level. In an otherwise healthy person, transfusion is not considered as long as the hemoglobin level exceeds **80 mmol/L** (8 g/dL) or the Hct level exceeds **0.24 volume fraction** (24%). In younger people who can safely and significantly increase their cardiac output, a Hct level of 18% may be acceptable. In an older individual with an already compromised oxygen-carrying capacity (caused by cardiopulmonary diseases), transfusion may be recommended when the Hct level is below 0.30 volume fraction or (30%).

INTERFERING FACTORS

- Abnormalities in RBC size may alter Hct values. Larger RBCs are associated with higher Hct levels because the larger RBCs constitute a greater percentage of the total blood volume.
- Extremely elevated white blood cell (WBC) counts decrease Hct level, which would falsely indicate anemia.
- Hemodilution and dehydration may affect the Hct level (see previous discussion).
- Pregnancy usually causes a slight decrease in Hct values because of chronic hemodilution.
- Living at high altitudes causes increases in Hct values as a result of a physiologic response to the decreased oxygen available.
- Hct values may not be reliable immediately after hemorrhage because the percentage of total blood volume composed of RBCs has not changed. Not until the total blood volume is replaced with fluids does the Hct level decrease.
- Drugs that may cause *decreases* in Hct levels include chloramphenicol and penicillin.

Clinical Priorities

- Normal Hct values vary according to gender and age.
- Pregnancy usually causes slight decreases in Hct values because of chronic hemodilution.
- The Hct (in percentage points) is usually three times the hemoglobin concentration (in grams per decilitre) when RBCs are of normal size and contain normal amounts of hemoglobin.
- In dehydration, the Hct value is artificially elevated. In overhydration, the value is decreased.

PROCEDURE AND PATIENT CARE

Before
- Explain the procedure to the patient.
- Inform the patient that no fasting is required.

During
- Collect a venous blood sample in a lavender-top tube; only 0.5 mL is required when capillary tubes are used.
- Avoid hemolysis.

After
- Apply pressure or a pressure dressing to the venipuncture site.
- Assess the venipuncture site for bleeding.

TEST RESULTS AND CLINICAL SIGNIFICANCE

▲ Increased Levels

Erythrocytosis: *The number of RBCs is increased. This can result from illnesses or as a physiologic response to external situations.*

Congenital heart disease: *Cyanotic heart diseases cause the partial pressure of oxygen (P_{O_2}) to be chronically low. In response, the RBCs increase in number. Therefore, the Hct increases.*

Polycythemia vera: *This is a result of the bone marrow's inappropriately producing great numbers of RBCs, which cause the Hct to increase.*

Severe dehydration (e.g., severe diarrhea, burns): *With depletion of extracellular fluid, the total blood volume decreases, but the number of RBCs stays the same. Therefore, the percentage of total blood volume that is taken up by the RBCs increases, and the Hct increases.*

Severe chronic obstructive pulmonary disease (COPD): *Chronic states of hypoxia cause stimulation of RBC production as a physiologic response to increased oxygen-carrying capacity. Therefore, the Hct increases.*

▼ Decreased Levels

Anemia: *This is the state in which RBC numbers are reduced. Because the Hct is an indirect reflection of RBC numbers, the Hct is also reduced. Many different types of diseases are associated with anemia.*

Hemoglobinopathy: *Patients with hemoglobin disorders or other blood dyscrasias have a reduced number and survival rate of RBCs. Therefore, the Hct is decreased.*

Cirrhosis: *This is a chronic state of fluid overload. The RBCs are diluted and constitute a smaller percentage of the total blood volume. Therefore, the Hct decreases.*

Hemolytic anemia (e.g., erythroblastosis fetalis, hemoglobinopathies, drug-induced hemolytic anemias, paroxysmal nocturnal hemoglobinuria): *The RBC survival rate is diminished in hemolytic anemia. The number of RBCs decreases; therefore, the Hct is decreased.*

Hemorrhage: *With active bleeding, the number of RBCs decreases; therefore, the Hct is decreased. It takes time (several hours), however, for the Hct to fall. Only when the blood volume is replenished with fluid does the Hct diminish.*

Dietary deficiency: *With certain vitamin or mineral deficiencies (e.g., iron), the RBC number or size is decreased. Therefore, the Hct is decreased.*

Bone marrow failure: *With reduced synthesis of the RBCs, the Hct decreases.*

Prosthetic valves: *The prosthetic valve causes mechanical trauma to the RBCs. RBC survival is diminished; therefore, RBC numbers diminish, and Hct decreases.*

Renal disease: *Erythropoietin is made in the kidneys and is a strong stimulant of RBC production. With a reduced level of erythropoietin, the RBC numbers diminish, and the Hct is decreased.*

Normal pregnancy: *In pregnancy, blood volume is normally increased because pregnant women are in a chronic state of overhydration. When pregnancy is combined with a relative "malnourished" state, the Hct is diminished by a decrease in the number of RBCs and in the percentage of total blood volume they constitute.*

Rheumatoid/collagen-vascular diseases (e.g., rheumatoid arthritis, lupus): *Chronic illnesses are associated with a reduced production of RBCs. Therefore, the Hct is decreased.*

Lymphoma,

Multiple myeloma,

Leukemia,

Hodgkin disease: *Hematologic cancers are often associated with bone marrow failure of RBC production. The number of RBCs diminishes, and the Hct decreases.*

RELATED TESTS

Hemoglobin (see following test p. 299). This is a measurement of the concentration of hemoglobin in the blood. It is closely associated with the RBC count and Hct value.

Red Blood Cell Count (p. 452). This is a measurement of the number of RBCs per cubic millimetre of blood. It is closely associated with the hemoglobin and Hct values.

Red Blood Cell Indices (p. 456). These indices are data about the size and hemoglobin content of the RBC.

Hemoglobin (Hb)

NORMAL FINDINGS

Adult male: **140–180 g/L** (14–18 g/dL)
Adult female: **120–160 g/L** (12–16 g/dL)
Pregnant female: **>110 g/L** (>11 g/dL)
Older adult: Values are slightly decreased.
Child/adolescent:
   Neonate (0-28 days): **140–240 g/L** (14–24 g/dL)
   Newborn (1–2 months): **120–200 g/L** (12–20 g/dL)
   2–6 months: **100–170 g/L** (10–17 g/dL)
   6 months to 1 year: **95–140 g/L** (9.5–14 g/dL)
   1–6 years: **95–140 g/L** (9.5–14 g/dL)
   6–18 years: **100–150 g/L** (10–15.5 g/dL)

Critical Values

<50 g/L (<5g/dL) or >200 g/L (>20 g/dL)

Age-Related Concerns

- Values in children are age specific; normal values vary throughout the first 18 years.
- Values are slightly decreased in older adults.

INDICATIONS

This test is a measure of the total amount of hemoglobin in the blood. It is used as a rapid indirect measurement of the red blood cell (RBC) count. It is repeated serially in patients with ongoing bleeding or as a routine part of the complete blood cell count (CBC). It is an integral part of the evaluation of anemic patients.

TEST EXPLANATION

The hemoglobin concentration is a measure of the total amount of hemoglobin in the peripheral blood. The test is normally performed as part of a CBC. Hemoglobin serves as a vehicle for oxygen and carbon dioxide transport. The oxygen-carrying capacity of the blood is determined by the hemoglobin concentration. Hemoglobin also acts as an important acid-base buffer system.

   As with the RBC count, normal values vary according to gender and age. Women tend to have lower values than do men, and hemoglobin values tend to decrease with age. The hemoglobin closely reflects the hematocrit and RBC values. The hematocrit in percentage points usually is approximately three times the hemoglobin concentration in grams per decilitre when RBCs are of normal size and contain normal amounts of hemoglobin.

Abnormal values indicate the same pathologic states as do abnormal RBC counts and abnormal hematocrit concentrations. Decreased levels indicate anemia (reduced number of RBCs). Increased levels can indicate erythrocytosis. In addition, however, changes in plasma volume are more accurately reflected by the hemoglobin concentration. Dilutional overhydration decreases the concentration, whereas dehydration tends to cause an artificially high value. Slight decreases in the values of hemoglobin and hematocrit during pregnancy reflect the expanded blood volume because pregnant women are in a chronic state of overhydration; the number of cells is actually increased during pregnancy. Hemoglobin is usually measured by an automated cell counter. There is very little variability (2% to 3%) with most well-kept machines.

Hemoglobin is made up of heme (iron surrounded by protoporphyrin) and globin consisting of an alpha- and a beta-polypeptide chain. Abnormalities in the globin structure are called *hemoglobinopathies* (e.g., sickle cell disease, hemoglobin C disease). Some diseases are caused by abnormalities in globin chain synthesis (such as thalassemia). In these diseases, the RBC counts can be low, the RBC survival rate can be diminished, and the RBC-carrying capacity can be reduced.

Too little hemoglobin puts a strain on the cardiopulmonary system to maintain good oxygen-carrying capacity. With critically low hemoglobin levels, affected patients are at great risk for angina, heart attack, heart failure, and stroke. When hemoglobin levels are too high because of increased numbers of RBCs, intravascular sludging occurs, leading to stroke and other organ infarction. Decisions concerning the need for blood transfusion are usually based on the hemoglobin or the hematocrit. In an otherwise healthy person, transfusion is not considered as long as the hemoglobin level exceeds **80 g/L (8 g/dL)** or the hematocrit level exceeds **0.24 volume fraction (24%)**. In younger people who can safely and significantly increase their cardiac output, a hemoglobin level of **60 g/L (6 g/dL)** may be acceptable. In an older adult with an already compromised oxygen-carrying capacity (cardiopulmonary diseases), transfusion may be recommended when the hemoglobin level is below **10 g/L (1g/dL)**.

INTERFERING FACTORS

- Slight hemoglobin decreases normally occur during pregnancy because of the dilution effect of the expanded blood volume.
- There is a slight diurnal variation in hemoglobin levels.
- Hemoglobin levels are highest at approximately 8 AM and are lowest at approximately 8 PM. The range may vary as much as **10 g/L (1 g/dL)**.
- Heavy smokers have higher hemoglobin levels than do nonsmokers.
- Living in high altitudes causes increased hemoglobin values as a result of a physiologic response to the decreased oxygen available at these high altitudes.

 Drugs that may cause *increases* in hemoglobin levels include gentamicin and methyldopa.

Drugs that may cause *decreases* in hemoglobin levels include antibiotics, antineoplastic drugs, aspirin, indomethacin (Indocid), rifampin, and sulphonamides.

✔ Clinical Priorities

- Dilutional overhydration decreases the hemoglobin concentration. Dehydration tends to cause an artificially high value.
- The hematocrit (in percentage points) is usually three times the hemoglobin concentration (in grams per decilitre) when RBCs are of normal size and contain a normal amount of hemoglobin.
- Living at high altitudes causes increased hemoglobin values as a result of a physiologic response to decreased oxygen levels.

PROCEDURE AND PATIENT CARE

Before
- Explain the procedure to the patient.
- Inform the patient that no fasting is required.

During
- Collect a venous blood sample in a lavender-top tube.
- Avoid hemolysis.
- On the laboratory slip, note whether the patient is taking any drugs that may affect test results.

After
- Apply pressure or a pressure dressing to the venipuncture site.
- Observe the venipuncture site for bleeding.

TEST RESULTS AND CLINICAL SIGNIFICANCE

▲ Increased Levels

Erythrocytosis: *The number of RBCs is increased as a result of illnesses or as a physiologic response to external situations (e.g., high altitude).*

Congenital heart disease: *Cyanotic heart diseases cause the partial pressure of oxygen (P_{O_2}) to be chronically low. In response, the RBCs increase in number. Therefore, the hemoglobin level increases.*

Severe chronic obstructive pulmonary disease: *Chronic states of hypoxia cause stimulation of RBC production as a physiologic response to increased oxygen-carrying capacity. Therefore, the hemoglobin level increases.*

Polycythemia vera: *This is a result of the bone marrow's inappropriately producing great numbers of RBCs. The hemoglobin increases accordingly.*

Severe dehydration (e.g., severe diarrhea, burns): *With depletion of extracellular fluid, the total blood volume decreases, but the number of RBCs stays the same. Therefore, the percentage of total blood volume that is composed of RBCs increases, and hemoglobin level increases.*

▼ Decreased Levels

Anemia: *This is a term given to the state associated with reduced RBC numbers. Because the hemoglobin is an indirect reflection of RBC numbers, the hemoglobin will also be reduced. Many different types of diseases are associated with anemia.*

Hemoglobinopathy: *Patients with hemoglobin disorders or other blood dyscrasias have reduced RBC number and RBC survival. Therefore the hemoglobin is decreased.*

Cirrhosis: *This is a chronic state of fluid overload. The RBCs are diluted and constitute a smaller percentage of the total blood volume. Therefore, the hemoglobin decreases.*

Hemolytic anemia (e.g., erythroblastosis fetalis, hemoglobinopathies, drug-induced hemolytic anemias, transfusion reactions, or paroxysmal nocturnal hemoglobinuria): *The RBC survival rate is diminished in hemolytic anemia. The number of RBCs decreases, and the hemoglobin decreases.*

Hemorrhage: *With active bleeding, the number of RBCs decreases and the hemoglobin level decreases. It takes time (several hours), however, for the hemoglobin level to fall. Only if the blood volume is replenished with fluid does the hemoglobin level diminish.*

Dietary deficiency: *With certain vitamin or mineral deficiencies (e.g., iron), the RBC number or size is decreased. Therefore, the hemoglobin level is decreased.*

Bone marrow failure: *With reduced synthesis of the RBCs, the hemoglobin level decreases.*

Prosthetic valves: *The prosthetic valve causes mechanical trauma to the RBCs. RBC survival rate is diminished. RBC numbers diminish, and hemoglobin level decreases.*

Renal disease: *Erythropoietin is made in the kidneys and is a strong stimulant of RBC production. With a reduced level of erythropoietin, the RBC numbers diminish, and the hemoglobin level is decreased.*

Normal pregnancy: *In pregnancy, blood volume is normally increased because pregnant women are in a chronic state of overhydration. When pregnancy is combined with a relative "malnourished" state, the hemoglobin level is diminished by a decrease in the number of RBCs and in the percentage of total blood volume they constitute.*

Rheumatoid/collagen-vascular diseases (e.g., rheumatoid arthritis, lupus, sarcoidosis): *Chronic illnesses are associated with reduced production of RBCs. Therefore, the hemoglobin level is decreased.*

Lymphoma,

Multiple myeloma,

Neoplasia,

Leukemia,

Hodgkin disease: *Hematologic cancers are often associated with bone marrow failure of RBC production. The number of RBCs diminishes, and the hemoglobin level decreases.*

Splenomegaly: *When a functioning spleen is enlarged, RBCs are sequestered and eliminated from the functioning vascular system.*

RELATED TESTS

Hematocrit (p. 295). This is the percentage of the total blood volume represented by the RBCs. It is closely associated with hemoglobin values and RBC count.

Red Blood Cell Count (p. 452). This is a measurement of the number of RBCs per cubic millimetre of blood. It is closely associated with hemoglobin and hematocrit values.

Red Blood Cell Indices (p. 456). These indices are data about the size and hemoglobin content of the RBC.

Hemoglobin Electrophoresis (Hb Electrophoresis)

NORMAL FINDINGS

Adult/older adult: percentage of total hemoglobin
  Hemoglobin A_1 (HbA$_1$): 95%–98%
  Hemoglobin A_2 (HbA$_2$): 2%–3%
  Fetal hemoglobin (HbF): 0.8%–2%
  Sickle cell hemoglobin (HbS): 0%
  Hemoglobin C (HbC): 0%
Child (HbF):
  Newborn (HbF): 50%–80%
  <6 months: <8%
  >6 months: 1%–2%

INDICATIONS

Hemoglobin electrophoresis is a test with which abnormal forms of hemoglobin (hemoglobinopathies) can be detected and quantified. This test is used to diagnose such conditions as sickle cell disease and thalassemia.

TEST EXPLANATION

Although many different hemoglobin variations have been described, the most common types are A_1, A_2, F, S, and C. Each major hemoglobin type is electrically charged to varying degrees. When the hemoglobin from lysed red blood cells (RBCs) is placed on electrophoresis paper in an electromagnetic field, the hemoglobin variants migrate at different rates and therefore spread apart from each other. The migration of the various forms of hemoglobin makes up a series of bands on the paper. The bands therefore correspond to the various forms of hemoglobin present. The pattern of bands is compared with normal and with well-known abnormal patterns. A diagnosis can then be made. Each band can be quantitated as a percentage of the total hemoglobin, which indicates the severity of any recognized abnormality.

The form HbA_1 constitutes the major component of hemoglobin in the normal RBC. HbA_2 is only a minor component (2% to 3%) of the normal hemoglobin total. HbF is the major hemoglobin component in the fetus but usually exists in only minimal quantities in the normal adult. Levels of HbF greater than 2% in patients older than 3 years are considered abnormal. HbF is able to transport oxygen when only small amounts of oxygen are available (as in fetal life). In patients requiring compensation for prolonged chronic hypoxia (as in congenital cardiac abnormalities), HbF may be found in increased levels to assist in the transport of the available oxygen.

HbS and HbC are abnormal forms of hemoglobin that occur predominantly in Black Canadians. Hemoglobin E occurs predominantly in people of Southeast Asian descent. HbS is associated with sickle cell disease and is a relatively insoluble variant. When little oxygen is available, it assumes a crescent (sickle) shape that greatly distorts the RBC structure. Vascular sludging is a consequence of the localized sickling and may lead to organ infarction. The duration of survival of sickled RBCs is diminished, and affected patients also have anemia. RBCs containing HbC have a decreased life span and are more readily lysed than normal RBCs. Mild to severe hemolytic anemia may result. The hemoglobin content of some common disorders affecting hemoglobin, as determined by electrophoresis, is listed in Table 2-29.

In some laboratories, high-performance liquid chromatography (HPLC) is used to identify and quantify hemoglobins. In HPLC, blood is passed through a filtered column under increased pressures, which results in separation of hemoglobins on the basis of chemical/physical characteristics. In some laboratories, HPLC is a simpler process than is electrophoresis.

TABLE 2-29	Hemoglobin Content of Some Common Disorders Affecting Hemoglobin					
Disorder	**HbA**	**HbA$_2$**	**HbF**	**HbS**	**HbH**	**HbC**
Sickle cell disease	0%	2%–3%	2%	95%–98%	0%	0%
Sickle cell trait	50%–65%	2%–3%	2%	35%–45%	0%	0%
Hemoglobin C disease	0%	2%–3%	2%	0%	0%	90%–100%
Third-generation alpha-thalassemia	65%–90%	2%–3%	0%	0%	5%–30%	0%
Beta-thalassemia major	0%	0%–15%	85%–100%	0%	0%	0%
Beta-thalassemia trait	50%–85%	4%–8%	1%–5%	0%	0%	0%

Hb, Hemoglobin.

INTERFERING FACTORS
- Blood transfusions within the previous 12 weeks may alter test results.

PROCEDURE AND PATIENT CARE
Before
- Explain the procedure to the patient.
- Inform the patient that no fasting is required.

During
- Collect a venous blood sample in a lavender-top tube.

After
- Apply pressure or a pressure dressing to the venipuncture site.
- Assess the venipuncture site for bleeding.

TEST RESULTS AND CLINICAL SIGNIFICANCE
▲ Increased Levels
Sickle cell disease,
Hemoglobin H disease,
Thalassemia major,
Sickle cell trait,
Thalassemia minor,
Hemoglobin C trait or disease,
Hemoglobin E trait or disease: *These hemoglobinopathies produce a specific hemoglobin electrophoresis pattern that is diagnostic for the respective disease.*

RELATED TEST
Hemoglobin (p. 299): This is a direct measurement of the hemoglobin that exists in the "average" RBC.

Hepatitis Virus Studies (Hepatitis-Associated Antigen [HAA], Australian Antigen)

NORMAL FINDINGS
Negative

INDICATIONS
This group of tests is used to diagnose and to identify the serologic type and a patient's current hepatitis status. It is important to diagnose and identify the type of hepatitis as soon as possible so that the patient can be immediately treated and appropriately isolated.

TEST EXPLANATION

Hepatitis is an inflammation of the liver caused by viruses, alcohol ingestion, drugs, toxins, or overwhelming bacterial sepsis. The three common viruses now recognized to cause disease are hepatitis A, hepatitis B, and hepatitis C (non-A/non-B) viruses. Hepatitis D and E viruses are much less common in Canada. Hepatitis D can infect the liver only by entering into a hepatitis B virus, which it uses as a carrying vehicle. Therefore, hepatitis D cannot cause disease unless patients have hepatitis B virus in their bloodstream in the active, chronic, or carrier forms. The various types of hepatitis cannot be differentiated on the basis of their clinical manifestation. The clinical manifestations are similar in that they all include low-grade fever, malaise, anorexia, and fatigue. They are most often associated with elevations of hepatocellular enzymes such as aspartate aminotransferase, alanine aminotransferase, and lactate dehydrogenase.

Disease caused by *hepatitis A virus* (HAV) was originally called *infectious hepatitis.* It has a short incubation period of 2 to 6 weeks and is highly contagious. During active infection, HAV is excreted in the stool and transmitted via oral-fecal contamination of food and drink. Most infections are not associated with symptoms severe enough to warrant medical evaluation. Immunoglobulins G and M (IgG and IgM) antibodies to HAV are routinely evaluated when HAV infection is suspected.

The first type of antibody to HAV is IgM antibody (HAV-Ab/IgM), which appears approximately 3 to 4 weeks after exposure or just before hepatocellular enzyme levels become elevated. These IgM levels usually return to normal in approximately 8 weeks. The second type of antibody to HAV is IgG (HAV-Ab/IgG), which appears approximately 2 weeks after the IgM level begins to increase, and it slowly returns to normal levels. The IgG antibody can remain detectable for more than 10 years after the infection. If the IgM antibody level is elevated in the absence of the IgG antibody, acute hepatitis is suspected. If, however, IgG antibody level is elevated in the absence of IgM elevation, a convalescent or chronic stage of HAV viral infection is indicated.

These antibodies may not be detectable soon after infection occurs, which can delay the investigation of the infectious outbreaks. The HAV virion can be detected directly by measuring HAV RNA in the sera of patients in whom acute infection is suspected.

Hepatitis B virus (HBV) is commonly known as *serum hepatitis.* It has a long incubation period (5 weeks to 6 months). HBV is most frequently transmitted by blood transfusion; however, it also can be contracted through exposure to other body fluids. HBV may cause a severe and unrelenting form of hepatitis that culminates in liver failure and death. The incidence is increased among blood transfusion recipients, homosexual men, patients receiving dialysis, transplant recipients, intravenous drug abusers, and patients with leukemia or lymphoma. Hospital personnel are also at increased risk for infection, mostly as a result of needlestick contamination.

HBV, also called the *Dane particle,* is made up of an inner core surrounded by an outer capsule. The outer capsule contains the *hepatitis B surface antigen* (HBsAg), formerly called *Australian antigen.* The inner core contains HBV core antigen (HBcAg). The hepatitis B e-antigen (HBeAg) is also found within the core. Antibodies to these antigens are called HBsAb, HBcAb, and HBeAb, respectively. The tests used to detect these antigens and antibodies (Table 2-30) are characterized as follows:

1. *Hepatitis B surface antigen* (HBsAg): This is the most frequently and easily performed test for hepatitis B, and it is the first test to yield abnormal results. HBsAg levels rise before the onset of clinical symptoms, peak during the first week of symptoms, and return to normal by the time jaundice subsides. The presence of HBsAg generally indicates active infection by HBV. If the level of this antigen persists in the blood, the patient is considered to be a carrier.
2. *Hepatitis B surface antibody* (HBsAb): This antibody appears approximately 4 weeks after the disappearance of the surface antigen and signifies the end of the acute infection phase. The

TABLE 2-30   Hepatitis Testing

Serologic Findings	Appearance After Infection	Disappearance After Disease	Application
HAV-Ab/IgM	4–6 wk	3–4 mo	Acute HAV infection
HAV-Ab/IgG	8–12 wk	10 yr	Previous HAV exposure/immunity
HBeAg	1–3 wk	6–8 wk	Acute HBV infection
HBeAb	4–6 wk	4–6 yr	Acute HBV infection ended
HBsAg	4–12 wk	1–3 mo	Acute HBV infection
HBsAb total	3–10 mo	6–10 yr	Previous HBV infection/immunity indicated
HBVcAb/IgM	2–12 wk	3–6 mo	Acute HBV infection
HBVcAb total	3–12 wk	Life	Previous HBV infection/convalescent stage
HCV-Ab/IgG	3–4 mo	2 yr	Previous HCV infection
HDV-Ag	1–3 days	3–5 days	Acute HDV infection
HDV-Ab/IgM	10 days	1–3 mo	Acute HDV infection
HDV-Ab total	2–3 mo	7–14 mo	Chronic HDV infection

Ab, Antibody; *Ag,* antigen; *cAB,* core antibody; *cAg,* core antigen; *eAb,* e-antibody; *e-Ag,* e-antigen; *HAV, HBV, HCV,* and *HDV,* hepatitis A, B, C, and D viruses; *IgG* and *IgM,* immunoglobulins G and M; *sAb,* surface antibody; *sAg,* surface antigen.

presence of HBsAb also signifies immunity to subsequent infection. Concentrated forms of this agent constitute the hyperimmune globulin given to patients who have come in contact with HBV-infected patients (e.g., contact by an inadvertent needlestick from a needle previously used on a patient with HBV infection). HBsAb is the antibody that denotes immunity after administration of hepatitis B vaccine.

3. *Hepatitis B core antigen* (HBcAg): No tests are currently available to detect this antigen.
4. *Hepatitis B core antibody* (HBcAb): This antibody appears approximately 1 month after infection with HBsAg, and its levels decline (although they remain elevated) over several years. HBcAb is also present in patients with chronic hepatitis. The HBcAb level is elevated during the time lag between the disappearance of HBsAg and the appearance of HBsAb. This interval is called the "core window." During the core window, HBcAb is the only detectable marker of a recent hepatitis infection.
5. *Hepatitis B e-antigen* (HBeAg): This antigen generally is not used for diagnostic purposes but rather as an index of infectivity. The presence of HBeAg is correlated with early and active disease, as well as with high infectivity in acute HBV infection. The persistent presence of HBeAg in the blood is predictive of the development of chronic HBV infection.
6. *Hepatitis B e-antibody* (HBeAb): This antibody indicates that an acute phase of HBV infection is almost or completely over and that the chance of infectivity is greatly reduced.

Hepatitis B DNA can be quantified by reverse-transcriptase polymerase chain reaction (RT-PCR) methods and is a direct measurement of the HBV viral load. A one- or two-log decrease in viral load means an antiviral therapy is working. A one- or two-log increase means an antiviral has stopped working and that viral resistance may have developed. High levels of HBV-DNA, ranging from 100 000 to more than 1 billion viral copies per millilitre, indicate a high rate of HBV replication. Low or undetectable levels, approximately 300 copies per millilitre or less, indicate an "inactive" infection. The World Health Organization established the international unit or copies per millilitre, written as "IU/mL" or "copies/mL," to measure HBV DNA. Detection of HBV DNA serves as an important finding that supplements serologic tests in a number of clinical settings. It is helpful in the early detection of HBV infection, in monitoring of disease, and in determining low levels of viremia in patients with nonreplicative HBV disease and chronic hepatitis. Because the intent of treatment is to eliminate HBV, accurate measurement of low viral load is very important.

HCV is transmitted in a manner similar to HBV. Most cases of hepatitis are caused by blood transfusion. HCV is found in as many as 8% of blood donors worldwide. The incubation period is 2 to 12 weeks after exposure. The clinical manifestations of the illness parallel those of HBV. However, unlike HBV infection, HCV infection is chronic in more than 60% of cases. Although the disease course is variable, it is slowly progressive. Twenty percent of patients with HCV infection develop cirrhosis and hepatocellular cancers associated with this chronic infection.

The screening test for detecting HCV infection is the detection of anti-HCV antibodies to HCV recombinant core antigen, *NS3* gene, NS4 antigen, and NS5 antigen. The antibodies can be detected within 4 weeks of infection. With HCV RNA testing, the HCV virion can be directly detected and quantitated (viral load). Like HBV DNA testing, HCV RNA viral load is quantitated by using RT-PCR methods and is usually expressed as U/mL or copies per mL. Although a higher viral load may not necessarily be a sign of more severe or more advanced disease, it is correlated with likelihood of responding to treatment. HCV RNA tests can also be used to monitor response to hepatitis C treatment.

HDV is known to cause *delta hepatitis.* As stated earlier, the HDV must enter the HBV to gain access to the liver and be infective. The patient must have HBV in the blood from a past or synchronously occurring infection. In Canada, this is most commonly transmitted through tainted blood. The HDV antigen can be detected by immunoassay within a few days after infection. The IgM and total antibodies to HDV are also detected early in the disease. A persistent elevation in levels of these antibodies indicates a chronic or carrier state.

HEV is an etiologic virus of short incubation. No antigen or antibody tests are currently widely available and accurate for the serologic identification of this infecting agent.

PROCEDURE AND PATIENT CARE

Before
- Explain the procedure to the patient.
- Inform the patient that no fasting is required.

During
- Collect a venous blood sample in a red-top tube.
- Usually a hepatitis profile that includes several HBV antigens and antibodies is performed.

After
- Apply pressure or a pressure dressing to the venipuncture site.
- Assess the venipuncture site for bleeding.
- Handle the specimen as if it were capable of transmitting hepatitis.
- Immediately discard the needle in the appropriate receptacle.
- Send the specimen to the laboratory promptly.
- Advise patients with suspected hepatitis that they should refrain from intimate contact with another person. Until the serologic results indicate otherwise, the patients should be considered infective.

TEST RESULTS AND CLINICAL SIGNIFICANCE

▲ Increased Levels

Hepatitis A,
Hepatitis B,
Hepatitis C,
Hepatitis D,
Hepatitis E: *These viral forms of hepatitis can exist in an acute, chronic, carrier, or chronic active phase.*

RELATED TESTS

Aspartate Aminotransferase (p. 130), Alanine Aminotransferase (p. 45), and Lactate Dehydrogenase (p. 339). Levels of these hepatocellular enzymes are elevated during the acute phase and chronic active phase of hepatitis.

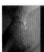

Hexosaminidase (Hexosaminidase A, Hex A, Total Hexosaminidase, Hexosaminidase A and B)

NORMAL FINDINGS

Hexosaminidase A: 7.5–9.8 U/L
Total hexosaminidase: 9.9–15.9 U/L
   Check with the laboratory because there is a wide variety of testing methods.

INDICATIONS

Hexosaminidase A testing is used to diagnose Tay-Sachs disease and to identify unaffected persons who may be carriers of this deadly genetic defect.

TEST EXPLANATION

Tay-Sachs disease is a lysosomal storage disease (GM_2 gangliosidosis) first characterized by loss of motor skills in infancy and early childhood. Death usually occurs by 4 to 8 years of age. Tay-Sachs disease is a result of a mutation in an autosomal recessive gene carried on chromosome 15. An affected person must inherit a defective gene from each parent to have Tay-Sachs disease. One per 25 Ashkenazi (Eastern European) Jews is a carrier for this genetic mutation. There are 80 different genetic mutations that inhibit the function of this important gene (p. 1139). This gene encodes the synthesis of an enzyme called *hexosaminidase*. Without this enzyme, lysosomes of GM_2 accumulate, particularly in the central nervous system.

   Two clinically important isoenzymes of hexosaminidase have been detected in the serum: hexosaminidase A (made up of one alpha subunit and one beta subunit) and hexosaminidase B (made up of two beta subunits). Any genetic mutation that affects the alpha unit causes a deficiency of hexosaminidase A, which results in Tay-Sachs disease. A mutation that affects the beta unit causes a deficiency in hexosaminidases A and B. Sandhoff disease, an uncommon variant of Tay-Sachs, occurs with deficiency of both of these enzymes. Other genetic mutations of this same gene can cause chronic GM_2-gangliosidosis, a disease similar to Tay-Sachs disease that becomes apparent later in life (adolescence).

Because Tay-Sachs disease is uniformly untreatable and fatal, a significant effort has gone into the development of biochemical testing to identify carriers of the genetic mutation (persons who carry one of the recessive defective genes). Hexosaminidase A levels have been found to be abnormally low in carriers, whereas hexosaminidase B levels are high. Therefore, testing for total hexosaminidase is not useful. A carrier has a 25% chance of having a child with Tay-Sachs disease if the other biologic parent is also a carrier. For such couples, pregnancy should occur only with thorough genetic counselling. In communities in which the Ashkenazi Jewish population is high, hexosaminidase A screening has been very effective in identifying carriers. Furthermore, hexosaminidase A is used to diagnose Tay-Sachs disease in infants and young children. Genetic testing (p. 1139) is useful for corroborating the identification of an affected person or a carrier.

If a couple at risk for producing offspring with Tay-Sachs disease chooses to proceed with pregnancy, amniocentesis (p. 660) can be performed. The amniotic fluid and/or cells obtained by chorionic villus sampling can be tested for hexosaminidase A. Cells obtained during amniocentesis can also be tested for the precise genetic mutation.

INTERFERING FACTORS
- Hemolysis of the blood sample can cause inaccurate test results.
- Pregnancy can cause markedly increased values. For this reason, blood tests are performed before, not during, pregnancy.
- Oral contraceptives can artificially increase levels.

PROCEDURE AND PATIENT CARE
Before
- Explain the procedure to the patient. Emphasize the importance of this test to Jewish couples of Eastern European ancestry who plan to have children. Explain that both biologic parents must carry the defective gene to transmit Tay-Sachs disease to their offspring.
- Professional genetic counselling should be provided to every person who considers undergoing this test.
- Patients should be made aware of the possible effects on their lives if hexosaminidase A levels are found to be reduced.
- Check with the laboratory with regard to withholding contraceptives.

During
- Collect a venous blood sample in a red-top tube. Avoid hemolysis.
- Note that pregnant women can be evaluated by amniocentesis (p. 660) or chorionic villus biopsy (p. 1134).
- Note that in infants, blood may be obtained by heelstick. For neonates, blood is often collected through the umbilical cord.

After
- If only one partner is a carrier, reassure the couple that their offspring cannot inherit Tay-Sachs disease.
- Arrange genetic counselling if both partners are carriers of Tay-Sachs disease and pregnancy is desired.

TEST RESULTS AND CLINICAL SIGNIFICANCE

▼ Decreased Hexosaminidase Level

Tay-Sachs disease: *The synthesis of hexosaminidase A is prevented by a genetic mutation in the gene encoded for production of the alpha unit of that enzyme. GM_2 gangliosides accumulate in neural tissue, causing neurologic and mental deterioration.*

▼ Decreased Hexosaminidase A and B Levels

Sandhoff disease: *The synthesis of hexosaminidases A and B is prevented by a genetic mutation in the gene that encodes for production of the beta unit of those enzymes. GM_2 gangliosides accumulate in neural tissue, causing neurologic and mental deterioration.*

RELATED TESTS

Genetic Testing (p. 1139). By testing for a mutation at the site of the gene known to be involved in Tay-Sachs disease, more definitive corroborative evidence of disease state and carrier status can be obtained.

Amniocentesis (p. 660). Through this technique, fetal cells and fluid can be obtained and tested for hexosaminidase A.

 HIV Serology (AIDS Serology, Acquired Immune Deficiency Serology, AIDS Screen, Human Immune Deficiency Virus [HIV] Antibody Test, Western Blot Test, p24 Antigen Capture Assay)

NORMAL FINDINGS

No evidence of human immunodeficiency virus (HIV) antigen or antibodies

INDICATIONS

These tests are used to detect HIV infection.

TEST EXPLANATION

There are two types of human immunodeficiency viruses: types 1 and 2. Type 1 is most prevalent in Canada, the United States, and Western Europe. Type 2 is limited mostly to Western African nations. Populations at high risk for acquired immune deficiency syndrome (AIDS) include sexually active homosexual men, bisexual men and women with multiple partners, intravenous drug abusers, persons receiving blood products containing HIV, and infants exposed to the virus during gestation and delivery.

Because of the medical and social significance of a positive result of the test for HIV antibody, test results must be accurate and their interpretation correct. Individuals can be said to have serologic evidence of HIV infection only after an enzyme immunoassay screening specimen is reactive and another test, such as the Western blot or immunofluorescence assay, validates the results. However, if a positive enzyme immunoassay result is not confirmed by the Western blot test or immunofluorescence, the overall result should not be considered negative. Repeated testing is required in 3 to 6 months. A person with positive HIV test results does not have AIDS until the patient develops the clinical features of diminished immune ability.

TABLE 2-31	Tests Used to Diagnose HIV Infection	
Test	**Detection**	**Indication**
ELISA (or enzyme immunoassay)	Antibodies to HIV	Screening test
Western blot	Antibodies to HIV	Confirmatory test after repeatedly reactive results of ELISA
Detuned ELISA	Antibodies to HIV	Used after Western blot to determine whether HIV infection is recent
p24 antigen capture assay	HIV-1 core protein	Used when Western blot is indeterminate
Oral mucosal transudate	Antibodies to HIV	Screening test
Urine test for HIV	Antibodies to HIV	Screening test
Home testing kits	Antibodies to HIV	Screening test
HIV viral load (see p. 314)	HIV RNA	Marker for diagnosis and progression of AIDS

AIDS, Acquired immune deficiency syndrome; *ELISA,* enzyme-linked immunosorbent assay; *HIV,* human immunodeficiency virus.

Enzyme immunoassay and enzyme-linked immunosorbent assay (ELISA) HIV serologic tests, which test for antibodies to HIV in serum or plasma, are the most widely used serologic tests for AIDS (Table 2-31). They are used for making a clinical diagnosis, screening donor blood and blood products, and testing individuals who believe they may be infected with HIV. Serologic tests detect antibodies to HIV. Because they do not detect viral antigens, they cannot detect infection in its earliest stage (before antibodies are formed). In a person who has been infected with HIV, seroconversion (positive findings of HIV antibodies) takes a period of time, usually within 2 to 12 weeks, but possibly as long as 6 months. This time is called the *window period.*

The sensitivity (i.e., probability that the test specimen will be reactive if it is truly positive) of the serologic tests are approximately 99% for blood from persons infected with HIV for 12 weeks or more. The probability of a false-negative result is remote except during the first few weeks after infection, before antibodies become detectable.

The specificity (probability that test specimen will be nonreactive if it is truly negative) of the serologic tests is approximately 99% for repeatedly nonreactive specimens or if potential exposure occurred more than 12 weeks earlier. False-positive results do occur but are rare. To increase the specificity of serologic tests further, a supplemental test (most often the Western blot test, immunofluorescent assay, or viral RNA test [p. 801]) is performed to validate repeatedly positive serologic test results.

The diagnostic tests described previously detect HIV infection on the basis of demonstration of antibodies to HIV. It has become possible to diagnose HIV infection by the direct detection of HIV RNA (see p. 310). The p24 antigen capture assay is an ELISA-type assay that detects the viral protein p24 in the peripheral blood of HIV-infected individuals, in which it exists either as a free antigen or complexed to anti-p24 antibodies. The p24 antigen may be detectable as early as 2 to 6 weeks after infection. The p24 antigen test can be used to assess the antiviral activity of anti-HIV therapies. The p24 antigen test can also be used to diagnose neonatal HIV infection, detect HIV infection before seroconversion, detect HIV in donor blood, and determine the progression of AIDS.

Oral fluids for the detection of antibodies to HIV have become available as an alternative to serum testing. These HIV-1 antibody tests entail the use of oral mucosal transudate, a serum-derived fluid that enters saliva from the gingival crevice and across oral mucosal surfaces. These tests compare favourably with serum tests with regard to reliability because they are based on the same serology–Western blot algorithm. The oral mucosal transudate tests for HIV involve a simple, safe, and noninvasive method of specimen collection and thus are an effective epidemiologic tool for HIV testing. In all the oral tests, a pretreated cotton pad is placed between the lower gums and the cheek. This pad is then sent to the central laboratory for antibody testing as described previously. It is hoped that these portable, user-friendly diagnostic tests will facilitate identification of greater numbers of infected individuals, with the ultimate goals of early identification, early treatment, and prevention of disease transmission.

Another noninvasive alternative to blood testing is urine testing for HIV. Only a spot urine collection is required. Testing urine for HIV antibodies is valuable, especially when venipuncture is inconvenient, difficult, or unacceptable. Insurance companies also commonly allow it. The sensitivity and specificity (accuracy) are somewhat less than those of the blood and oral fluid tests. This is also an enzyme immunoassay antibody test similar to blood enzyme immunoassay tests, and a follow-up confirmatory Western blot is needed for the same urine sample. Of importance is that all urine HIV tests detect antibodies and not the HIV particles. Urine does not contain the virus and is not a body fluid capable of spreading infection.

Rapid HIV testing results after high-risk exposures can be available in less than 1 hour. Like conventional HIV enzyme immunoassays, rapid HIV test results require confirmation if the specimen is reactive. There are several different types of rapid test involving either pinprick or oral mucosal transudate. All four tests are interpreted visually and require no instrumentation. HIV antigens are affixed to the test strip or membrane. If HIV antibodies are present in the specimen being tested, they bind to the affixed antigen. The test kit's colorimetric reagent binds to these immunoglobulins, creating an indicator that is visually detectable. Like conventional enzyme immunoassays, rapid HIV tests are screening tests. If performed correctly, they detect HIV antibodies with sensitivities similar to currently available enzyme immunoassays.

Home kits are now available that provide anonymous registration and pretest counselling through a toll-free call. Sample collection in the privacy of a patient's home, laboratory processing, and posttest counselling are components of this home-testing process. The procedure involves pricking a finger with a special device, placing drops of blood on a specially treated card, and then mailing the card in to be tested at a licenced laboratory. Test results are available to the patient (as described previously) through the Home Access Health Corporation, within 3 business days for the Express Kit and 7 days for the Standard Kit after shipment of the sample to the laboratory.

INTERFERING FACTORS

- False-positive results can occur in patients who have autoimmune disease, lymphoproliferative disease, leukemia, lymphoma, or syphilis or in alcoholic patients.
- False-negative results can occur in the early incubation stage or the end stage of AIDS. Tests for HIV antigen should be performed at each of these stages.

 Clinical Priorities

- Do not relay the test results over the telephone. News of positive results may have devastating consequences, including loss of job, insurance, relationships, and housing.
- Encourage patients with positive test results to inform their sexual partners so that the partners can be tested.
- Inform patients with positive test results that subsequent sexual contact will put partners at high risk for contracting AIDS.

PROCEDURE AND PATIENT CARE

Before

- Explain the procedure to the patient.
- Obtain informed consent as required by law.
- Inform the patient that no fasting or preparation is required.
- Maintain a nonjudgemental attitude toward the patient's sexual practices and allow the patient ample time to express his or her concerns regarding the results.

During

- Observe universal blood and body precautions. Wear gloves when handling blood products from all patients.
- For routine HIV testing, collect a venous blood sample in a red-top tube. The blood is usually sent to an outside laboratory for testing, although testing kits are becoming increasingly available in hospital laboratories and even in homes.
- If the patient wishes to remain anonymous, use a number with the patient's name; ensure that it is recorded accurately.
- Note that if the serologic specimen is reactive (i.e., test result is positive twice consecutively), the Western blot test must be performed on the same blood sample.
- If the Western blot test result is equivocal, collect a second serum specimen 2 to 4 months later for testing.

After

- Apply pressure or a pressure dressing to the venipuncture site.
- Assess the site for bleeding.
- Instruct the patient to observe the venipuncture site for infection. Patients with AIDS are immunocompromised and susceptible to infection.
- Follow the institution's policy regarding test result reporting.
- Do not give results over the telephone. News of positive results may have devastating consequences.
- Explain to the patient that a positive result of a Western blot test merely implies exposure to and presence of HIV within the body. It does not mean that the patient has clinical AIDS. Not all patients with positive results on an antibody test develop the disease.
- Encourage patients with positive test results to identify their sexual contacts so that those contacts can be informed and tested.
- Inform the patient that subsequent sexual contact will put new partners at high risk for contracting AIDS.
- Provide patient education regarding safe sexual practices.

TEST RESULTS AND CLINICAL SIGNIFICANCE

▲ Increased Levels

AIDS,

AIDS-related complex: *It is important to be aware that HIV infection occurs several years before development of AIDS. There is some evidence that the disease can be prevented with aggressive early treatment of HIV infection.*

RELATED TESTS

Cell Surface Immunophenotyping (p. 161). This test quantifies the number of CD4 and CD8 lymphocytes in an HIV-positive patient. These tests are predictive of the disease course and prognosis.

HIV Viral Load (see following test). This test is used to determine the amount of HIV viral load in the blood of an infected patient and is an accurate marker for prognosis and disease progression.

HIV Viral Load (HIV RNA)

NORMAL FINDINGS

Undetected

INDICATIONS

This test is used to determine the amount of human immunodeficiency virus (HIV) in the blood of an infected patient. This test is an accurate marker for prognosis, disease progression, response to antiviral treatment, and indication for antiretroviral prophylactic treatment.

TEST EXPLANATION

Quantitation of HIV viral load in the blood is used to detect HIV virus RNA in the blood of patients who are suspected of being infected with HIV. It is also used to follow the progression of acquired immune deficiency syndrome (AIDS). This information is used as an indicator for recommending the initiation and monitoring of antiretroviral treatment (Table 2-32). HIV viral load reflects a patient's response to antiviral therapy and indicates the course of the disease more

TABLE 2-32	Recommendations for Initiating and Monitoring Antiretroviral Therapy According to Layout Viral Load and CD4 Count			
CD4 Count: Cells/mm³ ($\times 10^5$/L)	Guidelines for Initiating Antiretroviral Therapy	MONITORING RESPONSE WITH HIV RNA VIRAL LOAD (COPIES/ML)		
		<20–75	<200	>200
350	Strong recommendation to start therapy	Optimal response	Low-level positive result	Virologic failure
350–500	Strong to moderate recommendation to start therapy	Optimal response	Low-level positive result	Virologic failure
>500	Moderate to optional recommendation to start therapy	Optimal response	Low-level positive result	Virologic failure
Symptomatic	Initiate therapy regardless of CD4 count when patient has symptoms HIV nephropathy, or hepatitis B co-infection	Optimal response	Low-level positive result	Virologic failue

HIV, Human immunodeficiency virus.

accurately than do any other tests, including CD4 T cell counts (see p. 161). HIV viral load testing is also used to monitor the effectiveness of treatment and to identify transplacental transmission of the HIV virus. Viral RNA testing is frequently used to test donor blood components.

HIV viral load is most accurately determined by quantifying the amount of genetic material of the virus in the blood. There are several different laboratory methods of measuring HIV viral load. It is important that the same method is used in monitoring the course of the disease in an individual patient. Because results vary according to the testing methods, it is important to know which method is used when initiation of treatment is under consideration. The most common method is to use a reverse-transcriptase polymerase chain reaction with gene amplification. This method can quantify RNA to ranges of less than 50 copies/mL.

In general, it is recommended that the baseline viral load be determined before therapy is initiated, after AIDS serologic testing (p. 315) yields positive results, and then preferably 2 to 4 weeks and not more than 8 weeks after treatment is initiated. Viral loads should be measured at 4- to 8-week intervals until the level falls below the assay's limit of detection. Monitoring should continue with testing every 3 to 4 months or as clinically indicated. Both CD4 and viral load tests provide data used to determine when to start antiviral treatment. The minimal change in viral load considered to be statically significant is $0.5 \log_{10}$ copies/mL change. Optimal viral suppression is usually defined as a viral load persistently below the level of detection (<20 to 75 copies/mL, depending on the assay used). However, it is not uncommon for successfully treated patients to have viral loads at less than 400 copies/mL. The AIDS Clinical Trial Group (ACTG) currently defines *virologic failure* as a confirmed viral load of less than 1000 copies/mL. It is important to recognize that a "nondetectable" result does not mean that the virus has been eradicated from the blood after treatment; it means that the viral load has fallen below the limit of detection by the test. A significant (greater than threefold) rise of viral load should warrant consideration of alteration in therapy.

INTERFERING FACTORS

- Incorrect handling and processing of the specimen can cause inconsistent results.
- Recent flu shots may temporarily increase viral levels.
- Concurrent infections can cause inconsistent results.
- Variable compliance to therapy may alter test results.

Clinical Priorities

- Do not give test results over the phone. News about increasing viral load results can have devastating consequences.
- Because test results vary according to the laboratory test method, it is important to use the same laboratory method for monitoring the course of the disease in individual patients.
- Viral load measurements are usually repeated after a patient starts or changes antiviral therapy. A significant rise in viral load warrants immediate re-evaluation of therapy.

PROCEDURE AND PATIENT CARE

Before
- Explain the procedure to the patient.
- Inform the patient that no fasting or preparation is required.
- Maintain a nonjudgemental attitude toward the patient's sexual practices. Allow the patient ample time to express his or her concerns regarding the results.

During

- Observe universal body and blood precautions. Wear gloves when handling blood products from all patients.
- Collect a blood sample in a lavender-top tube. If the test specimen is sent out, the plasma is separated out and at least 2.5 mL is frozen and sent.
- Never recap needles. Dispose of needles and syringes required for obtaining the blood specimen for HIV testing in a puncture-proof container designed for this purpose.

After

- Immediately transport the specimen to the laboratory.
- Specimens are often sent to a central laboratory.
- Apply pressure to the venipuncture site.
 Instruct the patient to observe the venipuncture site for infection. Patients with AIDS are immunocompromised and susceptible to infection.
- Do not give results over the telephone. News about increasing viral load may have devastating consequences.
- Encourage the patient to discuss his or her concerns regarding the prognostic information that may be obtained by these results.

TEST RESULTS AND CLINICAL SIGNIFICANCE

▲ Increased Levels

HIV infection: *In general, the level of HIV viral load parallels the course of HIV disease. Reduction in viral loads can be expected with successful therapy.*

RELATED TESTS

HIV Serology (p. 310). This test is used to diagnose HIV infection.

Cell Surface Immunophenotyping (p. 161). This test is used to measure CD4 lymphocyte counts. This is another marker for disease prognosis, response to treatment, and also an indicator for starting prophylactic antiretroviral treatment.

HLA-B27 Antigen (Human Lymphocyte Antigen B27, Human Leukocyte A Antigen, White Blood Cell Antigens, Histocompatibility Leukocyte A Antigen)

NORMAL FINDINGS

Negative

INDICATIONS

Human leukocyte antigen (HLA) testing is used to determine histocompatibility for organ or other tissue transplantation. These antigens are present with certain diseases, and so the test is used to support their diagnosis. HLA testing is also used in paternity investigations.

TEST EXPLANATION

The HLA antigens exist on the surface of white blood cells (WBCs) and on the surface of all nucleated cells in other tissues. These antigens can be detected most easily on the cell surface of lymphocytes. The presence or absence of these antigens is determined by the genes on chromosome 6. There are four genes at the specific locus. Each gene controls the presence or absence of HLA-A, HLA-B, HLA-C, and HLA-D. There is probably a fifth gene that is closely related to D and is called *DR*.

The HLA system of antigens has been used to indicate tissue compatibility with tissue transplantation. If the HLA antigens of the donor are not compatible with those of the recipient, the recipient will make antibodies to those antigens, which accelerates transplant rejection. Survival of the transplanted tissue is increased if HLA matching is achieved. Prior HLA sensitization causes antibodies to form in the blood of a transplant recipient and shortens the survival of red blood cells (RBCs) or platelets when they are transfused.

The HLA system has also been used to assist in the diagnosis of certain other diseases. For example, HLA-B27 is present in 80% of patients with Reiter's syndrome. When a patient presents with recurrent and multiple arthritic complaints, the presence of HLA-B27 supports the diagnosis of Reiter's syndrome. HLA-B27 is found in 5% to 7% of normal patients. Other HLA-disease associations are listed in Table 2-33.

Because HLA antigens are genetically determined, they are useful in paternity investigations. This is particularly helpful if the alleged father or the child has an unusual HLA genotype. A common HLA genotype in either the father or child increases the likelihood for many men to be the potential father of that child.

For this test, lymphocytes from the patient are extracted and incubated with anti–HLA-specific cytotoxic antibody. If the patient has the particular HLA antigen, a complex is formed on the cell surface. Serum complement is then added to the mixture, which kills the lymphocytes and aids in determining the titre of the HLA antigen.

TABLE 2-33   HLA and Diseases

Antigen	Disease
HLA-B27	Reiter's syndrome
	Ankylosing spondylitis
	Yersinia enterocolitica arthritis
	Anterior uveitis
	Graves' disease
HLA-B8	Celiac disease
	Chronic active hepatitis
	Multiple sclerosis
	Myasthenia gravis
	Dermatitis herpetiformis
HLA-B17	Psoriasis
HLA-Bw15 + HLA-B8	Juvenile diabetes
HLA-DR3 or HLA-DR4	Diabetes associated with beta cell autoantibodies
HLA-A3	Hemochromatosis
HLA-DR4	Rheumatoid arthritis
HLA-DR7, HLA-DRw3, HLA-B8	Gluten enteropathy

HLA, Human leukocyte antigen.

PROCEDURE AND PATIENT CARE

Before

X Explain the procedure to the patient.

X Inform the patient that no fasting or special preparation is required.

During

• Collect a venous blood sample in a green-top tube.

After

• Apply pressure or a pressure dressing to the venipuncture site.
• Assess the venipuncture site for bleeding.

TEST RESULTS AND CLINICAL SIGNIFICANCE

Positive for HLA Antigens

Ankylosing spondylitis,

Reiter's syndrome,

Yersinia enterocolitica arthritis,

Anterior uveitis,

Graves' disease,

Celiac disease/gluten enteropathy,

Chronic active hepatitis,

Multiple sclerosis,

Myasthenia gravis,

Dermatitis herpetiformis,

Psoriasis,

Juvenile diabetes/diabetes associated with beta cell autoantibodies,

Hemochromatosis,

Rheumatoid arthritis: *Specific HLA antigens are present in these diseases in varying frequencies. The association of these HLA antigens with the pathophysiologic process of these diseases is not known.*

Homocysteine (HCY)

NORMAL FINDINGS (PLASMA)

0–30 years: 4.6–8.1 *Mc*mol/L

30–59 years:

    Male: 6.3–11.2 *Mc*mol/L

    Female: 4.5–7.9 *Mc*mol/L

>59 years: 5.8–11.9 *Mc*mol/L

INDICATIONS

Homocysteine is an important predictor of coronary, cerebral, and peripheral vascular disease. When a strong familial predisposition or early-onset vascular disease is noted, homocysteine testing should be performed to determine whether genetic or acquired homocysteine excess exists.

Because elevated homocysteine levels are associated with deficiency in vitamin B_{12} or folate, this test is used for the detection and surveillance of malnutrition.

TEST EXPLANATION

Homocysteine is an intermediate amino acid formed during the metabolism of methionine. Increasing evidence suggests that elevation in blood levels of homocysteine may be an independent risk factor for ischemic heart disease, cerebrovascular disease, and peripheral arterial disease. Homocysteine appears to promote the progression of atherosclerosis by causing endothelial damage, promoting low-density lipoprotein (LDL) deposition, and promoting the growth of vascular smooth muscle. Screening for hyperhomocysteinemia (levels >15 Mcmol/L) should be considered in individuals with progressive and unexplained atherosclerosis despite normal lipoprotein levels and in the absence of other risk factors. It is also recommended in patients with an unusual family history of atherosclerosis, especially at a young age. A person with an elevated homocysteine level also has a five times higher risk than normal for stroke, dementia, and Alzheimer's disease. Elevated levels also appear to be a risk factor for osteoporotic fractures in older men and women.

Dietary deficiency of vitamin B_6, vitamin B_{12}, or folate is the most common nongenetic cause of elevated homocysteine levels. These vitamins are essential cofactors involved in the metabolism of homocysteine to methionine. Because of the relationship of homocysteine to these vitamins, homocysteine blood levels are helpful in the diagnosis of syndromes associated with deficiencies in these vitamins. In patients with megaloblastic anemia, homocysteine levels may be elevated before results of the more traditional tests become abnormal. Therefore, measuring homocysteine level as an indicator may result in earlier treatment and thus improvement of symptoms in patients with these vitamin deficiencies. Some practitioners recommend homocysteine testing in patients known to have poor nutritional status (alcoholic patients, patients who abuse drugs) and older adults.

Some researchers believe that elevations in homocysteine levels can be treated by administration of vitamin B_6, vitamin B_{12}, and folate. Several research reports recommend this vitamin therapy for homocysteine levels higher than 14 Mcmol/L. Whether this treatment will reduce the incidence of heart attacks remains to be seen.

Genetic defects encoding the synthesis of the enzymes responsible for the metabolism of homocysteine to cysteine or the remethylation of homocysteine to methionine are the most common familial cause of hyperhomocysteinemia. Affected children suffer from homocystinuria and experience very premature and accelerated atherosclerosis during childhood.

Both fasting and post–methionine loading levels of homocysteine can be measured. In most laboratories, total homocysteine concentrations are measured. A major disadvantage in homocysteine testing is that methods are not standardized.

With the more recent development of enzyme immunoassay, results have become more standardized. However, newer testing kits in which high-performance liquid chromatography is simplified with fluorescence detection are easy to use and accurate. In general, homocysteine levels lower than 12 Mcmol/L are considered optimal, levels from 12 to 15 Mcmol/L are borderline, and levels higher than 15 Mcmol/L are associated with high risk for vascular disease.

CONTRAINDICATIONS

- Elevated creatinine levels (in excess of 1.5 mg/dL) indicate malfunction of the kidneys, rendering them unable to filter methionine (a protein) effectively.

INTERFERING FACTORS

- Homocysteine levels may increase with age.
- Patients with renal impairment have elevated levels of homocysteine because of poor excretion of the protein.
- Men usually have higher levels of homocysteine than women do. This is probably because men have higher creatinine values and greater muscle mass.
- Patients with a low intake of B vitamins have higher levels of homocysteine. The B vitamins help to break down and recycle homocysteine.
- Smoking is associated with increased homocysteine levels.
- Drugs that may cause *increases* in homocysteine levels include carbamazepine, methotrexate, nitrous oxide, theophylline, and phenytoin.
- Drugs that are associated with *decreased* levels include folic acid, oral contraceptives, and tamoxifen.

PROCEDURE AND PATIENT CARE

Before

- Explain the procedure to the patient.
- Instruct the patient to fast for 10 to 12 hours before the test. Meats contain elevated levels of homocysteine.

During

- Obtain the fasting blood sample in a collection tube that contains ethylenediamine tetra-acetic acid (EDTA), heparin, or sodium citrate (blue-top or lavender-top tube).
- For methionine loading, the patient ingests approximately 100 mg/kg of methionine after fasting for 10 to 12 hours. A blood sample is obtained. Repeat blood samples are collected 2, 4, 8, 12, and 24 hours later to compare levels of B vitamins and amino acids in the plasma.

After

- In the laboratory, the blood should be spun down within 30 minutes to avoid false elevation caused by release of homocysteine from red blood cells (RBCs).
- Apply pressure or a pressure dressing to the venipuncture site.
- Assess the venipuncture site for bleeding.

TEST RESULTS AND CLINICAL SIGNIFICANCE

▲ Increased Levels

Cardiovascular disease,

Cerebrovascular disease,

Peripheral vascular disease: *As a direct effect of homocysteine on the vascular wall, intimal injury and plaque formation occur. Accentuated smooth muscle vascular constriction serves to further diminish the vessel lumen, thereby compounding the vascular occlusive results. Ischemic events in the cerebral, coronary, and peripheral tissues occur earlier, more severely, and more frequently.*

Cystinuria,

Vitamin B_6 or B_{12} deficiency,

Folate deficiency: *Deficient quantity of metabolic enzymes or metabolic cofactors (vitamin B_{12} or folate) diminishes metabolism of homocysteine. Blood levels and subsequently urine levels increase.*

Malnutrition: *Malnourished patients have low vitamin B_{12} and folate intake. Because these vitamins are essential to the metabolism of homocysteine, blood levels increase.*

RELATED TESTS

Vitamin B_{12} (p. 541) and Folic Acid (p. 256). Blood levels of these substances are easily determined. The results have an effect on levels of homocysteine.

Lipoprotein (p. 355), Cholesterol (p. 169), and Triglycerides (p. 523). These are important predictors of cardiac atherosclerotic risks.

Apolipoproteins (p. 116). This test is used to measure apolipoprotein levels. This may be a better indicator of atherogenic risks than is total high-density lipoprotein (HDL) or total LDL.

Human Placental Lactogen ([hPL], Human Chorionic Somatomammotropin [HCS])

NORMAL FINDINGS

Nonpregnant: **<0.5 *Mcg*/mL** (<0.5 mg/L)

Weeks of Pregnancy	hPL Concentration (*Mcg*/mL)*
Up to 20	0.05–1
Up to 22	1.5–3
Up to 26	2.5–5
Up to 30	4–6.5
Up to 34	5–8
Up to 38	5.5–9.5
Up to 42	5–7

*Conventional values are the same as the SI values but in milligrams per litre.

INDICATIONS

This test is used to evaluate the adequacy of the placenta in high-risk pregnancies.

TEST EXPLANATION

The human placenta produces several hormones that are homologous to hormones produced by the anterior pituitary gland. Human placental lactogen (hPL), whose task is to maintain the pregnancy, is structurally similar to both human prolactin and growth hormone. Not surprisingly, hPL demonstrates both lactogenic and growth-stimulating activity.

Serum levels of hPL rise very early in normal pregnancy and continue to increase until a plateau is reached at approximately the thirty-fifth week after conception. Assays for maternal serum levels of hPL are therefore useful in monitoring placental function. Measurements of hPL are also used in pregnancies complicated by hypertension, proteinuria, edema, postmaturity, placental insufficiency, or possible miscarriage.

A decreasing serum concentration of hPL is pathognomonic for a malfunction of the placenta that may cause intrauterine growth restriction, death of the fetus, or imminent miscarriage. Pregnant women experiencing hypertonia also have low serum concentrations of hPL. Because of the short biologic half-life of hPL in serum, the determination of hPL always provides a very accurate representation of the current situation.

Serum concentrations of hPL are increased in women suffering from diabetes mellitus and, because of the higher placental mass, in multiple pregnancies. In contrast to estriol, the hPL concentration depends on only the placental mass and not on the fetal function. The simultaneous determination of hPL and estriol can be helpful in the differential evaluation of the placental function.

No single endocrine test has proved to be effective in all cases. Of the current endocrine factors, serum unconjugated estriol (p. 240) appears to be the best predictor of fetal distress or well-being. However, interpretation of estriol values is limited because those values undergo short-term and daily fluctuations. When high-risk pregnancies are monitored, the decision to deliver should not be based on a single factor; rather, it should be based on the estriol values, hPL values, and the fetal heart rate in response to contractions or stress (p. 594).

Quantitative (and qualitative) analysis is performed by radial immunodiffusion. Enzyme-linked immunosorbent assay (ELISA) kits are available and yield accurate results.

INTERFERING FACTORS
• Prior nuclear medicine scans because they may affect the results of a radioimmunoassay.

PROCEDURE AND PATIENT CARE
Before
☒ Explain the procedure to the patient.
☒ Inform the patient that no fasting is required.

During
• Collect a venous blood sample in a red-top tube.
• On the laboratory slip, indicate the date of the most recent menstrual period.

After
• Apply pressure to the venipuncture site.
☒ Explain the possibility that serial testing is often required.

TEST RESULTS AND CLINICAL SIGNIFICANCE
▲ Increased Levels
Multiple pregnancies,
Placental site trophoblastic tumour,
Intact molar pregnancy,
Diabetes: *These diseases are commonly associated with increased placental mass and, as a result, increased hPL levels.*
Rh incompatibility

▼ Decreased Levels
Placental insufficiency,
Toxemia,

Pre-eclampsia,

Hydatidiform mole,

Choriocarcinoma: *All of these diseases are associated with a reduced function of the placenta. As a result, hPL level is reduced. The pathophysiologic mechanism underlying this finding is not clear.*

RELATED TESTS

Estrogen Fraction (p. 240). Estrogen fractions are an accurate predictor of the status of the placenta and fetus.

Fetal Contraction Stress Test (p. 594) and Fetal Nonstress Test (p. 597). These are tests of the adequacy of the fetal-placental unit.

Progesterone Assay (p. 429). Progesterone can be used to monitor the status of the placenta.

Human T-Cell Lymphotrophic Virus
(HTLV; HTLV I/II Antibody)

NORMAL FINDINGS

Negative

INDICATIONS

Testing for this virus is helpful in the diagnosis of certain types of leukemias.

TEST EXPLANATION

Several forms of HTLV, a human retrovirus, affect humans. The virus is endemic in southern Japan, the Caribbean islands, South America, and portions of Africa. HTLV-I is associated with T-cell leukemia/lymphoma in adults. HTLV-II is associated with hairy cell leukemia in adults. HTLV-I has also been linked to neurologic disorders such as tropical spastic paraparesis. It is possible, however, for a human to be infected with these viruses and yet not develop any malignancy or diseases.

The human immunodeficiency virus (HIV), which is known to be the cause of acquired immune deficiency syndrome (AIDS), is also a retrovirus; however, HTLV infection is not associated with AIDS. HTLV transmission is similar to HIV transmission (e.g., body fluid contamination, intravenous drug use, sexual contact, breast-feeding).

Most serologic tests for HTLV are performed with enzyme-linked immunosorbent assay (ELISA) techniques. Identification of antibodies to certain portions of the two viruses allows for specific diagnosis and differentiation of the two. Nucleic acid probes are also used at large testing laboratories.

PROCEDURE AND PATIENT CARE

Before

- Explain the procedure to the patient.
- Inform the patient that no fasting is required.

During

• Collect a venous blood sample in a red-top tube.

After

• Apply pressure or a pressure dressing to the venipuncture site.
• Assess the venipuncture site for bleeding.

TEST RESULTS AND CLINICAL SIGNIFICANCE

▲ Increased Levels

Acute HTLV infection,
Adult T-cell leukemia,
Hairy cell leukemia,
Tropical spastic paraparesis: *The pathophysiologic mechanism underlying the association of these illnesses with HTLV infection is not known.*

21-Hydroxylase Antibodies

NORMAL FINDINGS

<1 U/mL

INDICATION

This study is used to determine an autoimmune cause of Addison's disease.

TEST EXPLANATION

Chronic primary adrenal insufficiency (Addison's disease) is most commonly caused by the insidious autoimmune destruction of the adrenal cortex and is characterized by the presence of adrenal cortex autoantibodies in the serum. It can occur sporadically or in combination with other autoimmune endocrine diseases. This antibody may precipitate this disease. Measurement of this antibody is used in the investigation of causes of adrenal insufficiency.

PROCEDURE AND PATIENT CARE

Before

 Explain the procedure to the patient.
Tell the patient that no fasting is required.

During

• Collect a venous blood sample in a red-top tube.

After
• Apply pressure or a pressure dressing to the venipuncture site.

TEST RESULTS AND CLINICAL SIGNIFICANCE

Autoimmune adrenal insufficiency,
Autoimmune polyglandular syndrome: *These diseases are commonly associated with autoimmune-instigated antibodies.*

RELATED TESTS

Cortisol (p. 192). This blood test indicates the function of the adrenal gland. In Addison's disease this will be diminished.

Adrenocorticotropic Hormone (ACTH) (p. 34). This blood test helps in the diagnosis of Addison's disease and Cushing's syndrome.

Immunofixation Electrophoresis (IFE)

NORMAL FINDINGS

No monoclonal immunoglobulins identified

INDICATIONS

This test is used to identify more clearly whether a spike on the serum protein electrophoresis pattern (see p. 440) is monoclonal or whether quantitative immunoglobulin levels are elevated.

TEST EXPLANATION

In this technique, a monospecific antibody is placed in contact with gel after the proteins have been separated by electrophoresis. The resulting protein-antibody complexes are subsequently specifically stained for visualization after being precipitated out. The pathologist can then identify and classify specific immunoglobulin spikes. For example, multiple myeloma and Waldenström macroglobulinemia are characterized by monoclonal immunoglobulin spikes. Furthermore, both diseases are characterized by light chains in the urine immunofixation electrophoresis pattern; however, some patients with multiple myeloma have heavy chains in the urine. Polyclonal immunoglobulins are noted in chronic inflammatory processes, chronic liver diseases, and ongoing chronic infections.

This test is also used to monitor the course of the disease or treatment on patients with known monoclonal immunoglobulinopathies. For example, with successful treatment for neoplastic gammopathies, immunofixation electrophoresis can, on repetition, demonstrate reduction in the specific immunoglobulin. Furthermore, it can reveal whether the monoclonal spike is attributable to light chain or heavy chain components. This test is also helpful to define more clearly the immune status of a patient whose immune status may be compromised.

PROCEDURE AND PATIENT CARE

Before

𝄩 Explain the procedure to the patient.
𝄩 Inform the patient that no fasting or special preparation is required.

During

Blood

- Collect a venous blood sample in a red-top tube.
- On the laboratory slip, indicate whether the patient has received any vaccinations or immunizations within the previous 6 months.

Urine

𝄩 Instruct the patient to begin the 24-hour collection after the first morning void. Discard that first specimen.
𝄩 Instruct the patient to collect all urine passed during the next 24 hours.
- Note that it is not necessary to measure each urine specimen.
𝄩 Remind the patient to void before defecating so that the urine is not contaminated by feces.
𝄩 Instruct the patient not to put toilet paper in the collection container.
𝄩 Encourage the patient to drink fluids during the 24 hours unless this is contraindicated for medical purposes.
𝄩 Instruct the patient to void as close as possible to the end of the 24-hour period and to add this specimen to the collection.
- Place the 24-hour urine collection in a plastic container and keep it on ice.
- Apply pressure to the venipuncture site.

TEST RESULTS AND CLINICAL SIGNIFICANCE

▲ Increased Blood Monoclonal Immunoglobulins

Multiple myeloma,
Waldenström macroglobulinemia

▲ Increased Blood Polyclonal Immunoglobulin

Amyloidosis,
Autoimmune diseases,
Chronic infection/inflammation,
Chronic liver disease

▲ Increased Urine Monoclonal Immunoglobulins

Multiple myeloma,
Waldenström macroglobulinemia: *These and many other diseases are associated with particular gamma-globulin spikes that can be readily and specifically identified.*

RELATED TEST

Protein Electrophoresis (p. 440). This test is used to diagnose, evaluate, and monitor the disease course in patients with cancer (e.g., lymphoma, myeloma), intestinal/renal protein-wasting states, immune disorders, liver dysfunction, impaired nutrition, and chronic edematous states.

Immunoglobulin Electrophoresis (Gamma-Globulin Electrophoresis)

	Immunoglobulin G	
Age	g/L	(mg/dL)
Adult	5.65–17.65	(565–1765)
Child		
1 month	2.5–9.0	(250–900)
2–5 months	2.0–7.0	(200–700)
6–9 months	2.2–9.0	(220–900)
1 year	3.4–12.0	(340–1 200)
2–3 years	4.2–12.0	(420–1 200)
4–12 years	4.6–16.0	(460–1 600)

	Immunoglobulin A	
Age	g/L	(mg/dL)
Adult	0.85–3.85	(85–385)
Child		
1 month	0.01–0.04	(1–4)
2–5 months	0.04–0.8	(4–80)
6–9 months	0.08–0.8	(8–80)
1 year	0.15–1.10	(15–110)
2–3 years	0.18–1.50	(18–150)
4–12 years	0.25–3.5	(25–350)

	Immunoglobulin M	
Age	g/L	(mg/dL)
Adult	0.55–3.75	(55–375)
Child		
1 month	0.20–0.80	(20–80)
2–5 months	0.25–1.0	(25–100)
6–9 months	0.35–1.25	(35–125)
1–8 years	0.45–2.0	(45–200)
9–12 years	0.50–2.5	(50–250)

Immunoglobulins D and E: minimal in adults

INDICATIONS

This test is used to assist in the diagnosis and monitoring of therapeutic response in many disease states. It is often ordered if serum protein electrophoresis indicates a spike at the immunoglobulin level.

TEST EXPLANATION

Proteins in the blood are made up of albumin and globulin. Globulin consists of several types, one of which is gamma-globulin. Antibodies are made up of gamma-globulin protein and are called *immunoglobulins.* There are many classes of immunoglobulins (antibodies). Immunoglobulin G (IgG) constitutes approximately 75% of the serum immunoglobulins; therefore, it constitutes the majority of circulating blood antibodies. Maternal IgG can cross the placenta and provides effective immune protection of the newborn in the first few months of life. Immunoglobulin A (IgA) constitutes approximately 15% of the immunoglobulins within the body and is present primarily in the secretions of the respiratory and gastrointestinal tract, in saliva, in colostrum, and in tears. IgA is also present to a smaller degree in the blood. Immunoglobulin M (IgM) is responsible primarily for ABO blood grouping and rheumatoid factor, and yet it is involved in the immunologic reaction to many other infections (e.g., hepatitis, Gram-negative sepsis). Because IgM does not cross the placenta, an elevation of IgM level in the newborn indicates intrauterine infection such as rubella, cytomegalovirus, or a sexually transmitted disease. Immunoglobulin E (IgE) often mediates an allergic response and is measured to detect allergic diseases. Immunoglobulin D (IgD), which constitutes the smallest portion of the immunoglobulins, is rarely evaluated or detected.

Serum immunoelectrophoresis is used to detect and monitor the course of diseases, including hypersensitivity disorders, immune deficiencies, autoimmune diseases, chronic infections, multiple myeloma, chronic viral infections, and intrauterine fetal infections. For this test, the serum is placed on a slide containing agar gel, and an electric current is passed through the gel. Immunoglobulins are separated out and subjected to electrophoresis according to the quantity and difference in electric charge. Specific antisera are placed alongside the slide to identify the specific type of immunoglobulin present.

More commonly, *immunofixation electrophoresis* is used to identify pathologic processes related to immunoglobulins. In this technique, a monospecific antibody is placed in contact with the agar gel after the proteins have been separated by electrophoresis. The resulting protein-antibody complexes are specifically stained for visualization after being precipitated out. The pathologist can then identify and classify a specific immunoglobulin spike that indicates a monoclonal gammopathy, such as multiple myeloma or Waldenström macroglobulinemia. As treatment for neoplastic gammopathies succeeds, repeated immunofixation electrophoresis can demonstrate reduction in the specific immunoglobulin.

INTERFERING FACTORS

Drugs that may cause *increases* in immunoglobulin levels include dextran, hydralazine, isoniazid (INH), methadone, oral contraceptives, phenytoin (Dilantin), procainamide, steroids, tetanus toxoid and antitoxin, and therapeutic gamma-globulin.

PROCEDURE AND PATIENT CARE

Before

- Explain the procedure to the patient.
- Inform the patient that no fasting or special preparation is required.

During

- Collect a venous blood sample in a red-top tube.
- On the laboratory slip, indicate whether the patient has received any vaccinations or immunizations within the previous 6 months.

After

- Apply pressure or a pressure dressing to the venipuncture site.
- Observe the venipuncture site for bleeding.

TEST RESULTS AND CLINICAL SIGNIFICANCE

▲ Increased Immunoglobulin A Levels

Chronic liver diseases (e.g., primary biliary cirrhosis),

Chronic infections,

Inflammatory bowel disease: *The pathophysiologic mechanism underlying these observations is not well known.*

▼ Decreased Immunoglobulin A Levels

Ataxia,

Telangiectasia,

Congenital isolated deficiency: *These illnesses are caused by isolated IgA deficiency or combined immunoglobulin deficiencies.*

Hypoproteinemia (e.g., nephrotic syndrome, protein-losing enteropathies): *The hypoproteinemia that results from these diseases causes the IgA deficiency.*

Drug immunosuppression (steroids, dextran): *The production of IgA is diminished.*

Acquired immune deficiency syndrome (AIDS): *In this disease, a deficiency exists throughout the entire immune system. Levels of IgA and other immunoglobulins are diminished.*

▲ Increased Immunoglobulin G Levels

Chronic granulomatous infections (e.g., tuberculosis, Wegener granulomatosis, sarcoidosis),

Hyperimmunization reactions,

Chronic liver disease,

Multiple myeloma (monoclonal IgG type),

Autoimmune diseases (e.g., rheumatoid arthritis, Sjögren disease, systemic lupus erythematosus): *All the above conditions stimulate IgG synthesis. The pathophysiologic mechanism underlying this observation is not known.*

Intrauterine devices: *These devices work by creating a subclinical localized inflammatory reaction that is harmful to the sperm. Part of that reaction is the synthesis of IgG.*

▲ Decreased Immunoglobulin G Levels

Wiskott-Aldrich syndrome,

Agammaglobulinemia: *These diseases are a result of a genetic deficiency that results in inadequate synthesis of IgG and other immunoglobulins.*

AIDS: *In this disease, a deficiency exists throughout the entire immune system. Levels of IgG and other immunoglobulins are diminished.*

Hypoproteinemia (e.g., nephrotic syndrome, protein-losing enteropathies): *The hypoproteinemia that results from these diseases causes the IgG deficiency.*

Drug immunosuppression (steroids, dextran): *The production of IgG is diminished.*

Non-IgG multiple myeloma,

Leukemia: *IgG production is diminished because the bone marrow is taken over by tumour cells.*

▲ Increased Immunoglobulin M Levels

Waldenström macroglobulinemia: *This is a malignancy similar to myeloma in which IgM is secreted at high levels by the malignant lymphoplasm cells. It is very similar diagnostically to IgM myeloma.*

Chronic infections (e.g., hepatitis, mononucleosis, sarcoidosis): *These infections stimulate the humoral response and many of the immunoglobulins, including IgM.*

Autoimmune diseases (e.g., systemic lupus erythematosus, rheumatoid arthritis): *The pathophysiologic mechanism is not well known. It is assumed that these antibodies somehow contribute to the disease process.*

Acute infections: *IgM is the first immunoglobulin to respond to an infectious agent (viral, bacterial, parasitic).*

Chronic liver disorders (e.g., biliary cirrhosis): *The pathophysiologic mechanism is not well defined.*

▼ Decreased Immunoglobulin M Levels

Agammaglobulinemia: *This disease is a result of a genetic deficiency in which the synthesis of IgM and other immunoglobulins is inadequate.*

AIDS: *In this disease, a deficiency exists throughout the entire immune system. IgM and other immunoglobulins are diminished.*

Hypoproteinemia (e.g., nephrotic syndrome, protein-losing enteropathies): *The hypoproteinemia that results from these diseases causes the IgM deficiency.*

Drug immunosuppression (steroids, dextran): *The production of IgM is diminished.*

IgG or IgA multiple myeloma,

Leukemia: *IgM production is diminished because the bone marrow is taken over by tumour cells.*

▲ Increased Immunoglobulin E Levels

Allergy reactions (e.g., hay fever, asthma, eczema, anaphylaxis): *Allergic reactions stimulate the production of IgE antibodies.*

Allergic infections (e.g., *Aspergillus* species, parasites)

▼ Decreased Immunoglobulin E Levels

Agammaglobulinemia: *This can be specific for IgE or may include the deficiencies in the production of all the immunoglobulins.*

RELATED TESTS

Protein Electrophoresis (p. 440). This is a quantification of all the components that make up the serum proteins, including albumin and alpha$_1$-, alpha$_2$-, beta$_1$-, beta$_2$-, and gamma-globulins. This test can also detect abnormal proteins created by neoplasms and infections.

Prealbumin (p. 424). Prealbumin is a component of proteins. This test is a quantification of prealbumin and is used to assess a person's nutritional status. It is also used to indicate the status of liver function.

Immunofixation Electrophoresis (p. 325). This test is used to identify more clearly whether a spike on the serum protein electrophoresis pattern is monoclonal or when quantitative immunoglobulin levels are elevated.

Insulin Assay

NORMAL FINDINGS

Adult: **43–186 pmol/L** (6–26 µU/mL)
Newborn: **21–139 pmol/L** (3–20 µU/mL)

 Critical Values

>290 pmol/L (>30 µU/mL)

INDICATIONS

This test is used to diagnose insulinoma (tumours of the islets of Langerhans) and to evaluate abnormal lipid and carbohydrate metabolism; in the evaluation of patients with fasting hypoglycemia states and neoplasm differentiation; and to detect insulin resistance, which is associated with an increased risk of cardiovascular disease and diabetes.

TEST EXPLANATION

Insulin regulates blood glucose levels by facilitating the movement of glucose out of the bloodstream and into the cells. Insulin secretion is reactive primarily to the blood glucose level. Normally, as the blood glucose level increases, the insulin level is sensitive to that rise and it, too, increases; as the glucose level decreases, insulin release stops. Reduced insulin sensitivity is of major physiologic importance in clinical disorders such as type 2 diabetes, obesity, and other disease states affected by insulin-receptor alterations.

Some investigators believe that measurements of the ratio of the blood glucose and insulin levels in the same specimen obtained during the oral glucose tolerance test are more reliable than measurements of insulin levels alone. Combined with the oral glucose tolerance test, the insulin assay can show characteristic curves. For example, patients with juvenile diabetes have low fasting insulin levels and display flat glucose tolerance insulin curves because they have little or no increase in insulin levels. Patients who are mildly diabetic have normal fasting insulin levels and display glucose tolerance curves with a delayed rise.

Type 2 diabetes (adult onset) is characterized by an excess of insulin production in response to glucose tolerance testing. This hyper-response of insulin may precede hyperglycemia by many years, which allows the patient time and opportunity to take action (through diet management and lifestyle changes) to reduce the risk for outright diabetes.

Numerous calculations can be used to determine insulin resistance. One such calculation, the fasting Belfiore index, is as follows:

$$2 / \left[\text{Insulin} \left(\text{pmol} / \text{L} \right) \times \text{Glucose} \left(\text{mmol} / \text{L} \right) + 1 \right]$$

The extreme limits of the Belfiore index are a minimum of 0 (in cases of extreme maximum reduction in insulin sensitivity) and a maximum of 2 (in extreme supernormal insulin sensitivity).

INTERFERING FACTORS

- Most patients treated with insulin for diabetes develop insulin antibodies within a few months. These antibodies can interfere with insulin radioimmune assay results by competing with the insulin antibodies used in the insulin assay.
- Food intake and obesity may cause increases in insulin levels.
- Recent administration of radioisotopes may affect test results by interfering with the radioimmune assay method to detect insulin.
- Drugs that may cause *increases* in insulin levels include corticosteroids, levodopa, and oral contraceptives.

PROCEDURE AND PATIENT CARE

Before

- Explain the procedure to the patient.
- Keep the patient on NPO status (nothing by mouth) for 8 hours.

During

- Collect a venous blood sample in a red-top tube and pack it in a container of water and crushed ice.
- Avoid hemolysis.
- If the serum insulin level is measured during the glucose tolerance test, collect the blood sample before oral ingestion of the glucose load and at designated intervals after glucose ingestion (according to the laboratory's protocol).

After

- Apply pressure or a pressure dressing to the venipuncture site.
- Observe the venipuncture site for bleeding.
- Transport the specimen immediately to the laboratory.

TEST RESULTS AND CLINICAL SIGNIFICANCE

▲ Increased Levels

Insulinoma: *This is a tumour of the beta cells in the islets of Langerhans of the pancreas. It is diagnosed in patients who have hyperinsulinemia despite hypoglycemia. These patients have persistently high C-peptide levels despite glucose levels below 30 mg/dL. The amended Turner's insulin/glucose ratio exceeds 50.*

Cushing's syndrome: *Cortisol overproduction causes elevations in glucose level, which acts as a constant stimulant of insulin production.*

Acromegaly: *Growth hormone overproduction causes elevations in glucose level, which acts as a constant stimulant of insulin production.*

Obesity: *The insulin level is persistently high.*

Fructose or galactose intolerance: *These complex sugars cannot be metabolized normally and, like glucose, stimulate insulin production.*

▼ Decreased Levels

Diabetes: *Insulin-dependent diabetes is, in part, caused by lack of endogenous insulin.*

Hypopituitarism: *This disease is associated with reduced thyroid and adrenal function along with reduced growth hormone levels. This leads to reductions in glucose levels. Insulin production is diminished.*

RELATED TESTS

Glucose Tolerance (p. 276). This is a test of a patient's capability to handle a glucose load.

Glucose, Postprandial (p. 272). This is a timed glucose measurement after a carbohydrate meal.

C-Peptide (p. 197). This test is used to evaluate diabetic patients. It is also used to identify patients who secretly self-administer insulin.

Insulin Antibody Assay (p. 330). This test is used in the evaluation of insulin resistance. It is also used to identify type 1 diabetes. It is used when allergy to insulin is suspected.

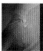 **Intrinsic Factor Antibody** (IF ab)

NORMAL FINDINGS

Negative

INDICATIONS

The intrinsic factor antibody is used to diagnose pernicious anemia. It is particularly helpful when the hematologic status is not completely clear.

TEST EXPLANATION

Pernicious anemia is one of the major causes of vitamin B_{12} deficiency and megaloblastic anemia. It is a disease of the stomach in which secretion of intrinsic factor is severely reduced or absent, resulting in malabsorption of vitamin B_{12}. In view of its association with a variety of antibodies, including anti–parietal cell antibody (see p. 102) and at least two types of anti–intrinsic factor antibody, pernicious anemia appears to be an autoimmune process. Antibodies to intrinsic factor are found in a very high percentage of children with juvenile pernicious anemia.

Approximately 50% to 75% of adult patients have intrinsic factor antibodies. There are two types of this antibody. Type I (blocking antibody), the more common, prevents the binding of vitamin B_{12} and intrinsic factor. Type II (binding antibody) is less specific for pernicious anemia and affects the binding of intrinsic factor in the ileum. The blocking antibody is extremely specific for pernicious anemia and is more sensitive than binding antibody. In the context of a low or borderline vitamin B_{12} result, in combination with other clinical and hematologic findings that are compatible with a diagnosis of vitamin B_{12} deficiency, the presence of intrinsic factor blocking antibody can be taken as confirmation of this diagnosis and, at the same time, as an indication of its cause. A negative result, on the other hand, cannot rule out the possibility of pernicious anemia because in nearly 50% of all patients with this disorder, blocking antibody is not demonstrable.

The diagnosis of pernicious anemia rarely necessitates vitamin B_{12} absorption testing (Schilling test, p. 862). Testing for anti–parietal cell antibodies and intrinsic factor antibodies is easier, quicker, and in most cases more accurate. Rapid testing can be performed easily with radioimmunoassay methods.

INTERFERING FACTORS

Intrinsic factor antibody levels are decreased if an injection of vitamin B_{12} is administered within 48 hours of testing. This is because the administration of vitamin B_{12} is also associated with other binding sites in addition to intrinsic factor, thus binding intrinsic factor antibody and lowering levels.

PROCEDURE AND PATIENT CARE

Before

- Explain the procedure to the patient.
- Inform the patient that no fasting or special preparation is required.
- Ensure that no vitamin B_{12} has been administered parenterally in the 48 hours before the test.

During

- Collect a venous blood sample in a red-top tube.

After

- Apply pressure or a pressure dressing to the venipuncture site.
- Check the venipuncture site for bleeding.

TEST RESULTS AND CLINICAL SIGNIFICANCE

▲ Increased Levels

Pernicious anemia: *Anti–intrinsic factor antibodies may destroy the parietal cell in the gastric antrum through complement-fixing antibodies against the parietal cell surface.*

RELATED TESTS

Schilling Test (p. 862). This test is used to evaluate the ability to absorb vitamin B_{12}. It is also used in the evaluation of patients with pernicious anemia. This test is no longer a major part of the diagnosis of pernicious anemia.

Anti–Parietal Cell Antibody (p. 102). This test is used to diagnose pernicious anemia serologically.

Vitamin B_{12} (p. 541). This test is a direct measurement of vitamin B_{12} serum levels, known to be reduced in pernicious anemia.

Iron Level, Total Iron-Binding Capacity, Transferrin, Transferrin Saturation (Fe, TIBC)

NORMAL FINDINGS

Iron

Adult:
  Male: **13–31 Mcmol/L** (75–175 Mcg/dL)
  Female: **5–29 Mcmol/L** (28–162 Mcg/dL)
Newborn:
  Male: **12.9–36.3 Mcmol/L** (72–203 Mcg/dL)
  Female: **13.4–42.1 Mcmol/L** (75–235 Mcg/dL)
Child 4–10 years:
  Male: **2.7–22.9 Mcmol/L** (15–128 Mcg/dL)
  Female: **5.0–21.8 Mcmol/L** (28–122 Mcg/dL)

Total Iron-Binding Capacity

Adult: **45–73 Mcmol/L** (250–410 Mcg/dL)
Newborn: **16.8–41.5 Mcmol/L** (94–232 Mcg/dL)

Transferrin

Adult male: **2.15–3.65 g/L** (215–365 mg/dL)
Adult female: **2.50–3.80 g/L** (250–380 mg/dL)
Newborn: **1.24–3.88 g/L** (124–388 mg/dL)
Child: **1.81–3.29 g/L** (181–329 mg/dL)

Transferrin Saturation

Male: 20%–50%
Female: 15%–50%

INDICATIONS

These tests are used to evaluate iron metabolism in patients when iron deficiency, overload, or poisoning is suspected.

TEST EXPLANATION

Serum Iron

Abnormal levels of iron are characteristic of many diseases, including iron-deficiency anemia and hemochromatosis. As much as 70% of the iron in the body is found in the hemoglobin of the red blood cells (RBCs). The other 30% is stored in the form of ferritin (see p. 248) and hemosiderin. Iron is supplied by the diet. Approximately 10% of the ingested iron is absorbed in the small intestine and transported to the plasma. In the plasma, the iron is bound to a globulin protein called *transferrin* and carried to the bone marrow for incorporation into hemoglobin. The serum iron determination is a measurement of the quantity of iron bound to transferrin.

Iron-deficiency anemia is a result of reduced levels of serum iron. It has many causes, including (1) insufficient iron intake, (2) inadequate gut absorption, (3) increased requirements (as in growing children and during late pregnancy), and (4) loss of blood (as in menstruation, bleeding peptic ulcer, colon neoplasm). Iron deficiency results in a decreased production of hemoglobin, which in turn results in small, pale (microcytic, hypochromic) RBCs. The mean corpuscular volume and mean corpuscular hemoglobin concentration (see p. 456) also decrease. A decreased serum iron level, an elevated total iron-binding capacity (TIBC), and a low transferrin saturation value are characteristics of iron-deficiency anemia.

Iron overload is called *hemochromatosis;* iron poisoning is called *hemosiderosis.* Excess iron is usually deposited in the brain, liver, and heart and causes severe dysfunction of these organs. Massive blood transfusions also may cause elevations in serum iron levels, although only transiently. Transfusions should be avoided before serum iron level is measured.

Because serum iron levels may vary significantly during the day, the blood specimen should be collected in the morning, especially when the results are used to monitor iron replacement therapy. The patient should refrain from eating for approximately 12 hours to avoid artificially high iron measurements caused by eating food with a high iron content.

TIBC and Transferrin

TIBC is a measurement of all proteins available for binding mobile iron. Transferrin represents the largest quantity of iron-binding proteins. Therefore, TIBC is an indirect but accurate measurement of transferrin. Ferritin is not included in TIBC, because it binds only stored iron. During iron overload, transferrin levels stay approximately the same or decrease, whereas the other less common iron-carrying proteins increase in number. In this situation, TIBC is less reflective of true transferrin levels. TIBC is increased in 70% of patients with iron deficiency.

Transferrin is a negative acute-phase reactant protein; therefore, in various acute inflammatory reactions, transferrin levels diminish. Transferrin levels are also diminished in patients with chronic illnesses such as malignancy, collagen-vascular diseases, or liver diseases. Hypoproteinemia is also associated with reduced transferrin levels. Pregnancy and estrogen therapy are associated with increased transferrin levels.

TIBC is usually measured by adding excess iron to the patient's serum. This saturates all the transferrin. The excess iron is then removed. The iron that is left is a direct measurement of TIBC and an indirect measurement of transferrin. Many laboratories do not perform TIBC measurements; in this case, transferrin is measured directly.

TIBC varies minimally with iron intake. TIBC is more a reflection of liver function (transferrin is produced by the liver) and nutrition than of iron metabolism. TIBC values often are used to monitor the course of patients receiving hyperalimentation.

TIBC and Transferrin Saturation

The percentage of transferrin and other mobile iron-binding proteins saturated with iron is calculated as the serum iron level divided by the TIBC:

$$\text{Transferrin saturation}\,(\%) = \frac{\text{Serum iron level} \times 100\%}{\text{TIBC}}$$

The normal value for transferrin saturation is 20% to 50%. Calculation of transferrin saturation is helpful in determining the cause of abnormal iron levels and TIBC. Transferrin saturation is decreased to below 15% in patients with iron-deficiency anemia. It is increased in patients with hemolytic, sideroblastic, or megaloblastic anemias and also in patients with iron overload or iron poisoning. Increased intake or absorption of iron (as in hemochromatosis) leads to elevations in iron levels. In such cases, the TIBC is unchanged; as a result, the percentage of transferrin saturation is very high.

Chronic illness (e.g., infections, neoplasia, cirrhosis) is characterized by a low serum iron level, decreased TIBC, and normal transferrin saturation. Pregnancy is characterized by high levels of protein, including transferrin. Because iron requirements are high, it is not unusual to find low serum iron levels, high TIBC, and a low percentage of transferrin saturation in late pregnancy.

CONTRAINDICATIONS

- Hemolytic diseases, because the iron content may be artificially high. The iron in the hemolyzed RBCs leaks out into the bloodstream.

INTERFERING FACTORS

- Recent blood transfusions may increase serum iron levels.
- Recent ingestion of a meal containing high iron content may increase serum iron levels.
- Hemolytic diseases may be associated with an artificially high iron content.
- Drugs that may cause *increases* in iron levels include chloramphenicol, dextran, estrogens, ethanol, iron preparations, methyldopa, and oral contraceptives.
- Drugs that may cause *decreases* in iron levels include adrenocorticotropic hormone (ACTH), cholestyramine, chloramphenicol, colchicine, deferoxamine, methicillin, and testosterone.
- Drugs that may cause *increases* in TIBC include fluorides and oral contraceptives.
- Drugs that may cause *decreases* in TIBC include ACTH and chloramphenicol.

PROCEDURE AND PATIENT CARE

Before

- Explain the procedure to the patient.
- Instruct the patient to fast for 12 hours before the blood test. Water is permitted during the fast.
- Assess the patient for a history of recent blood transfusion and recent meals high in iron content. Both may affect test results.

During

- Collect a venous blood sample in a red-top tube. The specimen should always be obtained by means of a 20-gauge or larger needle.
- Avoid hemolysis because the iron contained in the RBC will pour out into the serum and cause artificially high iron levels.

After

- Apply pressure or a pressure dressing to the venipuncture site.
- Assess the venipuncture site for bleeding.

TEST RESULTS AND CLINICAL SIGNIFICANCE

▲ Increased Serum Iron Levels

Hemosiderosis or hemochromatosis: *These two forms of iron deposits are created by serum iron excesses. They can be acquired or can result from a genetic defect in iron metabolism.*

Iron poisoning: *Increased iron intake increases serum iron levels.*

Hemolytic anemia: *The iron in the hemoglobin of the hemolyzed RBCs leaks out into the bloodstream.*

Massive blood transfusions: *There is approximately 1 mg of iron in each millilitre of packed RBCs.*

Hepatitis or hepatic necrosis: *The pathophysiologic mechanism underlying this observation is not well established.*

Lead toxicity: *The lead overload may displace the iron stores.*

▼ Decreased Serum Iron Levels

Insufficient dietary iron: *Because all body iron is from dietary intake, a persistent reduction in iron intake leads to reductions in serum levels.*

Chronic blood loss (irregular menses, uterine cancer, gastrointestinal cancer, inflammatory bowel disease, diverticulosis, urologic tract [hematuria] cancer, hemangioma, arteriovenous malformation): *Chronic blood loss depletes the iron because most of the iron in the body exists in the hemoglobin of the RBCs.*

Inadequate intestinal absorption of iron (e.g., malabsorption, short-bowel syndrome): *Because all body iron is from dietary intake, a persistent reduction in iron intake leads to reductions in serum levels.*

Pregnancy (late): *Fetal requirements deplete the mother's body store of iron.*

Iron-deficiency anemia: *This anemia results when iron and iron stores become depleted.*

Neoplasia: *Iron levels are depleted in these patients for several reasons.*

▲ Increased TIBC or Transferrin Levels

Estrogen therapy,

Pregnancy (late),

Polycythemia vera,

Iron-deficiency anemia: *The pathophysiologic mechanism underlying the observation in these conditions is not clear.*

▼ Decreased TIBC or Transferrin Levels

Malnutrition,

Hypoproteinemia: *Transferrin is a protein. Its levels can be expected to decrease as protein is depleted from the body.*

Inflammatory diseases,

Cirrhosis: *Transferrin is a negative acute-phase reactant protein; therefore, in various acute inflammatory reactions, transferrin levels diminish.*

Hemolytic anemia,

Pernicious anemia,

Sickle cell anemia: *These anemias are associated with elevations in iron levels and decreases in TIBC. The pathophysiologic mechanism underlying the latter is not clear.*

▲ Increased Transferrin Saturation or TIBC Saturation

Hemochromatosis or hemosiderosis,

Increased iron intake (oral or parenteral): *Increased iron levels saturate the transferrin.*

Hemolytic anemias: *The iron level is increased (see previous discussion). Increased iron levels saturate the transferrin.*

▼ **Decreased Transferrin Saturation or TIBC Saturation**

Iron-deficiency anemia,

Chronic illnesses (e.g., malignancy, other chronic illnesses): *Iron levels are low, and transferrin levels are increased.*

RELATED TEST

Ferritin (p. 248). This is a measure of iron stores and is the most accurate indicator of iron deficiency.

Ischemia-Modified Albumin (IMA)

NORMAL FINDINGS

<85 IU/mL

INDICATIONS

This test is performed on patients with chest pain to determine whether the pain is caused by cardiac ischemia.

TEST EXPLANATION

When albumin is exposed to an ischemic environment, its N-terminal is altered, which causes an alteration of the albumin called *ischemia-modified albumin* (IMA). The presence of IMA has become particularly helpful in identifying cardiac ischemia. When combined with troponin testing (p. 531), myoglobin testing (p. 378), and electrocardiography (p. 568), the diagnosis of an ischemic cardiac event can be corroborated or ruled out. IMA is produced continually during the period of ischemia. Blood levels appear and begin rising within 10 minutes of the initiation of the ischemic event and stay elevated for 6 hours after ischemia has resolved.

Normally, the N-terminal of albumin can easily bind heavy metals, such as cobalt. In contrast, IMA cannot bind cobalt. This distinction forms the basis for IMA testing. In the cobalt-binding test, cobalt is added to the patient's serum. Unbound cobalt levels are measured. Higher levels of unbound cobalt indicate greater concentrations of IMA, which in turn indicates the presence of cardiac ischemia.

IMA levels may also be elevated in patients with pulmonary embolus or acute stroke. False-positive findings can occur in other clinical circumstances such as advanced cancers, acute infections, and end-stage renal or liver disease.

PROCEDURE AND PATIENT CARE

Before

🖎 Explain the procedure to the patient.

🖎 Inform the patient that no food or fluid restrictions are required.

During

- Collect a venous blood sample in a yellow-top (serum separator) tube. This is usually done after the initial onset of chest pain, then 12 hours later, and then daily for 3 to 5 days.
- Rotate the venipuncture sites.

- On each laboratory slip, record the exact time and date of venipuncture. This aids in the interpretation of the temporal pattern of blood level elevations.

After
- Apply pressure or a pressure dressing to the venipuncture site.
- Observe the venipuncture site for bleeding.

TEST RESULTS AND CLINICAL SIGNIFICANCE

▲ Increased Levels
Myocardial ischemia,
Brain ischemia,
Pulmonary ischemia: *Myocardial ischemia produces free radicals that transform normal albumin into IMA.*

RELATED TESTS
Creatine Kinase (p. 201). Creatine phosphokinase MB levels are elevated early in myocardial injury. The usefulness of this finding is limited in patients who have had chest pain for more than 24 hours.

Myoglobin (p. 378). This protein is a nonspecific indicator of cardiac disease. However, it is also elevated with skeletal muscle disease or trauma.

Electrocardiography (p. 568). This is the electrical diagnostic test most commonly used to detect myocardial injury and infarction.

Troponins (p. 531). This test is a specific indicator of cardiac muscle injury. It is also helpful in predicting the possibility of future cardiac events.

 Lactate Dehydrogenase (LDH, Lactate Dehydrogenase)

NORMAL FINDINGS
Total Lactate Dehydrogenase Levels (serum)
Newborn: **160–450 IU/L** (160–450 U/L)
Infant: **100–250 IU/L** (100–250 U/L)
Child: **60–170 IU/L** (60–170 U/L)
Adult: **45–90 IU/L** (45–90 U/L)
>60 Years: **55–100 IU/L** (55–100 U/L)

Isoenzymes (Electrophoresis)
Adult/older adult:
  LDH-1: **0.17–0.27** (17%–27% of total)
  LDH-2: **0.27–0.37** (27%–37% of total)
  LDH-3: **0.18–0.25** (18%–25% of total)
  LDH-4: **0.03–0.08** (3%–8% of total)
  LDH-5: **0–0.05** (0%–5% of total)

INDICATIONS

Lactate dehydrogenase (LDH) is an intracellular enzyme used to support the diagnosis of injury or disease involving the heart, liver, red blood cells (RBCs), kidneys, skeletal muscle, brain, and lungs.

TEST EXPLANATION

LDH is found in the cells of many body tissues, especially the heart, liver, RBCs, kidneys, skeletal muscle, brain, and lungs. Because LDH is widely distributed through the body, the total LDH level is not a specific indicator of any one disease or of injury to any one organ. When disease or injury affects the cells containing LDH, the cells lyse and LDH is spilled into the bloodstream, in which it is identified in higher-than-normal levels. The blood LDH is a measure of total LDH. Actually, five separate fractions (isoenzymes) make up the total LDH. Each tissue contains a predominance of one or more LDH enzymes (Table 2-34).

The isoenzymes may be separated out by the use of electrophoresis or heat. When the blood specimen is heated to 60°C for 30 minutes, the heat-stable fractions 1 and 2 are separated out. Isoenzyme LDH-1 can also be detected by immunoassay, which is very accurate.

In general, isoenzyme LDH-1 is present mainly in the heart; LDH-2, primarily in the reticuloendothelial system; LDH-3, in the lungs and other tissues; LDH-4, in the kidneys, placenta, and pancreas; and LDH-5, mainly in the liver and striated muscle. In a healthy state, LDH-2 makes up the greatest percentage of total LDH.

Specific patterns of LDH isoenzymes are considered classic for certain diseases. For example:
- *Isolated elevation of LDH-1 level* (higher than LDH-2 level) indicates myocardial injury.
- *Isolated elevation of LDH-5 level* indicates hepatocellular injury or disease.
- *Elevation of LDH-2 and LDH-3 levels* indicates pulmonary injury or disease.
- *Elevation of all LDH* isoenzyme levels indicates multiorgan injury (e.g., myocardial infarction with heart failure, which cause pulmonary and hepatic congestion along with decreases in renal perfusion). Advanced malignancy and diffuse autoimmune inflammatory diseases such as lupus can also cause this pattern.

The serum LDH level rises within 24 to 48 hours after a myocardial infarction, peaks in 2 to 3 days, and returns to normal in approximately 5 to 10 days. Thus, the serum LDH level is especially useful in a delayed diagnosis of myocardial infarction (e.g., when the patient reports having had severe chest pain 4 days earlier). The LDH-1 level, of course, is a more sensitive and specific indicator of myocardial infarction than is the total LDH level. Its sensitivity alone is greater than 95%. The LDH-2 fraction level is normally higher than the LDH-1 fraction

TABLE 2-34 Lactate Dehydrogenase Isoenzymes in Tissue of Origin	
Tissue	**Lactate Dehydrogenase Isoenzyme**
Heart	1, 2
Red blood cell	1
Skeletal muscle	5
Lung	3, 2
Reticuloendothelial system	2
Kidney	4
Liver	5
Pancreas, placenta	4

level. Therefore, the normal ratio of LDH-1 to LDH-2 is less than 1. When the LDH-1 activity becomes greater than that of LDH-2, myocardial injury is strongly suspected. The reversal of the normal ratio is referred to as a "flipped LDH"; that is, the LDH-1/LDH-2 ratio of less than 1 is reversed. In acute myocardial infarction, the flipped LDH ratio usually appears in 12 to 24 hours and is present within 48 hours in approximately 80% of patients. When LDH-2 is greater than LDH-1 (a normal LDH-1/LDH-2 ratio), it is considered reliable evidence that myocardial infarction has not occurred. In the patient with chest pain because of angina only, the LDH is probably not elevated.

Clinical Priorities

- Because LDH is widely distributed throughout the body, the total LDH level is not a specific indicator of any disease or organ injury. Isoenzyme levels are more specific and helpful diagnostically.
- When LDH-1 level is greater than LDH-2 level, myocardial injury is strongly suspected. This situation may be referred to as a "flipped LDH."
- Isolated elevations of LDH-5 usually indicate hepatocellular injury or disease.
- Values vary markedly across the life span.

Of importance is that two diseases causing elevations in LDH levels may coexist and that one may obscure the other. For example, a patient who has one disease (e.g., pulmonary infarction or heart failure) may also be having an acute myocardial infarction. The elevation in LDH-1 level may be obscured by the elevation of LDH-2 or LDH-3 level. Some laboratories measure only the LDH-1 level by immunoassay. An elevated LDH level consisting of more than 40% LDH-1 is considered diagnostic of myocardial damage.

LDH is also measured in other body fluids. Elevated urine levels of total LDH indicate neoplasm or injury to the urologic system. When the LDH in an effusion (pleural, cardiac, peritoneal) is greater than 60% of the serum total LDH (i.e., ratio of effusion LDH to serum LDH > 0.6), the effusion is said to be an *exudate* and not a transudate.

INTERFERING FACTORS

- Hemolysis of blood causes the LDH to pour out of RBCs into the specimen blood and artificially elevate the LDH level.
- Strenuous exercise may cause elevation of total LDH and specifically LDH-1, LDH-2, and LDH-5 levels.
- Drugs that may cause *increases* in LDH levels include alcohol, anaesthetics, aspirin, clofibrate, fluorides, narcotics, and procainamide.
- Drugs that may cause *decreases* in LDH levels include ascorbic acid.

PROCEDURE AND PATIENT CARE

Before

- Explain the procedure to the patient.
- Inform the patient that no fasting is required.
- Inform the patient whether he or she will undergo frequent venipuncture for the evaluation of a myocardial infarction.

During

- Collect a venous blood sample in a red-top tube.
- On the laboratory slip, record the dates and times when blood was collected for an accurate evaluation of the temporal pattern of enzyme elevations.

After

- Apply pressure or a pressure dressing to the venipuncture site.
- Assess the venipuncture site for bleeding.

TEST RESULTS AND CLINICAL SIGNIFICANCE

▲ Increased Levels

Myocardial infarction: *Affected patients classically have significant elevations in levels of LDH-1 and, to a lesser degree, LDH-2.*

Pulmonary disease (e.g., embolism, infarction, pneumonia, heart failure): *Affected patients classically have significant elevations in LDH-2 and LDH-3 levels.*

Hepatic disease (e.g., hepatitis, active cirrhosis, neoplasm): *Affected patients classically have significant elevations in LDH-5 levels.*

RBC disease (e.g., hemolytic or megaloblastic anemia, RBC destruction from prosthetic heart valves): *Affected patients classically have significant elevations in LDH-1 levels.*

Skeletal muscle disease and injury (e.g., muscular dystrophy, recent strenuous exercises, muscular trauma): *Affected patients classically have significant elevations in LDH-5 levels.*

Renal parenchymal disease (e.g., infarction, glomerulonephritis, acute tubular necrosis, kidney transplant rejection): *Affected patients classically have significant elevations in LDH-1 levels.*

Intestinal ischemia and infarction: *Affected patients classically have significant elevations in LDH-5 levels.*

Neoplastic states,

Testicular tumours (seminoma, dysgerminomas): *Affected patients classically have significant elevations in LDH-1 levels.*

Lymphoma and other reticuloendothelial system (RES) tumours: *Affected patients classically have significant elevations in LDH-3 and LDH-2 levels.*

Advanced solid tumour malignancies: *Affected patients classically have significant elevations in levels of all LDH isoenzymes.*

Pancreatitis: *Affected patients classically have significant elevations in LDH-4 levels.*

Diffuse disease or injury (e.g., heat stroke, collagen disease, shock, hypotension): *Affected patients classically have significant elevations in levels of all LDH isoenzymes.*

RELATED TESTS

Aspartate Aminotransferase (p. 130), Gamma-Glutamyl Transpeptidase (p. 261), Alkaline Phosphatase (p. 53), and 5′-Nucleotidase (p. 389). These enzymes also exist predominantly in the liver.

Creatine Kinase (p. 201). Creatine phosphokinase is measured predominantly to evaluate heart and skeletal muscle.

Alanine Aminotransferase (p. 45). Measurement of this enzyme is similar to that of aspartate aminotransferase. This enzyme also exists predominantly in the liver.

Leucine Aminopeptidase (p. 351). This enzyme is specific to the hepatobiliary system. Diseases affecting that system cause elevation in levels of this enzyme.

Lactic Acid (Lactate)

NORMAL FINDINGS
Venous blood: **0.6–2.2 mmol/L** (5–20 mg/dL)
Arterial blood: **0.3–0.8 mmol/L** (3–7 mg/dL)

INDICATIONS
Measurement of lactic acid is helpful in documenting and quantifying the degree of tissue hypoxemia associated with shock or localized vascular occlusion. It is also a measurement of the success of treatment of those conditions.

TEST EXPLANATION
Under conditions of normal oxygen availability to tissues, glucose is metabolized to CO_2 and H_2O for energy. When oxygen to the tissues is diminished, anaerobic metabolism of glucose occurs, and lactate (lactic acid) is formed instead of CO_2 and H_2O. Compounding the problem of lactic acid buildup is that when the liver is hypoxic, it fails to clear the lactic acid. Lactic acid accumulates, causing lactic acidosis. Therefore, blood lactate level is a fairly sensitive and reliable indicator of tissue hypoxia. The hypoxia may be caused by local tissue hypoxia (e.g., mesenteric ischemia, extremity ischemia) or generalized tissue hypoxia (such as that which develops during shock). Lactic acid blood levels are used to document the presence of tissue hypoxia, determine the degree of hypoxia, and monitor the effect of therapy. Type I lactic acidosis is caused by diseases that increase lactate level but are not hypoxia related, such as glycogen storage diseases or liver diseases, or by drugs. Lactic acidosis resulting from hypoxia is classified as type II. Shock, convulsions, and extremity ischemia are the most common causes of type II lactic acidosis. Type III lactic acidosis is idiopathic and is most commonly observed in nonketotic patients with diabetes. The pathophysiologic mechanism underlying lactic acid accumulation in type III lactic acidosis is not known.

INTERFERING FACTORS
- The prolonged use of a tourniquet or clenching of hands increases lactate levels.
- Vigorous exercise can increase levels.
- Drugs that may *increase* lactic acid levels include aspirin, cyanide, ethanol, and nalidixic acid.

PROCEDURE AND PATIENT CARE
Before
- Explain the procedure to the patient.
- Inform the patient that no fasting is required.

During
- Instruct the patient to avoid clenching the hand before and while blood is being collected.
- Avoid the use of a tourniquet if possible.
- Collect a venous blood or arterial blood sample in a red-top tube.

After

- Apply pressure or a pressure dressing to the venipuncture site.
- Observe the venipuncture site for bleeding.

TEST RESULTS AND CLINICAL SIGNIFICANCE

▲ Increased Levels

Shock,

Tissue ischemia: *Anaerobic metabolism occurs in hypoxemic organs and tissues. As a result, lactic acid is formed, which causes increases in blood levels.*

Carbon monoxide poisoning: *Carbon monoxide binds hemoglobin more tightly than does oxygen. Therefore, no oxygen is available to the tissues for normal aerobic metabolism. Anaerobic metabolism occurs and lactic acid is formed, which results in increases in blood levels.*

Severe liver disease,

Genetic errors of metabolism: *Acquired and genetic diseases associated with inefficient aerobic glucose metabolism cause increased amounts of lactic acid to be synthesized. Therefore, blood levels rise.*

Diabetes mellitus (nonketotic): *Lactic acid levels rise in patients with poorly controlled diabetes probably because of inefficient aerobic glucose metabolism, which causes increased production of lactic acid.*

RELATED TEST

Arterial Blood Gases (p. 121). This is a measure of acid-base balance of the blood. An increased level of lactic acid is associated with metabolic acidosis.

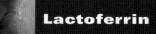

Lactoferrin

NORMAL FINDINGS

No lactoferrin detected

INDICATIONS

Lactoferrin is measured in order to diagnose inflammatory bowel diseases such as ulcerative colitis or Crohn's disease. It is also used as a screening test to determine the possibility of bacterial colitis.

TEST EXPLANATION

Lactoferrin is a glycoprotein expressed by activated neutrophils. The detection of lactoferrin in a fecal sample therefore serves as a surrogate marker for inflammatory white blood cells (WBCs) in the intestinal tract. WBCs in the stool are not stable and may be easily destroyed by temperature changes, delays in testing, and toxins within the stool. As a result, WBCs may not be detected by common microscopic methods. Lactoferrin assay has enabled the identification of inflammatory cells in the stool without the use of microscopy.

Detection of fecal lactoferrin allows for the differentiation of inflammatory and noninflammatory intestinal disorders in patients with diarrhea. Usually the test is used as a diagnostic aid to reveal active inflammatory bowel disease (such as Crohn's disease or ulcerative colitis) and rule out active irritable bowel syndrome, which is noninflammatory. Lactoferrin is also present in patients with bacterial enteritis such as that caused by *Shigella* organisms, *Salmonella* organisms, *Campylobacter jejuni,* and *Clostridium difficile.* Diarrhea caused by viruses and most parasites is not associated with elevations in lactoferrin levels. Lactoferrin testing is often used as a screening test for patients who may have bacterial enteritis. If the stool sample is negative for lactoferrin, it is unlikely that a stool culture will yield positive results.

The lactoferrin analyte may be qualitatively detected by two distinct methods: (1) a latex agglutination procedure (the most commonly used) and (2) a Microwell enzyme immunoassay procedure. The former method has been used primarily in the evaluation of patients with diagnoses of bacterial infectious gastroenteritis; the latter method was developed primarily as a diagnostic aid to distinguish between active inflammatory bowel disease and active noninflammatory irritable bowel syndrome.

INTERFERING FACTORS

- Delays in testing can interfere with test results: The stool specimen should be examined immediately. In some instances, a specific stool preservative–enteric transport media (Cary-Blair) can be used.
- Breast-feeding can affect test results: Because lactoferrin is a component of human breast milk, the test result is positive in breast-fed children and should not be used to evaluate neonates receiving breast milk. However, a human lactoferrin–specific antibody that does not cross-react with lactoferrin in cow's milk is used in the test.

PROCEDURE AND PATIENT CARE

Before
- Explain the procedure to the patient.
- Instruct the patient not to mix urine or toilet paper with the specimen.

During
- Stool is collected in a clean bedpan.
- Place at least 5 g of stool in a clean specimen container.

After
- Observe appropriate contamination precautions.
- Transfer the specimen to the laboratory immediately.
- Inform the patient that results are available in less than half an hour.

TEST RESULTS AND CLINICAL SIGNIFICANCE

Bacterial enteritis,
Acute Crohn's disease,
Acute ulcerative colitis: *Each of these diseases is associated with an inflammatory immune response of WBCs that causes positive lactoferrin results.*

RELATED TESTS

Stool Culture (p. 883). This test is used to identify the cause of bacterial enteritis.

Colonoscopy (p. 619). This is a commonly performed test to identify inflammatory bowel diseases such as ulcerative colitis and Crohn's disease.

Lactose Tolerance

NORMAL FINDINGS

Blood

Adult/older adult: rise in plasma glucose levels greater than **1.1 mmol/L** (20 mg/dL); no abdominal cramps or diarrhea

Breath

Higher than 50 ppm hydrogen increase over baseline

INDICATIONS

This test is used to identify patients who have lactose intolerance caused by lactase insufficiency, intestinal malabsorption, maldigestion, or bacterial overgrowth in the small intestine. This test is performed on adults who complain of diarrhea and in infants who have failure to thrive, persistent diarrhea, or vomiting.

TEST EXPLANATION

This test is performed to detect lactose intolerance. Lactose is a disaccharide typically found in dairy products; during digestion, lactose is broken down into glucose and galactose by the intestinal enzyme lactase. Because lactose-intolerant patients have an absence of lactase, lactose digestion does not occur. Likewise, patients with other causes of malabsorption or maldigestion also do not absorb lactose. Plasma glucose levels do not rise after ingestion of lactose, and the small bowel is flooded with a high lactose load. Bacterial catabolism of the lactose occurs within the intestine. This creates excess hydrogen ions and methane (flatus). It also has a strong cathartic effect. Symptoms of lactose intolerance include flatulence, abdominal cramping, abdominal bloating, diarrhea, and failure to thrive in infants. Although all adults have some degree of lactase reduction, severe lactose intolerance can occur in patients with inflammatory bowel disease, short-gut syndrome, and other malabsorption syndromes. Lactase deficiency can be congenital and become apparent in the newborn.

The incidence of primary lactose deficiency is higher than 50% in several ethnic groups, such as Mediterranean, Black African, and Asian populations. Northern European and North American white populations are the only groups generally able to maintain small-intestinal lactase activity throughout life.

In this test, a lactose load is given. If lactase is not present in sufficient quantities, lactose is not metabolized to glucose and galactose. Plasma levels of glucose do not rise as expected. Therefore, lower-than-expected serum glucose levels are suggestive of no absorption. In patients who have malabsorption without lactase deficiency, the blood glucose levels also fail to rise, not because the lactose was not broken down but because the glucose could not be absorbed. In these patients, the lactose tolerance test should be followed by a glucose tolerance test; that is, after a positive result of a lactose tolerance test, the patient returns and is given 25 g of a glucose/galactose preparation. A normal increase in glucose indicates that the patient can absorb glucose and that the problem is, indeed, lactase insufficiency.

There is also a breath assessment portion to this test in which the exhaled air is analyzed for hydrogen content. This is called the *lactose breath test* (or *hydrogen breath test*). The bacteria in the colon produce hydrogen when exposed to unabsorbed food, particularly the lactose-containing load that was not absorbed in the small intestine. Large amounts of hydrogen may also be produced when the colonic bacteria move back into the small intestine, a condition called *bacterial overgrowth of the small bowel.* In this instance, the bacteria are exposed to the lactose load, which has not had a chance to completely traverse the small intestine to be fully digested and absorbed. Large amounts of the hydrogen produced by the bacteria are absorbed into the blood flowing through the wall of the small intestine and colon. This hydrogen-containing blood travels to the lungs, where the hydrogen is released and exhaled in the breath in measurable quantities.

Before undergoing the lactose hydrogen breath test, individuals must fast for at least 12 hours. At the start of the test, the individual blows into a hydrogen analyzer. The individual then ingests a small amount of the test sugar (e.g., lactose, sucrose, sorbitol, fructose, or lactulose, depending on the purpose of the test). Additional samples of breath are collected and analyzed for hydrogen every 15 minutes for 1 to 5 hours. When intestinal transit is rapid, the test dose of nondigestible lactulose reaches the colon more quickly than normal, and therefore hydrogen is produced by the colonic bacteria soon after the sugar is ingested. When bacterial overgrowth of the small bowel is present, ingestion of lactulose results in two separate periods during the test in which hydrogen is produced: an earlier period caused by the bacteria in the small intestine and a later one caused by the bacteria in the colon.

INTERFERING FACTORS

- Enterogenous steatorrhea (i.e., malabsorption) diminishes absorption of glucose from the gut even if the lactose is broken down by normal levels of lactase.
- Strenuous exercise reduces the glucose levels and possibly leads to a false-positive result.
- Diabetic patients may have a rise in glucose levels that exceed **1 mmol/L** (20 mg/dL) despite lactase insufficiency.
- Smoking may increase blood glucose levels and lead to false-positive results.
- Ethnicity has a major effect on primary lactose deficiency.
- Antibiotics can *decrease* the bacteria in the intestine and may lead to false-negative breath test results. They should not be taken for 1 month before the test.

Age-Related Concerns

- Lactase deficiency may be the cause of vomiting, diarrhea, malabsorption, and failure to thrive in infants.
- Although older adults often have some degree of lactase reduction, severe lactose intolerance can occur in older patients with inflammatory bowel diseases and other malabsorption syndromes.

PROCEDURE AND PATIENT CARE

Before

 Explain the procedure to the patient. Inform the patient that four blood samples will be needed.

 Instruct the patient to fast for 8 hours before the test or as ordered by the physician.

Instruct the patient to avoid strenuous exercise for 8 hours before the test because it may factitiously affect the blood glucose level.

 Inform the patient that smoking is prohibited the day of the test. This may artificially increase the blood glucose level.

During

- Obtain a venous blood sample in a grey-top tube from the fasting patient.
- Provide a specified dose of lactose for the patient. Usually 100 g of lactose is diluted with 200 mL of water for ingestion by adults.
- Pediatric doses of lactose are based on weight.
- Collect three more blood samples 30, 60, and 120 minutes after the ingestion of lactose.

 Inform the patient that the only discomfort is the venipuncture; however, patients with lactase deficiency will have the symptoms previously described.

- If the breath test is being done, the exhaled air is evaluated for hydrogen content before ingestion of lactose and every 15 minutes thereafter. Hydrogen levels are recorded for 2 hours.

After

- Apply pressure or a pressure dressing to the venipuncture site.
- Observe the venipuncture site for bleeding.
- Note that patients with abnormal test results may require a monosaccharide tolerance test (e.g., glucose or galactose tolerance test).

TEST RESULTS AND CLINICAL SIGNIFICANCE

▼ Decreased Levels

Lactase insufficiency: *Lactase quantities are insufficient to break down the lactose load. Glucose is not absorbed, and serum glucose levels do not rise.*

Enterogenous diarrhea: *Despite normal breakdown of lactose, the glucose is not absorbed because of malabsorption disease of the gut. Serum glucose levels do not rise.*

RELATED TEST

Glucose Tolerance (p. 276). This test is used to assist in the diagnosis of diabetes mellitus. It is also used in the evaluation of patients with hypoglycemia. Because it differentiates the lactase-deficient patient from the patient with enterogenous malabsorption diarrhea, this test is helpful in the evaluation of patients suspected of having lactose intolerance.

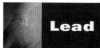

NORMAL FINDINGS

<0.48 mmol/L (<10 *Mcg*/dL)

❗ Critical Values

Pediatrics (≤15 years): ≥0.97 *Mcmol*/L (≥20 *Mcg*/dL)
Adults (≥16 years): ≥3.38 *Mcmol*/L (≥70 *Mcg*/dL)

INDICATIONS

This test is used to identify and monitor lead poisoning.

TEST EXPLANATION

Lead found in the environment is a heavy metal toxin. Although lead is now banned from household paints, it is still found in paint used before 1980. Lead is found in soil from areas adjacent to homes painted with lead-based paints. Water transported through lead or lead-soldered pipe will contain some lead, with higher concentrations found in water that is weakly acidic.

Lead inhibits aminolevulinic acid dehydratase and ferrochelatase, both of which catalyze synthesis of heme. The result is decreased hemoglobin synthesis and anemia. Lead also is an electrophile that avidly forms covalent bonds with the sulfhydryl group of cysteine in proteins. Thus proteins in all tissues exposed to lead will have lead bound to them. The most common sites affected are epithelial cells of the gastrointestinal tract and epithelial cells of the proximal tubule of the kidney. The brain is also a common depository for excess lead.

Signs and symptoms in adults may include a decline in mental status, muscle weakness, headaches, memory loss, mood disorders, and miscarriage or premature birth in pregnant women. Children may demonstrate irritability, anorexia, weight loss, and learning difficulties.

Lead poisoning is a preventable condition that results from environmental exposure to lead. This exposure, indicated by elevated blood lead levels, can result in permanent damage of almost all parts of the body. However, its effects are most pronounced on the central nervous system and kidneys, causing symptoms ranging from mild learning disabilities and behavioural problems to encephalopathy. Children less than 6 years of age are the most likely to be exposed and affected by lead. Blood lead levels are the best test for detecting and evaluating recent acute and chronic exposure. Blood lead samples are used to screen for exposure and to monitor the effectiveness of treatment. Lead in the human body can also be measured in blood, urine, bones, teeth, or hair. Blood tests are usually performed. Lead assay is performed on a quantitative inductively coupled plasma-mass spectrometer (hematofluorometry). If one test is elevated, it should be repeated.

At critically high levels, immediate medical evaluation is recommended and chelation therapy is considered when symptoms of lead toxicity are present. Although blood lead has the highest correlation with lead poisoning, lead can be detected in the urine, nails, and hair. These other specimens are used to corroborate blood analysis or document past lead exposure. If the hair is collected and segmented in a time sequence (based on length from root), the approximate time of exposure can be assessed.

PROCEDURE AND PATIENT CARE

Before

- Explain the procedure to the patient.
- Tell the patient that no fasting is required.

During

- Collect a venous blood in a royal blue–top tube. A tan-top (lead only) Becton-Dickinson tube can be used.
- A fingerstick can be performed to obtain nearly 1 mL of blood.
- In addition to the venous blood sample or the fingerstick, a few millilitres of EDTA whole blood can be collected.
- Usually the blood sample is sent to a central diagnostic laboratory. The results are available to the local hospital in 7 to 10 days.

After

• Apply pressure to the venipuncture site.

TEST RESULTS AND CLINICAL SIGNIFICANCE

Lead exposure: *This heavy metal still presents a risk of poisoning to inner-city children living near aging interior paint and lead water pipes.*

RELATED TESTS

Zinc Protoporphyrin (p. 557). This test is used to screen for lead poisoning.

Legionnaires' Disease Antibody

NORMAL FINDINGS

No *Legionella* antibody titre

INDICATIONS

This test is indicated in patients suspected to have legionnaires' disease and who have negative cultures and smears identifying *Legionella* infection.

TEST EXPLANATION

Legionnaires' disease was originally described as a fulminating pneumonia caused by *Legionella pneumophila,* a tiny, Gram-negative, rod-shaped bacterium. Nearly 50% of the clinical cases have been caused by serogroup type 1. This organism can also cause an influenza-like illness called *Pontiac fever.*

The diagnosis of legionnaires' disease can be made by culturing this organism from suspected infected fluid, such as blood, sputum, or pleural fluid, or from lung tissue. Sputum for this test is best obtained by transtracheal aspiration or from bronchial washings. However, growing this organism in culture is difficult. A negative culture result does not mean that the patient does not have legionnaires' disease. Another method of diagnosis is by directly identifying the organism in a microscopic smear of infected fluid with the use of direct fluorescent antibody methods. If positive, this allows for rapid identification of *Legionella* infection. However, this also is difficult because the concentration may not be high enough that the bacterium in the specimen is visible.

The most common and easiest method for diagnosis is detection of the antibody directed against the *Legionella* bacterium in the patient's blood. This is performed if the culture or direct fluorescent test results are negative. The indirect fluorescent antibody assay or enzyme-linked immunosorbent assay (ELISA) methods are commonly used. A presumptive diagnosis of legionnaires' disease can be made in a symptomatic person when a single antibody titre is 1:256 or higher. Another way to make the diagnosis is to perform the antibody test 1 and 3 weeks after the onset of symptoms. A fourfold rise in titre to at least 1:128 between the acute (1 week) and the convalescent (3 week) phases is diagnostic. Unfortunately, it may take 4 to 6 weeks for serologic tests to yield positive results. The patient would be seriously ill by then. *Legionella* antigens in the urine may be identified a few days after the onset of the clinical symptoms, but the sensitivity is very low (~30%).

PROCEDURE AND PATIENT CARE

Before

☒ Explain the procedure to the patient.
☒ Inform the patient that no fasting is required.

During

• Collect a venous blood sample in a red-top tube.

After

• Apply pressure or a pressure dressing to the venipuncture site.
• Observe the venipuncture site for bleeding.

TEST RESULTS AND CLINICAL SIGNIFICANCE

▲ Increased Levels

Legionnaires' disease

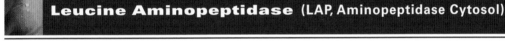

Leucine Aminopeptidase (LAP, Aminopeptidase Cytosol)

NORMAL FINDINGS

Blood

Male: **19.2–48.0 U/L** (80–200 U/mL)
Female: **18.0–44.4 U/L** (75–185 U/mL)

Urine

2–18 U/24 hr

INDICATIONS

This test is used for diagnosing liver disorders. It aids in the differential diagnosis for patients with high levels of alkaline phosphatase.

TEST EXPLANATION

Leucine aminopeptidase (LAP) is an intracellular enzyme that exists in the hepatobiliary system and, to a much smaller degree, in the pancreas and the small intestine. When disease or injury affects those organs, the cells lyse, and LAP is spilled into the bloodstream. Produced almost exclusively by the liver, LAP measurements are used in diagnosing liver disorders and in the differential diagnosis of increased levels of alkaline phosphatase. LAP levels tend to parallel alkaline phosphatase levels in hepatic disease. LAP is a sensitive indicator of cholestasis; however, unlike alkaline phosphatase levels, LAP levels remain normal in bone disease. LAP can be detected in both the blood and the urine. Patients with elevated serum LAP levels exhibit elevations in urine levels. When the urine LAP level is elevated, however, the blood level may have already returned to normal.

Levels of this enzyme were originally thought to be elevated during pregnancy and thus to serve as an indication of the viability of the fetal-placental unit. However, the enzyme found in pregnancy is immunochemically different from LAP.

INTERFERING FACTORS

- Pregnancy may cause increases in LAP values if LAP is tested by the enzyme method. Although there is not a quantitative increase in the "LAP-like" enzyme, its activity is increased. This causes an artificial increase in the LAP level on the enzyme test.
- Drugs that may cause *increases* in LAP levels include estrogens and progesterones.

PROCEDURE AND PATIENT CARE

Before

- Explain the procedure to the patient.
- Inform the patient that no fasting is required.

During

- Collect 7 to 10 mL of venous blood in a red-top tube.
- If a urine sample is needed, follow the procedure for a 24-hour urine collection (see p. 938).

After

- Apply pressure or a pressure dressing to the venipuncture site.
- Assess the venipuncture site for bleeding. Patients with liver dysfunction often have prolonged clotting times.

TEST RESULTS AND CLINICAL SIGNIFICANCE

▲ Increased Levels

Hepatobiliary disease (e.g., hepatitis, cirrhosis, hepatic necrosis, hepatic ischemia, hepatic tumour, hepatotoxic drugs, cholestasis, gallstones): *LAP is an enzyme that exists in the liver and biliary cells. Disease or injury of these tissues causes the cells to lyse. LAP spills into the bloodstream, and levels rise.*

RELATED TESTS

Creatine Kinase (p. 201). Creatine phosphokinase is measured in a similar manner as aspartate aminotransferase, and it exists predominantly in heart and skeletal muscle.

Alanine Aminotransferase (p. 45). This enzyme is also measured in a similar manner as AST, and it exists predominantly in the liver.

Lactate Dehydrogenase (p. 339). This is an intracellular enzyme whose measurements are used to support the diagnosis of injury or disease involving the heart, liver, red blood cells (RBCs), kidneys, skeletal muscle, brain, and lungs.

Aspartate Aminotransferase (p. 130), Gamma-Glutamyl Transpeptidase (p. 261), Alkaline Phosphatase (p. 53), and 5′-Nucleotidase (p. 389). These enzymes also exist predominantly in the liver.

NORMAL FINDINGS
0–160 U/L (values are method dependent)

INDICATIONS
This test is used in the evaluation of pancreatic disease.

TEST EXPLANATION
The most common cause of an elevated serum lipase level is acute pancreatitis. Lipase is an enzyme secreted by the pancreas into the duodenum to break down triglycerides into fatty acids. Like amylase, lipase appears in the bloodstream after damage to or disease affecting the pancreatic acinar cells.

Because lipase was thought to be produced only in the pancreas, elevated serum levels were considered to be specific to pathologic pancreatic conditions. It is now apparent that other conditions can be associated with elevations in lipase levels. Lipase is excreted through the kidneys; therefore, lipase levels are often elevated in patients with renal failure. Intestinal infarction or obstruction also can be associated with elevation in lipase levels. However, these elevations in nonpancreatic diseases are lower than 3 times the upper limit of normal, in comparison with pancreatitis, in which they are often 5 to 10 times higher than normal values. Other conditions such as cholangitis, mumps, cholecystitis, or peptic ulcer are more rarely associated with elevations in lipase levels.

In acute pancreatitis, elevations in lipase levels usually parallel those of serum amylase levels. The lipase levels usually rise a little later than amylase levels (24 to 48 hours after the onset of pancreatitis) and remain elevated for 5 to 7 days. Because they peak later and remain elevated longer than the serum amylase levels, serum lipase levels are more useful in the late diagnosis of acute pancreatitis. Lipase levels are less informative in more chronic pancreatic diseases (e.g., chronic pancreatitis, pancreatic carcinoma).

INTERFERING FACTORS
 Drugs that may cause *increases* in lipase levels include bethanechol, cholinergics, codeine, indomethacin, meperidine, methacholine, and morphine.
 Drugs that may cause *decreases* in lipase levels include calcium ions.

Clinical Priorities

- This test is useful in evaluating pancreatitis. Lipase elevations are often 5 to 10 times higher than normal values in pancreatitis.
- In acute pancreatitis, elevations in lipase levels usually parallel those of serum amylase levels. Because lipase levels peak later and remain elevated longer than amylase levels, they are more useful in the late diagnosis of acute pancreatitis.

PROCEDURE AND PATIENT CARE

Before

- Explain the procedure to the patient.
- Instruct the patient to remain on NPO status (nothing by mouth), except for water, for 8 to 12 hours before the test.

During

- Collect a venous blood sample in a red-top tube.

After

- Apply pressure or a pressure dressing to the venipuncture site.
- Observe the venipuncture site for bleeding.

TEST RESULTS AND CLINICAL SIGNIFICANCE

▲ Increased Levels

Pancreatic diseases (e.g., acute pancreatitis, chronic relapsing pancreatitis, pancreatic cancer, pancreatic pseudocyst): *Lipase exists in the pancreatic cell and is released into the bloodstream when disease or injury affects the pancreas.*

Biliary diseases (e.g., acute cholecystitis, cholangitis, extrahepatic duct obstruction): *Although the pathophysiologic mechanism underlying these observations is not well understood, it is suspected that lipase exists inside the cells of the hepatobiliary system. Disease or injury of these tissues causes the lipase to leak into the bloodstream and causes levels to be elevated.*

Renal failure: *Lipase is excreted by the kidneys. If excretion is poor, as in renal failure, lipase levels rise.*

Intestinal diseases (e.g., bowel obstruction, infarction): *Lipase exists in the mucosal cells lining the bowel (mostly in the duodenum). Injury through obstruction or ischemia causes the cells to lyse. Lipase leaks into the bloodstream, and levels rise.*

Salivary gland inflammation or tumour: *Like amylase, lipase exists in salivary glands, although to a much lesser degree. Tumours, inflammation, and obstruction of salivary ducts cause the cells to lyse. Lipase leaks into the bloodstream, and levels rise.*

Peptic ulcer disease: *The pathophysiologic mechanism underlying this observation is not well understood. In perforated peptic disease, the lipase in the gastrointestinal contents leaks into the peritoneum, where it is picked up by the bloodstream. Lipase levels rise.*

RELATED TEST

Amylase, Blood (p. 67). Amylase is another enzyme produced specifically in the pancreas. Disease affecting the pancreas also cause elevations in levels of this enzyme.

Lipoproteins (High-Density Lipoproteins [HDL, HDL-C], Low-Density Lipoproteins [LDL, LDL-C], Very-Low-Density Lipoproteins [VLDL], Lipoprotein Electrophoresis, Lipoprotein Phenotyping, Lipid Fractionation, Non-HDL Cholesterol)

NORMAL FINDINGS

High-Density Lipoprotein Levels

Adult: >0.91 mmol/L (<35 mg/dL)
  Low level/high risk: <0.91 mmol/L (<35 mg/dL)
  High level/low risk: ≥1.55 mmol/L (≥60 mg/dL)

Low-Density Lipoprotein Levels

Adult:
  Optimal: <3.4 mmol/L (<130 mg/dL)
  Near or above optimal: 2.59–3.34 mmol/L (100–129 mg/dL)
  Borderline high: 3.37–4.11 mmol/L (130–159 mg/dL)
  High: 4.14–4.90 mmol/L (160–189 mg/dL)
  Very high: ≥4.92 mmol/L (≥190 mg/dL)
Child: <2.85 mmol/L (<110 mg/dL)

Very-Low-Density Lipoprotein Levels

0.18–0.83 mmol/L (7–32 mg/dL)

INDICATIONS

Lipoproteins are considered accurate predictors of heart disease. As part of the lipid profile, these tests are performed to identify individuals at risk for developing heart disease and to monitor therapy if abnormalities are found (Box 2-8).

BOX 2-8	Blood Tests Used to Assess Risk for Coronary Vascular Disease

- Total cholesterol
- High-density cholesterol
- Low-density cholesterol
- Triglycerides
- Apolipoprotein B
- Lipoprotein (a)
- Apolipoprotein E genotyping
- Fibrinogen
- C-reactive protein
- Homocysteine
- Insulin, fasting

TEST EXPLANATION

Lipoproteins are proteins in the blood whose main purpose is to transport cholesterol, triglycerides, and other insoluble fats. They are measured as markers to indicate the levels of lipids within the bloodstream. Lipoproteins can be classified by their measured density.

General categories of lipoproteins, listed in order from larger and less dense (more fat than protein) to smaller and denser (more protein, less fat) are as follows:

- Chylomicrons: These carry triacylglycerol (fat) from the intestines to the liver, skeletal muscle, and adipose tissue.
- Very-low-density lipoproteins (VLDL): These carry (newly synthesized) triacylglycerol from the liver to adipose tissue.
- Intermediate-density lipoproteins (IDL): These are intermediate in size and density between VLDL and LDL. They are not usually detectable in the blood.
- Low-density lipoproteins (LDL): These carry cholesterol from the liver to cells of the body. They are sometimes referred to as the "bad cholesterol" lipoprotein.
- High-density lipoproteins (HDL): These collect cholesterol from the body's tissues (and vascular endothelium) and bring it back to the liver. Removing lipids from the endothelium (reverse cholesterol transport) provides protection against heart disease. Therefore, HDL is referred to as the "good cholesterol" lipoprotein.

The "lipid profile" usually includes measurements of total cholesterol (discussed separately on p. 169), triglycerides, HDL, LDL, and VLDL. Through the use of segmented gradient gel electrophoresis, lipoproteins can be subclassified to more accurately indicate cardiovascular risks and familial risks of heart disease. Levels of lipoproteins are genetically influenced; however, these levels can be altered by diet, lifestyle, and medications.

Clinical and epidemiologic studies have shown that total HDL cholesterol is an independent, inverse risk factor for coronary artery disease. Low levels (<1.036 mmol/L [<40 mg/dL]) are believed to increase a person's risk for coronary artery disease, whereas high levels (>1.55 mmol/L [>60 mg/dL]) are considered protective. When HDL and total cholesterol measurements are considered in a ratio (Table 2-35), the accuracy of predicting coronary artery disease is increased. The total cholesterol/HDL ratio should be at least 5:1; 3:1 is ideal.

Segmented gradient gel electrophoresis identified five subclasses of HDL (HDL-2a, -2b, -3a, -3b, and -3c), but only HDL-2b is cardioprotective. HDL-2b is the most efficient form of HDL in reverse cholesterol transport. Patients with low total HDL levels often have low levels of HDL-2b.

TABLE 2-35	Risk for Coronary Heart Disease According to Ratio of Cholesterol to High-Density Lipoproteins		
		RATIO OF TOTAL CHOLESTEROL TO HIGH-DENSITY LIPOPROTEINS	
Risk for Coronary Heart Disease		**Male**	**Female**
One-half average		3.4	3.3
Average		5.0	4.4
Two times average (moderate)		10.0	7.0
Three times average (high)		24.0	11.0

Data from Grundy, S. M., Cleeman, J. I., Merz, C. N., Brewer, H. B. Jr., Clark, L. T., Hunninghake, D. B., et al. (2004). Implications of recent clinical trials for the National Cholesterol Education Program Adult Treatment Panel III Guidelines. *Circulation, 110*(2), 227–239; and from Hackam, D. G., & Anand, S. S. (2004). Emerging risk factors for atherosclerotic vascular disease. *Journal of the American Medical Association, 290*(7), 932–940.

When levels of total HDL are between 40 and 60, cardioprotective levels of HDL-2b are minimal. However, when levels of total HDL are greater than 60, levels of HDL-2b predominate, and efficient reverse cholesterol transport takes place. This protects the coronary arteries from disease. The other subclasses of HDL are not capable of reverse cholesterol transport and therefore are not cardioprotective. Levels of HDL-2b can be increased by niacin supplements but not by statins (i.e., 3-hydroxymethyl-3-methylglutaryl–coenzyme A [HMG-CoA] reductase inhibitors [simvastatin, lovastatin]).

LDLs ("bad" cholesterol) are also cholesterol rich. However, most cholesterol carried by LDLs can be deposited into the lining of the blood vessels and is associated with an increased risk for arteriosclerotic heart and peripheral vascular disease. Therefore, high levels of LDLs are atherogenic. Target LDL levels vary according to the risk profile of the patient (Table 2-36). For example, the LDL cholesterol goal for persons with multiple (two or more) risk factors is less than 3.37 mmol/L (<130 mg/dL).

The LDL level can be calculated with a modified Friedwald formula:

$$LDL = \text{Total cholesterol level} - \left(\left[\text{Triglyceride level} \div 5\right] - \text{HDL level}\right)$$

TABLE 2-36 National Cholesterol Education Program Therapy 2011 Guidelines for LDL Cholesterol Goals and Cutpoints for Therapeutic Lifestyle Changes and Drug Therapy

Risk Category	LDL-C GOAL mmol/L	(mg/dL)	INITIATE TLC mmol/L	(mg/dL)	CONSIDER DRUG THERAPY mmol/L	(mg/dL)
High risk: CHD (10-year risk: >20%)	<2.59	(<100)	≥2.59	(≥100)	≥3.367	(130)
Drug therapy optional					2.59–3.34	(100–129)
Moderately high risk: 2+ risk factors (10-year risk: ≤20%)	<3.37	(<130)	≥3.37	(≥130)	≥3.37*	(≥130)*
Moderate risk: 2+ risk factors (10-year risk: <10%)	<3.37	(<130)	≥3.37	(≥130)	≥4.14	(≥160)
Lower risk: 0–1 risk factor	<4.14	(<160)	≥4.14	(≥160)	≥4.92	(≥190)
Drug therapy optional					4.24–4.89	(160–189)

Risk factors: cigarette smoking, hypertension, low levels of high-density lipoprotein (HDL) cholesterol, family history, and age. Ten-year risk: Data used to estimate risk for CHD (age, gender, HDL cholesterol, total cholesterol, systolic blood pressure, use of blood pressure medications) is from the Framingham Heart Study, a project of the National Heart, Lung and Blood Institute and Boston University.
CHD, Coronary heart disease; *LDL*, low-density lipoprotein; *LDL-C*, low density lipoprotein cholesterol; *TLC*, therapeutic lifestyle changes (reduced intake of saturated fats and cholesterol, drug therapy, increased fibre, weight reduction, and increased physical activity).
*10-year risk 10%–20%.

There are other formulas for deriving LDL, which may account for different sets of normal values. The calculations are inaccurate if the triglyceride levels exceed **10.36 mmol/L** (400 mg/dL). Laboratory chromogenic methods in which various detergents are used to separate out LDL allow for a more accurate measurement of LDL. In these methods, a unique detergent is used to solubilize only the non-LDL particles, and a second detergent solubilizes the remaining LDL particles, which are then measured by a chromogenic coupler that provides colour formation.

With the use of segmented gradient gel electrophoresis, LDL has been divided into seven classes on the basis of particle size. These subclasses include (from largest to smallest) LDL-I, LDL-IIa, LDL-IIb, LDL-IIIa, LDL-IIIb, LDL-IVa, and LDL-IVb. The most commonly elevated forms of LDL (LDL-IIIa and LDL-IIIb) are small enough to become inserted between the endothelial cells and cause atheromatous disease. The larger LDL particles (LDL-I, LDL-IIa, and LDL-IIb) cannot be inserted into the endothelial layer and therefore are not associated with increased risk for disease. LDL-IVa and LDL-IVb, however, are very small and are associated with aggressive arterial plaques that are particularly vulnerable to ulceration and vascular occlusion. Nearly all patients in whom LDL-IVa and LDL-IVb are found to constitute more than 10% of total LDL have vascular events within months.

LDL patterns can be identified, and they are associated with variable risks of coronary artery disease. LDL pattern A is observed in patients with mostly large LDL particles and does not carry increased risks for coronary artery disease. LDL pattern B is observed in patients with mostly small LDL particles and is associated with an increased risk for coronary artery disease. An intermediate pattern is noted in a large number of patients; they have small and large LDL particles and have an intermediate risk for coronary artery disease. LDL levels in such patients can be lowered with diet, exercise, and statins.

VLDLs, although carrying a small amount of cholesterol, are the predominant carriers of blood triglycerides. To a lesser degree, VLDLs are also associated with an increased risk for coronary artery disease because they can be converted to LDL by lipoprotein lipase in skeletal muscle. The VLDL value is sometimes expressed as a percentage of total cholesterol. Levels in excess of 25% to 50% are associated with increased risk for coronary disease.

The Adult Treatment Panel III of the National Cholesterol Education Program issued an evidence-based set of guidelines on cholesterol management. The goal for patients at high risk for major coronary events (those with known coronary artery disease or more than two risk factors) is an LDL level lower than **3.37 mmol/L** (<130 mg/dL). All Adult Treatment Panel reports have identified LDL cholesterol as the primary target of cholesterol-lowering therapy. Many prospective studies have shown that high serum concentrations of LDL cholesterol are a major risk factor for coronary heart disease (CHD). Moreover, lowering LDL cholesterol levels reduces the risk for major coronary events.

The World Health Organization adopted the Fredrickson classification of lipid disorders to identify particular lipoprotein patterns (phenotypes) that are associated with certain inherited or acquired diseases or syndromes. Fredrickson's classification (Table 2-37), through the use of electrophoresis, simply identifies which lipoproteins are raised.

Various methods are used to measure the lipoprotein classes. All require serum separation, usually by ultracentrifugation. In the past, lipoproteins were measured through the use of electrophoresis. Immunologic, catalase reagent, and chemical kits are now available for accurately quantifying lipoproteins.

INTERFERING FACTORS
- Smoking and alcohol ingestion decrease HDL levels.
- Binge eating can alter lipoprotein values.
- HDL values are dependent on age and sex.

TABLE 2-37   Primary Hyperlipidemias*

Class	Elevated Lipoprotein Level	Associated Clinical Disorders
I	Chylomicrons	Lipoprotein lipase deficiency, apolipoprotein CII deficiency, uncontrolled diabetes mellitus
IIa	LDL	Familial hypercholesterolemia, nephrosis, hypothyroidism, familial combined hyperlipidemia
IIb	LDL, VLDL	Familial combined hyperlipidemia
III	Intermediate-density lipoproteins	Dysbetalipoproteinemia, diabetes mellitus, alcoholism
IV	VLDL	Familial hypertriglyceridemia, familial combined hyperlipidemia, diabetes mellitus
V	Chylomicrons, VLDL	Diabetes, nephrosis, malnutrition

LDL, Low-density lipoprotein; *VLDL,* very-low-density lipoprotein.
*Fredrickson classification, adopted by the World Health Organization.

- HDL values, like cholesterol values, tend to decrease significantly for as long as 3 months after myocardial infarction.
- HDL values are elevated in patients with hypothyroidism and diminished in those with hyperthyroidism.
- High triglyceride levels can render LDL calculations inaccurate.
- Drugs that may cause alterations in lipoprotein levels include the following:
  - Beta blockers: increase triglyceride levels, decrease HDL cholesterol level, decrease LDL size, decrease HDL-2b level
  - Alpha-blockers: decrease triglyceride levels, increase HDL cholesterol level, increase LDL size, increase HDL-2b level
  - Dilantin: increases HDL cholesterol
  - Steroids: in general, increase triglyceride levels
  - Estrogens: increase triglyceride levels

Clinical Priorities

- Lipoproteins are considered to be predictors of heart disease. Blood levels should be collected after a 12- to 14-hour fast.
- HDL is often called "good cholesterol" because it removes cholesterol from the tissues and transports it to the liver for excretion. High levels are associated with a decreased risk for coronary heart disease.
- LDL is often called "bad cholesterol" because it carries cholesterol and deposits it into the peripheral tissues. High levels are associated with an increased risk for CHD.

Age-Related Concerns

Older adults (men older than 65 years and women older than 75 years) are at higher risk for developing CHD than are people in younger age groups. High LDL and low HDL levels can still predict the risk for developing CHD, but noninvasive testing for atherosclerosis can help confirm the presence of higher risk in older persons. For primary prevention, therapeutic lifestyle change is still the first line of therapy; however, LDL-lowering drugs can be considered when older persons are at a higher risk because of multiple risk factors of the presence of atherosclerosis.

Blood Studies

2

Cultural Considerations

According to the Canadian Ontario Survey on the Prevalence and Control of Hypertension (ON-BP), individuals of South Asian descent and Black individuals are three times more likely to be hypertensive than the general population and are more likely to develop CHD at a younger age. This study was the first Canadian population–based study to measure blood pressures and to determine hypertension rates among some of the most common ethnic groups in Canada (South Asians, East Asians, and Blacks). Black American individuals also have the highest overall CHD mortality rate and the highest rate of out-of-hospital coronary deaths of any ethnic group in the United States. Although the reasons for this are not clear, they can be attributed in part to a high prevalence of CHD risk factors such as hypertension, diabetes, smoking, obesity, and physical inactivity. Although the baseline risk for CHD varies somewhat in this group, the general recommendations for cholesterol management are no different from those for the general population.

PROCEDURE AND PATIENT CARE

Before
🖎 Instruct the patient to fast for 12 to 14 hours before the test. Only water is permitted during the fast.
🖎 Inform the patient that dietary indiscretion within the previous few weeks may influence lipoprotein levels.

During
• Collect a venous blood sample in a red-top tube.

After
• Apply pressure or a pressure dressing to the venipuncture site.
• Observe the venipuncture site for bleeding.
🖎 Instruct patients with high lipoprotein levels about diet, exercise, and appropriate body weight.

TEST RESULTS AND CLINICAL SIGNIFICANCE

▲ Increased HDL Levels
Familial HDL lipoproteinemia: *Affected patients are genetically predisposed toward having high HDL levels.*
Excessive exercise: *HDL levels can rise with chronic exercise for 30 minutes three times a week. When the exercise greatly exceeds that minimum, HDL levels can become significantly elevated.*

▼ Decreased HDL Levels
Metabolic syndrome: *This syndrome is associated with an atherogenic lipid profile that includes decreased HDL level, increased triglyceride levels, elevated fasting glucose level, high blood pressure, and abdominal obesity as measured by waist circumference.*
Familial low HDL: *Affected patients are genetically predisposed toward having low HDL levels. As a result, these patients are at high risk for CHD.*
Hepatocellular disease (e.g., hepatitis, cirrhosis): HDL is made in the liver. Without liver function, HDL is not made, and levels fall.
Hypoproteinemia (e.g., nephrotic syndrome, malnutrition): *With loss of proteins, HDL is not made, and levels fall. When the hypoproteinemia is severe, however, and oncotic pressures fall, the production of lipoproteins could be stimulated and actually rise. Elevation of HDL levels occurs only late in the disease.*

▲ Increased LDL and VLDL Levels

Familial LDL lipoproteinemia: *Affected patients are genetically predisposed toward having high LDL levels.*

Nephrotic syndrome: *The loss of proteins diminishes the plasma oncotic pressures. This appears to stimulate hepatic lipoprotein synthesis of LDL and possibly to diminish lipoprotein disposal of LDL.*

Glycogen storage diseases (e.g., von Gierke disease): *VLDL synthesis is increased and excretion is diminished. VLDL and LDL levels rise.*

Hypothyroidism: *VLDL and LDL catabolism is diminished. VLDL and LDL levels rise. This is a common cause of lipid abnormalities, especially among women.*

Alcohol consumption: *Hyperlipidemias are known to occur in persons who drink excessive quantities of alcohol. However, a genetic factor may also be associated with this observation.*

Chronic liver disease (e.g., hepatitis, cirrhosis): *The liver catabolizes LDL. Without that catabolism, blood levels increase.*

Hepatoma: *The normal inhibition of LDL synthesis by dietary fats does not occur. LDL synthesis continues unabated. LDL levels rise.*

Gammopathies (e.g., multiple myeloma): *High levels of gamma-globulins (immunoglobulins G and M) attach to the VLDL and LDL molecule and thereby decrease their catabolism.*

Familial hypercholesterolemia type IIa: *LDL receptors are altered, and LDL is produced at increased rates.*

Cushing's syndrome: *VLDL synthesis is increased. VLDL is converted to LDL.*

Apoprotein CII deficiency: *This genetic defect is associated with a deficiency of lipoprotein lipase. As a result, VLDL and other lipoproteins (chylomicrons) accumulate.*

▼ Decreased LDL and VLDL Levels

Familial hypolipoproteinemia: *Affected patients are genetically predisposed toward having low VLDL or LDL levels.*

Hypoproteinemia (e.g., malabsorption, severe burns, malnutrition): *Early in the course of this process, LDL levels are low. However, the LDL and VLDL levels can actually rise later.*

Hyperthyroidism: *Catabolism of LDL and VLDL is increased, and levels fall.*

RELATED TESTS

Cholesterol (p. 169). This is a measure of total cholesterol in the blood. It is a part of the lipid profile.

Triglycerides (p. 523). This is a measure of total triglyceride in the blood. It is a part of the lipid profile.

Apolipoproteins (p. 116). This test is used to measure apolipoprotein levels. This may be a better indicator of atherogenic risks than total HDL or total LDL.

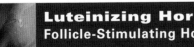

Luteinizing Hormone (LH, Lutropin) and **Follicle-Stimulating Hormone (FSH) Assay**

NORMAL FINDINGS

Values may vary depending on assay method.

Adult	Luteinizing Hormone (IU/L)	Follicle-Stimulating Hormone (IU/L)
Male	1.0–9.0	1.0–10.0
Female		
Follicular phase	2.0–10.0	1.37–9.9
Ovulatory peak	15.0–65.0	6.17–17.2
Luteal phase	1.0–12.0	1.09–9.2
Postmenopause	12.0–65.0	40–250

Child (Ages 6–10 Years)	Luteinizing Hormone (IU/L)	Follicle-Stimulating Hormone (IU/L)
Male	0.04–3.6	0.3–4.6
Female	0.03–3.9	0.68–6.7

INDICATIONS

Luteinizing hormone and follicle-stimulating hormone (FSH) levels are helpful in the confirmation of menopause. Furthermore, they are integral in the evaluation of suspected gonadal failure. Infertility evaluations also include these tests.

TEST EXPLANATION

Luteinizing hormone and FSH are glycoproteins produced in the anterior pituitary gland in response to stimulation by gonadotropin-releasing hormone (GnRH). GnRH is stimulated when circulating levels of estrogen (in women) or testosterone (in men) are low. Through a feedback mechanism, GnRH is stimulated by the hypothalamus, which in turn stimulates the production and release of luteinizing hormone and FSH. These two hormones then act on the ovary or testes. In girls and women, FSH stimulates the development of follicles in the ovary.

In boys and men, FSH stimulates Sertoli cell development. In girls and women, luteinizing hormone stimulates follicular production of estrogen, ovulation, and formation of a corpus luteum. In boys and men, luteinizing hormone stimulates testosterone production from the Leydig cells. In the end, estrogen or testosterone is produced, which in turn inhibits FSH and luteinizing hormone production. FSH is necessary for maturation of the ovaries and testes. FSH and luteinizing hormone are necessary for sperm production. In girls and women, these hormones are secreted differently at different times in the menstrual cycle. The midcycle peak of FSH is necessary for follicle/ovum formation. Luteinizing hormone also must peak at approximately that same time to stimulate ovulation or corpus luteal formation that could potentially support an embryo if fertilization were to occur.

Luteinizing hormone is secreted in a pulsatile manner. One specimen may not accurately indicate total body levels of this hormone. Often several specimens of blood are obtained 20 to 30 minutes apart, and either the blood is pooled or results of each are averaged. The variable nature of luteinizing hormone can be diminished by measuring it in a 24-hour urine sample. The disadvantage is that luteinizing hormone values can be artificially low because of dilution with large urine volumes. Spot urine tests have become very useful in the evaluation and treatment of infertility. Because luteinizing hormone is rapidly excreted into the urine, the plasma luteinizing hormone surge that precedes ovulation by 24 hours can be recognized quickly and easily. This is used to indicate the period when the woman is most fertile. The best time to obtain a urine specimen is between 11 AM and 3 PM. Usually the woman begins to test her urine on the 10th day after the onset of her menses and continues to do so daily. Home kits in which a colour change represents an end point are now marketed to make this process even more convenient.

These hormones are used in the evaluation of infertility. Performing a luteinizing hormone assay is an easy way to determine whether ovulation has occurred. A luteinizing hormone surge in blood levels indicates that ovulation has taken place. Under the influence of luteinizing hormone, the corpus luteum develops from the ruptured graafian follicle. Daily samples of serum luteinizing hormone at approximately the middle of the woman's cycle can detect the surge, which is thought to occur on the day of maximal fertility.

These assays also determine whether a gonadal insufficiency is primary (problem with the ovary or testicle) or secondary (caused by pituitary insufficiency, which results in reduced levels of FSH and luteinizing hormone). Elevated levels of FSH and luteinizing hormone in patients with gonadal insufficiency indicate primary gonadal failure, as may be seen in women with polycystic ovaries or during menopause. In secondary gonadal failure, luteinizing hormone and FSH levels are low as a result of pituitary failure or some other pituitary-hypothalamic impairment, stress, malnutrition, or physiologic delay in growth and sexual development.

FSH and luteinizing hormone assays are often performed to diagnose menopause. Luteinizing hormone is also used to study testicular dysfunction in men and to evaluate endocrine problems related to precocious puberty in children. These hormone assays can also help in the evaluation of disorders of sexual differentiation, such as Klinefelter's syndrome.

INTERFERING FACTORS

- Recent use of radioisotopes may affect test results if the testing method is radioimmunoassay.
- Human chorionic gonadotropin and thyroid-stimulating hormone may interfere with some immunoassay methods because of the similarities of part of the hormone molecule. Therefore, patients with human chorionic gonadotropin–producing tumours and those with hypothyroidism should be expected to have artificially high luteinizing hormone levels.
- Drugs that may *increase* levels of luteinizing hormone or FSH include anticonvulsants, cimetidine, clomiphene, digitalis, levodopa, naloxone, and spironolactone.
- Drugs that may *decrease* levels of luteinizing hormone include digoxin, estrogens, oral contraceptives, progesterones, steroids, testosterone, and phenothiazines.

Clinical Priorities

- Levels of FSH and luteinizing hormone vary in female patients according to phases in the menstrual cycle.
- These hormones are valuable in the evaluation of infertility. Daily samples of luteinizing hormone at approximately a woman's midcycle can detect the luteinizing hormone surge, which is thought to occur on the day of maximum fertility.
- Spot urine tests have become useful in evaluating and treating infertility. Home test kits are now available for detecting luteinizing hormone in the urine.
- FSH and luteinizing hormone assays are often performed to diagnose menopause so that hormone replacement therapy can be started.

PROCEDURE AND PATIENT CARE

Before

☒ Explain the procedure to the patient.
☒ Inform the patient that no food or fluid restrictions are needed.

During

Blood

- Collect a venous blood sample in a red-top tube.
- On the laboratory slip, indicate the date of the most recent menstrual period. Note whether the woman is postmenopausal.

Urine

- Collect a 24-hour specimen; a preservative may be used.
- Keep the specimen refrigerated during the collection period.
- Note that the patient may also perform luteinizing hormone assays at home by using a home urine test or a 24-hour urine test.
- If a spot urine test is performed, follow the directions accompanying the kit.

After

- Apply pressure or a pressure dressing to the venipuncture site.
- Assess the venipuncture site for bleeding.

TEST RESULTS AND CLINICAL SIGNIFICANCE

▲ Increased Levels

Gonadal failure (e.g., physiologic menopause, ovarian dysgenesis [Turner's syndrome], testicular dysgenesis [Klinefelter's syndrome], castration, anorchia, hypogonadism, polycystic ovaries, complete testicular feminization syndrome): *Levels of estrogen or testosterone decrease with gonadal failure. Through a feedback mechanism, FSH and luteinizing hormone secretion is stimulated maximally.*

Precocious puberty: *One cause of precocious puberty is oversecretion of FSH and luteinizing hormone.*

Pituitary adenoma: *Some pituitary adenomas secrete FSH or luteinizing hormone without regard to any feedback mechanism.*

▼ Decreased Levels

Pituitary failure: *FSH and luteinizing hormone are produced in the anterior pituitary gland. The first indication of pituitary failure is reduction of FSH and luteinizing hormone and the resulting gonadal failure.*

Hypothalamic failure: *GnRH is produced in the hypothalamus and stimulates FSH and luteinizing hormone production. Failure of that portion of the brain to produce GnRH causes reductions in FSH and luteinizing hormone levels.*

Stress,

Anorexia nervosa,

Malnutrition: *The pathophysiologic mechanism underlying these observations is not clear.*

Lyme Disease

NORMAL FINDINGS

Lyme antibody EIA (Lyme Index Value [LIV])
   <0.90 = negative
   0.91-1.09 = equivocal
   >1.10 = positive
Western Blot
   >5 different IgG antibodies reactive = positive
   >2 different IgM antibodies reactive = positive
PCR
   Negative

INDICATIONS

This test is used to diagnose Lyme disease.

TEST EXPLANATION

Lyme borreliosis is caused by the bacterium *Borrelia burgdorferi,* which comes from one of three families of spirochetes that belong to a phylum of distinctive Gram-negative bacteria. In Lyme disease, *B. burgdorferi* is transmitted by ixodid hard-bodied ticks that feed off rodents, birds, and deer. Songbirds migrating to Canada play a key role in the introduction and dispersal of several species of ticks that are infected with the *B. burgdorferi* spirochete. The black-legged hard-bodied tick, *Ixodes scapularis* (previously called the "deer tick"), is of particular interest because it specifically carries the *B. burgdorferi* spirochete. Areas in Canada known to have the disease are limited to the shores of Lake Erie, around Lake Ontario, Thousand Islands Park in Nova Scotia, southeastern Manitoba, and Gros Morne National Park in Newfoundland. Although these recognized areas are still limited, the incidence of Lyme disease in increasing in Canada.

These parasites attach to the skin of the host, take a blood meal, and drop off a few days later. Clinical presentation of Lyme disease can either be localized or disseminated. Characteristic of early localized disease is the presence of erythema migrans, a round or oval erythematous skin lesion with a bull's-eye pattern that develops at the site of the tick bite; it is usually present 7 to 14 days after the tick bite and should be ≥5 cm in largest diameter for a firm Lyme disease diagnosis. Disseminated disease that may affect the musculoskeletal, cardiac, or nervous system can follow erythema chronicum migrans (ECM) within days or weeks and is considered early-stage disseminated disease. Meningoencephalitis, cranial or peripheral neuropathies, myocarditis, atrioventricular nodal block, or arthritis are some of the inflammatory changes that may occur. Lyme carditis may overlap temporally with neurologic Lyme disease (late-stage disseminated disease).

Cultures of the erythema chronicum migrans can isolate the spirochete in 50% of the cases. However, the spirochete is difficult to culture and takes a long time to grow. Cultures of the blood or cerebrospinal fluid are even less helpful. The Public Health Agency of Canada recommends a two-tiered approach for blood testing for Lyme disease: screening blood samples with one test, and then continuing testing only on samples that are positive for Lyme disease. Currently, serologic studies are the most sensitive and specific tests for the detection of Lyme disease. Enzyme-linked immunosorbent assay (ELISA) is the best diagnostic test for Lyme disease. This test determines titres of specific IgM and specific IgG antibodies to the *B. burgdorferi* spirochete. Levels of specific IgM antibody peak during the third to sixth week after disease onset and then gradually decline.

Titres of specific IgG antibodies are generally low during the first several weeks of illness, reach maximal levels 4 to 6 months later during arthritis attacks, and often remain elevated for years. Early in the illness, the diagnosis usually can be determined from the gross appearance of erythema chronicum migrans and known exposure to an endemic area (woods with large populations of deer). Affected patients do not require antibody determination. In the absence of erythema chronicum migrans, however, Lyme disease can be confused with various viral infections. In such patients, a single titre of specific IgM antibody may suggest the correct diagnosis. Acute and convalescent sera can be tested to corroborate the diagnosis. Later in the illness, determination of specific IgG antibodies can differentiate Lyme disease from aseptic meningitis or unexplained cranial or peripheral nerve palsies.

Immunofluorescence testing is also performed but is less specific, as other spirochete disease (such as syphilis or leptospirosis) confounds results. The diagnosis of Lyme disease can be made with certainty only when both the clinical picture of the acute disease and the serologic results support the diagnosis. Without the clinical picture, serologic tests are often artificially positive and the diagnosis is incorrect. The Centers for Disease Control and Prevention (CDC) requires the following tests for the diagnosis to be made with certainty:

- Isolation of *B. burgdorferi* from an infected tissue or specimen
- Identification of IgM and IgG antibodies to *B. burgdorferi* in the blood or cerebrospinal fluid
- Acute and convalescent blood samples with significant positive antibody titres

Because of the high incidence of false-positive results on the ELISA for Lyme disease, it is now recommended that the diagnoses of all patients who have positive ELISA results for Lyme disease be confirmed by a Western blot–specific Lyme disease test. (This is very similar to the situation with human immune deficiency virus [HIV] infection, wherein all positive ELISA results are confirmed by the more specific and sensitive Western blot test.) In patients with suspected Lyme disease, the serologic test should be repeated if the initial test result is negative.

INTERFERING FACTORS

- Previous infection with *B. burgdorferi* can cause positive serologic results. Such patients no longer have Lyme disease.
- Other spirochete diseases (syphilis, leptospirosis) can cause false-positive results.

PROCEDURE AND PATIENT CARE

Before

- Explain the procedure to the patient.
- Inform the patient that no fasting or special preparation is required.

During

- Collect a venous blood sample in a red-top tube.

After
- Apply pressure or a pressure dressing to the venipuncture site.
- Assess the venipuncture site for bleeding.

TEST RESULTS AND CLINICAL SIGNIFICANCE
Lyme disease

Magnesium (Mg)

NORMAL FINDINGS
Adult: **0.65–1.05 mmol/L** (1.3–2.1 mEq/L)
Child: **0.70–0.85 mmol/L** (1.4–1.7 mEq/L)
Newborn: **0.70–1.0 mmol/L** (1.4–2 mEq/L/dL)

Critical Values
Tetany: **<0.6 mmol/L** (<1.2 mg/dL)
Central nervous system depression: **2.5–5 mmol/L** (5.0–10.0 mg/dL)
Coma and electrocardiographic changes: **2.5–7.5 mmol/L** (10–15 mg/dL)
Heart block: **15.0 mmol/L** (30 mg/dL)
Cardiac arrest: **17.0–20 mmol/L** (34–40 mg/dL)

INDICATIONS
This test is used to identify magnesium deficiency or overload.

TEST EXPLANATION
Most of the magnesium in the body is intracellular. Approximately 50% is in the bone. Most of the magnesium is bound to an adenosine triphosphatase (ATP) molecule and is important in phosphorylation of ATP (main source of energy for the body). Therefore, this electrolyte is critical in nearly all metabolic processes. Furthermore, magnesium acts as a cofactor that modifies the activity of many enzymes. Synthesis and metabolism of carbohydrate, protein, and nucleic acid depend on magnesium.

Most organ functions, including neuromuscular tissue, also depend on magnesium. It is important to monitor magnesium levels in patients with cardiac disease. Low magnesium levels may increase cardiac irritability and aggravate cardiac arrhythmias. Hypermagnesemia retards neuromuscular conduction and is demonstrated as slowing of cardiac conduction (widened PR and Q-T intervals with wide QRS), diminished deep-tendon reflexes, and respiratory depression.

As intracellular elements, body levels of potassium, magnesium, and calcium (in order of quantity) are closely linked. The intracellular electrical charge must be maintained. When the level of one of these positive electrically charged elements is low, another positively charged element is driven into the intracellular space to maintain electrical neutrality. Extracellular and blood levels of the second element therefore decrease. A total body reduction in one of those elements creates a comparable blood reduction in the others. Magnesium is closely related to calcium in that it increases the intestinal absorption of calcium. Magnesium is also important in calcium metabolism. Hypocalcemia often responds to magnesium replacement.

Magnesium deficiency occurs in patients who are malnourished because of malabsorption, maldigestion, or lack of food intake. This becomes especially significant in postoperative patients, who may not eat for 5 to 7 days and whose metabolism (and therefore the need for magnesium) is accelerated. Alcohol abuse increases magnesium loss in the urine. Moderate hypomagnesemia occurs with diabetes, hypoparathyroidism, hyperthyroidism, and hyperaldosteronism. Toxemia of pregnancy is also believed to be associated with reduced magnesium levels. Symptoms of magnesium depletion are mostly neuromuscular (i.e., weakness, irritability, tetany, electrocardiographic changes, delirium, and convulsions).

Increases in magnesium levels are most commonly associated with ingestion of magnesium-containing antacids. Most of the serum magnesium is excreted by the kidneys; therefore, chronic renal diseases also cause elevations in magnesium levels. In addition, several drug interactions can result in changes in magnesium levels. Because magnesium is an intracellular cation, hemolysis of the collected blood sample should be avoided. Hemolysis creates artificial elevations in levels of magnesium. Symptoms of increased magnesium levels include lethargy, nausea and vomiting, and slurred speech.

INTERFERING FACTORS

- Hemolysis should be avoided when this specimen is collected. Magnesium is an intracellular ion, and lysis of red blood cells (RBCs) causes the release of great quantities of magnesium into the blood and artificially elevates results.
- Blood samples should be collected with the patient in the prone position. The upright position can increase magnesium levels by 4%.
- Drugs that cause *increases* in magnesium levels include antacids, aminoglycoside antibiotics, calcium-containing medication, laxatives, lithium, loop diuretics, and thyroid medication.
- Drugs that cause *decreases* in magnesium levels include some antibiotics, diuretics, and insulin.

PROCEDURE AND PATIENT CARE

Before
- Explain the procedure to the patient.
- Inform the patient that no special diet or fasting is required.

During
- Collect a venous blood sample in a red-top or green-top tube.
- Avoid hemolysis.

After
- Apply pressure or a pressure dressing to the venipuncture site.
- Assess the venipuncture site for bleeding.

TEST RESULTS AND CLINICAL SIGNIFICANCE

▲ Increased Levels

Renal insufficiency: *Magnesium is excreted by the kidneys. In end-stage renal failure, excretion is reduced, and magnesium accumulates in the blood. See discussion under "Decreased Levels" regarding decreased magnesium levels in tubular diseases of the kidney.*

Addison's disease: *Aldosterone enhances magnesium excretion. With reduced aldosterone, magnesium excretion is diminished.*

Ingestion of magnesium-containing antacids or salts: *Magnesium is absorbed from the intestines. Blood levels rise.*

Hypothyroidism: *The pathophysiologic mechanism underlying this observation is not clear.*

▼ Decreased Levels

Malnutrition,

Malabsorption: *The major source of magnesium is dietary intake and absorption from the intestines. When either is inhibited, magnesium levels in the blood fall. In malabsorption, all fat-soluble vitamins are lost. Vitamin D levels diminish, and hypocalcemia follows. Magnesium levels therefore fall in the presence of the low calcium level (see Test Explanation).*

Hypoparathyroidism: *In this disease, calcium levels are reduced. Calcium enhances intestinal absorption of magnesium, and when calcium levels are low, magnesium is not well absorbed, and so blood levels diminish. In hyperparathyroidism, calcium levels are high, and magnesium levels increase.*

Alcoholism: *Ethanol increases magnesium losses in the urine.*

Chronic renal tubular disease: *Magnesium is reabsorbed in the renal tubule. Diseases affecting this area of the kidney (e.g., tubular necrosis) or drugs that are toxic to the renal tubule (e.g., aminoglycosides) allow increased losses of magnesium in the urine.*

Diabetic acidosis: *With treatment of this disease, magnesium levels fall. As insulin is given to these patients to drive glucose into the cells, blood levels of magnesium drop.*

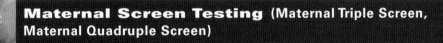

Maternal Screen Testing (Maternal Triple Screen, Maternal Quadruple Screen)

NORMAL FINDINGS

Low probability of fetal defects

INDICATIONS

This is a series of tests that are provided to pregnant women in early pregnancy as a screening test to identify potential birth defects or serious chromosomal/genetic abnormalities.

TEST EXPLANATION

These screening tests may indicate the potential for the presence of fetal defects (particularly trisomy 21 [Down syndrome] or trisomy 18). They may also indicate increased risk for neural tube defects (e.g., myelomeningocele, spina bifida) or abdominal wall defects (omphalocele or gastroschisis).

Several variations of this test are available:
- The double test is a measure of two markers: human chorionic gonadotropin (hCG; p. 426) and alpha-fetoprotein (p. 60).
- The triple test (maternal triple screen test) is a measure of three markers: hCG, alpha-fetoprotein, and estriol (p. 240). Alpha-fetoprotein is produced in the yolk sac and fetal liver. Unconjugated estriol and hCG are produced by the placenta.
- The quadruple test is a measure of four markers: hCG, alpha-fetoprotein, estriol, and inhibin A.
- The fully integrated screen test is a measure of alpha-fetoprotein, estriol, fetal nuchal translucency (p. 369), beta-hCG and total hCG, and pregnancy-associated plasma protein-A (PAPP-A).

The maternal triple screen test has become the standard. Testing of these three markers offers a 50% to 80% chance of detecting pregnancies with trisomy 21, in comparison with alpha-fetoprotein testing alone, which offers only a 30% chance of detection. These tests are most accurately performed during the second trimester of pregnancy, specifically between the fourteenth and twentieth weeks. The use of ultrasonography to accurately indicate gestational age improves the sensitivity and specificity of maternal serum screening.

First-trimester screening for genetic defects is now an option for pregnant women. This testing includes fetal nuchal translucency (see Pelvic Ultrasonography, p. 917) combined with the beta subunit of hCG (beta-hCG, p. 426), and PAPP-A. A low level of PAPP-A may indicate an increased risk for having a stillborn baby. The detection rates of these tests are comparable with those of standard second-trimester triple screening.

First-trimester screening offers several potential advantages over second-trimester screening. When test results are negative, maternal anxiety may be reduced earlier. If results are positive, it allows women to take advantage of first-trimester prenatal diagnosis by chorionic villus sampling at 10 to 12 weeks or early pregnancy amniocentesis. Detecting problems earlier in the pregnancy may allow women to prepare for a child with health problems. It also affords women greater privacy and less health risk if they elect to terminate the pregnancy.

When a fetus has trisomy 21, second-trimester absolute maternal serum levels of alpha-fetoprotein and unconjugated estriol are approximately 25% lower than normal levels, and maternal serum hCG is approximately two times higher than the normal hCG level. The results of the screening are expressed in "multiples of median" (MoM). Alpha-fetoprotein and unconjugated estrogen values during pregnancies with trisomy 21 are lower than those associated with normal pregnancies, which means that values below the mean are below 1 MoM. The hCG value for trisomy 21 is above 1 MoM. The MoM, fetal age, and maternal weight are used to calculate the possible risk for chromosomal abnormalities, such as trisomy 21. Specific computer programs used for this calculation have been developed. A composite estimate of the risk for trisomy 21 is reported to the clinician. A standard risk cutoff is used to determine when the screening test is considered "positive." Most laboratories use a risk cutoff of 1 per 270, which is equal to the second-trimester risk for trisomy 21 in a 35-year-old woman.

All of the maternal screening tests just described are discussed elsewhere in this book. For the sake of thoroughness, inhibin A and PAPP-A are discussed as follows.

Inhibin A is normally secreted by the granulosa cells in the ovaries and inhibits the production of follicle-stimulating hormone (FSH) by the pituitary gland. Inhibin A is a glycoprotein of placental origin in pregnancy similar to hCG. Levels in maternal serum remain relatively constant through the fifteenth to eighteenth weeks of pregnancy. Inhibin A is important in the control of fetal development. Maternal serum levels of inhibin A are twice as high in pregnancies affected by trisomy 21 as in unaffected pregnancies. The discovery of this fact led to the inclusion of inhibin A in the serum screening tests for trisomy 21 just described. Inhibin A concentrations are significantly lower in women with normal pregnancies than in women with pregnancies that result in spontaneous abortions. Furthermore, circulating concentrations of inhibin A appear to reflect tumour mass for certain forms of ovarian cancer. More accurate diagnostic testing is required if screening test results are abnormal.

PAPP-A is a product of the placenta and the endometrium. It is secreted into the maternal circulation during human pregnancy. Women with low blood levels of PAPP-A at 8 to 14 weeks of pregnancy have an increased risk for intrauterine growth restriction, trisomy 21, premature delivery, pre-eclampsia, and stillbirth. Levels of this protein rise rapidly in the first trimester of normal pregnancy. However, in a trisomy 21–affected pregnancy, serum levels are half those of unaffected pregnancies. Furthermore, low first-trimester levels of PAPP-A in maternal serum are associated with adverse fetal outcomes, including fetal death in utero and intrauterine growth restriction.

PROCEDURE AND PATIENT CARE

Before

☒ Explain the procedure to the patient.
☒ Allow the patient to express her concerns and fears regarding the potential for birth defects.

During

• Most of these tests can be performed with a venous blood sample in a red-top tube. Estriol and hCG can also be tested in a urine sample.

After

☒ Provide the results to the patient (and other family members as per patient desires) during a personal consultation.
☒ Allow the patient to express her concerns if the results are positive.
☒ Assist the patient in scheduling and obtaining more accurate diagnostic testing if the results are positive.

TEST RESULTS AND CLINICAL SIGNIFICANCE

Positive Serum Screening Tests

Trisomy 21,
Trisomy 18,
Neural tube defects,
Abdominal wall defects: *Increased serum markers are associated with potential for birth defects. Alpha-fetoprotein markers are decreased in trisomic chromosomal defects, however. Low levels of PAPP-A may be associated with stillbirth.*

RELATED TESTS

Alpha-Fetoprotein (p. 60). This test is one of the screening tests commonly performed to detect possible birth defects.

Pelvic Ultrasonography (p. 917). This test includes a description of fetal nuchal translucency, an accurate screening test for chromosomal abnormalities.

Human Placental Lactogen (p. 321). This is an accurate test to indicate the presence of fetal distress, disease, or growth restriction.

Metanephrine, Plasma Free

NORMAL FINDINGS

Normetanephrine: 18–111 pg/mL
Metanephrine: 12–60 pg/mL
   Results vary among laboratories.

INDICATIONS

This test is used to identify pheochromocytoma of the adrenal or extra-adrenal glands.

TEST EXPLANATION

Pheochromocytomas, although rarely a cause of hypertension, are dangerous tumours that should be investigated in large numbers of patients with hypertension. These tumours produce several catecholamines that can cause episodic or persistent hypertension that is unresponsive to treatment. The current diagnosis of pheochromocytoma depends on biochemical evidence of catecholamine production by the tumour. The best test to establish the diagnosis has not been determined.

Traditionally, urinary vanillylmandelic acid and catecholamine measurements (see p. 1009) were used. Urinary testing is not as sensitive as plasma testing. Because of the low prevalence of these tumours among the tested population and the inadequate sensitivity and specificity of urinary testing, diagnosis of pheochromocytoma was cumbersome and time consuming. The development of high-performance liquid chromatography has allowed for more sensitivity in measuring plasma-free metanephrine levels. In this blood test, the amounts of metanephrine and normetanephrine, which are metabolites of epinephrine and norepinephrine (two catecholamines), are measured.

The high sensitivity of plasma-free metanephrine testing provides a high negative predictive value to the test. This means that if the concentrations of the free metanephrines in the blood are normal, it is very unlikely that a patient has a pheochromocytoma. False-positive results do occur, although rarely. The diagnostic superiority of testing plasma metanephrines over testing plasma or urinary catecholamines and urinary vanillylmandelic acid is clear. In approximately 80% of patients with pheochromocytoma, the magnitude of increase in plasma-free metanephrines is so large that the tumour can be confirmed with close to 100% probability. Intermediate concentrations of normetanephrine and metanephrine are considered indeterminate.

Urinary testing may clarify indeterminate findings. However, plasma metanephrines and urine metanephrines must be compared with caution because different catecholamine metabolites are measured. Testing for some urinary catecholamines may be more specific than for plasma-free metanephrines, which means that false-positive results are less common with urinary testing.

When results are interpreted, the following facts may be helpful:
• In any sample in which the concentrations of *both* normetanephrine and metanephrine are less than the upper reference range limit, the result should be considered normal, and the presence of pheochromocytoma is highly unlikely.

- In any sample in which the concentration of *either* normetanephrine or metanephrine exceeds the limits of the respective upper reference range, the result should be considered elevated.
- Whenever the normetanephrine or metanephrine concentration exceeds the indeterminate range, the presence of pheochromocytoma is highly probable, and the tumour should be sought through imaging techniques.

INTERFERING FACTORS

- Levels of metanephrines may be increased by caffeine or alcohol.
- Vigorous exercise, stress, and starvation may cause increases in metanephrine levels.
- Drugs that may cause *increases* in metanephrine levels include epinephrine- or norepinephrine-containing drugs, levodopa, lithium, and nitroglycerin.
- Acetaminophen can interfere with high-performance liquid chromatography testing of metanephrines and should be avoided for 48 hours before the test.

PROCEDURE AND PATIENT CARE

Before
- Explain the procedure to the patient.
- Explain the dietary and medicinal restrictions.

During
- Identify and minimize factors contributing to patient stress and anxiety. Physical exertion and emotional stress may alter metanephrine test results.
- The patients may be asked to lie down and rest quietly for 15 to 30 minutes before sample collection.
- The blood sample may be collected while the patient is supine.
- Collect a venous blood sample in a chilled lavender-top or pink-top tube. Invert the tube to mix the blood with preservatives.

After
- Apply pressure to the venipuncture site.
- Send the specimen to the laboratory as soon as the test is completed.

TEST RESULTS AND CLINICAL SIGNIFICANCE

▲ Increased Levels

Pheochromocytoma: *This is a neuroendocrine tumour of the medulla of the adrenal glands (originating in the chromaffin cells) that secretes excessive amounts of catecholamines that are subsequently metabolized to metanephrines.*

RELATED TEST

Vanillylmandelic Acid and Catecholamines (p. 1009). This 24-hour urine test for vanillylmandelic acid and catecholamines is performed primarily to diagnose hypertension secondary to pheochromocytoma, neuroblastomas, and other rare adrenal tumours.

Methemoglobin (Hemoglobin M)

NORMAL FINDINGS

9.3–37.2 *Mc*mol/L (0.06–0.24 g/dL)
0.4%–1.5% of total hemoglobin

 Critical Values

>20%–70% of total hemoglobin: headaches, dizziness, fatigue, tachycardia
>70% of total hemoglobin: death

INDICATIONS

This test is used to identify methemoglobinemia in hypoxemic children and adults.

TEST EXPLANATION

Methemoglobin is continuously formed in the red blood cells (RBCs). During the production of normal adult deoxygenated hemoglobin, methemoglobin is reduced to normal adult deoxygenated hemoglobin by the reduced form of nicotinamide adenine dinucleotide (NADH). If oxygenation of the iron component in the protohemoglobin occurs without subsequent reduction to normal hemoglobin, excess methemoglobin accumulates. The iron form in methemoglobin is unable to combine with oxygen to carry the oxygen to the peripheral tissues. Therefore, the oxyhemoglobin dissociation curve is "shifted to the left," which results in cyanosis and hypoxia. Older adult, pediatric, or chronically hypoxemic patients are particularly sensitive to methemoglobin production.

Methemoglobinemia can be congenital or, more commonly, is acquired. Hemoglobin M disease is a genetic defect that results in a group of abnormal hemoglobins that are methemoglobins. Another genetic mutation can cause a deficiency in NADH methemoglobin reductase enzyme that is required to deoxygenate methemoglobin to normal adult hemoglobin. These forms of methemoglobinemia occur in infants, are usually severe, are not amenable to treatment, and are often fatal.

Acquired methemoglobinemia is a result of ingestion of nitrates (e.g., from well water), or drugs such as phenacetin, sulphonamides, isoniazid, local anaesthetics containing benzocaine, sulphonamide antibiotics, silver nitrate, and phenazopyridine (Pyridium). Several over-the-counter local anaesthetics used for toothache or hemorrhoidal pain contain benzocaine. The acquired form of the disease commonly occurs in older individuals and results in an acute crisis that is effectively treated with ascorbic acid or methylene blue.

INTERFERING FACTORS

- Tobacco use and carbon monoxide poisoning are associated with increased methemoglobin levels.
- Drugs that may cause *increases* in methemoglobin levels include some antibiotics, isoniazid, local anaesthetics, and sulphonamides.

PROCEDURE AND PATIENT CARE

Before

Ⅺ Explain the procedure to the patient.
Ⅺ Inform the patient that no fasting is required.

During

- Collect a venous blood sample in a green-top (heparin) tube.
- Methemoglobin is very unstable. Place the specimen tube in a container of water and crushed ice immediately after collection.
- Avoid hemolysis.

After

- Apply pressure to the venipuncture site.
- Be prepared to provide oxygen support and close monitoring in the event that the patient becomes increasingly hypoxic.

TEST RESULTS AND CLINICAL SIGNIFICANCE

Hereditary methemoglobinemia: *Cyanosis starts in early infancy. It is associated with hypoxemia and can be ameliorated with ascorbic acid and, in some cases, methylene blue.*

Acquired methemoglobinemia: *Associated with hypoxemia and can be improved with ascorbic acid and in some cases, methylene blue.*

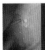

Mononucleosis Spot (Mononuclear Heterophil, Heterophil Antibody, Monospot)

NORMAL FINDINGS

Negative (<1:28 titre)

INDICATIONS

This is a rapid slide test designed to assist in the diagnosis of infectious mononucleosis.

TEST EXPLANATION

The mononucleosis test is performed to aid in the diagnosis of infectious mononucleosis, a disease caused by the Epstein-Barr virus (EBV). Usually young adults are affected by mononucleosis. The clinical presentation is fever, pharyngitis, lymphadenopathy, and splenomegaly. Approximately 2 weeks after the onset of the disease, many patients are found to have immunoglobulin M (IgM) heterophil antibodies in their serum that react against warm red blood cells (RBCs). When these antibodies are present in serial dilutions of greater than 1:56, infectious mononucleosis is probably present. However, false-positive results can occur in patients who have other diseases that cause elevation of heterophil antibodies: for example, lymphoma, systemic lupus erythematosus, Burkitt lymphoma, leukemia, and some gastrointestinal cancers. Burkitt lymphoma is strongly associated with EBV.

Several heterophil agglutination tests are available, but the most frequently performed is the rapid slide spot test (monospot test). Heterophil antibodies, normally present in most individuals, are produced in increased quantities in patients with infectious mononucleosis. These antibodies strongly and readily agglutinate horse RBCs. The spot slide test is performed by adding the patient's serum to horse RBCs on a slide. If agglutination occurs, heterophil antibodies are present in the patient's serum, which indicates an EBV infection. Approximately 30% of the cases of infectious mononucleosis are "heterophil antibody negative." When the diagnosis of infectious mononucleosis is still suspected, a repeat monospot test or EBV serologic test is done. The diagnosis of infectious mononucleosis must include the following criteria:

- Clinical presentation compatible with infectious mononucleosis
- Hematologic presentation compatible with infectious mononucleosis (lymphocytosis)
- Atypical lymphocytes in significant numbers
- Positive serologic test result for infectious mononucleosis

PROCEDURE AND PATIENT CARE

Before

 Explain the procedure to the patient.
 Inform the patient that no fasting or special preparation is required.

During

- Collect a venous blood sample in a red-top tube.

After

- Apply pressure or a pressure dressing to the venipuncture site.
- Observe the venipuncture site for bleeding.

TEST RESULTS AND CLINICAL SIGNIFICANCE

▲ Increased Levels

Infectious mononucleosis,
Chronic EBV infection,
Chronic fatigue syndrome,
Burkitt lymphoma,
Some forms of chronic hepatitis: *These diseases are often associated with abnormal quantities of heterophil agglutinating antibodies similar to those formed in patients with infectious mononucleosis.*

RELATED TEST

Epstein-Barr Virus Titre (p. 232). This is a more specific and sensitive test for EBV infections. It can also differentiate acute from chronic or old EBV infections.

Mycoplasma pneumoniae Antibodies, IgG and IgM

NORMAL FINDINGS

IgG

≤0.9 (negative)
0.91–1.09 (equivocal)
≥1.1 (positive)

IgM

≤0.9 (negative)
0.91–1.09 (equivocal)
≥1.1 (positive)

IgM by IFA

Negative (reported as positive or negative)

INDICATIONS

This test is used to support the clinical diagnosis of disease associated with *Mycoplasma pneumoniae*.

TEST EXPLANATION

Several diseases have been associated with the mycoplasmal pneumoniae infection, including pharyngitis, tracheobronchitis, pneumonia, and inflammation of the tympanic membrane. *Mycoplasma pneumoniae* accounts for approximately 20% of all cases of pneumonia. Classically it causes a disease that has been described as primary atypical pneumonia. The disease is of insidious onset with fever, headache, and malaise for 2 to 4 days before the onset of respiratory symptoms. Most patients do not require hospitalization. Symptomatic infections attributable to this organism most commonly occur in children and young adults. These infections may be associated with cold agglutinin syndrome (p. 184).

Positive IgM results are consistent with acute infection, although there may be some cross-reactivity associated with other mycoplasma infections. A single positive IgG result only indicates previous immunologic exposure. Negative results do not rule out the presence of *Mycoplasma pneumoniae*–associated disease because the specimen may have been drawn before the appearance of detectable antibodies. If a *Mycoplasma* infection is clinically suspected, a second specimen should be submitted at least 14 days later. The continued presence or absence of antibodies cannot be used to determine the success or failure of therapy.

After serologic combinations to identify IgG/IgM antibody complexes, serial dilutions are performed and the colour changes are measured photometrically. The colour intensity of the dilutions depends on the antibody concentration in the serum sample. The IgM complex can be identified by immunofluorescent assay (IFA).

PROCEDURE AND PATIENT CARE

Before

- Explain the procedure to the patient.
- Tell the patient that no fasting is required.

During

- Collect venous blood in a red-top tube.

After

- Apply pressure to the venipuncture site.
- Transport the specimen immediately to the laboratory. Avoid undue cooling of the specimen, which may lead to agglutination.

TEST RESULTS AND CLINICAL SIGNIFICANCE

Mycoplasma infection: *With the combination of positive antibodies and a compatible clinical picture, the diagnosis of* Mycoplasma *infection can be confidently made.*

RELATED TESTS

Cold Agglutinins (p. 184). This test identifies antibodies to RBCs that cause agglutination when exposed to cold temperatures. Although other diseases are also associated with the presence of these antibodies, *Mycoplasma* infections are considered predominant.

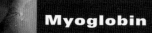

Myoglobin

NORMAL FINDINGS

1.0–5.3 nmol/L (<90 ng/mL)

INDICATIONS

This test is used in the early evaluation of a patient with suspected acute myocardial infarction. It is also used to assist in the diagnosis of disease or injury in skeletal muscle.

TEST EXPLANATION

Myoglobin is an oxygen-binding protein found in cardiac and skeletal muscle. Measurement of myoglobin provides an early index of damage to the myocardium, as occurs in myocardial infarction or reinfarction. Increases in levels, which indicate cardiac muscle injury or death, occur approximately 3 hours after infarction. Although this test is more sensitive than that for creatine phosphokinase isoenzymes, it is not as specific. Trauma, inflammation, or ischemic changes to the noncardiac skeletal muscles can also cause elevations in levels of myoglobin. The benefit of measuring myoglobin instead of creatine phosphokinase MB (see p. 201) is that myoglobin levels may become elevated earlier in some patients. This may prove beneficial because thrombolytic therapy should be started within the first 6 hours after a myocardial infarction.

As already mentioned, disease or trauma in the skeletal muscle also causes elevations in myoglobin levels. With sudden and severe muscle injury, myoglobin levels can become very high. Because myoglobin is excreted in the urine and is nephrotoxic, the levels must be monitored in such patients. Myoglobin can also be measured in the urine. To screen for myoglobin, the routine urine dipstick test for hemoglobin can be used.

INTERFERING FACTORS

- Recent administration of radioactive substances may affect test results determined by radioimmunoassay methods.
- Myoglobin levels can increase after intramuscular injections. Such an injection can cause localized muscle injury and instigate an inflammatory response, which could elevate myoglobin levels.

PROCEDURE AND PATIENT CARE

Before

- Explain the procedure to the patient.
- Inform the patient that no fasting is required.

During

- Collect a venous blood sample in a red-top tube.

After

- Apply pressure or a pressure dressing to the venipuncture site.
- Observe the venipuncture site for bleeding.

TEST RESULTS AND CLINICAL SIGNIFICANCE

▲ Increased Levels

Myocardial infarction: *Injury to cardiac muscle causes the cells to lyse and expel the myoglobin into the bloodstream.*

Skeletal muscle inflammation (myositis): *Injury to cardiac muscle causes the cells to lyse and expel the myoglobin into the bloodstream.*

Malignant hyperthermia,

Muscular dystrophy,

Skeletal muscle ischemia,

Skeletal muscle trauma,

Rhabdomyolysis: *All these diseases affect the skeletal muscles. This causes the muscle cells to lyse and expel the myoglobin into the bloodstream.*

Seizures: *Persistent seizure activity injures skeletal muscle tissue. This causes the muscle cells to lyse and expel the myoglobin into the bloodstream.*

▼ Decreased Levels

Polymyositis: *In some cases, antimyoglobin antibodies exist and diminish myoglobin levels in the blood.*

RELATED TESTS

Creatine Kinase (p. 201). Measurement of creatine phosphokinase is very useful in the evaluation of myocardial infarction.

Lactate Dehydrogenase (p. 339). Levels of this enzyme are also elevated when muscle tissue is injured.

Troponins (p. 531). This test is a specific indicator of cardiac muscle injury.

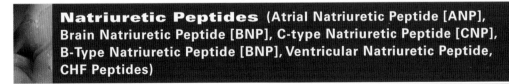

Natriuretic Peptides (Atrial Natriuretic Peptide [ANP], Brain Natriuretic Peptide [BNP], C-type Natriuretic Peptide [CNP], B-Type Natriuretic Peptide [BNP], Ventricular Natriuretic Peptide, CHF Peptides)

NORMAL FINDINGS

Atrial natriuretic peptide (ANP): **22–77 *Mcg*/L** (22–77 ng/mL)

Brain natriuretic peptide (BNP): **<100 *Mcg*/L** (<100 ng/mL)

C-type natriuretic peptide (CNP): to be determined

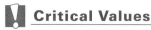 **Critical Values**

>100 *Mcg*/L (>100 ng/mL)

INDICATIONS

Natriuretic peptides are used to identify and stratify patients with heart failure (HF).

TEST EXPLANATION

Natriuretic peptides are neuroendocrine peptides that oppose the activity of the renin-angiotensin system. There are three major natriuretic peptides. ANP is synthesized in the cardiac atrial muscle. The main source of BNP is the cardiac ventricle, although it was initially found in porcine brain. C-type natriuretic peptide was first localized in the nervous system but later found to be produced by the endothelial cells. The cardiac peptides are continuously released by the heart muscle cells in low levels. However, the rate of release can be increased by a variety of neuroendocrine and physiologic factors, including hemodynamic load, to regulate cardiac preload and afterload. Because of these properties, BNP and ANP have been implicated in the pathophysiologic processes of hypertension, HF, and atherosclerosis. Both ANP and BNP are released in response to atrial and ventricular stretch, respectively, and cause vasorelaxation, inhibition of aldosterone secretion from the adrenal gland, and inhibition of renin from the kidney, thereby increasing natriuresis and causing reduction in blood volume. CNP has a vasorelaxation effect but does not stimulate natriuresis.

BNP, in particular, is strongly correlated to left ventricular pressures. As a result, BNP is a good marker for HF. BNP levels, by themselves, are more accurate than any historical or physical findings or laboratory values when heart failure is identified as the cause of dyspnea. The diagnostic accuracy of BNP at a cutoff of **100 *Mcg*/L** (100 ng/mL) was 83.4% in research studies.

The higher the levels of BNP are, the more severe the HF is. This test is used in urgent care settings to aid in the differential diagnosis of shortness of breath. If the BNP level is elevated, the shortness of breath is caused by HF. If BNP levels are normal, the shortness of breath has a pulmonary cause and not a cardiac cause. This is particularly helpful in evaluating shortness of breath in patients with cardiac and chronic lung disease.

Furthermore, BNP is a helpful prognosticator and is used in HF risk stratification. Patients with HF whose BNP levels do not rapidly return to normal after treatment have a significantly higher risk for mortality in the ensuing months than do those whose BNP levels rapidly normalize with treatment. In early rejection of heart transplants, BNP levels can be elevated. Measurement of plasma BNP concentration is evolving as a very efficient and cost-effective mass screening technique for identifying patients with various cardiac abnormalities. This measurement is important regardless of cause and degree of left ventricular systolic dysfunction that can potentially develop into obvious heart failure and carry a high risk for a cardiovascular event.

In some laboratories, BNP is measured as an *N-terminal fragment of pro–brain (B-type) natriuretic peptide [NT–pro-BNP]*. The clinical information provided by either the BNP or the NT–pro-BNP level is approximately the same, and the tests are used interchangeably. There is some evidence that NT–pro-BNP is a strong predictor of mortality among patients with acute coronary syndromes and may be a strong prognostic marker in patients with chronic coronary heart disease as well. NT–pro-BNP is a marker of long-term mortality in patients with stable coronary disease, and it provides prognostic information above and beyond that provided by conventional cardiovascular risk factors and the degree of left ventricular systolic dysfunction.

Screening diabetic patients for BNP elevation to determine the risk for cardiac diseases is becoming increasingly common because of the low cost of performing the test compared with echocardiography. It has been found that the incidence of death or severe cardiovascular problems was significantly higher for diabetic and nondiabetic patients whose NT–pro-BNP levels were in the top 20% of those tested. BNP level is also elevated in patients with prolonged systemic hypertension and in patients with acute myocardial infarction.

INTERFERING FACTORS

- BNP levels are generally higher in healthy women than in healthy men.
- BNP levels are higher in older patients.
- BNP levels are elevated in patients who have had cardiac surgery, and they remain elevated for 1 month postoperatively. This does not reflect the presence of CHF.
- There are several different methods of measuring BNP. Normal values vary regardless of whether the whole protein of a BNP fragment protein is measured.
- Nesiritide (Natrecor), a recombinant form of the endogenous human peptide used to treat HF, causes an *increase* in plasma BNP levels for several days.

PROCEDURE AND PATIENT CARE

Before

- Explain the procedure to the patient.
- Inform the patient that no fasting is required.

During

- Collect a venous blood sample in tube containing ethylenediamine tetra-acetic acid (EDTA) (usually a lavender-top tube).

After

- Apply pressure to the venipuncture site.
- Assess the venipuncture site for bleeding.
- Continue with aggressive medical care for suspected HF.

TEST RESULTS AND CLINICAL SIGNIFICANCE

▲ Increased Levels

Heart failure,
Myocardial infarction,
Systemic hypertension,
Heart transplant rejection,
Cor pulmonale: *These conditions are all associated with increased ventricular or atrial cardiac pressure. As a result, cardiac natriuretic peptides are secreted, which causes a relaxation of blood vessels (vasodilation), an increase in the excretion of sodium (natriuresis) and fluid (diuresis), and a decrease in injurious neurohormones (endothelin, aldosterone, angiotensin II). All of these actions work in concert on the vessels, heart, and kidneys to decrease the fluid load on the heart, allowing the heart to function better and improving cardiac performance.*

RELATED TEST

Chest Radiography (p. 1053). This test provides information about the heart, lungs, bony thorax, mediastinum, and great vessels.

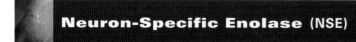

Neuron-Specific Enolase (NSE)

NORMAL FINDINGS

<8.6 Mcg/L

INDICATIONS

This test is used as a marker in patients with neuron-specific enolase-secreting tumours (e.g., carcinoids, small cell lung carcinoma [SCLC], neuroblastomas). It is also used as an auxiliary tool in the assessment of comatose patients: the higher the NSE level, the more injury to the central nervous system.

TEST EXPLANATION

NSE is a glycolytic enzyme that catalyzes the conversion of phosphoglycerate to phosphoenol pyruvate. It is present in neuronal, neuroendocrine, and amine precursor uptake decarboxylation (APUD) cells. NSE, in serum or cerebrospinal fluid (CSF), is often elevated in diseases, which results in neuronal destruction. Measurement of NSE in serum of CSF therefore can assist in the differential diagnosis of a variety of neuron-destructive and neurodegenerative disorders. NSE might also have utility as a prognostic marker in neuronal hypoxic injury.

Elevated NSE concentrations are observed in patients with neuroblastoma, pancreatic islet cell carcinoma, medullary thyroid carcinoma, pheochromocytoma, and other neural crest–derived or neuroendocrine tumours. NSE levels are frequently increased in patients with SCLC and infrequently in patients with non-SCLC. When increased, NSE can be used to monitor disease progression and management in SCLC. Levels of NSE occasionally can be elevated in benign disorders, such as pneumonia and benign hepatobiliary diseases.

NSE values can vary significantly among methods and assays. Serial follow-up should be performed with the same assay. If assays are changed, patients should have new baseline values. Immunometric assays are most commonly used.

INTERFERING FACTORS

- Hemolysis can lead to significant artifactual NSE elevations because erythrocytes contain NSE.

PROCEDURE AND PATIENT CARE

Before

- Explain the procedure to the patient.
- Tell the patient that no fasting is required.

During

- Collect a venous blood sample in a red-top tube.

After

- Apply pressure to the venipuncture site.

TEST RESULTS AND CLINICAL SIGNIFICANCE

▲ Increased Levels

Small cell lung cancer,

Neuroblastoma,

APUD-omas,

Creutzfeldt-Jakob disease: *Any neuronal based tumour or neuronal injured tissue will secrete excess NSE in the blood or CSF (if the disease affects the central nervous system). In doing so, NSE is a measure of tumour burden or neuronal injury or disease.*

RELATED TEST

Magnetic Resonance Imaging (p. 1148). This noninvasive diagnostic procedure provides invaluable information about the brain, central nervous system, bones, joints, breasts, and so on.

Neutrophil Antibody Screen (Granulocyte Antibodies, Polymorphonucleocyte Antibodies [PMN ab], Antigranulocyte Antibodies, Antineutrophil Antibodies, Neutrophil Antibodies)

NORMAL FINDINGS

Negative for neutrophil antibodies

INDICATIONS

This test is performed to identify antibodies to white blood cells (WBCs) if blood transfusion is associated with an immune reaction.

TEST EXPLANATION

Neutrophil antibodies are directed toward WBCs. They develop during blood transfusions. Patients who experience a transfusion reaction despite complete compatibility testing before blood administration should undergo a neutrophil antibody screen to determine whether WBC incompatibility is the source of the reaction. This test is most commonly a part of posttransfusion antibody screening, which is a battery of testing performed if a transfusion reaction is suspected (Boxes 2-9 and 2-10).

BOX 2-9	Symptoms of a Transfusion Reaction

- Fever
- Chills
- Rash
- Flank/back pain
- Bloody urine
- Fainting or dizziness

BOX 2-10   Adverse Transfusion Reactions

Immune Mediated
- Acute hemolytic reaction
- Delayed serologic reaction
- Febrile nonhemolytic reaction
- Allergic reaction
- Anaphylactic allergic reaction
- Acute lung injury

Non–Immune Mediated
- Fluid overload
- Hypothermia
- Iron and electrolyte overload
- Coagulation and immune dilution
- Infectious hepatitis
- Human immunodeficiency virus
- Cytomegalovirus
- Bacteria

Most commonly, the recipient has antibodies to the donor WBCs and experiences a fever during transfusion. More severe, however, is the reaction when the donor plasma contains antibodies to the recipient's WBCs. This nonhemolytic reaction can lead to severe transfusion reactions, including acute pulmonary failure (transfusion-related acute lung injury [TRALI]) and multiorgan system failure. The majority of TRALI cases can be triggered by passive transfer of human leukocyte antigen (HLA) or neutrophil-specific antibodies from the recipient to the donor. TRALI is the leading cause of transfusion-related mortality and accounts for 13% of all transfusion-related deaths.

INTERFERING FACTORS

- Recent administration of dextran may stimulate the induction of WBC antibodies.
- Recent administration of intravenous contrast media may stimulate the induction of WBC antibodies.
- Blood transfusion in the previous 3 months can instigate the induction of WBC antibodies to donor blood.

PROCEDURE AND PATIENT CARE

Before
- Explain the procedure to the patient.
- Inform the patient that no fasting is required.

During
- Collect a venous blood sample in a red-top or lavender-top tube.
- On the request slip, indicate that the patient has had a blood transfusion reaction.

After
- Apply pressure to the venipuncture site.

TEST RESULTS AND CLINICAL SIGNIFICANCE

Blood transfusion reaction: *In recipient's or donor's blood, a positive result indicates presence of neutrophil antibodies, which confirms that the transfusion reaction was a result of these antibodies.*

RELATED TESTS

Coombs Test, Direct (p. 188). This test is performed to identify hemolysis (lysis of red blood cells [RBCs]) or to investigate hemolytic transfusion.

Coombs Test, Indirect (p. 191). This test is used to detect antibodies against RBCs in the serum. It is most commonly used for screening potential blood recipients.

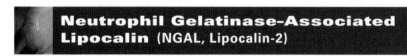

Neutrophil Gelatinase-Associated Lipocalin (NGAL, Lipocalin-2)

NORMAL FINDINGS

No rise in neutrophil gelatinase–associated lipocalin (NGAL) level from baseline. (Results vary according to testing methods.)

INDICATIONS

NGAL is a predictor for acute kidney injury (previously referred to as acute renal failure) and chronic kidney disease.

TEST EXPLANATION

There are no early markers for acute or chronic renal disease. Serum creatinine levels rise only after renal impairment and injury have become significant. The earlier renal disease or injury is identified, the more successfully it can be treated. Early treatment also helps to lessen the morbidity associated with the disease. This is particularly important in patients who have serious nonrenal disease (e.g., patients who have undergone heart surgery, renal transplant recipients, patients with sepsis). Severe acute kidney injury increases morbidity and mortality among such patients who are hospitalized.

NGAL is a member of the lipocalin family of proteins, which bind and transport small lipophilic molecules. NGAL is generally expressed in low concentrations from the renal tubules, but the concentration increases greatly in the presence of epithelial injury and inflammation. A marked elevation in NGAL level indicates that renal injury has occurred, and aggressive supportive treatment should be instituted. NGAL concentrations rise 48 hours before a rise in creatinine is noted. NGAL can be detected in both urine and blood within 2 hours of a renal insult.

NGAL can be measured in the urine, plasma, or serum samples with enzyme-linked immunosorbent assay (ELISA) kits. Results are available in less than 1 hour in a standard laboratory with conventional ELISA equipment. This is particularly helpful in an intensive care environment. By itself, the absolute baseline laboratory result is not as important as the succeeding results. Normal values vary according to which laboratory method is used and the patient's baseline glomerular filtration rate. NGAL varies inversely with the glomerular filtration rate. Urine or blood samples can also be analyzed with an established and validated enzyme immunoassay.

NGAL measurements are increasingly being used in a variety of clinical situations that may lead to acute kidney injury (e.g., during cardiac surgery, during kidney transplantation, in contrast nephropathy, in hemolytic uremic syndrome, and in the intensive care setting). It is also useful in conditions leading to chronic kidney disease (such as lupus nephritis, glomerulonephritis, obstruction, dysplasia, polycystic kidney disease, immunoglobulin A nephropathy, renal dysplasia, obstructive uropathy, and glomerular and cystic diseases).

PROCEDURE AND PATIENT CARE

Before

🗷 Explain the procedure to the patient.
🗷 Inform the patient that no fasting is required.

During

- Collect a venous blood sample in a red-top tube.
- Collect urine specimens at the same time each day, for consecutive days.

After

- Apply pressure or a pressure dressing to the venipuncture site.
- Observe the venipuncture site for bleeding.
- Results are compared with the test results of the previous day.

TEST RESULTS AND CLINICAL SIGNIFICANCE

▲ Increased Levels

Primary or secondary renal disease: *Levels of NGAL increase with renal injury.*

RELATED TESTS

Creatinine, Blood (p. 205). This is a late marker for impaired renal function.

Newborn Metabolic Screening

NORMAL FINDINGS

Negative

 Critical Values

Positive for any one of the tests

INDICATIONS

Newborn metabolic screening is the practice of testing every newborn for certain harmful or potentially fatal disorders that are not otherwise apparent at birth.

TEST EXPLANATION

Newborn screening tests take place before the newborn leaves the hospital. Infants are tested to identify serious or life-threatening (and, for the most part, preventable or treatable) diseases before symptoms begin. These diseases are usually rare. However, if they are not accurately diagnosed and treated, they can cause developmental delay, severe illness, and premature death in newborns. Many of these are metabolic disorders, often called *inborn errors of metabolism.* Other disorders that may be detected through screening are endocrine or hematologic. In most U.S. states and Canadian provinces, this testing is mandatory. More than 98% of all children born in the United States and Canada are tested for these disorders.

Within 48 hours of a child's birth, a sample of blood is obtained from a heelstick, and the blood is analyzed. The sample, called a *blood spot,* is tested at a reference laboratory. It is generally recommended that the sample be taken more than 24 hours after the birth. Some tests, such as the one for phenylketonuria (PKU), may not be as sensitive until the newborn has ingested an ample amount of the amino acid phenylalanine, which is a constituent of both human and cow's milk, and after the postnatal thyroid surge has subsided. This is generally after approximately 2 days.

With the use of *tandem mass spectrometry,* multiple blood tests can be performed quickly and efficiently. When directed to newborn blood screening, the use of these specialized instruments can detect abnormally elevated levels of proteins associated with certain metabolic disorders. They are capable of screening for more than 20 inherited metabolic disorders with a single test in only a few minutes. Tandem mass spectrometry is very accurate and can measure very small amounts of similar material with excellent precision. For example, tandem mass spectrometry for PKU (described as follows) has been shown to reduce the false-positive rate of findings for this disorder more than tenfold in comparison with the best alternative method available. The disorders listed as follows are the ones typically sought in newborn screening programs:

- PKU: An inherited disease, PKU is characterized by deficiency of the enzyme phenylalanine hydroxylase, which converts phenylalanine to tyrosine. Phenylalanine is an essential amino acid necessary for growth; however, any excess must be degraded by conversion to tyrosine. An infant with PKU lacks the ability to make this necessary conversion. Thus phenylalanine accumulates in the body and spills over into the urine. If the amount of phenylalanine is not restricted in infants with PKU, progressive developmental delay results. Affected patients must follow a low-phenylalanine diet throughout childhood and adolescence and perhaps into adult life. (Incidence of PKU in Canada is 1:15000 births.)
- Congenital hypothyroidism: In affected infants who do not receive treatment, growth and brain development are retarded. If the disorder is detected early, an infant can be treated with oral doses of thyroid hormone to enable normal development. (Incidence: 1 per 4000.)
- Galactosemia: Infants with galactosemia lack the enzyme that converts galactose into glucose, a sugar that the body is able to use. As a result, milk and other dairy products must be eliminated from the diet. Otherwise, galactose can build up and cause blindness, severe developmental delay, growth deficiency, and even death. (Incidence: 1 per 60000 to 1 per 80000.) Several less severe forms of galactosemia may be detected by newborn screening. These may not necessitate any intervention.
- Sickle cell disease: Sickle cell disease is an inherited blood disease in which red blood cells stretch into abnormal "sickle" shapes (see p. 476). This can cause episodes of pain, damage to vital organs (such as the lungs and kidneys), and even death. Young children with sickle cell anemia are especially prone to certain dangerous bacterial infections. The screening test can

also detect other disorders affecting hemoglobin (the oxygen-carrying substance in the blood). (Incidence in the United States: approximately 1 per 500 African American births and 1 per every 36 000 Hispanic births.)

- Biotinidase deficiency: Infants with this condition do not have enough biotinidase, an enzyme that recycles biotin (one of the B vitamins) in the body. This deficiency may cause seizures, poor muscle control, immune system impairment, hearing loss, developmental delay, coma, and even death. If the deficiency is detected early, however, problems can be prevented by biotin administration. (Incidences worldwide: profound deficiency, 1 per 112 271; partial deficiency, 1 per 129 282; combined profound and partial deficiency, 1 per 60 089.)
- Congenital adrenal hyperplasia: This is actually a group of disorders resulting in a deficiency of adrenal hormones. It can affect the development of the genitals and may cause death. Lifelong treatment through hormone supplementation manages the condition. (Incidence: 1 per 12 000.)
- Maple syrup urine disease (MSUD): Infants with MSUD are missing an enzyme needed to process the amino acids leucine, isoleucine, and valine (present in protein-rich foods such as milk, meat, and eggs) that are essential for the body's normal growth. When these are not processed properly, they can build up in the body, causing urine to smell like maple syrup or sweet, burnt sugar. These infants usually have little appetite and are extremely irritable. If not detected and treated early, MSUD can cause developmental delay, physical disability, and even death. A carefully controlled diet free of high-protein foods can prevent these outcomes. (Incidence: 1 per 250 000.)
- Homocystinuria: This metabolic disorder results from a deficiency in cystathionine β-synthase, responsible for the metabolism of methionine and homocysteine. If untreated, it can lead to dislocation of lenses of the eyes, developmental delay, skeletal abnormalities, and hypercoagulability. However, a special diet combined with dietary supplements may help prevent most of these problems. (Incidence: 1 per 50 000 to 1 per 150 000.)
- Tyrosinemia: Infants with this disorder cannot metabolize tyrosine. If it accumulates in the body, it can cause mild retardation, language skill difficulties, liver problems, and even death from liver failure. A special diet and sometimes liver transplantation are needed to treat the condition. Early diagnosis and treatment seem to offset long-term problems. (Incidence: not yet determined.)
- Cystic fibrosis: This is an inherited disorder expressed in the lung and gastrointestinal tract that causes cells to release thick mucus, which leads to chronic respiratory disease, problems with digestion, and poor growth. There is no known cure; treatment involves trying to prevent the serious lung infections associated with it and providing adequate nutrition. (Incidence: 1 per 2 000 White infants.)
- Toxoplasmosis: Toxoplasmosis is a parasitic infection that can be transmitted through the mother's placenta to a fetus. The disease-causing organism, which is found in undercooked meat, can invade the brain, eye, and muscle, possibly resulting in blindness and developmental delay. (Incidence: 1 per 1 000.)

These are not the only metabolic disorders that can be detected through newborn screening. Certain other rare disorders that can also be detected include Duchenne muscular dystrophy, human immunodeficiency virus (HIV) infection, and neuroblastoma. Hematologic disorders, such as glucose-6-phosphate dehydrogenase deficiency and thalassemia, can also be identified.

Most, but not all, U.S. states and Canadian provinces require newborns' hearing to be screened before they are discharged from the hospital. The hearing test involves placing a tiny earphone in the baby's ear and measuring his or her response to sound. A child develops critical speaking and language skills in the first few years of life, and if a hearing loss is discovered early, adverse developmental effects on language skills can be avoided.

INTERFERING FACTORS

- Premature infants may have false-positive results on newborn screening tests because of delayed development of liver enzymes.
- Tests on infants before they are 24 hours of age may yield false-negative results.
- Feeding problems (e.g., vomiting) may cause false-negative results.

PROCEDURE AND PATIENT CARE

Before
- Inform the parents about the purpose and method of the test.
- Assess the infant's feeding patterns before the test. An inadequate amount of protein ingested before the test can cause false-negative results.

During
- Place a few drops of blood from a heelstick in each circle on the filter paper.
- On the laboratory slip, document the infant's name, mother's name, hospital, current date and time, date and time of birth, and primary health care provider.

After
- Inform the parents that if test results are positive, they will be notified by their health care provider, and further testing or treatment will be recommended, depending on the particular condition.

TEST RESULTS AND CLINICAL SIGNIFICANCE

Metabolic diseases,
Endocrine diseases,
Hematologic diseases: *The detection of these disorders before they become clinically apparent may allow opportunities for treatment before significant mental or physical harm to the newborn occurs.*

5'-Nucleotidase

NORMAL FINDINGS

0.0–1.6 units at 37°C or 0.0–1.6 units at 37°C (SI units)

INDICATIONS

5'-Nucleotidase is measured to support the diagnosis of hepatobiliary obstructive disease. It is especially useful in helping confirm that an elevation in alkaline phosphatase level is the result of liver disease rather than disease of another tissue origin.

TEST EXPLANATION

5'-Nucleotidase is an enzyme specific to the liver. The 5'-nucleotidase level is elevated in patients with liver diseases, especially those associated with cholestasis. It provides information similar to that provided by alkaline phosphatase. However, alkaline phosphatase level is not specific to the liver. Diseases of the bone, sepsis, pregnancy, and other disease can produce alkaline phosphatase elevation. When the cause of an elevated alkaline phosphatase level is in doubt, a 5'-nucleotidase test is recommended. If levels of that enzyme are elevated along with the alkaline phosphatase level, the pathologic source is certainly the liver. If the 5'-nucleotidase level is normal when the alkaline phosphatase level is elevated, the pathologic source is outside the liver (bone, kidneys, spleen). Gamma-glutamyl transpeptidase is studied similarly, because it is also specific to the liver.

INTERFERING FACTORS

▰ Drugs that may cause *increases* in 5'-nucleotidase levels include hepatotoxic agents.

PROCEDURE AND PATIENT CARE

Before

𝑿 Explain the procedure to the patient.
𝑿 Inform the patient that no fasting is required.

During

- Collect a venous blood sample in a red-top tube.

After

- Apply pressure or a pressure dressing to the venipuncture site.
- Assess the venipuncture site for bleeding. Patients with liver dysfunction often have prolonged clotting times.

TEST RESULTS AND CLINICAL SIGNIFICANCE

▲ Increased Levels

Bile duct obstruction,
Cholestasis: *The 5'-nucleotidase test is most specific for pathologic conditions that cause intrahepatic or extrahepatic biliary obstruction.*
Hepatitis,
Cirrhosis,
Hepatic necrosis,
Hepatic ischemia,
Hepatic tumour,
Hepatotoxic drugs: *To a lesser degree, hepatocellular disease is associated with elevations in levels of this enzyme.*

RELATED TESTS

Gamma-Glutamyl Transpeptidase (p. 261). This is another enzyme that, when levels are elevated, specifically points to hepatic disease.

Alkaline Phosphatase (p. 53). This is an enzyme that exists in the liver and other organs. It is not specific to the liver.

 Osmolality, Blood (Serum Osmolality)

NORMAL FINDINGS

Adult/older adult: **285–295 mmol/kg** (285–295 mOsm/kg)
Child: **275–290 mmol/kg** (275–290 mOsm/kg)

Critical Values

<265 mmol/kg (<265 mOsm/kg)
>320 mmol/kg (>320 mOsm/kg)

INDICATIONS

This test is used to obtain information about fluid status and electrolyte imbalance. It is also helpful in evaluating illnesses involving antidiuretic hormone (ADH).

TEST EXPLANATION

Osmolality is the concentration of dissolved particles in blood. As the amount of free water in the blood increases or the amount of particles decreases, osmolality decreases. As the amount of water in the blood decreases or the amount of particles increases, osmolality increases. Osmolality increases with dehydration and decreases with overhydration.

An elaborate feedback mechanism controls osmolality. Increased osmolality stimulates secretion of ADH; this results in increased water reabsorption in the kidneys, more concentrated urine, and less concentrated serum. Low serum osmolality suppresses the release of ADH, which results in decreased water reabsorption and large amounts of dilute urine. The simultaneous measurement of blood osmolality and urine osmolality (see p. 972) helps in the interpretation and evaluation of problems involving osmolality.

The serum osmolality test is useful in evaluating fluid and electrolyte imbalance. The test is very helpful in evaluating patients with seizures, ascites, hydration status, acid-base balance, and suspected ADH abnormalities. Osmolality is also helpful in identifying the presence of organic acids, sugars, or ethanol. In these cases, there is an "osmolal gap," which represents the difference between what the osmolality should be—according to calculations of levels of serum sodium, glucose, and blood urea nitrogen (the three most important solutes in the blood)—and the osmolality as truly measured. If the "gap" is large, solutes such as organic acids (ketones) or unusually high levels of glucose or ethanol byproducts are suspected to be present. Finally, osmolality also plays an important role in toxicologic tests and workups for comatose patients. Values higher than **385 mmol/kg** (385 mOsm/kg) are associated with stupor in patients with hyperglycemia. When values of **400 to 420 mmol/kg** (400 to 420 mOsm/kg) are detected, grand mal seizures can occur. Values higher than **420 mmol/kg** (420 mOsm/kg) can be lethal.

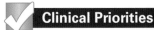
Clinical Priorities

- This test provides valuable information about fluid and electrolyte balance.
- Osmolality increases with dehydration and decreases with overhydration.
- The simultaneous measurement of blood and urine osmolality helps in interpreting and evaluating problems with fluid balance.

PROCEDURE AND PATIENT CARE

Before

☒ Explain the procedure to the patient.
☒ Inform the patient that no fasting is required.

During

- Collect a venous blood sample in a red-top tube.
- For newborns and infants, blood can be collected by means of a heelstick.

After

- Apply pressure or a pressure dressing to the venipuncture site.
- Observe the venipuncture site for bleeding.

TEST RESULTS AND CLINICAL SIGNIFICANCE

▲ Increased Levels

Hypernatremia,
Hyperglycemia,
Hyperosmolar nonketotic hyperglycemia,
Ketosis,
Azotemia: *All of these illnesses are associated with an increase in the number of particles dissolved in the blood.*
Dehydration: *Decreased replacement of ongoing water losses leads to dehydration and a rise in the serum osmolality.*
Mannitol therapy,
Ingestion of ethanol, methanol, or ethylene glycol: *These drugs stimulate free water loss from the kidneys and excretion in the urine. As a result, the serum osmolality is increased. Furthermore, byproducts of these drugs cause an increase in the number of solutes in the blood and thereby increase the osmolality.*
Uremia,
Diabetes insipidus,
Renal tubular necrosis,
Severe pyelonephritis: *These illnesses are associated with poor urine concentration. Free water is lost, and serum osmolality increases.*

▼ Decreased Levels

Overhydration: *The provision of free water above the ongoing losses creates a situation in which there is excess free water in the blood. Serum osmolality decreases.*
Syndrome of inappropriate ADH (SIADH) secretion: *Several illnesses can lead to this syndrome. ADH is inappropriately secreted despite factors that normally would inhibit its secretion. As a result, large quantities of water are reabsorbed by the kidneys. The serum becomes dilute, and osmolality decreases.*

Paraneoplastic syndromes associated with carcinoma (lung, breast, colon): *These cancers act as an autonomous ectopic source for the secretion of ADH. The pathophysiologic process is the same as described previously for SIADH.*

RELATED TESTS

Osmolality, Urine (p. 972). This is a measurement of the concentration of dissolved particles in the urine. When urine osmolality is measured with the serum osmolality, greater insight is obtained about problems of fluid balance.

Antidiuretic Hormone (p. 83). This is a direct measurement of ADH in the blood.

Antidiuretic Hormone Suppression (p. 85). This test is very helpful in the evaluation of ADH abnormalities.

Parathyroid Hormone (PTH, Parathormone)

NORMAL FINDINGS

Assay	Measurements Included in Assay	Normal Values (ng/L)*
PTH intact (whole)	Intact PTH	10–65
PTH N-terminal	N-terminal	8–24
	Intact PTH	
PTH C-terminal	C-terminal	
	Intact PTH	50–330
	Midmolecule	

*Conventional values are the same as the SI values but in picograms per millilitre.

INDICATIONS

Parathyroid hormone (PTH) is measured to assist in the evaluation of hypercalcemia or hypocalcemia. It is routinely monitored in patients with chronic renal failure.

TEST EXPLANATION

PTH is the only hormone secreted by the parathyroid gland in response to hypocalcemia. When calcium serum levels return to normal, PTH levels diminish. PTH is therefore one of the major factors affecting calcium metabolism. The PTH test is useful in establishing a diagnosis of hyperparathyroidism and distinguishing nonparathyroid from parathyroid causes of hypercalcemia. PTH levels are increased in patients with hyperparathyroidism (primary, secondary, or tertiary); in patients with nonparathyroid, ectopic PTH-producing tumours (pseudohyperparathyroidism); or as a normal compensatory response to hypocalcemia in patients with malabsorption or vitamin D deficiency.

Primary hyperparathyroidism is most often caused by a parathyroid adenoma and only rarely results from parathyroid cancer. Patients with primary hyperparathyroidism have high PTH and calcium levels. Secondary hyperparathyroidism is the exaggerated response of the parathyroid gland to kidney insensitivity to PTH in patients with chronic renal failure. Such patients have chronically low serum calcium levels in reaction to persistently high levels of phosphate that the kidney fails to excrete. In response to this chronically low calcium level, the parathyroid is constantly stimulated to produce PTH to attempt to maintain a normal calcium level. This response is called *secondary hyperparathyroidism.* Affected patients have high PTH and normal to slightly low calcium levels. On occasion, in a patient with chronic renal failure, the compensatory process is too strong, and autonomous PTH production becomes unnecessarily high, which leads to hypercalcemia. This process is called *tertiary hyperparathyroidism.* These patients have high PTH and high calcium levels.

It is important to measure serum calcium (see p. 152) simultaneously with PTH. Most laboratories have a PTH/calcium nomogram already made up, indicating what PTH level is considered normal for each calcium level.

PTH levels are decreased in patients with hypoparathyroidism or as a compensatory response to hypercalcemia in patients with metastatic bone tumours, sarcoidosis, vitamin D intoxication, or milk-alkali syndrome. Of course, surgical ablation of the parathyroid glands is another cause of hypoparathyroidism.

Whole (intact) PTH is metabolized to several different fragments, including an amino acid terminal (N-terminal), a midregion or midmolecule, and a carboxyl terminal (C-terminal). The intact PTH and the N-terminal are metabolically active. All these entities can be measured by immunoassay. The intact PTH and all fragments generally provide accurate information concerning the level of PTH in the blood. The intact PTH is probably most often tested because its measurement is most reliable.

INTERFERING FACTORS

- Recent injection of radioisotopes may interfere with this test if radioimmunoassay methods are used. However, radioimmunoassay is not frequently used to measure PTH fragments.
- Drugs that *increase* PTH level include anticonvulsants, isoniazid, lithium, phosphates, rifampin, and steroids.
- Drugs that *decrease* PTH level include cimetidine, pindolol, and propranolol.

✓ Clinical Priorities

- Results of this test are routinely monitored in patients with chronic renal failure. Such patients have chronically low serum calcium levels in reaction to persistently high phosphate levels that the kidneys fail to excrete.
- It is important to measure serum PTH and serum calcium levels at the same time. These values are important for a differential diagnosis. Most laboratories have PTH/calcium nomograms indicating normal PTH levels for each calcium level.
- PTH levels have diurnal variation: Levels are highest at approximately 2 AM and lowest at approximately 2 PM. Usually an 8 AM blood specimen is collected. If the patient works nights, the laboratory should be notified so that changes in the diurnal variation can be factored in.

PROCEDURE AND PATIENT CARE

Before

- Explain the procedure to the patient.
- Keep the patient on NPO status (nothing by mouth) except for water after midnight on the day of the test.

During

- Obtain a blood specimen at 8 AM because diurnal rhythm affects PTH levels. (If the patient works at night, check with the laboratory.) PTH levels are highest at approximately 2 AM and lowest at approximately 2 PM.
- Collect a venous blood sample in a red-top tube. Note that some laboratories require blood in an iced plastic syringe.
- Obtain a serum calcium level determination at the same time if it is ordered. The serum PTH and serum calcium levels are important for a differential diagnosis.

After

- On the laboratory slip, indicate the time the blood was collected, because the diurnal rhythm affects test results.
- Apply pressure or a pressure dressing to the venipuncture site.
- Check the venipuncture site for bleeding.
- Most PTH specimens are sent to a central laboratory. The specimen should be kept cold and transported on dry ice.

TEST RESULTS AND CLINICAL SIGNIFICANCE

▲ Increased Levels

Hyperparathyroidism secondary to adenoma or carcinoma of the parathyroid gland: *PTH is autonomously produced by the parathyroid gland. PTH levels are elevated.*

Non–PTH-producing tumours (paraneoplastic syndrome) commonly noted with lung, kidney, or breast carcinoma: *These tumours produce a "PTH-related protein" that acts like PTH and increases serum calcium. Because it is structurally similar to PTH, it is measured with PTH testing and produces an artificially high PTH result.*

Congenital renal defect: *The kidneys are congenitally unresponsive to "normal" quantities of PTH. As a result, the calcium level decreases despite normal quantities of PTH. The parathyroid consequently produces even greater quantities of PTH. This condition is also called* pseudohyperparathyroidism.

Hypocalcemia: *Elevation of PTH level is the result of a physiologic compensation for low serum calcium levels.*

Chronic renal failure: *Affected patients cannot excrete phosphates. As a result, serum calcium levels diminish. Elevation in PTH level is the result of a physiologic compensation for low serum calcium level. This is secondary hyperparathyroidism. On occasion, a patient with chronic renal failure develops parathyroid hyperplasia that causes PTH levels to exceed the amount required for physiologic homeostasis. This is tertiary hyperparathyroidism.*

Malabsorption syndrome: *Affected patients do not absorb calcium or fat-soluble vitamins such as vitamin D. Serum calcium levels fall. Elevation in PTH level is the result of a physiologic compensation for low serum calcium levels.*

Vitamin D deficiency and rickets: *Vitamin D is integral to the absorption of calcium from the gut. When levels are inadequate, serum calcium level decreases. Elevation of PTH level is the result of a physiologic compensation for low serum calcium levels.*

▼ Decreased Levels

Hypoparathyroidism caused by surgical ablation or immunoablation: *PTH is not produced at levels necessary to maintain normal calcium levels.*

Hypercalcemia: *Reduction in PTH level is a normal physiologic response to high serum calcium levels.*

Metastatic bone tumour: *Tumour in the bone can mobilize large quantities of calcium. Reduction in PTH level is a normal physiologic response to high serum calcium levels.*

Hypercalcemia of malignancy (most often with lung, breast, or lymphoma cancer): *For unknown reasons, serum calcium levels become very high in this type of cancer. Affected patients do not have bone metastasis or PTH-related proteins. Reductions in PTH level is a normal physiologic response to high serum calcium levels.*

Sarcoidosis: *Serum calcium levels may become elevated. Reduction in PTH level is a normal physiologic response to high serum calcium levels.*

Vitamin D intoxication: *Affected patients have high serum calcium levels because vitamin D stimulates maximal intestinal absorption of calcium. Reduction in PTH level is a normal physiologic response to high serum calcium levels.*

Milk-alkali syndrome: *Affected infants are given cooked whole milk that is very high in calcium. They develop high serum calcium levels. Reduction in PTH level is a normal physiologic response to high serum calcium levels.*

DiGeorge syndrome: *Children with this immunodeficiency also have hypocalcemia that may result from hypoparathyroidism.*

RELATED TESTS

Calcium, Blood (p. 152). This is a direct measurement of serum calcium. This test should be performed simultaneously with a PTH test to improve interpretation of PTH levels.

Phosphate, Phosphorus (p. 403). The phosphate test is a direct measurement of the inorganic phosphate levels in the serum, which are affected by PTH.

Partial Thromboplastin Time (PTT, Activated Partial Thromboplastin Time [aPTT])

NORMAL FINDINGS

Activated partial thromboplastin time (aPTT): 25–40 seconds
Partial thromboplastin time (PTT): 60–70 seconds
Patients receiving anticoagulant therapy: 1.5–2.5 times control value in seconds

 Critical Values

aPTT: >70 seconds
PTT: >100 seconds

INDICATIONS

The PTT test is used to assess the intrinsic system and the common pathway of clot formation. It is also used to monitor heparin therapy.

TEST EXPLANATION

Hemostasis and the coagulation system represent a homeostatic balance between factors encouraging clotting and factors encouraging clot dissolution. The first reaction of the body to active bleeding is blood vessel constriction. In small-vessel injury, this may be enough to stop bleeding. In large-vessel injury, hemostasis is required to form a clot that durably plugs the hole until healing can occur. The primary phase of the hemostatic mechanism involves platelet aggregation to blood vessel (see Figure 2-14, p. 181). Next, secondary hemostasis occurs. The first phase of reactions is called the *intrinsic system.* Factor XII and other proteins form a complex on the subendothelial collagen in the injured blood vessel. Through a series of reactions, activated factor XI (XIa) is formed and activates factor IX (IXa). In a complex formed by factors VIII, IX, and X, activated factor X (Xa) is formed.

At the same time, the *extrinsic system* is activated, and a complex is formed between tissue thromboplastin (factor III) and factor VII. Activated factor VII (VIIa) results. Factor VIIa can directly activate factor X. Alternatively, factor VIIa can activate factors IX and X together.

The final step is a common pathway in which prothrombin is converted to thrombin on the surface of the aggregated platelets. The main purpose of thrombin is to convert fibrinogen to fibrin, which is then polymerized into a stable gel. Factor XIII crosslinks the fibrin polymers to form a stable clot.

Almost immediately, three major activators of the fibrinolytic system act on plasminogen, which had previously been absorbed into the clot, to form plasmin. Plasmin causes the fibrin polymer to degenerate into fragments that are cleared by macrophages.

The PTT test is an evaluation of factors I (fibrinogen), II (prothrombin), V, VIII, IX, X, XI, and XII. When the PTT is combined with the prothrombin time, nearly all the hemostatic abnormalities can be recognized. When any of these factors exists in inadequate quantities, as in hemophilia A and B or consumptive coagulopathy, the PTT is prolonged. Because factors II, IX, and X are vitamin K–dependent factors, biliary obstruction—which precludes gastrointestinal absorption of fat and fat-soluble vitamins (e.g., vitamin K)—can reduce their concentration and thus prolong the PTT. Because coagulation factors are made in the liver, hepatocellular diseases also prolong the PTT.

Heparin has been found to inactivate prothrombin (factor II) and to prevent the formation of thromboplastin. These actions prolong the intrinsic clotting pathway for approximately 4 to 6 hours after each dose of heparin. Therefore, heparin is capable of providing therapeutic anticoagulation. The appropriate dosage of heparin can be monitored by the PTT. PTT test results are given in seconds along with a control value. The control value may vary slightly from day to day because of the reagents used.

Activators have been added to the PTT test reagents to shorten normal clotting time and provide a narrow normal range. This shortened time is called the *activated PTT* (aPTT). The normal aPTT is 30 to 40 seconds. The desired range for therapeutic anticoagulation is 1.5 to 2.5 times normal (e.g., 70 seconds). The aPTT specimen should be collected 30 to 60 minutes before the patient's next heparin dose is administered. If the aPTT is shorter than 50 seconds, therapeutic anticoagulation may not have been achieved and more heparin is needed. An aPTT longer than 100 seconds indicates that too much heparin is being given; serious spontaneous bleeding is a risk when the aPTT is this high. The effects of heparin can be reversed by the parenteral administration of 1 mg of protamine sulphate for every 100 units of the heparin dose.

Heparin's effect, unlike that of warfarin, is immediate and short-lived. When a thromboembolic episode (e.g., pulmonary embolism, arterial embolism, thrombophlebitis) occurs, immediate and complete anticoagulation is most rapidly and safely achieved through heparin administration. This drug is often given during cardiac and vascular surgery to prevent intravascular clotting during clamping of the vessels. Often, small doses of heparin (5000 U/mL subcutaneously every 12 hours) are given to prevent thromboembolism in patients at high risk. This dosage alters the PTT very little, and the risk for spontaneous bleeding is minimal.

INTERFERING FACTORS

 Drugs that may *prolong* PTT include antihistamines, ascorbic acid, chlorpromazine, heparin, and salicylates.

Clinical Priorities

- The PTT is used to monitor heparin therapy. Heparin's effect is immediate and short-lived.
- If too much heparin is given, its effects can be reversed by parenteral administration of protamine sulphate.
- Patients receiving heparin need to be evaluated for bleeding tendencies. Manifestations include bruising, petechiae, low-back pain, and bleeding gums. Blood may be detected in the urine and stool.

PROCEDURE AND PATIENT CARE

Before

- Explain the procedure to the patient.
- If the patient is receiving heparin by intermittent injection, plan to collect the blood specimen for the aPTT 30 minutes to 60 minutes before the patient receives the next dose of heparin.
- If the patient is receiving a continuous heparin infusion, collect the blood at any time.

During

- Collect a venous blood sample in one or two blue-top tubes.

After

- Apply pressure or a pressure dressing to the venipuncture site.
- Assess the venipuncture site for bleeding. Remember that if the patient is receiving anticoagulants or has coagulopathies, the bleeding time is increased.
- Assess the patient to detect possible bleeding. Check for blood in the urine and all other excretions, and assess the patient for bruises, petechiae, and bleeding gums.
- If severe bleeding occurs, reverse the anticoagulant effect of heparin by parenteral administration of protamine sulphate.

TEST RESULTS AND CLINICAL SIGNIFICANCE

▲ Increased Levels

Congenital clotting factor deficiencies (e.g., von Willebrand's disease, hemophilia, hypofibrinogenemia): *These hereditary illnesses are associated with very little, if any, of the respective clotting factors. As a result, the PTT is prolonged.*

Cirrhosis of liver,

Vitamin K deficiency: *The liver makes most of the clotting factors. For synthesis of some of those clotting factors, vitamin K is required. In the illnesses just listed, the clotting factors of the intrinsic system and common pathways are inadequate in quantity. As a result, the PTT is prolonged.*

Disseminated intravascular coagulation (DIC): *Key clotting factors involved in the intrinsic system are consumed.*

Heparin administration: *Heparin inhibits the intrinsic system at several points. As a result, the PTT is prolonged.*

Coumarin administration: *Although coumarin has a greater effect on the prothrombin time, it does inhibit the function of factors II, IX, and X. As a result, the PTT is prolonged.*

▼ Decreased Levels

Early stages of DIC: *Circulating procoagulants exist in the early stages of DIC. These act to shorten the PTT.*

Extensive cancer (e.g., ovarian, pancreatic, colon): *The pathophysiologic mechanism underlying this association is not well known.*

RELATED TESTS

Prothrombin Time (p. 446). This test is used to evaluate the adequacy of the extrinsic system and common pathway in the clotting mechanism.

Coagulating Factor Concentration (p. 177). This is a quantitative measurement of specific coagulation factors.

Parvovirus B19 Antibody

NORMAL FINDINGS

Negative for immunoglobulin M (IgM)– and immunoglobulin G (IgG)–specific antibodies to parvovirus B19

INDICATIONS

This test is performed on children who have vague symptoms of fever, arthralgias, and rash suggestive of erythema infectiosum. It is also becoming a part of routine testing for proposed organ donors.

TEST EXPLANATION

Parvoviruses include several species-specific viruses of animals. Parvovirus B19 is known to be a human pathogen. Many of the severe manifestations of parvovirus B19 viremia are related to the ability of the virus to infect and lyse red blood cell (RBC) precursors in the bone marrow. The name "B19" was derived from the code number of the human serum in which the virus was discovered.

Erythema infectiosum is the most common manifestation of parvovirus B19 infection and occurs predominantly in children. This pathogen is also referred to as *fifth disease,* because it was classified in the late nineteenth century as the fifth in a series of six exanthems of childhood. This infection is also sometimes referred to as "academy rash." The typical presentation is a self-limiting, mild illness with a low-grade fever, malar rash, and occasionally arthralgia. The rash usually begins on the face and may also develop on the arms and legs. Outbreaks of erythema infectiosum occur most often during the winter and spring months.

Parvovirus B19 has been associated with a number of other clinical problems:

- Flulike illness in association with joint inflammation, rash, and occasionally purpura in young adults.
- Hydrops fetalis and fetal loss in fewer than 10% of infected pregnant women.
- Transient aplastic crisis in patients with chronic hemolytic anemia. In immunocompromised patients (those with acquired immune deficiency syndrome [AIDS], organ donors), this virus can be so severe as to cause aplastic anemia and bone marrow failure. With increasing frequency, this antibody test is being used for all potential organ donors.
- Chronic severe anemia in patients with immunodeficiency caused by infection with human immune deficiency virus (HIV), congenital immunodeficiency, and acute lymphocytic leukemia during maintenance chemotherapy, and in recipients of bone marrow transplants.

Because of the spectrum of diseases caused by parvovirus B19, laboratory diagnosis has come into great demand. Serologic testing for parvovirus B19–specific IgM and IgG antibodies can be detected by enzyme-linked immunosorbent assay and indirect fluorescent antibody immunofluorescence methods. Acute infections can be documented from parvovirus B19–compatible symptoms and the presence of IgM antibodies that remain detectable up to a few months. Past infection or immunity is documented by the indefinite persistence of IgG antibodies. Fetal infection may be recognized by hydrops fetalis and the presence of parvovirus B19 DNA in amniotic fluid or fetal blood.

PROCEDURE AND PATIENT CARE

Before

- Explain the procedure to the patient.
- Inform the patient that no fasting or special preparation is required.

During

- Collect a venous blood sample according to the laboratory protocol.

After

- Apply pressure or a pressure dressing to the venipuncture site.
- Assess the venipuncture site for bleeding.
- Inform the patient that test results are normally available in approximately 2 to 3 days.

TEST RESULTS AND CLINICAL SIGNIFICANCE

▲ Increased Levels

Erythema infectiosum (fifth disease),

Joint arthralgia and arthritis: *These diseases are self-limiting and elevate antibodies through the course of viremia.*

Hydrops fetalis,

Fetal loss: *These obstetric disasters could be attributable to maternal infection with parvovirus.*

Transient aplastic anemia,

Chronic anemia,

Bone marrow failure: *These problems occur mostly in patients who are immunocompromised. In such patients, the viremia is much more significant. RBC precursors are target cells for the virus.*

Pheochromocytoma Suppression and Provocative Testing (Clonidine Suppression Test [CST], Glucagon Stimulation Test)

NORMAL FINDINGS

Glucagon Stimulation
Norepinephrine: <3 times the basal levels

Clonidine Suppression Test
Norepinephrine: >50% reduction in basal levels or <1 502 pmol/L (<500 pg/mL)
Epinephrine: >50% reduction in basal levels or <1 625 pmol/L (<275 pg/mL)

INDICATIONS

These tests are used to identify pheochromocytoma when catecholamine levels are not assuredly diagnostic.

TEST EXPLANATION

In patients with significantly high blood pressure that is refractory to treatment, the diagnosis of pheochromocytoma is often considered. Pheochromocytomas usually arise from the adrenal glands and are often difficult to detect. Pheochromocytomas release catecholamines (epinephrine, norepinephrine), which cause blood pressure to rise excessively and resist treatment. The definitive diagnosis of pheochromocytoma rests primarily on the demonstration of excessive catecholamine production, best achieved with a resting plasma catecholamine assay. When basal catecholamine plasma levels are excessive (norepinephrine >11 820 pmol/L [>2 000 pg/mL]) in nonstressed patients, the diagnosis of pheochromocytoma is certain. However, when basal levels are far less than 11 820 pmol/L (<2 000 pg/mL), the diagnosis of pheochromocytoma is far less certain. Plasma catecholamine levels are not often informative unless the blood specimen is obtained during a hypertensive paroxysm. Urine metanephrine levels (p. 1009) are best tested at times other than hypertensive episodes.

When the diagnosis of pheochromocytoma is not certain, suppression and provocative tests may be necessary. Measurements of plasma catecholamines (epinephrine and norepinephrine) are particularly useful during suppression or provocative tests.

Normally, glucagon (less commonly metoclopramide and naloxone) is used as a provocative agent. Glucagon stimulates the release of catecholamines. In the presence of pheochromocytoma, the agents can cause the tumour to release excessive catecholamines into the bloodstream. The glucagon stimulation test has been superseded by the clonidine suppression test because glucagon can provoke dangerous increases in blood pressure in patients with pheochromocytomas.

Clonidine is normally a potent suppressor of catecholamine production; however, it has little to no suppressive effect on catecholamines in patients with pheochromocytoma. Suppressive testing is much safer than provocative testing because there is no real chance of a hypertensive paroxysm. The clonidine suppression test is nearly 100% accurate.

POTENTIAL COMPLICATIONS

- Drowsiness during the clonidine suppression test
- Hypotension during the clonidine suppression test, especially in patients treated aggressively for hypertension

- Extremely high blood pressure during provocative testing: If a patient develops a sudden increase in blood pressure, intravenous medication may be administered in an attempt to control the blood pressure.

INTERFERING FACTORS

- False suppression with the clonidine suppression test may occur in patients with low basal catecholamine levels.
- Drugs that may cause *false-positive* results of suppression tests include antidepressants and beta blockers.

PROCEDURE AND PATIENT CARE

Before

- Explain the procedure to the patient.
- Identify and explain the medications being administered before the test.
- The patient must be reclining calmly for 30 minutes before the test.

During

- Collect a venous blood sample from an antecubital vein in a heparinized (green-top) tube for determination of basal catecholamine levels (epinephrine and norepinephrine).
- Monitor vital signs closely throughout the testing period.

Glucagon Provocation Test
- Administer a prescribed dose of glucagon intravenously.
- Two minutes later, obtain a blood specimen as described previously.
- Be prepared to treat a severe hypertensive episode.

Clonidine Suppression Test
- Administer a prescribed dose of clonidine orally.
- Three hours later, obtain a blood specimen as described previously.

After

- Monitor vital signs for at least 1 hour after conclusion of the procedure.

TEST RESULTS AND CLINICAL SIGNIFICANCE

Pheochromocytoma: *This is a rare catecholamine-secreting tumour of the adrenal gland derived from chromaffin cells. Such tumours that arise outside the adrenal gland are termed* extra-adrenal pheochromocytomas *or* paragangliomas. *They may precipitate life-threatening hypertension or cardiac arrhythmias.*

RELATED TEST

Vanillylmandelic Acid and Catecholamines (p. 1009). This 24-hour urine test is performed primarily to diagnose hypertension secondary to pheochromocytoma. It is also used to detect the presence of neuroblastomas and other rare adrenal tumours.

Phosphate, Phosphorus (PO₄, P)

NORMAL FINDINGS

Adult: **1.0–1.5 mmol/L** (3.0–4.5 mg/dL)
Older adult: slightly lower than adult values
Child: **1.3–2.3 mmol/L** (4.0–7.0 mg/dL)
Newborn: **1.4–3.0 mmol/L** (4.3–9.3 mg/dL)

 Critical Values

<0.32 mmol/L (<1 mg/dL)

INDICATIONS

This test is performed to assist in the interpretation of studies investigating parathyroid and calcium abnormalities. It is usually performed to measure phosphate levels and ensure that blood levels are adequate.

TEST EXPLANATION

Phosphorus in the body is in the form of a phosphate. The terms *phosphorus* and *phosphate* are used interchangeably throughout this and other discussions. Most of the phosphate in the body is a part of organic compounds. Only a small part of total body phosphate is inorganic phosphate (i.e., not part of another organic compound). The inorganic phosphate is measured when a "phosphate," "phosphorus," "inorganic phosphorus," or "inorganic phosphate" measurement is requested. Most of the body's inorganic phosphorus is intracellular and combined with calcium within the skeleton; however, approximately 15% of the phosphorus exists in the blood as a phosphate salt. The organic phosphate (not measured by this test) is used to synthesize part of the phospholipid compounds in the cell membrane, adenosine triphosphatase (ATP) for energy source in metabolism, nucleic acids, or enzymes (e.g., 2,3-diphosphoglycerate). The inorganic phosphate (measured in this test) contributes to electrical and acid-base homeostasis.

Dietary phosphorus is absorbed in the small bowel. The absorption is very efficient, and only rarely is hypophosphatemia caused by gastrointestinal malabsorption. Antacids, however, can bind phosphorus and decrease intestinal absorption. Renal excretion of phosphorus should equal dietary intake to maintain a normal serum phosphate level. Phosphate levels vary significantly during the day; values are lowest at approximately 10 AM and highest 12 hours later.

Phosphorus levels are determined by calcium metabolism, parathyroid hormone (PTH), renal excretion, and, to a lesser degree, intestinal absorption. Because calcium and phosphorus levels are inversely related, a decrease in one mineral results in an increase in the other. Therefore, serum phosphorus levels depend on calcium metabolism, and vice versa. The regulation of phosphate by PTH is such that PTH tends to decrease phosphate reabsorption in the kidneys. PTH and vitamin D, however, tend to stimulate phosphate absorption weakly within the gut.

INTERFERING FACTORS

- Recent carbohydrate ingestion, including intravenous glucose administration, causes decreased phosphorus levels, because phosphorus enters the cell with glucose.
- Laxatives or enemas containing sodium phosphate can *increase* phosphorus levels.
- Drugs that may cause *increases* in phosphorus levels include methicillin, steroids, some diuretics (furosemide and thiazides), and vitamin D (excessive).
- Drugs that may cause *decreases* in phosphorus levels include antacids, albuterol, anaesthesia agents, estrogens, insulin, oral contraceptives, and mannitol.

PROCEDURE AND PATIENT CARE

Before

- Explain the procedure to the patient.
- Keep the patient on NPO status (nothing by mouth) after midnight on the day of the test.
- If it is indicated, discontinue intravenous fluids with glucose for several hours before the test.

During

- Collect a venous blood sample in a red-top tube.
- Avoid hemolysis. Handle the tube carefully. Hemolysis can artificially elevate the phosphate level because phosphate is an intracellular ion. Cellular lysis of red blood cells (RBCs) causes the intracellular phosphate to spill into the blood.
- Use a heelstick to collect blood from infants.

After

- Apply pressure or a pressure dressing to the venipuncture site.
- Check the venipuncture site for bleeding.
- Take the specimen to the laboratory immediately.
- On the laboratory slip, indicate the time the blood was obtained.

TEST RESULTS AND CLINICAL SIGNIFICANCE

▲ Increased Levels (Hyperphosphatemia)

Hypoparathyroidism: *Renal reabsorption of phosphates is enhanced.*

Renal failure: *Renal excretion of phosphates is diminished.*

Increased dietary or intravenous intake of phosphorus: *Increased intake leads to transient elevations in phosphate levels.*

Acromegaly: *Renal reabsorption of phosphates is enhanced.*

Bone metastasis: *The phosphate stores in the bones are mobilized by the destructive bone tumours.*

Sarcoidosis: *Intestinal absorption of phosphates is increased because of the vitamin D effect produced by granulomatous infections.*

Hypocalcemia: *Calcium and phosphate levels are inversely related. When one is elevated, the other is low.*

Acidosis: *When the pH is reduced, phosphates are driven out of the cell and into the bloodstream as part of a buffering system.*

Rhabdomyolysis,

Advanced lymphoma or myeloma,

Hemolytic anemia: *Cell lysis associated with these diseases causes intracellular phosphate to pour out into the bloodstream. Phosphate levels rise.*

▼ Decreased Levels (Hypophosphatemia)

Inadequate dietary ingestion of phosphorus: *This is very rare, because phosphate reabsorption in the intestine is extremely efficient.*

Chronic antacid ingestion: *Antacids bind the phosphate in the intestine and preclude absorption.*

Hyperparathyroidism: *PTH increases urinary excretion of phosphates.*

Hypercalcemia: *Calcium and phosphate levels are inversely related. When one is elevated, the other is low.*

Chronic alcoholism: *The pathophysiologic mechanism underlying this observation is probably multifactorial. It may be in part nutritional and in part related to magnesium deficiency.*

Vitamin D deficiency (rickets): *Renal tubules fail to reabsorb phosphates.*

Treatment of hyperglycemia,

Plasminogen,

Hyperinsulinism (childhood): *Insulin tends to drive phosphates into the cells.*

Malnutrition: *Rarely is malnutrition a cause of phosphate deficiency, because phosphate is efficiently absorbed through the intestines. However, when malnutrition is associated with a deficiency of fat-soluble vitamins such as vitamin D, phosphate renal reabsorption is diminished. Phosphate levels decrease.*

Alkalosis: *Phosphate acts as a buffer. When pH increases, phosphate levels in the blood diminish because of an intracellular shift.*

Gram-negative sepsis

RELATED TESTS

Parathyroid Hormone (p. 393). This hormone raises serum phosphate and calcium levels.

Calcium, Blood (p. 152). This direct measurement of serum calcium should be performed simultaneously with phosphate measurements.

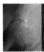

Phosphatidylinositol Antigen (PI-Linked Antigen)

NORMAL FINDINGS

RBCs
Type I (normal expression): 99%–100%
Type II (partial deficient): 0%–0.99%
Type III (deficient): 0%–0.01%
Granulocytes: 0%–0.01%
Monocytes: 0%–0.05%

INDICATIONS

The PI-linked antigen is useful for screening and confirming the diagnosis of paroxysmal nocturnal hemoglobinuria (PNH). It is also used to monitor the disease.

TEST EXPLANATION

Paroxysmal nocturnal hemoglobinuria (PNH) is an acquired hematologic disorder of the bone marrow stem cell that is characterized by nocturnal hemoglobinuria, chronic hemolytic anemia, thrombosis, and pancytopenia, and in some patients by acute or chronic myeloid malignancies.

These patients have dark urine caused by ongoing hemolysis. PNH appears to be a hematopoietic stem cell disorder that affects erythroid, granulocytic, and megakaryocytic cell lines. The abnormal cells in PNH have been shown to lack glycosylphosphatidylinositol (GPI)-linked proteins in RBCs and WBCs. Mutations in the *phosphatidylinositol glycan A* (*PIGA*) *gene* have been identified consistently in patients with PNH, thus confirming the biologic defect in this disorder.

Flow cytometric immunophenotyping of peripheral blood (WBC and RBC) is performed to determine the presence or absence of PI-linked antigens (CD14, FLAER, and/or CD59 antigens) using monoclonal antibodies directed against them. These proteins are absent on the cells of patients with PNH. Certain GPI-anchored proteins protect red blood cells from destruction; others are involved in blood clotting, whereas others are involved in fighting infection. Therefore the majority of the disease manifestations (i.e., hemolytic anemia, thrombosis, and infection) result from a deficiency of these GPI-anchored proteins.

Individuals without PNH have normal expression of all PI-linked antigens—CD14 (monocytes), CD16 (neutrophils and NK cells), CD24 (neutrophils), and CD59 (RBCs). Other GPI-linked antigens noted to be absent in PNH include CD55 and CD59. In addition, FLAER, a fluorescently labelled inactive variant of aerolysin, binds directly to the GPI anchor, and can be used to evaluate the expression of the GPI linkage.

PROCEDURE AND PATIENT CARE

Before
- Explain the procedure to the patient.
- Tell the patient that no fasting is required.

During
- Collect a venous blood sample in a yellow- (ACD) top tube.

After
- Apply pressure or a pressure dressing to the venipuncture site.

TEST RESULTS AND CLINICAL SIGNIFICANCE

▼ Decreased Levels
PNH: *These GPI-linked antigens are reduced or absent in patients with PNH. Determining which antigen is most significantly reduced will highlight the disease manifestations.*

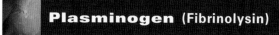

Plasminogen (Fibrinolysin)

NORMAL FINDINGS
2.4–4.4 units/mL is the range recommended by the Council on Thrombolytic Agents (CTA).

INDICATIONS
This test is used to diagnose suspected plasminogen deficiency in patients who experience multiple thromboembolic episodes.

TEST EXPLANATION

Plasminogen is a protein involved in the fibrinolytic process of dissolution of intravascular blood clots (see Figure 2-14, p. 181). Plasminogen is converted to plasmin by proteolytic cleavage. This reaction can be catalyzed by urokinase, streptokinase, or tissue plasminogen activator. Plasmin can destroy fibrin and dissolve clots. This fibrinolytic system helps maintain a normal homeostatic balance between coagulation and anticoagulation.

Plasminogen levels are occasionally measured during fibrinolytic therapy (for coronary and peripheral arterial occlusion) and are diminished. Decreased levels of plasminogen are also found in hyperfibrinolytic states (e.g., disseminated intravascular coagulation [DIC], primary fibrinolysis) because the plasminogen is used up. Because plasminogen is made in the liver, patients with cirrhosis or other severe liver diseases can be expected to have decreased levels. Rare hereditary deficiencies of this protein also exist. Decreased plasminogen levels greatly increase the risk for arterial or venous thrombosis.

Pregnancy and especially eclampsia are associated with increased levels of plasminogen. Patients with inflammatory conditions that may be associated with increased levels of C-reactive protein also may have concomitant mild elevations in levels of plasminogens, which are acute-phase reactant proteins.

PROCEDURE AND PATIENT CARE

Before

🖉 Explain the procedure to the patient.
🖉 Inform the patient that no fasting is required.

During

• Collect a venous blood sample in a blue-top tube containing sodium citrate.
• Avoid excessive agitation of the blood sample.

After

• Apply pressure or a pressure dressing to the venipuncture site.
• Assess the venipuncture site for bleeding, especially if the patient is suspected of having a hyperfibrinolytic process (e.g., DIC).

TEST RESULTS AND CLINICAL SIGNIFICANCE

▲ Increased Levels

Pregnancy: *The pathophysiologic mechanism underlying this observation is not well known. It may be related to amniotic proteins' gaining access to the maternal circulation.*

▼ Decreased Levels

Hyperfibrinolytic state (e.g., DIC, fibrinolysis),
Primary liver disease: *Plasminogen is made in the liver. In severe liver disease, plasminogen synthesis does not occur.*
Syndrome associated with hypercoagulation (e.g., venous and arterial clotting): *This syndrome can occur with many different types of diseases (e.g., colon cancer).*
Congenital deficiencies of plasminogen: *These rare deficiencies greatly increase the risk for thromboembolic episodes.*
Malnutrition: *In severe malnutrition, protein depletion is so severe that it interrupts plasminogen production.*

Plasminogen Activator Inhibitor 1 (PAI-1)

NORMAL FINDINGS

2–14 IU/mL (enzyme-linked immunosorbent assay [ELISA])
2–46 ng/mL (antigen assay)

INDICATIONS

Plasminogen activator inhibitor 1 (PAI-1) is the principal inactivator of the fibrinolytic system. High levels are associated with a number of atherosclerotic risk factors.

TEST EXPLANATION

PAI-1 is a protein that inhibits plasminogen activators. During fibrinolysis, tissue plasminogen activator converts plasminogen into plasmin. Plasmin plays a critical role in fibrinolysis by degrading fibrin (see Figure 2-14, p. 181). PAI-1 is the primary inhibitor of tissue plasminogen activator and other plasminogen activators in the blood. PAI-1 limits the production of plasmin and keeps fibrinolysis in check. High levels of PAI-1 are associated with an increased risk for arterial thrombosis as a result of inhibition of fibrinolysis. Low levels of PAI-1 are associated with an increased risk for bleeding in relation to excessive degradation of fibrin.

Patients with insulin resistance syndrome and diabetes mellitus tend to have increased PAI-1 levels. Increased levels are associated with an increased incidence of acute coronary syndrome. Levels are also increased in patients with acute and chronic coronary artery disease and in patients with restenosis after coronary angioplasty. Increased levels may reduce the effectiveness of antithrombolytic therapy.

INTERFERING FACTORS

- Because PAI-1 is an acute-phase reactant, it can become transiently elevated by infection, inflammation, or trauma.
- Levels increase during pregnancy.
- PAI-1 has a circadian rhythm in which the concentration is highest in the morning and lowest in the afternoon and evening.

PROCEDURE AND PATIENT CARE

Before

- Explain the procedure to the patient.
- Inform the patient that no fasting is required.

During

- Collect a venous blood sample in a blue-top tube. Discard the first several millilitres of blood if PAI-1 is the only test being performed. If multiple tests are being performed, fill the blue-top tube after any red-top tube.
- Gently invert the blood tube several times after collection.

After

- Apply pressure or a pressure dressing to the venipuncture site.
- Assess the venipuncture site for bleeding, especially if the patient has a bleeding disorder.
- Deliver the tube immediately to the laboratory.

TEST RESULTS AND CLINICAL SIGNIFICANCE

▲ Increased Levels

Acute coronary syndrome,
Coronary artery disease,
Restenosis after coronary angioplasty: *Inhibition of fibrinolysis increases the risk for thrombosis.*
Infection,
Inflammation,
Trauma: *PAI-1 is an acute-phase reactant and can be transiently elevated in these conditions.*
Pregnancy: *Pregnancy is associated with increases in levels of proteins, including PAI-1.*
Diabetes mellitus,
Insulin resistance syndrome: *The association of elevated PAI-1 with these diseases is observational. The pathophysiologic mechanism is unknown.*

▼ Decreased Levels

Bleeding disorders: *Excessive degradation of fibrin increases the risk for bleeding.*

RELATED TESTS

Plasminogen (p. 406). This test is used to diagnose suspected plasminogen deficiency in patients who experience multiple thromboembolic episodes.

C-Reactive Protein (p. 199). This measurement of an acute-phase reactant protein is used to indicate an inflammatory illness.

Platelet Aggregation

NORMAL FINDINGS

Vary according to platelet agonist used

INDICATIONS

This test is a measure of platelet function and aids in the evaluation of bleeding disorders.

TEST EXPLANATION

Platelet aggregation is important in hemostasis. A clump of platelets surrounds an area of acute blood vessel endothelial injury. Normal platelets adhere to this area of injury, and through a series of chemical reactions, they attract other platelets to the area. This is platelet aggregation, the first step in hemostasis. After this step, the normal coagulation factor cascade occurs. Certain diseases that affect either platelet number or function can inhibit platelet aggregation and thereby prolong bleeding times. Congenital syndromes, uremia, myeloproliferative disorders, and drugs are associated with abnormal platelet aggregation. If blood is passed through a heart-lung machine or a dialysis pump, platelets can be injured, and aggregation capability can be reduced.

Many agonists are used to stimulate platelet aggregation in the laboratory. Platelet aggregation is measured by determining the turbidity of platelet-rich plasma. As platelet aggregation is stimulated in vitro, turbidity decreases and light transmission through the specimen increases. This test is performed with an optical device called an *aggregometer.* Usually the patient's blood specimen is spun to a platelet-rich component. Next, an agonist to platelet aggregation—such as adenosine diphosphate, collagen, epinephrine, or ristocetin—is added. Turbidity is then measured within the aggregometer, and a curve indicating light transmission per unit of time is plotted. Normal curves have been identified for any one agonist that is used.

This is a very sensitive test, and it can be significantly affected by a number of variables:
1. Concentration of sodium citrate
2. Platelet count
3. Storage temperature
4. Concentration of the agonist addition
5. Reaction temperature
6. Degrees of lipemia, hemoglobinemia, or bilirubinemia

INTERFERING FACTORS

- Factors that may cause increases in platelet aggregation include blood storage temperature, hyperbilirubinemia, hemoglobinemia, hyperlipidemia, and platelet count.
- Drugs that may cause *decreases* in platelet aggregation include antiplatelet drugs (e.g., ticlopidine), aspirin, some antibiotics, beta blockers, clofibrate, dextran, ethanol, heparin, nonsteroidal anti-inflammatory drugs (NSAIDs), phenothiazines, tricyclic agents, theophylline, and warfarin sodium (Coumadin).

PROCEDURE AND PATIENT CARE

Before
- Explain the procedure to the patient.
- Inform the patient that no fasting is required.

During
- Collect a venous blood sample in a blue-top tube.
- On the laboratory request slip, indicate whether the patient is receiving any drugs that may interfere with platelet aggregation or has any diseases such as jaundice, hyperlipidemia, or hemolysis.

After
- Apply pressure or a pressure dressing to the venipuncture site.
- Assess the venipuncture site for bleeding.
- Remember that abnormalities in platelet aggregation can prolong bleeding time, and a significant hematoma at the venipuncture site may occur.

TEST RESULTS AND CLINICAL SIGNIFICANCE

Various congenital disorders (e.g., Wiskott-Aldrich syndrome, Bernard-Soulier syndrome, von Willebrand's disease): *Platelet aggregation is diminished in autosomal recessive diseases.*

Connective tissue disorder (e.g., systemic lupus erythematosus): *The pathophysiologic mechanism underlying these observations is not understood.*

Recent cardiopulmonary or dialysis bypass: *Platelets are injured as they are passing through this machinery. The injured platelets are less likely to function normally in regard to aggregation.*

Uremia: *Not only is the platelet number reduced in uremic patients but a reduced aggregation capability has also been observed.*

Various myeloproliferative diseases, including leukemia, myeloma, and dysproteinemia: *The pathophysiologic mechanism underlying these observations is not clear. It may be related to the effect of abnormal antibodies on the platelet membrane.*

Drugs (e.g., aspirin): *Drugs can have an immediate, and in some cases long-lasting, negative effect on platelet aggregation.*

Prolonged platelet aggregation

RELATED TESTS

Platelet Count (p. 416). This is a direct measurement of platelet number.

Platelet Antibody (see following test). This test identifies antibodies directed against platelets.

Platelet Volume, Mean (p. 419). This is a measurement of the size of the platelets. It is helpful in the evaluation of thrombocytopenia.

Platelet Antibody (Antiplatelet Antibody Detection)

NORMAL FINDINGS

No antiplatelet antibodies identified

INDICATIONS

This test is used to evaluate thrombocytopenia and confirm or rule out an immune-associated cause.

TEST EXPLANATION

Immune-mediated destruction of platelets may be caused either by autoantibodies directed against antigens located on the same person's platelets or by alloantibodies that develop after exposure to transfused platelets received from a donor. These antibodies are usually directed to an antigen on the platelet membrane, such as human leukocyte antigen (HLA; see p. 316) or platelet-specific antigen (PLA; e.g., PLA-1, PLA-2). Many different laboratory techniques can be used to demonstrate the antiplatelet antibodies. These tests can directly identify the immunoglobulin with the use of radioimmunoassay or immunofluorescence. Quantitative measurements are possible with cytofluorometry. Other tests identify complement binding on the affected platelet membrane. Most antiplatelet antibody testing is now performed with immunologic assays.

Antibodies directed to platelets cause early destruction of the platelets and subsequent thrombocytopenia. Different types of immunologic thrombocytopenia are as follows:

1. *Idiopathic thrombocytopenia purpura* is a term that describes a group of disorders characterized by immune-mediated destruction of the platelets within the spleen or other reticuloendothelial organs. Platelet-associated immunoglobulin G (IgG) antibodies are detected in 90% of affected patients.

2. *Posttransfusion purpura* is a rare syndrome characterized by the sudden onset of severe thrombocytopenia a few hours to a few days after transfusion of red blood cells (RBCs) or platelets. This is usually associated with an antibody to blood types AB, B, and O (ABO); HLA; or PLA antigens on the RBC. In most situations, the blood recipient has previously been sensitized to a PLA-1 antigen during previous transfusions or during previous pregnancy. Once these antibodies form, they destroy the donor's PLA-1–positive platelets and the recipient's PLA-1–negative platelets.

3. *Maternal-fetal platelet antigen incompatibility* (neonatal thrombocytopenia) occurs when the fetal platelets contain a PLA-1 antigen that is absent in the maternal platelets. As in Rh incompatibility, the mother's body creates anti–PLA-1 antibodies that cross the placenta and destroy the fetal platelets. The mother is not thrombocytopenic. Neonatal thrombocytopenia can also occur if the mother has idiopathic thrombocytopenia purpura autoantibodies that are passed through the placenta and destroy the fetal platelets.

4. *Drug-induced thrombocytopenia.* Although numerous drugs are known to induce autoimmune-mediated thrombocytopenia, heparin is the most common and causes heparin-induced thrombocytopenia (HIT). Two types of HIT, type I and II, may develop. Type I HIT is generally considered a benign condition and is not antibody mediated. In type II HIT, thrombocytopenia is usually more severe and is antibody mediated. Type II HIT is caused by an IgG antibody and usually occurs after 6 to 8 days of intravenous heparin therapy. Although platelet counts may be low, bleeding is unusual. Rather, paradoxical thromboembolism is the most worrisome complication and may be attributable to platelet activation caused by the antibody to the heparin/platelet factor 4 complex, which instigates platelet aggregation.

HIT occurs in approximately 1% to 5% of patients taking heparin for 5 to 10 days, and heparin-induced thrombosis occurs in one-third to one-half of those patients. Cessation of heparin therapy is mandatory, and alternative anticoagulation is initiated. The diagnosis is suspected on the basis of clinical symptoms, recent heparin administration, and low platelet counts. The diagnosis is confirmed by identifying *heparin-induced thrombocytopenia antibodies.* In this test, an enzyme-linked immunosorbent assay is used to detect HIT-specific antibodies to the heparin–platelet factor 4 complex. This assay can detect antibodies to IgG, immunoglobulin M, and immunoglobulin A, and it has a sensitivity of approximately 80% to 90%.

Other drugs known to cause antiplatelet antibodies include cimetidine, analgesics (salicylates, acetaminophen), antibiotics (cephalosporins, penicillin derivatives, sulphonamides), quinidine-like drugs, diuretics (e.g., chlorothiazide), digoxin, propylthiouracil, and disulphiram (Antabuse).

PROCEDURE AND PATIENT CARE

Before

- Explain the procedure to the patient.
- Inform the patient that no fasting is required.

During

- Collect a venous blood sample in a red-top tube. The amount of blood required depends on the initial platelet count.

After

- Apply pressure or a pressure dressing to the venipuncture site.
- Ensure adequate hemostasis in all patients with suspected thrombocytopenia.
- A platelet count is usually performed 1 to 2 hours after platelet transfusion. This not only documents the posttransfusion platelet count but also eliminates a large proportion of posttransfusion immune thrombocytopenia reactions.

TEST RESULTS AND CLINICAL SIGNIFICANCE

▲ Increased Levels

Immune thrombocytopenia,
Idiopathic thrombocytopenia purpura,
Neonatal thrombocytopenia,
Posttransfusion purpura,
Drug-induced thrombocytopenia: *The pathophysiologic mechanism underlying these diseases is described in the preceding "Test Explanation" section.*

RELATED TESTS

Platelet Count (p. 416). This is a direct measurement of platelet number.

Platelet Aggregation (p. 409). This is a test of platelet function.

Platelet Volume, Mean (p. 419). This is a measurement of the size of the platelets. It is helpful in the evaluation of thrombocytopenia.

Platelet Closure Time (Platelet Function Assay/Screen)

NORMAL FINDINGS

<175 seconds

INDICATIONS

Platelet closure time is used to identify platelet dysfunction in patients in whom a bleeding abnormality is suspected. This test can identify abnormalities in the ability of platelets to aggregate or instigate the hemostatic cascade. It is used for patients with a family or personal history of acute excessive bleeding.

TEST EXPLANATION

Platelet dysfunction may be acquired, inherited, or induced by platelet-inhibiting agents. It is clinically important to assess platelet function as a potential cause of a bleeding diathesis (epistaxis, menorrhagia, postoperative bleeding, or easy bruising). The most common causes of platelet dysfunction are related to uremia, liver disease, von Willebrand's disease, and exposure to agents such as acetylsalicylic acid (aspirin). Bleeding time had been the most common measurement performed to evaluate platelet function. However, testing for bleeding time is labour intensive and expensive, and its accuracy depends heavily on operator skills. Its results cannot be reproduced and quantified. Platelet aggregation studies (p. 409) have similar accuracy problems. As a result, more clinical laboratories are using the *platelet closure time* to accurately quantify platelet function. This test is often called a *platelet function screen*. Closure time can differentiate aspirin effects from other causes of platelet dysfunction.

Closure times are measured according to a system (platelet function analyzer) in which the process of platelet adhesion and aggregation after a vascular injury is simulated in vitro. Anticoagulated whole blood is passed over membranes at a standardized flow rate, which creates high shear rates that result in platelet attachment, activation, and aggregation on the membrane. A hole in the membrane is occluded when a stable platelet plug develops. The time required to obtain full occlusion of the hole is reported as the closure time in seconds.

This test is sensitive to platelet adherence and aggregation abnormalities and allows the discrimination of aspirin-like defects and intrinsic platelet disorder. Two membranes—one consisting of collagen/epinephrine and the other consisting of collagen/adenosine-5'-diphosphate (ADP), which is a potent platelet antiaspirin stabilizer—are used. The collagen/epinephrine membrane is used to detect platelet dysfunction induced by intrinsic platelet defects. Follow-up testing with the collagen/ADP membrane enables the discrimination of aspirin effects. Table 2-38 shows expected patterns observed with closure time in normal persons and in patients with various disorders.

This test can also be used to determine the presence of any resistance to the therapeutic effects of aspirin on platelets. Although aspirin remains a crucial and cost-effective therapy for the prevention and management of cardiovascular diseases, research findings suggest that a significant percentage of patients on a chronic aspirin regimen are "aspirin resistant" or do not achieve sufficient antiplatelet effects from aspirin. Previous studies have shown that aspirin resistance is associated with triple the risk for heart attack, stroke, and death. Once patients are tested and identified as aspirin resistant, physicians may opt for an alternative approach to therapy, which may include increasing the dosage of aspirin or placing the patient on another antiplatelet medication. Up to 27% of patients with coronary artery disease who use aspirin are resistant to its antiplatelet effects. Women, older adults, and those taking lower doses of aspirin are most likely to be aspirin resistant.

Enzyme-linked immunosorbent assay (ELISA) urine tests are now quick and easily performed to determine the effect of aspirin on the platelets. These *aspirin resistance tests* measure 11-dehydrothromboxane B_2, a stable thromboxane metabolite, in the urine. Aspirin's protective action is believed to be the result of its ability to inhibit the cyclooxygenase-1 pathway in the platelet that results in the generation of thromboxane A_2, initiating the blood clotting process.

TABLE 2-38	Platelet Closure Time		
Membrane Type	**Normal**	**Acetylsalicylic Acid Effect**	**Intrinsic Platelet Disorders**
Collagen/epinephrine membrane	Normal	Abnormal	Abnormal
Collagen/adenosine–5'-diphosphate membrane	Normal	Normal	Abnormal

Early research suggests that a positive test for aspirin resistance raises the possibility that the patient may be clopidogrel (Plavix) resistant as well.

INTERFERING FACTORS

▧ Aspirin and nonsteroidal antiarthritic agents (NSAIDs) can *increase* platelet closure time. These medications prevent blood from clotting by blocking the production of thromboxane A_2, a chemical that platelets produce that instigates platelet aggregation. Aspirin accomplishes this by inhibiting the enzyme cyclooxygenase-1 (COX-1), which produces thromboxane A_2.

▧ Thienopyridines can *increase* platelet closure time. When ADP attaches to ADP receptors on the surface of platelets, the platelets clump. The thienopyridines (e.g., ticlopidine and clopidogrel [Plavix]) block the ADP receptor, which prevents ADP from attaching to the receptor and the platelets from clumping.

PROCEDURE AND PATIENT CARE

Before

✍ Explain the procedure to the patient.

✍ Inform the patient that no fasting is required.

• Obtain a drug history to determine whether the patient has recently taken aspirin, anticoagulants, or any other medications that may affect test results.

During

• Collect a venous blood sample in a blue-top (citrate anticoagulated) tube.

After

• Apply pressure or a pressure dressing to the puncture site.

• Assess the puncture site for bleeding.

TEST RESULTS AND CLINICAL SIGNIFICANCE

▲ Prolonged Times or Increased Values

Myelodysplastic syndromes,

Myeloid leukemia,

Hereditary telangiectasia,

Myeloproliferative disorders,

Bernard-Soulier syndrome,

Glanzmann thromboasthenia,

Hermansky-Pudlak syndrome: *These diseases are associated with intrinsic platelet defects that cause platelet malfunction.*

von Willebrand's disease,

Collagen-vascular disease,

Cushing's syndrome,

Henoch-Schönlein syndrome,

Uremia,

Connective tissue disorder: *These diseases are characterized by a defect in the interaction of the platelet and the injured blood vessel, which renders the platelets unable to aggregate.*

RELATED TEST

Platelet Count (see following test). This is a quantitative measure of the number of circulating platelets. Thrombocytopenia is a common cause of excessive bleeding.

Platelet Count (Thrombocyte Count)

NORMAL FINDINGS

Adult/older adult: 150×10^9/L to 400×10^9/L ($150\,000$/mm^3 to $400\,000$/mm^3)
Child: 150×10^9/L to 400×10^9/L ($150\,000$/mm^3 to $400\,000$/mm^3)
Infant: 200×10^9/L to 475×10^9/L ($200\,000$/mm^3 to $475\,000$ mm^3)
Premature infant: 100×10^9/L to 300×10^9/L ($100\,000$/mm^3 to $300\,000$/mm^3)
Newborn: 150×10^9/L to 300×10^9/L ($150\,000$/mm^3 to $300\,000$/mm^3)

 Critical Values

$<50 \times 10^9$/L ($<50\,000$/mm^3) or $>1\,000 \times 10^9$/L (>1 million/mm^3)

INDICATIONS

The platelet count is an actual count of the number of platelets (thrombocytes) per cubic millilitre of blood. It is performed on patients who develop petechiae (small hemorrhages in the skin), spontaneous bleeding, increasingly heavy menses, or thrombocytopenia. It is used to monitor the course of the disease or therapy for thrombocytopenia or bone marrow failure.

TEST EXPLANATION

Platelets are formed in the bone marrow from megakaryocytes. They are small, round, nonnucleated cells whose main role is maintenance of vascular integrity. In blood vessel injury, hemostasis is required to form a clot that durably plugs the hole until healing can occur. The primary phase of the hemostatic mechanism involves platelet aggregation. From there, the platelets help initiate the coagulation factor cascade. The majority of platelets exist in the bloodstream. Twenty-five percent exist in the liver and spleen. Survival of platelets is measured in days (average of 7 to 9 days).

Platelet activity is essential to blood clotting. Counts of 150×10^9/L to 400×10^9/L ($150\,000$/mm^3 to $400\,000$/mm^3) are considered normal. Counts lower than 100×10^9/L ($<100\,000$/mm^3) are considered to indicate *thrombocytopenia; thrombocytosis* is said to exist when counts exceed 400×10^9/L ($>400\,000$/mm^3). *Thrombocythemia* is a term used to indicate a platelet count in excess of $1\,000 \times 10^9$/L (>1 million/mm^3). Vascular thrombosis with tissue or organ infarction is the major complication of thrombocythemia. The most common diseases associated with spontaneous thrombocytosis are iron-deficiency anemia and malignancy (leukemia, lymphoma, solid tumours such as that of the colon). Thrombocytosis may also occur with polycythemia vera and postsplenectomy syndromes. Even patients with elevated platelet counts can experience a bleeding tendency because the function (platelet aggregation) of those platelets may be abnormal. It is not uncommon for patients whose platelet counts exceed $1\,000 \times 10^9$/L (>1 million/mm^3) to experience spontaneous bleeding and thrombocytosis.

Spontaneous hemorrhage may occur with thrombocytopenia. If thrombocytopenia is severe, the platelets are often counted manually. Spontaneous bleeding is a serious danger when platelet counts fall below $20 \times 10^9/L$ (<20000/mm^3). Petechiae and ecchymosis also occur at that degree of thrombocytopenia. With counts exceeding $40 \times 10^9/L$ (>40000/mm^3), spontaneous bleeding rarely occurs, but bleeding from trauma or surgery may be prolonged.

Causes of thrombocytopenia include the following conditions:

1. Reduced production of platelets (secondary to bone marrow failure, infiltration of fibrosis, tumour, and other diseases)
2. Sequestration of platelets (secondary to hypersplenism)
3. Accelerated destruction of platelets (secondary to antibodies, infections, drugs, prosthetic heart valves)
4. Consumption of platelets (secondary to disseminated intravascular coagulation [DIC])
5. Platelet loss from hemorrhage
6. Dilution with large volumes of blood transfusions containing very few, if any, platelets

INTERFERING FACTORS

- Living in high altitudes may cause increases in platelet levels.
- Because platelets can clump together, automated counting is subject to at least a 10% to 15% error.
- Strenuous exercise may cause increases in platelet levels.
- Platelet levels may be decreased before menstruation.
- Drugs that may cause *increases* in platelet levels include estrogens and oral contraceptives.
- Drugs that may cause *decreases* in platelet levels include chemotherapeutic agents, chloramphenicol, colchicine, histamine-2–blocking agents (cimetidine, ranitidine [Zantac]), hydralazine, indomethacin, isoniazid (INH), quinidine, streptomycin, sulphonamides, thiazide diuretics, and tolbutamide (Sulfonylurea).

PROCEDURE AND PATIENT CARE

Before

- Explain the procedure to the patient.
- Inform the patient that no fasting is required.

During

- Collect a peripheral venous blood sample in a lavender-top tube.

After

- Apply pressure or a pressure dressing to the venipuncture site.
- Assess the venipuncture site for bleeding.
- If the results indicate that the patient has a serious platelet deficiency,
   1. Observe the patient for signs and symptoms of bleeding.
   2. Check for blood in the urine and all excretions.
   3. Assess the patient for bruises, petechiae, bleeding from the gums, epistaxis, and low-back pain.
   4. Reassess all venipuncture sites for signs of hematoma formation.

TEST RESULTS AND CLINICAL SIGNIFICANCE

▲ Increased Levels (Thrombocytosis)

Malignant disorders (leukemia, lymphoma, solid tumours such as of the colon): *The pathophysiologic mechanism underlying this observation is not known.*

Polycythemia vera: *This is hyperplasia of all the bone marrow cell lines, including platelets.*

Postsplenectomy syndrome: *The spleen normally extracts aging platelets from the bloodstream. With surgical splenectomy, that job is less effectively done by other organs (e.g., the liver). As a result, the platelet count increases.*

Rheumatoid arthritis: *The pathophysiologic mechanism underlying this observation is not known.*

Iron-deficiency anemia or following hemorrhagic anemia: *Iron is not needed for platelet production. Anemia causes maximal stimulation of cellular production by the marrow. Red blood cells (RBCs) may not be so easily produced in the presence of iron deficiency. Platelets, however, can easily respond even in the presence of iron deficiency.*

▼ Decreased Levels (Thrombocytopenia)

Hypersplenism: *The spleen normally extracts aging platelets from the bloodstream. An enlarged spleen, however, extracts more platelets, both aging and new. The platelet count diminishes.*

Hemorrhage: *Platelets are lost in the bleeding process. If they are not replaced by transfusion of platelets, the bone marrow takes some time (hours to days) to produce an adequate number of platelets. This problem is exacerbated with treatment that replenishes blood volume and RBC count. Such treatment dilutes the remaining platelets and further decreases the platelet count.*

Immune thrombocytopenia (e.g., idiopathic thrombocytopenia, neonatal, posttransfusion, or drug-induced thrombocytopenia): *Antibodies directed against antigens on the platelet cell membrane destroy the platelets, and the count decreases.*

Leukemia and other myelofibrosis disorders: *The bone marrow is replaced by neoplastic or fibrotic tissue. Megakaryocyte function and numbers diminish. Platelets are not produced, and the count drops.*

Thrombotic thrombocytopenia: *This disease and others such as HELLP syndrome (hemolysis, elevated liver enzyme levels, low platelet count) are highlighted by thrombocytopenia, hemolytic anemia, and other hematologic abnormalities.*

Graves' disease: *In a small number of these patients, thrombocytopenia occurs. The pathophysiologic mechanism underlying this observation is not known.*

Inherited disorders (e.g., Wiskott-Aldrich, Bernard-Soulier, Zieve syndromes): *The pathophysiologic mechanism underlying this observation is not known.*

DIC: *The pathophysiologic process of thrombocytopenia is not clear. In part, however, it is thought that ongoing thrombosis "consumes" the platelets in much the same way that coagulating factors are "consumed." DIC usually develops concurrently with other severe disease (e.g., Gram-negative sepsis) that can also produce thrombocytopenia.*

Systemic lupus erythematosus: *The pathophysiologic mechanism underlying this observation is not known.*

Pernicious anemia: *Unlike iron, vitamin B_{12} is necessary for platelet production. A deficiency of this vitamin or folate diminishes the production of platelets.*

Hemolytic anemia: *Often the same disease process that produces the hemolysis (e.g., hemolytic-uremic syndrome) also destroys the platelets. The platelet count falls.*

Cancer chemotherapy: *Cytotoxic drugs often affect the bone marrow. Platelets are not produced at adequate levels, and the count drops.*

Infection: *Bacterial, viral, and rickettsial infections can cause thrombocytopenia, especially when the patient is immunocompromised (e.g., as in acquired immune deficiency syndrome [AIDS]).*

RELATED TESTS

Platelet Aggregation (p. 409). This is a test of platelet function.

Platelet Antibody (p. 411). This test identifies antibodies directed against platelets.

Platelet Volume, Mean (see following test). This is a measurement of the size of the platelets. It is helpful in the evaluation of thrombocytopenia.

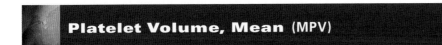

Platelet Volume, Mean (MPV)

NORMAL FINDINGS

7.4–10.4 fL (7.4–10.4 μm^3)

INDICATIONS

This test is helpful in the evaluation of platelet disorders, especially thrombocytopenia.

TEST EXPLANATION

The mean platelet volume (MPV) is a measure of the volume of a large number of platelets, determined by an automated analyzer. MPV is analogous to mean corpuscular volume (see p. 456) of red blood cells (RBCs).

The MPV varies with total platelet production. In cases of thrombocytopenia despite a normal reactive bone marrow (e.g., hypersplenism), the normal bone marrow releases immature platelets in an attempt to maintain a normal platelet count. These immature platelets are larger, and the MPV is increased. When bone marrow production of platelets is inadequate, the platelets that are released are small, and the MPV is low. Thus, the MPV is very useful in the differential diagnosis of thrombocytopenic disorders.

PROCEDURE AND PATIENT CARE

Before

- Explain the procedure to the patient.
- Inform the patient that no fasting is required.

During

- Collect a venous blood sample in a lavender-top tube.

After

- Apply pressure or a pressure dressing to the venipuncture site.
- Assess the venipuncture site for bleeding.
- If the patient is known to have a low platelet count,
  1. Observe the patient for signs and symptoms of bleeding.
  2. Check for blood in the urine and all excretions.
  3. Assess the patient for bruises, petechiae, bleeding of the gums, epistaxis, and low-back pain.

TEST RESULTS AND CLINICAL SIGNIFICANCE

▲ Increased Levels

Valvular heart disease,

Immune thrombocytopenia (e.g., idiopathic thrombocytopenia, neonatal, posttransfusion, or drug induced-thrombocytopenia),

Massive hemorrhage: *All these illnesses are characterized by thrombocytopenia and a normally reactive bone marrow that produces a great number of immature platelets in an attempt to maintain a normal platelet count. These immature platelets are large and increase the MPV.*

Vitamin B_{12} or folate deficiency: *Megaloblastic changes affect the megakaryocyte, just as the erythroid line is affected. The platelets that are produced are larger and may even be nucleated. The MPV is increased.*

Myelogenous leukemia: *Large, abnormal platelets are formed by neoplastic megakaryocytes if they are involved in the leukemic process. The MPV increases.*

▼ Decreased Levels

Aplastic anemia,

Chemotherapy-induced myelosuppression: *When bone marrow production of platelets is inadequate, the platelets that are released are small. MPV is reduced.*

Wiskott-Aldrich syndrome: *This syndrome is characterized by eczema, immune deficiency, thrombocytopenia, and small platelets.*

RELATED TESTS

Platelet Aggregation (p. 409). This is a test of platelet function.
  Platelet Antibody (p. 411). This test identifies antibodies directed against platelets.
  Platelet Count (p. 416). This is a direct measurement of the number of platelets.

Potassium, Blood (K)

NORMAL FINDINGS

Adult/older adult: **3.5–5.1 mmol/L (3.5–5.1 mEq/L)**
Child: **3.4–4.7 mmol/L (3.4–4.7 mEq/L)**
Infant: **4.1–5.3 mmol/L (4.1–5.3 mEq/L)**
Newborn: **3.7–5.9 mmol/L (3.7–5.9 mEq/L)**

Critical Values

Adult: **<2.5 mmol/L (<2.5 mEq/L) or >6.5 mmol/L (>6.5 mEq/L)**
Newborn: **<2.5 mmol/L (<2.5 mEq/L) or >8 mmol/L (>8 mEq/L)**

INDICATIONS

This test is routinely performed in most patients evaluated for any type of serious illness. Furthermore, because this electrolyte is so important to cardiac function, its measurement is a part of all complete routine evaluations, especially in patients who take diuretics or heart medications.

TEST EXPLANATION

Potassium is the major cation within the cell. The intracellular potassium concentration is approximately **150 mmol/L** (150 mEq/L), whereas the normal serum potassium concentration is approximately **4 mmol/L** (4 mEq/L). This ratio is the most important determinant in maintaining membrane electrical potential, especially in neuromuscular tissue. Because the serum concentration of potassium is so small, minor changes in concentration have significant consequences. Potassium is excreted by the kidneys. There is no reabsorption of potassium from the kidneys. Therefore, if potassium is not adequately supplied in the diet (or by intravenous administration in the patient who is unable to eat), serum potassium levels can drop rapidly.

Potassium is an important part of protein synthesis and maintenance of normal oncotic pressure and cellular electrical neutrality, as mentioned. It contributes to the metabolic portion of acid-base balance in that the kidneys can shift potassium for hydrogen ions to maintain a physiologic pH.

Serum potassium concentration depends on many factors:

1. *Aldosterone* (and, to a lesser extent, glucocorticosteroids). This hormone tends to increase renal losses of potassium.
2. *Sodium reabsorption.* As sodium is reabsorbed, potassium is lost.
3. *Acid-base balance.* Alkalotic states tend to lower serum potassium levels by causing a shift of potassium into the cell. Acidotic states tend to raise serum potassium levels by reversing that shift.

Symptoms of *hyperkalemia* include irritability, nausea, vomiting, intestinal colic, and diarrhea. The electrocardiogram may demonstrate peaked T waves, a widened QRS complex, and a depressed ST segment. Signs of *hypokalemia* are related to a decrease in contractility of smooth, skeletal, and cardiac muscles, which results in weakness, paralysis, hyporeflexia, ileus, increased cardiac sensitivity to digoxin, cardiac arrhythmias (dysrhythmias), flattened T waves, and prominent U waves. This electrolyte has profound effects on the heart rate and contractility. The potassium level should be monitored carefully in patients with uremia, Addison's disease, and vomiting and diarrhea and in patients taking steroid therapy and potassium-depleting diuretics. Potassium levels must also be closely monitored in patients taking digitalis-like drugs because cardiac arrhythmias may be induced by hypokalemia and digoxin.

Clinical Priorities

- Potassium has profound effects on the heart rate and contractility. Potassium levels must be monitored carefully in patients taking digitalis-like drugs and diuretics because cardiac arrhythmias may be induced by hypokalemia.
- Intravenous potassium may be indicated in order to prevent cardiac arrhythmias for hypokalemia in adults. The rate of potassium infusion is slow, to prevent irritation to the veins.
- Serum potassium levels are affected by acid-base balance. Alkalotic states lower potassium levels, and acidotic states raise levels.
- Hemolysis of blood during venipuncture or laboratory processing can cause elevations in potassium levels.

INTERFERING FACTORS

- Opening and closing of the hand with a tourniquet in place may increase potassium levels.
- Hemolysis of blood during venipuncture or during laboratory processing causes increases in potassium levels.
- Drugs that may cause *increases* in potassium levels include aminocaproic acid, antibiotics, antineoplastic drugs, captopril, epinephrine, heparin, histamine, isoniazid (INH), lithium, mannitol, potassium-sparing diuretics, potassium supplements, and succinylcholine.
- Drugs that may cause *decreases* in potassium levels include acetazolamide, salicylic acid, glucose infusions, amphotericin B, carbenicillin, cisplatin, diuretics (which cause potassium wasting), insulin, laxatives, lithium carbonate, penicillin G sodium (high doses), phenothiazines, salicylates (aspirin), and sodium polystyrene sulphonate (Kayexalate).

PROCEDURE AND PATIENT CARE

Before
- Explain the procedure to the patient.
- Inform the patient that no special diet or fasting is required.

During
- Instruct the patient to avoid opening and closing the hand after a tourniquet is applied.
- Collect a venous blood sample in a red-top or green-top tube.
- Avoid hemolysis.

After
- Apply pressure or a pressure dressing to the venipuncture site.
- Assess the venipuncture site for bleeding.
- Evaluate the patient with increased or decreased potassium levels for cardiac arrhythmias.
- Monitor patients taking digoxin and diuretics for hypokalemia.
- If it is indicated, administer resin exchanges (e.g., Kayexalate enema) to correct hyperkalemia.

TEST RESULTS AND CLINICAL SIGNIFICANCE

▲ Increased Levels (Hyperkalemia)

Excessive dietary intake,

Excessive intravenous intake: *Because the amount of potassium in the serum is so small, minimal but significant increases in potassium intake can cause elevations in the serum level.*

Acute or chronic renal failure: *This is the most common cause of hyperkalemia. Potassium excretion is diminished, and potassium levels rise.*

Addison's disease,

Hypoaldosteronism,

Aldosterone-inhibiting diuretics (e.g., spironolactone, triamterene): *Aldosterone is not excreted. Aldosterone enhances potassium excretion. Without that effect, potassium excretion is diminished, and potassium levels rise.*

Crush injury to tissues,

Hemolysis,

Transfusion of hemolyzed blood,

Infection: *Potassium exists in high levels in the cell. With cellular injury and lysis, the potassium within the cell is released into the bloodstream.*

Acidosis: *To maintain physiologic pH during acidosis, hydrogen ions are driven from the blood and into the cell. To maintain electrical neutrality, potassium is expelled from the cell. Potassium levels rise.*

Dehydration: *The potassium becomes more concentrated in dehydrated patients, and serum levels appear to be elevated. When the patient is rehydrated, potassium levels may in fact be reduced.*

▼ Decreased Levels (Hypokalemia)

Deficient dietary intake,

Deficient intravenous intake: *The kidneys cannot reabsorb potassium to compensate for the reduced potassium intake. Potassium levels decline.*

Burns,

Gastrointestinal disorders (e.g., diarrhea, vomiting, villous adenomas): *Excessive potassium is lost because of ongoing fluid and electrolyte losses, as described previously.*

Diuretics: *These medications act to increase renal excretion of potassium. This is especially important for patients who take diuretics and digitalis preparations for cardiac disease. Hypokalemia can exacerbate the ectopy that digoxin may instigate.*

Hyperaldosteronism: *Aldosterone enhances potassium excretion.*

Cushing's syndrome: *Glucocorticosteroids have an "aldosterone-like" effect, which is to enhance potassium excretion.*

Renal tubular acidosis: *Renal excretion of potassium is increased.*

Licorice ingestion: *Licorice has an "aldosterone-like" effect, which is to enhance potassium excretion.*

Alkalosis: *To maintain physiologic pH during alkalosis, hydrogen ions are driven out of the cell and into the blood. To maintain electrical neutrality, potassium is driven into the cell. Potassium levels fall.*

Insulin administration: *In patients with hyperglycemia, insulin is administered. Glucose and potassium are driven into the cell. Potassium levels drop.*

Glucose administration: *In a person without diabetes, insulin is secreted in response to glucose administration. Glucose and potassium are driven into the cell. Potassium levels drop.*

Ascites: *Renal blood flow is decreased as a result of reduced intravascular volume, which in turn results from the collection of fluid. The reduced blood flow stimulates the secretion of aldosterone, which increases potassium excretion. Furthermore, affected patients are often taking potassium-wasting diuretics.*

Renal artery stenosis: *Renal blood flow is reduced. The pathophysiologic process is as described for ascites.*

Cystic fibrosis: *In affected patients, potassium loss in secretions and sweat is increased.*

Trauma/surgery/burns: *The body's response to such injuries is mediated, in part, by aldosterone, which increases potassium excretion.*

RELATED TESTS

Sodium, Blood (p. 479), and Chloride, Blood (p. 167). These electrolytes are often measured at the same time as potassium. Metabolically, they are all intermingled.

Potassium, Urine (p. 976). This test is used to identify increased potassium excretion.

Prealbumin (PAB, Thyroxine-Binding Prealbumin [TBPA], Thyretin, Transthyretin)

NORMAL FINDINGS

Blood
Adult/older adult: **150–360 mg/L** (15–36 mg/dL)
Child:
<5 days: **60–210 mg/L** (6–21 mg/dL)
1–5 years: **140–300 mg/L** (14–30 mg/dL)
6–9 years: **150–330 mg/L** (15–33 mg/dL)
10–13 years: **220–360 mg/L** (22–36 mg/dL)
14–19 years: **220–450 mg/L** (22–45 mg/dL)

Prealbumin
Urine (24-hour): **0.28–45 mg/L** (<10–148 *Mcg*/L)

Cerebrospinal Fluid
Approximately 2% of total cerebrospinal fluid (CSF) protein

 Critical Values

Serum prealbumin levels **<107 mg/L** (<10.7 mg/dL) indicate severe nutritional deficiency.

INDICATIONS

This test is used to indicate a person's nutritional status. It is also used to indicate liver function status.

TEST EXPLANATION

Prealbumin is one of the major plasma proteins. Because prealbumin can bind thyroxine, it is also called *thyroxine-binding prealbumin.* However, the role of prealbumin is secondary to that of thyroxine-binding globulin in the transportation of triiodothyronine (T_3) and thyroxine (T_4). Prealbumin also plays a role in the transport and metabolism of vitamin A. Prealbumin is measured by immunoassay.

Because prealbumin levels in serum fluctuate more rapidly in response to alterations in synthetic rate than do those of other serum proteins, clinical interest in the quantification of serum prealbumin has centred on its usefulness as a marker of nutritional status. Its half-life of 1.9 days is much less than the 21-day half-life of albumin (see p. 440). Because of prealbumin's short half-life, it is a sensitive indicator of any change affecting protein synthesis and catabolism. Therefore, prealbumin measurement is frequently ordered to monitor the effectiveness of total parenteral nutrition.

Prealbumin levels are significantly reduced in hepatobiliary disease because of impaired prealbumin synthesis. Serum levels of prealbumin are better indicators of liver function than are albumin levels. Prealbumin is also a negative acute-phase reactant protein; serum levels decrease in inflammation, malignancy, and protein-wasting diseases of the intestines or kidneys. Because zinc is required for synthesis of prealbumin, levels are low with zinc deficiency. Levels of prealbumin are increased in Hodgkin disease and chronic kidney disease.

Because of the low quantity of prealbumin in the serum, this protein is not often visualized on serum protein electrophoresis. However, because prealbumin crosses the blood-brain barrier, it is found in the CSF and can be seen on CSF electrophoresis (see discussion of lumbar puncture on p. 676).

INTERFERING FACTORS

- Coexistent inflammation may make test result interpretation impossible.
- Drugs that may cause *increases* in prealbumin levels include anabolic steroids, androgens, estrogen, and prednisolone.
- Drugs that may cause *decreases* in prealbumin levels include amiodarone, estrogens, and oral contraceptives.

✓ Clinical Priorities

- Clinical interest in prealbumin has centred on its usefulness as a marker of nutritional status. Its half-life of 1.9 days is much less than the 21-day half-life of albumin.
- Prealbumin measurement is frequently indicated to monitor the effectiveness of total parenteral nutrition.
- Because prealbumin is a negative acute-phase reactant protein, serum levels may decrease with inflammatory processes and may make test result interpretation impossible.

PROCEDURE AND PATIENT CARE

Before

- Explain the procedure to the patient.
- Inform the patient that no food or fluid restrictions are required.
- If the patient is to collect a 24-hour urine specimen, provide a collection bottle.

During

- Collect a venous blood sample in a red-top tube.

After

- Apply pressure or a pressure dressing to the venipuncture site.
- Observe the venipuncture site for bleeding.
- Transport the 24-hour urine specimen to the laboratory promptly.
- Inform the patient how and when to obtain the results of this study.

TEST RESULTS AND CLINICAL SIGNIFICANCE

▲ Increased Levels

Some cases of nephrotic syndrome: *The major characteristic of the nephrotic syndrome is proteinuria that causes hypoproteinemia. Because prealbumin is made so rapidly, the percentage of prealbumin in the blood may be disproportionate when other proteins take somewhat longer to produce.*

Hodgkin disease: *The pathophysiologic mechanism underlying this observation is not known.*

Pregnancy: *The estrogen effect stimulates protein (prealbumin) synthesis.*

▼ Decreased Levels

Malnutrition,

Liver damage: *The synthesis of prealbumin is diminished.*

Burns: *Protein is lost acutely from the burn and chronically as a result of the constant loss of serum through the burn.*

Inflammation: *Prealbumin is a negative acute-phase reactant protein. Therefore, in the presence of inflammation, prealbumin levels diminish.*

RELATED TESTS

Protein Electrophoresis (p. 440). This is a quantification of all the components that make up the serum proteins, including albumin and alpha$_1$-, alpha$_2$-, beta$_1$-, beta$_2$-, and gamma-globulins. This test can also detect abnormal proteins created by neoplasms and/or infections.

Immunoglobulin Electrophoresis (p. 327). This is a quantification of the components that make up immunoglobulin, which is a gamma-globulin.

Pregnancy Tests (Human Chorionic Gonadotropin [hCG], Beta Subunit)

NORMAL FINDINGS

Qualitative

Negative; positive in pregnancy

Quantitative

Whole human chorionic gonadotropin (hCG):

Gestation (weeks)	Whole hCG (IU/L)*
<1	5–50
2	50–500
3	100–10 000
4	1 000–30 000
5	3 500–115 000
6–8	12 000–270 000
12	15 000–220 000

*Conventional values are the same as the SI values but in milli–international units per millilitre.

Male and nonpregnant female: <5

Beta subunit: Values depend on the method and test used

INDICATIONS

This test is used to diagnose pregnancy. It is also helpful in the monitoring of "high-risk" pregnancies and can be used as a tumour marker for certain cancers.

TEST EXPLANATION

All pregnancy tests are based on the detection of hCG, which is secreted by the placental tro-phoblast after the ovum is fertilized. This hormone appears in the blood and urine of pregnant women as early as 10 days after conception. In the first few weeks of pregnancy, hCG levels rise markedly, and serum levels are higher than urine levels. After approximately a month, hCG level is approximately the same in either specimen.

This hormone is a glycoprotein very similar to the pituitary proteins. Like other glyco-proteins, hCG is made up of two fractions: alpha and beta subunits. The alpha subunit is the same for all the glycoproteins. The beta subunit is unique to each. Therefore, the beta subunit for hCG is specific for hCG. The whole hCG molecule is metabolized into the alpha and beta subunits in the blood. They are then excreted by the kidneys into the urine. Whole hCG cross-reacts with pituitary hormones (especially luteinizing hormone). Therefore, testing for whole hCG is less specific, and the incidence of false-positive results (cross-reactions with luteinizing hormone) is high.

All pregnancy studies demonstrate the presence of hCG. Methods of pregnancy testing fall into three categories: immunologic tests, radioimmunoassay, and radioreceptor assays.

Immunologic Tests (Agglutination Inhibition Test [AIT]) (Blood and Urine)

Immunologic tests are performed with commercially prepared antibodies against the whole hCG molecule and can be completed within 2 minutes or 2 hours, depending on the method used. These immunologic tests have a high false-positive rate and usually do not yield positive results until approximately 28 days after the last menstrual period. The false-positive rate (lack of spec-ificity) is high because these antibodies are directed toward the whole hCG unit (alpha and beta subunits). The alpha subunit is the same for other pituitary hormones. This test often detects luteinizing hormone, which renders the result false-positive.

Immunologic testing for the beta subunit of hCG, however, has far better accuracy and a shorter time for yielding positive test results (18 days). With the development of monoclonal antibodies, current immunoassays can identify very small levels of hCG, and pregnancy can be detected 3 to 7 days after conception. Several immunologic tests are now commercially available to the public for testing. The patient's urine is tested, and its colour is compared with a standard containing a known small amount of hCG. If the colour matches that standard, pregnancy is confirmed. These tests take from 5 minutes to 2 hours to perform.

Radioimmunoassay (Serum)

Radioimmunoassay is a highly sensitive and reliable blood test for detection of the beta unit of hCG. In this test, maternal serum hCG and "test" hCG that has been radioactively bound to an antibody (labelled) compete for binding sites on a resin form. The higher the concentration of maternal hCG, the fewer the number of binding sites available for the radiolabelled test hCG.

This study requires a blood sample in a red-top tube; however, radioimmunoassay also may be performed with a urine test. The test can be completed in 1 to 5 hours. This test is so sensitive that pregnancy can be diagnosed before the first missed menstrual period.

Radioreceptor Assay (Serum)

The radioreceptor assay for serum hCG is highly sensitive and accurate. This test can be per-formed in 1 hour. The major advantage of this study is its reliability in diagnosing of early ges-tation in patients who request termination of pregnancy and in cases of individuals, especially those with infertility, who are anxious to confirm pregnancy. This study is 90% to 95% accurate 6 to 8 days after conception. Even the minute amounts of hCG secreted in an ectopic pregnancy can be measured with this study. This test is also used in assessment for early spontaneous abortion in patients who have difficulty maintaining early pregnancy: The ability of the patient's serum to inhibit the binding of radiolabelled hCG to receptors is measured.

Normally, hCG is not present in nonpregnant women, but in a very small number of women (<5%), hCG exists at very minute levels. The presence of hCG does not necessarily indicate a normal pregnancy. Ectopic pregnancy, hydatidiform mole of the uterus, and choriocarcinoma of the uterus can all produce hCG. Germ cell tumours (choriocarcinoma, embryonal cell cancers) of the testes or ovaries can produce hCG in men and nonpregnant women, respectively. Primary liver cell cancers (hepatoma) can also produce hCG. In these tumours, hCG is a valuable tumour marker to aid in tumour identification. For example, hCG is serially measured in patients with cirrhosis because such patients have a high chance of developing a hepatoma. If detected early enough, the tumour can be removed and the patient cured. Level of hCG is also used to monitor the therapy and disease progression and the regression of these tumours. When hCG levels are elevated in these patients, tumour progression must be suspected. Decreasing hCG levels indicate effectiveness of antitumour treatment.

INTERFERING FACTORS

- Tests performed too early in the pregnancy, before there is a significant hCG level, may yield false-negative results.
- Hematuria and proteinuria in the urine may cause false-positive results.
- Hemolysis of blood may interfere with test results.
- Urine pregnancy tests can vary according to the dilution of the urine. Levels of hCG may be undetectable in a dilute urine specimen but may be quite detectable on a concentrated urine specimen.
- Drugs that may cause *false-negative* urine results include diuretics (by causing dilute urine) and promethazine.
- Drugs that may cause *false-positive* results include anticonvulsants, antiparkinsonian drugs, hypnotics, and tranquilizers (especially promazine and its derivatives).

PROCEDURE AND PATIENT CARE

Before

- Explain the procedure to the patient.
- If a urine specimen is collected, give the patient a urine container the evening before the test so that she can provide a first-voided morning specimen. This specimen generally contains the greatest concentration of hCG.

During

- Collect the first-voided urine specimen for urine testing.
- Collect a venous blood sample in a red-top tube for serum testing.
- Avoid hemolysis.

After

- Apply pressure or a pressure dressing to the venipuncture site.
- Assess the venipuncture site for bleeding.
- Emphasize to the patient the importance of prenatal health care.

TEST RESULTS AND CLINICAL SIGNIFICANCE

▲ Increased Levels

Pregnancy,

Ectopic pregnancy: *Highest beta hCG levels (>30 000 IU/L) are recorded in pregnancy. Amounts are generally lowest in ectopic pregnancy.*

Hydatidiform mole of uterus,

Choriocarcinoma of uterus,

Germ cell (choriocarcinoma, teratomas, embryonal cell) tumours of testes or ovaries,

Other tumours (poorly differentiated tumours, such as hepatoma and lymphoma): *In these conditions, hCG is produced in variable amounts. The extent of tumour burden and ability to secrete hCG affect hCG levels. The findings in serial monitoring of hCG in these tumours are probably more important than the initial test result.*

▼ Decreased Levels

Threatened abortion,

Incomplete abortion,

Dead fetus: *All these conditions are associated with diminished viability of the placenta, which produces the hCG associated with pregnancy.*

Progesterone Assay

NORMAL FINDINGS*

Progesterone Level

Child

<9 years: **<0.6 nmol/L** (<0.18 ng/mL)

10–15 years: **<0.6 nmol/L** (<0.18 ng/mL)

Adult

Male: **0–1.3 nmol/L** (0–0.4 ng/mL)

Female:

   Follicular phase: **0.3–4.8 nmol/L** (0.1–1.5 ng/mL)

   Luteal phase: **8.0–89.0 nmol/L** (2.5–28.0 ng/mL)

   Postmenopausal: **<1.27 nmol/L** (<0.39 ng/mL)

Pregnancy (Trimester)

First: **23–139.9 nmol/L** (7.25–44.0 ng/mL)

Second: **62–262.3 nmol/L** (19.50–82.50 ng/mL)

Third: **206.7–728.2 nmol/L** (6.5–228.9 ng/mL)

---

*Considerable variation according to method used and laboratory. Measurements in nanograms per decilitre are by extraction/radioimmunoassay.

INDICATIONS

This test is used in the evaluation of women who are having difficulty becoming pregnant or maintaining a pregnancy. It is also used to monitor "high-risk" pregnancies.

TEST EXPLANATION

Progesterone acts primarily on the endometrium. It initiates the secretory phase of the endometrium in anticipation of implantation of a fertilized ovum. Normally, progesterone is secreted by the ovarian corpus luteum after ovulation. In pregnancy, progesterone is produced by the corpus luteum for the first few weeks. After that, the placenta begins to make progesterone. Both serum progesterone levels and the urine concentration of progesterone metabolites (pregnanediol) are significantly increased during the latter half of a normal ovulatory cycle. Progesterone levels provide information about the occurrence and timing of ovulation.

Because progesterone levels rise rapidly after ovulation, this study is useful in documenting whether ovulation has occurred and, if so, its exact time. This is very useful information in women who have difficulty becoming pregnant. A series of measurements can help pinpoint the day of ovulation. Plasma progesterone levels start to rise after ovulation, along with luteinizing hormone levels, and they continue to rise for approximately 6 to 10 days. The levels then fall and menstruation occurs. Blood samples collected at days 8 and 21 of the menstrual cycle normally show a large increase in progesterone levels in the latter specimen, which indicates that ovulation has occurred. Serum progesterone levels can provide comparable information and are sometimes measured in lieu of endometrial biopsy (see p. 756) to determine the phase of the menstrual cycle.

During pregnancy, progesterone levels normally rise because of the placental production of progesterone. Repeated assays can be used to monitor the status of the placenta in cases of "high-risk" pregnancy. Hormone assay for progesterone is used today to monitor progesterone supplementation in patients with an inadequate luteal phase, in order to maintain an early pregnancy.

INTERFERING FACTORS

- Recent use of radioisotopes may affect test results if the method of testing is radioimmunoassay.
- Hemolysis caused by rough handling of the sample may affect test results.
- Drugs that may *interfere* with test results include estrogen, clomiphene, and progesterone.

 Clinical Priorities

- Progesterone levels provide information about the occurrence and timing of ovulation. This is useful information for women who are having difficulty becoming pregnant.
- Hormone assays for progesterone are used to monitor progesterone supplementation in women with an inadequate luteal phase, in order to maintain an early pregnancy.
- During pregnancy, progesterone levels normally rise because of placental production of progesterone. Repeated assays can be used to monitor placental states in "high-risk" pregnancies. Values decrease when placental viability is threatened.

PROCEDURE AND PATIENT CARE

Before
- Explain the procedure to the patient.
- Inform the patient that no fasting is required.

During
- Collect a venous blood sample in a red-top tube.
- On the laboratory slip, indicate the date of the patient's most recent menstrual period.

After
- Apply pressure or a pressure dressing to the venipuncture site.
- Assess the venipuncture site for bleeding.

TEST RESULTS AND CLINICAL SIGNIFICANCE

▲ Increased Levels

Ovulation: *This occurs with the normal development of a corpus luteum, which makes progesterone.*

Pregnancy: *A healthy placenta produces progesterone to maintain the pregnancy.*

Luteal cysts of ovary: *The corpus luteum produces progesterone in the nonpregnant state and in the early stages of pregnancy. Cysts can also produce progesterone for prolonged periods of time.*

Hyperadrenocorticalism,

Adrenocortical hyperplasia: *Adrenal cortical hormones are secreted at increased rates. 17-Hydroxyprogesterone is a precursor of these cortical hormones.*

Choriocarcinoma of ovary: *This tumour produces progesterone.*

Molar pregnancy: *Hydatidiform mole can produce progesterone, although at lower levels than does the corpus luteum in pregnancy.*

▼ Decreased Levels

Pre-eclampsia,

Toxemia of pregnancy,

Threatened abortion,

Placental failure,

Fetal death: *All of these obstetric emergencies are associated with decreased placental viability. Progesterone is made by the placenta during pregnancy. Values decrease when placental viability is threatened.*

Ovarian neoplasm: *Ovarian epithelial cancers can destroy the functional ovarian tissue. Progesterone levels may decrease.*

Amenorrhea,

Ovarian hypofunction: *Without ovulation, a corpus luteum does not develop. Progesterone is not secreted, and progesterone and pregnanediol levels are lower than expected.*

RELATED TEST

Pregnanediol (p. 978). Pregnanediol is a catabolic metabolite of progesterone that is excreted via the kidneys into the urine.

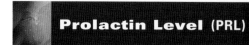

Prolactin Level (PRL)

NORMAL FINDINGS

Adult male: **1–20** *Mcg*/L (1–20 ng/mL)
Adult female: **1–25** *Mcg*/L (1–25 ng/mL)
Pregnant female: **20–400** *Mcg*/L (20–400 ng/mL)

INDICATIONS

Prolactin levels are used to diagnose and monitor prolactin-secreting pituitary adenomas.

TEST EXPLANATION

Prolactin is a hormone secreted by the anterior pituitary gland (adenohypophysis). In women, prolactin promotes lactation. Its role in men has not been demonstrated. Prolactin secretion is controlled by prolactin-inhibiting and prolactin-releasing factors secreted by the hypothalamus. Thyroid-releasing hormone can also stimulate prolactin production. During sleep, prolactin levels increase twofold to threefold, attaining circulating levels that can be equal to the high levels observed in pregnant women. With breast stimulation, pregnancy, nursing, stress, or exercise, a surge of this hormone occurs. Prolactin is elevated in patients with prolactin-secreting pituitary acidophilic or chromophobic adenomas. To a lesser extent, moderately high prolactin levels have been observed in women with secondary amenorrhea (i.e., postpubertal), galactorrhea, primary hypothyroidism, polycystic ovary syndrome, and anorexia. Paraneoplastic tumours (e.g., lung cancer) may cause ectopic secretion of prolactin as well. In general, very high prolactin levels are more likely to be related to pituitary adenoma than to other causes.

The prolactin level is helpful in diagnosing and monitoring pituitary adenomas. Successful treatment is associated with a reduction in serum prolactin levels. The success of treatment can be monitored through repeated measurements of prolactin levels. Several prolactin stimulation (with thyroid-releasing hormone or chlorpromazine) and suppression (with levodopa) tests have been designed to help differentiate pituitary adenoma from other causes of prolactin overproduction.

INTERFERING FACTORS

- Stress from illness, trauma, or surgery or even the fear of a blood test can elevate prolactin levels. In patients who are fearful of venipuncture, it is best to place a saline lock and collect the blood specimen 2 hours later.
- Drugs that may cause *increases* in prolactin values include antihistamines, estrogens, histamine antagonists, monoamine oxidase inhibitors, opiates, oral contraceptives, phenothiazines, reserpine, and verapamil.
- Drugs that may cause *decreases* in prolactin values are clonidine, dopamine, ergot alkaloid derivatives, and levodopa.

PROCEDURE AND PATIENT CARE

Before

- Explain the procedure to the patient.
- Inform the patient that no fasting or special preparation is required.
- Inform the patient that this blood sample should be collected in the morning.
- Record the use of any medication that may affect results.

During

- Obtain a venous blood sample in a red-top tube.
- Transfer the specimen to the laboratory as soon as possible. If a delay occurs, the specimen should be placed in a container of water and crushed ice.

After

- Apply pressure or a pressure dressing to the venipuncture site.
- Assess the venipuncture site for bleeding.

TEST RESULTS AND CLINICAL SIGNIFICANCE

▲ Increased Levels

Galactorrhea: *Voluminous galactorrhea can be caused by elevations in prolactin levels. A small-volume nipple discharge is quite common and not pathologic unless it is bloody.*

Amenorrhea: *Patients who have had normal menses and then stop having menses may be found to have elevated prolactin levels. Many are subsequently found to have prolactin-secreting pituitary adenomas.*

Prolactin-secreting pituitary tumour: *Most of these are benign adenomas of the acidophilic type.*

Infiltrative diseases of hypothalamus and pituitary stalk (e.g., granuloma, sarcoidosis),

Metastatic cancer of pituitary gland: *The pathologic destruction of the hypothalamus or pituitary gland can destroy the prolactin-inhibiting regulatory mechanisms.*

Hypothyroidism: *Patients with hypothyroidism because of thyroid failure have elevated thyroid-releasing hormone levels. Thyroid-releasing hormone also stimulates prolactin production.*

Paraneoplastic syndrome: *These cancers are associated with ectopic production of prolactin.*

Stress (e.g., anorexia nervosa, surgery, strenuous exercise, trauma, severe illness): *The pathophysiologic mechanism underlying these observations is not known.*

Empty sella syndrome: *In affected patients, a large sella turcica is noted on radiographs, but a pituitary adenoma is not apparent; however, many such patients have elevated prolactin levels.*

Polycystic ovary syndrome: *The pathophysiologic mechanism underlying this observation is not well known.*

Renal failure: *Affected patients probably have reduced clearance of prolactin.*

▼ Decreased Levels

Pituitary apoplexy (Sheehan's syndrome): *Women who have severe hemorrhage after obstetric delivery experience circulatory collapse. Their pituitary glands become infarcted. Prolactin levels are diminished along with other pituitary hormones.*

Pituitary destruction by tumour (craniopharyngioma): *Any disease that destroys the pituitary gland is associated with reduced prolactin levels.*

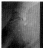

Prostate-Specific Antigen (PSA)

NORMAL FINDINGS

Normal: **0–4** *Mcg*/L (0–4 ng/mL)
Low: **0–2.5** *Mcg*/L (0–2.5 ng/mL)
Normal to moderately elevated: **2.6–10** *Mcg*/L (2.6–10 ng/mL)
Moderately elevated: **10–19.9** *Mcg*/L (10–19.9 ng/mL)
Significantly elevated: **20** *Mcg*/L (20 ng/mL) or greater

INDICATIONS

This test is used as a screening method for early detection of prostatic cancer. When the prostate-specific antigen (PSA) test is combined with a rectal examination, nearly 90% of clinically significant cancers can be detected. This test is also used to monitor the disease after treatment.

TEST EXPLANATION

PSA is a glycoprotein found in high concentrations in the prostatic lumen. Significant barriers such as prostate glandular tissue and vascular structure are interposed between the prostatic lumen and the bloodstream. These protective barriers can be broached when disease such as cancer, infection, or benign hypertrophy is present. PSA can be detected in all men; however, levels are greatly increased in patients with prostatic cancer.

Elevated PSA levels are associated with prostate cancer. Levels greater than **4** *Mcg*/L (4 ng/mL) have been found in more than 80% of men with prostate cancer. The higher the levels are, the greater the tumour burden is. The PSA assay is also a sensitive test for monitoring response to therapy. Successful surgery, radiation, or hormone therapy helps markedly reduce the PSA blood level. Significant elevation in PSA subsequently indicates the recurrence of prostatic cancer. PSA is more sensitive and specific than other prostatic tumour markers, such as prostatic acid phosphatase. Also, measurements of PSA are more accurate than those of prostatic acid phosphatase in monitoring response to therapy and recurrence of tumour after therapy.

Prostate Canada advises men to get a PSA test in their 40s to determine a baseline and then "know their number" to establish future risk of developing prostate cancer. At or over the age of 70, the decision to be tested is based on individual factors such as health status and life expectancy. PSA testing should be performed in conjunction with the digital rectal examination, because the combination of the two tests is more sensitive for diagnosis than either one alone.

Any abnormal values should be closely monitored with the frequency of testing to be determined by the physician.

Some patients with early prostate cancer do not have elevated levels of PSA. Of equal importance is that PSA levels above 4 are not always associated with cancer. The PSA is limited by a lack of specificity within the "diagnostic grey zone" of **4–10** *Mcg*/L (4–10 ng/mL). PSA levels also may be minimally elevated in patients with benign prostatic hypertrophy and prostatitis. In an effort to increase the accuracy of PSA testing, other measures of PSA (Box 2-11) have been proposed.

BOX 2-11	Strategies for Enhancing PSA Specificity

- Volume-adjusted PSA
- PSA density
- Age-specific PSA
- Percentage of free PSA

PSA, Prostate-specific antigen.

- *PSA velocity:* PSA velocity is the change in PSA levels over time. A sharp rise in the PSA level raises the suspicion of cancer and may indicate a fast-growing cancer. Men who have a PSA velocity higher than **0.35 *Mcg*/L** (>0.35 ng/mL) per year have a higher relative risk for dying of prostate cancer than do men who have a PSA velocity lower than **0.35 *Mcg*/L** (<0.35 ng/mL) per year.
- *Age-adjusted PSA* (Table 2-39): Age is an important factor in increasing PSA levels. Men younger than 50 years should have a PSA level below **2.4 *Mcg*/L** (<2.4 ng/mL), whereas a PSA level up to **6.5 *Mcg*/L** (6.5 ng/mL) would be considered normal for men in their 70s.
- *PSA density:* PSA density is the relationship of the PSA level to the size of the prostate. The use of PSA density to interpret PSA results is controversial because cancer might be overlooked in a man with an enlarged prostate. PSA density is an adjustment in which the PSA measurement is divided by the gland volume. Several formulas have been created to partially correct for gland volume. One such volume-adjusted formula is as follows:

$$\text{Predicted PSA} = 0.12 \times \text{Gland volume (in cubic centimetres)} \text{ as determined by ultrasonography}$$

Free versus attached PSA: PSA circulates in the blood in two forms: free or bound to a protein molecule. In benign prostate conditions (such as benign prostatic hypertrophy), more free PSA is present, whereas in cancer, more of the bound form is produced. If a man's bound PSA level is high but his free PSA level is not, the presence of cancer is more likely. When the proportion of free PSA is less than 25%, the likelihood of cancer is high (Table 2-40).

- *Alteration of PSA cutoff level:* Some researchers have suggested lowering the cutoff levels that determine whether a PSA measurement is normal or elevated. For example, a number of studies have used cutoff levels of **2.5 to 3.0 *Mcg*/L** (2.5–3.0 ng/mL) rather than **4.0 *Mcg*/L** (4.0 ng/mL).

TABLE 2-39	Age-Specific Reference Ranges for Serum Prostate-Specific Antigen

Age Range (Years)	REFERENCE RANGE, *Mcg*/L (ng/mL)		
	Black Men	**White Men**	**Japanese Men**
40–49	0.0–2.0	0.0–2.5	0.0–2.0
50–59	0.0–4.0	0.0–3.5	0.0–3.0
60–69	0.0–4.5	0.0–4.5	0.0–4.0
70–79	0.0–5.5	0.0–6.5	0.0–5.0

TABLE 2-40	Probability of Cancer According to Percentage of Free PSA
Percentage of Free PSA	**Probability of Cancer (%)**
0–10	56
10–15	28
15–20	20
20–25	16
>25	8

PSA, Prostate-specific antigen.

- *Protein patterns:* Patterns of prostate proteins are being studied to determine whether biopsy is necessary when the PSA level is slightly elevated or when the digital rectal examination reveals abnormalities. *Prostatic specific membrane antigen* may, with further study, represent an excellent marker for prostate cancer. It is more frequently present than PSA in more advanced cancer. Another protein of interest is *early prostate cancer antigen* (EPCA). Unlike the PSA, this protein is not found in normal prostate cells. Instead, EPCA occurs in relatively large amounts only in prostate cancer cells. Early research findings suggest that EPCA may be more accurate than PSA in identifying prostate cancer. Furthermore, EPCA levels are significantly higher in patients whose cancers spread outside the prostate than in those with disease confined to the gland. The EPCA-1 test is tissue based, and the EPCA-2 test is blood based. Patients with an EPCA-2 cutoff level of **30 *Mcg*/L (30 ng/mL)** or higher are considered to be at risk for prostate cancer.

PSA is used in the staging prostate cancer. When PSA levels are lower than 10 ng/mL, disease is most likely to be localized and to respond well to local therapy (radical prostatectomy or radiation therapy). Routine metastatic staging tests are generally not required for men with clinically localized prostate cancer when the PSA is lower than **20 *Mcg*/L (<20 ng/mL)**.

PSA measurement is used for follow-up in men after treatment for prostate cancer. Periodic PSA testing should follow any form of treatment for prostate cancer because PSA levels can indicate need for further treatment. After curative radical prostatectomy or radiation therapy, PSA levels should probably be **0 to 0.5 *Mcg*/L (0–0.5 ng/mL)**. The pattern of PSA level elevation after local therapy for prostate cancer can help distinguish between local recurrence and distant spread. Patients with elevated PSA levels more than 24 months after local treatment and with a PSA doubling time after 12 months are likely to have recurrence.

PSA can be measured by electrochemiluminescent immunoassay, immunohistochemistry, or radioimmunoassay. Newer, comparably accurate chemical tests are being used to improve the worldwide use of PSA screening testing.

INTERFERING FACTORS

- Rectal examinations are well known to artificially elevate prostatic acid phosphatase levels, and they may also minimally elevate the PSA level. To avoid this problem, the PSA should be collected before rectal examination of the prostate or several hours afterward.
- Prostatic manipulation by biopsy or transurethral resection of the prostate causes significant elevations in the PSA levels. The blood test should be done before surgery or 6 weeks after manipulation.
- Ejaculation of semen within 24 hours before blood testing is associated with elevated PSA levels.

- Recent urinary tract infection or prostatitis can cause elevations of PSA values as much as five times higher than baseline for as long as 6 weeks.
- Finasteride (Propecia, Proscar) and diethylstilbestrol (DES) may cause *decreases* in levels of PSA.

PROCEDURE AND PATIENT CARE

Before
- Explain the procedure to the patient.
- Inform the patient that no fasting is required.

During
- Collect a venous blood sample in a red-top tube.
- The use of the percentage of free PSA mandates strict sample handling not required with the total PSA. Appropriate sample handling is necessary for accurate and consistent assay performance. Check with the laboratory for specific guidelines.

After
- Apply pressure or a pressure dressing to the venipuncture site.
- Observe the venipuncture site for bleeding.

TEST RESULTS AND CLINICAL SIGNIFICANCE

▲ Increased Levels

Prostate cancer,
Benign prostatic hypertrophy,
Prostatitis: *The PSA in the cytoplasm of the diseased prostate is expelled into the bloodstream, and PSA levels are elevated.*

RELATED TEST

Prostatic Acid Phosphatase (p. 30). This is another tumour marker for prostate cancer. It is less specific and less sensitive than the PSA test, and its use is diminishing.

Protein C, Protein S

NORMAL FINDINGS

Protein S: 60%–130% of normal activity
Protein C: 70%–150% of normal activity
    Protein C level decreases with age and in women.

INDICATIONS

This test identifies deficiencies in protein C, protein S, or both. This is part of the evaluation of patients with coagulation disorders.

TEST EXPLANATION

The plasma coagulation system is carefully balanced between thrombosis and fibrinolysis. This precise homeostatic regulation is important. The "protein C–protein S" system is an important inhibitor of coagulation. Protein S is a vitamin K–dependent plasma glycoprotein synthesized in the liver, and it functions as a cofactor with protein C in the inactivation of factors Va and VIIIa (see Figure 2-14, p. 181). This inhibitory function of protein C is enhanced by protein S.

In the circulation, protein S exists in two forms: a free form and a complex form bound to complement protein C4b. Only the free form has cofactor activity.

Inherited protein S deficiency manifests as an autosomal dominant trait; manifestations of thrombosis are observed in both heterozygous and homozygous genetic deficiencies of protein S. In the rare inherited homozygous or compound heterozygous state, protein C deficiency is associated with severe life-threatening neonatal purpura fulminans or massive venous thrombosis. The inherited heterozygous state of protein C deficiency is most frequently associated with deep-vein thrombosis in the lower limb but also may manifest in other venous locations. Heterozygous protein C deficiency is usually asymptomatic until after puberty.

Acquired deficiencies (e.g., vitamin K deficiency) may cause spontaneous intravascular (usually venous) thrombosis. Other diseases that could instigate deficiencies in these proteins include septic shock; disseminated intravascular coagulation (DIC); liver disease; preterm delivery; acute inflammation; acute thrombosis; and administration of warfarin and some chemotherapy agents.

Furthermore, dysfunctional forms of other proteins result in a hypercoagulable state. In addition, nearly 50% of hypercoagulable states are caused by the presence of a form of factor V (factor V–Leiden) that is resistant to protein C inhibition.

When protein C is tested, protein S activity should also be tested because the decrease in activity of protein C may be the result of decreased activity of protein S. In addition, when protein C activity is decreased, protein C resistance (presence of factor V–Leiden, p. 246) should be tested.

These proteins are vitamin K–dependent and are decreased in patients who take warfarin (Coumadin), those who have liver diseases, and those who are severely malnourished. Complement 4 (C4) binding protein can inactivate protein S. Therefore, diseases that increase C4 binding proteins (such as autoimmune diseases and other inflammatory diseases) are associated with acquired protein S deficiency and may precipitate hypercoagulation events.

Several test kits are available for the measurements of these proteins. Enzyme-linked immunosorbent assay (ELISA), chromogenic, and clotting methods are variably used.

INTERFERING FACTORS

- Levels of protein C may be decreased in the postoperative state.
- Pregnancy or the use of exogenous sex hormones is associated with decreases in levels of proteins C and S. These low levels of protein S in pregnancy do not cause thrombosis by themselves.
- The concentration of citrate in the collection tube varies and can affect activity results.

PROCEDURE AND PATIENT CARE

Before

🖉 Explain the procedure to the patient.
🖉 Inform the patient that fasting is not usually required unless it is ordered by the physician.

During

- Collect a venous blood sample in a blue-top tube. If more than one blood specimen is to be obtained, collect the blood for proteins C or S second to avoid contamination with tissue thromboplastin that may occur in the first tube. If only blood for protein C or S is being obtained, collect blood in a red-top tube first (and throw it away) and then collect the blood for this study in a blue-top tube (two-tube method of blood collection).
- Place the tube in a mixture of water and crushed ice.

After

- Apply pressure to the venipuncture site.
🖉 If the patient is found to have a deficiency in either protein, encourage the patient's family to be tested because they may be similarly affected.

TEST RESULTS AND CLINICAL SIGNIFICANCE

▼ Decreased Levels

Inherited deficiency of protein C or protein S: *Protein S or C defect that may not be recognized until adulthood.*

DIC,

Hypercoagulable states,

Pulmonary emboli,

Arterial or venous thrombosis: *These thrombotic diseases, when recurrent, may be the result of a deficiency in protein C or S.*

Vitamin K deficiency: *Proteins C and S are dependent on vitamin K for their synthesis. If vitamin K is not available because of malnutrition, biliary disease, or malabsorption, these proteins are not produced in adequate levels. Because several coagulation factors are also vitamin K–dependent, a hypercoagulable event may not occur.*

Sickle cell disease: *This condition alone does not produce a thrombophilic state.*

Autoimmune diseases,

Inflammation: *These proteins may be consumed in the inflammatory process.*

Warfarin (Coumadin)–induced skin necrosis: *This occurs in the feet, buttocks, thighs, breasts, upper extremities, and genitalia. The lesions usually begin as maculopapular lesions several days after initiation of warfarin treatment and progress into bullous, hemorrhagic, necrotic lesions. Patients with protein C deficiency are at high risk for warfarin-induced skin necrosis during initiation of therapy with warfarin. Approximately one-third of patients with warfarin-induced skin necrosis have protein C deficiency.*

RELATED TEST

Disseminated Intravascular Coagulation Screening (p. 225). This group of tests is indicated for patients with coagulopathies, such as DIC.

Protein (Protein Electrophoresis, Albumin, Globulin, Total Protein)

NORMAL FINDINGS

Adult/Older Adult

Total protein: **60–80 g/L** (6.0–8.0 g/dL)
Albumin: **35–55 g/L** (3.5–5.5 g/dL)
Globulin: **23–34 g/L** (2.3–3.4 g/dL)
Alpha$_1$-globulin: **1–3 g/L** (0.1–0.3 g/dL)
Alpha$_2$-globulin: **6–10 g/L** (0.6–1 g/dL)
Beta-globulin: **7–11 g/L** (0.7–1.1 g/dL)

Children

Total Protein
Premature infant: **42–76 g/L** (4.2–7.6 g/dL)
Newborn: **46–74 g/L** (4.6–7.4 g/dL)
Infant: **60–67 g/L** (6–6.7 g/dL)
Child: **62–80 g/L** (6.2–8 g/dL)

Albumin
Premature infant: **30–42 g/L** (3–4.2 g/dL)
Newborn: **35–54 g/L** (3.5–5.4 g/dL)
Infant: **44–54 g/L** (4.4–5.4 g/dL)
Child: **40–59 g/L** (4–5.9 g/dL)

INDICATIONS

Evaluation and fractionation of serum proteins are performed to diagnose, assess, and monitor the disease course in patients with cancer (e.g., lymphoma, myeloma), intestinal/renal protein-wasting states, immune disorders, liver dysfunction, impaired nutrition, and chronic edematous states.

TEST EXPLANATION

Proteins are constituents of muscle, enzymes, hormones, transport vehicles, hemoglobin, and several other key functional and structural entities within the body. They are the most significant component contributing to the osmotic pressure within the vascular space. This osmotic pressure keeps fluid within the vascular space, minimizing extravasation of fluid.

Total serum protein is a combination of prealbumin, albumin, and globulins. *Albumin* is a protein that is formed within the liver. It constitutes approximately 60% of the total protein. The major effect of albumin within the blood is to maintain colloidal osmotic pressure. Furthermore, albumin transports important blood constituents such as drugs, hormones, and enzymes. Albumin is synthesized within the liver and is therefore a measure of hepatic function. When disease affects the hepatocyte, the cell loses its ability to synthesize albumin. The serum albumin level is thereby greatly decreased. Because the half-life of albumin is 12 to 18 days, however, severe impairment of hepatic albumin synthesis may not be recognized until after that period.

Globulins are the key building block of antibodies. Their role in maintaining osmotic pressure is far less significant than that of albumin. Alpha$_1$-globulins are mostly alpha$_1$-antitrypsin. Some transporting proteins, such as thyroid and cortisol-binding globulin, also contribute to this electrophoretic zone. Alpha$_2$-globulins include serum haptoglobins (which bind hemoglobin during hemolysis), ceruloplasmin (a carrier for copper), prothrombin, and cholinesterase (an enzyme used in the catabolism of acetylcholine). Beta$_1$-globulins include lipoproteins, transferrin, plasminogen, and complement proteins; beta$_2$-globulins include fibrinogen. Gamma-globulins are the immune globulins (antibodies) (see p. 327). To a lesser degree, globulins also act as transport vehicles.

Serum albumin and globulin levels are measures of nutrition. Malnourished patients, especially after surgery, have a greatly decreased level of serum proteins. Patients with burns and patients who have protein-losing enteropathies and uropathies have low levels of protein despite normal synthesis. Pregnancy, especially in the third trimester, is usually associated with reduced total protein levels.

In some diseases, albumin level is selectively diminished, and globulin levels are normal or increased to maintain a normal total protein level. For example, in collagen vascular diseases (e.g., systemic lupus erythematosus), capillary permeability is increased. Albumin, a molecule much smaller than globulin, is selectively lost into the extravascular space. Chronic liver diseases are similarly associated with low albumin, high globulin, and normal total protein levels. In these diseases, the liver cannot produce albumin, but adequate amounts of globulin are made in the reticuloendothelial system. In both collagen vascular disease and chronic liver disease, the albumin level is low, but the total protein level is normal because of increased globulin levels. These changes, however, can be detected through measurement of the albumin/globulin ratio. This ratio normally exceeds 1.0. The diseases just described, which selectively affect albumin levels, are associated with lower ratios. Total protein levels, particularly the globulin fraction, are increased in multiple myeloma and other gammopathies. Of importance is that the albumin fraction of the total protein can be factitiously elevated in dehydrated patients.

In most laboratories, simple chromogenic methods are used to measure the total protein and albumin levels in the serum. These are often part of multichannel testing screens. Electrophoresis can separate the various components of blood protein into bands or zones according to their electrical charge. A densitometer or similar instrument can quantify these bands (Figure 2-20). Several well-established electrophoretic patterns have been identified and are associated with specific diseases (Table 2-41). Normally, the pattern specific to immunoglobulins is polyclonal (i.e., many components make up the group of immunoglobulins). When the pattern of immunoglobulins changes to a large monoclonal spike (indicating an overabundance of one type of immunoglobulin), infection, allergy, or neoplasm such as myeloma is suspected.

Protein electrophoresis can also be performed with urine to classify certain renal protein-losing nephropathies. Again, certain patterns may be specific for certain disease.

Bence-Jones proteins are associated with multiple myeloma. Affected patients have monoclonal spikes in the beta- or gamma-globulin zone. Lipoid nephrosis causes the kidneys to leak small particles of protein, such as albumin. Therefore, a spike is expected in the albumin zone of the electrophoretic pattern.

Electrophoresis can be performed in several different methods. Each is an attempt to improve the specificity of the test. These various methods include radial immunodiffusion, immunonephelometry, immunofluorometry, and radioimmunoassay. These methods involve measuring the exact quantity of each protein rather than providing a vague measurement quantity for each "type" of protein. Sensitivity and specificity can be even further improved with the use of immunoelectrophoresis or immunofixation, which can further separate out abnormal proteins that may contribute to each zone spike.

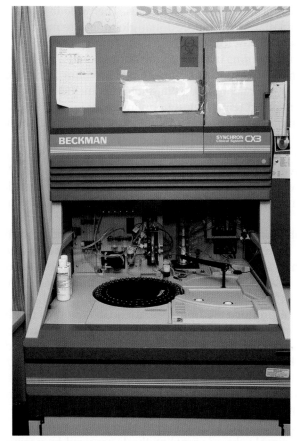

Figure 2-20 Equipment used to perform serum protein electrophoresis.

In most health care centres, when the protein electrophoresis is abnormal, *immunofixation electrophoresis* is performed. In this technique, a monospecific antibody is placed in contact with the gel after the proteins have been separated. The resulting protein-antibody complexes are subsequently specifically stained for visualization. The pathologist then makes an interpretation by comparing reference protein electrophoretic patterns with the patient's pattern. Immunofixation electrophoresis has become particularly useful for the identification of various monoclonal gammopathies such as multiple myeloma or Waldenström macroglobulinemia (see p. 440).

INTERFERING FACTORS

Prolonged application of tourniquet can increase both fractions of total proteins.

Sampling of peripheral venous blood proximal to the site of intravenous administration can result in an inaccurately low protein level. Likewise, massive intravenous infusion of crystalloid fluid can result in acute hypoproteinemia.

▨ Drugs that can cause *increases* in protein levels include anabolic steroids, androgens, corticosteroids, dextran, growth hormone, insulin, phenazopyridine, and progesterone.

▨ Drugs that can cause *decreases* in protein levels include ammonium ions, estrogens, hepatotoxic drugs, and oral contraceptives.

TABLE 2-41   Protein Electrophoresis Patterns in Specific Diseases

Electrophoresis Pattern	Interpretation	Disease
Acute reaction	↓ Albumin ↑ Alpha$_2$-globulin	Acute infections, tissue necrosis, burns, surgery, stress, myocardial infarction
Chronic inflammatory	Slightly ↓ albumin Slightly ↑ gamma-globulin Normal alpha$_2$-globulin	Chronic infection, granulomatous diseases, cirrhosis, rheumatoid-collagen diseases
Nephrotic syndrome	↓↓ Albumin ↑↑ Alpha$_2$-globulin Normal to ↑ beta-globulin	Nephrotic syndrome
Far-advanced cirrhosis	↓ Albumin ↑ Gamma-globulin Incorporation of beta- and gamma-globulin peaks	Far-advanced cirrhosis
Polyclonal gamma-globulin elevation	↑↑ Gamma-globulin with a broad peak	Cirrhosis, chronic infection, sarcoidosis, tuberculosis, endocarditis, rheumatoid-collagen disease
Hypogammaglobulinemia	↓ Gamma-globulin with normal other globulin levels	Light-chain multiple myeloma
Monoclonal gammopathy	Thin spikes in gamma globulin	Myeloma, macroglobulinemia, gammopathies

↓, Decreased; ↑, increased; ↓↓, greatly decreased; ↑↑, greatly increased.

PROCEDURE AND PATIENT CARE

Before
- Explain the procedure to the patient.
- Inform the patient that no fasting or preparation is required.

During
Blood
- Collect a venous blood sample in a red-top tube.

Urine
- Collect a first-voided morning specimen or a 24-hour specimen (preferred).
- No preservative is required as long as the specimen is kept refrigerated.

After
Blood
- Apply pressure or a pressure dressing to the venipuncture site.
- Observe the venipuncture site for bleeding.

TEST RESULTS AND CLINICAL SIGNIFICANCE

▲ Increased Albumin Levels
Dehydration: *As intravascular volume diminishes, albumin concentration measurements must increase mathematically.*

▼ Decreased Albumin Levels

Malnutrition: *Lack of amino acids available for building proteins contributes to this observation. The liver dysfunction (albumin synthesis) associated with malnutrition probably also contributes to the lowering of albumin levels.*

Pregnancy: *Albumin levels progressively decrease until delivery.*

Liver disease (e.g., hepatitis, extensive metastatic tumour, cirrhosis, hepatocellular necrosis): *The liver is the site of synthesis of albumin. If production of albumin is inadequate, levels can be expected to fall.*

Protein-losing enteropathies (e.g., malabsorption syndromes such as Crohn's disease, sprue, Whipple's disease): *Large volumes of protein are lost from the intestines because absorption is inadequate. Albumin levels therefore fall.*

Protein-losing nephropathies (e.g., nephrotic syndrome, nephrosis): *Large volumes of albumin can be lost through the kidneys. This loss may be selective for albumin (lipoid nephrosis) or may involve all components of proteins (glomerulonephritis).*

Third-space losses (e.g., ascites, third-degree burns): *Large amounts of albumin can be lost in the serum that weeps from chronic open burns. Albumin readily accumulates in the peritoneum of patients with ascites.*

Overhydration: *As the blood volume increases, albumin concentration measurements decrease mathematically.*

Increased capillary permeability (e.g., collagen-vascular diseases such as systemic lupus erythematosus): *Albumin can seep out of the microvascular spaces in the tissues and cause edema, or it can seep into the kidneys and cause proteinuria. The serum albumin level decreases.*

Inflammatory disease: *Diseases associated with inflammation, necrosis, infarction, or burns cause an increase in acute-phase reactant proteins, mostly globulins. Therefore, the globulin component of proteins increases and the albumin component decreases.*

Familial idiopathic dysproteinemia: *In this genetic disease, albumin level is significantly reduced (and globulin levels are increased).*

▲ Increased Alpha$_1$-Globulin Levels

Inflammatory disease: *Alpha$_1$-antitrypsin is an acute-phase reactant protein, levels of which are increased in diseases associated with inflammation, in necrosis, in infarction, in malignancy, or in burns.*

▼ Decreased Alpha$_1$-Globulin Levels

Juvenile pulmonary emphysema: *These patients have a genetic decrease or absence of this enzyme, which is important to normal pulmonary function.*

▲ Increased Alpha$_2$-Globulin Levels

Nephrotic syndrome: *This probably represents a response to albumin reduction caused by protein-wasting nephropathies. However, the pathophysiologic process is not well defined.*

Inflammatory disease: *Haptoglobin and ceruloplasmin are alpha$_2$-globulins. These proteins are acute-phase reactant proteins whose levels are increased in diseases associated with inflammation, in necrosis, in infarction, in malignancy, or in burns.*

▼ Decreased Alpha$_2$-Globulin Levels

Hemolysis: *Haptoglobin is an alpha$_2$-globulin, and its levels are decreased when hemolysis occurs (see* p. 289).

Wilson disease: *Ceruloplasmin is an alpha$_2$-globulin. Its levels are decreased in Wilson disease (see* p. 165).

Hyperthyroidism: *The pathophysiologic mechanism underlying this observation is not known.*

Severe liver dysfunction: *Haptoglobin is an alpha$_2$-globulin that is made in the liver. Its levels are decreased when liver function is inadequate (see p. 289).*

▲ Increased Beta-Globulin Levels

Hypercholesterolemia (which can occur by itself or in association with biliary cirrhosis, hypothyroidism, or nephrosis): *Beta-lipoprotein is a beta-globulin, and its levels are increased in hypercholesterolemia (see p. 169).*

Iron-deficiency anemia: *Transferrin is a beta-globulin, and its levels are increased in this form of anemia (see p. 334).*

▼ Decreased Beta-Globulin Levels

Malnutrition: *Transferrin is a beta-globulin, and its levels are decreased in malnutrition.*

▲ Increased Gamma-Globulin Levels

Multiple myeloma,

Waldenström macroglobulinemia: *These cancers are characterized by production of gamma-globulin from neoplastic plasma cells or lymphocytes. The total gamma-globulin zone may not be increased, but a monoclonal spike in one portion is often observed.*

Chronic inflammatory disease (e.g., rheumatoid arthritis, systemic lupus erythematosus): *These diseases are associated with autoantibodies, and affected patients exhibit a gamma-globulin spike.*

Malignancy (e.g., Hodgkin disease, lymphoma, leukemia): *These diseases may be associated with elevated levels of gamma-globulins.*

Hyperimmunization: *A small spike can occur in the immunoglobulin A (IgA) portion of the gamma band.*

Cirrhosis: *Most patients have gamma-globulin spikes and some have beta-globulin spikes in association with this disease. The pathophysiologic process is not well known.*

Acute and chronic infection: *Infection is associated with an antibody response and therefore with an increase in levels of immunoglobulins (gamma-globulins).*

▼ Decreased Gamma-Globulin Levels

Genetic immune disorders: *Numerous immune deficiencies are associated with reduced levels or absence of immunoglobulins.*

Secondary immune deficiency: *Several conditions (e.g., steroid use, nephrotic syndrome, severe Gram-negative infection, lymphoma, leukemia) are associated with deficient levels of immunoglobulins.*

RELATED TESTS

Immunofixation Electrophoresis (p. 325). This test is used to more clearly identify whether a spike on the serum protein electrophoresis test (p. 440) is monoclonal or when quantitative immunoglobulin levels are elevated.

Immunoglobulin Electrophoresis (p. 327): This is a quantification of the components that make up immunoglobulins, which are gamma-globulins.

Prealbumin (p. 424): This is a quantification of prealbumin, which is a component of proteins. This test is used to indicate the level of a patient's nutritional status. It is also used to indicate the status of liver function.

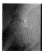

Prothrombin Time (PT, Pro-Time, International Normalized Ratio [INR])

NORMAL FINDINGS*

11.0–12.5 seconds; 85%–100%
Full anticoagulant therapy: >1.5–2.0 times control value in seconds; 20%–30%
Normal international normalized ratio (INR): 0.9–1.1

 Possible Critical Values

Prothrombin time: >20 seconds (for individuals not taking anticoagulants)
INR: >3.6 (for patients on anticoagulants)

INDICATIONS

The prothrombin time is used to evaluate the adequacy of the extrinsic system and common pathway in the clotting mechanism.

TEST EXPLANATION

The hemostasis and coagulation system is a homeostatic balance between factors that encourage clotting and factors that encourage clot dissolution. The first reaction of the body to active bleeding is blood vessel constriction. In small-vessel injury, this may be enough to stop bleeding. In large-vessel injury, hemostasis is required to form a clot that durably plugs the hole until healing can occur. The primary phase of the hemostatic mechanism involves platelet aggregation to the blood vessel (see Figure 2-14, p. 181). Next, secondary hemostasis occurs. The first phase of reactions is called the *intrinsic system*. Factor XII and other proteins form a complex on the subendothelial collagen in the injured blood vessel. Through a series of reactions, activated factor XI (XIa) is formed and activates factor IX (IXa). In a complex formed by factors VIII, IX, and X, activated factor X (Xa) is formed.

At the same time, the *extrinsic system* is activated, and a complex is formed between tissue thromboplastin (factor III) and factor VII (which is exposed after cellular injury). Activated factor VII (VIIa) results. Factor VIIa can directly activate factor X. Alternatively, factor VIIa can activate factors IX and X together.

In the third reaction, factor X is activated by the proteases formed by the two prior reactions and by activated factor IX. This reaction is a common pathway that provides the link between the intrinsic and the extrinsic systems. In the fourth and final reaction, prothrombin is converted into thrombin by activated factor X in the presence of factor V, phospholipid, and calcium.

Thrombin not only converts fibrinogen to fibrin in "clot stabilization" but also stimulates platelet aggregation and activates factors V, VIII, and XIII. Once fibrin is formed, it is then polymerized into a stable gel. Factor XIII crosslinks the fibrin polymers to form a stable clot.

Almost immediately, three major activators of the fibrinolytic system act on plasminogen, which was previously absorbed into the clot, to form plasmin. Plasmin degenerates the fibrin polymer into fragments, which are cleared by macrophages.

The prothrombin time is a measure of the clotting ability of factors I (fibrinogen), II (prothrombin), V, VII, and X (i.e., the extrinsic system and common pathway). When quantities of these clotting factors are deficient, the prothrombin time is prolonged. Many diseases and drugs are associated with decreases in levels of these factors:

---

*Findings depend on reagents used for prothrombin time.

1. *Hepatocellular liver disease* (e.g., cirrhosis, hepatitis, and neoplastic invasive processes). Factors I, II, V, VII, IX, and X are produced in the liver. With severe hepatocellular dysfunction, synthesis of these factors does not occur, and serum concentrations of these factors are decreased.

2. *Obstructive biliary disease* (e.g., bile duct obstruction secondary to tumour or gallstones or intrahepatic cholestasis secondary to sepsis or drugs). As a result of the biliary obstruction, the bile necessary for fat absorption fails to enter the gut, and fat malabsorption results. Vitamins A, D, E, and K are fat soluble and also are not absorbed. Because the synthesis of factors II, VII, IX, and X depends on vitamin K, these factors are not adequately produced, and serum concentrations fall. *Hepatocellular liver disease* can be differentiated from obstructive biliary disease by determination of the patient's response to parenteral administration of vitamin K. If the prothrombin time returns to normal after 1 to 3 days of vitamin K administration (usual dose is 2.5 to 10 mg intramuscularly and may be repeated in 6 to 8 hours), the patient probably has obstructive biliary disease that is causing vitamin K malabsorption. If, however, the prothrombin time does not return to normal with the vitamin K injections, the patient probably has severe hepatocellular disease and the liver cells are incapable of synthesizing the clotting factors no matter how much vitamin K is available.

3. *Coumarin ingestion.* The coumarin derivatives dicumarol and warfarin (Coumadin, Panwarfin) are used to prevent coagulation in patients with thromboembolic disease (e.g., pulmonary embolism, thrombophlebitis, arterial embolism). These drugs interfere with the production of vitamin K–dependent clotting factors, which results in a prolongation of prothrombin time, as already described. The adequacy of coumarin therapy can be monitored by following the patient's prothrombin time. For anticoagulation, the INR typically should be between 2.0 and 3.0 for patients with atrial fibrillation and between 3.0 and 4.0 for patients with mechanical heart valves. However, the ideal INR must be individualized for each patient (Table 2-42).

Prothrombin time test results were traditionally given in seconds, along with a control value. The control value usually varied somewhat from day to day because the reagents used varied. The patient's prothrombin time value was supposed to be approximately equal to the control value. Some laboratories reported prothrombin time values as percentages of normal activity because the patient's results were compared with a curve representing normal clotting time. A normal prothrombin time result was 85% to 100%.

To establish uniform prothrombin time results for physicians in different parts of the country and the world, the World Health Organization (Longstaff et al., 2010) recommended that prothrombin time results include the use of the *international normalized ratio* (INR) value. The

TABLE 2-42	Preferred International Normalized Ratio According to Indication for Anticoagulation	
Indication		**Preferred INR**
Prophylaxis of deep-vein thrombosis		2.0–3.0
Orthopedic surgery		2.0–3.0
Deep-vein thrombosis		2.0–3.0
Atrial fibrillation		2.0–3.0
Pulmonary embolism		2.0–3.0
Prosthetic valve prophylaxis		3.0–4.5

INR, International normalized ratio.

reported INR results are independent of the reagents or methods used. Many hospitals now report prothrombin time times in both absolute and INR numbers. Factors such as weight, body mass index, age, diet, and concurrent medications are known to affect warfarin dose requirements during anticoagulation therapy.

Warfarin interferes with the regeneration of reduced vitamin K from oxidized vitamin K in the vitamin K oxidoreductase (VKOR) complex. A gene for the major subunit of VKOR, called *VKORC1,* has been recently identified and may explain up to 44% of the variance in warfarin dose requirements. Furthermore, warfarin is metabolized in part by the cytochrome P450 enzyme CYP2C9. The *CYP2C9*2* and *CYP2C9*3* genetic mutations have been shown to decrease the enzyme activity of these metabolizing enzymes, which has led to warfarin sensitivity and, in serious cases, bleeding complications. A warfarin metabolism genetic test is available that can identify any mutations in the *VKORC1 CYP2C9*2,* or *CYP2C9*3* genes. With this information, an algorithm has been developed to be more accurate than prothrombin time for warfarin dosing.

Coumarin derivatives are slow acting, but their action may persist for 7 to 14 days after discontinuation of the drug. The action of a coumarin drug can be reversed in 12 to 24 hours by slow parenteral administration of vitamin K (phytonadione). The administration of plasma reverses the coumarin effect even more rapidly. The action of coumarin drugs can be enhanced by drugs such as aspirin, quinidine, sulpha, and indomethacin. Barbiturates, chloral hydrate, and oral contraceptives cause increases in coumarin drug binding and may therefore decrease the effects of coumarin drugs.

INTERFERING FACTORS

- Alcohol intake can prolong PT times. Alcohol diminishes liver function. Many factors are made in the liver. Lesser quantities of coagulation factors result in prolonged PT times.
- A diet high in fat or leafy vegetables may shorten PT times. Absorption of vitamin K is enhanced. Vitamin K–dependent factors are made at increased levels, thereby shortening PT times.
- Diarrhea or malabsorption syndromes can prolong PT times. Vitamin K is malabsorbed, and as a result, factors II, VII, IX, and X are not made.
- Drugs that may cause *increases* in levels include allopurinol, salicylic acid, barbiturates, beta-lactam antibiotics, chloral hydrate, cephalothin, chloramphenicol, cholestyramine, cimetidine, clofibrate, colestipol, ethyl alcohol, glucagon, heparin, methyldopa, neomycin, oral anticoagulants, propylthiouracil, quinidine, quinine, salicylates, and sulphonamides.
- Drugs that may cause *decreases* in levels include anabolic steroids, barbiturates, chloral hydrate, digitalis, diphenhydramine, estrogens, oral contraceptives, and vitamin K.

PROCEDURE AND PATIENT CARE

Before

- Explain the procedure to the patient.
- Inform the patient that no fasting is required.
- If the patient is receiving warfarin, obtain the blood specimen before the patient is given the daily dose of warfarin. The daily dose may be increased, decreased, or kept the same, depending on the prothrombin time test results for that day.

During

- Collect a venous blood sample in a blue-top tube.
- On the laboratory slip, list any drugs the patient is taking that may affect test results.

After

- Apply pressure or a pressure dressing to the venipuncture site.
- Assess the venipuncture site for bleeding. Remember that hemostasis is delayed if the patient is taking warfarin or if the patient has any coagulopathies.
- If the prothrombin time is greatly prolonged, evaluate the patient for bleeding tendencies (i.e., check for blood in the urine and all excretions and assess the patient for bruises, petechiae, and low-back pain). Back pain may be a symptom of retroperitoneal bleeding.
- If severe bleeding occurs, the anticoagulant effect of warfarin can be reversed by the slow parenteral administration of vitamin K (phytonadione). If coagulation must be returned to near normal more quickly, plasma can be administered.
- Because of drug interactions, instruct the patient not to take any medication unless drugs are specifically ordered by the physician.

 Home Care Responsibilities

- Warfarin (Coumadin) levels are regulated by prothrombin time and INR values.
- Inform patients to evaluate themselves for bleeding tendencies. Patients should assess themselves for bruises, petechiae, low-back pain, and bleeding gums. Blood may be detected in the urine and stool.
- Because of many drug interactions, instruct patients receiving warfarin (Coumadin) therapy not to take any other medications unless the drugs are approved by their physician.

TEST RESULTS AND CLINICAL SIGNIFICANCE

▲ Increased Levels (Prolonged Prothrombin Time)

Liver disease (e.g., cirrhosis, hepatitis): *Coagulation factors are made in the liver. In liver disease, synthesis is inadequate, and the prothrombin time is increased.*

Hereditary factor deficiency: *A genetic defect causes a decrease in a coagulation factor. The prothrombin time is increased. Factors II, V, VII, or X could be similarly affected.*

Vitamin K deficiency: *Vitamin K–dependent factors (II, VII, IX, X) are not made. The prothrombin time is therefore increased.*

Bile duct obstruction: *Fat-soluble vitamins, including vitamin K, are not absorbed. Vitamin K–dependent factors (II, VII, IX, X) are not made. The prothrombin time is therefore increased.*

Coumarin ingestion: *Synthesis of the vitamin K–dependent coagulation factors is inhibited. The prothrombin time is therefore increased.*

Disseminated intravascular coagulation: *Coagulation factors are consumed in the intravascular coagulation process. The prothrombin time is increased.*

Massive blood transfusion: *Coagulation is inhibited by the anticoagulant in the banked blood. Furthermore, with massive bleeding, the factors are diluted out by the "factor-poor" banked blood.*

Salicylate intoxication

RELATED TESTS

Partial Thromboplastin Time (p. 396). This test is used to evaluate the intrinsic system and the common pathway of clot formation. It is most commonly used to monitor heparin therapy.

Coagulating Factor Concentration (p. 177). This is a quantitative measurement of specific coagulation factors.

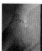

QuantiFERON-TB Gold (QFT, QFT-G, TB Gold test, TB Blood Test)

NORMAL FINDINGS

Negative

INDICATIONS

The QuantiFERON-TB (QFT) test is used to diagnose active tuberculosis infection in patients recently exposed to or suspected to have tuberculosis infection.

TEST EXPLANATION

The QFT test is a whole-blood test for use as an aid in diagnosing *Mycobacterium tuberculosis* infection. The diagnosis of active or latent tuberculosis still requires additional testing (such as a chest radiograph, sputum smear, and culture). QFT testing is a diagnostic aid in which a component of cell-mediated immune reactivity to *M. tuberculosis* is measured, much like the tuberculin skin testing (TST; see p. 1168). Unlike TST, however, this test does not cause a hypersensitivity response in patients with prior bacille Calmette-Guérin vaccination. Furthermore, in comparison with TST, QFT results are not subject to reader bias and error. As with TST, false-negative QFT results can occur in anergic patients.

QFT testing cannot differentiate active from latent tuberculosis infection. Its use in latent infection is being studied. Because QFT testing involves the use of tuberculosis-specific antigens—in comparison with TST, in which nonspecific purified protein derivative (PPD) antigens are used—QFT testing is more accurate and specific. QFT results are available in 24 hours. Because this test is an in vitro test that never exposes the patient to its antigenic proteins, QFT never generates a "booster" false-positive response. Furthermore, because a second patient visit for skin reading is not necessary, QFT testing is an attractive alternative to TST. QFT testing can be used for serial surveillance testing less than 12 months after a negative PPD test result, if the initial QFT result is negative.

QFT testing is used in the same scenarios as is TST. These include contact investigations, evaluation of recent immigrants, and sequential-testing surveillance programs for infection control, such as those for health care workers.

In this enzyme-linked immunosorbent assay (ELISA), blood samples are mixed with synthetic PPD antigens (ESAT-6 and CFP-10). After incubation of the blood with these antigens for 16 to 24 hours, interferon-gamma (IFN-γ) from sensitized lymphocytes is measured. If patients are infected with *M. tuberculosis*, their lymphocytes release large quantities of IFN-γ in response to contact with the tuberculosis antigens.

Because of a suppressed IFN-γ response, the QFT result may be artificially negative in patients with advanced tuberculosis. The QFT test (unlike some skin tests) does not account for anergy and may yield inaccurately negative findings in immunosuppressed patients. The sensitivity and rate of indeterminate results with QFT is diminished in immunocompromised persons with human immunovirus (HIV) infection, those with acquired immune deficiency syndrome (AIDS), those currently receiving treatment with immunosuppressive drugs, those with selected hematologic disorders, and those with certain malignancies. These conditions or treatments are known or suspected to decrease responsiveness to the TST, and they might also decrease production of IFN-γ in the QFT assay. As with a negative TST result, negative QFT results alone might be insufficient to rule out tuberculosis infection in these persons.

PROCEDURE AND PATIENT CARE

Before

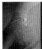 Explain the procedure to the patient or the family.

During

- Collect 1 mL whole blood in each of three Cellestis QuantiFERON-TB Gold collection tubes.
- Immediately after collection, mix each specimen vigorously by shaking the tube up and down 10 times to ensure that the entire inner surface of the tube has been coated with blood.

After

- Apply pressure or a pressure dressing to the venipuncture site.
- Incubate the blood tubes upright at 37°C for 16 to 24 hours (within 16 hours of collection).
- If the patient's results are positive, educate the patient about the necessary follow-up studies, such as chest radiography and sputum cultures.

TEST RESULTS AND CLINICAL SIGNIFICANCE

▲ Increased Levels

Tuberculosis infection: *Patients with active or dormant tuberculosis infections have elevated QFT levels unless the tuberculosis is so advanced as to cause immunodeficiency.*

RELATED TESTS

Tuberculin Skin Testing (p. 1168). This skin test is performed on patients in whom tuberculosis infection is suspected.

Tuberculosis Culture (p. 798). This is the "gold standard," most sensitive test for diagnosing mycobacterial infection.

Rabies-Neutralizing Antibody

NORMAL FINDINGS

<1:16

INDICATIONS

This test is performed after vaccination to document seroprotection in animal care workers. It is also used to determine exposure to rabies and in the diagnosis of rabies.

TEST EXPLANATION

Identification and documentation of the presence of rabies-neutralizing antibody is important for veterinary health care workers and others who are at risk or may have been exposed to the rabies virus. This test is performed on individuals who are at great risk for animal bites (veterinarians and their staff, zoo workers, people who work with animals in laboratories) and on those who have received the human diploid cell rabies vaccine (HDCV). A rabies titre higher than 1:16 is considered protective.

Rabies antibody is also used in diagnosing rabies in patients suspected of being exposed to the virus. A fourfold rise in antibody titre over several weeks in a person not previously exposed to the HDCV indicates rabies exposure. If the patient has received HDCV and has been bitten by an animal suspected of having rabies infection, a very high antibody titre may support the diagnosis. The presence of antibody in the cerebrospinal fluid is also supportive of the diagnosis because the cerebrospinal fluid usually contains no antibodies after the HDCV vaccine, but it does contain antibodies after a bite from a rabies-infected animal. In patients who may have been exposed to rabies, the human rabies immune globulin is given after the antibody titres have been obtained. If feasible, half the dose of the human rabies immune globulin should be administered to thoroughly infiltrate the area around the bite, and then the other half administered as an intramuscular injection into the deltoid muscle of the upper arm, or the lateral thigh muscle. At the same time, the first of the HDCV injections are administered to begin vaccination. Four subsequent intramuscular injections are administered over the next 28 days. The rabies antibody levels may increase in approximately 10 days, but protective levels may not be present for several weeks. Postexposure protocols are followed to determine the proper handling of the patient and animal, depending on the real risk that the animal is infected.

The rabies antibody has traditionally been identified by the direct fluorescent antibody method. More recently, immunofluorescence has been used.

PROCEDURE AND PATIENT CARE

Before

- Explain the procedure to the patient.
- Inform the patient that no fasting or special preparation is required.

During

- Collect a venous blood sample in a red-top tube.

After

- Apply pressure or a pressure dressing to the venipuncture site.
- Assess the venipuncture site for bleeding.

TEST RESULTS AND CLINICAL SIGNIFICANCE

Exposure to rabies vaccine: This causes a relatively low titre of 1:16 or greater.

Recent bite exposure to rabies virus: This causes a progressive rise in titre to levels of 1:200 to 1:160 000.

Active rabies in patient or animal: Antibody titres are extremely high in patients who present with encephalitis and brain stem dysfunction. Such patients rarely recover from the disease.

Red Blood Cell Count (RBC Count, Erythrocyte Count)

NORMAL FINDINGS

RBC × 10^{12}/L (million/mm^3)
Adult/older adult:
Male: 4.7–6.2 × 10^{12}/L
Female: 4.2–5.4 × 10^{12}/L

Child:
    2–8 weeks: **4.0–6.0 × 10^{12}/L**
    2–6 months: **3.5–5.5 × 10^{12}/L**
    6 months–1 year: **3.5–5.2 × 10^{12}/L**
    1–6 years: **4.0–5.5 × 10^{12}/L**
    6–18 years: **4.0–5.5 × 10^{12}/L**
Newborn: **4.8–7.1 × 10^{12}/L**

INDICATIONS

The red blood cell (RBC) count is closely related to the hemoglobin (p. 299) and hemato-crit (p. 295) levels and represents different ways of evaluating the number of RBCs in the peripheral blood. This count is repeated serially in patients with ongoing bleeding or as a routine part of the complete blood cell count. It is an integral part of the evaluation of anemic patients.

TEST EXPLANATION

This test is a count of the number of circulating RBCs in $1\,mm^3$ of peripheral venous blood. The RBC count is routinely performed as part of a complete blood cell count. Within each RBC are molecules of hemoglobin that enable the transport and exchange of oxygen to the tissues and carbon dioxide from the tissues. RBCs are produced by the erythroid elements in the bone marrow. Under the stimulation of erythropoietin, RBC production is increased. Normally, RBCs survive in the peripheral blood for approximately 120 days. During that time, they are transported through the bloodstream. In the smallest capillaries, RBCs must fold and bend to conform to the size of these tiny vessels. Toward the end of an RBC's life, the cell membrane becomes less pliable; the aged RBC is then lysed and extracted from the circulation by the spleen. Abnormal RBCs have a shorter life span and are extracted earlier. Intravascular RBC trauma, such as that caused by artificial heart valves or peripheral vascular atherosclerotic plaques, also shortens the RBC's life span. Enlargement of the spleen, such as that caused by portal hypertension or leukemia, may inappropriately destroy and remove normal RBCs from the circulation.

Normal RBC values vary according to gender and age. Women tend to have lower values than men, and RBC counts tend to decrease with age. When the value is decreased by more than 10% of the expected normal value, the patient is said to be anemic. Low RBC values have many causes:
1. Hemorrhage (as in gastrointestinal bleeding or trauma)
2. Hemolysis (as in glucose-6-phosphate dehydrogenase deficiency, spherocytosis, or secondary splenomegaly)
3. Dietary (iron or vitamin B_{12}) deficiency
4. Genetic aberrations (such as sickle cell disease or thalassemia)
5. Ingestion of drugs (such as chloramphenicol, hydantoin, or quinidine)
6. Marrow failure (as in fibrosis, leukemia, or antineoplastic chemotherapy)
7. Chronic illness (such as tumour or sepsis)
8. Other organ failure (as in renal disease)

RBC counts can be physiologically increased as a result of the body's requirements for greater oxygen-carrying capacity (e.g., at high altitudes). Diseases that produce chronic hypoxia (e.g., congenital heart disease) also provoke this physiologic increase in RBCs. Polycythemia vera is a neoplastic condition causing uncontrolled production of RBCs.

Like the hemoglobin and hematocrit values, the RBC count can be altered by many factors other than RBC production. For instance, in dehydrated patients, the total blood volume is lower; therefore, the RBCs are more concentrated, and the RBC count per litre is artificially high. Likewise, in overhydrated patients, the blood concentration is diluted, and the RBC count is artificially low. In most hospitals and laboratories, the RBC count is performed by an automated counting machine with an error range of approximately 4% to 5%.

INTERFERING FACTORS

- Normally, the RBC count decreases during pregnancy as a result of normal body fluid increases that dilute the blood. Also, an element of nutritional deficiency that is often associated with pregnancy may play a role in the anemia of pregnancy.
- At high altitudes for prolonged periods, the RBC counts rise as a physiologic response to the decreased oxygen available at these altitudes.
- Hydration status: As stated previously, dehydration factitiously increases the RBC count, and overhydration factitiously decreases the RBC count.
- Drugs that may cause *increases* in RBC levels include gentamicin and methyldopa.
- Drugs that may cause *decreases* in RBC levels include chloramphenicol, erythropoietin, hydantoin, and quinidine.

PROCEDURE AND PATIENT CARE

Before
- Explain the procedure to the patient.
- Inform the patient that no fasting is required.

During
- Collect a venous blood sample in a lavender-top tube.
- Thoroughly mix the blood with the anticoagulant by tilting the tube.
- Avoid hemolysis.

After
- Apply pressure or a pressure dressing to the venipuncture site.
- Observe the venipuncture site for bleeding.

TEST RESULTS AND CLINICAL SIGNIFICANCE

▲ Increased Levels

Erythrocytosis: *The number of RBCs increases as a result of illnesses or as a physiologic response to external situations (e.g., high altitude).*

Congenital heart disease: *Cyanotic heart diseases cause chronically low partial pressure of oxygen (P_{O_2}). In response, the RBCs increase in number.*

Severe chronic obstructive pulmonary disease: *In chronic states of hypoxia, RBC production is stimulated as a physiologic response to increase oxygen-carrying capacity.*

Polycythemia vera: *This is a result of the bone marrow's producing inappropriately great numbers of RBCs.*

Severe dehydration (e.g., severe diarrhea or burns): *With depletion of extracellular fluid, the total blood volume decreases, but the number of RBCs stays the same. Because the blood is more concentrated, the number of RBCs per litre is increased.*

Hemoglobinopathies,

Thalassemia trait: *Because abnormal hemoglobin has decreased oxygen-carrying capacity, more RBCs may be produced in order to increase oxygen-carrying capacity.*

▼ Decreased Levels

Anemia: *This is a state associated with reduced RBC numbers. Many different types of diseases are associated with anemia.*

Hemoglobinopathy: *Patients with hemoglobin disorders or other blood dyscrasias may have reduced RBC number and life span.*

Cirrhosis: *This is a chronic state of fluid overload. The RBCs are diluted, and the number of RBCs per litre is reduced.*

Hemolytic anemia (as in erythroblastosis fetalis, hemoglobinopathies, drug-induced reactions, transfusion reactions, paroxysmal nocturnal hemoglobinuria): *The RBC life span is diminished in hemolytic anemia. The number of RBCs also decreases.*

Hemorrhage: *With active bleeding, the number of RBCs decreases. It takes time (several hours), however, for the RBC count to fall. Only if the blood volume is replenished with fluid does the RBC count diminish.*

Dietary deficiency: *With certain vitamin or mineral deficiencies (e.g., of iron or vitamin B_{12}), the RBC size or number is decreased.*

Bone marrow failure: *This results in reduced synthesis of RBCs.*

Prosthetic valves: *Prosthetic valves cause mechanical trauma to RBCs. The RBC life span is shortened, and RBC numbers diminish.*

Renal disease: *Erythropoietin is made in the kidneys and is a strong stimulant of RBC production. When levels of erythropoietin are reduced, the RBC numbers diminish.*

Normal pregnancy: *Normally, blood volume increases during pregnancy because pregnant women are in a chronic state of overhydration. In combination with a relative "malnourished" state, the RBC count per litre of blood is diminished.*

Rheumatoid/collagen-vascular diseases (e.g., rheumatoid arthritis, lupus, sarcoidosis): *Production of RBCs is reduced in chronic illnesses.*

Lymphoma,

Multiple myeloma,

Leukemia,

Hodgkin disease: *Hematologic cancers are often associated with bone marrow failure of RBC production.*

RELATED TESTS

Hematocrit (p. 295). This is the percentage of the total blood volume that is composed of the RBCs. It is closely associated with the hemoglobin value and the RBC count.

Hemoglobin (p. 299). This is the total amount of hemoglobin in the peripheral blood. It is closely associated with the RBC count and hematocrit value.

Red Blood Cell Indices (see following test). These indices provide information about the size and hemoglobin content of the RBC.

Red Blood Cell Indices (RBC Indices, Mean Corpuscular Volume [MCV], Mean Corpuscular Hemoglobin [MCH], Mean Corpuscular Hemoglobin Concentration [MCHC], Blood Indices, Erythrocyte Indices, Red Blood Cell Distribution Width [RDW])

NORMAL FINDINGS

Mean Corpuscular Volume (MCV)
Adult/older adult/child: **76–100 fL** ($76–100\,mm^3$)
Newborn: **96–108 fL** ($96–108\,mm^3$)

Mean Corpuscular Hemoglobin (MCH)
Adult/older adult/child: **27–31 pg**
Newborn: 32–34 pg

Mean Corpuscular Hemoglobin Concentration (MCHC)
Adult/older adult/child: **32–36 g/dL** (32%–36%)
Newborn: **32–33 g/dL** (32%–33%)

Red Blood Cell Distribution Width (RDW)
Adult: varies between 11%–14.5%

INDICATIONS

The red blood cell (RBC) indices provide information about the size (mean corpuscular volume [MCV] and RBC distribution width [RDW]), weight, colour (mean corpuscular hemoglobin [MCH]), and hemoglobin concentration (mean corpuscular hemoglobin concentration [MCHC]) of RBCs. This test is useful in classifying anemias.

TEST EXPLANATION

This test is routinely performed as part of an automated complete blood cell count. The results of the RBC, hematocrit, and hemoglobin tests (see pp. 452, 295, and 299 respectively) are necessary for calculating the RBC indices. When anemia is investigated, it is helpful to categorize the anemia according to the RBC indices, as shown in Box 2-12. Cell size is indicated by the terms *normocytic, microcytic,* and *macrocytic.* Hemoglobin content is indicated by the terms *normochromic, hypochromic,* and *hyperchromic.* Additional information about the RBC size, shape, colour, and intracellular structure is described in the blood smear study (see p. 738).

Mean Corpuscular Volume
The MCV is a measure of the average volume, or size, of a single RBC and is therefore used in classifying anemias. MCV is derived by dividing the hematocrit by the total RBC count:

$$MCV\,(fL) = \frac{Hematocrit\,(\%) \times 10}{RBC\,(10^{12}/L\,)}$$

Normal values vary according to age and gender. When the MCV value is increased, the RBC is said to be abnormally large, or *macrocytic.* This occurs most frequently in megaloblastic

| BOX 2-12 | Categorization of Anemia According to Red Blood Cell Indices |

Normocytic,* Normochromic† Anemia
- Iron deficiency (detected early)
- Chronic illness (e.g., sepsis, tumour)
- Acute blood loss
- Aplastic anemia (e.g., chloramphenicol toxicosis)
- Acquired hemolytic anemias (e.g., from a prosthetic cardiac valve)

Microcytic‡, Hypochromic§ Anemia
- Iron deficiency (detected late)
- Thalassemia
- Lead poisoning

Microcytic, Normochromic Anemia
- Renal disease (because of the loss of erythropoietin)

Macrocytic,¶ Normochromic Anemia
- Vitamin B_{12} or folic acid deficiency
- Hydantoin ingestion
- Chemotherapy
- Some myelodysplastic syndromes
- Myeloid leukemia
- Ethanol toxicity
- Thyroid dysfunction

*Normal RBC size.
†Normal colour (normal hemoglobin content).
‡Smaller-than-normal RBC size.
§Paler-than-normal colour (decreased hemoglobin content).
¶Larger-than-normal RBC size.
RBC, Red blood cell.

anemias (e.g., vitamin B_{12} or folic acid deficiency). When the MCV value is decreased, the RBC is said to be abnormally small, or *microcytic.* This is associated with iron-deficiency anemia or thalassemia. A significant number of patients who have disorders associated with a variation in MCV may, in fact, not have an abnormality in MCV. For example, only 65% of patients with iron-deficiency anemia have reduced MCV. Furthermore, the normal values for MCV and all the other RBC indices vary considerably. Each laboratory must develop its own normal index values.

Mean Corpuscular Hemoglobin

The MCH is a measure of the average amount (weight) of hemoglobin within an RBC. MCH is derived by dividing the total hemoglobin concentration by the number of RBCs:

$$MCH(pg) = \frac{Hemoglobin(g/dL) \times 10}{RBC(10^{12}/L)}$$

Because macrocytic cells generally have more hemoglobin and microcytic cells have less hemoglobin, the causes of these values closely resemble those of the MCV value. This has been documented with the use of automated counting instruments. The MCH adds very little information to the other indices.

Mean Corpuscular Hemoglobin Concentration. The MCHC is a measure of the average concentration or percentage of hemoglobin within a single RBC. MCHC is derived by dividing the total hemoglobin concentration by the hematocrit:

$$MCHC(g/dL) = \frac{Hemoglobin(g/dL)}{Hematocrit(\%)}$$

When values are decreased, the cell has a deficiency of hemoglobin and is said to be *hypochromic* (frequently observed in iron-deficiency anemia and thalassemia). When values are normal, the anemia is said to be *normochromic* (e.g., hemolytic anemia). RBCs cannot be considered hyperchromic because only 3.7 g/L (37 g/dL) of hemoglobin can fit into the RBC. Alteration in RBC shape (spherocytosis, acute transfusion reactions, erythroblastosis fetalis) may cause automated counting machines to indicate MCHC levels above normal.

Red Blood Cell Distribution Width

The RDW is an indication of the variation in RBC size. It is calculated by a machine from the MCV and RBC values. Variations in the width of the RBCs may be helpful when certain types of anemia are classified. The RDW is essentially an indicator of the degree of *anisocytosis,* a blood disorder characterized by RBCs of variable and abnormal size.

The newer electronic cell-counting machines are able to sort out RBCs according to size and compare those sizes with a histogram. Normally, all the RBCs are approximately the same size with very little variation. The resulting histogram has a single narrowed peak. Certain diseases change the size of some of the RBCs, whereas the less abnormal RBCs are less affected. For example, with folic acid deficiency or iron deficiency, the newer RBCs are more significantly affected than the older cells and therefore are of significantly different size. The resulting histogram thus has multiple peaks, which indicate large numbers of cells at variable sizes.

INTERFERING FACTORS

- Abnormal RBC size may affect the MCH and MCHC.
- Extremely elevated white blood cell counts ($>50 \times 10^9$/L [$>50000\,mm^3$]) may increase the MCV and MCH indices when processed by automated counters.
- Large RBC precursors, such as reticulocytes (see p. 465), cause MCV to be abnormally high. This commonly occurs in response to anemias when the bone marrow is not diseased.
- Marked elevation in lipid levels (**>200 g/L** [$>2000\,mg/dL$]) causes automated cell counters to indicate high hemoglobin levels. Measurements of MCV, MCHC, and MCH are artificially high.
- The presence of cold agglutinins also artificially elevates MCHC, MCH, and MCV.
- Drugs that may cause *increases* in MCV results include azathioprine, phenytoin, and zidovudine.

PROCEDURE AND PATIENT CARE

Before
- Explain the procedure to the patient.
- Inform the patient that no fasting is required.

During
- Collect a venous blood sample in a lavender-top tube.
- Avoid hemolysis.

After

- Apply pressure or a pressure dressing to the venipuncture site.
- Assess the venipuncture site for bleeding.
- Transport the specimen to the hematology laboratory, in which the blood is passed through automated machines that calculate the RBC indices.

TEST RESULTS AND CLINICAL SIGNIFICANCE

▲ Increased Mean Corpuscular Volume

Pernicious anemia (vitamin B_{12} deficiency),
Folic acid deficiency: *These are the most common causes of macrocytic anemia. These vitamin deficiencies may be caused by malnutrition, malabsorption, competitive parasites, or enzyme deficiencies that impair utilization of these vitamins.*
Antimetabolite therapy: *This form of chemotherapy for cancer treatment and, in lesser doses, for arthritis treatment acts as vitamin B_{12} and folate inhibitors and can cause macrocytic anemia.*
Alcoholism: *Increased MCV in this case is probably related to malnutrition.*
Chronic liver disease: *The pathophysiologic mechanism underlying this observation is multifactorial and includes poor nutrition, erythropoietin alterations, and the effects of chronic illness.*

▼ Decreased Mean Corpuscular Volume

Iron-deficiency anemia,
Thalassemia,
Anemia of chronic illness: *These are the most common diseases associated with microcytosis.*

▲ Increased Mean Corpuscular Hemoglobin

Macrocytic anemias: *The MCH is increased if the size of the RBC is large.*

▼ Decreased Mean Corpuscular Hemoglobin

Microcytic anemia,
Hypochromic anemia: *The MCH is decreased if the size of the RBC is small or the hemoglobin is diminished.*

▲ Increased Mean Corpuscular Hemoglobin Concentration

Spherocytosis: *The automated cell counter's false perception of an elevation in the MCHC is caused by a variation in the shape of the RBC. The RBC can hold only 37 g/dL of hemoglobin. "Real" hyperchromatism cannot exist.*
Intravascular hemolysis: *This is caused by free hemoglobin in the blood. The automated counter incorporates the free hemoglobin into its calculations.*
Cold agglutinins: *Cold agglutinins cause the misperception of increased MCV and decreased hematocrit. The automated machine calculates an artificially high MCHC.*

▼ Decreased Mean Corpuscular Hemoglobin Concentration

Iron-deficiency anemia,
Thalassemia: *These are the most common causes of hypochromatism. Thalassemia minor (heterozygous) may not be clinically evident except in measurements of RBC count, MCV, and MCHC.*

▲ Increased RBC Distribution Width

Iron-deficiency anemia,
B_{12} vitamin or folate-deficiency anemia: *Increased variation in RDW is caused by a combination of factors in these diseases. RBC fragmentation alters RBC size and shape. Furthermore, new cells produced*

when the deficiency was most severe are markedly different in size and shape than the older RBCs that were produced before the deficiencies were as severe.

Hemoglobinopathies (e.g., sickle cell disease or protein C disease): *Fragmentation increases RDW variation. Furthermore, different RBCs have different amounts of pathologic hemoglobin and therefore are affected by fragmentation to varying degrees.*

Hemolytic anemias: *Fragmentation increases RDW variation.*

Posthemorrhagic anemias: *The bone marrow's response to bleeding is to release RBCs prematurely into the bloodstream. These RBCs are larger than mature RBCs and contribute to RDW variation.*

RELATED TESTS

Hematocrit (p. 295). This is the percentage of the total blood volume taken up by the RBCs. It is closely associated with the hemoglobin value and the RBC count.

Hemoglobin (p. 299). This is the total amount of hemoglobin in the peripheral blood. It is closely associated with the RBC count and hematocrit value.

Red Blood Cell Count (p. 452). This is the number of RBCs $\times 10^{12}$/L. It is closely associated with the hemoglobin and hematocrit values.

Renin Assay, Plasma (Plasma Renin Activity [PRA], Plasma Renin Concentration [PRC])

NORMAL FINDINGS

Plasma Renin Assay

Adult/Older Adult

Upright position, sodium depleted (sodium-restricted diet):
  20–39 years: **2.9–24 Mcg/L/hr** (2.9–24 ng/mL/hr)
  >40 years: **2.9–10.8 Mcg/L/hr** (2.9–10.8 ng/mL/hr)
Upright position, sodium replaced (normal-sodium diet):
  20–39 years: **0.1–4.3 Mcg/L/hr** (0.1–4.3 ng/mL/hr)
  >40 years: **0.1–3 Mcg/L/hr** (0.1–3 ng/mL/hr)

Child

0–3 years: **<16.6 Mcg/L/hr** (<16.6 ng/mL/hr)
3–6 years: **<6.7 Mcg/L/hr** (<6.7 ng/mL/hr)
6–9 years: **<4.4 Mcg/L/hr** (<4.4 ng/mL/hr)
9–12 years: **<5.9 Mcg/L/hr** (<5.9 ng/ml/hr)
12–15 years: **<4.2 Mcg/L/hr** (<4.2 ng/mL/hr)
15–18 years: **<4.3 Mcg/L/hr** (<4.3 ng/mL/hr)

Renal Vein

Renin ratio of involved kidney to uninvolved kidney: <1.4

INDICATIONS

Plasma renin activity (PRA) is measured to evaluate hypertension. It is helpful in the differential diagnosis of aldosteronism.

TEST EXPLANATION

Renin is an enzyme released by the juxtaglomerular apparatus of the kidney into the renal veins in response to hyperkalemia, sodium depletion, decreased renal blood perfusion, or hypovolemia. Renin activates the renin-angiotensin system, which produces angiotensin II, a powerful vasoconstrictor that also stimulates aldosterone production from the adrenal cortex. Angiotensin and aldosterone increase the blood volume, blood pressure, and serum sodium (Figure 2-21). After release of renin from the kidney into the bloodstream, angiotensinogen, an alpha$_2$-globulin that is made in the liver, is converted into angiotensin I. This is then converted into angiotensin II in the lungs.

Renin is not actually measured in this test. (In research laboratories, renin can be directly measured with great difficulty.) The PRA test actually measures, by radioimmunoassay, the rate of angiotensin I generation per unit time. This is a commonly used renin assay. The plasma renin concentration is used to measure the maximum renin effect. This is useful in patients who are pregnant or have estrogen-induced increased protein levels. The PRA and the plasma renin concentration tests are very difficult to perform. Most assays are performed at central laboratories. The specimen must be collected under ideal circumstances, handled by the local laboratory correctly, and transferred to the central laboratory in a timely manner. Even then, results may vary significantly.

The PRA is a screening procedure for the detection of essential, renal, or renovascular hypertension. The PRA may be supplemented by other tests, such as the renal vein renin assay. A determination of the PRA and a measurement of the plasma aldosterone level are used in the differential diagnosis of primary versus secondary hyperaldosteronism (Table 2-43). In primary hyperaldosteronism (adrenal adenoma overproducing aldosterone or Conn syndrome), aldosterone production is increased in association with decreased renin activity. In secondary hyperaldosteronism (caused by renovascular occlusive disease or primary renal disease), levels of plasma renin are increased.

Renal vein assays for renin are used to diagnose and lateralize renovascular hypertension (hypertension that is related to inappropriately high renin levels from a diseased kidney or a hypoperfused kidney). A radiopaque dye is injected into the inferior vena cava in order to outline the renal veins. A catheter is placed into each renal vein, and blood is withdrawn from

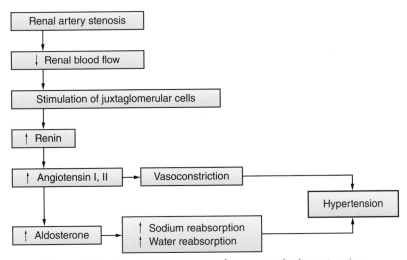

Figure 2-21 Physiologic process of renovascular hypertension.

TABLE 2-43   **Differential Diagnosis According to Renin Level and Aldosterone Risk**

Disease	Renin (PRA) Level	Aldosterone Risk
Conn syndrome	Low	High
Renal artery stenosis (or occlusion)	High	High
Primary renal disease	High	High
Increased sodium intake	Low	Low
Sodium restriction	High	High
Hypokalemia	Low	Low
Sodium-losing diuretic therapy	High	High
Addison's disease	High	Low
Cushing's syndrome	Low	High
Essential hypertension	Low	Normal

each vein. PRA is determined in each sample. If hypertension is caused by renal artery stenosis or renal disease, the renin level in the renal vein of the affected kidney should be 1.4 or more times greater than that in the unaffected kidney. If the levels are the same, the hypertension is not caused by a renovascular source. This finding is very helpful in determining whether a stenosis observed on a renal angiogram is significantly contributing to hypertension. Any stenosis identified on an arteriogram would not be considered severe enough to cause renin-related hypertension if renin levels from the affected kidney were not at least 1.4 times those of the opposite kidney. In this case, another cause of the patient's elevated blood pressure should be considered.

The *renin stimulation* test can be performed to more clearly diagnose and distinguish primary and secondary hyperaldosteronism. In this test, PRA is obtained while the patient is in the recumbent position and on a low-sodium diet and then repeated while the patient is standing erect. In primary hyperaldosteronism, the blood volume is greatly expanded. A change in position or reduced sodium intake does not result in decreased renal perfusion or sodium level. Therefore, renin levels do not increase. In secondary hyperaldosteronism (or normal persons with essential hypertension), the renal perfusion decreases while the patient is in the upright position, and sodium levels do decrease with decreased sodium intake. Therefore, renin levels increase.

The PRA is assessed as part of the *captopril test* (a screening test for renovascular hypertension). Patients with renovascular hypertension have greater decreases in blood pressure and increases in PRA after administration of angiotensin-converting enzyme (ACE) inhibitors than do patients with essential hypertension. In the captopril test, the patient receives an oral dose of captopril (ACE inhibitor) after a baseline PRA test, and blood pressure is then measured. Subsequent blood pressure measurements and a repeat PRA test at 60 minutes are used for interpretation of the findings. This screening procedure is excellent for determining the need for a more invasive radiographic evaluation (such as digital subtraction renal arteriography [p. 1026] or bilateral renal arteriography [p. 1026]).

CONTRAINDICATIONS

• Allergy to shellfish or iodinated dye, because of potential allergic reaction to the radiopaque dye during renal vein renin assay

POTENTIAL COMPLICATIONS

- Allergic reactions to iodinated dye can occur during the renal vein renin assay. The reaction may vary from mild flushing, itching, and urticaria to severe, life-threatening anaphylaxis (evidenced by respiratory distress, drop in blood pressure, shock). In the unusual event of anaphylaxis, the patient may be treated with diphenhydramine (Benadryl), steroids, and epinephrine. Oxygen and endotracheal equipment should be on hand for immediate use.

INTERFERING FACTORS

- Renin is increased during pregnancy by virtue of increases in levels of substrate proteins concomitantly present in the serum during testing.
- Renin is increased with reduced sodium intake. Reduction in sodium intake acts as a direct stimulant of renin production.
- Renin is increased by ingestion of large amounts of licorice. Licorice has an aldosterone-like effect. This increases sodium reabsorption in the kidney and raises blood pressure, which in turn inhibits renin production.
- There is diurnal variation in renin production: Values are higher early in the day.
- Renin levels are increased when the patient is in an upright position. The upright position normally decreases renal perfusion because the blood pools in the veins of the lower extremities. This decreased renal perfusion is a strong stimulant of renin production. Renin levels are decreased in the recumbent position for the same reason (i.e., renal perfusion is increased in the recumbent position, and renin levels diminish).
- Drugs that cause *increases* in levels of renin include ACE inhibitors, antihypertensives, diuretics, estrogens, oral contraceptives, and vasodilators.
- Drugs that cause *decreases* in renin levels include beta blockers, clonidine, and potassium.

Clinical Priorities

- There is diurnal variation in renin production: Renin levels are higher in the morning. Therefore, a morning blood sample is usually collected.
- Renin levels are affected by body position: Levels are higher in the upright position and decreased in the recumbent position.
- Renin levels are increased with reduced sodium intake, because reduced sodium levels are a stimulant of renin production.

PROCEDURE AND PATIENT CARE

Before

- Explain the procedure to the patient.
- Instruct the patient to maintain his or her usual diet but with a restricted amount of sodium (~3 g/day) for 3 days before the test.
- Instruct the patient to discontinue medications (e.g., diuretics, steroids, antihypertensives, vasodilators, oral contraceptives) and to avoid licorice for 2 to 4 weeks before the test, as ordered by the physician.
- Plan to collect a morning sample, because renin values are higher in the morning.
- For stimulation tests, instruct the patient to significantly reduce sodium intake (and to supplement the diet with potassium) for 3 days before the test.

During

- Usually perform the test with the patient in an upright position.
- For the stimulation test, collect the blood while the patient is in the recumbent and upright positions.
- Ensure that the patient stands or sits upright for 2 hours before the blood is collected.
- If a recumbent sample is ordered, have the patient remain in bed in the morning until the blood sample has been obtained.
- It is best to release the tourniquet immediately before obtaining the blood specimen because stasis can lower renin levels.
- Collect a venous blood sample in a chilled lavender-top tube with ethylenediamine tetra-acetic acid (EDTA) as an anticoagulant. Heparin can artificially decrease results.

After

- Apply pressure or a pressure dressing to the venipuncture site.
- Observe the venipuncture site for bleeding.
- Inform the patient that his or her usual diet and medications may be resumed.
- Gently invert the blood tube to allow adequate mixing of the blood sample and the anticoagulant.
- On the laboratory slip, record the patient's position, dietary status, and time of day.
- Place the tube of blood in a mixture of water and crushed ice, and send it immediately to the laboratory.
- In the laboratory, the blood is centrifuged, and the serum is frozen.

TEST RESULTS AND CLINICAL SIGNIFICANCE

▲ Increased Levels

Essential hypertension: *A small percentage of affected patients have renin hypertension.*

Malignant hypertension: *A large percentage of affected patients with aggressive hypertensive episodes have secondary hyperaldosteronism (usually because of renal vascular occlusion or stenosis).*

Renovascular hypertension: *Renal artery stenosis or occlusion decreases the renal blood flow, which is a strong stimulant of renin production.*

Chronic renal failure: *Diseases of the kidney can stimulate the production of renin.*

Sodium-losing gastrointestinal disease (vomiting or diarrhea): *Affected patients develop hyponatremia, which is a strong stimulant of renin production.*

Addison's disease: *Affected patients have hyponatremia, which is a strong stimulant of renin production.*

Renin-producing renal tumour: *Tumours of the juxtaglomerular apparatus, which are rare, can produce renin.*

Bartter syndrome: *This syndrome is associated with potassium wasting in the kidney, high renin levels, and high aldosterone levels. It is caused by a tubular defect in sodium reabsorption.*

Cirrhosis: *Affected patients have increased total body water, which dilutes sodium. Sodium levels are chronically low, which is a stimulant of renin production.*

Hyperkalemia: *This is a direct stimulant of renin production.*

Hemorrhage: *Any form of hypotension (including cardiogenic or septic shock) is associated with a reduction in the renal blood flow, which is a strong stimulant of renin production.*

▼ Decreased Levels

Primary hyperaldosteronism: *This is usually caused by an adrenal adenoma, and aldosterone levels are high. Aldosterone inhibits further renin production.*

Steroid therapy: *Glucocorticosteroids also have an aldosterone effect, which acts to increase serum sodium levels, decrease potassium levels, and increase blood volume. These responses all tend to diminish renin levels.*

Congenital adrenal hyperplasia: *An enzyme defect in cortisol synthesis causes an accumulation of cortisol precursors, some of which have strong aldosterone-like activity. These act to increase serum sodium levels, decrease potassium levels, and increase blood volume, all of which tend to diminish renin levels.*

RELATED TEST

Aldosterone (p. 48). This is a direct measurement of aldosterone level. It is used to evaluate hypertension and aldosteronism.

Reticulocyte Count (Retic Count)

NORMAL FINDINGS

Reticulocyte Count

Adult/older adult/child: 0.5%–2% of total number of RBCs
Infant: 0.5%–3.1% of total number of RBCs
Newborn: 2.5%–6.5% of total number of RBCs

Reticulocyte Index

1.0

INDICATIONS

The reticulocyte count is an indication of the ability of the bone marrow to respond to anemia and make RBCs. It is used to classify and monitor therapy for anemias.

TEST EXPLANATION

The reticulocyte count is a test for determining bone marrow function and evaluating erythropoietic activity. This test is also useful in classifying anemias. A reticulocyte is an immature red blood cell (RBC) that can be readily identified under a microscope on a peripheral blood smear stained with Wright or Giemsa stain. It is an RBC that still has some microsomal and ribosomal material left in the cytoplasm. It sometimes takes a few days for that material to be cleared from the cell. The bloodstream normally contains a small number of reticulocytes.

The reticulocyte count gives an indication of RBC production by the bone marrow. Increased reticulocyte counts indicate that the marrow is releasing an increased number of RBCs into the bloodstream, usually in response to anemia. A normal or low reticulocyte count in a patient with anemia indicates that the marrow response to the anemia is inadequate and the low production of RBCs may be contributing to or the cause of the anemia (as in aplastic anemia, iron deficiency, vitamin B_{12} deficiency, depletion of iron stores). An elevated reticulocyte count in combination with a normal hemogram indicates increased RBC production in compensation for an ongoing loss of RBCs (hemolysis or hemorrhage).

Because the reticulocyte count is a percentage of the total number of RBCs, a normal to low number of reticulocytes can appear high in an anemic patient because the total number of mature RBCs is low. To determine whether a reticulocyte count indicates an appropriate erythropoietic (RBC marrow) response in patients with anemia and a decreased hematocrit, the reticulocyte index is calculated as follows:

$$\text{Reticulocyte index} = \text{Reticulocyte count}(\%) \times \frac{\text{Patient's hematocrit}}{\text{Normal hematocrit}}$$

The reticulocyte index in a patient with a good marrow response to the anemia should be 1.0. If it is below 1.0, even when the reticulocyte count is elevated, the bone marrow response is inadequate in its ability to compensate (as seen in iron deficiency, vitamin B_{12} deficiency, marrow failure). In these clinical situations, if iron or vitamin B_{12} is administered, the reticulocyte count rises significantly to the point that the index equals or exceeds 1.0.

INTERFERING FACTORS

- Pregnancy may cause an increase in reticulocyte count.
- Howell-Jolly bodies are blue stippling material in the RBC that appear in severe anemia or hemolytic anemia. The RBCs that contain Howell-Jolly bodies look like reticulocytes and can be miscounted by some automated counter machines as reticulocytes; as a result, the number of reticulocytes is artificially high.

PROCEDURE AND PATIENT CARE

Before

🖋 Explain the procedure to the patient.
🖋 Inform the patient that no fasting is required.

During

- Collect a venous blood sample in a lavender-top tube.

After

- Apply pressure or a pressure dressing to the venipuncture site.
- Observe the venipuncture site for bleeding.

TEST RESULTS AND CLINICAL SIGNIFICANCE

▲ Increased Levels

Hemolytic anemia (e.g., immune hemolytic anemia, hemoglobinopathies, hypersplenism, trauma from a prosthetic heart valve): *The RBC life span is decreased, and RBCs are destroyed at a faster rate than normal. The bone marrow attempts to compensate for the shortened RBC life span by producing large numbers of RBCs, some of which are immature RBCs (reticulocytes).*

Hemorrhage (3 to 4 days later): *In response to significant blood loss, the bone marrow attempts to compensate by producing large numbers of RBCs, some of which are immature RBCs (reticulocytes).*

Hemolytic disease of the newborn: *Immune-mediated destruction of RBCs reduces RBC life span. The bone marrow attempts to compensate for the shortened RBC life span by producing large numbers of RBCs, some of which are immature RBCs (reticulocytes).*

Treatment for deficiency in iron, vitamin B$_{12}$, or folate: *After replacement treatment for anemia caused by nutritional deficiency, the marrow responds by increasing production of RBCs, some of which are immature RBCs (reticulocytes).*

▼ Decreased Levels

Pernicious anemia and folic acid deficiency,

Iron-deficiency anemia: *These nutritional deficiencies suppress marrow production of RBCs, including reticulocytes.*

Aplastic anemia,

Radiation therapy,

Malignancy,

Marrow failure,

Adrenocortical hypofunction,

Anterior pituitary hypofunction: *The bone marrow fails to produce RBCs and reticulocytes.*

Chronic diseases: *In patients with chronic diseases, bone marrow production of RBCs and reticulocytes is reduced.*

RELATED TESTS

Hemoglobin (p. 299) and Hematocrit (p. 295). These are indirect measurements of the RBCs.
Red Blood Cell Count (p. 452). This is a direct count of the total number of RBCs.

Rheumatoid Factor (RF, Rheumatoid Arthritis [RA] Factor)

NORMAL FINDINGS

Negative (<60 IU/mL by nephelometric testing)
Older adult patients may have slightly increased values.

INDICATIONS

The rheumatoid factor test is useful in the diagnosis of rheumatoid arthritis.

TEST EXPLANATION

Rheumatoid arthritis is a chronic inflammatory disease that affects most joints, especially the metacarpal and phalangeal joints, the proximal interphalangeal joints, and the wrists; however, any synovial joint can be involved. The British Columbia Ministry of Health Advisory Committee (2012) has defined criteria for the diagnosis of rheumatoid arthritis:

• Morning stiffness lasting longer than 30 minutes
• Painful swelling of at least three joints
• Involvement of joints of the hands and feet
• Duration of at least 4 weeks

In this disease, abnormal immunoglobulin G (IgG) antibodies produced by lymphocytes in the synovial membranes act as "antigens." Other IgG and immunoglobulin M (IgM) antibodies in the patient's serum react with the crystallizable fragment component of the abnormal synovial antigenic IgG to produce immune complexes. These immune complexes activate the complement system and other inflammatory systems to cause joint damage. The reactive IgM and sometimes IgG and immunoglobulin A (IgA) make up what is called the *rheumatoid factor*. IgG and IgA can also react to the synovial "IgG antigen." Tissues other than the joints—including blood vessels, lungs, nerves, and heart—may also be involved in the autoimmune inflammation.

Tests for rheumatoid factor are directed toward identification of the IgM antibodies. The exact role, if any, that rheumatoid factor plays in the pathophysiologic process of the disease is not well known. Approximately 80% of patients with rheumatoid arthritis have positive rheumatoid factor titres. For the titre to be considered positive, rheumatoid factor must be found in a dilution of greater than 1:80; when rheumatoid factor is found in titres of less than 1:80, diseases such as systemic lupus erythematosus, scleroderma, and other autoimmune conditions should be considered. Although the normal value is "no rheumatoid factor identifiable at low titres," rheumatoid factor is present in a very low titre in a small number of normal patients. Furthermore, a negative rheumatoid factor titre does not exclude the diagnosis of rheumatoid arthritis. When the nephelometric testing procedure is used, the normal value is considered to be less than 60 IU/mL. Rheumatoid factor is not a useful disease marker because it does not disappear in patients who are experiencing a remission of symptoms.

There are many serologic methods for detecting rheumatoid factor. The sheep cell agglutination test and the latex fixation test were most easily performed in the past. Better quantitation is now obtained by nephelometry. In the sheep cell agglutination test, rabbit IgG is placed on the sheep red blood cells (RBCs). When this is mixed with the patient's serum (which has been serially diluted), visual agglutination occurs if any rheumatoid factor is present. In the latex fixation test, human IgG is placed on a synthetic latex particle and mixed with the patient's serum. Visual agglutination is then detected if rheumatoid factor is present (Figure 2-22).

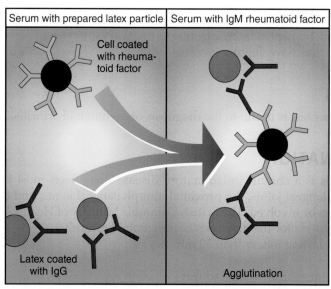

Serum with prepared latex particle	Serum with IgM rheumatoid factor
Cell coated with rheumatoid factor	
Latex coated with IgG	Agglutination

Figure 2-22 Appearance of a positive result for rheumatoid factor in the sheep cell agglutination test (*left*) and the latex test (*right*). *IgG,* Immunoglobulin G; *IgM,* immunoglobulin M.

Other autoimmune diseases (see Table 2-7, p. 100), such as systemic lupus erythematosus or Sjögren syndrome, also may cause a positive result in a rheumatoid factor test. Rheumatoid factor is also occasionally observed in patients with tuberculosis, chronic hepatitis, infectious mononucleosis, and subacute bacterial endocarditis.

INTERFERING FACTORS
- In older adults, testing often yields false-positive results.
- Hemolysis or lipemia can be associated with false-positive results.

PROCEDURE AND PATIENT CARE
Before
- Explain the procedure to the patient.
- Inform the patient that no fasting or other preparation is required.

During
- Collect a venous blood sample in a red-top tube.

After
- Apply pressure or a pressure dressing to the venipuncture site.
- Observe the venipuncture site for bleeding.

TEST RESULTS AND CLINICAL SIGNIFICANCE
▲ Increased Levels
Rheumatoid arthritis,
Other autoimmune disease (e.g., systemic lupus erythematosus, Sjögren syndrome, scleroderma),
Chronic viral infection,
Subacute bacterial endocarditis,
Tuberculosis,
Chronic active hepatitis,
Dermatomyositis,
Infectious mononucleosis,
Leukemia,
Biliary cirrhosis,
Syphilis,
Renal disease: *The pathophysiologic mechanism underlying these observations is not known.*

RELATED TESTS
Anti-DNA Antibody (p. 88), Anti-SS-A, Anti–SS-B, and Anti–SS-C Antibody (p. 107), Anti–Extractable Nuclear Antigen (p. 89), and Antinuclear Antibody (p. 98). These antibodies are also present in some cases of rheumatoid arthritis.

Rubella Antibody (German Measles, Hemagglutination Inhibition [HAI])

NORMAL FINDINGS

Method	Result	Interpretation
Hemagglutination inhibition	<1:8	No immunity to rubella
	>1:20	Immunity to rubella
Latex agglutination	Negative	No immunity to rubella
Enzyme-linked immunosorbent assay (ELISA) immunoglobulin M (IgM)	<0:9 IU/mL	No infection
	>1.1 IU/mL	Active infection
ELISA immunoglobulin G (IgG)	<7 IU/mL	No immunity to rubella
	>10 IU/mL	Immunity to rubella

 Critical Values

Evidence of susceptibility in pregnant women with recent exposure to rubella

INDICATIONS

Screening for rubella antibodies is performed to detect immunity to rubella (the causative agent for German measles). This is important for pregnant women or health care providers working with pregnant women. It is also used to diagnose rubella in newborns, children, and adults.

TEST EXPLANATION

These tests detect the presence of IgG or IgM antibodies, or both, to rubella. Their levels become elevated a few days to a few weeks (depending on the method of testing) after the onset of the rash. IgM tends to disappear after approximately 6 weeks. IgG, however, persists at low but detectable levels for years (Table 2-44).

Levels of these antibodies become elevated in patients with active rubella infection or with past infections. Since 2000, children have received rubella vaccine to prevent the effects of the disease and to minimize infection. Rubella testing documents immunity to rubella. Rubella immunity testing is suggested for all health care providers. Of most importance, however, is that testing is performed to verify the presence or absence of rubella immunity in pregnant women, because congenital rubella infection in the first trimester of pregnancy is associated with congenital abnormalities (heart defects, brain damage, deafness), spontaneous abortion, or stillbirth.

TABLE 2-44	Rubella Antibody Testing

Indication	Antibody
Evaluate immune status	IgG
Identify active infection	IgM or IgG, acute and convalescent
Identify congenital infection	IgM

IgG, Immunoglobulin G; *IgM*, immunoglobulin M.

The acronym *TORCH*—toxoplasmosis, other, rubella, cytomegalovirus, and herpes—is applied to infections with recognized detrimental effects on the fetus. The effects on the fetus may be direct or indirect (e.g., precipitating spontaneous abortion or premature labour). Included in the category of "other" are infections (e.g., syphilis). All tests for infections are discussed separately.

If the woman's titre is greater than 1:10 to 1:20, she is not susceptible to rubella. If the woman's titre is 1:8 or less, she has little or no immunity to rubella. Pregnant women should be strongly advised to stay away from small children, especially those with symptoms of an upper respiratory tract infection (prodromal symptoms of rubella). In addition, all health care providers associated with maternal and child care should be screened for rubella. Immunization, if required, is not performed during pregnancy but should be completed before pregnancy or after delivery in nonimmune women.

A change in the hemagglutination inhibition titre (a measure of IgG and IgM) from the acute phase to the chronic phase in a patient with a rash is the most useful method of demonstrating that the rash is related to a rubella infection. With a rubella rash, diagnosis of rubella is confirmed by obtaining an acute sample (~3 days after the onset of the rash) and a convalescent sample (~2 to 3 weeks later). A fourfold increase in the acute to convalescent titres indicates that the rash was caused by an active rubella infection. Alternatively, in a pregnant woman with a rash suspected to be from rubella, an IgM antibody titre can be measured. If the titre is positive, recent infection has occurred. IgM titres appear 1 to 2 days after onset of the rash and disappear 5 to 6 weeks after infection.

Antirubella antibody testing is also used to diagnose rubella in infants (congenital rubella). Rubella is suspected in infants of low birth weight. Although IgG antibodies can be passed from mother to fetus, IgM antirubella antibodies cannot pass through the placenta. If an infant has IgM antibodies, acute congenital or newborn rubella is suspected. Antibody testing is often used in children with congenital abnormalities that may have resulted from congenital rubella infection. This test is also recommended for anyone with a rash that may be related to rubella.

The hemagglutination inhibition method tests for IgG and IgM. The latex agglutination test detects only IgG and is often used as a simple screen for immunity. ELISA methods for detecting IgG and IgM are now the standard for rubella testing. They are more accurate testing methods, and antibody quantities can be determined.

PROCEDURE AND PATIENT CARE

Before
🖎 Explain the purpose of the test to the patient.

During
• Collect a venous blood sample in a red-top tube.

After
• Apply pressure or a pressure dressing to the venipuncture site.
• Assess the venipuncture site for bleeding.
🖎 Inform the patient when to return for a follow-up hemagglutination inhibition test of the titre, if it is indicated.

TEST RESULTS AND CLINICAL SIGNIFICANCE

Active rubella infection
Previous rubella infection leading to immunity

Rubeola Antibody

NORMAL FINDINGS
Negative

INDICATIONS
This test is used to diagnose rubeola infection (measles). It is currently used more commonly to document immunity to infection by prior vaccination or clinical disease.

TEST EXPLANATION
Rubeola is an RNA paramyxovirus that is known to cause the measles (which is different from German measles; see preceding section on rubella antibody). Upper respiratory symptoms, fever, conjunctivitis, a rash, and Koplik spots on the buccal mucosa are hallmarks of the disease. Since the 1970s, children have been vaccinated to prevent this disease. Although it is usually a self-limiting disease, the virus can easily be spread (by respiratory droplets) to nonimmune pregnant women and cause preterm delivery or spontaneous abortion.

Testing for rubeola includes serologic identification of antibodies to immunoglobulins G and M (IgG and IgM) through indirect immunofluorescence. The presence of IgG represents a previous infection. The presence of IgM indicates an acute infection. A fourfold rise in IgM titre indicates a current infection.

This test is used to diagnose measles in patients with a rash or viral syndrome when the diagnosis cannot be made clinically. Of more importance, however, is that this test is used to establish and document immunity: active (by previous measles infection) or passive (by previous vaccination). Populations commonly tested to document immunity include college students, health care providers, and pregnant women.

PROCEDURE AND PATIENT CARE
Before
🖋 Explain the purpose of the test to the patient.

During
• Collect a venous blood sample in a red-top tube.

After
• Apply pressure to the venipuncture site.
🖋 Inform the patient when to return for a follow-up measurement of rubeola titre, if it is indicated.
🖋 If the results are negative for immunity, recommend immunization. For women of childbearing age, vaccination should precede future pregnancy.

TEST RESULTS AND CLINICAL SIGNIFICANCE
Active rubeola infection: *Affected patients may not have the "classical" clinical signs of measles, and diagnosis can be made with certainty through the identification of IgM antibodies in the patient's serum.*

Previous rubeola infection leading to immunity: *Affected patients have IgG antibodies but not IgM antibodies. They are protected from the disease because of previous active infection or vaccination.*

RELATED TEST

Rubella Antibody (p. 470). This test is used to diagnose German measles and to document immunity to it.

Septin 9 DNA Methylation Assay (Methylated Septra 9, mSEPT9, ColoVantage)

NORMAL FINDINGS

0.0005–50 ng DNA

INDICATIONS

This test is used to screen asymptomatic patients for colorectal cancer. Its use as a screening modality has not been established, but its main benefit may be in the early detection of colorectal cancer in patients who refuse colonoscopy or stool testing.

TEST EXPLANATION

More than half of Canadians aged 50 to 74 years are up to date in their CDC screening (55.2%), which means that almost half are not up to date. This precludes the opportunity for the early detection of an intestinal cancer. Recently a blood test for the detection of methylated DNA from the septin 9 (SEPT9) gene has been developed that, when positive, is very sensitive for the presence of a colorectal cancer. Using real-time methylated PCR, septin can be isolated and quantified from extracted nucleic acid in the plasma. This test has been validated in several clinical studies and shows a strong association between detection of mSEPT9 in blood plasma and the presence of colorectal cancer. Although more expensive than stool for occult blood testing, this real-time PCR laboratory blood test outperforms the stool test without the unpleasantness of a stool collection and may improve compliance for screening for colorectal cancer. Although the SEPT9 methylated DNA test may perform comparably to colonoscopy in detecting CRCs, it lacks the advantage of being potentially able to remove any precancerous polyps, thereby decreasing subsequent risks of cancer. Furthermore, SEPT9 does not perform well for adenoma detection.

A positive test result means that there is an increased likelihood for the presence of a colorectal cancer or polyp. Individuals with positive test results are encouraged to undergo a diagnostic colonoscopy. Not all individuals with colorectal cancer will have a positive test result. Therefore individuals with a negative result should follow usual colorectal cancer screening guidelines.

PROCEDURE AND PATIENT CARE

Before

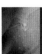 Explain the procedure to the patient.

Tell the patient that no fasting or special preparations are required.

During
- Collect a venous blood sample in a lavender (EDTA) tube.

After
- Apply pressure to the venipuncture site.

TEST RESULTS AND CLINICAL SIGNIFICANCE

▲ Increased Levels

Colorectal cancer,

Colorectal polyps: *Although it is clear that CRC screening reduces mortality by detecting the disease in its earliest stages when it is most effectively treated, only 55.2% of Canadians age 50 to 74 years are up to date in their CDC screening. Reasons for not having a colonoscopy include the time-consuming nature of the procedure and concern about invasiveness. In addition to the challenges of patient compliance with stool testing, such as the requirement for multiple samples and the handling of specimens, the performance of these tests is quite variable. Newer stool-based tests such as the immunochemical FOBT (FIT) have demonstrated sensitivity for adenoma detection.*

RELATED TESTS

Colonoscopy (p. 619). This is an endoscopic study of the entire colon and rectum that is the most effective screening study for the detection of early colorectal cancer.

Stool for Occult Blood (p. 885). Testing the stool for occult blood or DNA is an alternative accurate method of screening for early colorectal cancer.

Apt Test (p. 876). This is a method of identifying blood in newborn stool and differentiating the newborn's from the mother's blood.

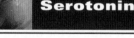

Serotonin (5-Hydroxytryptamine, 5-HT) and Chromogranin A

NORMAL FINDINGS

Chromogranin A ($\leq$225 ng/mL)
Serotonin: : ($\leq$230 ng/mL)

INDICATIONS

This test is used in conjunction with, or as an alternative to, 5-HIAA (p. 961) or serum chromogranin A measurements as a first-line test in the diagnosis of carcinoid syndrome or symptoms such as flushing. It is also used to monitor patients with known or treated carcinoid tumours.

TEST EXPLANATION

Serotonin is synthesized from the essential amino acid tryptophan chiefly in the gastrointestinal enterochromaffin cells (EC-cells). Many different stimuli can release serotonin from EC-cells. After it is secreted, in concert with other gut hormones, serotonin increases GI blood flow, motility, and fluid secretion. On first pass through the liver, 30% to 80% of serotonin is metabolized, predominantly to 5-hydroxyindoleacetic acid (5-HIAA), which is then excreted by the kidneys.

The main diseases that may be associated with measurable increases in serotonin are neuroectodermal tumours, in particular tumours arising from EC-cells. These tumours are collectively referred to as *carcinoids*. They are subdivided into *foregut carcinoids*, arising from respiratory tract, stomach, pancreas, or duodenum (approximately 15% of cases); *midgut carcinoids*, occurring in the jejunum, ileum, or appendix (approximately 70% of cases); and *hindgut carcinoids*, which are found in the colon or rectum (approximately 15% of cases). In patients with more advanced tumours, serotonin is elevated in nearly all patients with midgut tumours, but only in approximately 50% of those with foregut carcinoids, and in no more than 20% of individuals with hindgut tumours. Foregut and hindgut tumours often have low or absent serotonin.

Carcinoids display a spectrum of aggressiveness with no clear distinguishing line between benign and malignant. The majority of carcinoid tumours do not cause significant clinical symptoms. Most symptoms are caused by elevated serotonins (carcinoid syndrome). The carcinoid syndrome consists of flushing, diarrhea, right-sided valvular heart lesions, and bronchoconstriction. The carcinoid syndrome is usually caused by midgut tumours. Because midgut tumours drain into the liver, nearly all of the serotonin is metabolized on first pass. Carcinoid symptoms, therefore, do not usually occur until liver or other distant metastases have developed that bypass the hepatic metabolism.

Diagnosis of carcinoid tumours with symptoms suggestive of carcinoid syndrome rests on measurements of serum serotonin, urinary 5-HIAA (p. 961), and serum chromogranin A (a peptide that is cosecreted alongside serotonin by the neuroectodermal cells). Metastasizing midgut carcinoid tumours usually produce blood or serum serotonin concentrations greater than 1 000 ng/mL. Only a minority of patients with carcinoid tumours will have elevated serotonin blood levels because the liver rapidly metabolizes the serotonin. It is usually impossible to diagnose small carcinoid tumours (>95% of cases) without any symptoms suggestive of carcinoid syndrome by measurement of serotonin, 5-HIAA, or chromogranin A. It is only after carcinoid tumours metastasize that serotonins become detectable because the blood that drains the metastatic carcinoid tumours carries serotonin from the metastatic tumours but does not pass through the liver for metabolism. In most cases, if a person has true carcinoid syndrome symptoms, serotonin levels are significantly elevated. If none of three analytes are elevated, carcinoids can be excluded as a cause of those symptoms.

Disease progression can be monitored in patients with serotonin-producing carcinoid tumours by measurement of serotonin or chromogranin A in the blood. However, at levels greater than approximately 5 000 ng/mL, there is no longer a linear relationship between tumour burden and blood serotonin levels. Urinary 5-HIAA and serum chromogranin A continue to increase in proportion to the tumour burden.

Chromogranin A also acts as a useful diagnostic marker for other neuroendocrine neoplasms, including carcinoids, pheochromocytomas, neuroblastomas, medullary thyroid carcinomas, some pituitary tumours, functioning and nonfunctioning islet-cell tumours, and other amine precursor uptake and decarboxylation (APUD) tumours. It can also serve as a sensitive means for detecting residual or recurrent disease in treated patients. Carcinoid tumours, in particular colon and rectal carcinoids, almost always secrete chromogranin A. Other neuroendocrine tumours, such as small cell carcinoma of the lung or prostate carcinoma, may also display elevated chromogranin A levels.

After being extracted from the serum by reversed-phase solid-phase extraction, serotonin is analyzed using liquid chromatography/tandem mass spectrometry and quantified using a stable isotope-labelled internal standard. Chromogranin A is measured in a homogeneous automated immunofluorescent assay. This assay uses technology based on time-resolved amplified cryptae emission.

INTERFERING FACTORS

- Drugs that may cause *increased* serotonin levels include lithium, MAO-inhibitors, methyldopa, morphine, and reserpine.
- Drugs that may *decrease* serotonin levels include selective serotonin reuptake inhibitors (e.g., fluoxetine).
- Drugs that may cause *increased* chromogranin A levels include proton pump inhibitors (e.g., omeprazole) and should be discontinued 2 weeks before testing.

PROCEDURE AND PATIENT CARE

Before

- Explain the procedure to the patient.
- Tell the patient that no fasting or special preparations are required.

During

- Collect venous blood in a red-top tube and deliver to the laboratory as soon as possible. Because most circulating 5-HT is contained in platelets, the preferred specimens for measurement either include all or most of the platelets (i.e., whole blood and platelet-rich plasma) or consist of serum from completely clotted specimens, a process that releases nearly all 5-HT from platelets.
- Note that testing is usually performed at a reference laboratory.

After

- Apply pressure to the venipuncture site.

TEST EXPLANATION AND CLINICAL SIGNIFICANCE

▲ Increased Levels

Carcinoid tumours,

Neuroendocrine tumours,

Pheochromocytoma,

Small cell lung cancer: *These tumours are associated with increased replication of enterochromaffin cells, which produced these proteins that are then detected in the blood. For primary intestinal carcinoid tumours, elevated levels of these proteins may only occur with metastatic disease.*

RELATED TESTS

5-Hydroxyindoleacetic Acid (p. 961). This urinary test measures the quantity of 5-hydroxyindoleacetic acid, a metabolite of serotonin that is excreted in the urine. Its use is similar to serotonin and chromogranin A.

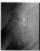

Sickle Cell Screen (Sickle Cell Preparation, Sickledex, Sickle-Cell Hemoglobin [HbS])

NORMAL FINDINGS

Negative

INDICATIONS

This test is used to screen for sickle cell disease or trait.

TEST EXPLANATION

Both sickle cell disease (homozygosity for hemoglobin S [HbS]) and sickle cell trait (heterozygosity for HbS) can be detected by this study. Sickle cell disease results from a genetic homozygous defect and is caused by the presence of HbS instead of hemoglobin A (Figure 2-23). In the United States, 5% to 10% of Black people have sickle cell trait, but fewer than 1% have sickle cell disease.

When HbS becomes deoxygenated, it tends to bend in such a way that the red blood cell (RBC) assumes a sickle shape. These sickled RBCs cannot pass freely through the capillaries, and thus they cause plugging of the microvascular tree. This may compromise the blood supply to various organs. HbS is found in varying quantities (8% to 10%) of the Black population.

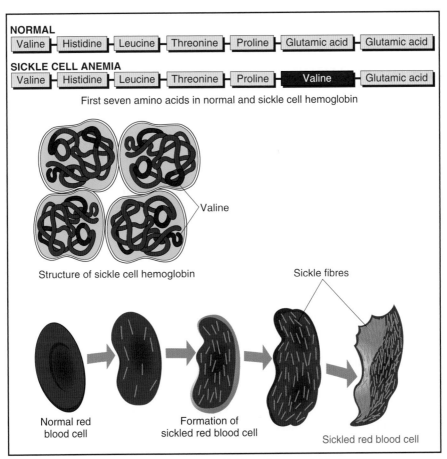

NORMAL

| Valine | Histidine | Leucine | Threonine | Proline | Glutamic acid | Glutamic acid |

SICKLE CELL ANEMIA

| Valine | Histidine | Leucine | Threonine | Proline | Valine | Glutamic acid |

First seven amino acids in normal and sickle cell hemoglobin

Valine

Structure of sickle cell hemoglobin

Sickle fibres

Normal red blood cell   Formation of sickled red blood cell   Sickled red blood cell

Figure 2-23 Sickle cell disease. Sickle cell hemoglobin (HbS) is produced by a recessive allele of the gene encoding the beta chain of hemoglobin. It represents a change in a single amino acid from a glutamic acid to valine at the sixth position in the chain. In the folded beta chain, the sixth position contacts the alpha chain, and the amino acid change causes the hemoglobin to aggregate into long chains, which alters the shape of the cell.

Blood Studies

2

The routine peripheral blood smear of patients with sickle cell disease does not contain sickled RBCs unless hypoxemia is present. In the sickle cell preparation, a deoxygenating agent (e.g., 2% sodium metabisulphite) is added to the patient's blood. If 25% or more of the patient's hemoglobin is of the S variant, the cells assume the crescent (sickle) shape, and the test result is positive. If no sickling occurs, the test result is negative. In the more commonly performed solubility blood tests (e.g., Sickledex), a dithionate is added to the patient's blood. HbS then precipitates out. A negative test result indicates that the patient has no or very little (<10%) HbS. These tests cannot differentiate between sickle cell disease and trait. With sickle cell disease, 80% to 100% of the hemoglobin is the S variant. With the trait, 20% to 40% of the hemoglobin is the S variant. Other less common hemoglobin variants (HbC–Harlem) also may cause sickling.

This test is only a screening test, and its sensitivity varies according to the method used by the laboratory. The definitive diagnosis of sickle cell disease or trait is made by hemoglobin electrophoresis (p. 302) or high-pressure liquid chromatography (p. 304), in which HbS can be identified and quantified. Immunofluorescence methods with monoclonal antibodies are also being used to quantify HbS.

INTERFERING FACTORS

- Any blood transfusions within 3 to 4 months before the sickle cell test may cause false-negative results because the donor's normal Hb may dilute the recipient's abnormal HbS.
- Polycythemia may cause false-negative results.
- Infants less than 3 months of age may have false-negative results, because even infants with sickle cell disease have a significant amount of fetal hemoglobin in their RBCs at that age. Fetal hemoglobin does not cause sickling. After 6 months of age, the HbS variant increases in numbers in these infants. It is then that the test yields positive results.
- Drugs that may cause *false-negative results* include phenothiazines.

PROCEDURE AND PATIENT CARE

Before

- Explain the procedure to the patient or patient's parent or caregiver.
- Inform the patient that no fasting is required.

During

- Collect a venous blood sample in a lavender-top tube.

After

- Apply pressure or a pressure dressing to the venipuncture site.
- Check the venipuncture site for bleeding.
- If the test result is positive, hemoglobin electrophoresis should be performed.
- If the test result is positive, offer the family genetic counselling. A patient with one recessive gene (heterozygous) is said to have sickle cell trait. A patient with two recessive genes (homozygous) has sickle cell disease.
- Inform patients with sickle cell disease that they should avoid situations in which hypoxia may occur (e.g., strenuous exercise, air travel in unpressurized aircraft, travel to high-altitude regions).

TEST RESULTS AND CLINICAL SIGNIFICANCE

▲ Increased Levels

Sickle cell trait,

Sickle cell disease: *In these clinical situations, more than 25% of the hemoglobin is the S variant. Sickling then occurs.*

RELATED TEST

Hemoglobin Electrophoresis (p. 302). This test can identify and measure HbS. Sickle cell disease can be differentiated from the trait.

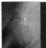

Sodium, Blood (Na)

NORMAL FINDINGS

Adult/older adult: **136–145 mmol/L** (136–145 mEq/L)
Child: **136–145 mmol/L** (136–145 mEq/L)
Infant: **134–150 mmol/L** (134–150 mEq/L)
Newborn: **134–144 mmol/L** (134–144 mEq/L)

 Critical Values

<**120 mmol/L** (<120 mEq/L) or >**160 mmol/L** (>160 mEq/L)

INDICATIONS

This test is a part of the routine laboratory evaluation of most patients. It is one of the tests automatically performed when measurement of "serum electrolytes" is requested. This test is used to evaluate and monitor fluid balance, electrolyte balance, and therapy.

TEST EXPLANATION

Sodium is the major cation in the extracellular space, in which serum levels are approximately 140 mmol/L (140 mEq/L). The concentration of sodium intracellularly is only 5 mEq/L. Therefore, sodium is a major determinant of extracellular osmolality. The sodium content in the blood is a result of a balance between dietary sodium intake and renal excretion. Nonrenal sodium losses (e.g., sweat) normally are minimal.

Many factors regulate sodium balance. Aldosterone causes conservation of sodium by stimulating the kidneys to reabsorb sodium and by decreasing renal losses. Natriuretic hormone, or third factor, is stimulated by increased sodium levels. This hormone decreases renal absorption and increases renal losses of sodium. Antidiuretic hormone (ADH; also called *vasopressin*), which controls the reabsorption of water at the distal tubules of the kidney, affects sodium serum levels by dilution or concentration.

Physiologically, water and sodium are closely interrelated. As free body water is increased, serum sodium is diluted, and the concentration may decrease. The kidneys compensate by conserving sodium and excreting water. If free body water were to decrease, the serum sodium concentration would rise; the kidneys would then respond by conserving free water. Aldosterone,

ADH, and natriuretic hormone all assist in these compensatory actions of the kidneys to maintain appropriate levels of free water.

The average sodium intake needed to maintain sodium balance for adults is 1 300 mg per day. Symptoms of *hyponatremia* may begin when sodium levels are below **125 mmol/L** (<125 mEq/L). The first symptom is weakness. When sodium levels fall below **115 mmol/L** (<115 mEq/L), confusion and lethargy occur and may progress to stupor and coma if levels continue to decline. Symptoms of *hypernatremia* include dry mucous membranes, thirst, agitation, restlessness, hyper-reflexia, mania, and convulsions.

INTERFERING FACTORS

- Recent trauma, surgery, or shock may cause increases in sodium levels because renal blood flow is decreased. Renin and angiotensin (see p. 460) stimulate the secretion of aldosterone, which stimulates increased renal absorption of sodium.
- Drugs that may cause *increases* in sodium levels include anabolic steroids, antibiotics, carbenicillin, clonidine, corticosteroids, cough medicines, estrogens, laxatives, methyldopa, and oral contraceptives.
- Drugs that may cause *decreases* in sodium levels include angiotensin-converting enzyme (ACE) inhibitors, captopril, carbamazepine, diuretics, haloperidol, heparin, nonsteroidal anti-inflammatory drugs, sodium-free intravenous fluids, sulphonylureas, triamterene, tricyclic antidepressants, and vasopressin.

PROCEDURE AND PATIENT CARE

Before
- Explain the procedure to the patient.
- Inform the patient that no food or fluid restrictions are necessary.

During
- Collect a venous blood sample in a red-top or green-top tube.
- If the patient is receiving an intravenous infusion, obtain the blood from the opposite arm.

After
- Apply pressure or a pressure dressing to the venipuncture site.
- Assess the venipuncture site for bleeding.

TEST RESULTS AND CLINICAL SIGNIFICANCE

▲ Increased Levels (Hypernatremia)

Increased Sodium Intake

Increased dietary intake: *If sodium (usually in the form of dietary salt) is ingested at high quantities without adequate free water, hypernatremia occurs.*

Excessive sodium in intravenous fluids: *The normal kidneys can excrete approximately 450 to 500 mmol (450 to 500 mEq) of sodium per day. If intake of sodium exceeds that amount in a patient without ongoing sodium losses or a prior sodium deficit, sodium levels can be expected to rise.*

Decreased Sodium Loss

Cushing's syndrome: *Corticosteroids have an aldosterone-like effect. See descriptions of Addison's disease in the section on adrenocorticotropic hormone (p. 34).*

Hyperaldosteronism: *Aldosterone stimulates the kidneys to absorb sodium at the level of the renal tubule.*

Excessive Free Body Water Loss

Gastrointestinal loss (without rehydration): *If free water is lost, residual sodium becomes more concentrated.*

Excessive sweating: *Although sweat does contain some sodium, most is free water. This causes the serum sodium to become more concentrated. If the water loss is replaced without any sodium, sodium dilution and hyponatremia can occur.*

Extensive thermal burns: *If the burn is extensive, serum and a great amount of free water are lost through the open wounds. Sodium becomes more concentrated. As fluid is replaced and the body physiologically responds by stimulating ADH, sodium can be diluted, and hyponatremia may occur.*

Diabetes insipidus: *The deficiency of ADH and the inability of the kidney to respond to ADH cause large free water losses. Sodium becomes concentrated.*

Osmotic diuresis: *With osmotic diuresis (excluding hyperglycemia; see descriptions of hyperglycemia in the following test section), water may be lost at a rate that exceeds sodium loss. In those situations, sodium levels increase as a result of greater concentration. If, however, free water is therapeutically provided, sodium levels may become dilute, and hyponatremia may occur.*

▼ Decreased Levels (Hyponatremia)

Decreased Sodium Intake

Deficient dietary intake: *Sodium intestinal absorption is highly efficient. Sodium deficiency is rare.*

Deficient sodium in intravenous fluids: *If intravenous fluid replacement provides sodium at a level less than minimal physiologic losses or less than ongoing losses, residual sodium becomes diluted.*

Increased Sodium Loss

Addison's disease: *Aldosterone and corticosteroid hormone levels are inadequate. Sodium is not reabsorbed by the kidneys and is lost in the urine.*

Diarrhea, vomiting, or nasogastric aspiration: *Sodium in the gastrointestinal contents is lost with the fluid. Hyponatremia is magnified if intravenous fluid replacement does not contain adequate amounts of sodium.*

Intraluminal bowel loss (ileus, mechanical obstruction): *Great amounts of extracellular fluid are forced into the lumen of the dilated bowel. This fluid contains sodium. Hyponatremia is magnified if intravenous fluid replacement does not contain adequate amounts of sodium.*

Diuretic administration: *Many diuretics work by inhibiting sodium reabsorption by the kidney. Sodium levels can diminish.*

Chronic renal insufficiency: *The kidneys lose their reabsorptive capabilities. Large quantities of sodium are lost in the urine.*

Large-volume aspiration of pleural or peritoneal fluid: *Sodium concentration in these fluids is the same as serum concentration. The aspiration of these fluids is compensated by secretion of ADH, which acts to increase renal absorption of free water. Sodium becomes diluted.*

Increased Free Body Water

Excessive oral water intake: *Psychogenic polydipsia can dilute sodium.*

Hyperglycemia: *High levels of glucose in the blood can result in an osmotic effect in which the glucose pulls free water from the extracellular space and thus dilutes sodium. Also with hyperglycemia, sodium ketotic salts are lost in the urine. Sodium levels diminish further.*

Excessive intravenous water intake: *When intravenous therapy provides less sodium than maintenance and ongoing losses, sodium is diluted. If sodium-free intravenous therapy is given to a patient who has a significant sodium deficit, sodium dilution occurs with rehydration.*

Heart failure,

Peripheral edema: *These conditions are associated with increased free water retention. Sodium is diluted.*

Ascites,

Peripheral edema,

Pleural effusion,

Intraluminal bowel loss (ileus or mechanical obstruction): *These conditions are associated with third-space losses of sodium.*

Syndrome of inappropriate or ectopic secretion of ADH: *Oversecretion of ADH stimulates the kidneys to reabsorb free water. Sodium is diluted.*

RELATED TESTS

Sodium, Urine (p. 980). This measurement of sodium in the urine is helpful in assessing sodium and water balance.

Aldosterone (p. 48). More than any other hormone, aldosterone has a significant effect on sodium blood levels.

Antidiuretic Hormone (p. 83). By affecting free body water excretion, sodium levels become diluted or concentrated.

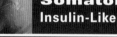

Somatomedin C (Insulin-Like Growth Factor 1 [IGF-1], Insulin-Like Growth Factor Binding Proteins [IGF BP])

NORMAL FINDINGS

Adult: **5.5–14.4 nmol/L** (42–110 ng/mL)
Child:

Age (Years)	Female, nmol/L (ng/mL)	Male, nmol/L (ng/mL)
1–3	**1.6–17.5** (12–135)	**2.2–15** (17–116)
4–6	**1.7–22.8** (13–176)	**2.7–20.8** (21–160)
7–9	**6.9–32.9** (53–253)	**8.4–26.9** (65–207)
10–12	**9.8–46.3** (75–357)	**9.0–25.4** (69–196)
13–15	**8.6–44.7** (66–344)	**10.4–52.5** (80–404)
16–18	**12.8–47.3** (99–364)	**12.5–49.7** (96–383)

INDICATIONS

Somatomedin C is a screening test to identify patients with growth hormone deficiency, pituitary insufficiency, and acromegaly. These levels depend on the levels of growth hormone.

TEST EXPLANATION

Growth hormone, or somatotropin, is secreted by the acidophil cells in the anterior pituitary gland and plays a central role in modulating growth from birth until the end of puberty. Growth hormone is secreted through an elaborate feedback mechanism. The hypothalamus secretes growth hormone–releasing hormone, which stimulates growth hormone release from the pituitary gland. Growth hormone exerts its effects on many tissues through a group of peptides called *somatomedins*. The most commonly tested somatomedin is somatomedin C, which is produced by the liver and has its major effect on cartilage. High levels of somatomedins stimulate the production of somatostatin from the hypothalamus. Somatostatin inhibits further secretion of growth hormone from the pituitary gland.

Growth hormone is secreted during sleep, and secretion is stimulated by exercise and ingestion of protein and in response to hypoglycemia. As a result of these and other factors that can cause great variation in growth hormone secretion, normal and abnormal results of random growth hormone assays may overlap significantly. To diminish the common variations in growth hormone secretion, screening for insulin-like growth factor 1 (IGF-1) or somatomedin C provides a more accurate reflection of the mean plasma concentration of growth hormone. IGF-1 is particularly helpful in the evaluation of acromegaly. Virtually no patient with a normal IGF-1 level has acromegaly. IGF-1 is not helpful in evaluating patients with growth hormone deficiency because levels are affected by nutritional status, liver and thyroid function, and age. These proteins are not affected by the time of day or food intake as is growth hormone, because they circulate bound to proteins that are durable and long lasting. As a result, there is no overlap between normal and abnormal results of somatomedin C testing.

Somatomedin C is produced by the liver. Values in girls and women are higher than in boys and men (by approximately 15%). Values are also higher in children than in adults. Normally there is a large increase during the pubertal growth spurt.

Levels of somatomedin C depend on levels of growth hormone. As a result, somatomedin levels are low when growth hormone levels are deficient. (See discussion of growth hormone for causes of and diseases associated with growth hormone deficiency.) Nonpituitary causes of reduced somatomedin C include malnutrition, severe chronic illnesses, severe liver disease, hypothyroidism, and Laron-type dwarfism. The test method used is radioimmunoassay, immunochemiluminometric assay, or radioreceptor assay.

When somatomedin C levels are abnormally low, a growth stimulation test must demonstrate abnormally reduced or absent growth hormone in order to confirm the diagnosis of growth hormone deficiency. The causes of short stature and the initial tests for patients with short stature are listed in Box 2-13 and Table 2-45, respectively.

BOX 2-13   Causes of Short Stature

- Growth hormone deficiency
- Gonadal dysgenesis
- Russell-Silver dwarfism
- Hypothyroidism
- Pseudohypoparathyroidism
- Laron-type dwarfism
- Cushing's syndrome
- Bone/cartilage dysplasia
- Idiopathic causes

TABLE 2-45	Initial Tests for Patients With Short Stature
Test	**Reason for Test**
Thyroxine	Rule out hypothyroidism
Somatomedin C	Rule out GH deficiency
GH	Rule out GH deficiency
GH stimulation	Rule out GH deficiency
Radiographs of wrists	Document growth retardation
Calcium (serum levels)	Rule out pseudohypoparathyroidism
Phosphate (serum levels)	Rule out rickets
Bicarbonate (serum levels)	Rule out renal tubular acidosis
Blood urea nitrogen (BUN)	Rule out renal failure
Complete blood cell count	Rule out anemia or nutritional or chronic disorders
Erythrocyte sedimentation rate	Rule out inflammatory bowel diseases
Chromosomal karyotype	Rule out chromosomal abnormalities (gonadal dysgenesis)

GH, Growth hormone.

INTERFERING FACTORS

- A radioactive scan performed a week before the test may affect test results because somatomedin C is often measured by radioimmunoassay. Results may be confounded by the prior administration of radioisotopes.
- Estrogens may cause decreases in somatomedin C levels.

PROCEDURE AND PATIENT CARE

Before

- Explain the procedure to the patient.
- Inform the patient that an overnight fast before the test is preferred unless otherwise ordered by physician.

During

- Collect a venous blood sample in a red-top tube.

After

- Apply pressure or a pressure dressing to the venipuncture site.
- Assess the venipuncture site for bleeding.

TEST RESULTS AND CLINICAL SIGNIFICANCE

▲ Increased Levels

Gigantism,
Acromegaly: *These two syndromes are caused by excess growth hormone levels, which increase somatomedin C level.*
Stress,
Major surgery,
Hypoglycemia,

Starvation,

Deep-sleep state,

Exercise: *These conditions stimulate growth hormone secretion, which increases somatomedin C levels.*

Hypoglycemia: *Hypoglycemia stimulates growth hormone, which stimulates somatomedin C production.*

▼ Decreased Levels

Growth hormone deficiency: *Somatomedin C production is dependent on growth hormone levels.*

Pituitary insufficiency: *Growth hormone is produced in the pituitary gland. Diseases, tumours, ischemia, and trauma to the pituitary or hypothalamus cause growth hormone deficiency. Somatomedin C production is dependent on growth hormone levels.*

Dwarfism: *This is a result of deficiencies in growth hormone and somatomedin C in children.*

Laron-type dwarfism: *This syndrome is associated with growth hormone receptor resistance. Somatomedin C secretion does not occur.*

Hyperglycemia: *Elevated glucose levels inhibit growth hormone and somatomedin C secretion.*

Failure to thrive: *This is a result of deficiencies in growth hormone and somatomedin C in infants.*

Delayed sexual maturity: *This is a result of deficiencies in growth hormone and somatomedin C in adolescents.*

Malnutrition,

Malabsorption,

Anorexia nervosa: *These diseases lead to hypoproteinemia. Because somatomedin C is a protein, levels are reduced with hypoproteinemia.*

Severe liver disease: *Somatomedin C is made in the liver. With severe liver disease, somatomedin levels fall.*

Hypothyroidism: *Somatomedin C levels fall in hypothyroid patients.*

RELATED TESTS

Growth Hormone Stimulation (p. 287). This is a test designed to stimulate the secretion of growth hormone. It is required to accurately make the diagnosis of growth hormone deficiency.

Growth Hormone (p. 284). This is a direct quantitative assay for growth hormone.

Squamous Cell Carcinoma Antigen (SCC Antigen)

NORMAL FINDINGS

≤2.2 ng/mL

INDICATIONS

This test is used to determine the stage and prognosis of squamous cell carcinomas. It is also used to monitor the treatment of carcinomas and a variety of nonmalignant conditions.

TEST EXPLANATION

Squamous cell carcinoma (SCC) antigen is a glycoprotein that is expressed in normal epithelium and epithelial tissues. Although the neutral forms of SCC normally remain inside the cell, acidic SCC antigen is released and often elevated in patients who have squamous cell carcinomas or other nonmalignant squamous cell lesions. It can occur in several cancers (e.g., uterine, cervical, oral cavity, esophageal, lung, anal canal, skin). SCC antigen may be involved in the malignant behaviour of squamous cell cancers. Consequently, serum concentrations of SCC antigen can be used to monitor various SCCs after surgical removal. Concentrations that remain persistently elevated or begin to increase following tumour removal suggest persistent or recurrent disease. There may be an association between serum SCC antigen concentrations and tumour stage, size, and tumour aggressiveness.

A variety of nonmalignant benign diseases of the skin (e.g., eczema, erythrodermic epidermitis, pemphigus, and psoriasis), lungs (e.g., TB, adult respiratory distress syndrome, sarcoidosis, presence of pleural effusion), and other common conditions may result in increased serum concentrations of SCC antigen. Thus SCC antigen results alone should not be interpreted as evidence of the presence or absence of malignant disease.

PROCEDURE AND PATIENT CARE

Before

- Explain the procedure to the patient.
- Tell the patient that no fasting is required.

During

- Collect a venous blood sample in a red-top tube.
- The blood sample may be sent to a central diagnostic laboratory and results may not be available for 7 to 10 days.

After

- Apply pressure or a pressure dressing to the venipuncture site.

TEST RESULTS AND CLINICAL SIGNIFICANCES

▲ Increased Values

Squamous cell carcinoma: *Cancers of the cervix, head, neck, esophagus, lung, anus, and skin are associated with increased SSC antigen.*
Dermatitis,
Pulmonary disease: *Benign diseases are associated with increased levels of SSC antigen, but to a lesser extent than squamous cell carcinoma.*

RELATED TEST

Carcinoembryonic Antigen (p. 159). This is a tumour marker used in evaluating several cancers.

Syphilis Detection (Serologic Test for Syphilis [STS], Venereal Disease Research Laboratory [VDRL], Rapid Plasma Reagin [RPR], Fluorescent Treponemal Antibody [FTA])

NORMAL FINDINGS

Negative or nonreactive

INDICATIONS

These serologic tests are used to diagnose and to document successful therapy of syphilis.

TEST EXPLANATION

Syphilis is caused by the spirochete *Treponema pallidum*. The disease is divided into four stages: acute, secondary, latent, and tertiary. The acute stage is marked by the development of a chancre on the skin near the infection (usually the genitalia). The chancre develops approximately 3 to 6 weeks after inoculation and lasts for approximately 4 to 6 weeks. The secondary stage is highlighted by a rash (often on the soles and palms) and generalized lymphadenopathy. This stage lasts for approximately 3 months. The latent stage represents a period of disease inactivity and can last for 5 years. Some patients are cured of the infection during this stage. Many go into the tertiary stage marked by central nervous system, cardiovascular, and ocular signs and symptoms.

The immunologic tests for syphilis detect antibodies to *T. pallidum*. Two groups of antibodies are sought. The first group of tests detects the presence of a nontreponemal antibody called *reagin*, which reacts to phospholipids in the body (which are probably similar to lipids in the membrane of *T. pallidum*). The second group of tests detects antibodies directed against the *Treponema* organism itself. The nontreponemal antibody tests are grouped as serologic screening tests for syphilis and are relatively nonspecific. These antibodies are most often detected by the Wassermann test or the Venereal Disease Research Laboratory (VDRL) test. A more sensitive nontreponemal test is the rapid plasma reagin (RPR) test. The VDRL and RPR tests, by virtue of their testing for a nonspecific antibody, have high false-positive (or cross-reactive) rates. The VDRL test yields positive results approximately 2 weeks after the patient's inoculation with *T. pallidum* and returns to normal after adequate treatment. The test result is positive in nearly all primary and secondary stages of syphilis and in two-thirds of patients with tertiary syphilis.

If the VDRL or RPR test result is positive, the diagnosis must be confirmed by the more specific *Treponema* test, such as the fluorescent treponemal antibody absorption test (FTA-ABS). This test, which reacts to a specific treponemal antibody, is more accurate than the VDRL and RPR tests and yields positive results approximately 4 to 6 weeks after inoculation. To improve its specificity, non–*T. pallidum* antibodies are absorbed out of the patient's serum before the serum is added to the *T. pallidum*–impregnated slide. Anti–gamma-globulin antibodies that are fluorescent are then added to the slide. If anti–*T. pallidum* antibodies exist in the patient's serum, they react to the *T. pallidum* on the slide, and the fluorescent anti–gamma-globulin antibodies that were subsequently added attach to the patient's serum antibody–*T. palladium* complex and make it visible under the fluorescent microscope. The FTA-ABS test is required before the syphilis can be diagnosed with certainty. A microhemagglutination test is also available and is comparable in accuracy with the "standard criterion" FTA-ABS test. Enzyme-linked immunosorbent assay (ELISA) methods are also available for serologic testing for syphilis.

BOX 2-14   **Causes of False-Positive Results of the VDRL and RPR Tests**

- Malaria
- Typhus
- Leptospirosis
- Cat-scratch fever
- Leprosy
- Hepatitis
- Mononucleosis
- Periarteritis nodosa
- Systemic lupus erythematosus
- Acute viral or bacterial infections
- Lymphogranuloma venereum
- Hypersensitivity reactions
- Mycoplasmal pneumonia
- Recent vaccinations

RPR, Rapid plasma reagin; *VDRL,* Venereal Disease Research Laboratory.

If the VDRL or RPR test result is positive and the FTA-ABS result is negative, other diseases that can cause positive results on screening serologic syphilis tests must be sought (Box 2-14).

Screening for syphilis is usually performed during the first prenatal checkup of pregnant women with the VDRL test. Syphilis, if untreated, may cause spontaneous abortion, stillbirth, or premature labour. The effect on the fetus can be CNS damage, hearing loss, or death. In patients who have symptoms compatible with primary syphilis, an FTA-ABS test is recommended. Congenital syphilis is difficult to distinguish from the passive immunity provided by a mother who has syphilis. However, in congenital syphilis, the FTA-ABS result of the infant is usually much higher than the mother's. The acronym *TORCH*—toxoplasmosis, other, rubella, cytomegalovirus, and herpes—has been applied to infections with recognized detrimental effects on the fetus. The effects on the fetus may be direct or indirect (e.g., precipitating spontaneous abortion, premature labour). Included in the category of "other" are infections (e.g., syphilis). All tests for infections are discussed separately.

In general, serologic test results return to normal after successful treatment for syphilis. The earlier the disease is treated, the sooner those results return to normal. In the early primary stage, the serologic test results may become negative in 2 to 4 months after successful antibiotic treatment. It may take longer than 1 year for the patient's status to convert to seronegative when later stages of the disease are treated. When treatment is begun in the tertiary stage, the patient's status may never convert to seronegative. Testing should be performed routinely to document successful therapy.

INTERFERING FACTORS

- Excessive hemolysis and gross lipemia may cause false-positive results of the serologic test for syphilis (STS).
- Excess chyle in the blood may cause false-positive STS test results. Testing should be performed after at least an 8-hour fast.
- Recent ingestion of alcohol may cause false-positive STS test results. Alcohol should be avoided for 24 hours before the test.

- Many conditions cause false-positive results when VDRL and RPR tests are used (see Box 2-14).
- If the patient is tested too soon after inoculation and before antibodies have developed, the test results may be artificially negative. The test should be repeated in 2 months, or the patient should be treated despite the negative test results, if clinical suspicion is high.

> ### Clinical Priorities
>
> - If the patient is tested too soon after inoculation and before antibodies have developed, the tests may be artificially negative.
> - Because the FTA-ABS test is for a specific treponemal antibody, it is more accurate than the VDRL and RPR tests. The FTA-ABS test result becomes positive approximately 4 to 6 weeks after inoculation.
> - Screening for syphilis is usually performed during the first prenatal checkup of pregnant women with the VDRL test.

PROCEDURE AND PATIENT CARE

Before
- Explain the procedure to the patient.
- Check with the laboratory regarding food and alcohol fasting requirements, and advise the patient accordingly.

During
- Collect a venous blood sample in a red-top tube.

After
- Apply pressure or a pressure dressing to the venipuncture site.
- Check the venipuncture site for bleeding.
- If the test result is positive, instruct the patient to inform recent sexual contacts so they can be evaluated.
- If the test result is positive, ensure that the patient receives the appropriate antibiotic therapy.
- If a screening serologic test result is positive, a more specific antitreponemal test is necessary to confirm the diagnosis.

TEST RESULTS AND CLINICAL SIGNIFICANCE

Positive Results
Syphilis

Testosterone (Total Testosterone Serum Level)

NORMAL FINDINGS

Free testosterone:
  Male: 9.5–30 nmol/L (275–875 ng/dL)

Female: **0.8–2.6 nmol/L** (23–875 ng/dL)
Percentage of total testosterone:
Male: 1.0%–2.7%
Female: 0.5%–1.8%
Total testosterone:

Age	Male, nmol/L (ng/dL)	Female, nmol/L (ng/dL)
7 mo to 9.8 yr (Tanner Stage I)	**<0.1–0.4** (<3–10)	**<0.1–0.4** (<3–10)
9.8–14.5 yr (Tanner Stage II)	**0.6–5.3** (18–150)	**0.3–1.0** (7–28)
10.7–15.4 yr (Tanner Stage III)	**3.5–11.2** (100–320)	**0.5–1.2** (15–35)
11.8–16.2 yr (Tanner Stage IV)	**7.0–21.7** (200–620)	**0.5–1.1** (13–32)
12.8–17.3 yr (Tanner Stage V)	**12.3–34.0** (350–970)	**0.7–1.3** (20–38)
20 yr and older	**9.75–38.0** (280–1 080)	**0.52–2.43** (<70)

INDICATIONS

Testosterone levels are used to evaluate ambiguous sex characteristics, precocious puberty, virilizing syndromes in girls and women, and infertility in men. This test can also be used as a tumour marker for rare tumours of the ovary and testicle.

TEST EXPLANATION

Androgens include dehydroepiandrosterone (DHEA), androstenedione, and testosterone. The adrenal glands produce DHEA in the process of making cortisol and aldosterone. DHEA is also produced de novo by the testes or the ovaries. DHEA is the precursor of androstenedione, which is the precursor of testosterone (and estrogen).

Testosterone levels vary by stage of maturity (indicated by Tanner stage). Serum concentrations of testosterone in both sexes during the first week of life average approximately **1.0 nmol/L** (25 ng/dL). In male infants, values increase sharply in the second week to a maximum mean ~**5.3 nmol/L** (~175 ng/dL) at approximately 2 months, which lasts until approximately 6 months of age. In female infants, values decrease in the first week and remain low throughout early childhood. Levels increase during puberty to adult values.

In boys and men, most of the testosterone is made by the Leydig cells in the testicles; this accounts for 95% of the circulating testosterone in men. In girls and women, approximately half of the testosterone is made by the conversion of DHEA to testosterone in the peripheral fat tissue. Another 30% is made by the same conversion of DHEA in the adrenal gland, and 20% is made directly by the ovaries.

Approximately 60% of circulating testosterone binds strongly to sex hormone–binding globulin, which is also called *testosterone-binding globulin.* Most of the remaining testosterone is bound loosely to albumin, and approximately 2% is free or unbound. The unbound portion is the active component. In most assays for testosterone, measurements are of the total testosterone (i.e., bound and unbound portions). The free testosterone can be measured in conditions in which the testosterone-binding proteins may be altered (obesity, cirrhosis, thyroid disorders). Free testosterone is estimated in this test by an indirect method: equilibrium ultrafiltration. It can be reported as a percentage of total testosterone or as an absolute number.

Boys and men have a biofeedback mechanism that starts in the hypothalamus. Gonadotropin-releasing hormone (GnRH) induces the pituitary to produce luteinizing hormone (called *interstitial cell–stimulating hormone* in boys and men) and follicle-stimulating hormone (FSH). Luteinizing hormone stimulates the Leydig cells to produce testosterone. FSH stimulates the Sertoli cells to produce sperm. Testosterone then acts to inhibit further secretion of GnRH.

Physiologically, testosterone stimulates spermatogenesis and influences the development of male secondary sexual characteristics. Overproduction of this hormone in young boys may cause precocious puberty. Such overproduction can be caused by testicular, adrenal, or pituitary tumours. Overproduction of this hormone in girls and women causes masculinization, which is manifested as amenorrhea and excessive growth of body hair (hirsutism). Ovarian and adrenal tumours/hyperplasia and medications (e.g., danazol) are all potential causes of masculinization in girls and women. Reduced levels of testosterone in men suggest hypogonadism or Klinefelter's syndrome.

Several testosterone stimulation tests can be performed to more accurately evaluate hypogonadism. Human chorionic gonadotropin, clomiphene, and GnRH can be used to stimulate testosterone secretion.

Methods used for the measurement of testosterone include radioimmunoassay and extraction chromatography. There is a slight diurnal variation in the secretion of testosterone. Levels are maximal at approximately 7 AM and minimal at approximately 8 PM.

INTERFERING FACTORS

- Drugs that may cause *increases* in testosterone levels include alcohol, anticonvulsants, barbiturates, estrogens, and oral contraceptives.
- Drugs that may cause *decreases* in testosterone levels include alcohol, androgens, dexamethasone, diethylstilbestrol, digoxin, ketoconazole, phenothiazine, spironolactone, and steroids.

PROCEDURE AND PATIENT CARE

Before
- Explain the procedure to the patient.
- Inform the patient that no fasting is required.
- Because testosterone levels are highest in the early morning hours, blood should be collected in the morning.

During
- Collect a venous blood sample in a red-top tube.

After
- Apply pressure or a pressure dressing to the venipuncture site.
- Assess the venipuncture site for bleeding.

TEST RESULTS AND CLINICAL SIGNIFICANCE

▲ Increased Levels (Male)

Idiopathic sexual precocity: *This is usually because of oversecretion of luteinizing hormone, which stimulates the testicles to produce testosterone.*

Pinealoma: *This is a hypothalamic tumour that produces an increased quantity of GnRH, which stimulates the pituitary gland to produce luteinizing hormone, which in turn stimulates the testicles to produce testosterone.*

Encephalitis: *This viral infection of the CNS can stimulate the hypothalamus to produce an increased quantity of GnRH, which stimulates the pituitary gland to produce luteinizing hormone, which in turn stimulates the testicles to produce testosterone.*

Congenital adrenal hyperplasia: *An enzyme deficiency in the production of cortisol causes an accumulation of large amounts of DHEA. DHEA is a precursor of androstenedione, which is a precursor of testosterone.*

Adrenocortical tumour: *Neoplasm involving the adrenal gland can cause the gland to produce large amounts of testosterone or DHEA. DHEA is a precursor of androstenedione, which is a precursor of testosterone.*

Testicular or extragonadal tumour: *Leydig cell tumours can produce testosterone, which can cause precocious puberty in boys. However, no spermatogenesis occurs because production of gonadotropin hormones does not occur and is, in fact, inhibited.*

Hyperthyroidism: *Affected patients have elevated levels of bound testosterone because of elevated levels of sex hormone–binding globulin proteins. This causes elevation of the total testosterone levels.*

Testosterone resistance syndromes: *Affected patients resist the effect of testosterone on tissue. In response, higher levels of testosterone are secreted.*

▼ Decreased Levels (Male)

Klinefelter's syndrome: *Affected patients have an extra X chromosome (XXY). This syndrome is associated with primary testicular failure.*

Cryptorchidism: *These patients usually have normal testosterone levels, but on occasion, testicles that fail to descend into the scrotum can be atrophic.*

Primary and secondary hypogonadism: *Infection, tumour, and congenital abnormalities are all possible causes of primary (testicular) or secondary (pituitary) failure.*

Trisomy 21: *The pathophysiologic processes of this genetic defect are not defined.*

Orchiectomy: *Both testicles must have been removed. Surgical removal of just one testicle does not cause deficiency in testosterone levels.*

Hepatic cirrhosis: *Affected patients have reduced protein levels and therefore have reduced amounts of bound testosterone, which makes up most of the total testosterone that is measured.*

▲ Increased Levels (Female)

Ovarian tumour: *Arrhenoblastoma is an uncommon ovarian tumour that can produce testosterone.*

Adrenal tumour: *Neoplasms involving the adrenal gland can cause the gland to produce large amounts of testosterone or DHEA. DHEA is a precursor of androstenedione, which is a precursor of testosterone. Hirsutism in girls and women is common with these tumours.*

Congenital adrenocortical hyperplasia: *An enzyme deficiency in the production of cortisol causes an accumulation of large amounts of DHEA. DHEA is a precursor of androstenedione, which is a precursor of testosterone. In girls, this can result in pseudohermaphroditism (ambiguous genitalia).*

Trophoblastic tumour: *These tumours (hydatidiform mole, choriocarcinoma) produce human chorionic gonadotropin, which can stimulate the production of testosterone.*

Polycystic ovaries: *This syndrome is associated with obesity, hirsutism, and amenorrhea. Affected patients have increased testosterone levels. The pathophysiologic process is not well defined.*

Idiopathic hirsutism: *The pathophysiologic mechanism underlying this observation is not known.*

RELATED TEST

Androstenediones (p. 69). Androstenedione testing is used in the diagnosis of virilizing syndromes, especially in girls.

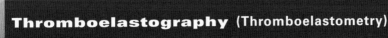

Thromboelastography (Thromboelastometry)

NORMAL FINDINGS

5.3–12.4 dynes/cm^2

 Critical Values

>12.4 dynes/cm^2

INDICATIONS

This test is performed to evaluate the coagulation system. It is used to do the following:
- Identify potential hypercoagulable states
- Identify potential accelerated fibrinolysis
- Assess platelet and coagulating factor function

TEST EXPLANATION

Hemostasis is a well-regulated process in which the blood forms localized clots when the integrity of the vascular system is breached. Trauma, infection, and inflammation all activate the blood's clotting system, which depends on the interaction of two separate systems: enzymatic proteins (clotting factors, intrinsic and extrinsic systems) and platelets. The two systems work in concert to plug defects in the broken vessels. The clots that form in this process need to be of sufficient strength to resist dislodgement. If a particular clotting factor is dysfunctional or absent, as in hemophilia, an insufficient amount of fibrin forms. Similarly, massive consumption of clotting factors in a trauma situation decreases the amount of fibrin formed. Inadequate numbers of platelets resulting from trauma, surgery, or chemotherapy also decrease platelet aggregation, as do genetic disorders, uremia, or medication therapy. Ultimately, reduced fibrin formation or platelet aggregation results in clots of inadequate tensile strength. This hypocoagulable state is associated with excessive bleeding. Conversely endothelial injury, stasis, cancer, genetic diseases, or other hypercoagulable states lead to thrombosis formation causing thromboembolic events.

In this test whole blood is rapidly transferred to a cuvette. Clot-activating catalysts may be added to speed up the process. The cuvette is rotated as a clot forms in a machine. The fibrin in the clot creates fluid resistance that is determined by a sensor transducer (also placed within the cuvette) that converts the tensile strength of the clot to an electronic signal displayed on a graph. Thrombosis time and lysis time can be calculated and is reported as a coagulation index. This test is able to represent all global analysis of the hemostatic function from initial thrombin generation to clot lysis. When plotted on a graph, specific patterns can be identified, including normal, hemophilia, thrombocytopenia, decreased platelet function, increased fibrinolysis, and hypercoagulation.

This test is used to identify patients who are hypercoagulable and may experience a thromboembolic phenomenon when immobile (e.g., after surgery or trauma). It is particularly helpful in cardiac surgery and liver transplantation. It is also used to determine hyperfibrinolysis. Finally this shows the complete evaluation of platelet function. Usually three separate tracings using different reagents can determine the percent of platelet inhibition instigated by heparin, aspirin, and antiplatelet drugs (Plavix, Ticlid). This test correlates better with operative bleeding than does bleeding time, closure time (p. 413), or thromboxane levels. With the present instrumentation, point of service (e.g., in the operating room) testing can be performed.

INTERFERING FACTORS

Drugs that may cause *decreased* thromboelastography include antiplatelet drugs (e.g., ticlopidine), some antibiotics, aspirin, beta blockers, clofibrate, dextran, ethanol, heparin, nonsteroidal anti-inflammatory drugs (NSAIDs), phenothiazines, tricyclics, theophylline, and warfarin sodium (Coumadin).

PROCEDURE AND PATIENT CARE

Before
- Explain the procedure to the patient.
- Tell the patient that no fasting is required.

During
- Collect a venous blood sample in a red-top tube.
- If the patient is receiving any drugs that may interfere with normal coagulation or has any diseases such as jaundice, hyperlipidemia, or hemolysis, this should be listed on the laboratory request slip.
- Immediately transfer the specimen to the laboratory.

After
- Apply pressure or a pressure dressing to the venipuncture site.
- Assess the venipuncture site for bleeding.
- Remember that abnormalities in platelet aggregation can prolong bleeding time, and a significant hematoma at the venipuncture site may occur.

TEST RESULTS AND CLINICAL SIGNIFICANCE

Hypocoagulability
Factor deficiency,
Anticoagulation,
Thrombocytopenia,
Platelet function abnormalities,
Increased fibrinolysis: *All are associated with a fibrin clot with reduced tensile strength. Very succinct graph patterns can identify and differentiate these abnormalities.*

Hypercoagulability
Factor V-Leiden,
Protein S/C abnormality,
Genetic hypercoagulability,
Idiopathic hypercoagulability: *All are associated with an early fibrin clot. Again, very succinct graph patterns can be identified to differentiate these abnormalities.*

RELATED TESTS

Platelet Aggregation (p. 409). This is a measure of the abilities of the platelets to aggregate.

Platelet Function Assay (p. 413). This is a measure of platelet function.

Platelet Count (p. 416). This is an account of the number of thromboses.

Coagulating Factor Concentration (p. 177). These tests measure the quantity of each specific factor.

Factor V-Leiden (p. 246). This is an inherited abnormality affecting the coagulation cascade.

Protein C, Protein S (p. 437). These are important inhibitors of the coagulation system.

Plasminogen (p. 406). This protein is involved in the fibrinolytic process.

 Thrombosis Indicators (Fibrin Monomers [Fibrin Degradation Products (FDPs)], Fibrin Split Products (FSPs)], Fibrinopeptide A [FPA], Prothrombin Fragment 1+2 [F1+2])

NORMAL FINDINGS

Fibrin degradation products (FDPs): **<10 mg/dL** (<10 *Mcg*/mL)

Fibrinopeptide A:

Male: 0.4–2.6 mg/mL

Female 0.7–3.1 mg/mL

Prothrombin fragment 1+2 (F1+2): **7.4–103** *Mcg*/L (0.2–2.8 nmol/L)

Critical Values

FDP **>40 mg/dL** (>40 *Mcg*/mL)

INDICATIONS

FDPs, fibrinopeptide A, and F1+2 are identified and used to document that fibrin clot formation and, therefore, thrombosis is occurring. These tests support the diagnosis of disseminated intravascular coagulation. They also provide an indication about the effectiveness of anticoagulation therapy. In addition, they are used to support the diagnosis of and monitor treatment for hypercoagulable states.

TEST EXPLANATION

F1+2 is liberated when prothrombin is converted to thrombin in reaction 4 of secondary hemostasis (see Figure 2-14, p. 181). These fragments are evaluated primarily to indicate thrombosis. F1+2 levels are also significantly increased in patients with leukemia, severe liver disease, and after myocardial infarction. Patients with elevated F1+2 concentration before the beginning of heparin therapy show decreases after 1 day of therapy. For patients in the stable phase of oral anticoagulant therapy, decreasing F1+2 concentrations are noted with increasing international normalized ratios. F1+2 determination is thus particularly helpful in monitoring anticoagulant therapy.

Fibrinopeptide A is made up of two small peptide chains removed from the N-terminal segment of the alpha chains of fibrinogen during its conversion to fibrin. It is released into the bloodstream by that reaction during the blood coagulation process and is therefore a measure of thrombosis.

Measurement of FDPs provides a direct indication of the activity of the fibrinolytic system. The fibrinolytic system plays an important role in balancing clot formation and clot dissolution. Clot formation stimulates the activation of three major activators of the fibrinolytic system. These in turn act on plasminogen, which was previously absorbed into the clot, to form plasmin. Plasmin degenerates the fibrin polymer of the clot into fragments, the FDPs (X, D, E, Y). These products are usually cleared by macrophages. If present in increased quantities, they can have an anticoagulant effect by inhibiting fibrinogen conversion to fibrin and by interrupting fibrin polymerization to tighten the clot.

When present in large amounts, FDPs indicate increased fibrinolysis, as occurs in thrombotic states. The thrombosis stimulates the activation of the fibrinolytic system. Other diseases can secondarily activate the fibrinolytic system and elevate FDP levels. These may include extensive malignancy, tissue necrosis, and Gram-negative sepsis. Thrombolytic therapy for myocardial infarction, for example, is associated with increased levels of FDPs. Streptokinase or urokinase stimulates the conversion of plasminogen to plasmin. The plasmin splits the fibrinogen polymer into FDPs, as discussed previously.

These products of hemostasis and fibrinolysis may also be present in elevated levels in patients with extensive malignancy, tissue necrosis, and Gram-negative sepsis.

INTERFERING FACTORS

- Traumatic venipunctures may increase fibrinopeptide A levels.
- Surgery or massive trauma is associated with increased levels of thrombosis indicators because of the thrombosis that is instigated by surgery.
- Menstruation may be associated with increased FDP levels.
- The presence of rheumatoid factor may cause levels of thrombosis indicators to be artificially high.
- Drugs that may cause *increases* in levels of thrombosis indicators include barbiturates, heparin, streptokinase, and urokinase.
- Drugs that may cause *decreases* in levels of thrombosis indicators include warfarin (Coumadin) and other oral anticoagulants.

PROCEDURE AND PATIENT CARE

Before

- Explain the procedure to the patient.
- Inform the patient that no fasting is required.
- Avoid prolonged use of a tourniquet.

During

- Collect the sample before initiating heparin therapy.
- Collect a venous blood sample in a small blue-top tube or in the colour-top tube designated by the laboratory.
- Avoid excessive agitation of the blood sample.

After

- Apply pressure to the venipuncture site.
- Note that it is best to place the blood in a mixture of water and crushed ice and take it immediately to the hematology laboratory.

- On the laboratory slip, list any drugs that the patient is taking that may cause elevations in levels of thrombosis indicators.

TEST RESULTS AND CLINICAL SIGNIFICANCE

▲ Increased Levels

Disseminated intravascular coagulation,

Heart or vascular surgery,

Thromboembolism,

Thrombosis,

Advanced malignancy,

Severe inflammation,

Postoperative states,

Massive trauma: *These diseases or states are all associated with increased thrombosis or fibrinolysis, or both.*

Deficiency in protein S and protein C: *The "protein C–protein S" system is an important inhibitor of coagulation. With deficiencies in these proteins, thrombosis proceeds without inhibition.*

Antithrombin III deficiency: *Antithrombin III competes with activated coagulation proteins and blocks their biologic activity. Even mild reductions in this protein are therefore associated with markedly increased thrombosis.*

▼ Decreased Levels

Anticoagulation therapy: *Reduction in thrombosis is associated with a reduction in all the proteins that are products of that biologic system.*

RELATED TEST

Disseminated Intravascular Coagulation Screening (p. 225). This is a group of commonly used tests to diagnose disseminated intravascular coagulation.

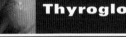

Thyroglobulin (Tg, Thyrogen-Stimulated Thyroglobulin)

NORMAL FINDINGS

Age	Male (*Mc*g/L)*	Female (*Mc*g/L)*
0–11 months	0.6–5.5	0.5–5.5
1–11 years	0.6–50.1	0.5–52.1
≥12 years	0.5–53.0	0.5–43.0

*Conventional values are the same as the SI values but in nanograms per millilitre.

INDICATIONS

This test is primarily used as a tumour marker for well-differentiated thyroid cancer.

TEST EXPLANATION

Thyroglobulin is the protein precursor of thyroid hormone and is made by normal well-differentiated benign thyroid cells or thyroid cancer cells. Because thyroglobulin is normally only made by thyroid cells, it is useful for evaluating the presence or absence of thyroid cells, especially after surgery for thyroid cancer. In the treatment of well-differentiated thyroid cancers, it is important to remove as much thyroid tissue as possible so that adjunctive radioactive iodine treatment is delivered not to residual thyroid gland tissue in the neck but instead to any metastatic thyroid cells. If postoperative thyroglobulin levels are low, very little thyroid tissue remains.

Thyroglobulin is also used as a tumour marker in these postoperative patients. Thyroglobulin is a marker of disease activity and the volume of thyroid tumour. Ideally, the thyroglobulin levels are low or undetectable after treatment (usually surgery followed by therapy with radioactive iodine). Rising levels herald tumour recurrence and progression. Thyroglobulin levels may be elevated both in thyroid cancer and in a large number of benign thyroid conditions. Therefore, an increased thyroglobulin level alone in a patient is not sensitive or specific for the diagnosis of thyroid cancer. A simple examination of the thyroid or a thyroid biopsy can produce significant elevations in the circulating blood level of thyroglobulin. Similarly, patients with thyroid inflammation can have very high levels of thyroglobulin. In some patients with anti–thyroglobulin antibodies (see p. 113), testing may demonstrate inaccurate thyroglobulin levels.

After thyroidectomy, thyroid hormone replacement is required for normal metabolic function. Because of thyroid hormone replacement therapy, thyroid-stimulating hormone (TSH) levels are usually very low, and endogenous stimulation of any residual thyroid cells is minimal in these patients. As a result, levels of thyroglobulin and thyroid endogenous thyroid hormones are low. In the past, in order to stimulate thyroglobulin production in these patients for cancer surveillance testing, thyroid hormone was temporarily discontinued for as much as 6 weeks until the body was depleted of any thyroid hormone. TSH was then maximally stimulated and was able to stimulate the production of thyroglobulin from any thyroid cells. If there were any functioning thyroid cancer cells, thyroglobulin levels would be elevated. During the time of thyroid hormone withdrawal, the patient was very uncomfortable, lethargic, tired, and slow.

Testing with thyrotropin alfa (Thyrogen) stimulation has eliminated the need for withdrawal of thyroid hormone medications and provides a safe and effective method of elevating TSH levels so that even minimal levels of thyroglobulin can be detected. This allows patients to undergo periodic thyroid cancer follow-up evaluation while avoiding the often debilitating side effects of hypothyroidism caused by withdrawal of hormone medication. Thyrogen is a highly purified recombinant source of human TSH. Thyrogen raises serum TSH levels and thereby stimulates thyroglobulin production. Normal thyroid remnant and well-differentiated thyroid tumours display a greater (>10-fold) serum thyroglobulin response to TSH stimulation. If after thyroid surgery, Thyrogen-stimulated thyroglobulin levels are elevated, either a significant amount of normal thyroid gland was left in the neck or metastatic disease exists. If Thyrogen-stimulated thyroglobulin levels are elevated after postoperative therapeutic administration of iodine-131 (^{131}I; given to destroy any residual thyroid tissue in the neck), metastatic disease certainly exists, and further treatment is required.

Thyrogen stimulation is also used for patients undergoing ^{131}I whole-body scanning for metastatic thyroid cancer. In the past, as with thyroglobulin testing, affected patients had to discontinue the thyroid hormone replacement regimen so that their endogenous TSH levels would rise and stimulate any metastatic thyroid cancer cells to pick up ^{131}I, so that the cancer cells would be detected on a nuclear scan of the body. Now, with the use of Thyrogen, the ill effects of hormone withdrawal are not experienced.

INTERFERING FACTORS

- Thyroglobulin levels are decreased in less well-differentiated thyroid cancers.
- Thyrogen stimulation of thyroglobulin levels is less effective in patients whose tumours do not have TSH receptors or whose tumours cannot make thyroglobulin.
- Thyroglobulin autoantibodies cause either underestimation or overestimation of serum thyroglobulin measurements made by immunometric assay and radioimmunoassay methods, respectively.

Clinical Priorities

- Thyroid cancer is the most common endocrine cancer and occurs in all age groups.
- The incidence of thyroid cancer is rising faster than that of other cancers among women.
- Thyroid cancer may recur in up to 30% of patients, even decades after initial diagnosis.

PROCEDURE AND PATIENT CARE

Before

- Explain the procedure to the patients.
- Inform the patient that no fasting is required.
- Determine whether the patient is to have a whole-body nuclear scan along with the thyroglobulin blood test.

During

- Collect a venous blood sample in a gold-top (serum separator) tube.
- If Thyrogen stimulation is to be used:
  1. Administer Thyrogen intramuscularly to the buttock every 24 hours for two or three doses as ordered by the physician.
  2. Collect blood in a gold-top (serum separator) tube 3 days after the last Thyrogen dose.
- For radioiodine imaging:
  1. The nuclear medicine technologist administers radioiodine 24 hours after the final Thyrogen injection.
  2. Scanning is usually performed 48 hours after radioiodine administration. Whole-body images are acquired for a minimum of 30 minutes or should contain a minimum of 140 000 counts.
  3. Scanning for single (spot) images of body regions may be performed.

After

- Apply pressure or a pressure dressing to the venipuncture site.
- Assess the venipuncture site for bleeding.

TEST RESULTS AND CLINICAL SIGNIFICANCE

▲ Increased Levels

Residual thyroid tissue in the neck,
Metastatic thyroid cancer: *Normal thyroid cells and well-differentiated thyroid cancer cells make thyroglobulin as a precursor to thyroid hormone.*

RELATED TEST

Anti–Thyroglobulin Antibody (p. 113). Although this antibody is used primarily to identify patients with thyroiditis, its presence can affect thyroglobulin test results.

Thyroid-Stimulating Hormone (TSH, Thyrotropin)

NORMAL FINDINGS

Adult: **0.4–4.8 mIU/L** (0.4–4.8 mIU/L)
Newborn: **3–18 mIU/L** (3–18 µIU/mL)
Umbilical cord: **3–12 mIU/L** (3–12 µIU/mL)
  Values vary among laboratories.

 Critical Values

<0.1 mIU/L is an indication of primary hypertension or exogenous thyrotoxicosis. Patients with levels <0.1 mIU/L are also at a high risk for atrial fibrillation and stroke.

INDICATIONS

This test is used to diagnose primary hypothyroidism and to differentiate it from secondary (pituitary) and tertiary (hypothalamus) hypothyroidism.

TEST EXPLANATION

The concentration of TSH (also called thyrotropin) aids in differentiating primary from secondary hypothyroidism. Pituitary TSH secretion is stimulated by hypothalamic thyroid-releasing hormone (TRH). Low levels of triiodothyronine (T_3) and thyroxine (T_4) are the underlying stimuli for TRH and TSH production. Therefore, a compensatory elevation of TRH and TSH levels occurs in patients with primary hypothyroid states, such as surgical or radioactive thyroid ablation; in patients with burned-out thyroiditis, thyroid agenesis, idiopathic hypothyroidism, or congenital cretinism; and in patients taking antithyroid medications.

In secondary or tertiary hypothyroidism, the function of the pituitary gland or hypothalamus, respectively, is faulty as a result of tumour, trauma, or infarction. Therefore, TRH and TSH cannot be secreted, and plasma levels of these hormones are near zero despite the stimulation that occurs with low T_3 and T_4 levels.

The TRH stimulation test is sometimes used to stimulate low levels of TSH in order to differentiate primary from secondary hypothyroidism in cases in which TSH level is low. However, this test is not commonly used because extremely low levels of TSH can be identified with the use of immunoassays.

The TSH test is used to monitor exogenous thyroid replacement or suppression as well. The goal of thyroid replacement therapy is to provide an adequate amount of thyroid medication so that TSH secretion is in the "low normal range," indicating a euthyroid state. The goal of thyroid suppression is to completely suppress the thyroid gland and TSH secretion by providing excessive thyroid medication. This treatment is used to diminish the size of a thyroid goitre. The dose of medication is given to keep the TSH level less than **2 mIU/L** for replacement. Even lower TSH levels are preferred if thyroid suppression is the clinical goal.

This test is also used to detect primary hypothyroidism in newborns with low screening T_4 levels. TSH and T_4 levels are frequently measured to differentiate pituitary and thyroid dysfunction. A decreased T_4 level and a normal or elevated TSH level can indicate a thyroid disorder. A decreased T_4 level with a decreased TSH level can indicate a pituitary disorder.

INTERFERING FACTORS

- Recent radioisotope administration may affect test results.
- Severe illness may cause decreases in TSH levels.
- There is a diurnal variation in TSH levels. Basal levels occur at approximately 10 AM and highest levels ($\sim$ two to three times basal levels) occur at approximately 10 PM.
- Drugs that may cause *increases* in levels include antithyroid medications, lithium, potassium iodide, and TSH injection.
- Drugs that may cause *decreases* in levels include aspirin, heparin, nonsteroidal antiarthritics, dopamine, steroids, and T_3.

Clinical Priorities

- This test is useful for differentiating primary hypothyroidism from secondary (pituitary) and tertiary (hypothalamus) hypothyroidism. Elevations of TSH occur in patients with primary hypothyroid states. In contrast, plasma levels of TSH are near zero in patients with secondary and tertiary hypothyroidism.
- This test may be used to detect primary hypothyroidism in newborns with low screening T_4 levels.
- TSH levels are subject to a diurnal variation. Basal levels occur at approximately 10 AM and highest levels occur at approximately 10 PM.

PROCEDURE AND PATIENT CARE

Before
- Explain the procedure to the patient.
- Inform the patient that no food or drink restrictions are necessary.

During
- Collect a venous blood sample in a red-top tube.
- Use a heelstick to obtain blood from newborns.

After
- Apply pressure or a pressure dressing to the venipuncture site.
- Assess the venipuncture site for bleeding.

TEST RESULTS AND CLINICAL SIGNIFICANCE

▲ Increased Levels
Primary hypothyroidism (thyroid dysfunction),
Thyroiditis,

Thyroid agenesis,

Congenital cretinism,

Large doses of iodine,

Radioactive iodine injection,

Surgical ablation of thyroid,

Severe and chronic illnesses: *In these diseases, inadequate thyroid hormone levels act as a potent stimulant for the release of TSH from the anterior pituitary. TSH levels rise accordingly. In some cases, however, TSH level may be diminished.*

Pituitary TSH-secreting tumour: *In this very rare tumour, TSH levels are increased.*

▼ Decreased Levels

Secondary hypothyroidism (pituitary or hypothalamus dysfunction): *Diseases of the hypothalamus diminish the capability of the hypothalamus to secrete TRH, which is the major determinant of TSH production and secretion. Diseases of the pituitary gland diminish pituitary production of TSH.*

Hyperthyroidism: *Increased levels of thyroid hormones inhibit the release of TSH.*

Suppressive doses of thyroid medication: *When thyroid medication (e.g., Synthroid) is administered (usually to shrink a goitre), TSH levels fall because of inhibition by the thyroid medication.*

Factitious hyperthyroidism: *This condition occurs when patients take thyroid medication without prescription. These medications act to inhibit TSH production.*

RELATED TESTS

Thyroid-Stimulating Immunoglobulins (p. 504). Long-acting thyroid stimulator (LATS) and other thyroid-stimulating immunoglobulins are measured to support the diagnosis of Graves' disease, especially when the differential diagnosis is complex.

Thyrotropin-Releasing Hormone (p. 506). This test assists in the evaluation of patients with hyperthyroidism and hypothyroidism. It is especially helpful in the differential diagnosis of hypothyroidism.

Triiodothyronine Uptake (p. 528). This test is an indirect measurement of total T_4.

Thyroid-Stimulating Hormone Stimulation (see following test p. 503). This test is also used to differentiate primary from secondary (and tertiary) hypothyroidism.

Thyroxine-Binding Globulin (p. 509). This major thyroid hormone protein carrier is measured in the evaluation of patients who have abnormal total thyroxine (T_4) and triiodothyronine (T_3) levels. When this test is performed concurrently with a T_4/T_3 test, T_4 and T_3 levels can be interpreted more easily.

Thyroxine, Total (p. 516). This is one of the first tests performed to assess thyroid function. It is used to evaluate thyroid function and to monitor replacement and suppressive medical therapy.

Triiodothyronine (p. 525). A T_3 is used to evaluate thyroid function, primarily in order to diagnose hyperthyroidism. It is also used to monitor thyroid replacement and suppressive medical therapy.

Thyroxine Index, Free (p. 514). This test is used to evaluate thyroid function. It corrects for changes in thyroid hormone–binding serum proteins that can affect total T_4 levels. It is also used to diagnose hyperthyroidism and hypothyroidism.

Thyroxine, Free (p. 511). This test is used to evaluate thyroid function in patients who may have protein abnormalities that could affect total T_4 levels. It is used to evaluate thyroid function and to monitor replacement and suppressive medical therapy.

Anti–Thyroglobulin Antibody (p. 113). This test is used primarily for the differential diagnosis of thyroid diseases, such as Hashimoto thyroiditis and chronic lymphocytic thyroiditis (in children).

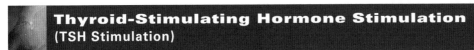

Thyroid-Stimulating Hormone Stimulation
(TSH Stimulation)

NORMAL FINDINGS

Increased thyroid function with administration of exogenous thyroid-stimulating hormone (TSH)

INDICATIONS

This test is used to differentiate primary from secondary (and tertiary) hypothyroidism.

TEST EXPLANATION

The TSH stimulation test is used to differentiate primary (thyroid) hypothyroidism from secondary (hypothalamic-pituitary) hypothyroidism. Normal individuals and patients with hypothalamic-pituitary hypothyroidism are capable of increasing thyroid function when exogenous TSH is administered. However, patients with primary hypothyroidism, because of disease in the thyroid, are not; their thyroid gland is inadequate and cannot function no matter how much stimulation it receives. Patients with less than a 10% increase in radioactive iodine uptake or less than a 1.5-Mcg/dL rise in thyroxine (T_4) level are considered to have primary hypothyroidism. If the hypothyroidism is caused by inadequate pituitary secretion of TSH or hypothalamic secretion of thyroid-releasing hormone, the radioactive iodine uptake should increase at least 10% and the T_4 level should rise 1.5 Mcg/dL or more. This is characteristic of secondary hypothyroidism.

PROCEDURE AND PATIENT CARE

Before

- Explain the procedure to the patient.
- Obtain measurements of baseline levels of radioactive iodine uptake or T_4 as indicated.
- Inform the patient that no fasting is required.

During

- Administer the prescribed dose of TSH intramuscularly for 3 days.
- Repeat the measurement of radioactive iodine uptake or T_4 as indicated.

After

- Apply pressure or a pressure dressing to the venipuncture site.
- Assess the venipuncture site for bleeding.

TEST RESULTS AND CLINICAL SIGNIFICANCE

▲ Increased Levels

Primary hypothyroidism (thyroid dysfunction),
Thyroiditis,
Thyroid agenesis,
Congenital cretinism,
Large doses of iodine,
Radioactive iodine injection,

Surgical ablation of thyroid,

Severe and chronic illnesses: *In these conditions, the thyroid is unable to increase T₄ levels or radioactive iodine uptake no matter how significant the stimulation, because the disease involves the thyroid itself.*

Secondary hypothyroidism (pituitary or hypothalamus dysfunction): *The thyroid is capable of producing T₄ and radioactive iodine uptake, but the pituitary-hypothalamic stimulation is inadequate for appropriate stimulation of those functions. When TSH is administered, T₄ and radioactive iodine uptake increase significantly.*

RELATED TESTS

Thyroid-Stimulating Immunoglobulins (see following test p. 504). Long-Acting Thyroid Stimulator (LATS) and other thyroid-stimulating immunoglobulins are measured to support the diagnosis of Graves' disease, especially when the differential diagnosis is complex.

Thyrotropin-Releasing Hormone (p. 506). This test assists in the evaluation of patients with hyperthyroidism and hypothyroidism. It is especially helpful in the differential diagnosis of hypothyroidism.

Thyroid-Stimulating Hormone (p. 500). This test is used to diagnose primary hypothyroidism and to differentiate it from secondary (pituitary) and tertiary (hypothalamus) hypothyroidism.

Triiodothyronine Uptake (p. 528). This test is an indirect measurement of total T_4.

Thyroxine-Binding Globulin (p. 509). This major thyroid hormone protein carrier is measured for evaluation of patients who have abnormal total thyroxine (T_4) and triiodothyronine (T_3) levels. When this test is performed concurrently with a T_4/T_3 test, the T_4 and T_3 levels can be interpreted more easily.

Thyroxine, Total (p. 516). This is one of the first tests performed to assess thyroid function. It is used to evaluate thyroid function and to monitor replacement and suppressive medical therapy.

Triiodothyronine (p. 525). A T_3 is used to evaluate thyroid function primarily in order to diagnose hyperthyroidism. It is also used to monitor thyroid replacement and suppressive medical therapy.

Thyroxine Index, Free (p. 514). This test is used to evaluate thyroid function. It corrects for changes in thyroid hormone–binding serum proteins that can affect total T_4 levels. It is also used to diagnose hyperthyroidism and hypothyroidism.

Thyroxine, Free (p. 511). This test is used to evaluate thyroid function in patients who may have protein abnormalities that could affect total T_4 levels. It is used to evaluate thyroid function and to monitor replacement and suppressive medical therapy.

Anti–Thyroglobulin Antibody (p. 113). This test is used primarily for the differential diagnosis of thyroid diseases, such as Hashimoto thyroiditis and chronic lymphocytic thyroiditis (in children).

Thyroid-Stimulating Immunoglobulins
(TSI, Long-Acting Thyroid Stimulator [LATS], Thyroid-Binding Inhibitory Immunoglobulin [TBII], Thyrotropin Receptor Antibody)

NORMAL FINDINGS

Thyroid-stimulating immunoglobulins: <130% of basal activity
Thyroid-binding inhibitory immunoglobulin: <10% of basal activity

INDICATIONS

These immunoglobulins are measured to support the diagnosis of Graves' disease, especially when the differential diagnosis is complex.

TEST EXPLANATION

The nomenclature for various assays for thyroid-stimulating hormone (TSH) receptors is confusing. The characterizations of these hormones demonstrate that they act very similarly but are thought to be different because of the different animal test systems used to identify the various antibodies. Thyroid-stimulating immunoglobulins represent a group of immunoglobulin G (IgG) antibodies directed against the thyroid cell receptor for TSH. The autoimmune complexes then act to stimulate (or, in some patients, inhibit) the release of thyroid hormones from the thyroid cells. These immunoglobulins, present in 90% of patients with Graves' disease, play a major role in the pathogenesis of that disease. In some cases, thyroid-stimulating immunoglobulins are inhibitory and have been demonstrated in patients with Hashimoto thyroiditis.

The use of these antibodies is helpful in the evaluation of patients for whom the diagnosis of Graves' disease is hampered by conflicting data (such as subclinical Graves' hyperthyroidism or euthyroidism with ophthalmopathy). In these patients, the antibodies help determine and support the diagnosis of Graves' disease.

The effect of these antibodies on the thyroid may be long lasting, and titres do not decrease until nearly 1 year after successful treatment of the thyroid disease. However, measurement of these antibodies may be helpful in identifying remission from or relapse of Graves' disease after treatment. Because thyroid-stimulating immunoglobulins can cross the placenta, they may be found in neonates whose mothers have Graves' disease. These infants experience hyperthyroidism for as long as 4 to 8 months. This syndrome must be identified and treated early.

INTERFERING FACTORS

• Recent administration of radioactive iodine may affect test results.

PROCEDURE AND PATIENT CARE

Before
⋈ Explain the procedure to the patient.
⋈ Inform the patient that no fasting or special preparation is required.

During
• Collect a venous blood sample in a red-top or gold-top tube.
• If the patient has received radioactive iodine in the preceding 2 days, notify the laboratory.
• Handle the blood sample gently. Hemolysis may interfere with interpretation of test results.

After
• Apply pressure to the venipuncture site.

TEST RESULTS AND CLINICAL SIGNIFICANCE

▲ Increased Levels
Malignant exophthalmos,
Graves' disease,

Hashimoto thyroiditis: In these forms of hyperthyroidism, the disease process has an autoimmune element. IgG antibodies are present in most cases. These antibodies can act to stimulate or inhibit thyroid function.

RELATED TESTS

Triiodothyronine Uptake (p. 528). This test is an indirect measurement of total T_4.

Thyrotropin-Releasing Hormone (see following test p. 506). This test assists in the evaluation of patients with hyperthyroidism and hypothyroidism. It is especially helpful in the differential diagnosis of hypothyroidism.

Thyroid-Stimulating Hormone (p. 500). This test is used to diagnose primary hypothyroidism and to differentiate it from secondary (pituitary) and tertiary (hypothalamus) hypothyroidism.

Thyroid-Stimulating Hormone Stimulation (p. 503). This test is also used to differentiate primary from secondary (and tertiary) hypothyroidism.

Thyroxine-Binding Globulin (p. 509). This major thyroid hormone protein carrier is measured for evaluation of patients who have abnormal total thyroxine (T_4) and triiodothyronine (T_3) levels. When this test is performed concurrently with a T_4/T_3 test, the T_4 and T_3 levels can be interpreted more easily.

Thyroxine, Total (p. 516). This is one of the first tests performed to assess thyroid function. It is used to evaluate thyroid function and to monitor replacement and suppressive medical therapy.

Triiodothyronine (p. 525). A T_3 test is used to evaluate thyroid function, primarily in order to diagnose hyperthyroidism. It is also used to monitor thyroid replacement and suppressive medical therapy.

Thyroxine Index, Free (p. 514). This test is used to evaluate thyroid function. It corrects for changes in thyroid hormone–binding serum proteins that can affect total T_4 levels. It is also used to diagnose hyperthyroidism and hypothyroidism.

Thyroxine, Free (p. 511). This test is used to evaluate thyroid function in patients who may have protein abnormalities that could affect total T_4 levels. It is used to evaluate thyroid function and to monitor replacement and suppressive medical therapy.

Anti–Thyroglobulin Antibody (p. 113). This test is primarily used for the differential diagnosis of thyroid diseases, such as Hashimoto thyroiditis and chronic lymphocytic thyroiditis (in children).

Thyrotropin-Releasing Hormone (TRH, **Thyrotropin-Releasing Factor [TRF])**

NORMAL FINDINGS

Prompt rise in serum thyroid-stimulating hormone (TSH) level to approximately twice the baseline value in 30 minutes after an intravenous bolus of thyrotropin-releasing hormone (TRH)

Clinical Condition	Baseline TSH Level (μIU/mL)	TSH Level After Stimulation[*]
Euthyroid	<10	>2
Hyperthyroid	<10	<2
Primary hypothyroid (thyroid)	>10	>2
Secondary hypothyroid (pituitary)	<10	<2
Tertiary hypothyroid (hypothalamus)	<10	>2

[*]Stimulated TSH (times the baseline) is measured 30 minutes after the intravenous injection of TRH.

INDICATIONS

This test assists in the evaluation of patients with hyperthyroidism and hypothyroidism. It is especially helpful in the differential diagnosis of hypothyroidism.

TEST EXPLANATION

The TRH test is performed to assess the anterior pituitary gland with regard to its secretion of TSH in response to an intravenous injection of TRH. After the TRH injection, the normally functioning pituitary gland should secrete TSH (and prolactin). In hyperthyroidism, the TSH level increases either slightly or not at all because pituitary TSH production is suppressed by the inhibitory effect of excess circulating thyroxine (T_4) and triiodothyronine (T_3) on the pituitary gland. A normal result is considered reliable evidence for excluding the diagnosis of thyrotoxicosis. Since the development of a very sensitive radioimmunoassay for TSH, the TRH stimulation test is no longer necessary for diagnosing hyperthyroidism. However, it still has a role in the evaluation of pituitary deficiency.

In addition to assessing the responsiveness of the anterior pituitary gland, this test aids in the detection of primary, secondary, and tertiary hypothyroidism. In primary hypothyroidism (thyroid gland failure), the increase in the TSH level is two or more times the normal result. With secondary hypothyroidism (anterior pituitary failure), no TSH response occurs. Tertiary hypothyroidism (hypothalamic failure) may be diagnosed from a delayed rise in the TSH level. Multiple injections of TRH may be needed to induce the appropriate TSH response in this case.

The TRH test also may be useful in differentiating primary depression, bipolar psychiatric illness, and secondary types of depression. In primary depression, the TSH response is blunted in most patients, whereas patients with other types of depression have a normal TRH-induced TSH response.

INTERFERING FACTORS

- The normal response may be exaggerated in women.
- The normal response may be less than expected in older adults.
- Pregnancy may increase the TSH response to TRH.
- Drugs that may modify the TSH response include antithyroid drugs, aspirin, corticosteroids, estrogens, levodopa, and T_4.

PROCEDURE AND PATIENT CARE

Before
- Explain the procedure to the patient.
- Instruct the patient to discontinue thyroid preparations for 3 to 4 weeks before the TRH test, if it is indicated.
- Assess the patient for medications currently being taken.
- Inform the patient that no fasting or sedation is required.

During
- Administer an intravenous bolus of TRH.
- Obtain venous blood samples at intervals and measure TSH levels.

After
- Apply pressure or a pressure dressing to the venipuncture site.
- Assess the venipuncture site for bleeding.
- On the laboratory slip, indicate whether the patient is pregnant.

TEST RESULTS AND CLINICAL SIGNIFICANCE

▲ Increased Levels

Hyperthyroidism: *Because the pituitary gland is already maximally suppressed by the high levels of T_3 and T_4, pituitary response to TRH is blunted and baseline levels are less than double.*

Primary hypothyroidism (thyroid disease): *Because the TSH is already stimulated by the lack of T_3 and T_4, stimulation is maximized by the TRH and stimulated TSH is more than double the baseline.*

Secondary hypothyroidism (pituitary disease): *Because the diseased pituitary is unable to produce TSH, no matter how significant the stimulation, TSH does not double after TRH stimulation.*

Tertiary hypothyroidism (hypothalamus): *The pituitary is functioning normally. If TRH is provided exogenously, the pituitary gland responds normally and produces twice the TSH level.*

Psychiatric primary depression: *In most patients with primary depression, the TSH response is blunted, whereas patients with other types of depression have a normal TRH-induced TSH response.*

RELATED TESTS

Thyroid-Stimulating Hormone (p. 500). This test is used to diagnose primary hypothyroidism and to differentiate it from secondary (pituitary) and tertiary (hypothalamus) hypothyroidism.

Thyroid-Stimulating Hormone Stimulation (p. 503). This test is also used to differentiate primary from secondary (and tertiary) hypothyroidism.

Thyroxine-Binding Globulin (see following test p. 509). This major thyroid hormone protein carrier is measured for evaluation of patients who have abnormal total thyroxine (T_4) and triiodothyronine (T_3) levels. When this test is performed concurrently with a T_4/T_3 test, the T_4 and T_3 levels can be interpreted more easily.

Thyroxine, Total (p. 516). This is one of the first tests performed to assess thyroid function. It is used to evaluate thyroid function and to monitor replacement and suppressive medical therapy.

Triiodothyronine (p. 525). A T_3 test is used to evaluate thyroid function, primarily in order to diagnose hyperthyroidism. It is also used to monitor thyroid replacement and suppressive medical therapy.

Thyroxine Index, Free (p. 514). This test is used to evaluate thyroid function. It corrects for changes in thyroid hormone-binding serum proteins that can affect total T_4 levels. It is used to diagnose hyperthyroidism and hypothyroidism.

Thyroxine, Free (p. 511). This test is used to evaluate thyroid function in patients who may have protein abnormalities that could affect total T_4 levels. It is used to evaluate thyroid function and to monitor replacement and suppressive medical therapy.

Thyroid-Stimulating Immunoglobulins (p. 504). Long-acting thyroid stimulator (LATS) and other thyroid-stimulating immunoglobulins are measured to support the diagnosis of Graves' disease, especially when the differential diagnosis is complex.

Anti–Thyroglobulin Antibody (p. 113). This test is used primarily for the differential diagnosis of thyroid diseases, such as Hashimoto thyroiditis and chronic lymphocytic thyroiditis (in children).

Triiodothyronine Uptake (p. 528). This test is an indirect measurement of total T_4.

Thyroxine-Binding Globulin (TBG, Thyroid-Binding Globulin)

NORMAL FINDINGS

	Male, mg/L (mg/dL)	Female, mg/L (mg/dL)
1–5 days of age	22–42 (2.2–4.2)	22–42 (2.2–4.2)
1–11 months of age	16–36 (1.6–3.6)	17–37 (1.7–3.7)
1–9 years of age	12–28 (1.2–2.8)	15–27 (1.5–2.7)
10–19 years of age	14–26 (1.4–2.6)	14–30 (1.4–3.0)
≥20 years of age	17–36 (1.7–3.6)	17–36 (1.7–3.6)
Oral contraceptives	—	15–55 (1.5–5.5)
Pregnancy (third trimester)	—	47–59 (4.7–5.9)

INDICATIONS

This test is a measure of thyroxine-binding globulin (TBG), the major thyroid hormone protein carrier. It is used in the evaluation of patients who have abnormal total thyroxine (T_4) and triiodo-thyronine (T_3) levels. When performed concurrently with a T_4/T_3 test, the T_4 and T_3 levels can be interpreted more easily.

TEST EXPLANATION

Assays of T_4 and T_3 are measures of total T_4 and T_3 levels; that is, they are a measure of bound and unbound thyroid hormones. Most of these hormones are bound to TBG. The unbound or "free T_4/T_3" is the metabolically active hormone. Certain illnesses are associated with elevated or decreased TBG levels. With increased TBG levels, more T_4 and T_3 are bound to that protein. Less free, metabolically active T_4 and T_3 are available. TSH is stimulated to produce higher levels of T_4 and T_3 to compensate. T_4 and T_3 levels increase but do not cause hyperthyroidism because the increase is merely a compensation for the increased TBG. When the total T_4 level is elevated, the clinician must ascertain whether that elevation is caused by an elevation in TBG level or is an independent elevation in T_4 level alone in association with hyperthyroidism. Other indirect measurements of TBG include thyroid hormone-binding ratio (see p. 528).

The most common causes of elevations in TBG level are pregnancy, hormone replacement therapy, or use of oral contraceptives. TBG levels are also elevated in some cases of porphyria and in infectious hepatitis. Decreases in TBG level are commonly associated with other causes of hypoproteinemia (e.g., nephrotic syndrome, gastrointestinal malabsorption, malnutrition).

INTERFERING FACTORS

- Previous administration of diagnostic radioisotopes may confound test results if TBG is measured by radioimmunoassay.
- Drugs that cause *increases* in TBG include estrogens, methadone, oral contraceptives, and tamoxifen.
- Drugs that cause *decreases* in TBG include androgens, danazol, phenytoin, propranolol, and steroids.

PROCEDURE AND PATIENT CARE

Before

✗ Explain the procedure to the patient.
✗ Inform the patient that no fasting is required.

During

- Collect a venous blood sample in a red-top tube.
- On the laboratory slip, list any drugs that the patient is taking that may affect test results.

After

- Apply pressure or a pressure dressing to the venipuncture site.
- Assess the venipuncture site for bleeding.

TEST RESULTS AND CLINICAL SIGNIFICANCE

▲ Increased Levels

Pregnancy (and estrogen-replacement therapy, estrogen-producing tumours): *Levels of all proteins, including TBG, are increased with increased estrogen levels.*
Infectious hepatitis: *The pathophysiologic mechanism underlying this observation is not well known.*
Genetic increase of TBG level: *A genetic variation that causes elevation in TBG levels is rare.*
Acute intermittent porphyria: *The pathophysiologic mechanism underlying this observation is not well known.*

▼ Decreased Levels

Protein-losing enteropathy,
Protein-losing nephropathy,
Malnutrition: *Proteins whose levels are decreased include TBG.*
Testosterone-producing tumours: *Testosterone decreases TBG levels.*
Ovarian failure: *With reduced estrogens (e.g., menopause), TBG level is reduced.*
Major stress: *Major stress is often associated with low levels of proteins, including TBG.*

RELATED TESTS

Thyroid-Stimulating Immunoglobulins (p. 504). Long-acting thyroid stimulator (LATS) and other thyroid-stimulating immunoglobulins are measured to support the diagnosis of Graves' disease, especially when the differential diagnosis is complex.

Thyrotropin-Releasing Hormone (p. 506). This test assists in the evaluation of patients with hyperthyroidism and hypothyroidism. It is especially helpful in the differential diagnosis of hypothyroidism.

Thyroid-Stimulating Hormone (p. 500). This test is used to diagnose primary hypothyroidism and to differentiate it from secondary (pituitary) and tertiary (hypothalamus) hypothyroidism.

Thyroid-Stimulating Hormone Stimulation (p. 503). This test is also used to differentiate primary from secondary (and tertiary) hypothyroidism.

Triiodothyronine Uptake (p. 528). This test is an indirect measurement of total T_4.

Thyroxine, Total (p. 516). This is one of the first tests performed to assess thyroid function. It is used to diagnose thyroid function and to monitor replacement and suppressive medical therapy.

Triiodothyronine (p. 525). A T_3 test is used to evaluate thyroid function, primarily in order to diagnose hyperthyroidism. It is also used to monitor thyroid replacement and suppressive medical therapy.

Thyroxine Index, Free (p. 514). This test is used to evaluate thyroid function. It corrects for changes in thyroid hormone-binding serum proteins that can affect total T_4 levels. It is also used to diagnose hyperthyroidism and hypothyroidism.

Thyroxine, Free (see following test). This test is used to evaluate thyroid function in patients who may have protein abnormalities that could affect total T_4 levels. It is used to evaluate thyroid function and to monitor replacement and suppressive medical therapy.

Anti–Thyroglobulin Antibody (p. 113). This test is used primarily for the differential diagnosis of thyroid diseases, such as Hashimoto thyroiditis and chronic lymphocytic thyroiditis (in children).

Thyroxine, Free (FT$_4$)

NORMAL FINDINGS

Ages 0–4 days: **26–77 pmol/L** (2–6 ng/dL)
Ages 2 weeks to 20 years: **10–26 pmol/L** (0.8–2 ng/dL)
Adult: **13–27 pmol/L** (1.0–2.1 ng/dL)

INDICATIONS

The free thyroxine (FT_4) level is measured to evaluate thyroid function in patients who may have protein abnormalities that could affect total thyroxine (T_4) levels. It is used to diagnose thyroid function and to monitor replacement and suppressive medical therapy.

TEST EXPLANATION

Thyroid hormone is made up of T_4 and triiodothyronine (T_3). Over 90% of thyroid hormone is made up of T_4. As much as 99% of T_4 is bound to proteins (thyroxine-binding globulin [TBG] and albumin). Only 1% to 5% of total T_4 is unbound or "free." FT_4 is the metabolically active thyroid hormone. In measurements of total T_4, the bound and the unbound portions are calculated.

Abnormalities in protein levels can have a significant effect on the total T_4 results. Pregnancy and hormone replacement therapy increase TBG levels and cause T_4 levels to be artificially elevated, which suggests that hyperthyroidism exists although, in fact, the patient has normal thyroid function. If the FT_4 level is measured in these patients, it is normal, which indicates that FT_4 is a more accurate indicator of thyroid function than total T_4. Likewise, when TBG level is reduced (as in hypoproteinemia), the total T_4 is also reduced, which is suggestive of hypothyroidism. Measurements of FT_4 indicate normal levels and thereby imply that the abnormal total T_4 measurement is merely a result of the reduced TBG level and not a result of hypothyroidism.

This test is used to determine thyroid function, especially when the patient has concurrent clinical problems that may alter protein blood levels. FT_4 levels higher than normal indicate hyperthyroid states, and subnormal values are seen in hypothyroid states. This test is performed by direct dialysis extraction of FT_4 and measured by radioimmunoassay. There are significant laboratory variations in results and testing quality. The free thyroxine index may be a better indication of true thyroid function.

INTERFERING FACTORS

- Neonates have higher FT_4 levels than do older children and adults.
- Prior use of radioisotopes can alter test results, if the method used to determine free T_4 levels is radioimmunoassay.
- Exogenously administered T_4 causes elevations in FT_4 measurements.
- Drugs that cause *increases* in FT_4 levels include aspirin, danazol, heparin, and propranolol.
- Drugs that cause *decreases* in FT_4 levels include furosemide, methadone, phenytoin, and rifampicin.

Clinical Priorities

- This test is used to evaluate thyroid function in patients who may have protein abnormalities that could affect total T_4 levels.
- High FT_4 levels indicate hyperthyroidism, and low FT_4 levels indicate hypothyroidism.

PROCEDURE AND PATIENT CARE

Before

- Explain the procedure to the patient.
- Evaluate the patient's medication history.
- If it is indicated, instruct the patient to stop taking exogenous T_4 medication 1 month before the test.
- Inform the patient that no fasting is required.

During

- Collect a venous blood specimen in a red-top tube.

After

- Apply pressure or a pressure dressing to the venipuncture site.
- Assess the venipuncture site for bleeding.

TEST RESULTS AND CLINICAL SIGNIFICANCE

▲ Increased Levels

Primary hyperthyroid states (e.g., Graves' disease, Plummer disease, toxic thyroid adenoma): *The thyroid produces increased amounts of T_4 despite lack of TSH stimulation.*

Acute thyroiditis: *The thyroid secretes increased amounts of T_4 during the acute inflammatory stages of thyroiditis (e.g., Hashimoto thyroiditis). However, in the latter stages, the thyroid may become "burned out," and the patient may develop hypothyroidism.*

Factitious hyperthyroidism: *Patients who self-administer T_4 have elevated levels. Many patients believe they will feel more energetic or will lose weight faster if they take T_4.*

Struma ovarii: *Ectopic thyroid tissue in the ovary or anywhere can produce excess T_4.*

▼ Decreased Levels

Hypothyroid states (e.g., cretinism, surgical ablation, myxedema): *The thyroid in these diseases cannot produce an adequate amount of T_4 despite the stimulation provided.*

Pituitary insufficiency: *The pituitary gland produces an insufficient amount of thyrotropin. As a result, the thyroid is not stimulated to produce T_4.*

Hypothalamic failure: *The hypothalamus produces an insufficient amount of TRH. As a result, the pituitary does not produce thyrotropin, and the thyroid is not stimulated to produce T_4.*

Iodine insufficiency: *Iodine is the basic raw material for T_4. Without iodine, T_4 cannot be produced. With the introduction of iodide in most table salts, iodine insufficiency has become rare in the United States and Canada.*

Nonthyroid illnesses (e.g., renal failure, Cushing's disease, cirrhosis, surgery, advanced cancer): *The pathophysiologic mechanism underlying these observations is not well known.*

RELATED TESTS

Thyroid-Stimulating Immunoglobulins (p. 504). Long-acting thyroid stimulator (LATS) and other thyroid-stimulating immunoglobulins are measured to support the diagnosis of Graves' disease, especially when the differential diagnosis is complex.

Thyrotropin-Releasing Hormone (p. 506). This test assists in the evaluation of patients with hyperthyroidism and hypothyroidism. It is especially helpful in the differential diagnosis of hypothyroidism.

Thyroid-Stimulating Hormone (p. 500). This test is used to diagnose primary hypothyroidism and to differentiate it from secondary (pituitary) and tertiary (hypothalamus) hypothyroidism.

Thyroid-Stimulating Hormone Stimulation (p. 503). This test is also used to differentiate primary from secondary (and tertiary) hypothyroidism.

Thyroxine-Binding Globulin (p. 509). This major thyroid hormone protein carrier is measured for evaluation of patients who have abnormal total thyroxine (T_4) and triiodothyronine (T_3) levels. When this test is performed concurrently with a T_4/T_3 test, the T_4 and T_3 levels can be interpreted more easily.

Thyroxine, Total (p. 516). This is one of the first tests performed to assess thyroid function. It is used to evaluate thyroid function and to monitor replacement and suppressive medical therapy.

Triiodothyronine (p. 525). A T_3 test is used to evaluate thyroid function, primarily in order to diagnose hyperthyroidism. It is also used to monitor thyroid replacement and suppressive medical therapy.

Triiodothyronine Uptake (p. 528). This test is an indirect measurement of total T_4.

Thyroxine Index, Free (see following test). This test is used to evaluate thyroid function. It corrects for changes in thyroid hormone–binding serum proteins that can affect total T_4 levels. It is also used to diagnose hyperthyroidism and hypothyroidism.

 Clinical Priorities

- The diagnostic value of measuring the FT_4 index is that it is not affected by TBG abnormalities. Therefore, it is correlated more closely with hormonal status than are the T_4 and T_3 tests.
- The FT_4 index is determined by a mathematical calculation involving the T_3 uptake and the T_4 values. This calculation corrects the estimated total T_4 assay for the effects of TBG protein abnormalities.
- A high FT_4 index calculation suggests hyperthyroidism. Low levels suggest hypothyroidism.

Anti–Thyroglobulin Antibody (p. 113). This test is used primarily for the differential diagnosis of thyroid diseases, such as Hashimoto thyroiditis and chronic lymphocytic thyroiditis (in children).

Thyroxine Index, Free (FTI, T$_7$, FT$_4$ Index, FT$_4$ I)

NORMAL FINDINGS

13–27 pmol/L (1.0–2.1 ng/dL)
Adult index: 1.5–4.5 U (these are arbitrary units)
    Check with the laboratory for normal values.

INDICATIONS

This test is used to evaluate thyroid function. It corrects for changes in thyroid hormone-binding serum proteins that can affect total thyroxine (T$_4$) levels. It is used to diagnose hyperthyroidism and hypothyroidism.

TEST EXPLANATION

The free thyroxine (FT$_4$) index study measures the amount of FT$_4$, which is only 1% of the total T$_4$. FT$_4$ is the unbound T$_4$ that enters the cell and is metabolically active. The diagnostic value of measuring the FT$_4$ index is that it is not affected by thyroxine-binding globulin (TBG) abnormalities; therefore, it is correlated more closely with the true hormonal status than total T$_4$ or triiodothyronine (T$_3$) determinations. To determine the FT$_4$ index, T$_3$ uptake (p. 528) is measured and multiplied by the measured T$_4$. This simple mathematical computation corrects the estimated total T$_4$ level for the effects of TBG protein alterations. If TBG level is increased, the T$_3$ uptake decreases and corrects for the increase in T$_4$ associated with the increased TBG level. However, when the TBG level is normal and the T$_4$ level is elevated, the FT$_4$ level is increased, which indicates true hyperthyroidism. Therefore, the FT$_4$ index yields the same information as the FT$_4$ radioimmunoassay.

This index is useful in diagnosing hyperthyroidism and hypothyroidism, especially in patients with abnormalities in TBG levels. High FT$_4$ index calculations suggest hyperthyroidism; low FT$_4$ index values suggest hypothyroidism. The FT$_4$ index study also aids in the evaluation of the thyroid status of pregnant women and patients who have abnormal TBG levels as a result of treatment with certain drugs (e.g., estrogen, phenytoin, salicylates).

INTERFERING FACTORS

• See factors affecting T$_4$ on p. 516 and T$_3$ uptake on p. 525.

PROCEDURE AND PATIENT CARE

Before
 Explain the procedure to the patient.
• Obtain the T$_4$ value and T$_3$ uptake ratio.

During
- Multiply the T_3 uptake value by the T_4 value to obtain the FT_4 index:
  $FT_4 \text{ index} = T_4 \text{ (total)} \times T_3 \text{ uptake (\%)} \div 100$

After
- Apply pressure or a pressure dressing to the venipuncture site.
- Check the venipuncture site for bleeding.

TEST RESULTS AND CLINICAL SIGNIFICANCE

▲ Increased Levels

Primary hyperthyroid states (e.g., Graves' disease, Plummer disease, toxic thyroid adenoma): *The thyroid produces increased amounts of T_4 despite lack of TSH stimulation.*

Acute thyroiditis: *The thyroid secretes increased amounts of T_4 during the acute inflammatory stages of thyroiditis (e.g., Hashimoto thyroiditis). However, in the latter stages, the thyroid may become "burned out," and the patient may develop hypothyroidism.*

Factitious hyperthyroidism: *Patients who self-administer T_4 have elevated levels. Many patients believe they will feel more energetic or will lose weight faster if they take T_4.*

Struma ovarii: *Ectopic thyroid tissue in the ovary or anywhere can produce excess T_4.*

▼ Decreased Levels

Hypothyroid states (e.g., cretinism, surgical ablation, myxedema): *The thyroid in these diseases cannot produce an adequate amount of T_4 despite the stimulation provided.*

Pituitary insufficiency: *The pituitary gland produces an insufficient amount of thyrotropin. As a result, the thyroid is not stimulated to produce T_4.*

Hypothalamic failure: *The hypothalamus produces an insufficient amount of thyrotropin-releasing hormone. As a result, the pituitary gland does not produce thyrotropin, and the thyroid is not stimulated to produce T_4.*

Iodine insufficiency: *Iodine is the basic raw material for T_4. Without iodine, T_4 cannot be produced. With the introduction of iodide in most table salts, iodine insufficiency has become rare in the United States and Canada.*

RELATED TESTS

Thyroid-Stimulating Immunoglobulins (p. 504). Long-acting thyroid stimulator (LATS) and other thyroid-stimulating immunoglobulins are measured to support the diagnosis of Graves' disease, especially when the differential diagnosis is complex.

Thyrotropin-Releasing Hormone (p. 506). This test assists in the evaluation of patients with hyperthyroidism and hypothyroidism. It is especially helpful in the differential diagnosis of hypothyroidism.

Thyroid-Stimulating Hormone (p. 500). This test is used to diagnose primary hypothyroidism and to differentiate it from secondary (pituitary) and tertiary (hypothalamus) hypothyroidism.

Thyroid-Stimulating Hormone Stimulation (p. 503). This test is also used to differentiate primary from secondary (and tertiary) hypothyroidism.

Thyroxine-Binding Globulin (p. 509). This major thyroid hormone protein carrier is measured for evaluation of patients who have abnormal total thyroxine (T_4) and triiodothyronine (T_3) levels. When this test is performed concurrently with a T_4/T_3 test, the T_4 and T_3 levels can be interpreted more easily.

Thyroxine, Total (see following test). This is one of the first tests done for assessing thyroid function. It is used to evaluate thyroid function and to monitor replacement and suppressive medical therapy.

Triiodothyronine (p. 525). A T_3 test is used to evaluate thyroid function, primarily in order to diagnose hyperthyroidism. It is also used to monitor thyroid replacement and suppressive medical therapy.

Thyroxine Index, Free (p. 514). This test is used to evaluate thyroid function. It corrects for changes in thyroid hormone–binding serum proteins that can affect total T_4 levels. It is also used to diagnose hyperthyroidism and hypothyroidism.

Triiodothyronine Uptake (p. 528). This test is an indirect measurement of total T_4.

Anti–Thyroglobulin Antibody (p. 113). This test is used primarily for the differential diagnosis of thyroid diseases, such as Hashimoto thyroiditis and chronic lymphocytic thyroiditis (in children).

Thyroxine, Total (T_4, Thyroxine Screen)

Age	Male, nmol/L (*Mcg*/dL)	Female, nmol/L (*Mcg*/dL)
1–30 days	**76–276** (5.9–21.5)	**81–276** (6.3–21.5)
31 days to 1 year	**82–179** (6.4–13.9)	**63–176** (4.9–13.7)
1–3 years	**90–169** (7.0–13.1)	**91–180** (7.1–14.1)
4–6 years	**79–162** (6.1–12.6)	**93–180** (7.2–14.0)
7–12 years	**86–172** (6.7–13.4)	**79–156** (6.1–12.1)
13–15 years	**62–148** (4.8–11.5)	**75–144** (5.8–11.2)
16–18 years	**76–148** (5.9–11.5)	**67–170** (5.2–13.2)

NORMAL FINDINGS

Child:

    Adult male: **51–154 nmol/L** (4–12 *Mcg*/dL)
    Adult female: **64–154 nmol/L** (5–12 *Mcg*/dL)
    Adult >60 years: **64–142 nmol/L** (5–11 *Mcg*/dL)

 ## Critical Values

Adult:

At **<26 nmol/L** (<2.0 *Mcg*/dL), myxedema coma is possible
At **>258 nmol/L** (>20 *Mcg*/dL), thyroid storm is possible
Newborn: **<90 nmol/L** (<7 *Mcg*/dL)

INDICATIONS

This is one of the first tests performed to assess thyroid function. It is used to diagnose thyroid function and to monitor replacement and suppressive medical therapy.

✓ **Clinical Priorities**

- This test is used to diagnose thyroid function and to monitor replacement or suppressive medical therapy.
- This is a very reliable test of thyroid function. However, because thyroxine (T_4) is bound to serum proteins (such as TBG), T_4 levels are affected by levels of carrier proteins. Carrier proteins can be measured by the triiodothyronine (T_3) resin uptake test. This helps in interpreting results.
- Newborns are screened with T_4 tests to detect hypothyroidism. A heelstick is used to collect the blood. Developmental delay can be prevented with early diagnosis.

TEST EXPLANATION

Thyroid hormones are produced when tyrosine incorporates organic iodine to form monoiodotyrosine. This complex picks up another iodine molecule and becomes diiodotyrosine. Two diiodotyrosine molecules combine to form tetraiodothyronine (also called T_4 *thyroid hormone*). If a diiodotyrosine molecule combines with a monoiodotyrosine molecule, triiodothyronine (also called T_3 *thyroid hormone*) is formed. T_4 makes up nearly all of thyroid hormone; T_3 makes up less than 10% of thyroid hormone. Nearly all of T_4 and T_3 is bound to protein. Thyroxine-binding globulin (TBG) binds most of T_3 and T_4. Albumin and prealbumin bind the rest. The unbound or "free" hormone is metabolically active. T_4 can be measured by radioimmunoassay or enzyme-linked immunosorbent assay techniques. The serum T_4 test is a measure of total T_4 (i.e., bound and free T_4).

Thyrotropin-releasing hormone (TRH) is secreted in the hypothalamus. This stimulates the anterior pituitary to secrete thyrotropin (thyroid-stimulating hormone [TSH]). TSH stimulates the thyroid to secrete thyroid hormone. The increased levels of T_3 and T_4 inhibit further production of TRH.

The serum T_4 study is a direct measurement of the total amount of T_4 present in the patient's blood. Levels higher than normal indicate hyperthyroid states, and subnormal values are observed in hypothyroid states. Newborns are screened with T_4 tests to detect hypothyroidism. Developmental delay can be prevented with early diagnosis.

This is a very reliable test of thyroid function; however, results are affected by TBG level. Because T_4 is bound by serum proteins such as TBG, any increase in levels of these proteins (as in pregnant women and patients taking oral contraceptives) causes factitious elevations in levels of T_4 (and T_3). Therefore, levels of these carrier proteins (e.g., TBG) are concomitantly measured (by T_3 resin uptake studies). Furthermore, T_3 resin results must be considered when the T_4 test results are interpreted.

INTERFERING FACTORS

- T_4 levels may be increased after iodinated contrast radiographic studies.
- Pregnancy causes increases in T_4 levels.
- Drugs that may cause *increases* in T_4 levels include amphetamines, clofibrate, estrogens, heroin, iodinated contrast media, iodine, methadone, and oral contraceptives.
- Drugs that may cause *decreases* in levels include anabolic steroids, androgens, anti-inflammatory agents, antithyroid drugs (e.g., propylthiouracil), barbiturates, furosemide, nonsteroidal lithium, phenytoin, and propranolol.

PROCEDURE AND PATIENT CARE

Before
- Explain the procedure to the patient.
- Evaluate the patient's medication history.
- If it is indicated, instruct the patient to stop taking exogenous T_4 medication 1 month before the test.
- Inform the patient that no fasting is required.

During

Adult
- Collect a venous blood sample in a red-top tube.

Newborn
- Perform a heelstick to obtain blood.
- Thoroughly saturate the circles on the filter paper with blood.
- Note that prompt collection and processing are crucial for the early detection of hypothyroidism.
- Note that the optimal collection time is 2 to 4 days after birth.
- All newborns should be screened before discharge (regardless of age), however, because of the consequences of delayed diagnosis.

After
- Apply pressure or a pressure dressing to the venipuncture site.
- Assess the venipuncture site for bleeding.

TEST RESULTS AND CLINICAL SIGNIFICANCE

▲ Increased Levels

Primary hyperthyroid states (e.g., Graves' disease, Plummer disease, toxic thyroid adenoma): *The thyroid produces increased amounts of T_4 despite lack of TSH stimulation.*

Acute thyroiditis: *The thyroid secretes increased amounts of T_4 during the acute inflammatory stages of thyroiditis (e.g., Hashimoto thyroiditis). However, in the latter stages, the thyroid may become "burned out," and the patient may develop hypothyroidism.*

Familial dysalbuminemic hyperthyroxinemia: *Affected patients have a genetically defective form of albumin that binds T_4 unusually tightly. As a result, the bound portion of T_4 increases. The patient is not hyperthyroid because the protein-bound T_4 is not metabolically active.*

Factitious hyperthyroidism: *Patients who self-administer T_4 have elevated levels. Many patients believe they will feel more energetic or will lose weight faster if they take T_4.*

Struma ovarii: *Ectopic thyroid tissue in the ovary or anywhere can produce excess T_4.*

TBG increase (e.g., as occurs in pregnancy, hepatitis, congenital hyperproteinemia): *Because the T_4 assay measures total bound and unbound T_4, any condition associated with elevated TBG levels causes an elevation of T_4 levels.*

▼ Decreased Levels

Hypothyroid states (e.g., cretinism, surgical ablation, myxedema): *The thyroid in these diseases cannot produce an adequate amount of T_4 despite the stimulation provided.*

Pituitary insufficiency: *The pituitary produces an insufficient amount of thyrotropin. As a result, the thyroid is not stimulated to produce T_4.*

Hypothalamic failure: *The hypothalamus produces an insufficient amount of TRH. As a result, the pituitary does not produce thyrotropin, and the thyroid is not stimulated to produce T_4.*

Protein malnutrition and other protein-depleted states (e.g., nephrotic syndrome): *When the protein source is reduced, TBG and albumin levels decrease. Because the T_4 assay measures hormone bound to these proteins, T_4 can be expected to be reduced.*

Iodine insufficiency: *Iodine is the basic raw material for T_4. Without iodine, T_4 cannot be produced. With the introduction of iodide in most table salts, iodine insufficiency is rare in the United States and Canada.*

Nonthyroid illnesses (e.g., renal failure, Cushing's disease, cirrhosis, surgery, advanced cancer): *The pathophysiologic mechanism underlying these observations is not well known. It may be related in part to a depletion of thyroid-binding proteins associated with severe medical illnesses.*

RELATED TESTS

Thyroid-Stimulating Immunoglobulins (p. 504). Long-acting thyroid stimulator (LATS) and other thyroid-stimulating immunoglobulins are measured to support the diagnosis of Graves' disease, especially when the differential diagnosis is complex.

Thyrotropin-Releasing Hormone (p. 506). This test assists in the evaluation of patients with hyperthyroidism and hypothyroidism. It is especially helpful in the differential diagnosis of hypothyroidism.

Thyroid-Stimulating Hormone (p. 500). This test is used to diagnose primary hypothyroidism and to differentiate it from secondary (pituitary) and tertiary (hypothalamus) hypothyroidism.

Thyroid-Stimulating Hormone Stimulation (p. 503). This test is also used to differentiate primary from secondary (and tertiary) hypothyroidism.

Thyroxine-Binding Globulin (p. 509). This major thyroid hormone protein carrier is measured for evaluation of patients who have abnormal total thyroxine (T_4) and triiodothyronine (T_3) levels. When this test is performed concurrently with a T_4/T_3 test, the T_4 and T_3 levels can be interpreted more easily.

Triiodothyronine Uptake (p. 528). This test is an indirect measurement of total T_4.

Triiodothyronine (p. 525). A T_3 test is used to evaluate thyroid function, primarily in order to diagnose hyperthyroidism. It is also used to monitor thyroid replacement and suppressive medical therapy.

Thyroxine Index, Free (p. 514). This test is used to evaluate thyroid function. It corrects for changes in thyroid hormone–binding serum proteins that can affect total T_4 levels. It is also used to diagnose hyperthyroidism and hypothyroidism.

Thyroxine, Free (p. 511). This test is used to evaluate thyroid function in patients who may have protein abnormalities that could affect total T_4 levels. It is used to evaluate thyroid function and to monitor replacement and suppressive medical therapy.

Anti–Thyroglobulin Antibody (p. 113). This test is used primarily for the differential diagnosis of thyroid diseases, such as Hashimoto thyroiditis and chronic lymphocytic thyroiditis (in children).

Toxoplasmosis Antibody Titre

NORMAL FINDINGS

Immunoglobulin G (IgG) titres <1:16: no previous infection
IgG titres of 1:16–1:256: prevalent in the general population
IgG titres >1:256: suggestive of recent infection
Immunoglobulin M (IgM) titres >1:256: indicative of acute infection

INDICATIONS

These serologic tests are used to diagnose acute toxoplasmosis in immunosuppressed patients, pregnant women, and newborns. Immunity obtained from prior infection (e.g., fetal infection) is also confirmed by this test.

TEST EXPLANATION

Toxoplasmosis is a protozoan disease caused by *Toxoplasma gondii,* which is found in humans and many animals (especially cats). Humans become infected by eating poorly cooked or raw meat. Exposure to feces of cats or other infected material can cause infection. Infected humans are most often asymptomatic. When symptoms occur, this disease is characterized by central nervous system lesions, which may lead to blindness, brain damage, and death. The condition may occur congenitally or sometime after birth. Estimates suggest that as many as one-third of Canadians have been exposed to toxoplasmosis, as determined by positive antibody titres. As mentioned, most acutely infected pregnant women are symptom free, and the best way to diagnose infection is by antibody testing.

The presence of antibodies before pregnancy indicates prior exposure and chronic asymptomatic infection. The presence of these antibodies probably ensures protection against congenital toxoplasmosis in the child. Fetal infection occurs if the mother acquires toxoplasmosis after the fetus's conception and passes it to the fetus through the placenta. Repeat testing of pregnant patients with low or negative titres may be done before the twentieth week and before delivery to identify antibody converters and determine appropriate therapy (e.g., therapeutic abortion at 20 weeks, treatment during the remainder of the pregnancy, or treatment of the newborn).

Hydrocephaly, microcephaly, chronic retinitis, and convulsions are complications of congenital toxoplasmosis. Congenital toxoplasmosis is diagnosed when the antibody levels are persistently elevated or a rising titre is found in the infant 2 to 3 months after birth.

The acronym *TORCH*—toxoplasmosis, other, rubella, cytomegalovirus, and herpes—has been applied to infections with recognized detrimental effects on the fetus. The effects on the fetus may be direct or indirect (e.g., precipitating spontaneous abortion or premature labour). Included in the category of "other" are infections (e.g., syphilis). All tests for infections are discussed separately.

Because of the difficulty in growing *Toxoplasma* organisms in culture, the best way to diagnose this disease is by serologic testing. A commonly used test is the indirect fluorescent antibody test. With this technique, IgM and IgG can be detected together or separately. The IgM titre rises approximately 1 week after inoculation, peaks in approximately 2 to 3 months, and declines to undetectable levels in approximately 1 year. The IgG titre begins to rise approximately 2 weeks after inoculation, peaks in approximately 2 to 3 months, and declines to low but persistent levels in approximately 6 months. Low titres of IgG especially indicate past infection and protection from passing acute infection to a fetus. High or rapidly rising titres of either IgM or IgG indicate acute infection in the adult or newborn. Hemagglutination is another more easily performed method of detecting IgG antibodies to *T. gondii*. This test is often used to screen new mothers. Enzyme-linked immunosorbent assay (ELISA) and radioimmunoassay are other techniques to identify antibodies.

Elevated numbers of IgM antibodies, IgG titres greater than 1:1 000, or a fourfold rise in IgG antibodies indicates an acute *T. gondii* infection. Low but significant titres of IgG indicate past infection. High, nonrising titres indicate acute infection more than 3 to 12 months before the test.

INTERFERING FACTORS

- Rheumatoid factor or antinuclear antibodies can cause false-positive results.
- Other active congenital infections can cause false-positive results.

PROCEDURE AND PATIENT CARE

Before

✐ Explain the procedure to the patient.

During

- Collect a venous blood sample in a red-top tube.
- On the laboratory slip, indicate whether the patient is pregnant or has been exposed to cats.

After

- Apply pressure or a pressure dressing to the venipuncture site.
- Assess the venipuncture site for bleeding.

TEST RESULTS AND CLINICAL SIGNIFICANCE

▲ Increased Levels

Toxoplasmosis

Transferrin Receptor Assay

NORMAL FINDINGS

Adult male: **2–5.0 g/L** (250–500 mg/dL)
Adult female: **1.9–4.4 g/L** (190–440 mg/dL)
Results vary depending on the testing method.

INDICATIONS

Serum transferrin receptor (TfR) concentration is used to differentiate iron-deficiency anemia from the anemia of chronic disease or other "iron-low" anemias, particularly in children.

TEST EXPLANATION

Both iron metabolism and transport are altered in chronic and critical illness. Differentiation of the anemia of chronic disease (also called *anemia of inflammation* or *anemia of aging*) from iron-deficiency anemia may be difficult, and the results of conventional laboratory assessment of iron stores may not be definitive. The most valuable iron store marker in distinguishing these two entities is the TfR concentration.

TfR is a cell surface protein found on most cells, especially those with a high requirement for iron, such as immature erythroid and malignant cells. Its function is to internalize absorbed iron into target cells. The TfR level is increased when erythropoiesis is enhanced (as often occurs in iron deficiency). The concentration of cell surface–transferrin receptor is carefully regulated by transferrin receptor messenger RNA, according to the internal iron content of the cell and its individual iron requirements. Iron-deficient cells contain increased numbers of receptors, whereas receptor numbers are downregulated in iron-replete cells.

TABLE 2-46 **Tests Used to Evaluate Iron Status**

Measurement	Aspect Tested	Iron Deficiency Anemia	Anemia of Chronic Disease	Iron Deficiency and Anemia of Chronic Disease
Ferritin	Changes in iron stores	Low	High	Normal or high
Total iron-binding capacity	Changes in iron status	High	Low	Normal or high
Serum iron	Changes in iron status	Low	Low	Low
Soluble transferrin receptor	Changes in iron status	High	Normal	High

The mean TfR concentration in patients with iron-deficiency anemia is increased in comparison with that in patients with anemia secondary to chronic critical illnesses. TfR is also useful in distinguishing iron-deficiency anemia from situations that are commonly encountered in childhood, adolescence, and during pregnancy when iron stores are uniformly low to absent. In these situations, iron-deficient erythropoiesis is not necessarily present, and TfR levels are not elevated. Finally, in situations in which iron-deficiency anemia coexists with anemia of chronic disease, transferrin receptor concentrations increase as a secondary response to the underlying iron deficiency, thus precluding the need for a bone marrow examination.

In general, to increase sensitivity and specificity, the measurement of serum soluble transferrin receptor should be performed in combination with other tests of iron status, including ferritin level, total iron-binding capacity, and serum iron level (Table 2-46). Calculation of the ratio of transferrin receptor to log ferritin concentration provides an even higher sensitivity and specificity for the detection of Fe deficiency.

The principal method for measurement of soluble transferrin receptor (TfR) is immunoturbidimetry with a commercially available clinical analyzer. Latex-bound anti-TfR antibodies react with the antigen in the sample to form an antigen-antibody complex. After agglutination, this is measured turbidimetrically.

INTERFERING FACTORS

- Individuals who live at high altitudes have a reference range that extends 6% higher than the upper level of the reference interval for TfR.
- Results are related to ethnicity. Individuals of African descent can be expected to have higher levels.
- Drugs that may cause *increases* in TfR levels include recombinant human erythropoietin.

PROCEDURE AND PATIENT CARE

Before

- Explain the procedure to the patient.
- Inform the patient that no fasting is required.

During

- Collect a venous blood sample in a red-top, green-top, or lavender-top tube (depending on laboratory preferences or techniques).

After
- Apply pressure to the venipuncture site.
- Assess the venipuncture site for bleeding.

TEST RESULTS AND CLINICAL SIGNIFICANCE

▲ Increased Serum Transferrin Receptor Levels

Iron-deficiency anemia: *TfR receptors are affected by intracellular stores of iron. Low intracellular iron levels instigate (through messenger RNA stimulus) TfR proliferation.*

▼ Decreased Serum Transferrin Receptor Levels

Hemochromatosis: *Elevations in iron stores diminish TfR levels.*

RELATED TESTS

Ferritin (p. 248). This is the most sensitive test for determining iron-deficiency anemia.

Serum Iron Level, Total Iron-Binding Capacity, and Transferrin Saturation (p. 334). These tests of iron status and storage are critical in the diagnosis of iron-deficiency anemia.

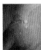

Triglycerides (TGs)

NORMAL FINDINGS

Adult/older adult:
   Male: **0.45–1.71 mmol/L** (40–150 mg/dL)
   Female: **0.40–1.52 mmol/L** (35–135 mg/dL)
Children:

Age (Years)	Male, mmol/L (mg/dL)	Female, mmol/L (mg/dL)
0–3	**0.31–1.41** (27–125)	**0.31–1.41** (27–125)
4–6	**0.36–1.31** (32–116)	**0.36–1.31** (32–116)
7–9	**0.32–1.46** (28–129)	**0.32–1.46** (28–129)
10–11	**0.27–1.55** (24–137)	**0.44–1.58** (39–140)
12–13	**0.27–1.64** (24–145)	**0.42–1.47** (37–130)
14–15	**0.38–1.86** (34–165)	**0.43–1.52** (38–135)
16–19	**0.38–1.58** (34–140)	**0.42–1.58** (37–140)

 Critical Values

>5.6 mmol/L (>500 mg/dL)

INDICATIONS

Triglyceride measurements identify the risk of developing coronary heart disease. This test is part of a lipid profile that includes the measurement of cholesterol and lipoproteins. This test is also performed on patients with suspected fat metabolism disorders.

TEST EXPLANATION

Triglycerides are a form of fat in the bloodstream. They are transported by very-low-density lipo-proteins (VLDLs) and low-density lipoproteins (LDLs). Triglycerides are produced in the liver; glycerol and other fatty acids are used as building blocks. Triglycerides act as a storage source for energy. When triglyceride levels in the blood are high, they are deposited in the fatty tissues. Triglycerides constitute most of the fat in the body and are a part of a lipid profile that also evaluates cholesterol and lipoprotein. A lipid profile is performed to assess the risk of coronary and vascular disease.

INTERFERING FACTORS

- Ingestion of fatty meals may cause elevations in triglyceride levels.
- Ingestion of alcohol may cause elevated levels of triglycerides by increasing the production of VLDL.
- Pregnancy may cause increases in levels.
- Drugs that may cause *increases* in triglyceride levels include cholestyramine, estrogens, and oral contraceptives.
- Drugs that may cause *decreases* in triglyceride levels include ascorbic acid, asparaginase, clofibrate, colestipol, fibrates, and statins.

PROCEDURE AND PATIENT CARE

Before

- Explain the procedure to the patient.
- Instruct the patient to fast for 12 to 14 hours before the test. Only water is permitted during the fast.
- Instruct the patient not to drink alcohol for 24 hours before the test.
- Inform the patient that dietary indiscretion for as much as 2 weeks before this test will influence results.

During

- Collect a venous blood sample in a red-top tube.

After

- Apply pressure or a pressure dressing to the venipuncture site.
- Assess the venipuncture site for bleeding.
- On the laboratory slip, mark the patient's age and gender.
- Instruct patients with increased triglyceride levels about diet, exercise, and appropriate weight.

TEST RESULTS AND CLINICAL SIGNIFICANCE

▲ Increased Levels

Glycogen storage disease (von Gierke disease): *Synthesis of VLDL (triglyceride-carrying proteins) is increased, whereas catabolism is decreased. Triglyceride levels in the blood increase.*

Familial hypertriglyceridemia: *This is a genetic predisposition to elevations in triglyceride levels.*

Apoprotein C-II deficiency: *This congenital disease is associated with lipoprotein lipase deficiency. Triglycerides accumulate.*

Hyperlipidemias: *As lipids in the blood increase, so does triglyceride, the major blood lipid.*

Hypothyroidism: *Catabolism of triglycerides is diminished.*

High-carbohydrate diet: *Excess carbohydrates are converted into triglycerides, and blood levels of tri-glycerides rise.*

Poorly controlled diabetes: *In diabetic patients, synthesis of triglyceride-carrying VLDL is increased and catabolism is decreased. Therefore, triglyceride blood levels increase.*

Nephrotic syndrome: *The loss of proteins diminishes the plasma oncotic pressures. This appears to stim-ulate hepatic lipoprotein synthesis of VLDL and LDL. Also, lipoprotein disposal may be diminished.*

Chronic renal failure: *Insulin levels are high in affected patients, because insulin is excreted by the kid-neys. Insulin increases lipogenesis and causes triglyceride levels to increase. Also, affected patients have a deficiency in lipoprotein lipase that clears the blood of triglycerides.*

▼ Decreased Levels

Malabsorption syndrome: *In affected patients, fat from the diet is malabsorbed. As triglyceride is the major component of dietary fat, triglyceride levels can be expected to fall in response to poor gastroin-testinal absorption.*

Abetalipoproteinemia: *In affected patients, not only is fat malabsorbed but also synthesis of apoprotein B (triglyceride-carrying lipoproteins) is defective. Triglyceride blood levels are low.*

Malnutrition: *Affected patients have diminished fat in the diet. As triglyceride is the major component of dietary fat, triglyceride levels can be expected to fall.*

Hyperthyroidism: *The catabolism of VLDL, the main triglyceride-carrying lipoprotein, is increased. Therefore, triglyceride blood levels diminish.*

RELATED TESTS

Cholesterol (p. 169). This is a measure of total cholesterol in the blood. It is a part of the lipid profile.

Lipoproteins (p. 355). These proteins play an important role in the transport of lipids in the bloodstream. They, too, have been measured in the assessment of risk for coronary heart disease.

Triiodothyronine (Radioimmunoassay [T$_3$ by RIA], Free T$_3$)

NORMAL FINDINGS

Adult : **1.1–2.9 mmol/L** (70–190 ng/dL)
Child:

Age	Male, pmol/L (ng/dL)	Female, pmol/L (ng/dL)
1–3 days	**2.2–7.4** (0.14–0.48)	**2.2–8.3** (0.14–0.54)
4–30 days	**2.2–8.4** (0.14–0.55)	**2.3–7.7** (0.15–0.50)
1–12 months	**3.1–10.6** (0.20–0.69)	**3.8–10.0** (0.25–0.65)
1–5 years	**3.7–10.3** (0.24–0.67)	**4.6–9.2** (0.30–0.60)
6–10 years	**4.4–9.2** (0.29–0.60)	**4.1–9.5** (0.27–0.62)
11–15 years	**4.8–9.1** (0.31–0.59)	**4.0–8.8** (0.26–0.57)
16–18 years	**5.4–8.8** (0.35–0.57)	**4.3–8.0** (0.28–0.52)

INDICATIONS

Triiodothyronine (T_3) measurement is used to evaluate thyroid function. It is used primarily to diagnose hyperthyroidism. It is also used to monitor thyroid replacement and suppressive medical therapy.

TEST EXPLANATION

Thyroid hormones are produced when tyrosine incorporates organic iodine to form monoiodotyrosine. This complex picks up another iodine molecule and becomes diiodotyrosine. Two diiodotyrosine molecules combine to form tetraiodothyronine (also called T_4 *thyroid hormone*). If a diiodotyrosine molecule combines with a monoiodotyrosine molecule, triiodothyronine (also called T_3 *thyroid hormone*) is formed. A large proportion of T_3 is formed in the liver by conversion of thyronine (T_4) to T_3. Like the T_4 test, the serum T_3 test is an accurate indicator of thyroid function. T_3 is less stable than T_4 because it is much less tightly bound to serum proteins than is T_4. Only approximately 7% to 10% of thyroid hormone is composed of T_3, and 70% of that T_3 is bound to proteins (thyroxine-binding globulin [TBG] and albumin). Only minute quantities are unbound, or "free." The free T_3 is metabolically active. Furthermore, measurement of free T_3 is not subject to the effects that alterations of serum proteins have on the total T_3, which is described in this test. This test measures the total bound and unbound (free) T_3. In general, when the T_3 level is below normal, the patient is in a hypothyroid state.

Other severe nonthyroid diseases can decrease T_3 levels by diminishing the conversion of T_4 to T_3 in the liver. This makes T_3 levels less useful in indicating hypothyroid states. Furthermore, there is considerable overlap between hypothyroid states and normal thyroid function. Because of this, T_3 levels are used primarily to assist in the diagnosis of hyperthyroid states. An elevated T_3 level indicates hyperthyroidism, especially when the T_4 level is also elevated. In a rare form of hyperthyroidism called T_3 *toxicosis*, the T_4 level is normal and the T_3 level is elevated.

In the hypothalamus, thyrotropin-releasing hormone (TRH) is secreted. This stimulates the anterior pituitary gland to secrete thyrotropin (thyroid-stimulating hormone [TSH]). TSH stimulates the thyroid to secrete thyroid hormone. The increased levels of T_3 and T_4 inhibit further production of TRH.

Clinical Priorities

- The T_3 test is used primarily to diagnose hyperthyroidism.
- T_3 level is less useful in the diagnosis of hypothyroidism because other nonthyroid diseases can decrease T_3 levels by decreasing the conversion of T_4 to T_3 in the liver.
- This test is not the same as the T_3 resin uptake test.

This test is performed by direct dialysis extraction of both bound T_3 and free T_3, which are measured by radioimmunoassay. This test is not the same as the T_3 uptake test and should not be confused with it.

INTERFERING FACTORS

- Radioisotope administration before the test may alter the results, if this test is performed by radioimmunoassay methods.

- Total T_3 values are increased in pregnancy because serum protein levels are increased at that time. Free T_3, however, is not affected by protein levels.
- Drugs that may cause *increases* in levels include estrogen, methadone, and oral contraceptives.
- Drugs that may cause *decreases* in levels include anabolic steroids, androgens, phenytoin (Dilantin), propranolol (Inderal), reserpine, and salicylates (high dose).

PROCEDURE AND PATIENT CARE

Before

- Explain the procedure to the patient.
- Determine whether the patient is taking any exogenous T_3 medication, because this will affect test results.
- Withhold drugs that may affect results (with physician's approval).
- Inform the patient that no fasting is required.

During

- Collect a venous blood sample in a red-top tube.

After

- Apply pressure or a pressure dressing to the venipuncture site.
- Observe the venipuncture site for bleeding.

TEST RESULTS AND CLINICAL SIGNIFICANCE

▲ Increased Levels

Primary hyperthyroid states (e.g., Graves' disease, Plummer disease, toxic thyroid adenoma): *The thyroid produces increased amounts of T_3 despite lack of TSH stimulation.*

Acute thyroiditis: *The thyroid secretes increased amounts of T_3 during the acute inflammatory stages of thyroiditis (e.g., Hashimoto thyroiditis). However, in the latter stages, the thyroid may become "burned out," and the patient may develop hypothyroidism.*

Factitious hyperthyroidism: *Patients who self-administer T_3 have elevated levels. Many patients believe they will feel more energetic or will lose weight faster if they take T_3.*

Struma ovarii: *Ectopic thyroid tissue in the ovary or anywhere else can produce excess T_3.*

TBG increase (e.g., as occurs in pregnancy, hepatitis, congenital hyperproteinemia): *Because the T_3 assay measures total bound and unbound T_3, any condition associated with elevated TBG causes elevation of T_3. Free T_3 levels are not elevated, however.*

▼ Decreased Levels

Hypothyroid states (e.g., cretinism, surgical ablation, myxedema): *The thyroid in these diseases cannot produce an adequate amount of T_3 despite the stimulation provided.*

Pituitary insufficiency: *The pituitary gland produces an insufficient amount of thyrotropin. As a result, the thyroid is not stimulated to produce T_3.*

Hypothalamic failure: *The hypothalamus produces an insufficient amount of TRH. As a result, the pituitary gland does not produce thyrotropin, and the thyroid is not stimulated to produce T_3.*

Protein malnutrition and other protein-depleted states (e.g., nephrotic syndrome): *When the protein source is reduced, TBG and albumin levels decrease. Because the T_3 assay measures hormones bound to these proteins, T_3 levels may be reduced. Free T_3 levels are unaffected by serum protein changes.*

Iodine insufficiency: *Iodine is the basic raw material for T_3. Without iodine, T_3 cannot be produced. With the introduction of iodine in most table salts, iodine insufficiency has become rare in the United States and Canada.*

Nonthyroid illnesses (e.g., renal failure, Cushing's disease, cirrhosis, surgery, advanced cancer): *The pathophysiologic mechanism underlying these observations is not well known. It may be related in part to a depletion of T_4-binding proteins, which is associated with severe medical illnesses. T_3 levels are more significantly affected by these diseases than are T_4 levels.*

Hepatic diseases: *Because a large proportion of T_3 is made by conversion of T_4 in the liver, severe liver dysfunction may affect T_3 levels. Often, however, other peripheral tissues take over T_3 synthesis by T_4 conversion.*

RELATED TESTS

Thyroid-Stimulating Immunoglobulins (p. 504). Long-acting thyroid stimulator (LATS) and other thyroid-stimulating immunoglobulins are measured to support the diagnosis of Graves' disease, especially when the differential diagnosis is complex.

Thyrotropin-Releasing Hormone (p. 506). This test assists in the evaluation of patients with hyperthyroidism and hypothyroidism. It is especially helpful in the differential diagnosis of hypothyroidism.

Thyroid-Stimulating Hormone (p. 500). This test is used to diagnose primary hypothyroidism and to differentiate it from secondary (pituitary) and tertiary (hypothalamus) hypothyroidism.

Thyroid-Stimulating Hormone Stimulation (p. 503). This test is also used to differentiate primary from secondary (and tertiary) hypothyroidism.

Thyroxine-Binding Globulin (p. 509). This major thyroid hormone protein carrier is measured for evaluation of patients who have abnormal total thyroxine (T_4) and triiodothyronine (T_3) levels. When this test is performed concurrently with a T_4/T_3 test, the T_4 and T_3 levels can be interpreted more easily.

Thyroxine, Total (p. 516). This is one of the first tests performed to assess thyroid function. It is used to evaluate thyroid function and to monitor replacement and suppressive medical therapy.

Triiodothyronine Uptake (see following test). This test is an indirect measurement of total T_4.

Thyroxine Index, Free (p. 514). This test is used to evaluate thyroid function. It corrects for changes in thyroid hormone–binding serum proteins that can affect total T_4 levels. It is used to diagnose hyperthyroidism and hypothyroidism.

Thyroxine, Free (p. 511). This test is used to evaluate thyroid function in patients who may have protein abnormalities that could affect total T_4 levels. It is used to evaluate thyroid function and to monitor replacement and suppressive medical therapy.

Anti–Thyroglobulin Antibody (p. 113). This test is used primarily for the differential diagnosis of thyroid diseases, such as Hashimoto thyroiditis and chronic lymphocytic thyroiditis (in children).

Triiodothyronine Uptake (T₃ Uptake, Resin Triiodothyronine Uptake Test [RT₃ Units, T₃ RU], Thyroid Hormone–Binding Ratio [THBR])

NORMAL FINDINGS

24%–34% uptake

INDICATIONS

Along with thyroxine (T_4), this test is used to evaluate thyroid function. Before direct T_4 assay was developed, this test was used as an indirect measurement of T_4. It is also an indirect measurement of the quantity of thyroid hormone–binding proteins.

TEST EXPLANATION

This test was originally called the *triiodothyronine (T_3) uptake.* Because it is not a measurement of T_3 but rather a measurement of the amount of unsaturated thyroid-binding sites on protein (thyroxine-binding globulin [TBG] and thyroid-binding prealbumin), the term *thyroid hormone–binding ratio* (THBR) has been adopted.

This test is actually an indirect measurement of total T_4. In this test, radioactive T_3 is added to the patient's serum along with a hormone-binding resin. The number of protein-binding sites available for the radioactive T_3 depends primarily on the amount of T_4 already occupying those sites, because T_4 represents most of the thyroid hormone that is bound to protein. The lower the T_4 levels are, the more radioactive T_3 binds on the serum proteins and less on the hormone-binding resin. The higher the T_4 levels are, the less radioactive T_3 can bind to serum proteins and the more that is available to bind to the resin. Therefore, the higher the resin uptake, the higher the T_4 level, and the lower the resin uptake, the lower the T_4 level. As may be expected, the THBR depends not only on the T_4 level but also on the amount of thyroid hormone–binding proteins, specifically TBG. As TBG level increases, the THBR decreases. Likewise, as TBG level decreases, THBR increases, if T_4 level stays the same. Therefore, it is important to measure the T_4 level and the THBR together, as shown in Table 2-47.

Pregnancy, oral contraceptives, and some genetic disorders tend to inappropriately increase the quantity of these carrying proteins. As a result, T_4 and T_3 levels may be artificially elevated, but the patient may have normal thyroid function. Similarly, androgenic hormones, concurrent serious illness, and nephrotic syndromes tend to lower the quantity of these proteins, causing artificially low T_3 and T_4 levels in euthyroid patients.

The T_3 uptake test is useful for the diagnosis of hypothyroidism or hyperthyroidism. This test is also used with the T_4 test to provide the free T_4 index. It is important to note that the radioactive T_3 units test is not a measurement of serum T_3. With the increasing availability of direct assay for T_3, T_4, and TBG, this test is used less frequently.

THBR levels consistent with hypothyroidism are not too different from low normal levels. This test is less than 60% accurate in indicating hypothyroidism.

TABLE 2-47	Results of Thyroid Hormone–Binding Ratio and Thyroxine With Clinical Diagnoses	
THBR	**Thyroxine Level**	**Clinical Diagnosis**
Increased	Increased	Hyperproteinemia (e.g., pregnancy, estrogen)
Increased	Decreased	Hypothyroidism
Decreased	Increased	Hyperthyroidism
Decreased	Decreased	Hypoproteinemia (e.g., protein wasting)

THBR, Thyroid hormone–binding ratio.

INTERFERING FACTORS

- Recent radioisotope scans before the blood collection may affect test results, if radioactive-labelled T_3 is used in this test method.
- Severe acidosis may increase THBR. The pathophysiologic process is not known.
- Drugs that may cause *increases* in TBG and thyroxine-binding prealbumin levels include anabolic steroids, heparin, phenytoin (Dilantin), salicylates (high dose), thyroid agents, and warfarin (Coumadin).
- Drugs that may cause *decreases* in levels include antithyroid agents, clofibrate, estrogen, oral contraceptives, and thiazides.

PROCEDURE AND PATIENT CARE

Before
- Explain the procedure to the patient.
- Inform the patient that no fasting is required.

During
- Collect a venous blood sample in a red-top tube.
- On the laboratory slip, list any drugs that the patient is taking that may affect test results.

After
- Apply pressure or a pressure dressing to the venipuncture site.
- Assess the venipuncture site for bleeding.

TEST RESULTS AND CLINICAL SIGNIFICANCE

▲ Increased Levels

Hyperthyroidism: *With increased production of T_4 and T_3, blood levels rise. Fewer TBG-binding sites are available for the radioactive T_3, which then binds an increased percentage of resin sites.*

Hypoproteinemia (e.g., protein malnutrition, protein-losing enteropathy, nephropathy): *Fewer TBG-binding sites are available for the radioactive T_3, which then binds an increased percentage of resin sites.*

Familial dysalbuminemic hyperthyroxinemia: *Affected patients have a genetically defective form of albumin that binds T_4 unusually tightly. Fewer binding sites are available for the radioactive T_3, which then binds an increased percentage of resin sites.*

Nonthyroid conditions (e.g., renal failure, Cushing's disease, cirrhosis, surgery, advanced cancer): *The pathophysiologic mechanism underlying these observations is not well known. It may be related in part to a depletion of thyroid-binding proteins, which is associated with severe medical illnesses. Fewer protein binding sites are available for radioactive T_3, which then binds an increased percentage of resin sites.*

Factitious hyperthyroidism: *Patients who self-administer T_4 have elevated levels. Fewer TBG-binding sites are available for the radioactive T_3, which then binds an increased percentage of resin sites.*

Struma ovarii: *Ectopic thyroid tissue in the ovary or anywhere can produce excess T_4. Fewer TBG-binding sites are available for the radioactive T_3, which then binds an increased percentage of resin sites.*

▼ Decreased Levels

An increase in TBG level (e.g., as occurs in pregnancy, hepatitis, congenital hyperproteinemia): *More protein-binding sites are available for radioactive T_3; therefore, less radioactive T_3 is bound to the resin.*

Hypothyroid states (e.g., cretinism, surgical ablation, pituitary insufficiency, hypothalamic failure, myxedema): *The thyroid in these diseases does not produce an adequate amount of T_4. T_4 levels are decreased. More protein-binding sites are available for radioactive T_3 binding, and less is bound to the resin.*

Hepatitis and cirrhosis: *These illnesses are associated with elevated TBG. Therefore, more protein-binding sites are available for radioactive T_3, and less radioactive T_3 is bound to the resin.*

RELATED TESTS

Thyroid-Stimulating Immunoglobulins (p. 504). Long-acting thyroid stimulator (LATS) and other thyroid-stimulating immunoglobulins are measured to support the diagnosis of Graves' disease, especially when the differential diagnosis is complex.

Thyrotropin-Releasing Hormone (p. 506). This test assists in the evaluation of patients with hyperthyroidism and hypothyroidism. It is especially helpful in the differential diagnosis of hypothyroidism.

Thyroid-Stimulating Hormone (p. 500). This test is used to diagnose primary hypothyroidism and to differentiate it from secondary (pituitary) and tertiary (hypothalamus) hypothyroidism.

Thyroid-Stimulating Hormone Stimulation (p. 503). This test is also used to differentiate primary from secondary (and tertiary) hypothyroidism.

Thyroxine-Binding Globulin (p. 509). This major thyroid hormone protein carrier is measured for evaluation of patients who have abnormal total thyroxine (T_4) and triiodothyronine (T_3) levels. When this test is performed concurrently with a T_4/T_3 test, the T_4 and T_3 levels can be interpreted more easily.

Thyroxine, Total (p. 516). This is one of the first tests performed to assess thyroid function. It is used to evaluate thyroid function and to monitor replacement and suppressive medical therapy.

Triiodothyronine (p. 525). A T_3 test is used to evaluate thyroid function, primarily in order to diagnose hyperthyroidism. It is also used to monitor thyroid replacement and suppressive medical therapy.

Thyroxine Index, Free (p. 514). This test is used to evaluate thyroid function. It corrects for changes in thyroid hormone–binding serum proteins that can affect total T_4 levels. It is also used to diagnose hyperthyroidism and hypothyroidism.

Thyroxine, Free (p. 511). This test is used to evaluate thyroid function in patients who may have protein abnormalities that could affect total T_4 levels. It is used to evaluate thyroid function and to monitor replacement and suppressive medical therapy.

Anti–Thyroglobulin Antibody (p. 113). This test is used primarily for the differential diagnosis of thyroid diseases, such as Hashimoto thyroiditis and chronic lymphocytic thyroiditis (in children).

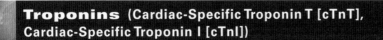

Troponins (Cardiac-Specific Troponin T [cTnT], Cardiac-Specific Troponin I [cTnI])

NORMAL FINDINGS

Cardiac troponin T: **<0.1 *Mcg*/L** (<0.1 ng/mL)
Cardiac troponin I: **<0.35 *Mcg*/L** (<0.35 ng/mL)

INDICATIONS

This test is performed on patients with chest pain to determine whether the pain is caused by cardiac ischemia. It is a specific indicator of cardiac muscle injury. It is also helpful in predicting the possibility of future cardiac events.

TEST EXPLANATION

Cardiac troponins are biochemical markers for cardiac disease. This test is used to assist in the evaluation of patients with suspected acute coronary ischemic syndromes. In addition to improving the diagnosis of acute ischemic disorders, troponins are also valuable for early risk stratification in patients with unstable angina. They can be used to predict the likelihood of future cardiac events.

Troponins are proteins that exist in skeletal and cardiac muscle and that regulate the calcium-dependent interaction of myosin with actin for the muscle contractile apparatus. Cardiac troponins can be distinguished from skeletal troponins by the use of monoclonal antibodies or enzyme-linked immunosorbent assay (ELISA). There are two cardiac-specific troponins: cardiac troponin T (cTnT), and cardiac troponin I (cTnI).

Because of their extraordinarily high specificity for myocardial cell injury, cardiac troponins are very informative in the evaluation of patients with chest pain. Use of their measurements is similar to that of creatine phosphokinase MB (CPK-MB; see p. 201). However, cardiac troponins have several advantages over CPK-MB. Cardiac troponins are more specific for cardiac muscle injury. CPK-MB levels can be elevated with severe skeletal muscle injury, with brain or lung injury, or in renal failure. Cardiac troponin levels are nearly always normal in noncardiac muscle diseases. Cardiac troponins become elevated sooner and remain elevated longer than does CPK-MB. This expands the time window of opportunity for diagnosis and thrombolytic treatment of myocardial injury. Finally, cTnT and cTnI are more sensitive to muscle injury than CPK-MB. That is most important in evaluating patients with chest pain.

Cardiac troponin levels become elevated as early as 3 hours after myocardial injury. Levels of cTnI may remain elevated for 7 to 10 days after myocardial infarction, and cTnT levels may remain elevated for up to 14 days. Measurement of these troponins is preferable to measurement of lactate dehydrogenase (see p. 339) and its isoenzymes in patients who seek medical attention more than 24 to 48 hours after the onset of symptoms. However, if reinfarction is considered, troponin levels are not informative because they could be elevated just from the first ischemic event. Each cardiac monitor has its specific use, depending on the time from onset of chest pain to the time of presentation to the hospital.

Troponins can be detected by monoclonal antibody immunoassay, by ELISA, and by monoclonal "sandwich" antibody qualitative testing. The test results with the first two laboratory techniques listed are available after approximately 2 hours. The "sandwich" technique is performed at the bedside in approximately 20 minutes, and results are read visually, much in the same way as a glucometer. Because of this fast turnaround time, this blood test is extremely useful. The earlier myocardial injury is detected, the more rapidly treatment directed toward revascularization can begin. The earlier revascularization occurs, the less myocardial muscle is injured.

Cardiac troponins are used in the following cardiac clinical situations:

1. Evaluation of patients with unstable angina. Such patients can be treated in one of two ways on the basis of information from cardiac troponins. If cardiac troponin levels are normal, no myocardial injury has occurred, and there is no lasting cardiac dysfunction. If cardiac troponin levels are elevated, muscle injury has occurred. Thrombolytic therapy may be indicated because patients with this latter situation are at great risk for a subsequent cardiac event (infarction or sudden death).

2. Detection of reperfusion associated with coronary recanalization. A "washout" or second peak of cardiac troponin levels accurately indicates reperfusion by way of recanalization or coronary angioplasty.
3. Estimation of myocardial infarction size. Late (4 weeks) cardiac troponin levels are inversely related to left ventricular ejection fraction. These late elevations in cardiac troponin levels are related to degradation of the contractile apparatus.
4. Detection of perioperative myocardial infarction. The use of CPK-MB determinations in the diagnosis of myocardial infarction after surgery is difficult because of the frequent increase in levels of this enzyme, which is associated with skeletal muscle injury during surgery. Cardiac troponin levels are not affected by skeletal muscle injury.
5. Evaluation of the severity of pulmonary emboli. Elevated troponin levels may indicate more severe disease and the need for thrombolytic therapy.
6. Heart failure. Persistently elevated troponin levels indicate continued ventricular strain.

INTERFERING FACTORS

- Troponin T levels are artificially *elevated* in dialysis patients.

PROCEDURE AND PATIENT CARE

Before

🖐 Explain the procedure to the patient.
🖐 Discuss with the patient the need and reason for frequent venipuncture in diagnosing myocardial infarction.
🖐 Inform the patient that no food or fluid restrictions are necessary.

During

- Collect a venous blood sample in a yellow-top (serum separator) tube. This is usually done initially and 12 hours later, followed by daily testing for 3 to 5 days and possibly weekly for 5 to 6 weeks.
- Rotate the venipuncture sites.
- On each laboratory slip, record the exact time and date of venipuncture. This aids in the interpretation of the temporal pattern of enzyme elevations.
- If a qualitative immunoassay is to be done at the patient's bedside, whole blood is obtained in a micropipette and placed in the sample well of the testing device. A red or purple colour in the "read" zone indicates that 0.2 Mcg/L (0.2 ng/mL) or more of cardiac troponin is present in the patient's blood.

After

- Apply pressure or a pressure dressing to the venipuncture site.
- Observe the venipuncture site for bleeding.

TEST RESULTS AND CLINICAL SIGNIFICANCE

▲ Increased Levels

Myocardial injury,
Myocardial infarction: *This myocardial intracellular protein becomes available to the bloodstream after myocardial cell death because of ischemia. Blood levels therefore rise. Normally, no troponins can be detected in the blood.*

RELATED TESTS

Creatine Kinase (p. 201). Elevation of the CPK-MB level in this blood test is closely linked to myocardial muscle. It is elevated early in myocardial injury. Its usefulness is limited in patients who have had chest pain for more than 24 hours.

Myoglobin (p. 378). This protein is a nonspecific indicator of cardiac disease. However, it is also elevated with skeletal muscle disease or trauma.

Electrocardiography (p. 568). This is the electrodiagnostic test most commonly used to detect myocardial injury and infarction.

Urea Nitrogen, Blood (Blood Urea Nitrogen [BUN], Serum Urea Nitrogen)

NORMAL FINDINGS

Adult: **2.9–8.2 mmol/L** (8–23 mg/dL)
Older adult: may be slightly higher than adult
Child: **1.8–6.4 mmol/L** (5–18 mg/dL)
Infant: **1.8–6.0 mmol/L** (5–17 mg/dL)
Newborn: **0.7–4.6 mmol/L** (2–13 mg/dL)
Umbilical cord: **7.5–14.3 mmol/L** (21–40 mg/dL)

 Critical Values

>35 mmol/L (>100 mg/dL) indicates serious impairment of renal function

INDICATIONS

Blood urea nitrogen (BUN) is an indirect and rough measurement of renal function and glomerular filtration rate (if normal liver function exists). It is also a measurement of liver function. The test is performed on patients undergoing routine laboratory testing. It is usually performed as a part of a multiphasic automated testing process.

TEST EXPLANATION

The BUN is a measure of the amount of urea nitrogen in the blood. Urea is formed in the liver as the end product of protein metabolism and digestion. During ingestion, protein is broken down into amino acids. In the liver, these amino acids are catabolized and free ammonia is formed. The ammonia molecules are combined to form urea, which is then deposited in the blood and transported to the kidneys for excretion. Therefore, the BUN level is directly related to the metabolic function of the liver and the excretory function of the kidneys. It serves as an index of the function of these organs. Patients who have elevated BUN levels are said to have azotemia or be azotemic.

Nearly all renal diseases cause an inadequate excretion of urea, which causes the blood concentration to rise above normal. If the disease is unilateral, however, the unaffected kidney can compensate for the diseased kidney, and the BUN level may not become elevated. The BUN level also increases in conditions other than primary renal disease. In prerenal azotemia, the BUN level is elevated as a result of pathologic conditions that affect urea nitrogen accumulation before it reaches the kidneys. Such conditions include shock, dehydration, heart failure, and excessive protein catabolism. Another cause of prerenal azotemia is gastrointestinal bleeding, in which variable and sometimes significant amounts of blood are leaked into the intestinal tract. The proteins in the blood and blood cells are digested and converted to urea. As the marked increase in intestinal urea is absorbed, the BUN level increases, sometimes significantly. *Postrenal azotemia* is caused by pathologic conditions that affect urea nitrogen accumulation after it reaches the kidneys. Examples of such conditions include ureteral and urethral obstruction.

The synthesis of urea depends on the liver. Patients with severe primary liver disease have a decreased BUN level. With combined liver and renal disease (as in hepatorenal syndrome), the BUN level can be normal because poor hepatic functioning results in decreased formation of urea and is not an indicator that renal excretory function is adequate.

The BUN level is interpreted in conjunction with results of the creatinine test. These tests are referred to as *renal function studies.* The BUN/creatinine ratio is a good measurement of kidney and liver function. The normal adult range is 6 to 25; 15.5 is the optimal value.

INTERFERING FACTORS

- Changes in protein intake may affect BUN levels. Low-protein diets decrease BUN level if caloric intake is maintained with carbohydrates. High-protein diets or alimentary tube feeding is associated with elevated BUN levels.
- To some degree, muscle mass determines BUN levels. Women and children tend to have lower BUN levels than do men.
- Advanced pregnancy may cause increases in levels as a result of high protein metabolism.
- Gastrointestinal bleeding can cause increases in BUN levels.
- Overhydration and underhydration affect BUN levels. In overhydrated patients, BUN tends to be diluted and levels are lower. In dehydrated patients, BUN tends to be concentrated and levels are higher.
- Drugs that may cause *increases* in BUN levels include allopurinol, aminoglycosides, cephalosporins, chloral hydrate, cisplatin, furosemide, guanethidine, indomethacin, methotrexate, methyldopa, nephrotoxic drugs (e.g., aspirin, amphotericin B, bacitracin, carbamazepine, colistin, gentamicin, methicillin, neomycin, penicillamine, polymyxin B, probenecid, vancomycin), propranolol, rifampin, spironolactone, tetracyclines, thiazide diuretics, and triamterene.
- Drugs that may cause *decreases* in levels include chloramphenicol and streptomycin.

✓ Clinical Priorities

- Almost all renal diseases cause an inadequate excretion of urea, which causes the BUN level to rise. Because the synthesis of urea depends on the liver, severe liver disease can cause a decrease in BUN level. Therefore, the BUN level is directly related to the metabolic function of the liver and the excretory function of the kidney.
- Changes in protein intake can affect BUN levels. Low-protein diets can decrease the BUN level, and high-protein diets can increase BUN levels.
- Hydration status can also affect levels. Overhydration dilutes the BUN and causes lower levels. Dehydration tends to concentrate the BUN and cause higher levels.

PROCEDURE AND PATIENT CARE

Before
☒ Explain the procedure to the patient.
☒ Inform the patient that no fasting is required.

During
- Collect a venous blood sample in a red-top tube.
- Avoid hemolysis.

After
- Apply pressure or a pressure dressing to the venipuncture site.
- Observe the venipuncture site for bleeding.

TEST RESULTS AND CLINICAL SIGNIFICANCE

▲ Increased Levels
Prerenal causes,

Hypovolemia,

Shock,

Burns,

Dehydration: *With reduced blood volume, renal blood flow is diminished. Therefore, renal excretion of BUN is decreased, and BUN levels rise.*

Heart failure,

Myocardial infarction: *With reduced cardiac function, renal blood flow is diminished. Therefore, renal excretion of BUN is decreased, and BUN levels rise.*

Gastrointestinal bleeding,

Excessive protein ingestion (alimentary tube feeding): *Blood or feeding supplements overload the gut with protein. Urea is formed at a higher rate, and BUN accumulates.*

Excessive protein catabolism,

Starvation: *As protein is broken down to amino acids at an accelerated rate, urea is formed at a higher rate, and BUN accumulates.*

Sepsis: *For a host of reasons, renal blood flow and primary renal function are reduced. BUN levels rise.*

Renal disease (e.g., glomerulonephritis, pyelonephritis, acute tubular necrosis),

Renal failure,

Nephrotoxic drugs: *Primary renal diseases are all associated with reduced excretion of BUN.*

Ureteral obstruction from stones, tumour, or congenital anomalies,

Bladder outlet obstruction from prostatic hypertrophy or cancer or bladder/urethral congenital anomalies: *Obstruction of the flow of urine causes reduction in BUN excretion, and BUN levels rise.*

Postrenal azotemia

▼ Decreased Levels
Liver failure: *BUN is made in the liver from urea. Reduced liver function is associated with reduced BUN levels.*

Overhydration because of fluid overload in the syndrome of inappropriate antidiuretic hormone secretion (SIADH): *BUN is diluted by fluid overload.*

Negative nitrogen balance (e.g., malnutrition, malabsorption): *With protein depletion, urea production is reduced; therefore, BUN level is reduced.*

Pregnancy: *Early pregnancy is associated with increased water retention and BUN dilution.*
Nephrotic syndrome: *This syndrome is associated with protein loss in the urine. With protein depletion, BUN level is reduced.*

RELATED TESTS

Creatinine, Blood (p. 205). This is a more accurate test of renal function that is not dependent on liver function.
Creatinine Clearance (p. 208). This is another more accurate test of renal function.

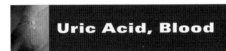
Uric Acid, Blood

NORMAL FINDINGS

Adult
Male: 240–501 *Mc*mol/L (4.0–8.5 mg/dL)
Female: 160–430 *Mc*mol/L (2.7–7.3 mg/dL)
Older adult: Values may be slightly increased.
Child: 150–320 *Mc*mol/L (2.5–5.5 mg/dL)
Newborn: 120–370 *Mc*mol/L (2.0–6.2 mg/dL)

 Critical Values

>710 *Mc*mol/L (>12 mg/dL)

INDICATIONS

This test is used in the evaluation of gout or recurrent urinary calculus.

TEST EXPLANATION

Uric acid is a nitrogenous compound that is the final breakdown product of purine (a DNA building block) catabolism. Seventy-five percent of uric acid is excreted by the kidney and 25% by the intestinal tract. When uric acid levels are elevated (hyperuricemia), the patient may have gout. Gout is a form of arthritis caused by deposition of uric acid crystals in periarticular tissue. Soft-tissue deposits of uric acid (tophi) can also develop. Uric acid can become supersaturated in the urine and crystallize to form kidney stones that can block the ureters.

Uric acid is made primarily in the liver. The blood level is determined by the rate of synthesis by the liver and the rate of excretion by the kidneys. Uric acid level varies somewhat with age and sex.

Causes of hyperuricemia can be overproduction or decreased excretion of uric acid (e.g., kidney failure). Overproduction of uric acid may occur in patients with a catabolic enzyme deficiency that stimulates purine metabolism, or in patients with cancer, in whom purine and DNA turnover is great. Many causes of hyperuricemia are undefined and are therefore considered idiopathic.

INTERFERING FACTORS

- Stress may cause increases in uric acid levels.
- Radiographic contrast agents increase uric acid excretion and may cause decreases in levels.
- High-protein infusion (especially glycine), as in total parental nutrition, may cause increases in uric acid, which is a breakdown product of glycine.
- Drugs that may cause *increases* in levels include alcohol, ascorbic acid, aspirin (low dose), caffeine, cisplatin, diazoxide, epinephrine, ethambutol, levodopa, methyldopa, nicotinic acid, phenothiazines, and theophylline.
- Drugs that may cause *decreases* in levels include allopurinol, aspirin (high dose), azathioprine, clofibrate, corticosteroids, diuretics, estrogens, glucose infusions, guaifenesin, mannitol, probenecid, and warfarin.

PROCEDURE AND PATIENT CARE

Before

- Explain the procedure to the patient.
- Instruct the patient with regard to the institution's requirements regarding fasting. (Some authorities recommend that the patient fast.)

During

- Collect a venous blood sample in a red-top tube.

After

- Apply pressure or a pressure dressing to the venipuncture site.
- Assess the venipuncture site for bleeding.

TEST RESULTS AND CLINICAL SIGNIFICANCE

▲ Increased (Hyperuricemia)

Increased Production of Uric Acid

Increased ingestion of purines: *Nucleic acid content is high in such foods as liver, sweetbreads, kidney beans, and anchovies.*

Genetic inborn error in purine metabolism: *The most common such error is an X-linked disorder that causes an increase in levels of an enzyme; this leads to increased synthesis of purines and therefore an increased amount of purine breakdown products, including uric acid. A second type of genetic error is a deficiency of an enzyme that produces RNA and DNA from building blocks of those substances. When levels of this enzyme are deficient, these building blocks accumulate and are broken down to uric acid, which is then present in high levels in the blood.*

Metastatic cancer,

Multiple myeloma,

Leukemias,

Cancer chemotherapy: *Rapid cell destruction associated with rapidly growing cancers (with high cell turnover), especially after chemotherapy for rapidly growing tumours, causes the cells to lyse and spill their nucleic acids into the bloodstream. These free nucleic acids are converted to uric acid in the liver. Levels of uric acid increase.*

Hemolysis: *Both the nucleic acid and adenosine triphosphate (ATP) in the red blood cell (RBC) are spilled into the bloodstream when hemolysis occurs. These free nucleic acids are converted to uric acid in the liver. Levels of uric acid increase.*

Rhabdomyolysis (e.g., heavy exercise, burns, crush injury, epileptic seizure, myocardial infarction): *Muscle cell lysis leads to excessive muscle ATP levels (uric acid is a breakdown product of ATP) in the blood. Uric acid levels increase.*

Decreased Excretion of Uric Acid

Idiopathic: *This is the most common cause of hyperuricemia. For unknown reasons, affected patients have reduced uric acid clearance in the kidneys. As a result, uric acid accumulates in the blood. Patients with gout excrete less than half the uric acid in their urine that normal persons do.*

Chronic renal disease: *The pathophysiologic explanation for why affected patients cannot excrete uric acid in appropriate quantities is not completely clear. The reason may be decreased glomerular filtration only, but other mechanisms seem to be at work as well.*

Acidosis (ketotic [diabetic or starvation] or lactic): *Decreased renal tubular secretion of uric acid in the urine causes reduced excretion of uric acid. Furthermore, keto acids (as occur in diabetic or alcoholic ketoacidosis) may compete with uric acid for tubular excretion and may cause decreases in uric acid excretion. Uric acid levels increase in the blood.*

Hypothyroidism,

Toxemia of pregnancy,

Hyperlipoproteinemia: *The pathophysiologic mechanism underlying these observations is not well defined.*

Alcoholism: *Alcohol consumption causes accelerated breakdown of ATP in the liver, which increases uric acid production. The chronic acidosis from excessive alcohol ingestion decreases renal tubular secretion of uric acid into the urine. Both lead to hyperuricemia.*

Shock or chronic blood volume depletion states: *The increased tubular reabsorption of water and electrolytes causes increased tubular reabsorption of uric acid.*

▼ Decreased Levels

Wilson disease,

Fanconi's syndrome,

Lead poisoning: *Wilson disease and accompanying Fanconi's syndrome are associated with increased uric acid renal excretion. Heavy metal poisoning is also associated with this observation.*

Yellow atrophy of liver: *With severe liver dysfunction, uric acid is not made, and levels in the blood are low.*

RELATED TEST

Uric Acid, Urine (p. 989). This test is used to evaluate uric acid levels in the urine and is used in the evaluation of patients with nephrolithiasis.

Uroporphyrinogen-1-Synthase

NORMAL FINDINGS

81.9–129.6 U/mol of hemoglobin (1.27–2.00 mU/g of hemoglobin)

INDICATIONS

This test is used to identify persons at risk for porphyria. It is also used to diagnose porphyria in the acute and latent stages.

TEST EXPLANATION

Porphyria is a group of genetic disorders characterized by an accumulation of porphyrin products in the liver or red blood cell (RBC). Liver porphyrias are much more common. Symptoms of liver porphyrias include abdominal pain, neuromuscular signs and symptoms, constipation, and occasionally psychotic behaviour. This group of disorders results from enzymatic deficiencies in the synthesis of heme (a portion of hemoglobin). Acute intermittent porphyria is the most common form of liver porphyria; this is caused by a deficiency in uroporphyrinogen-1-synthase (also called *porphobilinogen deaminase*). This enzyme is necessary for erythroid cells to make heme.

Most patients with acute intermittent porphyria have no symptoms (latent phase) until the acute phase is precipitated by surgery, infection, a low-calorie diet, or certain drugs (Box 2-15). The acute phase is highlighted by symptoms of abdominal and muscular pain, nausea, vomiting, hypertension, mental symptoms (anxiety, insomnia, hallucinations, paranoia), sensory loss, and urinary retention. Hemolytic anemia also may occur with these acute attacks. These acute symptoms are associated with increased serum and urine levels of porphyrin precursors (see urine tests for aminolevulinic acid [p. 955], porphyrins and porphobilinogens [p. 974]).

This enzyme is significantly reduced during the acute and latent phases of this disorder. It is important to identify this disease process because acute bouts of porphyria are occasionally fatal. The acute phase can be avoided by controlling factors that can precipitate the acute symptoms.

PROCEDURE AND PATIENT CARE

Before

- Explain the procedure to the patient.
- Inform the patient that no fasting is required.

During

- Collect a peripheral venous blood sample in a lavender-top tube.
- Because this test is based on the hemoglobin measurement, measure the patient's hemoglobin level at the same time.

BOX 2-15	Drugs That Precipitate Acute Porphyria	
- Barbiturates	- Estrogens/progestins	- Chlordiazepoxide
- Sulphonamides	- Valproic acid	- Phenylbutazone
- Succinimides	- Methyldopa	- Amphetamines
- Carbamazepine	- Theophylline	- Meprobamate
- Phenytoin	- Danazol	- Glutethimide
- Ergots	- Alcohol	- Arsenic

After

- Apply pressure or a pressure dressing to the venipuncture site.
- Assess the venipuncture site for bleeding.
- Blood samples should be stored frozen during laboratory transfer to avoid an artificial decrease in enzyme level.
- On the laboratory slip, indicate whether the patient is having symptoms of acute porphyria.

TEST RESULTS AND CLINICAL SIGNIFICANCE

▼ Decreased Levels

Acute intermittent porphyria

RELATED TESTS

Delta-Aminolevulinic Acid, Urine (p. 955). This test is used to diagnose porphyria. It is also used in the evaluation of children with subclinical lead poisoning.

Porphyrins and Porphobilinogens (p. 974). This is a quantitative measurement of porphyrins and porphobilinogen in the urine. This test helps define the porphyrin pattern that can classify the type of porphyria.

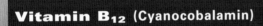

Vitamin B$_{12}$ (Cyanocobalamin)

NORMAL FINDINGS

Vitamin B$_{12}$: **118–701 pmol/L** (160–950 pg/mL)
Urinary methylmalonic acid (UMMA): <3.6 Mcmol/L

INDICATIONS

This test measures the amount of vitamin B$_{12}$ in the blood. It is used to identify the cause of megaloblastic anemia and to evaluate malnourished patients.

TEST EXPLANATION

Vitamin B$_{12}$ is necessary for conversion of the inactive form of folate to the active form. This reaction is vital for the synthesis of nucleic acids and amino acids. This is most notable in the formation and function of red blood cells (RBCs). Vitamin B$_{12}$ deficiency, like folic acid deficiency, causes anemia. The RBCs formed in the presence of these deficiencies become large and megaloblastic. These RBCs cannot conform to the size of small capillaries; instead, they fracture and hemolyze. The shortened life span ultimately leads to anemia. RBCs are not the only blood cells affected. Other marrow cells are also affected; for example, neutrophils may be giant-sized and segmented, and platelets may be large and nucleated. It may take 6 to 18 months of vitamin B$_{12}$ depletion before anemia develops.

Meats, eggs, and dairy products are the main source of vitamin B$_{12}$. In the stomach, gastric acid detaches vitamin B$_{12}$ from its binding proteins. Intrinsic factor, necessary for vitamin B$_{12}$ absorption in the small intestine, is made in the stomach mucosa. Without intrinsic factor, vitamin B$_{12}$ cannot be absorbed. Deficiency of intrinsic factor is the most common cause of vitamin B$_{12}$ deficiency (pernicious anemia). The next most common cause of vitamin B$_{12}$ deficiency is lack of gastric acid to separate the ingested vitamin B$_{12}$ from its binding proteins. A third cause of vitamin B$_{12}$ deficiency is malabsorption that results from diseases of the small terminal ileum.

Serum vitamin B$_{12}$ level is a measurement of recent vitamin B$_{12}$ ingestion. More prolonged vitamin B$_{12}$ deficiency is better and more easily assessed with UMMA measurement. Elevated serum UMMA levels are direct measures of tissue vitamin B$_{12}$ activity. The active form of vitamin B$_{12}$ is essential in the intracellular conversion of L-methylmalonyl coenzyme A (MMA CoA) to succinyl coenzyme A. Without vitamin B$_{12}$, MMA CoA metabolism is diverted to make large quantities of L-methylmalonyl. L-Methylmalonyl is then excreted by the kidneys.

UMMA is measured by mass spectrometry in a random spot urine specimen. The UMMA value is normalized to urine creatinine to correct for urine dilution. The urinary L-methylmalonyl–creatinine ratio test is more accurate than the serum L-methylmalonyl level because it indicates tissue–cellular vitamin B$_{12}$ deficiency.

INTERFERING FACTORS

- Chloral hydrate is known to cause *increases* in vitamin B$_{12}$ levels.
- Drugs known to cause *decreases* in vitamin B$_{12}$ levels include alcohol, aminoglycosides, salicylic acid, anticonvulsants, colchicine, and oral contraceptives.

PROCEDURE AND PATIENT CARE

Before

- Explain the procedure to the patient.
- Inform the patient that no fasting is usually required. (Determine whether the laboratory requires fasting, and instruct the patient accordingly.)
- Instruct the patient not to consume alcoholic beverages before the test as ordered by physician.
- Collect the specimen before starting vitamin B$_{12}$ therapy.

During

- Collect a venous blood sample in a red-top tube.

After

- Apply pressure or a pressure dressing to the venipuncture site.
- Assess the venipuncture site for bleeding.
- Transport the blood immediately to the laboratory after collection.

TEST RESULTS AND CLINICAL SIGNIFICANCE

▲ Increased Levels

Leukemia,
Polycythemia vera: *The pathophysiologic mechanism underlying these observations is not well known.*
Severe liver dysfunction,
Myeloproliferative disease: *In these illnesses, levels of transcobalamin (a vitamin B$_{12}$ carrier protein) are increased, producing an artificially high vitamin B$_{12}$ level.*

▼ **Decreased Levels**

Pernicious anemia: *Intrinsic factor, necessary for vitamin B_{12} absorption, is deficient.*

Malabsorption syndromes (e.g., inflammatory bowel disease, sprue, Crohn's disease): *Absorption of vitamin B_{12} is inadequate.*

Intestinal worm infestation: *There is competition for vitamin B_{12} in the gut. Very little vitamin B_{12} is left for absorption.*

Atrophic gastritis,

Zollinger-Ellison syndrome,

Large proximal gastrectomy: *Intrinsic factor, necessary for vitamin B_{12} absorption, is deficient because the mucosal gastric cells necessary for production of intrinsic factor are absent.*

Resection of terminal ileum: *Vitamin B_{12} is absorbed at the terminal portion of the ileum. Without that piece of intestine, vitamin B_{12} cannot be absorbed.*

Achlorhydria: *Gastric acid is necessary to separate vitamin B_{12} from binding proteins. Without gastric acid, vitamin B_{12} stays bound and cannot be absorbed from the intestine.*

Pregnancy: *Vitamin B_{12} deficiency in pregnancy is probably caused by a combination of inadequate intake and increased demand placed by the fetus on the maternal source of folic acid.*

Vitamin C deficiency,

Folic acid deficiency: *The pathophysiologic mechanism underlying these observations is not clear.*

RELATED TESTS

Folic Acid (p. 256). This is a measurement of serum folic acid level. Folic acid level should always be determined when vitamin B_{12} levels are measured. The clinical symptoms of either deficiency are the same.

Schilling Test (p. 862). This test assists in the determination of the cause of vitamin B_{12} deficiency.

Complete Blood Cell Count and Differential Count (p. 187). This group of tests is performed routinely and can reveal megaloblastic anemia.

Vitamin D (25-Hydroxyvitamin D)

NORMAL FINDINGS

Total 25-hydroxyvitamin D: **75–200 nmol/L** (30–80 ng/mL)

INDICATIONS

Vitamin D levels are used to ensure that postmenopausal women have adequate vitamin D levels to absorb dietary calcium. Because of the increased number of research investigations of the role of vitamin D in osteoporosis and cancer prevention, this blood test is being performed in increasing numbers of patients.

TEST EXPLANATION

Vitamin D is a fat-soluble vitamin. The two major forms of vitamin D are vitamin D_2 (or ergocalciferol) and vitamin D_3 (or cholecalciferol). The term *vitamin D* also refers to the "hydroxy-" metabolites of these substances. Vitamin D_2 is provided by dietary sources. Because only fish is naturally rich in vitamin D, most of the vitamin D_2 intake in the industrialized world is from fortified products, such as milk, soy milk, and breakfast cereals or supplements.

Vitamin D_3 is produced in skin exposed to sunlight, specifically ultraviolet B radiation. In this scenario, 7-dehydrocholesterol reacts with ultraviolet B light at wavelengths between 270 and 300 nm to produce vitamin D_3. These wavelengths are present in sunlight at sea level when the ultraviolet index is greater than 3. These wavelengths occur on a daily basis within the tropics, daily during the spring and summer seasons in temperate regions, and almost never within the Arctic Circle. Adequate amounts of vitamin D_3 can be made in the skin after only 10 to 15 minutes of sun exposure at least 2 times per week to the face, arms, hands, or back without sunscreen. Melanin functions as a light filter in the skin. Individuals with higher skin melanin content require more time in sunlight to produce the same amount of vitamin D than do individuals with lower melanin content.

Once vitamin D is produced in the skin or consumed in food, it is converted in the liver and kidneys to form 1,25-dihydroxyvitamin D ($1,25[OH]_2D$), the physiologically active form of vitamin D. After this conversion, the hormonally active form of vitamin D is released into the circulation. After binding to a carrier protein in the plasma (vitamin D–binding protein), it is transported to various target organs. The hormonally active form of vitamin D mediates its biologic effects by binding to the vitamin D receptor, which is located principally in the nuclei of target cells. The binding of D_3 to the vitamin D receptor allows the vitamin D receptor to act as a transcription factor that modulates the gene expression of transport proteins (such as TRPV6 and calbindin), which encourage calcium absorption in the intestine. Vitamin D receptor activation in the intestines, bones, kidneys, and parathyroid gland cells leads to the maintenance of calcium and phosphorus levels in the blood.

Vitamin D regulates the calcium and phosphorus levels in the blood by promoting their absorption from food in the intestines, and by promoting reabsorption of calcium in the kidneys. This enables normal mineralization of bone needed for bone growth and bone remodelling.

Vitamin D inhibits parathyroid hormone secretion from the parathyroid gland. Vitamin D promotes the immune system by increasing phagocytosis, antitumour activity, and other immunomodulatory functions.

Vitamin D deficiency can result from inadequate dietary intake, inadequate sunlight exposure, malabsorption syndromes, liver or kidney disorders, or by a number of metabolic hereditary disorders. Deficiency results in impaired bone mineralization and leads to bone softening diseases (rickets in children and osteomalacia in adults). Vitamin D deficiency may also contribute to the development of osteoporosis.

Vitamin D receptor is thought to be involved in cell proliferation, apoptosis, and differentiation. This involvement may have some influence on the observations that vitamin D deficiencies are associated with cancers in the colon, breast, and pancreas. Several reports indicate a beneficial correlation between vitamin D intake and prevention of cancer. Vitamin D deficiency is associated with an increase in high blood pressure and cardiovascular risk. Vitamin D also affects the immune system through vitamin D receptor expressed in monocytes and activated T and B cells.

Vitamin D levels can be measured in the blood. Usually 25-hydroxyvitamins D_2 and D_3 are measured and added to obtain the total 25-hydroxyvitamin D level. Therapy is based on the measurement of total hydroxyvitamin D levels. Levels below **50 nmol/L** (<20 ng/mL) indicate a vitamin D deficiency. D levels between **50 and 70 nmol/L** (20 and 30 ng/mL) suggest insufficiency. Levels higher than **70 nmol/L** (>30 ng/mL) are optimal (Table 2-48). Dietary guidelines have recommended that older adults, individuals with dark skin, and those exposed to insufficient ultraviolet radiation (i.e., sunlight) consume extra vitamin D from vitamin D–fortified foods (such as milk), supplements, or both. Fish liver oils and eggs have naturally high levels of vitamin D.

TABLE 2-48 Clinical Features and Associated Blood Levels

nmol/L (ng/mL)	Clinical Features
<27.5 (<11)	Associated with vitamin D deficiency and rickets in infants and young children
<25–37 (<10–15)	Generally considered inadequate for bone and overall health
≥70 (≥30)	Proposed by some authorities as desirable for overall health and disease prevention, although a government-sponsored expert panel concluded that data are insufficient to support these higher levels
Consistently >499 (>200)	Considered potentially toxic, leading to hypercalcemia and hyperphosphatemia, although human data are limited; in an animal model, concentrations ≤400 ng/mL (≤1 000 nmol/L) demonstrated no toxicity.

TABLE 2-49 Adequate Intakes for Vitamin D

Age	Child	Male	Female
Birth to 13 years	5 Mcg (200 IU)		
14–18 years		5 Mcg (200 IU)	5 Mcg (200 IU)
19–50 years		5 Mcg (200 IU)	5 Mcg (200 IU)
51–70 years		10 Mcg (400 IU)	10 Mcg (400 IU)
≥71 years		15 Mcg (600 IU)	15 Mcg (600 IU)

Vitamin D requirements increase with age, and the ability of skin to convert 7-dehydrocholesterol to D$_3$ decreases. At the same time, the ability of the kidneys to convert vitamin D$_2$ to its active form also decreases with age, prompting the need for increased vitamin D supplementation in older adults (Table 2-49). Other individuals particularly at risk for vitamin D deficiency are as follows:
- Breast-fed infants because human milk alone does not have adequate vitamin D levels
- Individuals with limited sun exposure, such as homebound individuals and those living in northern latitudes (such as Indigenous people and residents of Newfoundland and Labrador)
- Women who wear long robes and head coverings for religious reasons
- Individuals with occupations that prevent sun exposure
- Individuals with a body mass index (BMI) of 30 or higher because vitamin D$_2$ is trapped in the subcutaneous fat and cannot get into the bloodstream
- Individuals who have a reduced ability to absorb dietary fat because, as a fat-soluble vitamin, vitamin D requires some dietary fat in the gut for absorption
- Individuals with liver or renal disease because they cannot convert vitamin D to its active metabolic forms

Vitamin D toxicity can cause nonspecific symptoms such as nausea, vomiting, poor appetite, constipation, weakness, weight loss, confusion, and heart rhythm abnormalities (associated with hypercalcemia). The use of calcium and vitamin D supplements by postmenopausal women to decrease the risk of osteoporosis has been associated with a 17% increase in the risk of kidney stones.

INTERFERING FACTORS

▮ Corticosteroid drugs can *decrease* vitamin D levels by reducing calcium absorption.

▮ The weight-loss drug orlistat and the cholesterol-lowering drug cholestyramine can *decrease* vitamin D levels by reducing the absorption of vitamin D and other fat-soluble vitamins.

▮ Barbiturates and phenytoin *decrease* vitamin D levels by increasing hepatic metabolism of vitamin D to inactive compounds.

PROCEDURE AND PATIENT CARE

Before

✗ Explain the test to the patient.

✗ Inform the patient that fasting is not necessary.

• Obtain a list of medications the patient is taking, including supplements and over-the-counter preparations.

During

• Collect a venous blood sample in a red-top or green-top tube.

After

• Apply pressure or a pressure dressing to the venipuncture site.

• Assess the site for bleeding.

✗ If the patient has a vitamin D deficiency, educate him or her about dietary food sources and about the importance of sunlight.

TEST RESULTS AND CLINICAL SIGNIFICANCE

▲ Increased Levels

Williams syndrome: *This is a rare genetic disorder characterized by mild to moderate developmental delay or learning difficulties, a distinctive facial appearance, and a particular personality that combines overfriendliness and high levels of empathy with anxiety. The most significant medical problem associated with Williams syndrome is cardiovascular disease caused by narrowed arteries. Williams syndrome is also associated with elevated blood levels of calcium and elevated vitamin D levels in infancy.*

Excess dietary supplements: *With increased oral ingestion of vitamin D, blood levels can rise to toxic levels.*

▼ Decreased Levels

Rickets,

Osteomalacia,

Osteoporosis: *Vitamin D encourages the absorption of calcium from the intestines. Bone matrix formation depends on adequate levels of calcium.*

Gastrointestinal malabsorption syndromes: *Vitamin D is a fat-soluble vitamin that is not absorbed in diseases of maldigestion or malabsorption.*

Renal disease,

Hepatic disease: *Diseases affecting the metabolic function of the liver and kidneys inhibit the conversion of vitamin D to its active form, 1,25-dihydroxyvitamin D.*

Familial hypophosphatemic rickets (X-linked hypophosphatemic rickets): *This is a disease caused by a mutation in the* PHEX *gene on the X chromosome. Affected patients experience high levels of phosphaturia that is resistant to vitamin D therapy.*

Acute inflammatory disease: *Because inflammation leads to the increased conversion of 25-hydroxyvitamin D into 1,25-hydroxyvitamin D, 25-hydroxyvitamin D (total) levels are decreased.*

Inadequate dietary intake: *With decreased oral ingestion of vitamin D, blood levels can fall to insufficient or deficient levels.*

Inadequate exposure to sunlight: *With decreased exposure to adequate sunlight, endogenous production of vitamin D levels can fall to insufficient or deficient levels.*

RELATED TESTS

Calcium, Blood (p. 152). This test is used to evaluate parathyroid function and calcium metabolism.

Bone Densitometry (p. 1041). This test determines bone mineral content and density to diagnosis osteoporosis.

Phosphate, Phosphorus (p. 403). This test assists in the interpretation of the results of investigations of parathyroid and calcium abnormalities.

West Nile Virus Testing

NORMAL FINDINGS

Negative for West Nile antibody

INDICATIONS

Testing for West Nile virus (WNV) is indicated when the flulike symptoms occur in an area in which the virus exists. In other areas, testing is performed only when the disease has progressed to one of the more complicated syndromes as discussed subsequently.

TEST EXPLANATION

WNV is an RNA virus of the Flaviviridae family. Reservoir hosts include birds (especially crows and jays) and farm animals (particularly horses). The vector is the common mosquito, which carries the virus from the hosts to humans. WNV is not transmitted from human to human. Before 1999, this disease was mostly limited to the African continent. Since then, every U.S. state has reported cases of the disease. In the United States, WNV is most common during peak mosquito season (July through October). In Canada, the peak season is from mid-April until the first hard frost in late September or October. In 2010, there were confirmed cases in only three provinces in Canada (Ontario, Saskatchewan, and British Columbia).

Common symptoms of this infection are flulike and include fever, lethargy, headache, neck and body aches, and a skin rash. This disease can progress to encephalitis, aseptic meningitis, and an atypical form of Guillain-Barré acute flaccid paralysis.

Front-line testing entails measurement of immunoglobulin M (IgM) antibodies to flaviviruses and is not specific to WNV. In nearly all infected patients, this antibody is measurable approximately 10 days after symptoms start. If the front-line test for IgM is positive and the symptoms fulfill the U.S. Centers for Disease Control and prevention (CDC) criteria, the diagnosis of WNV can be made and treatment altered. This is especially true if the patient lives in or has travelled to an area that is known to harbour WNV.

If the front-line testing yields positive results, confirmatory tests may be carried out (especially in areas in which the WNV has not been previously known to exist; see Table 7-3, p. 801). This testing is more important for public health officials and researchers. Confirmatory tests may include the following:

- A second IgM serologic test on convalescing serum 3 to 4 weeks later. A fourfold rise in antibody levels would be confirmatory.
- Direct detection of WNV RNA by nucleic acid amplification testing (plaque reduction neutralization test performed by the CDC). WNV can be transmitted through donated blood or blood components. For that reason, WNV testing for WNV antibodies is routinely performed on all donated blood. WNV diseases can be prevented by applying insect repellent containing diethyltoluamide (DEET) to exposed skin and clothing.

INTERFERING FACTORS

- Other *Flavivirus* infections, such as St. Louis encephalitis virus, cause elevations in serologic values, especially when combined total immunoglobulin M and IgG are tested.

PROCEDURE AND PATIENT CARE

Before
✗ Explain the procedure to the patient and family.

During
- Blood: Obtain a venous blood sample in a red-top tube.
- Cerebrospinal fluid: During lumbar puncture (see p. 676), 1 to 2 mL is reserved in a sterile tube until bacteriologic specimens are found to be negative. Then the reserved specimen is sent out for testing.

After
- Although there is no treatment specific for WNV, these patients may need acute medical/nursing support for neurologic and respiratory sequelae.
✗ Explain to patient and family that testing is carried out at only a few centres and the specimen must be sent out.
✗ Explain that results may not be available for 2 weeks.

TEST RESULTS AND CLINICAL SIGNIFICANCE

West Nile virus infections: *Most infected individuals have no symptoms. Approximately 25% may develop a mild fever; head and body aches occur approximately 3 to 15 days after inoculation by a mosquito. Some patients may even have a rash or enlarged lymph nodes.*

White Blood Cell Count and Differential Count
(WBC and Differential, Leukocyte Count, Neutrophil Count, Lymphocyte Count, Monocyte Count, Eosinophil Count, Basophil Count)

NORMAL FINDINGS

Total White Blood Cells (WBCs)

Adult/child >2 years: **3.5–12.0 × 10⁹/L** (3500–12000/mm³)

Child ≤2 years: **6.2–17 × 10⁹/L** (6200–17000/mm³)

Newborn (0–6 weeks): **9–30 × 10⁹/L** (9000–30000/mm³)

Differential Count

	Percentage (%)	× 10⁹/L	Absolute (per mm³)
Neutrophils	55–70	**3.0–5.8**	300–5800
Lymphocytes	20–40	**1.5–3.0**	1500–3000
Monocytes	2–8	**0.3–0.5**	300–500
Eosinophils	1–4	**0.0–0.25**	50–250
Basophils	0.5–1.0	**0.01–0.05**	15–50

 Critical Values

WBCs **<2.5 × 10⁹/L** (<2500/mm³) or **>30 × 10⁹/L** (>30000/mm³)

INDICATIONS

The measurement of the total and differential WBC counts is a part of all routine laboratory diagnostic evaluations. It is especially helpful in the evaluation of patients with infection, neoplasm, allergy, and immunosuppression (Box 2-16).

Age-Related Concerns

- The WBC values tend to be age related.
- The total number of WBCs is unchanged with the aging process; however, their function deteriorates as a person ages.
- Normal newborns and infants tend to have higher WBC values than do adults.
- It is not uncommon for older adults to fail to respond to infection by the absence of leukocytosis. In older adults, the WBC count may not increase even in the presence of a severe bacterial infection.

TEST EXPLANATION

The WBC count has two components. The first is a count of the total number of WBCs in 1 mm³ of peripheral venous blood. The other component, the differential count, measures the percentage of each type of leukocyte present in the same specimen. An increase in the percentage of one type of leukocyte means a decrease in the percentage of another. Neutrophils and lymphocytes make up 75% to 90% of the total leukocytes. These leukocyte types can be identified easily by their struc-

BOX 2-16	Precautions for Immunocompromised Patients

- Observe protective isolation:
  - Wash hands before entering room.
  - Wear mask, gown, and gloves.
  - Restrict visitations.
  - Prohibit visitation by individuals with infections (viral, fungal bacterial).
- Avoid bacteremia from patient's own bacterial flora:
  - Do not measure temperatures rectally.
  - Do not perform rectal examinations or administer rectal enemas.
  - Do not allow patient to floss teeth.
- Avoid bacterial contamination from foods:
  - Serve the patient only foods from newly opened packages.
  - Do not give the patient fresh fruits and vegetables.
  - Ensure that all the patient's foods are cooked.
- Avoid infection by administration of intramuscular injections, if possible.
- Observe the patient closely for infections or fever.

ture on a peripheral blood smear (see p. 738) or by automated counters. The total leukocyte count has a wide range of normal values, but many diseases may induce abnormal values.

An increased total WBC count (leukocytosis; WBC count $>10 \times 10^9$/L [$>10\,000\,\text{mm}^3$]) usually indicates infection, inflammation, tissue necrosis, or leukemic neoplasia. Trauma or stress, either emotional or physical, may increase the WBC count. In some infections, especially sepsis, the WBC count may be extremely high and reach levels associated with leukemia. This is called a *leukemoid* reaction and resolves quickly as the infection is successfully treated.

A decreased total WBC count (leukopenia; WBC count $<4 \times 10^9$/L [$<4\,000\,\text{mm}^3$]) occurs in many forms of bone marrow failure (e.g., after antineoplastic chemotherapy or radiation therapy, marrow infiltrative diseases, overwhelming infections, dietary deficiencies, autoimmune diseases).

The major function of WBCs is to fight infection and react against foreign bodies or tissues. Five types of WBCs may easily be identified on a routine blood smear. These cells, in order of frequency, are neutrophils, lymphocytes, monocytes, eosinophils, and basophils. All of these WBCs arise from the same "pluripotent" stem cell within the bone marrow as the RBC (Figure 2-24). Beyond this origin, however, each cell line differentiates separately. Most mature WBCs are then deposited into the circulating blood.

WBCs are categorized as granulocytes and nongranulocytes. Granulocytes include neutrophils, basophils, and eosinophils. Because of their multilobed nuclei, neutrophils are sometimes referred to as *polymorphonuclear leukocytes* (PMNs or "polys"). The normal ranges for absolute counts depend on age, sex, and ethnicity. For example, the normal range for absolute neutrophils for Black men is $1.4–7.0 \times 10^9$/L ($1\,400–7\,000\,\text{mm}^3$).

The most common granulocytes, *neutrophils,* are produced in 7 to 14 days, and exist in the circulation for only 6 hours. The primary function of the neutrophil is phagocytosis (killing and digestion of bacterial microorganisms). Acute bacterial infections and trauma stimulate neutrophil production, which results in an increased WBC count. When neutrophil production is significantly stimulated, neutrophils often enter the circulation prematurely. These immature forms are called *band* or *stab cells.* This occurrence, referred to as a "shift to the left" in WBC production, is indicative of an ongoing acute bacterial infection.

Basophils (also called *mast cells*) and especially *eosinophils* are involved in allergic reactions. They are capable of phagocytosis of antigen-antibody complexes. As the allergic response

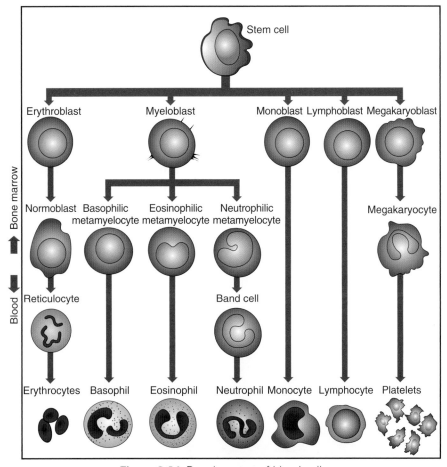

Figure 2-24 Development of blood cells.

diminishes, the eosinophil count decreases. Eosinophils and basophils do not respond to bacterial or viral infections. The cytoplasm of basophils contains heparin, histamine, and serotonin. Basophils infiltrate the tissue (e.g., in the form of hives in the skin) involved in the allergic reaction and serve to further the inflammatory response.

Nongranulocytes (mononuclear cells) include lymphocytes and monocytes (the count also includes histiocytes). They have no cytoplasmic granules and have a small, single, rounded nucleus. *Lymphocytes* are categorized as two types: T cells (mature in the thymus) and B cells (mature in the bone marrow). T cells are involved primarily with cellular-type immune reactions, whereas B cells participate in humoral immunity (antibody production). T cells are the killer cells, suppressor cells, and T_4 helper cells (see "Cell Surface Immunophenotyping," p. 161). The primary function of lymphocytes is to fight chronic bacterial infection and acute viral infections. The differential count does not involve counting the T and B cells separately; rather, it is a count of the combination of the two.

Monocytes are phagocytic cells capable of fighting bacteria in a similar way that neutrophils do. Through phagocytosis, they remove necrotic debris and microorganisms from the blood. The monocytes produce interferon, which is the body's endogenous immunostimulant. Monocytes can be produced more rapidly, however, and can spend a longer time in the circulation than do the neutrophils.

The WBC and differential count are routinely measured as part of the complete blood cell count (see p. 187) (Figure 2-25). Serial WBC counts and differential counts have both diagnostic and prognostic value. For example, a persistent increase in the WBC count (and particularly the neutrophils) may indicate worsening of an infectious process (e.g., appendicitis). A reduction in WBC count to the normal range from a previously elevated range indicates resolution of an infection. A dramatic decrease in the WBC count below the normal range may indicate bone marrow failure. In patients receiving chemotherapy, a reduced WBC count may contraindicate further chemotherapy.

The absolute count is calculated by multiplying the differential count (%) by the total WBC count. For example, the absolute neutrophil count is helpful in determining the patient's real risk for infection. It is calculated by multiplying the WBC count by the percent of neutrophils and percent of bands, that is:

Absolute neutrophil count = WBC × (%Neutrophils + % Bands)

If the absolute neutrophil count is below $1 \times 10^9/L$ (<1 000 mm^3), the patient may need to be placed in protective isolation because he or she could be severely immunocompromised (see Box 2-16, p. 550) and is at great risk for infection.

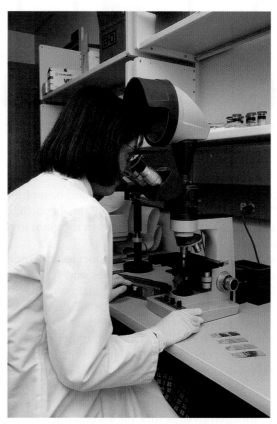

Figure 2-25 Medical technologist conducting a microscopic examination of white blood cells (WBCs).

INTERFERING FACTORS

- Eating, physical activity, and stress may cause an increase in WBC count and could alter the differential values.
- Pregnancy (final month) and labour may be associated with increases in WBC levels.
- Patients who have undergone splenectomy have a persistent mild to moderate elevation of WBC counts.
- The WBC count tends to be lower in the morning and higher in the late afternoon.
- The WBC count tends to be age related. Normal newborns and infants tend to have higher WBC counts than do adults. It is not uncommon for older adults to fail to respond to infection by the absence of leukocytosis. In fact, in older adults, the WBC count may not increase even in the presence of a severe bacterial infection.
- Drugs that may cause *increases* in WBC levels include adrenaline, allopurinol, aspirin, chloroform, epinephrine, heparin, quinine, steroids, and triamterene.
- Drugs that may cause *decreases* in WBC levels include antibiotics, anticonvulsants, antihistamines, antimetabolites, antithyroid drugs, arsenicals, barbiturates, chemotherapeutic agents, diuretics, and sulphonamides.

Clinical Priorities

- An increased WBC count (leukocytosis) usually indicates infection, inflammation, tissue necrosis, or leukemic neoplasia.
- Serial WBC and differential counts have both diagnostic and prognostic value. For example, a persistent increase in the WBC count may indicate a worsening of an infectious process (e.g., appendicitis).
- A drastic decrease in WBCs below the normal range may indicate bone marrow failure.

PROCEDURE AND PATIENT CARE

Before
- Explain the procedure to the patient.
- Inform the patient that no fasting is required.

During
- Collect a venous blood sample in a lavender-top tube.

After
- Apply pressure or a pressure dressing to the venipuncture site.
- Check the venipuncture site for bleeding.

TEST RESULTS AND CLINICAL SIGNIFICANCE

▲ Increased WBC Count (Leukocytosis)

Infection: *WBCs are integral to initiating and maintaining the body's defence mechanism against infection.*

Leukemic neoplasia or other myeloproliferative disorders: *These neoplastic cells are produced by the marrow and are released into the bloodstream.*

Other malignancy: *Advanced non–bone marrow cancers (e.g., lung) are associated with leukocytosis. The pathophysiologic mechanism underlying this observation is not defined.*

Trauma, stress, or hemorrhage: *The WBC count is probably under hormonal influence (e.g., epinephrine). However, the pathophysiologic mechanism underlying this observation is not defined.*

Tissue necrosis,

Inflammation: *The pathophysiologic mechanism underlying these observations is complex, including the recognition of necrotic or normal tissue as "foreign" so that a WBC response is instituted.*

Dehydration: *Not only is dehydration a stress that, by itself, increases the WBC count, but also the WBC count increases because of hemoconcentration.*

Thyroid storm: *The WBC count is probably influenced by thyroid hormones. Marked increases in levels of these hormones could be associated with an increased WBC count.*

Steroid use: *Glucocorticosteroids stimulate WBC production.*

▼ Decreased WBC Count (Leukopenia)

Drug toxicity (e.g., cytotoxic chemotherapy; see also drugs that decrease the WBC count),
Bone marrow failure,
Overwhelming infections,
Dietary deficiency (e.g., vitamin B_{12} deficiency, iron deficiency),
Congenital bone marrow aplasia,
Bone marrow infiltration (e.g., myelofibrosis): *These conditions are associated with all different forms of bone marrow failure whereby WBC production is reduced.*
Autoimmune disease: *The pathophysiologic mechanism underlying this observation is not known.*
Hypersplenism: *The spleen more aggressively extracts WBCs from the bloodstream.*

Changes in Differential Count

Table 2-50 lists causes of increases and decreases in the differential count.

RELATED TESTS

Cell Surface Immunophenotyping (p. 161). This test is used to detect the progressive depletion of CD4 T lymphocytes, which is associated with an increased likelihood of clinical complications from acquired immunodeficiency syndrome (AIDS). Test results can indicate whether a patient with AIDS is at risk for developing opportunistic infections.

Blood Smear (p. 738). The peripheral blood smear is a direct microscopic analysis of the cellular components of the blood.

TABLE 2-50	Causes of Abnormalities in the White Blood Cell Differential Count	
Type of White Blood Cell	**Elevated**	**Decreased**
Neutrophils	Neutrophilia	Neutropenia
	Physical or emotional stress	Aplastic anemia
	Acute suppurative infection	Dietary deficiency
	Myelocytic leukemia	Overwhelming bacterial infection
	Trauma	(especially in older adults)
	Cushing's syndrome	Viral infections (e.g., hepatitis,
	Inflammatory disorders (e.g.,	influenza, measles)
	rheumatic fever, thyroiditis,	Radiation therapy
	rheumatoid arthritis)	Addison's disease
	Metabolic disorders (e.g.,	Drug therapy: myelotoxic drugs (as
	ketoacidosis, gout, eclampsia)	in chemotherapy)

TABLE 2-50	Causes of Abnormalities in the White Blood Cell Differential Count—cont'd	

Type of White Blood Cell	Elevated	Decreased
Lymphocytes	Lymphocytosis Chronic bacterial infection Viral infection (e.g., mumps, rubella) Lymphocytic leukemia Multiple myeloma Infectious mononucleosis Radiation Infectious hepatitis	Lymphocytopenia Leukemia Sepsis Immunodeficiency diseases Lupus erythematosus Later stages of human immunodeficiency virus infection Drug therapy: adrenocorticosteroids, antineoplastics Radiation therapy
Monocytes	Monocytosis Chronic inflammatory disorders Viral infections (e.g., infectious mononucleosis) Tuberculosis Chronic ulcerative colitis Parasites (e.g., malaria)	Monocytopenia Aplastic anemia Hairy cell leukemia Drug therapy: prednisone
Eosinophils	Eosinophilia Parasitic infections Allergic reactions Eczema Leukemia Autoimmune diseases	Eosinopenia Increased adrenosteroid production
Basophils	Basophilia Myeloproliferative disease (e.g., myelofibrosis, polycythemia rubra vera) Leukemia	Basopenia Acute allergic reactions Hyperthyroidism Stress reactions

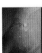

D-Xylose Absorption (Xylose Tolerance)

NORMAL FINDINGS

Age	60-Minute Plasma Value	120-Minute Plasma Value	Urine Value
Child	>1.0 mmol/L (>15 mg/dL)	>1.3 mmol/L (>20 mg/dL)	>16%–33% of 5-g dose
Adult	>1.3 mmol/L (>20 mg/dL)	>1.6 mmol/L (>25 mg/dL)	>16% of 5-g dose

INDICATIONS

This test is used to evaluate the absorptive capability of the intestines. It is used in the evaluation of patients with suspected malabsorption.

TEST EXPLANATION

D-Xylose is a monosaccharide that is easily absorbed by the normal intestines. In patients with malabsorption, intestinal D-xylose absorption is diminished, and as a result, blood levels and urine excretion are reduced. D-Xylose is the monosaccharide chosen for the test because it is not metabolized by the body. Serum levels directly reflect intestinal absorption.

This monosaccharide is also measured because absorption does not require pancreatic or biliary exocrine function. Its absorption is directly determined by the absorptive function of the small intestine. This test is used to differentiate diarrhea caused by maldigestion (pancreatic/biliary dysfunction) and diarrhea caused by malabsorption (sprue, Whipple's disease, Crohn's disease). It is also used to quantitate the degree of malabsorption to monitor therapy.

In this test, the patient is asked to drink a fluid containing a prescribed amount of D-xylose. Blood and urine levels are subsequently evaluated. Excellent gastrointestinal absorption is documented by high blood levels and good urine excretion of D-xylose. Poor intestinal absorption is marked by low blood levels and poor urine excretion.

CONTRAINDICATIONS

- Dehydration, because the dose of D-xylose can cause diarrhea and may precipitate hypovolemia in affected patients

INTERFERING FACTORS

- Abnormal kidney function, because affected patients may not be able to excrete the D-xylose. The urine measurement for D-xylose should not be performed, and the interpretation should be based on only the blood test results.
- Drugs that may affect test results include aspirin, atropine, and indomethacin.

PROCEDURE AND PATIENT CARE

Before

- Explain the procedure to the patient.
- Instruct the adult patient to fast for 8 hours before the test. Drinking water is permitted during the fast and, in fact, should be encouraged.
- Inform the pediatric patient or the parents that the patient should fast for at least 4 hours before the test, unless otherwise ordered by physician.

During

- Collect a venous blood sample in a red-top tube before the patient ingests the D-xylose.
- Collect a first-voided morning urine specimen and send it to the laboratory.
- Ask the patient to take the prescribed dose of D-xylose dissolved in 8 oz of water. Record the time of ingestion.
- Calibrate pediatric doses according to the patient's body weight.
- Repeat venipunctures to obtain blood in exactly 2 hours for an adult and 1 hour for a child.
- Collect urine for a designated time, usually 5 hours, in a dark bottle. Refrigerate the urine during the collection period.
- Observe the patient for nausea, vomiting, and diarrhea, which may occur as side effects of D-xylose ingestion.

Instruct the patient to remain in a restful position. Intense physical activity may alter the digestive process and affect the test results.

After

- Apply pressure or a pressure dressing to the venipuncture site.
- Observe the venipuncture site for bleeding.
- Provide the patient with food or drink and inform the patient that he or she may resume normal activity after completion of the study.

TEST RESULTS AND CLINICAL SIGNIFICANCE

▼ Decreased Levels

Malabsorption caused by sprue, lymphatic obstruction, enteropathy (e.g., radiation), Crohn's disease, or Whipple's disease: *The D-xylose is not absorbed in these patients; therefore, blood and urine levels are not as normally expected.*

Short-bowel syndrome: *Because of the lack of absorptive surface, absorption of D-xylose does not occur. Therefore, blood and urine levels are not as normally expected.*

RELATED TEST

Small Bowel Follow-Through (p. 1109). This is a radiographic test that visualizes the mucosa of the small intestine. Patients with Crohn's disease and other malabsorption syndromes may have obvious abnormal findings.

Zinc Protoporphyrin (ZPP)

NORMAL FINDINGS

0–69 µmol ZPP/mol heme

INDICATIONS

ZPP is a screening test for lead poisoning and iron deficiency anemia.

TEST EXPLANATION

ZPP is used in screening for iron deficiency anemia or lead poisoning. It is also used in monitoring the treatment/interventions of chronic lead poisoning. ZPP is found in red blood cells when heme production is inhibited by lead toxicity. Lead prevents iron, but not zinc, from attaching to the protoporphyrin. Or, if there is iron deficiency, instead of incorporating a ferrous ion to form heme, protoporphyrin (the immediate precursor of heme) incorporates a zinc ion, forming ZPP. In addition to lead poisoning and iron deficiency, zinc protoporphyrin levels can be elevated as the result of a number of other conditions (e.g., sickle cell anemia). Because of this lack of specificity, ZPP is not commonly used as a screening test for lead poisoning.

The fluorescent properties of ZPP in intact red cells allow the ZPP/heme molar ratio to be measured quickly, at low cost, and in a small sample volume. However, it is more commonly measured using a hematofluorometer, which is able to measure the ZPP/heme ratio.

PROCEDURE AND PATIENT CARE

Before
🖉 Instruct the patient to fast for 12 hours before the blood test. Water is permitted.

During
- Collect a venous blood sample in a royal blue–, tan-, lavender-, or pink-top tube.
- Indicate on the laboratory slip any drugs that may affect test results.

After
- Apply pressure to the venipuncture site.

TEST RESULTS AND CLINICAL SIGNIFICANCE

▲ Increased Levels
Lead poisoning,

Vanadium exposure: *Lead and a few other heavy metals inhibit the action of the enzyme ferrochelatase, which facilitates the uptake of iron into protoporphyrin IX in the production of hemoglobin. As a result, zinc is taken up by the protoporphyrin and incorporated into ZPP. Increased ZPP is noted.*

Iron deficiency,

Anemia of chronic illness,

Sickle cell anemia,

Sideroblastic anemia: *When iron is deficient or hemoglobin synthesis outstrips iron availability, zinc is preferentially taken up by protoporphyrin IX in the production of hemoglobin. As a result, zinc is taken up by the protoporphyrin and incorporated into ZPP. Increased ZPP is noted.*

RELATED TESTS
Lead (p. 348). This is a measure of lead in the blood.

Iron Level and Total Iron Binding Capacity (p. 334). This is a measure of iron in the blood.

Transferrin Receptor Assay (p. 521). This test is used to help differentiate the various causes of iron deficiency anemia.

CHAPTER 3

Electrodiagnostic Tests

NOTE: *Throughout this chapter, SI units are presented in* boldface colour, *followed by conventional units in parentheses.*

OVERVIEW

TESTS

OVERVIEW

REASONS FOR PERFORMING ELECTRODIAGNOSTIC STUDIES

Most electrodiagnostic studies involve the use of electrical activity and electronic devices to evaluate disease or injury to a specified area of the body. The electrical impulses can be generated spontaneously or can be stimulated. For example, in electrocardiography, spontaneous electrical impulses generated by the heart during the cardiac cycle are recorded. In electromyography, the electrical impulses are stimulated by an electrical shock applied to the body. In the caloric study, nystagmus is induced by irrigating the ear canal with water to determine the normal functioning of the cranial nerves. The electrical activity is usually detected by electrodes placed on the body. The electrodes are attached to instruments for receiving and recording electrical impulses. Table 3-1 lists the various areas of the body that can be evaluated by electrodiagnostic studies. Refer to agency protocols for specific procedural care for patients undergoing electrodiagnostic studies.

TABLE 3-1   Body Areas Evaluated in Electrodiagnostic Studies

Name of Test	Evaluation
Caloric study	Cranial nerve VIII
Cardiac stress	Cardiac muscle
Contraction stress (fetal)	Fetal viability
Electrocardiography	Cardiac muscle and conduction system
Electroencephalography	Brain
Electromyography	Neuromuscular system
Electroneurography	Peripheral nerves
Electronystagmography	Oculovestibular reflex pathway
Electrophysiologic studies	Cardiac conduction system
Evoked potential studies	Sensory pathways of the eyes, ears, and peripheral nerves
Holter monitoring	Cardiac rhythm
Nonstress (fetal)	Fetal viability
Pelvic floor sphincter electromyography	Urinary or fecal continence

PROCEDURAL CARE FOR ELECTRODIAGNOSTIC STUDIES

Before

- Explain the procedure to the patient.
- Obtain baseline values for comparison during and after the test.
- Explain food restrictions, if they are indicated. For example, caloric studies necessitate fasting to reduce the possibility of nausea and vomiting. On the other hand, fasting would affect electroencephalography results by causing hypoglycemia.
- Determine whether there are any drug restrictions. Sedatives may adversely affect most test results.
- Because of its stimulating effect, caffeine ingestion is restricted before most studies.
- Most of these studies are considered noninvasive, and a consent form is not required.

During

- For most tests, a type of electrode is applied to some part of the patient's body to record electrical activity.
- Some tests (such as electromyography) entail some type of electrical stimulation. The patient may feel slight discomfort if electrical stimulation is applied.
- Instruct the patient to remain still during testing. Any movement can alter test results.

After

- Monitor the patient for a return to pretest baseline activity.
- Some studies may cause nausea and vomiting. The patient should rest until these symptoms subside.
- If any sedative was given, safety precautions should be in effect—for example, side rails up, call bell in reach.

POTENTIAL COMPLICATIONS OF ELECTRODIAGNOSTIC STUDIES

Most tests in this category have few potential complications. Those mentioned as follows apply to specific tests and are grouped accordingly.

Cardiac Stress Testing
Cardiac arrhythmias
Severe angina
Fainting
Myocardial infarction
Hypotension

Contraction Stress Test
Premature labour

REPORTING OF RESULTS
Many of these tests are performed by technicians. Test results are available after interpretation by a physician.

Caloric Study (Oculovestibular Reflex Study)

NORMAL FINDINGS
Nystagmus with irrigation

INDICATIONS
This test is used to evaluate the function of cranial nerve VIII. It also can indicate disease in the temporal portion of the cerebrum.

TEST EXPLANATION
Caloric studies are used to evaluate the vestibular portion of cranial nerve VIII by irrigating the external auditory canal with hot or cold water. This is usually part of a complete neurologic examination. Stimulation with cold water normally causes rotary nystagmus (involuntary rapid eye movement) away from the ear being irrigated; hot water induces nystagmus toward the side of the ear being irrigated. If the labyrinth is diseased or cranial nerve VIII is not functioning (e.g., from tumour compression), no nystagmus is induced. This study aids in the differential diagnosis of abnormalities that may occur in the vestibular system, brain stem, or cerebellum. When results are inconclusive, electronystagmography (p. 584) may be performed.

CONTRAINDICATIONS
- Perforated eardrum. Cold air may be substituted for the fluid, although this method is less reliable.
- Acute disease of the labyrinth (e.g., Ménière syndrome). The test can be performed when the acute attack subsides.

Clinical Priorities

- This study aids in evaluating the vestibular portion of cranial nerve VIII.
- During this test, the external auditory canal is irrigated with hot or cold water to induce nystagmus.
- Most patients experience nausea and dizziness during this test. Patients with a decreased level of consciousness should be safely positioned to avoid potential aspiration from vomiting.

INTERFERING FACTORS

Drugs such as sedatives and antivertigo agents can alter test results.

PROCEDURE AND PATIENT CARE

Before

- Explain the procedure to the patient.
- Withhold solid foods for 24 hours before the test to reduce the incidence of vomiting.
- Inform the patient that he or she will probably experience nausea and dizziness during the test. If the patient has a decreased level of consciousness, position the patient safely to avoid potential aspiration from vomiting.

During

- Although the exact procedures for caloric studies vary, a typical test includes the following steps:
    1. Before the test, the patient is examined for the presence of nystagmus, postural deviation (Romberg sign), and past-pointing (the inability to place a finger on a specific part of the body, such as touch the tip of the nose). This examination provides the baseline values for comparison during the test.
    2. The ear canal should be examined and cleaned by a physician before the test to ensure that the water will flow freely to the middle ear area.
    3. The ear on the suspected side is irrigated first because the patient's response may be minimal.
    4. After an emesis basin is placed under the ear, the irrigation solution is directed into the external auditory canal until the patient complains of nausea and dizziness, or nystagmus is observed. This usually occurs in 20 to 30 seconds.
    5. If after 3 minutes no symptoms occur, the irrigation is stopped.
    6. The patient is tested again for nystagmus, past-pointing, and the Romberg sign.
    7. After approximately 5 minutes, the procedure is repeated on the other side.
- This procedure is usually performed by a physician or technician in approximately 15 minutes.

After

- Usually, place the patient on bed rest for approximately 30 to 60 minutes until nausea or vomiting subsides.
- Ensure patient safety with regard to dizziness.

TEST RESULTS AND CLINICAL SIGNIFICANCE

Inflammation, infarction, or tumour in the brain stem,

Inflammation, infarction, or tumour in the cerebellum,

Vestibular or cochlear inflammation or tumour,

Acoustic neuroma,

Neuritis or neuropathy of cranial nerve VIII: *These diseases involve the central nervous system from the vestibular/cochlear end organ to the temporal area of the cerebrum.*

RELATED TEST

Electronystagmography (p. 584). During this test, nystagmus is stimulated in a manner similar to that described for caloric studies. The direction, velocity, and amplitude of the nystagmus are recorded through the use of electrodes.

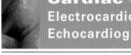

Cardiac Stress Testing (Stress Testing, Exercise Testing, Electrocardiographic Stress Testing, Nuclear Stress Testing, Echocardiographic [Echo] Stress Testing)

NORMAL FINDINGS

Ability of patient to obtain and maintain maximal heart rate of 85% for predicted age and gender with no cardiac symptoms or electrocardiographic change

No cardiac muscle wall dysfunction

INDICATIONS

Stress testing is conducted in the following situations:

1. To evaluate chest pain in a patient with suspected coronary disease (On occasion, a patient has significant coronary stenosis that is not apparent during normal physical activity. If, however, the pain can be reproduced with exercise, coronary occlusion may be present.)
2. To determine the safe limits of exercise during a cardiac rehabilitation program or to assist patients with cardiac disease in maintaining good physical fitness
3. To detect labile or exercise-related hypertension
4. To detect intermittent claudication in patients with suspected vascular occlusive disease in the extremities (which may manifest as leg muscle cramping during the exercise)
5. To evaluate the effectiveness of treatment in patients who take antianginal or antiarrhythmic medications
6. To evaluate the effectiveness of cardiac intervention (such as bypass grafting or angioplasty)

TEST EXPLANATION

Stress testing is a noninvasive study that provides information about the patient's cardiac function. In stress testing, the heart is stressed in some way. The heart is then evaluated during the stress. Changes indicating ischemia point to coronary occlusive disease. By far the most commonly used method of stress is exercise (usually on a treadmill). Chemical stress methods are becoming more common because of their safety and better accuracy. A third method, less frequently used, is pacer stress (Box 3-1).

BOX 3-1	Commonly Used Methods of Stressing the Heart

- Exercise
  - Bicycle
  - Treadmill
- Chemical
  - Adenosine
  - Dipyridamole
  - Dobutamine
  - Stimulatory drugs
  - Vascular dilation drugs
- Pacing
  - Cardiac pacemaker

During *exercise stress testing,* the electrocardiogram (ECG), heart rate, and blood pressure are monitored while the patient engages in some type of physical activity (stress). Two methods of stress testing are pedalling a stationary bicycle and walking on a treadmill. In testing with the stationary bicycle, the pedalling tension is slowly increased to increase the heart rate. In testing with the treadmill test, the speed and grade of incline are increased. The treadmill test is the most frequently used because it is the most easily standardized and its results are most reproducible (Figure 3-1). The cardiologist determines the various grades of exercise in attendance according to estimates of cardiac function capabilities.

The usual goal of the exercise stress testing is to increase the heart rate to just below maximal levels of the "target heart rate zone."

The target heart rate for the stress test is usually 80% to 90% of the maximal heart rate. The test is usually discontinued if the patient reaches that target heart rate or if any symptoms or changes on the ECG develop. The maximal heart rate is determined by referring to a chart that takes into account the patient's maximum heart rate and age (e.g., 220 minus the patient's age)

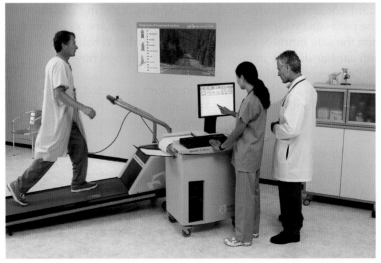

Figure 3-1 A patient taking an exercise stress test while a nurse and the attending cardiologist monitor the electrocardiographic response.

and gender. The normal maximal heart rate for adults varies from 150 to 200 beats/minute; in patients taking calcium channel blockers and sympathetic blockers, the maximal heart rate is lower than expected.

Exercise stress testing is based on the principle that occluded arteries are unable to meet the heart's increased demand for blood during the testing. This may become obvious with symptoms (e.g., chest pain, fatigue, dyspnea, tachycardia, cardiac arrhythmias [dysrhythmias], fall in blood pressure) or with changes on the ECG (e.g., ST-segment variance >1 mm, increasing premature ventricular contractions, other rhythm disturbances). An advantage of stress testing is that these symptoms can be stimulated and identified in a safe environment. In addition to the electrodiagnostic method of cardiac evaluation, nuclear scanning or echocardiography, which are more sensitive and accurate also can evaluate the stressed heart. Findings of ischemia are discussed in the section "Test Results and Clinical Significance."

When exercise stress testing is not advisable or the patient is unable to exercise to a level adequate to stress the heart (patients with an orthopedic, arthritic, neurologic, or pulmonary limitation), chemical stress testing is recommended. Chemical stress testing is being used increasingly because of its accuracy and ease of performance. Although chemical stress testing causes fewer physiologic changes than does exercise testing, it is safer and more controllable. Dipyridamole (Persantine) is a coronary vasodilator. If one coronary artery is significantly occluded, the coronary blood flow is diverted to the opened vessels. This causes a "steal syndrome" away from the stenotic or occluded coronary vessel; that is, the dipyridamole-induced vascular dilation "steals" the blood from the ischemic areas and diverts it to the open, dilated coronary vessels. Caution must be taken, however, because this can precipitate angina or myocardial infarction. This test should be performed only with a cardiologist in attendance. Intravenous aminophylline can reverse the effect of dipyridamole. Adenosine works similarly to dipyridamole.

Dobutamine is another chemical that can stress the heart. To stimulate heart muscle function, progressively greater amounts of dobutamine must be administered over 3-minute intervals. The normal heart muscle increases its contractility (wall motion). Ischemic muscle has no augmentation. In time, the ischemic area becomes hypokinetic, whereas infarcted tissue is akinetic. In chemical stress testing, the stressed heart is evaluated by nuclear scanning or echocardiography.

Pacing is another method of stress testing. In patients with permanent pacemakers, the rate of capture can be increased to a rate that would be considered a cardiac stress. The heart is then evaluated electrodiagnostically or with nuclear scanning or echocardiography.

As indicated in Box 3-2, the methods of evaluating the heart are nuclear scanning, echocardiography, and electrophysiologic parameters. Echocardiography is becoming the method of choice for urgent and elective cardiac evaluation, with or without stress testing.

Stress testing is discontinued when any of the criteria noted in Box 3-3 occur.

 Age-Related Concerns

- A decreased heart rate, reduced myocardial contractility, and decreased cardiac output are all age-related physiologic changes that can affect an older adult's response to the stress test. A normal maximum heart rate for adults ranges from 150 to 220 beats/minute.
- An older adult's heart rate does not increase as quickly with exercise, nor does it decrease as rapidly after exercise, as does a younger adult's heart rate. It is therefore important to allow adequate time after the stress test for the older adult to recover and for the heart rate to return to that in a resting state.

BOX 3-2	Commonly Used Methods of Cardiac Evaluation During Stress Testing

- Cardiac nuclear scanning (p. 817)
- Echocardiography (p. 906)
- Electrophysiologic parameters: electrocardiogram (ECG), blood pressure, and heart rate

BOX 3-3	Criteria for Discontinuation of an Exercise Stress Test

- Abnormal electrocardiographic changes
- Attainment of maximal performance
- Chest pain
- Cyanosis
- Ectopy
  - Flipped T waves
  - ST changes
- Excessive heart rate changes: tachycardia or bradycardia
- Excessive hypertension or hypotension
- Leg claudication
- Severe shortness of breath
- Syncope

CONTRAINDICATIONS

- Unstable angina, because stress may induce an infarction
- Severe aortic valvular heart disease (especially stenotic lesions), because stress tolerance is quite low and easily reached
- Inability to participate in an exercise program because of impaired lung or motor function; however, affected patients can undergo chemical stress testing
- Recent myocardial infarction; however, limited stress testing may be performed
- Severe heart failure
- Severe claudication and inability to walk adequately to stress the heart; however, affected patients can undergo chemical stress testing
- Severe left main coronary artery disease

POTENTIAL COMPLICATIONS

- Fatal cardiac arrhythmias (e.g., bradycardia, tachycardia, syncope, atrial fibrillation, ventricular tachycardia, ventricular fibrillation)
- Severe angina
  - Severe shortness of breath
- Myocardial infarction
- Fainting
  - Cyanosis
  - Leg claudication

INTERFERING FACTORS

- Heavy meals before the test can divert blood to the gastrointestinal tract.
- Nicotine from smoking can cause coronary artery spasm.
- Caffeine blocks the effect of dipyridamole.
- Medical problems such as hypertension, valvular heart disease (especially of the aortic valve), severe anemia, hypoxemia, and chronic pulmonary disease can affect results.
- Left ventricular hypertrophy may affect test results.
- The ECG is not a reliable indicator of ischemia in patients with left bundle branch block.
- Drugs that can *affect* test results include beta blockers (e.g., propranolol [Inderal]), calcium channel blockers, digoxin, and nitroglycerin.

PROCEDURE AND PATIENT CARE (FOR EXERCISE STRESS TESTING AND ELECTRODIAGNOSTIC MONITORING)

Before

- Explain the procedure to the patient.
- Instruct the patient to abstain from eating, drinking, and smoking for 4 hours before the test.
- Inform the patient about the risks of the test, and obtain informed consent.
- Instruct the patient to bring comfortable clothing and athletic shoes for exercise. Slippers are not acceptable.
- If any medications should be discontinued before the test, inform the patient accordingly.
- Obtain a pretest ECG.
    - Emergency resuscitation equipment should be available during testing (e.g., oxygen, crash cart).
- Apply and secure appropriate electrodes for the ECG.

During

- Note that a physician usually is present during stress testing.
- After the patient begins to exercise, adjust the treadmill machine settings to apply increasing levels of stress at specific intervals. It is helpful to encourage and provide emotional support to the patient at each level of increased stress.
- Encourage patients to report any symptoms.
- Record the patient's vital signs for baseline values. Monitor the blood pressure during the testing.
- Note that during the test, the electrocardiographic tracing and vital signs are monitored continuously.
- Terminate the test if the patient complains of chest pain, exhaustion, dyspnea, fatigue, or dizziness.
- Note that testing usually takes approximately 45 minutes.
- Inform the patient that the physician in attendance usually interprets the results and will explain them to the patient.

After

- Place the patient in a comfortable position (e.g., supine) to rest after the test.
- Monitor the electrocardiographic tracing and record vital signs at poststress intervals until recordings and values return to pretest levels.
- Remove electrodes and paste.

TEST RESULTS AND CLINICAL SIGNIFICANCE

Coronary artery–occlusive disease: *Subclinical coronary artery–occlusive disease often becomes evident with stress testing.*

Exercise-related hypertension or hypotension: *The blood pressure is higher or lower than what is considered normal for the level of exercise.*

Intermittent claudication: *As with the coronary system, peripheral vascular stenosis or occlusion may not become evident until the legs are stressed as in an exercise stress test.*

Abnormal cardiac rhythms such as ventricular tachycardia or supraventricular tachycardia: *Ectopy may not occur or become symptomatic until the patient is stressed.*

RELATED TESTS

Cardiac Nuclear Scanning (p. 817). This test is used to evaluate the heart during stress testing.
Echocardiography (p. 906). This test is also used to evaluate the heart during stress testing.

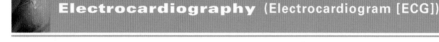

Electrocardiography (Electrocardiogram [ECG])

NORMAL FINDINGS

Normal heart rate (60–100 beats/minute), rhythm, and wave deflections (see Figure 3-3)

INDICATIONS

This electrodiagnostic test records the electrical impulses that stimulate the heart to contract. It is used to evaluate arrhythmias, conduction defects, myocardial injury and damage, hypertrophy (both left and right), and pericardial diseases. It is also used to assist in the diagnosis of other noncardiac conditions such as electrolyte abnormalities, drug level abnormalities, and pulmonary diseases.

TEST EXPLANATION

The ECG is a graphic representation of the electrical impulses that the heart generates during the cardiac cycle. These electrical impulses are conducted to the body's surface, and detected by electrodes placed on the patient's limbs and chest. The monitoring electrodes detect the electrical activity of the heart from a variety of spatial perspectives. The electrocardiographic lead system is composed of several electrodes that are placed on each of the four extremities and at varying sites on the chest. Each combination of electrodes is called a *lead*.

A 12-lead ECG provides a comprehensive view of the flow of the heart's electrical currents in two different planes. There are six limb leads (combination of electrodes on the extremities) and six chest leads (corresponding to six sites on the chest).

The limb leads provide a *frontal* plane view that bisects the body, whereby impulses from the front of the body are recorded separately from those of the back. The chest leads provide a *horizontal* plane view that bisects the body, whereby impulses from the top of the body are recorded separately from those from the bottom (Figure 3-2). Leads I, II, and III are considered the *standard limb leads*. Lead I records the difference in electrical potential between the left arm and the right arm. Lead II records the electrical potential between the right arm and the left leg. Lead III reflects

A Frontal plane

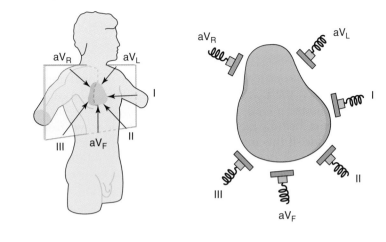

B Horizontal plane

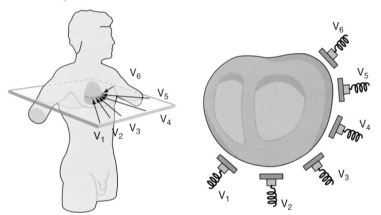

Figure 3-2 Planes of reference. **A,** The frontal plane. **B,** The horizontal plane.

the difference between the left arm and the left leg. The right leg electrode is an inactive ground in all leads. There are three *augmented limb leads:* aV_R (right arm), aV_L (left arm), and aV_F (left foot or leg). The augmented leads record the electrical potential between the centre of the heart and the right arm (aV_R), the left arm (aV_L), and the left leg (aV_F). The six standard *chest,* or *precordial, leads* (V_1, V_2, V_3, V_4, V_5, V_6) are recorded by placing electrodes at six different positions on the chest, surrounding the heart. (The exact locations of the leads are described in the section "Procedure and Patient Care.")

In general, leads II, III, and aV_F transmit information from the inferior portion of the heart. Leads aV_L and I transmit information from the lateral portion of the heart. Leads V_2 to V_4 transmit information from the anterior portion of the heart.

The ECG is recorded on special paper with a graphic background of horizontal and vertical lines for rapid measurement of time intervals (X coordinate) and voltages (Y coordinate). Time duration is measured by vertical lines 1 mm apart, each representing 0.04 second. Voltage is measured by horizontal lines 1 mm apart. A distance of five 1-mm squares represents 0.5 mV.

The normal electrocardiographic pattern is composed of waves that were originally designated arbitrarily by the letters P, Q, R, S, and T. The Q, R, and S waves are grouped together and described as the QRS complex. The significance of the waves and the time intervals are described as follows and are illustrated in Figure 3-3.

P wave. This represents atrial electrical depolarization associated with atrial contraction. It represents electrical activity associated with the spread of the original impulse from the sinoatrial node through the atria. If the P waves are absent or altered, the cardiac impulse originates outside the sinoatrial node.

PR interval. This represents the time required for the impulse to travel from the sinoatrial node to the atrioventricular node. If this interval is prolonged, a conduction delay exists in the atrioventricular node (e.g., a first-degree heart block). A shortened PR interval indicates that the impulse reached the ventricle through a "shortcut" (as in Wolff-Parkinson-White syndrome).

QRS complex. This represents ventricular electrical depolarization associated with ventricular contraction. This complex consists of an initial downward (negative) deflection (Q wave), a large upward (positive) deflection (R wave), and a small downward deflection (S wave). A widened QRS complex indicates abnormal or prolonged ventricular depolarization time (as in a bundle branch block).

ST segment. This represents the period between the completion of depolarization and the beginning of repolarization of the ventricular muscle. This segment may be elevated or depressed in transient muscle ischemia (e.g., angina) or in muscle injury (as in the early stages of myocardial infarction).

T wave. This represents ventricular repolarization (i.e., return to neutral electrical activity).

QT interval. This represents the time between the onset of ventricular depolarization and the end of ventricular depolarization. This interval varies with age, sex, heart rate, and medications.

U wave. This deflection follows the T wave and is usually quite small. It represents repolarization of the Purkinje fibres within the ventricles.

Through the analysis of these wave forms and time intervals, valuable information about the heart may be obtained. The ECG is used primarily to identify abnormal heart rhythms (arrhythmias, or dysrhythmias) and to diagnose acute myocardial infarction, conduction defects, and ventricular hypertrophy. Of importance is that the ECG may be normal, even in the presence of heart disease, if the heart disorder does not affect the electrical activity of the heart.

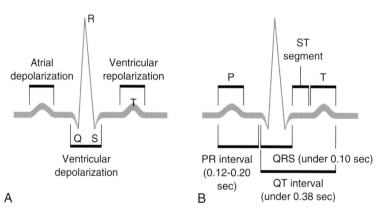

Figure 3-3 **A,** Normal electrocardiographic deflections during depolarization and repolarization of the atria and ventricles. **B,** Principal electrocardiographic intervals between the P wave, QRS complex, and T wave.

For some patients at high risk for malignant ventricular dysrhythmias, a *signal-averaged ECG* (SAECG) can be obtained. This test averages several hundred QRS waveforms to detect late potentials that are likely to lead to ventricular dysrhythmias. The SAECG has been a useful precursor to electrophysiologic study (p. 587) because it can identify ventricular tachycardia in patients with unexplained syncope. The SAECG can be performed at the patient's bedside in 15 to 20 minutes and must be ordered separately from a standard ECG.

Microvolt T-wave alternans (MTWA) testing reveals T wave alternans (variations in the vector and amplitude of the T waves) on electrocardiographic signals as small as one-millionth of a volt. MTWA is defined as an alteration in the structure of the T wave in an every-other-beat pattern. It has long been associated with ventricular arrhythmias and sudden death. T wave alternans is linked to the rapid onset of ventricular tachyarrhythmias.

MTWA testing is significant in the clinical context because it helps stratify risk with regard to the need for an implantable cardiac defibrillator. Patients whose MTWA test results are negative have a very low risk for sudden cardiac death and are less likely to require implantable cardiac defibrillators than are those whose test results are positive. In this test, high-fidelity electrocardiographic leads are placed on the patient's chest during an exercise test. The goal is to get the patient walking fast enough to get the heart rate in the range of 105 to 110 beats/minute, but no higher. Minute changes in T waves are measured and recorded via computer analysis.

INTERFERING FACTORS

- Inaccurate placement of the electrodes
- Electrolyte imbalances
- Poor contact between the skin and the electrodes
- Movement or muscle tremors (twitching) during the test
- Ingestion of drugs that can affect results, including barbiturates, digitalis, and quinidine

Age-Related Concerns

- The prevalence of atrial fibrillation increases with age, as does the prevalence of a decrease in resting heart rate and a reduction in the maximum heart rate.

PROCEDURE AND PATIENT CARE

Before

- Explain the procedure to the patient.
- Inform the patient that no food or fluid restriction is necessary.
- Assure the patient that the flow of electric current is from the patient. He or she will feel nothing during this procedure.
- Expose only the patient's chest, arms, and lower legs. Keep the abdomen and thighs adequately covered.

During

- Note the following procedural steps:
  1. The skin areas designated for electrode placement are prepared with alcohol swabs to remove skin oil or debris. Sometimes the skin is shaved if the patient has a large amount of hair.
  2. Prelubricated leads are applied to ensure electrical conduction between the skin and the electrodes.

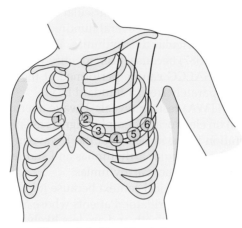

Figure 3-4 Chest lead placement.

3. The four limb leads are usually held in place by clamps attached to the electrodes that can easily be opened and applied to the electrode on the extremity.
4. Many cardiologists recommend that arm electrodes be placed on the upper arm because fewer muscle tremors are detected there.
5. The chest leads are applied one at a time, three at a time, or six at a time, depending on the type of electrocardiographic machine used. These leads are positioned as follows (Figure 3-4):
   V_1: in the fourth intercostal space at the right sternal border
   V_2: in the fourth intercostal space at the left sternal border
   V_3: midway between V_2 and V_4
   V_4: in the fifth intercostal space at the midclavicular line
   V_5: at the left anterior axillary line at the level of V_4 horizontally
   V_6: at the left midaxillary line at the level of V_4 horizontally
- Note that cardiac technicians, nurses, or physicians perform this procedure in less than 5 minutes at the bedside or in the cardiology clinic.
- Instruct the patient that although this procedure causes no discomfort, he or she must lie still in the supine position without talking while the ECG is recorded.

After
- Remove the electrodes from the patient's skin, and wipe off the electrode gel.
- Indicate on the ECG strip or request slip whether the patient was experiencing chest pain during the study. The pain may be correlated with an arrhythmia on the ECG.

TEST RESULTS AND CLINICAL SIGNIFICANCE

Arrhythmia (dysrhythmia): *Arrhythmias can start in an atrium or in a ventricle. They can cause the heart to speed up (tachyarrhythmias) or to slow down (bradyarrhythmias). With serious arrhythmias, cardiac output can fall significantly, causing the patient to lose consciousness (syncope). Often the patient may experience palpitations during some arrhythmias. Most arrhythmias are asymptomatic, however.*

Acute myocardial infarction,

Myocardial ischemia,

Old myocardial infarction: *Acute myocardial muscle damage is often seen as elevations in the ST segment or as inverted T waves. The presence of old myocardial infarctions (or areas of dead muscle tissue) manifests as deep Q waves on the ECG. The ECG should be one of the first tests to be performed on an adult patient who complains of chest pain.*

Conduction defects,

Conduction system disease,

Wolff-Parkinson-White syndrome: *The number and type of conduction defects are too great to discuss within the scope of this book. Some conduction defects slow the normal conduction of electrical voltage through the heart (e.g., bundle branch block). Some (e.g., Wolff-Parkinson-White syndrome) speed up the electrical conduction.*

Ventricular hypertrophy: *As a result of prolonged strain on the left ventricle (e.g., aortic stenosis), the thickened myocardium produces large R waves in V_5 and V_6 and large S waves in V_1.*

Cor pulmonale,

Pulmonary embolus: *The right-sided heart strain associated with acute pulmonary diseases (e.g., embolism) is called* acute cor pulmonale. *The classic electrocardiographic finding is the "$S_1Q_3T_3$" pattern, which is the presence of an S wave in lead I, a Q wave in lead III, and T wave inversion in lead III. Many times, however, there may be no changes other than tachycardia in association with pulmonary emboli.*

Electrolyte imbalance: *Each electrolyte abnormality is associated with different changes in the ECG (Table 3-2).*

Pericarditis: *The findings of pericarditis on an ECG are classical for that disease: widespread elevations of the ST segments involving most of the leads (except aVR) and normal QRS complexes. When effusion is associated with the pericarditis, the voltages are diminished throughout.*

RELATED TESTS

Echocardiography (p. 906). This is another method of imaging the heart with the use of ultrasonography.

Cardiac Nuclear Scanning (p. 817). This is a nuclear method of cardiac imaging.

TABLE 3-2	Electrolyte Abnormalities and Associated Electrocardiographic Abnormalities	
Electrolyte Abnormality	**Electrocardiographic Abnormality**
Increased calcium level: **>2.75 mmol/L**	Prolonged PR interval Shortened QT interval
Decreased calcium level: **<2.25 mmol/L**	Prolonged QT interval
Increased potassium level: **>5 mmol/L**	Narrowed, elevated T waves Atrioventricular conduction changes Widened QRS complex
Decreased potassium level: **<3.5 mmol/L**	Prolonged U wave Prolonged QT interval

Electroencephalography (Electroencephalogram [EEG])

NORMAL FINDINGS

Normal frequency, amplitude, and characteristics of brain waves

INDICATIONS

This electrodiagnostic test is performed to identify and evaluate patients with seizures. Pathologic conditions involving the brain cortex (such as tumours, infarction) can also be detected.

TEST EXPLANATION

The EEG is a graphic recording of the electrical activity of the brain. Electrodes are placed on the scalp, overlying multiple areas of the brain, to detect and record electrical impulses within the brain. This study is invaluable in the investigation of epileptic states, in which the focus of seizure activity is characterized by rapid, spiking waves seen on the graph. Patients with cerebral lesions (e.g., tumours, infarctions) have abnormally slow EEG waves, depending on the size and location of the lesion. Because this study reveals the overall electrical activity of the brain, it can be used to evaluate trauma and drug intoxication and also to determine cerebral death in comatose patients.

The EEG also can be used to monitor the electrophysiologic effects of cerebral blood flow during surgical procedures. For example, during carotid endarterectomy, the carotid vessel must be temporarily occluded. When this surgery is performed with the patient under general anaesthesia, the EEG can be used for the early detection of cerebral tissue ischemia, which would indicate that continued carotid occlusion will result in a cerebrovascular accident (stroke) syndrome. Temporary shunting of the blood during the surgery is then required.

Electrocorticography (ECoG) is a form of EEG performed during craniotomy in which electrodes are placed directly on the exposed surface of the brain to record electrical activity from the cerebral cortex. ECoG is currently considered to be the "gold standard" for defining epileptogenic zones before attempts at surgical interruption are carried out. This procedure is invasive.

The same information can be obtained by a noninvasive brain imaging technique called *magnetoencephalography* (MEG). In MEG, the magnetic fields produced by electrical activity in the brain are measured with an extremely sensitive device called a *superconducting quantum interference device* (SQID). The data obtained with MEG are commonly used to assist neurosurgeons in localizing pathologic processes or defining sites of origin of epileptic seizures. MEG is also used in localizing important adjacent cortical areas for surgical planning in patients with brain tumours or intractable epilepsy. Such localization enables the surgeon to identify and preserve important nearby cortical tissue, the injury of which would cause grave neurologic defects (such as blindness, aphasia, or loss of sensation).

INTERFERING FACTORS

- Fasting may cause hypoglycemia, which could modify the EEG pattern.
- Ingesting caffeine (e.g., in coffee, tea, cocoa, cola) interferes with the test results.
- Body and eye movements during the test can cause changes in the brain wave patterns.

- Lights (especially bright or flashing) can alter test results.
- There may be electrical interference from equipment (e.g., cardiac monitors).
- Hypothermia can alter results.
- Drugs that may *affect* test results include sedatives.

✔ Clinical Priorities

- The patient should not be in the fasting state during this test. Hypoglycemia could modify the EEG pattern.
- Stimulants (such as caffeine) should not be taken before the test because they may affect test results.
- Sleep may need to be shortened if a sleep EEG is attempted.

PROCEDURE AND PATIENT CARE

Before

- Explain the procedure to the patient.
- Assure the patient that this test cannot "read the mind" or detect senility.
- Assure the patient that the flow of electrical activity is *from* the patient. He or she will not feel anything during the test.
- Instruct the patient to wash his or her hair the night before the test. No oils, sprays, or lotion should be used.
- Check whether the physician wants the patient to discontinue any medications before the study. (Anticonvulsants should be taken unless the physician instructs otherwise.)
- If sleeping time should be shortened the night before the test, instruct the patient accordingly. If a sleep EEG is attempted at the time of testing, adults may not be allowed to sleep more than 4 or 5 hours and children not more than 5 to 7 hours.
- Do not administer any sedatives or hypnotics before the test because they will cause abnormal waves on the EEG.
- Instruct the patient not to fast before the study. Fasting may cause hypoglycemia, which could alter test results.
- Instruct the patient not to drink any coffee, tea, cocoa, cola, or other caffeinated drink on the morning of the test because of their stimulating effect.
- Instruct the patient that he or she needs to remain still during the test. Any movement, including opening the eyes, creates interferences and alters the EEG recording.
- Inform the patient that he or she needs to arrange for transportation after the procedure because he or she will not be permitted to drive.

During

- Note the following procedural steps:
  1. The EEG is usually performed in a specially constructed room that is shielded from outside disturbances.
  2. The patient is placed in a supine position on a bed or in a reclining position on a chair.
  3. Sixteen or more electrodes are applied to the scalp with electrode gel in a specified pattern (as determined by the international *10–20 system* of applying scalp electrodes) over both sides of the head, covering the prefrontal, frontal, temporal, parietal, and occipital areas (Figures 3-5 and 3-6). In some laboratories, the electrodes are tiny needles superficially placed in the skin of the scalp.

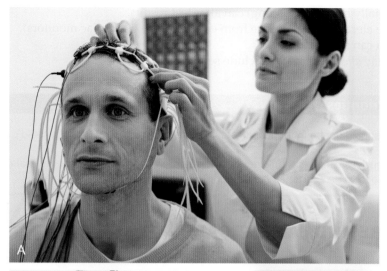

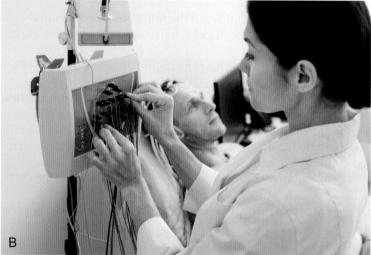

Figure 3-5 Electroencephalography (EEG). Routine EEG takes approximately 1¼ hours. The actual test lasts approximately 30 minutes. Electrodes are attached to the patient's head **(A)** with the wires leading to corresponding areas on the equipment **(B)** for recording brain wave activity.

4. One electrode may be applied to each earlobe for grounding.
5. After the electrodes are applied, the patient is instructed to lie still with his or her eyes closed.
6. The technician continuously observes the patient during the EEG recording for any movements that could alter results.
7. Approximately every 5 minutes, the recording is interrupted to permit the patient to move if he or she desires.

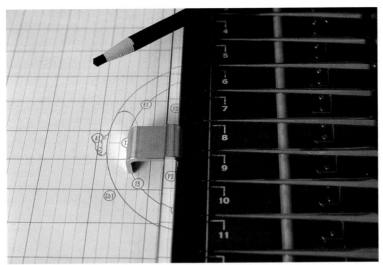

Figure 3-6 Equipment used to record brain waves during electroencephalography (EEG).

- In addition to the resting EEG, note that the following *activating procedures* can be performed:
  1. The patient is *hyperventilated* (asked to breathe deeply 20 times a minute for 3 minutes) to induce alkalosis and cerebral vasoconstriction, which can activate otherwise hidden abnormalities.
  2. *Photostimulation* is performed by flashing a light at variable speeds over the patient's face with the patient's eyes opened or closed. Photostimulated seizure activity may be seen on the EEG.
  3. A *sleep* EEG may be performed to aid in the detection of some abnormal brain waves that occur only when the patient is sleeping (e.g., as in frontal lobe epilepsy). The sleep EEG is performed after the patient orally ingests a sedative or hypnotic. A recording is performed while the patient is falling asleep, while the patient is asleep, and while the patient is waking.
- Note that this study is performed by an EEG technician in approximately 45 minutes to 2 hours.
- Inform the patient that no discomfort is associated with this study, other than possibly missing sleep.

After

- Help the patient remove the electrode gel using warm water and a mild soap if necessary.
- Instruct the patient to shampoo the hair.
- Ensure safety precautions until the effects of any sedatives have worn off. Keep the bed's side rails up.
- Remind the patient who has had a sleep EEG not to drive.

TEST RESULTS AND CLINICAL SIGNIFICANCE

Seizure disorders (e.g., epilepsy): *The EEG can detect major, minor, and focal motor seizures only when they are occurring. Between seizures, the EEG may be normal.*

Brain tumour,

Brain abscess,

Intracranial hemorrhage,

TABLE 3-3	Medical Standards for Neurologic Determination of Death	

Recommendations	Criteria	Clinical Symptoms
Minimum clinical criteria	Established cause capable of causing neurologic death	Acute neurologic event: stroke, transection of the spinal cord
	Deep unresponsive coma	Absence of spinal reflexes
	Absence of brain stem reflexes	Absence of gag reflexes and cough reflexes, and bilateral absence of motor responses, corneal response, pupillary responses, vestibulo-ocular responses
	Absent respiratory test based on apnea test	
	Absence of confounding factors	Confounding factors must be treated and corrected if possible
No confounding factors	Unresuscitated shock	Acute renal failure
	Hypothermia with core temperature <34° C	Hypothermia
	Severe metabolic disorders (PO$_4$, Ca, and Mg imbalances)	Drug overdose
	Severe liver and renal dysfunction	
Minimum temperature	≥34°C	Core body temperature of 34°C or lower is the minimum criterion for neurologic determination of death
Apnea testing	Thresholds of the apnea test are met and documented by arterial blood gas measurement and continuous observation or respiratory effort	Paco$_2$ of ≥60 mm Hg Paco$_2$ rises to ≥20 mm Hg above the pre–apnea test level pH of <7.28 Lack of respiratory efforts throughout the test

Recommendations from the Canadian Council for Donation and Transplantation.
Paco$_2$, Partial pressure of arterial carbon dioxide.

Cerebral infarct: *Most diseased areas of the brain exhibit localized slowing of brain waves.*

Cerebral death: *Cerebral death is total cessation of brain blood flow and function while the patient is being ventilated. The EEG is flat; that is, there is no electrical activity. Table 3-3 lists the standard criteria for the neurologic determination of brain death. EEG is no longer recommended as an ancillary test for determining brain death.*

Encephalitis: *Diffuse global slowing of brain waves may be noted on the EEG.*

Narcolepsy: *Sleep waves are noted during what are normally waking hours.*

Metabolic encephalopathy: *This may be drug induced or may occur with hypoxia (e.g., after a cardiac arrest), hypoglycemia, or other metabolic disorders. The EEG usually shows diffuse slowing of electrical activity.*

RELATED TESTS

Evoked Potential Studies (p. 589). These tests are used to evaluate specific areas of the cortex that receive incoming stimuli from the eyes, ears, and lower- or upper-extremity sensory nerves.

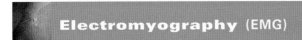

Electromyography (EMG)

NORMAL FINDINGS

No evidence of neuromuscular abnormalities

INDICATIONS

This test is used in the evaluation of patients with diffuse or localized muscle weakness. In combination with electroneurography, electromyography (EMG) can identify primary muscle diseases and differentiate them from primary neurologic pathologic conditions.

TEST EXPLANATION

By placing a recording electrode into a skeletal muscle, a clinician can monitor the electrical activity of a patient's skeletal muscle in a way very similar to electrocardiography. The electrical activity is displayed on an oscilloscope as an electrical wave form. An audio electrical amplifier can be added to the system so that both the appearance and sound of the electrical potentials can be analyzed and compared simultaneously. EMG is used to detect primary muscular disorders, as well as muscular abnormalities caused by other system diseases (e.g., nerve dysfunction, sarcoidosis, paraneoplastic syndrome).

Spontaneous muscle movement, such as fibrillation and fasciculation, can be detected during EMG. When evident, these rapid wave forms indicate injury or disease of the nerve innervating that muscle or spastic myotonic muscle disease. Reduced amplitude (size) of the electrical wave form is indicative of a primary muscle disorder (e.g., polymyositis, muscular dystrophies, various myopathies). A progressive decrease in amplitude of the electrical wave form during contraction is a classical sign of myasthenia gravis. The number of muscle fibres able to contract decreases with peripheral nerve damage. This study is usually done in conjunction with electroneurography (p. 582) and also may be called *electromyoneurography.*

A physical therapist, a psychiatrist, or a neurologist performs EMG in approximately 30 to 60 minutes. Because of the small needle size, the procedure is nearly painless.

CONTRAINDICATIONS

- Anticoagulant therapy, because the electrodes may induce intramuscular bleeding
- Extensive skin infection, because the electrodes may penetrate the infected skin and spread the infection to the muscle

POTENTIAL COMPLICATION

- In rare cases, hematoma at the needle insertion site

INTERFERING FACTORS

- Edema, hemorrhage, or thick subcutaneous fat can interfere with the transmission of electrical waves to the electrodes and alter test results.
- Patients with excessive pain may produce false results.

Clinical Priorities

- This test cannot be performed on patients receiving anticoagulation therapy because the electrodes may induce bleeding.
- Slight discomfort may occur with insertion of the needle electrodes into the muscle.
- If ordered, levels of serum enzymes (such as aspartate aminotransferase, lactic dehydrogenase, creatine phosphokinase) should be measured 5 to 10 days after EMG because penetration of the muscle may cause misleading elevations in the enzyme levels.

PROCEDURE AND PATIENT CARE

Before

- Explain the procedure to the patient. Allow the patient to express concerns, and allay those concerns.
- Obtain informed consent if it is required by the institution.
- Fasting is not usually required; however, some facilities may restrict the use of stimulants (coffee, tea, cocoa, cola, cigarettes) for 2 to 3 hours before the test. Instruct the patient accordingly.
- If serum enzymes (e.g., aspartate aminotransferase, creatine phosphokinase, lactic dehydrogenase) are to be measured, the specimen should be drawn before EMG or 5 to 10 days afterward because the penetration of the muscle by the electrodes may cause misleading elevations in levels of these enzymes, which can be produced by the muscle tissue.
- Premedication or sedation is usually avoided because of the need for the patient's cooperation.

During

- Note the following procedural steps:
  1. This study is usually conducted in an EMG laboratory. The laboratory may be specially designed (with copper-lined walls) to minimize extraneous electrical activity.
  2. The patient's position and the position of the electrode depend on the muscle being studied.
  3. A tiny needle that acts as a recording electrode is inserted into the muscle being examined (Figure 3-7) or overlying the nerve itself.
  4. A reference electrode is placed nearby on the skin surface.
  5. The patient is asked to keep the muscle at rest.
  6. The oscilloscope display is viewed for any evidence of spontaneous electrical activity, such as fasciculation or fibrillation.
  7. The patient is asked to contract the muscle slowly and progressively.

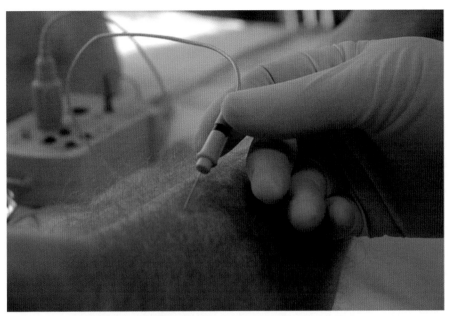

Figure 3-7 Needle inserted in the forearm of a patient undergoing electromyography (EMG). Because of the tiny needle size, the procedure is nearly painless.

8. The electrical waves produced are examined for their number, form, and amplitude. This is how the muscular component of the test is evaluated.
9. Next, a nerve innervating a particular muscle group is stimulated, and the resulting muscle contraction is examined as described in step 8. This is how the nerve portion of the neuromuscular component is evaluated.

After
- Observe the needle site for hematoma or inflammation.
- Provide pain medication if needed.

TEST RESULTS AND CLINICAL SIGNIFICANCE

Polymyositis: *This disease is evidenced by fast, small, spontaneous waveforms (myotonia), caused by hyperirritability of the muscle membrane.*

Muscular dystrophy,

Myopathy,

Traumatic injury: *These primary muscle diseases are manifested by decreased electrical activity and amplitude. Even with nerve stimulation, little or no activity is observed. This indicates weakened muscle tissue.*

Hyperadrenalism,

Hypothyroidism: *These endocrine diseases are marked by decreased electrical activity in both amplitude and frequency. This indicates that muscle tissue is weakened.*

Paraneoplastic syndrome (e.g., lung cancer),

Sarcoidosis: *These two diseases can be associated with ectopic production of adrenocorticotropic hormone. As in hyperadrenalism, decreased electrical activity in both amplitude and frequency is noted. This indicates that muscle tissue is weakened.*

Guillain-Barré syndrome,

Myasthenia gravis,

Peripheral nerve injury, entrapment, or compression,

Spinal cord injury or disease,

Acetylcholine blockers (e.g., curare, snake venom),

Multiple sclerosis,

Diabetic neuropathy,

Anterior poliomyelitis,

Muscle denervation,

Amyotrophic lateral sclerosis: *The presence of these neurologic diseases and injuries is indicated by reduced muscle electrical activity with spontaneous contraction. With electrical stimulation, the electrical activity within the muscle is more normal.*

RELATED TEST

Electroneurography (see following test). This is similar to EMG except that the integrity of the peripheral nerves is evaluated. This test is often performed with EMG.

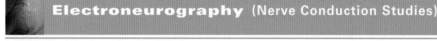

Electroneurography (Nerve Conduction Studies)

NORMAL FINDINGS

No evidence of peripheral nerve injury or disease

Conduction velocity is usually decreased in older adults.

INDICATIONS

This test is performed to identify peripheral nerve injury in patients with localized or diffuse weakness, to differentiate primary peripheral nerve disease from muscular injury, and to document the severity of injury in legal cases. It also is used to monitor the nerve injury and response to treatment.

TEST EXPLANATION

Electroneurography (nerve conduction studies) allows the detection and location of peripheral nerve injury or disease. When an electrical impulse is initiated at one site (proximal) of a nerve and the time required for that impulse to travel to a second site (distal) of the same nerve is recorded, the conduction velocity of any impulse in that nerve can be determined. This study is usually performed in conjunction with electromyography (p. 579) and is also called *electromyoneurography*.

The normal value for conduction velocity varies from one nerve to another. Such values also vary between individuals. It is always best to compare the conduction velocity of the suspected side with that of the contralateral nerve conduction velocity. In general, a range of normal conduction velocity is approximately 50 to 60 m/sec.

Traumatic transection or contusion of a nerve usually causes maximal slowing of conduction velocity in the affected side in comparison with the normal side. Neuropathies, both local and generalized, also cause a slowing of conduction velocity. A velocity greater than normal does not indicate a pathologic condition.

Because conduction velocity may require contraction of a muscle as an indication of an impulse arriving at the recording electrode, primary muscular disorders may cause an artificially slow nerve conduction velocity. To eliminate this "muscular" variable, the muscle group with the suspected pathologic disorder should be examined before nerve conduction studies are performed. This muscular variable can be evaluated by measuring distal latency (i.e., the time required for stimulation of the distal end of the nerve to cause muscular contraction). Once the distal latency is calculated, the nerve conduction study is then performed normally by stimulating the proximal portion of the nerve bundle. Conduction velocity can then be determined by the following equation:

$$\text{Conduction velocity (in metres per second)} = \left\{ \frac{\text{Distance (in metres)}}{\text{Total latency} - \text{Distal latency}} \right\}$$

This test takes approximately 15 minutes and is performed by a physiatrist or a neurologist. This test may be uncomfortable because a mild shock is required for nerve impulse stimulation.

INTERFERING FACTORS

- Severe pain may lead to false results.

PROCEDURE AND PATIENT CARE

Before
- Explain the procedure to the patient. Allow the patient to express concerns, and allay those concerns.
- Obtain informed consent if required by the institution.
- Inform the patient that no fasting or sedation is usually required.

During
- Note the following procedural steps:
  1. This test can be performed in a nerve conduction laboratory or at the patient's bedside.
  2. The patient's position depends on the area of suspected peripheral nerve injury or disease.
  3. A recording electrode is placed on the skin overlying a muscle innervated solely by the relevant nerve.
  4. A reference electrode is placed nearby.
  5. All skin-to-electrode connections are ensured through the use of electrode gel.
  6. A shock-emitting device at an adjacent location stimulates the nerve.
  7. The time between nerve impulse and muscular contraction (distal latency) is measured in milliseconds on an electromyograph machine.
  8. The nerve is similarly stimulated at a location proximal to the area of suspected injury or disease.
  9. The time required for the impulse to travel from the site of initiation to muscle contraction (total latency) is recorded in milliseconds.
  10. The distance between the site of stimulation and the recording electrode is measured in centimetres.
  11. Conduction velocity is converted to metres per second and is computed as in the previous equation.

After

• Remove the electrode gel from the patient's skin.

TEST RESULTS AND CLINICAL SIGNIFICANCE

Peripheral nerve injury or disease,

Carpal tunnel syndrome,

Herniated disc disease,

Poliomyelitis,

Diabetic neuropathy: *With peripheral nerve injury, nerve conduction is reduced. Treatment of the nerve entrapment can improve the nerve function and conduction.*

Myasthenia gravis,

Guillain-Barré syndrome: *These diseases affect the spinal cord and, to a lesser degree, the peripheral nerves. The extent to which the peripheral nerve is diseased is correlated with the extent of abnormality of the nerve conduction velocity.*

RELATED TEST

Electromyography (p. 579). This test is often performed simultaneously with electroneurography to determine distal latency (muscular contraction) and to identify muscular disorder as a contributing cause of weakness.

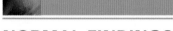

Electronystagmography (ENG, Electrooculography)

NORMAL FINDINGS

Normal nystagmus response

Normal oculovestibular reflex

INDICATIONS

Electronystagmography is used to evaluate patients with vertigo and to differentiate organic from psychogenic vertigo. With this test, pathologic conditions of the central nervous system (cerebellum, brain stem, cranial nerve VIII) can be differentiated from peripheral (vestibular-cochlear) pathologic conditions. If a known lesion exists, electronystagmography can identify the site of the lesion. This test is also used to evaluate unilateral deafness.

TEST EXPLANATION

Electronystagmography is used to evaluate nystagmus (involuntary rapid eye movement) and the muscles controlling eye movement. By measuring changes in the electrical field around the eye, this study can make a permanent recording of eye movement, whether at rest, with a change in head position, or in response to various stimuli. The test delineates the presence or absence of nystagmus, which is caused by the initiation of the oculovestibular reflex. Nystagmus should occur when initiated by positional, visual, or caloric (p. 561) stimuli. In caloric studies, nystagmus is usually determined visually, whereas in electronystagmography, the direction, velocity, and degree of nystagmus can be recorded. If nystagmus does not occur with stimulation, the vestibular-cochlear apparatus, cerebral cortex (temporal lobe), auditory nerve, or brain stem is abnormal. Tumours, infection, ischemia, and degeneration can cause such abnormalities. The pattern of nystagmus, in combination with the entire clinical picture, helps in the differentiation between central and peripheral vertigo. This test is used in the differential diagnosis of lesions in the vestibular system, brain stem, and cerebellum.

This test also may help evaluate unilateral hearing loss and vertigo. Unilateral hearing loss may be related to middle ear problems or nerve injury. If the patient experiences nystagmus with stimulation, the auditory nerve is working, and hearing loss can be attributed to an abnormality of the middle ear.

CONTRAINDICATIONS

- Perforated eardrums, which should not be subjected to water irrigation
- Presence of a pacemaker

INTERFERING FACTORS

- Blinking of the eyes can alter test results.
- Drugs that can alter results include antivertigo agents, sedatives, and stimulants.

Clinical Priorities

- Various procedures are used to instigate nystagmus, such as pendulum tracking, changing head position, and changing gaze position.
- Sedatives, stimulants, and antivertigo drugs can alter test results.
- Food should not be eaten before this test, in order to reduce the possibility of vomiting.

PROCEDURE AND PATIENT CARE

Before

- Explain the procedure to the patient.
- Instruct the patient not to apply facial makeup before the test because electrodes will be taped to the skin around the eyes.
- Instruct the patient not to eat solid food for 24 hours before the test, in order to reduce the likelihood of vomiting.
- Instruct the patient not to drink caffeine or alcoholic beverages for approximately 24 to 48 hours (as ordered) before the test.
- Inform the patient that nausea and vomiting may occur during the test.
- Check with the physician about withholding any medications that could interfere with the test results.

During

- Note the following procedural steps:
  1. This procedure is usually performed in a darkened room with the patient seated or lying down on an examining table.
  2. If there is any wax in the ear, it is removed.
  3. Electrodes are taped to the skin around the eyes (Figure 3-8).

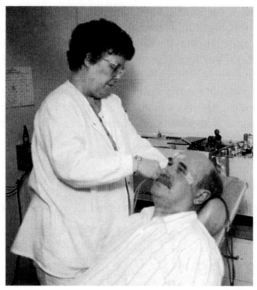

Figure 3-8 Electrodes are applied to a patient's face, near the eyes, in preparation for electronystagmography.

4. Various procedures are used to instigate nystagmus, such as pendulum tracking, changing head position, changing gaze position, and caloric studies (p. 561).
5. Several recordings are made with the patient at rest and with the patient demonstrating responses to various procedures (e.g., blowing air into the ear, irrigating the ear with water).
6. Nystagmus response is compared with the expected ranges, and the results are recorded as "normal," "borderline," or "abnormal."
• Note that this procedure is performed by a physician or audiologist in approximately 1 hour.

After
• Consider prescribing bed rest until nausea, vertigo, or weakness subsides.

TEST RESULTS AND CLINICAL SIGNIFICANCE

Brain stem lesions,

Cerebellum lesions,

Injury to cranial nerve VIII: *Tumours, infection, or degeneration of the central nervous system can be diagnosed, localized, and differentiated from peripheral vestibular diseases.*

Vestibular system lesions: *Infection is the most common pathologic condition affecting the peripheral vestibular system.*

Congenital disorder,

Demyelinating disease: *The demyelinating disorders (such as multiple sclerosis) are usually central, whereas the congenital disorders are usually peripheral.*

RELATED TEST

Caloric Study (p. 561). This is a test in which nystagmus is instigated by warm or cold water (or air) and the presence or absence of nystagmus is observed.

Electrophysiologic Study (EPS, Cardiac Mapping)

NORMAL FINDINGS

Normal conduction intervals, refractive periods, and recovery times

INDICATIONS

Electrophysiologic study is a method of studying evoked potentials within the heart. It is used to evaluate patients with syncope, palpitations, or arrhythmias. It is used to identify the location of conduction defects that cause abnormal electroconduction and arrhythmias. It can also be used to monitor responses to antiarrhythmic therapy. Through electrophysiologic study, the area known to induce arrhythmias can be obliterated by radiofrequency waves.

TEST EXPLANATION

In this invasive procedure, fluoroscopic guidance is used to place multiple-electrode catheters through a peripheral vein and into the right atrium or right ventricle (or both) or, less often, through an artery into the left atrium or left ventricle (or both). With close cardiac monitoring, the electrode catheters are used to pace the heart and potentially induce arrhythmias (dysrhythmias). Defects in the heart conduction system can then be identified; arrhythmias that are otherwise not apparent also can be induced, identified, and treated. To assess the effectiveness of antiarrhythmic drugs (e.g., lidocaine, phenytoin, quinidine), the electrical threshold needed to induce arrhythmias can be determined.

Electrophysiologic study can also be therapeutic. With the use of radiofrequency waves, sites with documented low thresholds for induction of arrhythmias can be obliterated to stop the arrhythmias.

CONTRAINDICATIONS

- Patient's inability to cooperate
- Acute myocardial infarction

POTENTIAL COMPLICATIONS

- Cardiac arrhythmias leading to ventricular tachycardia or fibrillation
- Perforation of the myocardium
- Catheter-induced embolic cerebrovascular accident (stroke) or myocardial infarction
- Peripheral vascular problems
- Hemorrhage
- Phlebitis at the venipuncture site

INTERFERING FACTORS

Drugs that may *interfere* with test results include analgesics, sedatives, and tranquilizers.

Clinical Priorities

- In this procedure, fluoroscopic guidance is used to place electrode catheters into the heart to pace the heart and to induce arrhythmias. The effectiveness of antiarrhythmic drugs can be evaluated.
- After this procedure, the patient is kept on bed rest for approximately 6 to 8 hours to allow the blood vessel access site to seal.
- After this procedure, the patient is carefully monitored for arrhythmias and hypotension.

PROCEDURE AND PATIENT CARE

Before

- Instruct the patient to fast for 6 to 8 hours before the procedure. Fluids are usually permitted until 3 hours before the test.
- Obtain an informed consent from the patient.
- Encourage the patient to verbalize any fears regarding this test, and allay those fears.
- Shave and prepare the catheter insertion site.
- Collect a blood sample to measure potassium or drug levels, if indicated.
- Obtain peripheral intravenous access for the administration of drugs.

During

- Note the following procedural steps:
  1. After the patient is transported to the cardiac catheterization laboratory, electrocardiographic leads are attached.
  2. The catheter insertion site, usually the femoral artery or vein, is prepared and draped in a sterile manner.
  3. Under fluoroscopic guidance, the catheter is passed to the atrium and ventricle.
  4. Baseline surface intracardiac electrocardiograms are recorded.
  5. Various parts of the cardiac electroconduction system are stimulated by atrial or ventricular pacing.
  6. Mapping of the electroconduction system and its defects is performed by measuring evoked potentials.
  7. Arrhythmias (dysrhythmias) are identified.
  8. Drugs may be administered to assess their efficacy in preventing arrhythmias induced by the electrophysiologic study.
  9. Because dangerous arrhythmias can be prolonged, equipment for cardioversion must be available for immediate use.
  10. Not only are vital signs and the heart monitored, but also the patient is constantly engaged in light conversation in order to assess mental status and consciousness.
- Note that this procedure is performed by a cardiologist within a darkened cardiac catheterization laboratory in approximately 1 to 4 hours.
- Inform the patient that he or she may experience palpitations, light-headedness, or dizziness when arrhythmias are induced. The patient should report these sensations to the physician. For most patients, this experience produces anxiety.
- Inform the patient that discomfort from catheter insertion is minimal.

After

- Keep the patient on bed rest for approximately 6 to 8 hours.
- Apply pressure to the catheter insertion site. Evaluate the venous access site for swelling and bleeding.
- Monitor the patient's vital signs for at least 2 to 4 hours for hypotension and arrhythmias (dysrhythmias). Additional monitoring is especially important for certain medications that the patient received during the test. For example, if the patient received quinidine, he or she should be monitored for hypotension and abdominal cramping.
- Continue cardiac monitoring to identify arrhythmias. Transfer to a monitored unit may be necessary.
- Cover the area with sterile dressings if the electrical catheter is left in place for subsequent studies.

TEST RESULTS AND CLINICAL SIGNIFICANCE

Electroconduction defects,
Cardiac arrhythmia,
Sinoatrial node defects (e.g., sick sinus syndrome),
Atrioventricular node defects and heart blocks,
Inducible arrhythmias (e.g., ventricular tachycardia and Wolff-Parkinson-White syndrome): *These arrhythmias and others can be determined by electrophysiologic study. (Before these studies were available, the site and actual presence could only be guessed.) Furthermore, areas of arrhythmia inducement can be obliterated by burning the tissue with radiofrequency waves.*
Vasomotor syncope syndrome

RELATED TEST

Electrocardiography (p. 568). This is the only other mechanism available to identify and locate the source of arrhythmia.

Evoked Potential Studies (EP Studies, Evoked Brain Potentials, Evoked Responses, Visual-Evoked Responses [VERs], Auditory Brain Stem–Evoked Potentials [ABEPs], Somatosensory-Evoked Responses [SERs])

NORMAL FINDINGS

No neural conduction delay

INDICATIONS

Evoked potential studies are indicated for patients who have a suspected sensory deficit but are unable to indicate or are unreliable in indicating recognition of a stimulus. These may include infants, comatose patients, or patients who are unable to communicate. These tests are used to evaluate specific areas of the cortex that receive incoming stimulus from the eyes, ears, and lower or upper extremities' sensory nerves. They are used to monitor natural progression or treatment of deteriorating neurologic diseases (e.g., multiple sclerosis).

TEST EXPLANATION

Evoked potential studies focus on changes and responses in brain waves that are evoked from stimulation of a sensory pathway. The study of evoked potentials grew out of early work with electroencephalography (EEG; p. 574). Whereas EEG is a measure of "spontaneous" brain electrical activity, the sensory evoked potential study is a measure of minute voltage changes produced in response to a specific stimulus, such as a light pattern, an audible click, or a shock. In contrast to EEG, which records signals that reach amplitudes of up to 50 to 100 mV, evoked potential signals are usually less than 5 mV. Because of this, they can be detected only with an averaging computer. The computer averages out (or cancels) unwanted random waves to sum the evoked response that occurs at a specific time after a stimulus is delivered.

Evoked potential studies enable the clinician to measure and assess the entire sensory pathway, from the peripheral sensory organ all the way to the brain cortex (recognition of the stimulus). Clinical abnormalities are usually detected by an increase in latency, which is the delay between the stimulus and the wave response. Normal latency times are calculated according to body size, position of the body where the stimulus is applied, conduction velocity of axons in the neural pathways, number of synapses in the system, location of nerve generators of evoked potential components (brain stem or cortex), and presence of pathologic conditions of the central nervous system. Conduction delays indicate damage or disease anywhere along the neural pathway from the sensory organ to the cortex.

Sensory stimuli used for the evoked potential study can be visual, auditory, or somatosensory. The choice of sensory stimulus depends on what sensory system is suspected to be diseased (e.g., questionable blindness, deafness, or numbness). The choice of sensory stimulus may also depend on the area of brain in which abnormality is suspected. (Auditory stimuli are used to check the brain stem and temporal lobes of the brain; visual stimuli are used to test the optic nerve, central neural visual pathway, and occipital portions of the brain; somatosensory stimuli are used to check the peripheral nerves, spinal cord, and parietal lobe of the brain.) Increased latency (i.e., abnormally prolonged period from the time of stimulus to the time of recognition on brain EEG) indicates a pathologic condition of the sensory organ or the specific neural pathway, as described previously (Table 3-4).

Visual-evoked responses (VERs) are usually instigated by a strobe light flash, a reversible checkerboard pattern (Figure 3-9), or retinal stimuli. A visual stimulus to the eye causes an electrical response in the occipital area that can be recorded with EEG-like electrodes placed on the scalp overlying the vertex and on the occipital lobes. Ninety percent of patients with multiple sclerosis exhibit abnormal latencies in VERs, a phenomenon attributed to demyelination of nerve fibres. In addition, patients with other neurologic disorders (e.g., Parkinson's disease) show an abnormal latency with VERs. The degree of latency seems to be correlated with the disease severity. Results also may be abnormal in patients with lesions of the optic nerve, optic tract, visual centre of the brain, and the eye itself. Absence of binocularity, which is a neurologic developmental disorder in infants, can be detected and evaluated by VERs. Eyesight problems or blindness can be detected in infants through VERs or electroretinography. This test also can be used during eye surgery to provide a warning of possible damage to the optic nerve. Infants' gross visual acuity can even be checked through the use of VERs.

Auditory brain stem–evoked potentials (ABEPs) are usually stimulated by clicking sounds to evaluate the central auditory pathways of the brain stem (Figure 3-10). Either ear can be evoked to detect lesions in the brain stem that involve the auditory pathway without affecting hearing. One of the most successful applications of ABEPs has been screening newborns of low birth weight and other infants for hearing disorders. Recognition of deafness enables infants to be fitted with

TABLE 3-4	Overview of Evoked Potential Studies		
Type of Evoked Potential	**Targeted Area of Brain or Nervous System**	**Stimulus**	**Examples of Clinical Applications**

Visual-evoked response (VER)	Optic nerve
	Central neural
	  visual pathway
	Occipital area
		Strobe light flash
		Reversible
		  checkerboard
		Retinal stimuli
			Multiple sclerosis
			Parkinson's disease
			Optic nerve lesions
			Blindness
			Gross visual acuity
			  in infants

Auditory brain stem–evoked potentials (ABEP)	Brain stem Temporal lobe	Clicking sounds	Brain stem lesions Hearing disorder in infants Brain tumours

Somatosensory-evoked responses (SER)	Peripheral nerves
	Spinal cord
	Parietal lobe
		Sensory stimulus
		  to an area of
		  the body
			Spinal cord injuries
			Head injury
			Malingering
			Monitoring response
			  to treatment for
			  multiple sclerosis

3 Electrodiagnostic Tests

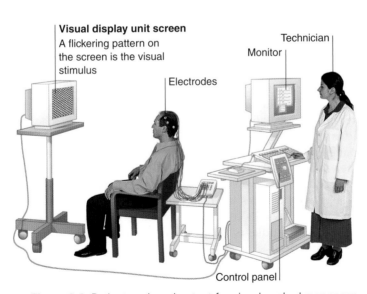

Figure 3-9 Patient undergoing test for visual-evoked responses. The patient is asked to concentrate on the yellow dot in the middle of the screen while the checkerboard pattern moves. Usually a patch is placed over one eye at a time. The room is darkened for the actual procedure.

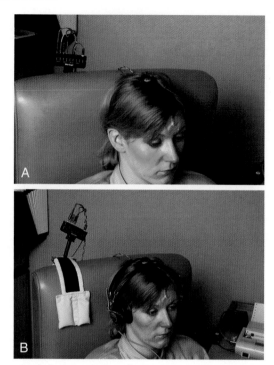

Figure 3-10 Patient undergoing test for auditory brain stem–evoked potentials (ABEPs).

corrective devices as early as possible. Use of these devices before affected children learn to speak helps prevent speech abnormalities. ABEPs also have great therapeutic implications in the early detection of brain tumours in the posterior fossa.

Somatosensory-evoked responses (SERs) are usually initiated by sensory stimulus to an area of the body. The examiner then measures the time it takes for the current of the stimulus to travel along the nerve to the cortex of the brain. SERs are used to evaluate patients with spinal cord injuries and to monitor spinal cord functioning during spinal surgery. SERs are also used to monitor treatment of diseases (e.g., multiple sclerosis), to evaluate the location and extent of areas of brain dysfunction after head injury, and to pinpoint tumours at an early stage. In addition, these tests can be used to identify malingering or hysterical numbness. The latency is normal in these patients despite the patients' assertions that they are experiencing numbness.

One of the main benefits of evoked potential studies is their objectivity: Voluntary patient response is not needed. Thus, evoked potential studies are useful with nonverbal and uncooperative patients. This objectivity enables the distinction of organic from psychogenic problems, which is invaluable in settling lawsuits concerning workers' compensation insurance. The projected future of evoked potential studies is that they will aid in diagnosing and monitoring mental disorders and learning disabilities.

PROCEDURE AND PATIENT CARE

Before

- Explain the procedure to the patient.
- Instruct the patient to shampoo his or her hair before the test.
- Inform the patient that no fasting or sedation is required.

During

- Note that the position of the electrode depends on the type of evoked potential study to be performed:
  1. VERs are elicited with the use of a strobe light, a checkerboard pattern, or retinal stimuli. Electrodes placed on the scalp along the vertex and the cortex lobes detect the responses.
  2. ABEPs are elicited by clicking noises or tone bursts delivered via earphones. The responses are detected by scalp electrodes placed along the vertex and on each earlobe.
  3. SERs are elicited with the use of electrical stimuli applied to nerves at the wrist (medial nerve) or the knee (peroneal nerve). The response is detected by electrodes placed over the sensory cortex of the opposite hemisphere on the scalp.
- Note that this study is performed by a physician or technician in less than 30 minutes.
- Inform the patient that little or no discomfort is associated with this study.

After

- Remove the electrode gel used for the adherence of the electrodes.

TEST RESULTS AND CLINICAL SIGNIFICANCE

Prolonged Latency for Visual-Evoked Responses

Parkinson's disease,

Demyelinating diseases (e.g., multiple sclerosis): *Diseases affecting the peripheral and central nervous systems prolong VER latency.*

Optic nerve damage: *In the absence of a functioning optic nerve, the stimulus cannot reach the cortex. VER latency is prolonged or absent.*

Ocular disease or injury,

Blindness: *Without visual sensory functioning, the stimulus cannot reach the cortex; therefore, stimulus recognition does not occur.*

Optic tract disease,

Occipital lobe tumour or cerebrovascular accident: *Unilateral or bilateral latency may be noted in diseases in which occipital cortical tissue is compressed or destroyed.*

Absence of binocularity,

Visual field defects: *These defects are caused by disorders such as congenital or acquired diseases, infections, and tumours.*

Prolonged Latency for Auditory Brain Stem–Evoked Potentials

Demyelinating diseases (e.g., multiple sclerosis): *In demyelinating diseases, the function and integrity of the peripheral and central nervous systems are destroyed. Latency is prolonged.*

Tumour (acoustic neuroma): *Such tumours grow where cranial nerve VIII passes under the temporal lobe. Destruction of the nerve by compression prolongs latency.*

Cerebrovascular accident (stroke),

Temporal lobe cortex,

Brain stem: *Infarctions of either portion of the brain cause ABEP latency to be prolonged. The brain stem is an important part of the reflex auditory mechanism.*

Auditory nerve damage: *If the auditory nerve is not functioning, the stimulus cannot reach the cortex. ABEP latency is therefore prolonged or absent.*

Deafness: *Without auditory sensory functioning, the stimulus cannot reach the cortex. Stimulus recognition does not occur. The test can, however, be performed with vibratory stimuli, which bypass the function of the inner ear.*

Abnormal Latency for Somatosensory-Evoked Responses

Spinal cord injury,

Cervical disc disease,

Spinal cord demyelinating diseases: *Because the spinal cord is the path by which the stimulus reaches the cortex, diseases affecting the spinal cord cause latency to be prolonged.*

Peripheral nerve injury, transection, or disease: *The somatic stimulus must travel by way of sensory peripheral nerves to the spinal cord. Diseases that affect the function of these nerves cause latency to be prolonged.*

Parietal cortical tumour or cerebrovascular accident: *Unilateral or bilateral latency may be noted in diseases in which parietal cortical tissue is compressed or destroyed.*

RELATED TEST

Electroencephalography (p. 574). This electrodiagnostic test is used to detect large electrical waves generated by the cortical structures of the brain and to identify areas of seizure activity or wave slowing that are indicative of specific pathologic conditions.

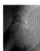

Fetal Contraction Stress Test (CST, Oxytocin Challenge Test [OCT])

NORMAL FINDINGS

Negative

INDICATIONS

The fetal contraction stress test (CST) is a method to evaluate the viability of a fetus. It documents the ability of the placenta to provide an adequate blood supply to the fetus. The fetal CST can be used to evaluate any high-risk pregnancy in which fetal well-being may be threatened. These pregnancies include those marked by diabetes, hypertensive disease of pregnancy (toxemia), intrauterine growth restriction, Rh-factor sensitization, history of stillbirth, postmaturity, or low estriol levels.

TEST EXPLANATION

The fetal CST, frequently called the *oxytocin challenge test,* is a relatively noninvasive test of fetoplacental adequacy used in the assessment of high-risk pregnancy. Other tests used to evaluate the fetoplacental unit are listed in Box 3-4. For the fetal CST, a temporary stress in the form of uterine contractions is initiated by the intravenous administration of oxytocin. An external fetal heart monitor assesses the reaction of the fetus to the contractions. Uterine contractions cause transient impediment of placental blood flow. If the placental reserve is adequate, the maternal-fetal oxygen transfer is not significantly compromised during the contractions and the fetal heart rate (FHR) remains normal (a negative test result). The fetoplacental unit can then be considered adequate for the next 7 days.

If the placental reserve is inadequate, the fetus does not receive enough oxygen during the contraction. This results in intrauterine hypoxia and late deceleration of the FHR. The test result is considered *positive* if consistent, persistent, late decelerations of the FHR occur with two or

BOX 3-4	Tests Used in the Evaluation of the Fetoplacental Unit

- Alpha-fetoprotein measurement
- Amniocentesis
- Biophysical profile
- Contraction stress test
- Estriol excretion measurement
- Fetoscopy
- Nonstress test
- Obstetric ultrasonography
- Pregnanediol measurement

more uterine contractions. Uterine hyperstimulation causes false-positive results in 10% to 30% of fetuses. Thus, positive test results warrant a complete review with other studies (e.g., amniocentesis) before the pregnancy is terminated by delivery.

The test result is considered to be *unsatisfactory* if it cannot be interpreted (e.g., because of hyperstimulation of the uterus, excessive movement of the mother, or deceleration of unknown meaning [not associated with contractions]). In the case of unsatisfactory results, other means of evaluation (ultrasonography or amniocentesis) should be considered.

Two advantages of the fetal CST are that it can be performed at any time and that its results are available shortly afterward. Although this test can be performed reliably at 32 weeks of gestation, it usually is performed after 34 weeks. The fetal CST can induce labour, and a fetus at 34 weeks is more likely to survive an unexpected induced delivery than is a fetus at 32 weeks. The fetal nonstress test (p. 597) is the preferred test in almost every instance and can be performed more safely at 32 weeks; the fetal CST if necessary can then follow it 2 weeks later. The fetal CST may be performed weekly until delivery.

A noninvasive, alternative method of performing the fetal CST is called the *breast stimulation* or *nipple stimulation technique*. Stimulation of the woman's nipple causes nerve impulses to the hypothalamus that trigger the release of oxytocin into her bloodstream. This causes uterine contractions and may eliminate the need for intravenous administration of oxytocin. Uterine contractions are usually satisfactory after 15 minutes of nipple stimulation (gentle twisting of the nipples). Advantages of this technique include the ease of performing the test, shorter duration of the study, and elimination of the need to start, monitor, and stop intravenous infusions. If sufficient contractions do not result from nipple stimulation, the standard fetal CST procedure is followed.

The fetal CST is performed safely on an outpatient basis in the labour and delivery unit, where qualified nurses and necessary equipment are available. A nurse performs the test, but a physician should also be available. The duration of this study is approximately 2 hours. The discomfort associated with the fetal CST may consist of mild labour contractions. Breathing exercises are usually sufficient to control any discomfort.

CONTRAINDICATIONS

- Pregnancy with multiple fetuses, because the myometrium is under greater tension and, with stimulation, premature labour is more likely to be induced
- Premature rupture of membranes, because labour may be stimulated by the fetal CST
- Placenta previa, because vaginal delivery may be induced

- Abruptio placentae, because the placenta may separate from the uterus as a result of the oxytocin-induced uterine contractions
- Previous hysterotomy, because the strong uterine contractions may cause uterine rupture
- Previous vertical or classic Caesarean section, because the strong uterine contractions may cause uterine rupture (The test can be performed, however, if it is carefully monitored and controlled.)
- Pregnancies of less than 32 weeks, because early delivery may be induced by the procedure

POTENTIAL COMPLICATIONS
- Premature labour

INTERFERING FACTORS
- Hypotension may cause false-positive results.

Clinical Priorities

- The blood pressure needs to be carefully monitored during this test to avoid hypotension, which may diminish fetal blood flow and cause a false-positive test result.
- This test is usually performed after 34 weeks' gestation because it could induce labour.
- The breast stimulation technique is an alternative method of performing the fetal CST that eliminates the need for intravenous administration of oxytocin.

PROCEDURE AND PATIENT CARE

Before
- Explain the procedure to the patient.
- Obtain informed consent from the patient for the procedure.
- Teach the patient breathing and relaxation techniques.
- Record the patient's blood pressure and the FHR before the test; these measurements are baseline values.
- If the fetal CST is performed on an elective basis, the patient may be kept on NPO status (nothing by mouth) in case labour occurs.

During
- Note the following procedural steps:
  1. After the patient empties her bladder, place her in a semi-Fowler's position and tilted slightly to one side to avoid vena caval compression by the enlarged uterus.
  2. Check patient's blood pressure every 10 minutes to avoid hypotension, which may diminish placental blood flow and lead to a false-positive test result.
  3. Place an external fetal monitor over the patient's abdomen to record the fetal heart tones. Attach an external tocodynamometer to the abdomen at the fundal region to monitor uterine contractions.
  4. Record the output of the fetal heart tones and uterine contractions on a two-channel strip recorder.
  5. Monitor baseline FHR and uterine activity for 20 minutes.
  6. If uterine contractions are detected during this pretest period, withhold oxytocin and monitor the response of the fetal heart tone to spontaneous uterine contractions.

7. If no spontaneous uterine contractions occur, administer oxytocin (Pitocin) by intravenous infusion pump.
8. Increase the rate of oxytocin infusion until the patient is having moderate contractions; then record the FHR pattern.
9. After the oxytocin infusion is discontinued, continue FHR monitoring for another 30 minutes until the uterine activity has returned to its preoxytocin state. The body metabolizes oxytocin in approximately 20 to 25 minutes.

After

- Monitor the patient's blood pressure and the FHR.
- Discontinue the intravenous line, and assess the site of needle entry for bleeding.

TEST RESULTS AND CLINICAL SIGNIFICANCE

Fetoplacental inadequacy: *Any disease, trauma, or alteration in the fetoplacental unit causes deceleration of the FHR. Such conditions include those with maternal causes, placental causes, or fetal diseases (or severe genetic defects).*

RELATED TEST

Fetal Nonstress Test (see following test). This is a preferred method of evaluating the fetoplacental unit. This test is performed in a manner similar to that described for the fetal CST except that oxytocin is not used.

Fetal Nonstress Test (NST, Fetal Activity Determination)

NORMAL FINDINGS

"Reactive" fetus (heart rate acceleration in association with fetal movement)

INDICATIONS

The fetal nonstress test is a method of evaluating the viability of a fetus. It documents the placenta's ability to provide adequate blood supply to the fetus. The fetal nonstress test can be used to evaluate any high-risk pregnancy in which fetal well-being may be threatened. Such pregnancies include those characterized by maternal diabetes, maternal hypertensive disease of pregnancy (toxemia), intrauterine growth restriction, Rh-factor sensitization, history of stillbirth, postmaturity, or low estriol levels.

TEST EXPLANATION

The fetal nonstress test is a noninvasive study that monitors acceleration of the fetal heart rate (FHR) in response to fetal movement. This FHR acceleration reflects the integrity of the central nervous system and fetal well-being. Fetal activity may be spontaneous, induced by uterine contraction, or induced by external manipulation. Oxytocin stimulation is not used. Fetal response is characterized as "reactive" or "nonreactive." The fetal nonstress test indicates that the fetus is reactive when, with fetal movement, two or more FHR accelerations are detected, each of which must be at least 15 beats/minute for 15 seconds or more within any 10-minute period. The test is 99% reliable in indicating fetal viability and negates the need for the fetal contraction stress test (CST; p. 594). If the test reveals that the fetus is nonreactive (i.e., no FHR acceleration occurs with fetal movement) within 40 minutes, the mother is a candidate for the fetal CST. A 40-minute test period is used because this is the average duration of the sleep-wake cycle of the fetus. The cycle may vary considerably, however.

The fetal nonstress test is useful in screening high-risk pregnancies and in determining which patients may require the fetal CST. A fetal nonstress test is now routinely performed before the fetal CST to avoid the complications associated with oxytocin administration. No complications are associated with the fetal nonstress test.

Clinical Priorities

- A fetal nonstress test is routinely performed before the fetal CST to avoid the complications associated with oxytocin administration.
- Fetal activity is enhanced by a high maternal serum glucose level. Therefore, the mother should eat before this study.
- If this test indicates that the fetus is nonreactive, further testing (such as the fetal CST) is indicated to evaluate fetal health.

PROCEDURE AND PATIENT CARE

Before
- Explain the procedure to the patient.
- Encourage the patient to verbalize her fears. The necessity for the study usually raises realistic fears in expectant mothers.
- If the patient is hungry, instruct her to eat before the fetal nonstress test is begun. Fetal activity is enhanced when the maternal serum glucose level is high.

During
- After the patient empties her bladder, place her in the Sims' position.
- Place an external fetal monitor on the patient's abdomen to record the FHR. The patient can indicate fetal movement by pressing a button on the fetal monitor whenever she feels the fetus move. The FHR and fetal movement are concomitantly recorded on a two-channel strip graph.
- Observe the fetal monitor for FHR accelerations associated with fetal movement.
- If the fetus is quiet for 20 minutes, stimulate fetal activity by external methods, such as rubbing or compressing the patient's abdomen, ringing a bell near the abdomen, or placing a pan on the abdomen and hitting the pan.
- Note that a nurse performs the fetal nonstress test in approximately 20 to 40 minutes in the physician's office or a hospital unit.
- Inform the patient that no discomfort is associated with the fetal nonstress test.

After
- If the results indicate that the fetus is nonreactive, calmly inform the patient that she is a candidate for the fetal CST. Provide appropriate education.

TEST RESULTS AND CLINICAL SIGNIFICANCE

Nonreactive fetus: *This result alone does not indicate fetal distress, but when it is combined with results of other noninvasive tests such as fetal CST, biophysical profile, alpha-fetoprotein measurement, pregnanediol measurement, and obstetric ultrasonography, fetal health can be accurately determined.*

RELATED TEST

Fetal Contraction Stress Test (p. 594). This test is frequently called the *oxytocin challenge test*. It is a relatively noninvasive test of fetoplacental adequacy used in the assessment of high-risk pregnancy.

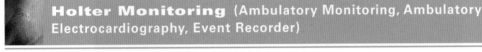

Holter Monitoring (Ambulatory Monitoring, Ambulatory Electrocardiography, Event Recorder)

NORMAL FINDINGS

Normal sinus rhythm

INDICATIONS

Holter monitoring is used to record a patient's heart rate and rhythm for 1 or more days. It is indicated for patients who experience syncope, palpitations, atypical chest pains, or unexplained dyspnea.

TEST EXPLANATION

Holter monitoring is a continuous recording of the electrical activity of the heart. This can be performed for periods of up to 72 hours. With this technique, an electrocardiogram (ECG) is recorded continuously on magnetic tape during unrestricted activity, rest, and sleep. The Holter monitor is equipped with a clock that enables accurate time monitoring on the ECG tape. The patient is asked to carry a diary and record daily activities, as well as any cardiac symptoms that may develop during the period of monitoring (Figure 3-11).

Most Holter units are equipped with an "event marker." This is a button that the patient can push when he or she experiences symptoms such as chest pain, syncope, or palpitations. This type of monitor is referred to as an *event recorder.* Many monitors store the rhythm that immediately precedes activation of the recorder. The patient should be instructed to record the reason why he or she pushed the button so that the clinician evaluating the recording can determine whether the event is correlated with any changes in the recording. Stored information can be transmitted by telephone to a recording station.

The Holter monitor is used primarily to identify suspected cardiac rhythm disturbances and to determine whether these disturbances are correlated with symptoms such as dizziness, syncope, palpitations, or chest pain. The monitor is also used to assess pacemaker function and the effectiveness of antiarrhythmic medications (Figure 3-12).

After completion of the determined time period, usually 24 to 72 hours, the Holter monitor is removed from the patient and the recording is played back at high speed. The electrocardiographic tracing is usually interpreted by computer, which can detect any significant abnormal

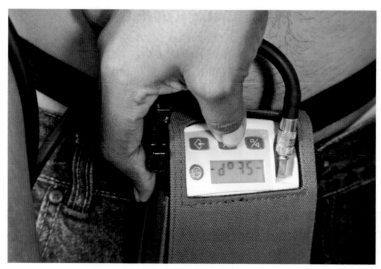

Figure 3-11 Patient wearing Holter monitor.

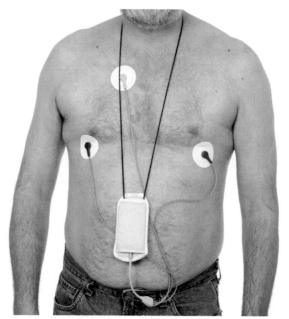

Figure 3-12 Equipment for ambulatory electrocardiography (Holter monitoring).

waveform patterns that occurred during the testing. Two different computer printouts can be generated. The first is generated from an "event recording," in which representative tracings during noted events are printed out. Tracings demonstrating maximum and minimum heart rates are also printed. A report then can be generated regarding the frequency and severity of abnormal cardiac events, especially in relation to the patient's symptoms. The second type of report is generated from a "full disclosure recording," in which all the beats are printed out and are scanned by a technologist, who looks for aberrant waveforms. These aberrations are then provided to the cardiologist for review.

Implantable loop recorders are used when long-term monitoring is required. These recorders are implanted subcutaneously through a small incision. They record electrocardiographic tracings continuously or only when purposefully activated by the patient. The recording device can be automatically activated by a predefined arrhythmia that triggers device recording. If nothing irregular happens, the information is subsequently erased. But if an arrhythmia does occur, the device locks it in and saves it to memory. Implantable loop recorders can provide a diagnosis in many patients with unexplained syncope or presyncope.

CONTRAINDICATIONS

- Patients' inability to cooperate with maintaining the lead placement
- Patients' inability to maintain an accurate diary of significant activities or events

INTERFERING FACTORS

- Interruption in the electrode contact with the skin

PROCEDURE AND PATIENT CARE

Before

- Explain the procedure to the patient.
- Instruct the patient about care of the Holter monitor.
- Inform the patient about the necessity of ensuring good contact between the electrodes and the skin.
- Teach the patient how to maintain an accurate diary. Stress the need to record activities and significant symptoms.
- Instruct the patient to note in the diary any interruption in Holter monitoring.
- Assure the patient that the electrical flow is coming *from* the patient and that he or she will not experience any electrical stimulation from the machine.
- Instruct the patient not to bathe during the period of cardiac monitoring.
- Instruct the patient to minimize the use of electrical devices (e.g., electric toothbrushes, shavers), which may cause artificial changes in the electrocardiographic tracing.

During

- Prepare the sites for electrode placement with alcohol (this is usually done in the cardiology department by a technologist).
- Securely place the gel and electrodes at the appropriate sites. The chest and abdomen are usually the most appropriate locations for limb-lead electrode placement. The precordial leads also may be placed.
- Usually, do not use the extremities for electrode placement, in order to minimize alterations in tracing that occur with normal physical activity.
- Encourage the patient to call if he or she has any difficulties.
- Use a tight undershirt or netlike dressing to hold the leads in place.

After

- Gently remove the tape and other paraphernalia securing the electrodes.
- Wipe the patient clean of electrode gel.
- Inform the patient that the Holter monitoring interpretation will be available in a few days.

TEST RESULTS AND CLINICAL SIGNIFICANCE

Cardiac arrhythmia (dysrhythmia): *Tachycardia or bradycardia may be noted and may be a cause of syncope. Frequent premature beats may be identified.*

Ischemic changes: *If a patient experiences unusual pain symptoms during a particular exercise, a monitor can be applied and that particular exercise performed. If the pain occurs and associated ischemic changes are noted on the ECG monitor, the diagnosis of angina can be made even though the pain is atypical.*

RELATED TEST

Electrocardiography (p. 568). This is an electrodiagnostic test of the heart taken at one particular time, whereas Holter monitoring continually records electrocardiographic data during the entire monitoring period.

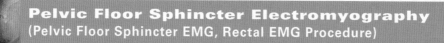

Pelvic Floor Sphincter Electromyography
(Pelvic Floor Sphincter EMG, Rectal EMG Procedure)

NORMAL FINDINGS

Increased electromyographic signal during bladder filling
Silent electromyographic signal on voluntary micturition
Increased electromyographic signal at the end of voiding
Increased electromyographic signal with voluntary contraction of the anal sphincter

INDICATIONS

This test is used to document pelvic diaphragm muscle weakness or paralysis. It is performed most often in patients who have urinary or fecal incontinence. The pathologic condition causing the muscle weakness can be muscular or neurologic.

TEST EXPLANATION

In this urodynamic test, electrodes are placed on or in the pelvic floor musculature to evaluate the neuromuscular function of the urinary or anal sphincter. The main benefit of this study is to evaluate the external sphincter (skeletal muscle) activity during voiding. This test is also used to evaluate the bulbocavernosus reflex and voluntary control of external sphincter or pelvic floor muscles. Pelvic floor sphincter electromyography (EMG) also aids in the investigation of functional or psychologic disturbances of voiding. Fecal incontinence caused by muscular dysfunction can also be identified by rectal sphincter EMG.

Three electrodes are used for this procedure. Recordings may be made from surface electrodes or needle electrodes within the muscle; surface electrodes are most often used. These electrodes allow for observation of and change in the muscle activity before and during voiding.

Patient cooperation is essential. If the patient does not cooperate, the interpretation of the test results will be difficult. A urologist, psychiatrist, or neurologist performs this study in less than 30 minutes. This study is slightly more uncomfortable than urethral catheterization.

CONTRAINDICATIONS

• Patients' inability to cooperate during the procedure

PROCEDURE AND PATIENT CARE

Before

✗ Explain the procedure to the patient.
✗ Inform the patient that cooperation is essential.

During

- Note the following procedural steps:
  1. Two electrodes are placed at the 2-o'clock and 10-o'clock positions on the perianal skin to monitor the pelvic floor musculature during voiding.
  2. The third electrode is usually placed on the thigh and serves as a ground.
  3. Electrical activity is recorded with the bladder empty and the patient relaxed.
  4. To evaluate reflex activity, the patient is asked to cough, and the urethra and trigone are stimulated by gentle tugging on an inserted Foley catheter (bulbocavernosus reflex).
  5. To evaluate voluntary activity, the patient is asked to contract and relax the sphincter muscle.
  6. The bladder is filled with sterile water at room temperature at a rate of 100 mL/minute.
  7. The electromyographic responses to filling and detrusor hyperreflexia (if present) are recorded.
  8. Finally, when the bladder is full and with the patient in a voiding position, the filling catheter is removed, and the patient is asked to urinate. Normally, the electromyographic signals build during bladder filling and cease promptly on voluntary micturition, remaining silent until the pelvic floor contracts at the end of voiding.
  9. The electrical waves produced are examined for their number, amplitude, and form.

After

- If needle electrodes were used, observe the needle site for hematoma or inflammation.

TEST RESULTS AND CLINICAL SIGNIFICANCE

Neuromuscular dysfunction of the lower urinary sphincter,
Pelvic floor muscle dysfunction of the anal sphincter: *With overly relaxed pelvic musculature, the frequency and amplitude of the electrical waveform are diminished. This is most commonly seen in older women who have had significant muscle stretching during childbirth. It is also seen in patients who have neurologic injury to the nerves innervating the pelvic muscles. The resultant weakness can affect the posterior portion of the pelvic sling and cause anal incontinence. It can affect the anterior portion of the pelvic muscle and cause cystocele, uterine prolapse, urinary incontinence, or a combination of these conditions.*

RELATED TESTS

Electromyography (p. 579). This test is used to diagnose peripheral muscle pathologic conditions. In theory, electromyography and pelvic floor sphincter EMG are similar.

Urine Flow Studies (p. 729). This test is often performed at the same time to evaluate incontinent patients.

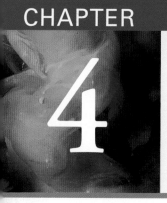

4 Endoscopic Studies

NOTE: *Throughout this chapter, SI units are presented in* **boldface colour,** *followed by conventional units in parentheses.*

OVERVIEW

TESTS

OVERVIEW
INDICATIONS FOR ENDOSCOPY

Endoscopy is a general term referring to the inspection of the internal body organs and cavities through the use of an endoscope. Endoscopic procedures are named for the organ or body area to be visualized or treated. Table 4-1 provides an overview of body areas viewed through endoscopy.

   In addition to direct observation, endoscopy enables biopsy of suspicious tissue, removal of polyps, injection of variceal blood vessels, and the performance of many surgical procedures, as indicated in Box 4-1. Furthermore, areas of stricture within a lumen of a hollow viscus can be dilated and a stent placed during endoscopy.

TABLE 4-1	Types of Endoscopy and Areas of Visualization
Type	**Area of Visualization**
Arthroscopy	Joints
Bronchoscopy	Larynx, trachea, bronchi, and alveoli
Colonoscopy	Rectum and colon
Colposcopy	Vagina and cervix
Cystoscopy	Urethra, bladder, ureters, and prostate
Enteroscopy	Upper colon and small intestines
Endoscopic retrograde cholangiopancreatography (ERCP)	Pancreatic and biliary ducts
Esophagogastroduodenoscopy (EGD)	Esophagus, stomach, duodenum
Fetoscopy	Fetus
Gastroscopy (part of EGD)	Stomach
Genitourinary endoscopy	Bladder and urethra
Hysteroscopy	Uterus
Laparoscopy	Abdominal cavity
Mediastinoscopy	Mediastinal lymph nodes
Sigmoidoscopy	Anus, rectum, sigmoid colon
Sinus endoscopy	Sinus cavities
Thoracoscopy	Pleura and lung
Transesophageal echocardiography (TEE)	Heart

BOX 4-1	Endoscopic Surgical Procedures

Laparoscopy
- Cholecystectomy
- Hiatal hernia repair
- Inguinal hernia repair
- Video-assisted colectomy
- Nephrectomy

Pelviscopy
- Oophorectomy
- Video-assisted hysterectomy
- Tubal ligation
- Oophoropexy
- Ovarian cystectomy

Thoracoscopy
- Wedge lung resection
- Video-assisted lung resection

Arthroscopy
- Meniscus removal or repair
- Ligamentous repair
- Tendon repair
- Tendon release (carpal tunnel)

Sinus Endoscopy
- Drainage of sinuses

Endoscopic Studies

4

BOX 4-1   **Endoscopic Surgical Procedures—cont'd**

Cystoscopy
- Transurethral resection of prostate
- Transurethral resection of superficial bladder tumours
- Removal of ureteral and bladder calculi
- Retrograde cystoscopy
- Ureteral stent placement

Esophagogastroduodenoscopy (EGD)
- Dilation of lumen strictures
- Placement of esophageal stents

Endoscopic Retrograde Cholangiopancreatography (ERCP)
- Stent placement in the pancreatobiliary tree

Fetoscopy
- Placement of central nervous system shunts

INSTRUMENTATION

An endoscope is a tubular instrument with a light source and a viewing lens for observation. The endoscope can be inserted through a body orifice (e.g., the rectum) or through a small incision (e.g., as in arthroscopy). There are two basic types of endoscopes: rigid and flexible. *Rigid metal endoscopes* were the first type available and are still used in operative endoscopy (e.g., arthroscopy). *Flexible fibreoptic endoscopes* are most often used in pulmonary and gastrointestinal (GI) endoscopy. An example of a flexible fibreoptic endoscope used in esophagogastroduodenoscopy is shown in Figure 4-1. This type of endoscope enables the transmission of images over flexible, light-carrying bundles of glass wires. The endoscope contains one or more accessory lumens for

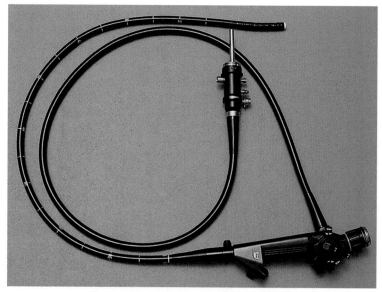

Figure 4-1 Endoscope used to perform esophagogastroduodenoscopy.

the insertion of water or medication or for the suctioning of debris. Also, instruments can be inserted through the accessory lumens of the endoscope for the following purposes:
- To obtain biopsy specimens (with forceps or brushes)
- To coagulate blood vessels (with laser beams)
- To remove tissue (with laser beams)

Endoscopic procedures are most often performed with the use of a video chip in the tip of a camera that is placed over the viewing lens. The image is then transmitted in colour to a nearby television monitor (Figure 4-2). This enables other people in the room to observe the procedure and more actively provide assistance. In many situations, endoscopy eliminates the need for open surgery.

PROCEDURAL CARE FOR THE PATIENT UNDERGOING ENDOSCOPY
Pulmonary and Gastrointestinal Endoscopy

Endoscopic procedures are generally considered invasive. Preparation and care of the patient are similar to those for most minor surgical procedures. General principles are described in this section. Detailed descriptions are included in this chapter for each individual test.

Before
- Explain the test preparation.
- Preparation varies with the type of endoscopy to be performed. For example, gastroscopy requires that the patient be kept on NPO status (nothing by mouth) for 8 to 12 hours before the procedure, in order to prevent vomiting and aspiration.

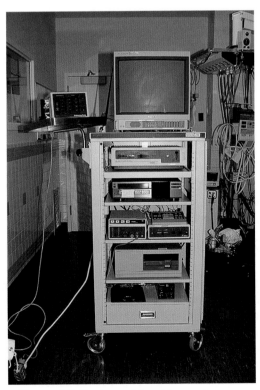

Figure 4-2 Equipment for video endoscopy.

- Dentures should be removed, and the presence of loose teeth should be noted and recorded.
- For colonoscopy, the bowel must be cleansed and free of fecal material to allow adequate visualization of the mucosa.
- GI endoscopy should precede barium contrast studies. Barium can coat the GI mucosa and preclude adequate visualization of the mucosa.
- Baseline laboratory tests (e.g., measurement of hemoglobin, hematocrit, electrolyte levels) should be performed, especially if a surgical procedure or biopsy may be needed.
- A thorough history concerning bleeding tendencies and allergies should be obtained before the procedure.
- Because GI endoscopy has the potential to expose the patient to contamination, intravenous antibiotics are recommended for patients who have cardiac valvular disease (to prevent endocarditis) and for patients who have prosthetic joints (to prevent bacterial seeding of the joint).

During

- Endoscopic procedures are performed preferably in a specially equipped endoscopy room or in the operating room. However, in cases of emergency, endoscopy can be performed at the patient's bedside.
- Because the patient is under sedation during the procedure, resuscitative equipment should be available.
- Room air is instilled into the bowel during GI endoscopy to maintain patency of the bowel lumen and to allow better visualization of the mucosa. If cautery is to be used, the air is exchanged for carbon dioxide to prevent ignition of oxygen or methane inside the bowel.
- Because air insufflation is used, the patient may experience gas pains during the procedure and after the procedure.
- Any surgical or biopsy procedures can be performed.

After

- Specific postprocedure interventions are determined by the type of endoscopic examination performed. All GI procedures can be potentially complicated by perforation and bleeding. See the discussions of potential complications.
- These procedures entail the use of sedation for the patient. Safety precautions should be observed until the effects of the sedatives have worn off. A family member or friend should drive the patient home after the test.
- After lower GI tract endoscopy, the patient may complain of rectal discomfort. A warm tub bath may be soothing.
- Usually the patient is kept on NPO status for 2 hours after pulmonary endoscopy or upper GI tract endoscopy. Ensure that the swallowing mechanism and cough reflex have returned to normal before allowing the patient to consume fluids or food.

OPERATIVE ENDOSCOPY AND GENITOURINARY ENDOSCOPY
Before

- These procedures usually necessitate general anaesthesia. Furthermore, complications of operative endoscopy may necessitate open surgical treatment. Therefore, the patient must be prepared for general anaesthesia and the possibility of open surgery. Routine preoperative care and teaching must be performed.
- The area to be examined should be shaved to remove hair if preferred by the surgeon.
- Because genitourinary endoscopy has the potential to expose the patient to contamination, intravenous antibiotics are recommended for patients who have cardiac valvular disease (to prevent endocarditis) and for patients who have prosthetic joints (to prevent bacterial seeding of the joint).

During

- During laparoscopy, CO_2 is instilled into the peritoneal cavity. If not all the CO_2 is allowed to escape after the procedure, this may cause significant gas pains and shoulder pain postoperatively.
- During cystoscopy, water is used to distend the bladder to allow visualization of the bladder mucosa. Accurate measurement of intake and output is difficult.
- The appropriate surgical procedure is performed as indicated in each test.

After

- Patients undergoing endoscopic surgical procedures should be monitored in the same way as any postsurgical patient.

POTENTIAL COMPLICATIONS OF ENDOSCOPY

Specific complications depend on the type of endoscopic procedure performed. The following guidelines apply to most types of endoscopy.

Perforation of Organ or Cavity

Examine the abdomen for evidence of colon perforation. Assess for abdominal distension, tenderness, and pain.

Persistent Bleeding From a Biopsy Site

Assess the vital signs. Watch for a decrease in blood pressure and an increase in pulse rate. Inspect body secretions (such as stool, urine, sputum) for blood.

Respiratory Depression as a Result of Oversedation

Carefully assess the patient for respiratory depression. Naloxone (Narcan) may be used to reverse the effects of opiates, such as meperidine (Demerol). Flumazenil (Romazicon) may be used to reverse the effects of benzodiazepines, such as diazepam (Valium) and midazolam (Versed).

Infections and Transient Bacteremia

This is a special concern with cystoscopy. Patients must drink a lot of fluids to maintain a constant flow of urine in order to prevent stasis and accumulation of bacteria in the bladder. Observe also for signs and symptoms of sepsis, which include elevated temperature, flushing, chills, hypotension, and tachycardia.

Aspiration After Evaluation of Upper Airway or Upper Gastrointestinal Tract

Instruct the patient not to eat or drink anything until tracheal anaesthesia has worn off and the gag reflex has returned, usually in 2 hours.

Cardiovascular Problems

Arrhythmias and even myocardial infarction can result. Vasovagal-induced bradycardia can be treated with atropine.

Age-Related Concerns

- Dysphagia is a common problem for adults aged 65 years and older. Patients undergoing endoscopic examinations who present with dysphagia may be at higher risk for complications such as perforation and aspiration.
- An anatomic cricopharyngeal protrusion is clearly associated with the aging process, and that protrusion can be a physical barrier that affects normal swallowing and can pose a risk during endoscopy.

REPORTING OF RESULTS

Most results are observed directly by the physician performing the procedure. Tissue samples for biopsy or culture need to be sent to the laboratory for evaluation. Results are discussed with the patient as soon as the effect of any sedation has worn off. However, because the sedation has an amnesic effect, the patient may later not recall this discussion. If possible, a written reminder of the physician's findings and instructions should be provided to the patient.

Arthroscopy

NORMAL FINDINGS

Normal ligaments, menisci, and articular surfaces of the joint

INDICATIONS

In arthroscopy, a specially designed endoscope is used to examine the interior of a joint.

TEST EXPLANATION

Arthroscopy is a highly accurate test because it enables direct visualization of an anatomic site (Figure 4-3). Although this technique can help visualize many joints of the body, it is most often used to evaluate the knee for injury to the meniscus cartilage or ligament. It is also used in the differential diagnosis of acute and chronic disorders of the knee (e.g., arthritic inflammation vs. injury).

Physicians can now perform corrective surgery on the knee through the use of the endoscope. Meniscus removal, spur removal, ligamentous repair, and biopsy are but a few of the procedures that are performed through the arthroscope itself. Arthroscopy is a safe, convenient alternative to open surgery (arthrotomy) because surgery is performed with the use of small trocars that are placed into the joint. Surgical manoeuvres are carried out under direct vision of the camera that is attached to the arthroscope. Because a large incision is avoided, recovery is faster and more comfortable.

Arthroscopy is also used to monitor the progression of disease and the effectiveness of therapy. Visual findings may be recorded by attaching a video camera to the arthroscope. Joints that can be evaluated by the arthroscope include the tarsal, ankle, knee, hip, carpal, wrist, shoulder, and

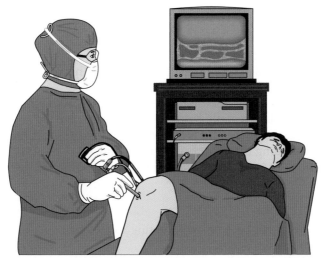

Figure 4-3 Illustration of arthroscopy. The arthroscope is placed within the joint space of the knee. In video arthroscopy, water is used to distend the joint space, a light source helps visualize the contents of the joint, and a television monitor projects the image. Other trocars are used for access of the joint space for other operative instruments.

temporomandibular joints. Synovial fluid can be obtained for fluid analysis (see Arthrocentesis with Synovial Fluid Analysis, p. 668).

This procedure is performed in the operating room by an orthopedic surgeon in approximately 30 minutes to 2 hours. Patients receiving a local anaesthetic have transient discomfort from the injection of the anaesthetic and the pressure of the tourniquet. A thumping sensation may be felt as the arthroscope is inserted into the joint. The joint may be painful and slightly swollen for several days or weeks, depending on the extent of surgery performed.

CONTRAINDICATIONS

- Ankylosis, because it is almost impossible to manoeuvre the instrument into a joint stiffened by adhesions
- Local skin or wound infections, because of the risk of sepsis
- Recent arthrography, because some residual inflammation remains after the injection of the contrast dye

POTENTIAL COMPLICATIONS

- Infection
- Hemarthrosis
- Swelling
- Thrombophlebitis
- Joint injury
- Synovial rupture

PROCEDURE AND PATIENT CARE

Before

- ✗ Explain the procedure to the patient.
- Ensure that the physician has obtained written consent for this procedure.
- Follow the routine preoperative procedure of the institution.
- ✗ Keep the patient on NPO status (nothing by mouth) after midnight on the day of the test because general anaesthesia is usually required.
- ✗ Advise the patient to use crutches after arthroscopy until he or she can walk without limping. Instruct the patient regarding the appropriate crutch gait.
- Shave the hair in the area 6 inches above and below the joint before the test (as ordered).

During

- Place the patient on his or her back on an operating room table.
- Note the following procedural steps:
  1. A general anaesthetic is usually administered to diminish pain and to allow for complete relaxation of the muscles around the knee.
  2. The leg is carefully scrubbed, elevated, and wrapped with an elastic bandage from the toes to the lower thigh to drain as much blood from the leg as possible.
  3. A tourniquet is placed on the patient's leg. If the tourniquet is not used, a fluid solution (usually saline) is instilled into the patient's knee immediately before insertion of the arthroscope to distend the knee and to help reduce bleeding.
  4. The foot of the table is lowered so that the patient's knee is at a 45-degree angle.
  5. A small incision is made in the skin around the knee.
  6. The arthroscope (a lighted instrument) is inserted into the joint space to visualize the inside of the knee joint.
  7. Although the entire joint can be viewed from one puncture site, additional punctures for better visualization and surgical manoeuvres are often necessary.
  8. After the area is examined, biopsy or appropriate surgery can be performed.
  9. Before removal of the arthroscope, the joint is irrigated. Steroids are sometimes injected to decrease inflammation. Pressure is then applied to the knee to remove the irrigating solution.
  10. After a few stitches are placed into the skin, a pressure dressing is applied over the incision site.

After

- Assess the patient's neurologic and circulatory status.
- Assess vital signs and observe the patient for signs of infection, including fever, swelling, increased pain, and redness or drainage at the incision site.
- ✗ Instruct the patient to elevate the knee when sitting and to avoid overbending the knee so that swelling is minimized.
- ✗ Inform the patient that he or she can usually walk with the assistance of crutches; however, this depends on the extent of the procedure and the physician's protocol. A referral may be made for physical therapy.
- ✗ Advise the patient to minimize use of the joint for several days.
- Examine the incision site for bleeding.
- ✗ Instruct the patient to apply ice to reduce pain and swelling.
- ✗ Inform the patient that the sutures will be removed in approximately 7 to 10 days.

Home Care Responsibilities

- Teach the patient to walk on crutches.
- Educate the patient about signs of bleeding into the joint (significant swelling, increasing pain, or joint weakness).
- Teach the patient to observe for signs of infection of the joint (fever, swelling, redness about the joint, and increasing pain).
- Educate the patient about signs of phlebitis. This is not uncommon in a person immobilized by joint pain. The involved leg may become swollen, painful, and edematous.
- Instruct the patient not to drive until driving is approved by the physician.
- Advise the patient to apply ice at home to minimize the normal swelling that may occur around the involved joint.

TEST RESULTS AND CLINICAL SIGNIFICANCE

Torn cartilage: *Either meniscus (in the knee) is fractured. The fracture may further injure the underlying joint surface.*

Torn ligament: *Ligaments support the joint. Injury to a ligament weakens joint stability.*

Patellar disease,

Patellar fracture: *Fracture, inflammation, and malformation can be visualized with knee arthroscopy.*

Chondromalacia: *Disease or structural damage to the cartilaginous joint surfaces can cause joint pain and dysfunction.*

Osteochondritis dissecans: *Injury to the joint surfaces can occur as a result of joint fragments in the joint space.*

Cyst (e.g., Baker): *A synovial cyst behind the knee may result from herniation of synovial fluid into the soft tissue surrounding the knee.*

Synovitis: *This is an inflammation of the lining of the joint.*

Rheumatoid arthritis,

Degenerative arthritis: *Destruction of the articular surfaces causes inflammation in the joint.*

Trapped synovium: *Synovial tissue can become trapped between two bones of the joint, causing pain and inflammation.*

RELATED TESTS

Arthrocentesis with Synovial Fluid Analysis (p. 668). In this procedure, a needle is inserted into the joint space to obtain synovial fluid for analysis.

Arthrography. This radiographic test of the joint space provides information about anatomic and disease abnormalities affecting the joint.

Magnetic Resonance Imaging (p. 1148). In this scanning technique, placement of the patient in a magnetic field provides valuable information.

Bronchoscopy

NORMAL FINDINGS

Normal larynx, trachea, bronchi, and alveoli

INDICATIONS

In bronchoscopy, the larynx, trachea, and bronchi are visualized directly through either a flexible fibreoptic bronchoscope or a rigid bronchoscope.

TEST EXPLANATION

♣ There are many diagnostic and therapeutic uses for bronchoscopy. *Diagnostic* uses of bronchoscopy include the following:

1. Direct visualization of the tracheobronchial tree for abnormalities (e.g., tumours, inflammation, strictures)
2. To obtain specimens for microbiology and histology
3. To evaluate a persistent or unexplained cough, wheezing, and hoarseness
4. To assess hemoptysis, unresolved lung abscess, pneumonia, atelectasis, airway involvement in burn patients, and bronchial abnormalities
5. To evaluate trachea and lungs prior to and after surgical procedures, radiation therapy, and chemotherapy
6. Aspiration of "deep" sputum for culture and sensitivity tests and for cytologic determinations
7. Direct visualization of the larynx for identification of vocal cord paralysis, if it is present; with pronunciation of "eeee," the cords should move toward the midline.

Therapeutic uses of bronchoscopy include the following:

1. Aspiration of retained secretions in patients with airway obstruction or postoperative atelectasis
2. Control of bleeding within the bronchus
3. Treat strictures and insert stents
4. Removal of foreign bodies, mucus plugs, and excessive secretions
5. Brachytherapy (endobronchial radiation therapy in which an iridium wire is placed via the bronchoscope)
6. Palliative laser obliteration of bronchial neoplastic obstruction

The rigid bronchoscope is a wide-bore metal tube that enables visualization of only the larger airways. It is used mainly for the removal of large foreign bodies. Its use has radically diminished since the advent of the flexible fibreoptic bronchoscope.

Because of its smaller size and its flexibility, the flexible fibreoptic bronchoscope has increased the diagnostic reach to the smaller bronchi. It also has accessory lumens through which cable-activated instruments can be used for removing biopsy specimens of pathologic lesions (Figure 4-4). In addition, the collection of bronchial washings (obtained by flushing the airways with saline solution), pulmonary toilet, and the instillation of anaesthetic agents can be carried out through these extra lumens. Double-sheathed, plugged protected brushes also can be passed through this accessory lumen. Specimens for cytologic and bacteriologic study can be obtained with these brushes. This allows more accurate determination of pulmonary infectious agents. Needles or biopsy forceps can be placed through the bronchoscope to obtain biopsy specimens from tissue immediately adjacent to the bronchi. Laser therapy can now be performed through the bronchoscope to burn out endotracheal lesions.

Bronchoscopy is performed in approximately 30 to 45 minutes by a physician, usually a pulmonary specialist or a surgeon. The patient usually feels no discomfort. It is recommended that all bronchoscopies be performed in a negative pressure isolation room, which has a lower pressure than adjacent areas, preventing air from flowing out of the isolation room. If bronchoscopy is performed under fluoroscopy, guidelines for radiation safety should be followed. In some facilities an anaesthesiologist may assist with the procedure, and capnography monitoring may be used.

Laryngoscopy is often performed through a short bronchoscope to allow inspection of the larynx and perilaryngeal structures. An otorhinolaryngologic surgeon most commonly performs this test. Cancers, polyps, inflammation, and infections of those structures can be identified. The vocal cord motion can also be evaluated. Anaesthesiologists use laryngoscopy to visualize the vocal cord structures when intubation for general anaesthesia is difficult. In this instance, the

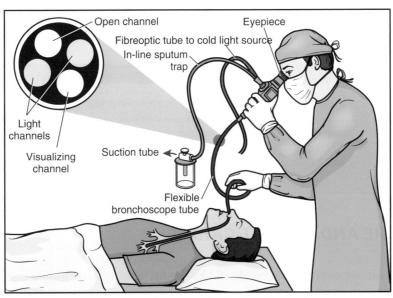

Figure 4-4 Illustration of the use of a flexible fibreoptic bronchoscope. The four channels consist of two channels that provide a light source, one vision channel, and one open channel that accommodates instruments or allows administration of an anaesthetic or oxygen.

laryngoscope is shaped very much like a rigid bronchoscope; it is routinely used to visualize the vocal cords directly with retraction of the anterior portion of the neck during intubation. This endoscopic laryngoscope, however, is attached to a camera that projects the image of the vocal cords onto a monitor.

CONTRAINDICATIONS

- Hypercapnia and severe shortness of breath, which preclude interruption of high-flow oxygen (bronchoscopy, however, can be performed through a special oxygen mask or an endotracheal tube so that the patient can receive oxygen if required)
- Acute asthmatic episode
- Hypoxia, unless patient is intubated
- Respiratory failure requiring high FiO_2
- Severe tracheal stenosis, which may make it difficult to pass the bronchoscope

POTENTIAL COMPLICATIONS

- Fever
- Bronchospasm
- Hemorrhage (after biopsy)
- Hypoxemia
- Pneumothorax
- Infection
- Laryngospasm

- Aspiration
- Cardiac arrest

 Age-Related Concerns

- A child's respiratory tract is constantly changing until approximately 12 years of age. As a result, the thyroid, cricoid, and tracheal cartilages are immature in the infant and child and may collapse easily when the neck is flexed during bronchoscopy. The tracheal airway is also shorter and narrower than an adult's airway. The bronchoscope can significantly decrease the available space for the child to breathe, and the risk of hypoxemia during the procedure is higher in a child than in an adult.

PROCEDURE AND PATIENT CARE

Before

- Emergency resuscitation equipment should be readily available, including equipment for endotracheal intubation and defibrillation.
- Explain the procedure to the patient. Allow the patient to verbalize any concerns, and allay those fears.
- Obtain the patient's informed consent for this procedure.
- Obtain baseline vital signs, oximetry levels, cardiac rhythm. Oxygen levels should be maintained at 90% or above.
- Verify the patient has been NPO (nothing by mouth) for 4 to 8 hours before the test to reduce the risk of aspiration.
- Instruct the patient to perform good mouth care to minimize the risk of introducing bacteria into the lungs during the procedure.
- Remove and safely store the patient's dentures, glasses or contact lenses, and hearing aids before the preprocedural medications are administered.
- Administer the preprocedure medications as ordered, which may include conscious sedation, medications to reduce oral secretions, and a local anaesthetic to numb the gag reflex.
- Reassure the patient that he or she will be able to breathe during this procedure.
- Instruct the patient not to swallow the local anaesthetic sprayed into the throat.
- Provide a basin for expectoration of the anaesthetic.
- All individuals assisting with the procedure must wear appropriate PPE, including a fitted N95 mask, eye goggles/face shield, gown, and gloves.

During

- All patients undergoing bronchoscopy require monitoring by a Registered Nurse or qualified health care provider including monitoring O_2 saturation, vital sign, level of consciousness, and skin colour, warmth, and dryness.
- Note the following procedural steps for *fibreoptic bronchoscopy:*
  1. The patient's nasopharynx and oropharynx are anaesthetized topically with lidocaine spray before the insertion of the bronchoscope. A bite block may be used.
  2. The patient is placed in the sitting or supine position, and the bronchoscope is inserted through the nose or mouth and into the pharynx (Figure 4-5).
  3. After the bronchoscope passes into the larynx and through the glottis, more lidocaine is sprayed into the trachea to prevent the cough reflex.

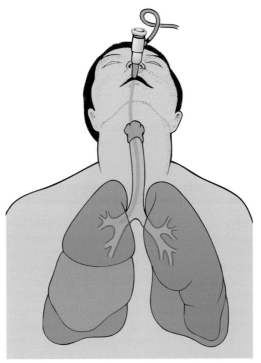

Figure 4-5 Illustration of bronchoscopy. A bronchoscope is inserted through the trachea and into the bronchus.

4. The bronchoscope is passed farther—well into the trachea, bronchi, and the first- and second-generation bronchioles—for systematic examination of the bronchial tree.
5. Biopsy specimens and washings are obtained if a pathologic condition is suspected.
6. If bronchoscopy is performed for pulmonary toilet (removal of mucus), each bronchus is aspirated until clear.
7. Monitor the patient's oxygen saturation to ensure that the patient is well oxygenated. Many patients undergoing this procedure have pulmonary diseases that already compromise their oxygenation. When a bronchoscope is placed, breathing may be further impaired.

After

- Instruct the patient not to eat or drink anything until the tracheobronchial anaesthesia has worn off and the gag reflex has returned, usually in approximately 2 hours.
- Postprocedure, it is recommended the patient is transferred to a negative pressure room for monitoring until discharge criteria are met. During transportation the patient should wear an appropriate barrier mask as determined by the facility policies.
- A full respiratory assessment should be conducted and then checked every 15 minutes until stable and ready for discharge.
- Adhere to the agency's conscious sedation policies.
- Observe the patient's sputum for hemorrhage if biopsy specimens were removed. A small amount of blood streaking may occur and is normal for several hours. Large amounts of bleeding can cause a chemical pneumonitis.
- Observe the patient closely for evidence of impaired respiration or laryngospasm. The vocal cords may go into spasms after intubation.

◌ Inform the patient that postbronchoscopy fever often develops within the first 24 hours.

• If a tumour is suspected, collect a postbronchoscopy sputum sample for a cytologic determination.

◌ Inform the patient that warm saline gargles and lozenges may be helpful if the throat becomes sore.

• Note that a chest radiograph may be ordered to identify a pneumothorax if a deep biopsy specimen was obtained.

◌ Instruct the patient on limitations after conscious sedation, such as driving or operating heavy equipment.

Home Care Responsibilities

• If conscious sedation is used, provide written discharge instructions as per agency policy, which may include the following: information on the medications administered during the procedure; alerting the patient that balance, coordination, and clear thinking may be affected; recommending the patient not sign any legal documents for 24 hours and not consume alcohol; start with clear fluids and progress as tolerated; and notify physician or go to emergency if they experience extreme sleepiness or fainting or have any concerns.
• Suggest that the patient gargle with saline or soothing mouthwash to minimize throat soreness.
• Fever is not uncommon after bronchoscopy. High persistent fever should be reported immediately.
• Bronchospasm or laryngospasm should be reported immediately to emergency personnel.
• Inform the patient that biopsy or culture reports will be available in 2 to 7 days.

TEST RESULTS AND CLINICAL SIGNIFICANCE

Inflammation: *Bronchitis is readily obvious with this method. Culture specimens can be obtained to identify infections.*

Strictures: *Strictures can be identified and sometimes dilated with this technique.*

Cancer: *Neoplasm of the larynx, bronchus, or lung can be identified, and a biopsy can be performed. The extent of the tumour and its resectability can sometimes be determined. The amount of lung that must be removed can be estimated at bronchoscopy. Laser energy can be delivered to diminish the intraluminal size of the tumour. Iridium radiation strips can be positioned accurately at bronchoscopy.*

Hemorrhage: *Hemorrhage can be identified and sometimes controlled by this technique. The source of the hemorrhage can be determined.*

Foreign body: *Often foreign bodies can be removed by fibreoptic flexible bronchoscopy. Large-bore rigid bronchoscopy may be required.*

Abscess: *Pockets of infection can be diagnosed and drained by bronchoscopy. Good culture specimens can be obtained.*

Infection: *Infections can be identified and culture specimens can be obtained to provide information for treatment. Difficult-to-grow organisms can be better cultured by this technique. This is especially helpful for tuberculosis, fungal infections, and* Pneumocystis jiroveci *infections.*

RELATED TESTS

Computed Tomography, Chest (p. 1068). This test can visualize the pulmonary, bronchial, and mediastinal structure but cannot identify a specific disease process.

Chest Radiography (p. 1053). This test is important in the complete evaluation of the pulmonary and cardiac systems.

NORMAL FINDINGS

Normal rectum, colon, and distal small bowel

INDICATIONS

In this test, the rectum, colon, and small bowel are visualized directly. Colonoscopy is used to diagnose suspected pathologic conditions of these organs. It is recommended for patients who have had a change in bowel habits, obvious or occult blood in the stool, or who have abdominal pain. It is also used as a surveillance tool for patients who have had colorectal cancer, inflammatory bowel disease, or polyposis.

TEST EXPLANATION

With fibreoptic colonoscopy, the entire colon from anus to cecum (and often a portion of terminal ileum) can be examined in most patients. Table 4-2 lists types of gastrointestinal (GI) endoscopy. As with sigmoidoscopy (p. 651), benign and malignant neoplasms, polyps, mucosal inflammation, ulceration, and sites of active hemorrhage can be visualized. Diseases such as cancer, polyps, ulcers, and arteriovenous malformations also can be visualized. Biopsy specimens of cancers, polyps, and sites of inflammatory bowel diseases can be taken through the colonoscope with cable-activated instruments. Sites of active bleeding can be coagulated with the use of laser, electrocoagulation, and injection of sclerosing agents.

This test is recommended for patients who have Hemoccult-positive stools, abnormal findings on sigmoidoscopy, lower GI tract bleeding, or a change in bowel habits. This test is also recommended for patients who are at high risk for colon cancer. Such patients include those with a strong personal or family history of colon cancer, polyps, or ulcerative colitis. Colonoscopy is also used for colorectal screening in patients who have no symptoms or increased risks for cancer. The Canadian Cancer Society recommends colorectal screening as a part of routine medical care for all patients, even when no symptoms are present. The recommendations for screening are summarized in Table 4-3.

A physician trained in GI endoscopy performs the test in approximately 30 to 60 minutes. It is usually performed in an endoscopy suite or the operating room. Because the patient is heavily sedated, the patient experiences very little discomfort.

See p. 623 for a discussion of a virtual colonoscopy.

TABLE 4-2	Types of Gastrointestinal Endoscopy
Endoscopy	**Portion of Bowel Examined**
Anoscopy	Anus and distal rectum
Colonoscopy	Anus, rectum, and entire colon
Proctoscopy	Rectum
Sigmoidoscopy	
Rigid	Anus, rectum, and sigmoid colon to a distance of 25 cm
Flexible	Anus, rectum, and sigmoid colon to a distance of 60 cm

TABLE 4-3	Canadian Cancer Society Recommendations for Colorectal Cancer Screening
Recommendations	**<50 Years** Screen only if patient is at high risk (e.g., family history, inflammatory bowel disease, benign polyps of colon or rectum) Individual plan should be developed in consultation with physician
Stool tests	**≥50 Years** Stool tests every 2 years Fecal occult blood testing (see p. 885) Fecal immunochemical testing (see p. 885)
Follow-up after a positive result of stool test	Sigmoidoscopy Colonoscopy Double-contrast barium enema Virtual colonoscopy with computerized tomography

From Canadian Cancer Society's Steering Committee on Cancer Statistics. (2011). *Canadian cancer statistics 2011: Featuring colorectal cancer.* Toronto: Author.

CONTRAINDICATIONS

- Patient's inability to cooperate, because, as in all studies that require technical finesse, patient cooperation is essential for successful completion of the test
- Unstable medical conditions, because this test necessitates sedation, which may induce hypotension in medically unstable patients
- Profuse bleeding from the rectum, because the viewing lens will become covered with blood clots, preventing visualization of the lower intestinal tract
- Suspected perforation of the colon, because the air insufflated during colonoscopy may worsen the fecal peritoneal soilage
- Toxic megacolon, which may worsen with the test preparation
- Colon anastomosis within the previous 14 to 21 days, because the anastomosis may break down with significant insufflation of carbon dioxide

 Age-Related Concerns

- With patients older than 65 years, caution should be observed because of the dehydration and exhaustion that may result from the test preparation. It may be helpful for another individual to stay with the older adult patient if this test is performed on an outpatient basis.

POTENTIAL COMPLICATIONS

- Bowel perforation
- Persistent bleeding from a biopsy site
- Respiratory depression as a result of oversedation

INTERFERING FACTORS

- If bowel preparation is poor, the stool may immediately obstruct the lens and preclude adequate visualization of the colon.
- Active bleeding may obstruct the lens system and preclude adequate visualization of the colon.

Clinical Priorities

- Patients need to drink large amounts of fluids to prevent dehydration from the test preparation.
- It is recommended that the patient drink the complete gallon of the glycol preparation within 4 hours.
- Nausea and vomiting should indicate immediate cessation of the preparation procedure.
- Patients with valvular heart disease should receive prophylactic antibiotics before the test.

PROCEDURE AND PATIENT CARE

Before

- Explain the procedure to the patient.
- Fully inform the patient about the risks of this procedure, and obtain the patient's informed consent for the procedure.
- Instruct the patient in the appropriate bowel preparation. One type is the 2-day bowel preparation, in which clear liquids are consumed for 2 days, along with a strong cathartic such as magnesium citrate and bisacodyl (Dulcolax). On the day of examination, an enema is given. A 1-day preparation involving a clear liquid diet and using a glycol bowel preparation (CoLyte) is more widely used. After the procedure the patient ingests 4 L of polyethylene glycol–electrolyte solution (CoLyte), enemas are not usually needed.
- The 4 L should be consumed within 4 hours, if possible.
- Lemonade powder may be added to the glycol cathartic to improve its flavour.
- Avoid an oral bowel preparation in patients with upper GI tract obstruction, with suspected acute diverticulitis, or who have undergone recent bowel resection surgery.
- Assure patients that they will be appropriately draped to avoid unnecessary embarrassment.
- Administer appropriate preprocedure sedation, usually meperidine (Demerol) and midazolam (Versed). Atropine is often ordered to minimize secretions.

During

- Note the following procedural steps:
  1. Intravenous access is obtained, through which the sedative is administered.
  2. After a rectal examination indicates adequate bowel preparation, the patient is sedated.
  3. The patient is placed in the lateral decubitus position, and the colonoscope is placed into the rectum.
  4. Under direct visualization, the colonoscope is directed to the cecum. Often a significant amount of manipulation is required to obtain this position.
  5. As in all types of endoscopy, room air is insufflated to distend the bowel for better visualization.
  6. Complete examination of the large bowel is performed.
  7. Polypectomy, biopsy, and other endoscopic surgery are performed after appropriate visualization.
  8. When the laser or coagulator is used, the air is removed and carbon dioxide is used as an insufflating agent to avoid explosion.

4   Endoscopic Studies

After

 Explain to the patient that air has been insufflated into the bowel. The patient may experience flatulence or gas pains.

- Examine the patient's abdomen for evidence of colon perforation (abdominal distension and tenderness).
- Assess the patient's vital signs. Watch for a decrease in blood pressure and an increase in pulse rate as indications of hemorrhage.
- Inspect the stools for gross blood.
- Notify the physician if the patient develops increased pain or significant GI bleeding.
- Allow the patient to eat when fully alert if there is no evidence of bowel perforation.

 Encourage the patient to drink large amounts of fluids when intake is allowed. This will make up for the dehydration associated with the bowel preparation.

Home Care Responsibilities

- Instruct the patient to report increasing abdominal pain, which may indicate bowel perforation.
- Instruct the patient to report frequent, bloody bowel movements, which may indicate poor hemostasis if biopsy or polypectomy was performed.
- Instruct the patient to report abdominal bloating and inability to pass flatus, which may indicate colon obstruction if a neoplasm was identified.
- Advise the patient to report weakness and dizziness, which may indicate orthostasis and hypovolemia because of dehydration.
- Advise the patient to report fever and chills, which may indicate a bowel perforation.

TEST RESULTS AND CLINICAL SIGNIFICANCE

Colon cancer: *The appearance is of a red, friable, fleshy tumour concentrically involving the mucosa of the bowel.*

Colon polyp: *This is a tumour that protrudes from only one part of the mucosa of the bowel. Some cancers and most polyps can be removed with the colonoscope. A biopsy specimen can be obtained from neoplasms.*

Inflammatory bowel disease (e.g., ulcerative colitis or Crohn's disease): *The mucosa of the bowel is red, friable, and thickened. Patients with ulcerative colitis are at great risk for the development of cancer over time. These patients should undergo colonoscopy frequently to identify any cancer or precancerous conditions.*

Arteriovenous malformations: *These are small red dots on the mucosa of the bowel. They are a common source of bleeding in adults, especially those with aortic sclerosis and valvular disease. These lesions can be fulgurated by electrocautery through the colonoscope.*

Hemorrhoids: *These are excess fleshy tissue immediately inside the anus.*

Diverticulosis: *This is the presence of diverticula, which are outpouchings in the wall of the colon. Recognition of these abnormalities is important, but they usually do not necessitate surgical therapy.*

Ischemic or postinflammatory stricture: *This is a fibrotic narrowing of the bowel lumen. Stricture may occur after any injury to the bowel. It is a result of fibrosis and scarring that follow an acute insult to the bowel.*

RELATED TESTS

Barium Enema (p. 1033). This is another form of visualization of the bowel. It is not as accurate as colonoscopy.

Computed Tomography, Abdomen (p. 1059). Virtual colonoscopy is a noninterventional method of examining the entire colon through computed tomography. Positron emission tomography (PET) scan (p. 849) may be added to the computed tomographic scan and will add accuracy to this form of colon examination.

Colposcopy

NORMAL FINDINGS
Normal vagina and cervix

INDICATIONS
Colposcopy is used to identify malignant and premalignant lesions of the vagina and cervix. It is helpful in the more thorough evaluation of abnormal findings on Papanicolaou (Pap) smears.

TEST EXPLANATION
Colposcopy provides an in situ macroscopic examination of the vagina and the cervix with a colposcope, which is a macroscope with a light source and a magnifying lens (Figure 4-6). With this procedure, tiny areas of dysplasia, carcinoma in situ, and invasive cancer that would be missed by the naked eye can be visualized, and biopsy specimens can be obtained. The study is performed on patients with abnormal vaginal epithelial patterns, cervical lesions, or suspect Pap

Endoscopic Studies

4

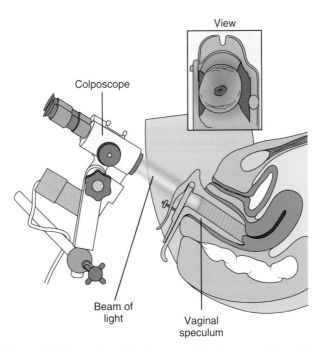

Figure 4-6 Illustration of colposcopy. A colposcope is used to evaluate patients with an abnormal finding on a Papanicolaou smear and a grossly normal cervix.

smear results and on women who were exposed to diethylstilbestrol in utero. It may be a sufficient substitute for cone biopsy (removal and examination of a cone of tissue from the cervix) in evaluating the cause of abnormal cervical cytologic findings (Table 4-4).

Colposcopy is useful only in identifying a suspicious lesion. Definitive diagnosis requires biopsy of the tissue. One of the major advantages of this procedure is that the biopsy can be directed to the area most likely to be truly representative of the lesion. In a biopsy performed without colposcopy, the specimen may not necessarily be representative of the lesion's true pathologic condition, and thus the risk of missing a serious lesion is significant.

The patient needs to have diagnostic conization in the following instances:

1. Colposcopy and endocervical curettage do not explain the problem or match the cytologic findings of the Pap smear within one grade.
2. The entire transformation zone (between squamous and columnar epithelium) is not seen. This area is also called the *endocervix,* in which many cancers can originate.
3. The lesion extends up the cervical canal beyond the vision of the colposcope.

The need for up to 90% of cone biopsies is eliminated with examination by an experienced colposcopist. Endocervical curettage may routinely accompany colposcopy to detect unseen lesions in the endocervical canal.

A physician, a nurse practitioner, or a physician's assistant performs colposcopy in approximately 5 to 10 minutes. Some women complain of pressure pain from the vaginal speculum, and momentary discomfort may be felt if biopsy specimens are obtained. If a mild sedative does not ameliorate the discomfort, a paracervical block can be established.

CONTRAINDICATIONS

- Heavy menstrual flow

POTENTIAL COMPLICATIONS

- Infectious cervicitis
- Hemorrhage
- Vasovagal reaction

TABLE 4-4	Gynecologic Procedures	
Test	**Advantage**	**Disadvantage(s)**
Colposcopy	Enables evaluation of the vagina and cervix	Cannot help with evaluation of the endocervix High false-positive rate
Cone biopsy of the cervix	Enables evaluation of the cervix and endocervix	Cannot help with evaluation of the endometrium
Hysteroscopy	Enables evaluation of the endometrium	Cannot help with evaluation of the cervix and endocervix
Papanicolaou (Pap) smear	Enables evaluation of the cervix, endocervix, and endometrium	Misses important pathologic conditions of cervix, endocervix, and endometrium and may overread inflammation Cannot help with localizing the lesion

INTERFERING FACTORS

- Failure to cleanse the cervix of foreign materials (e.g., creams, medications) may impair visualization.

PROCEDURE AND PATIENT CARE

Before

- Explain the procedure to the patient.
- Obtain the patient's informed consent for this procedure if it is required by the institution.

During

- Note the following procedural steps:
    1. The patient is placed in the lithotomy position, and a vaginal speculum is used to expose the vagina and cervix. Endocervical curettage is performed to minimize any dropping of endocervical cells onto the external surface of the cervix.
    2. After a cervical sample is obtained for cytologic study, the cervix is cleansed with a 3% acetic acid solution to remove excess mucus and cellular debris. The acetic acid also accentuates the difference between normal and abnormal epithelial tissues: abnormal cells turn white.
    3. The colposcope is focused on the cervix, which is then carefully examined. Photographs and rough sketches of the cervix may be created.
    4. Usually the entire lesion can be outlined, and the most atypical areas can be selected for biopsy specimen removal.
    5. A biopsy can be performed at this time on any abnormality.

After

The cervix is cleaned with normal saline solution, and hemostasis is ensured.

- Inform the patient that she may have vaginal bleeding if biopsy specimens were taken. Suggest that she wear a sanitary pad or tampon.
- Instruct the patient to abstain from intercourse and not to insert anything (except a tampon) into the vagina until healing of the biopsy site is confirmed.
- Inform the patient when and how to obtain the results of this study.

TEST RESULTS AND CLINICAL SIGNIFICANCE

Dysplasia: *This is visible as a white, sharply bordered lesion after acetic acid is applied.*
Carcinoma in situ: *This is visible as a pink or reddened well-circumscribed punctate lesion.*
Invasive cancer: *This lesion is noted by its disarray of blood vessels and a mass effect in the cervix.*

RELATED TESTS

Cervical Biopsy (p. 749). A biopsy of the cervix is performed to more accurately identify and treat premalignant and superficial malignant lesions of the cervix.

Papanicolaou Smear (p. 774). This is a smear of the cells that have been shed by the cervix and uterus. Early detection of cancer of the uterus and cervix can be accomplished by routine use of this test.

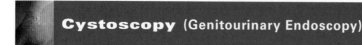

NORMAL FINDINGS

Normal structure and function of the urethra, bladder, ureters, and prostate (in male patients)

INDICATIONS

This endoscopic test is used to evaluate patients with suspected pathologic conditions involving the urethra, bladder, and lower ureters. It is also used to obtain biopsy specimens and to treat pathologic conditions related to those structures. This procedure is commonly performed for patients with the following problems:

- Hematuria
- Recurrent or resistant urinary tract infections
- Urinary symptoms of dysuria, frequency, urinary retention, inadequate urinary stream, urgency, and incontinence

TEST EXPLANATION

Cystoscopy provides direct visualization of the urethra and bladder through the transurethral insertion of a cystoscope into the bladder (Figure 4-7). Cystoscopy is used *diagnostically* to allow the following:

1. Direct inspection and biopsy of the prostate, bladder, and urethra
2. Collection of a separate urine specimen directly from each ureter by the placement of ureteral catheters

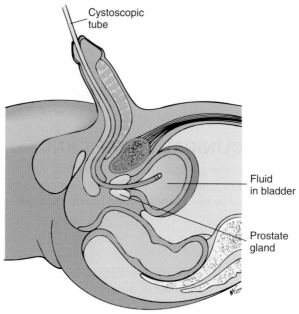

Figure 4-7 Illustration of cystoscopic examination of the male bladder.

3. Measurement of bladder capacity and determination of ureteral reflux
4. Identification of bladder and ureteral calculi
5. Placement of ureteral catheters (Figure 4-8) for retrograde pyelography (p. 1102)
6. Identification of the source of hematuria

Cystoscopy is used *therapeutically* to provide the following:
1. Resection of small, superficial bladder tumours (transurethral resection of the bladder)
2. Removal of foreign bodies and stones
3. Dilation of the urethra and ureters
4. Placement of stents to drain urine from the renal pelvis
5. Coagulation of bleeding areas
6. Implantation of radium seeds into a tumour
7. Resection of hypertrophied or malignant prostate gland overgrowth (transurethral resection of the prostate)
8. Placement of ureteral stents for identification of ureters during pelvic surgery

The cystoscope consists primarily of an obturator and a telescope. The obturator is used to insert the cystoscope atraumatically. After the cystoscope is within the bladder, the obturator is removed and the telescope is passed through the cystoscope. The lens and lighting system of the telescope permit adequate visualization of the lower genitourinary tract. Transendoscopic instruments, such as forceps, scissors, needles, and electrodes, are used when needed.

Genitourinary endoscopy is an endoscopic procedure that visualizes the bladder and urethra. It is more comprehensive than cystoscopy because it includes a detailed visualization of the urethra. This test is important in the evaluation of hematuria, chronic infection, suspected stones, and radiographic filling defects. On inspection of the urethra, inflammation or structural causes of obstruction (e.g., stricture, neoplasia, prostatic hypertrophy) may be visible. If the obstruction is

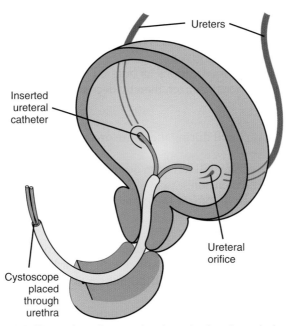

Figure 4-8 Illustration of ureteral catheterization through the cystoscope. Note the ureteral catheter inserted into the right orifice. The left ureteral catheter is ready to be inserted.

functional rather than structural (e.g., detrusor–bladder neck dyssynergia), no site of obstruction is demonstrated by endoscopy.

Although diagnostic cystoscopy is usually performed in the operating room with the patient under general anaesthesia, it can be performed in the urologist's office in approximately 10 minutes. A flexible cystoscope is used for this. The urethra is anaesthetized with an anaesthetic gel. The only discomfort felt is when the cystoscope passes through the sphincter. When a rigid scope is to be used for diagnostic or therapeutic cystoscopy, general or spinal anaesthesia is used.

POTENTIAL COMPLICATIONS

- Perforation of the bladder
- Sepsis resulting from seeding of the bloodstream with bacteria from infected urine
- Hematuria
- Urinary retention

PROCEDURE AND PATIENT CARE

Before

- Explain the procedure to the patient.
- Obtain the patient's informed consent for this procedure.
- If enemas are ordered to clear the bowel, assist the patient as needed, and record the results.
- Encourage the patient to drink fluids the night before the procedure to maintain a continuous flow of urine for collection and to prevent multiplication of bacteria that may be introduced during this technique.
- If the procedure will be done with a local anaesthetic, small volumes of liquids may be acceptable.
- If the procedure will be performed with the patient under general anaesthesia, follow routine precautions. Keep the patient on NPO status (nothing by mouth) after midnight on the day of the test. Intravenous fluids may be given.
- Administer the preprocedural medications as ordered 1 hour before the study. Sedatives decrease the spasm of the bladder sphincter, thereby decreasing the patient's discomfort.

During

- Instruct the patient to lie very still during the entire procedure to prevent trauma to the urinary tract.
- Inform the patient that he or she will have the desire to void as the cystoscope passes the bladder neck and with bladder distension.
- When local anaesthesia is used, inform the patient of the associated discomfort (much more than with urethral catheterization).
- Note the following procedural steps:
  1. Cystoscopy is performed in the operating room or in the urologist's office.
  2. The patient is placed in the lithotomy position with his or her feet in stirrups.
  3. The external genitalia are cleansed with an antiseptic solution such as povidone-iodine (Betadine).
  4. A local anaesthetic gel is instilled into the urethra if the patient is not under general anaesthesia.
  5. The cystoscope is inserted, and the bladder is distended with saline.
  6. The desired diagnostic or therapeutic studies are performed.

- When the procedure is completed, bed rest should be prescribed for a short time.
- Note that if genitourinary endoscopy is performed, the urethra will also be evaluated.
- This procedure is performed in approximately 25 minutes by a urologist.

After

- Instruct the patient not to walk or stand alone immediately after the legs have been removed from the stirrups. The orthostasis that may result from standing erect may cause dizziness and fainting.
- Assess the patient's ability to void for at least 24 hours after the procedure if the patient is hospitalized. Urinary retention may be secondary to edema caused by instrumentation.
- Note the urine colour. Pink-tinged urine is common. The presence of bright red blood or clots should be reported to the urologist.
- Monitor the patient for complaints of back pain, bladder spasms, urinary frequency, and burning on urination. Warm sitz baths and mild analgesics may be ordered and given. Sometimes belladonna and opium (B&O) suppositories are given to relieve bladder spasms. Warm, moist heat to the lower abdomen may help relieve pain and promote muscle relaxation.
- The first few times the patient voids after cystoscopy, a burning sensation is felt in the urethra. This may be intense. Encourage men to urinate while sitting to avoid a vagal reaction related to severe dysuria.
- Encourage increased intake of fluids. Dilution of urine decreases dysuria. Fluids also maintain a constant flow of urine to prevent stasis and the accumulation of bacteria in the bladder.
- Check and record the patient's vital signs as ordered. Watch for a decrease in blood pressure and an increase in pulse rate as indications of hemorrhage.
- Observe for signs and symptoms of sepsis (elevated temperature, flushing, chills, decreased blood pressure, increased pulse rate).
- Note that antibiotics are occasionally ordered 1 day before and continuing through 3 days after the procedure to reduce the incidence of bacteremia that may occur with instrumentation of the urethra and bladder.
- Encourage the patient to use cathartics, especially after cystoscopic surgery. Increases in intra-abdominal pressure caused by constipation may initiate severe lower urologic bleeding.
- If postprocedure irrigation is ordered, use an isotonic solution containing mannitol, glycine, or sorbitol to prevent fluid overhydration in the event that any of the irrigation is absorbed through opened venous sinuses in the bladder.
- If a catheter is left in after the procedure, provide catheter care instructions.

Home Care Responsibilities

- Instruct the patient to watch for signs of urinary retention for 24 to 48 hours: a distended bladder, mild to severe abdominal discomfort, and dribbling urinary leakage overflow.
- Advise the patient to watch for signs of bleeding. Pink urine is normal; clots are not.
- Instruct the patient to report symptoms of increasing lower abdominal pain immediately.
- Recommend the use of warm sitz baths or B&O suppositories to reduce bladder spasms.
- Encourage the patient to drink large amounts of fluids.
- Instruct the patient to report fever, shaking chills, or prolonged dysuria, which are possible signs of urinary tract infection.
- Stress the importance of taking postprocedure antibiotics if they are ordered.

Endoscopic Studies

4

TEST RESULTS AND CLINICAL SIGNIFICANCE

Lower urologic tract tumour: *Bladder cancers or polyps are seen as red friable tumours arising from the mucosa. Sometimes noninvasive tumours can be completely removed with the cystoscope.*

Stones in the ureter or bladder: *These can be retrieved through endourologic surgery. If the stones are too large for retrieval, they can be fractured mechanically, with laser, or with ultrasonography.*

Prostatic hypertrophy: *This benign lesion occludes the urethra. Removal of the portion of the prostate blocking the urethra (by transurethral resection of the prostate) resolves the obstruction.*

Prostate cancer: *This malignant lesion can obstruct the urethra. Removal of the portion of the prostate cancer that is blocking the urethra (by transurethral resection of the prostate) resolves the obstruction. In the older adult, this is not an aggressive tumour.*

Inflammation of the bladder and urethra: *Reddening and thickening of the bladder mucosa indicates chronic infection. This may be present because of urethral stricture, bladder diverticula, or inadequate bladder function.*

Urethral, ureteral, or vesical stricture: *A fibrous obstruction of the urethra or ureteral opening into the bladder indicates stricture, which is usually benign.*

RELATED TESTS

Cystometry (p. 713). This is a test of bladder function and capacity.

Cystography (p. 1075). This is a radiographic study of the bladder. It is used to identify bladder tumours, leaks, or fistulas.

Ductoscopy (Mammary Ductoscopy)

NORMAL FINDINGS

No tumour or premalignant changes

INDICATIONS

In ductoscopy, the breast ducts in women who have nipple discharge are visualized directly. The accuracy and diagnostic potential of this test depend on the experience of the surgeon and the patient's anatomy.

TEST EXPLANATION

Most breast cancers start in the cells that line the milk ducts within the breast. In mammary ductoscopy, a "miniaturized endoscope" is used to get a closer look at the lining of milk ducts of the breast and provide access for biopsy or retrieval of cells lining the ducts.

The mammary ductoscope consists of a tiny outer sheath with an external diameter only barely larger than that of a piece of thread. The sheath has two channels. In one channel, the camera light source is inserted. In the other channel, water is injected to dilate the ducts for better visibility. A video endoscopic camera is attached, and the images are projected on a television monitor through a video system (Figure 4-9). The ductoscope is then advanced to the smallest branches of the milk ducts.

With the use of this technique, breast diseases, including cancers, can be found at their very earliest stages. Ductoscopy can identify cancers so small that mammography, ultrasonography,

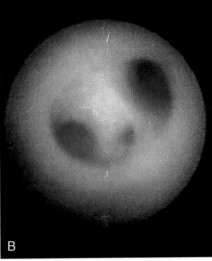
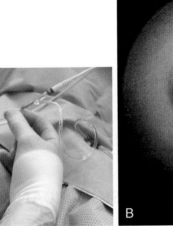

Figure 4-9 Mammary ductoscopy. **A,** Ductoscope is passed into the breast nipple. **B,** Image of normal ducts in the breast.

and even magnetic resonance imaging (MRI) cannot reveal them. With this technique, premalignant changes can be identified and treated in an attempt to prevent breast cancer. Mammary ductoscopy is used as a diagnostic technique in women with nipple discharge.

Ductal lavage (p. 673) is a technique used to obtain and identify premalignant atypical cells from breast ducts in patients who are considered at high risk for cancer and who have no evidence of breast malignancy on mammogram or ultrasonography. Ductoscopy is used to look into these ducts in the hopes of identifying the causes of those changes (e.g., intraductal papillomas or early cancers) in these ducts and possibly delivering ablative therapies to eradicate them.

INTERFERING FACTORS

- Inability to access the duct precludes performance of this endoscopic procedure.

PROCEDURE AND PATIENT CARE

Before

- Explain the procedure to the patient.
- Ensure that the results of the breast examination and the mammogram are normal.
- Obtain the patient's informed consent for this procedure.
- If the procedure is to be performed with the patient under general anaesthesia, keep the patient on NPO status (nothing by mouth) for at least 8 hours.
- If the procedure is to be performed with local anaesthesia, apply a topical anaesthetic to the nipple area for approximately 30 to 60 minutes before the test.

During

- Note the following procedural steps:
  1. The breast is massaged to promote the discharge of nipple fluid. This helps to visually identify the ductal orifice in the nipple for endoscopy.

2. The ductal opening in the nipple is gently dilated with tiny dilators of increasing sizes, and the mammary sheath containing the ductoscope is inserted and advanced under direct visualization as saline is injected to dilate the branches of the duct for visualization.
3. The ductoscopy findings can be video-recorded.
4. If any disease is identified, the surgeon can use the ductoscope for directed surgical removal.
5. Ductal washings can also be obtained by aspiring some of the fluid for microscopic analysis.

- This procedure is usually performed in approximately 30 minutes by a surgeon in the office.

After

Instruct the patient to contact the physician if she develops any redness, breast pain, or fever, which may indicate mastitis.

TEST RESULTS AND CLINICAL SIGNIFICANCE

Invasive ductal cancer: *This is usually evident only from complete obstruction of the breast ducts.*
Noninvasive ductal cancer,
Atypical ductal hyperplasia: *These diseases are evident from changes in the epithelial lining of the breast ducts.*
Papilloma: *This is a small polyploid tumour projecting into the breast duct lumen.*

RELATED TEST

Breast Ductal Lavage (p. 673). In this procedure, the breast ducts are flushed. Cells are obtained for cytologic study to identify malignant or premalignant cells.

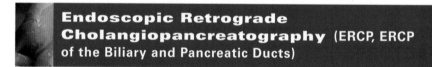

Endoscopic Retrograde Cholangiopancreatography (ERCP, ERCP of the Biliary and Pancreatic Ducts)

NORMAL FINDINGS

Normal size of biliary and pancreatic ducts
No obstruction or filling defects within the biliary or pancreatic ducts

INDICATIONS

This test is used in the evaluation of the patient with jaundice. It is also used to evaluate patients with unexplained upper abdominal pain or pancreatitis.

TEST EXPLANATION

With the use of a fibreoptic endoscope, endoscopic retrograde cholangiopancreatography (ERCP) provides radiographic visualization of the bile and pancreatic ducts. This is especially useful in patients with jaundice. If those ducts are partially or totally obstructed, characteristics of the obstructing lesion can be demonstrated. Stones, benign strictures, cysts, ampullary stenosis, anatomic variations, and malignant tumours can be identified. Only ERCP and percutaneous transhepatic cholangiography (PTHC) can provide direct radiographic visualization of the biliary and pancreatic ducts. PTHC (p. 1097) is an invasive procedure with significant morbidity; ERCP is associated with much less morbidity but must be performed by an experienced endoscopist.

Incision of the papillary muscle in the ampulla of Vater can be performed through the endoscope at the time of ERCP. This incision widens the distal common duct so that common bile duct gallstones can be removed. Stents can be placed through bile ducts with strictures during ERCP, which allow the bile of jaundiced patients to be internally drained. Pieces of tissue and brushings of the common bile duct can be obtained by ERCP for pathologic review.

Manometric studies of the sphincter of Oddi and pancreatobiliary ducts can be performed at the time of ERCP. These are used to investigate unusual functional abnormalities of these structures.

CONTRAINDICATIONS

- Patient's inability to cooperate, because cannulation of the ampulla of Vater requires that the patient lie very still
- Endoscopic inaccessibility of the ampulla of Vater because of previous upper gastrointestinal (GI) tract surgery (e.g., patients who have undergone gastrectomy and whose duodenum containing the ampulla is surgically separated from the stomach)
- Esophageal diverticula, because the endoscope can fall into a diverticulum and perforate its wall
- Presence of known acute pancreatitis, because ERCP can worsen this inflammation

POTENTIAL COMPLICATIONS

- Perforation of the esophagus, stomach, or duodenum
- Gram-negative sepsis, which results from introduction of bacteria through the biliary system and into the blood; this usually occurs in patients who have obstructive jaundice
- Pancreatitis, which results from pressure of the dye injection
- Aspiration of gastric contents into the lungs
- Respiratory arrest as a result of oversedation

INTERFERING FACTORS

- The presence of barium within the abdomen—as a result of a previous upper GI radiographic series or barium enema radiographic studies—precludes adequate visualization of the biliary and pancreatic ducts.

PROCEDURE AND PATIENT CARE

Before

- Explain the procedure to the patient.
- Obtain the patient's informed consent for this procedure.
- Inform the patient that breathing will not be compromised by the insertion of the endoscope.
- Keep the patient on NPO status (nothing by mouth) after midnight on the day of the test.
- Administer appropriate premedication (e.g., midazolam [Versed] and atropine), if it is ordered.

During

- Note the following procedural steps:
  1. A kidney, ureter, and bladder (KUB) radiograph of the abdomen (see Figure 12-16) is taken to ensure that any barium from previous studies will not obscure visualization of the bile duct.
  2. The patient is placed in the supine position or on the left side.
  3. The patient is usually sedated with a narcotic and a sedative/hypnotic.
  4. The pharynx is sprayed with a local anaesthetic (lidocaine) to inactivate the gag reflex and to lessen the discomfort caused by the passage of the endoscope.
  5. A side-viewing fibreoptic duodenoscope is inserted through the oral pharynx, passed through the esophagus and stomach, and inserted into the duodenum (Figure 4-10). A bite block may be used.
  6. Glucagon is often administered intravenously to minimize the spasm of the duodenum and to improve visualization of the ampulla of Vater. Simethicone may be instilled to diminish any bubbles present that may inhibit visualization of the ampulla.
  7. Through the accessory lumen within the endoscope, a small catheter is passed through the ampulla and into the common bile or pancreatic ducts.
  8. Radiographic dye is injected, and radiographic images are taken.
- This test is usually performed in approximately 1 hour by a physician trained in endoscopy. The radiologist interprets the radiographs.
- 🖉 Inform the patient that no discomfort is associated with the dye injection but that minimal gagging may occur during the initial introduction of the endoscope into the oral pharynx.

After

- 🖉 Do not allow the patient to eat or drink until the gag reflex returns to prevent aspiration.
- Observe the patient closely for development of abdominal pain, nausea, and vomiting. This may herald the onset of ERCP-induced pancreatitis.

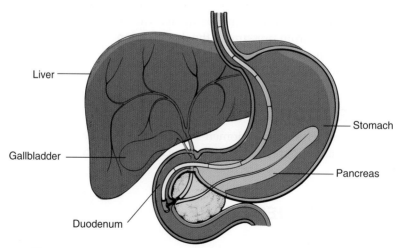

Figure 4-10 Illustration of endoscopic retrograde cholangiopancreatography (ERCP). The fibreoptic endoscope is passed into the duodenum. Note that at the end of the fibreoptic endoscope, there is a small catheter being advanced into the biliary duct.

- Observe safety precautions until the effects of the sedatives have worn off.
- Monitor the patient for signs of respiratory depression. Medication (e.g., naloxone [Narcan]) should be available to counteract serious respiratory depression. Resuscitative equipment should also be available for immediate use.
- Assess the patient for signs and symptoms of septicemia, which may indicate the onset of ERCP-induced cholangitis.

 Inform the patient that he or she may be hoarse and have a sore throat for several days. Drinking cool fluids and gargling will help to relieve some of this soreness.

Home Care Responsibilities

- Soreness in the throat is expected. A soothing mouthwash gargle may help.
- Instruct the patient to notify the physician immediately if abdominal pain increases or if nausea or vomiting occurs. These may be the early signs of pancreatitis or gastroduodenal perforation.
- Instruct the patient to notify the physician immediately of fever or shaking chills. These may indicate possible cholangitis.
- Encourage the patient to eat lightly for the next 12 to 24 hours.

TEST RESULTS AND CLINICAL SIGNIFICANCE

Tumour, strictures, or gallstones of the common bile duct: *These conditions are obvious in the presence and character of the filling defect noted in the dye-filled duct.*

Sclerosing cholangitis,

Biliary sclerosis: *These conditions appear as a long area of strictures involving, but not limited to, the extrahepatic ducts.*

Cysts of the common bile duct: *These congenital cysts appear as large balloon-like dilations of any portion of the extrahepatic ducts.*

Tumour, strictures, or inflammation of the pancreatic duct: *Some tumours of the pancreas appear as large cystic structures involving and leading from the pancreatic duct. Most pancreatic tumours, however, appear as a localized narrowing of the pancreatic duct with a dilated duct distal to the narrowing. Strictures and inflammation usually involve the entire duct with very little duct dilation beyond the narrowing.*

Pseudocyst of the pancreatic duct: *This condition results from pancreatic duct injury (usually after severe pancreatitis). The pancreatic juices leak out of the duct and into the peripancreatic tissue. A cyst is formed that communicates with the main pancreatic duct.*

Chronic pancreatitis: *This condition may appear in the form of multiple small partial strictures involving multiple short segments of the pancreatic duct with dilation of the duct in between the strictures. This appearance is of a string of beads along the duct.*

Anatomic biliary or pancreatic duct variations: *Variable pathologic and nonpathologic anomalies can occur. Usually no symptoms are caused by these abnormalities.*

Cancer of the duodenum or ampulla: *These cancers are quite obvious as friable tumour masses emanating from the mucosa of those regions.*

RELATED TEST

Percutaneous Transhepatic Cholangiography (p. 1097). In this test, the liver is percutaneously punctured with a needle, and a catheter is threaded into the biliary duct radical. Dye is injected, and the biliary tree can be visualized radiographically.

Esophagogastroduodenoscopy (EGD, Upper Gastrointestinal [UGI] Endoscopy, Gastroscopy)

NORMAL FINDINGS

Normal esophagus, stomach, and duodenum

INDICATIONS

In this test, the lumen of the esophagus, stomach, and duodenum are visualized directly. Esophagogastroduodenoscopy (EGD) is used to evaluate patients with the following:

- Dysphagia
- Weight loss
- Early satiety
- Upper abdominal pain
- "Ulcer symptoms" or dyspepsia
- Alcoholism and suspected varices
- Results of barium swallow or upper gastrointestinal (GI) radiographic study that are suggestive of a pathologic condition

TEST EXPLANATION

EGD enables direct visualization of the upper gastrointestinal (GI) tract by means of a long, flexible, fibreoptic-lighted endoscope. The lumen of the esophagus, stomach, and duodenum are examined for tumours, varices, mucosal inflammations, hiatal hernias, polyps, ulcers, and obstructions. The endoscope has up to three channels. The first channel is used for viewing, the second for insufflation of air and aspiration of fluid, and the third for passing cable-activated instruments to obtain a biopsy sample of suspected pathologic tissue. Probes also can be passed through the third channel to allow coagulation or injection of sclerosing agents to areas of active GI bleeding. A laser beam can pass through the endoscope to perform endoscopic surgery (e.g., obliteration of tumours or polyps, control of bleeding), and the fibreoptics of endoscopy are so refined that video images and still pictures can be taken.

Endoscopy enables the clinician not only to evaluate the esophagus, stomach, and duodenum, but also, with the use of an extra-long fibreoptic endoscope, to visualize and perform a biopsy of tissue in the upper small intestinal tract. This procedure is referred to as *enteroscopy* (Table 4-5).

TABLE 4-5	Endoscopy of the Gastrointestinal Tract
Endoscopic Procedure	**Area Evaluated**
Esophagoscopy	Esophagus
Gastroscopy	Esophagus and stomach
Esophagogastroduodenoscopy (EGD)	Esophagus, stomach, and duodenum
Enteroscopy	Esophagus, stomach, duodenum, and upper jejunum
Panendoscopy	Esophagus, stomach, duodenum, upper jejunum and colon (per colonoscopy)
Endoscopic retrograde cholangiopancreatography (ERCP)	Duodenum, ampulla, and pancreatobiliary ducts

Abnormalities of the small intestine, such as arteriovenous malformations, tumours, enteropathies (e.g., celiac disease), and ulcerations, can be diagnosed with enteroscopy.

In *capsule endoscopy,* a capsule containing a miniature camera is used to record images of the entire digestive tract, particularly the small intestine. This capsule is approximately the size of a large vitamin tablet and contains a colour video camera, a radiofrequency transmitter, four light-emitting diode (LED) beams, and enough battery power to take 50 000 colour images during an 8-hour passage through the digestive tract. It moves through the digestive tract naturally with the aid of peristaltic activity. During the 6- to 10-hour examination, the images are continuously transmitted to special antenna pads placed on the body and captured on a recording device approximately the size of a portable radio that is worn around the patient's waist. After the examination, the patient returns to the physician's office, and the recording device is removed. The stored images are transferred to a computer workstation, in which they are transformed into a digital movie that the physician can later examine on the computer monitor.

Patients are not required to retrieve and return the video capsule to the physician. It is disposable and expelled normally and effortlessly with the next bowel movement. The most common reason for performing capsule endoscopy is to search for a cause of bleeding from the small intestine. It may also be useful for detecting polyps, inflammatory bowel disease (Crohn's disease), ulcers, and tumours of the small intestine.

Besides being much more sensitive and specific than an upper GI radiographic series in diagnosing diseases of the esophagus, stomach, and duodenum, EGD also can be used therapeutically. An experienced endoscopist can often control active GI tract bleeding by electrocoagulation, laser coagulation, or the injection of sclerosing agents, such as alcohol. Also, with the endoscope, benign and malignant strictures can be dilated to re-establish patency of the upper GI tract. Biliary stents and a percutaneous gastrostomy tube can be placed with the use of EGD. The role of endoscopic surgery is expanding as a result of its dramatic success and minimal morbidity.

CONTRAINDICATIONS

- Patient's inability to cooperate fully, because, as in all studies that require technical finesse, patient cooperation is essential for successful, safe, and accurate test completion
- Severe upper GI tract bleeding, because blood clots will cover the viewing lens and prevent adequate visualization; however, lavage and aspiration of the stomach to clear the blood clots will allow EGD to be performed
- Esophageal diverticula, because the endoscope can easily fall into the diverticulum and perforate the wall of the esophagus
- Suspected perforation, which can be worsened by the insufflation of pressurized air into the GI tract
- Recent surgery in the upper GI tract surgery, because the pressure of the required air insufflation may lead to anastomotic disruption

POTENTIAL COMPLICATIONS

- Perforation of the esophagus, stomach, and duodenum
- Bleeding from a biopsy site
- Pulmonary aspiration of gastric contents
- Oversedation from the medication administered during the test
- Hypotension induced by the sedative medication: Usually the patient already has some significant hypovolemia or dehydration
- Local intravenous phlebitic reaction to the injection of sclerosing sedative medication

INTERFERING FACTORS

- Food in the stomach may interfere with the visualization of the digestive tract.
- Excessive GI tract bleeding may interfere with visualization of the digestive tract.

 Age-Related Concerns

- Older adults (aged ≥65 years) have a higher chance of having a Zenker diverticulum above the upper esophageal sphincter than do younger adults (≤65 years). It is important to be aware of this when EGD is performed, because the tip of the endoscope could be misplaced into the diverticulum, rather than the esophagus, and cause a perforation.
- In older adults, the motility of the esophagus declines and the resting pressure of the lower esophageal sphincter increases. These developments may increase the difficulty of inserting and advancing the endoscope.
- Older adults are also more likely to have several health problems and to be taking various medications; thus, their risk for complications from the anaesthesia, if it is required, is higher.

PROCEDURE AND PATIENT CARE

Before

- Explain the procedure to the patient.
- Inform the patient that the test is mildly uncomfortable.
- Obtain the patient's informed consent for this procedure if it is required by the institution.
- Instruct the patient to abstain from eating as of midnight the day of the test.
- Reassure the patient that this test is not painful. Inform the patient that the throat will be anaesthetized with a spray to depress the gag reflex.
- Encourage the patient to verbalize fears. Provide emotional support.
- Remove the patient's dentures and eyewear before testing.
- Remind the patient that he or she will not be able to speak during the test but that respiration will not be affected.
- Instruct the patient not to bite down on the endoscope.
- Instruct the patient in appropriate oral hygiene because the tube will be passed through the mouth.

During

- Note the following procedural steps:
  1. The patient is placed on the endoscopy table in the left lateral decubitus position.
  2. The throat is topically anaesthetized with viscous lidocaine (Xylocaine) or another anaesthetic spray. This is to decrease the gag reflex caused by passage of the endoscope.
  3. The patient is usually sedated. This minimizes anxiety and allows the patient to relax.
  4. The endoscope is gently passed through the mouth and into the esophagus; once in the esophagus, visualization can be performed. A bite block may be used.
  5. Room air is insufflated to distend the upper GI tract for adequate visualization.
  6. The esophagus, stomach, and duodenum are evaluated.
  7. During enteroscopy, the upper small bowel is visualized, and a biopsy is performed if needed.

8. Biopsy or any endoscopic surgery is performed under direct visualization.

9. At the completion of direct inspection and surgery, the excess air and GI tract secretions are aspirated through the scope.

• Note that the test, which takes approximately 20 to 30 minutes, is performed in the endoscopy laboratory by a physician trained in GI endoscopy.

After

✗ Inform the patient that he or she may have hoarseness or a sore throat after the test.

✗ Withhold any fluids until the patient is completely alert and the swallowing reflex returns to normal, usually in 2 to 4 hours.

• Observe the patient's vital signs. Evaluate the patient for bleeding, fever, abdominal pain, dyspnea, or dysphagia.

✗ Remind the patient that he or she may experience some postendoscopic bloating, belching, and flatulence.

• Observe safety precautions until the effects of the sedatives have worn off.

✗ Inform the patient that the sedation may cause some retrograde and antegrade amnesia for a few hours.

 Home Care Responsibilities

• Soreness in the throat is expected after EGD. A soothing mouthwash may help.
• Instruct the patient to notify the physician immediately if bleeding, fever, abdominal pain, dyspnea, or dysphagia occurs.
• Inform the patient that it is normal to have some bloating, belching, and flatulence after the procedure.

TEST RESULTS AND CLINICAL SIGNIFICANCE

Tumours (benign or malignant) of the esophagus, stomach, or duodenum: *These appear as red, friable ulcers or masses in the mucosa of the respective organ. Such tumours can obstruct, bleed, or perforate.*

Esophageal diverticula: *These are outpouchings of the esophagus at the level of the cricopharyngeal muscle or the diaphragm.*

Hiatal hernia: *In this condition, a portion of the stomach is above the diaphragm (seen as an extrinsic compression of the lower esophagus).*

Esophagitis, gastritis, duodenitis: *Inflammation is characterized by reddened, friable mucosa without ulcer or mass.*

Gastroesophageal varices: *These are submucosal vessels that protrude into the lumen of the distal esophagus and stomach and indicate a reversal of portal blood flow because of hepatic cirrhosis.*

Peptic ulcer: *This benign, acid-induced ulcer usually occurs in the duodenum but may occur in the distal stomach. It is small to moderate in size and is seen in the mucosa of the organ.*

Peptic stricture and subsequent scarring: *After healing of an ulcer or inflammation, scarring and stricture can form and partially obstruct the lumen of the organ involved (usually the esophagus).*

Endoscopic Studies

4

Extrinsic compression by a cyst or tumour outside the upper GI tract: *Tumours, cysts, or enlarged organs can compress the upper GI tract. This compression appears as a convex narrowing involving the organ being evaluated.*

Source of upper GI tract bleeding: *Ulcers, tumours, varices, arteriovenous malformations, inflammation, and bleeding can be identified and often treated by EGD.*

RELATED TESTS

Barium Swallow (p. 1038) and Upper Gastrointestinal Tract Radiography (p. 1117). These radiographic contrast studies are also performed to evaluate the upper GI tract. They are not as accurate as EGD. Furthermore, biopsy and therapy cannot be performed with the radiographic studies, but they can be performed with EGD.

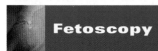

Fetoscopy

NORMAL FINDINGS

No fetal distress or diseases seen
No hematologic abnormalities noted

INDICATIONS

Fetoscopy is indicated for any woman who is at risk for delivery of a baby with a significant birth defect. It is used also to perform corrective surgery on the fetus when possible.

TEST EXPLANATION

Fetoscopy is an endoscopic procedure that allows direct visualization of the fetus via the insertion of a tiny, telescope-like instrument through the abdominal wall and into the uterine cavity (Figure 4-11). Through direct visualization, a severe malformation, such as a neural tube defect, may be diagnosed. During the procedure, fetal blood samples to detect congenital blood disorders (e.g., hemophilia, sickle cell anemia) can be drawn from a blood vessel in the umbilical cord for biochemical analysis. Fetal skin biopsy also can be performed to detect primary skin disorders. Fetoscopic surgery (e.g., placement of central nervous system shunts) is increasingly performed.

Fetoscopy is performed at approximately 18 weeks' gestation. At this time, the vessels of the placental surface are of adequate size, and the fetal parts are readily identifiable. A therapeutic abortion would not be as hazardous at this time as it would be if it were done later in the pregnancy. An ultrasound examination is usually performed the day after the procedure to confirm the adequacy of the amniotic fluid and fetal viability.

POTENTIAL COMPLICATIONS

- Spontaneous abortion
- Premature delivery
- Amniotic fluid leak
- Intrauterine fetal death
- Amnionitis

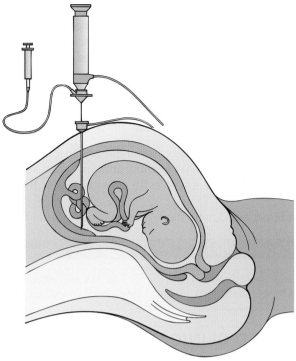

Figure 4-11 Illustration of fetoscopy for fetal blood sampling.

Clinical Priorities

- Ultrasound examination is performed before the procedure to identify a safe area to enter the uterine cavity.
- After the test, a patient who is Rh negative should receive Rho(D) immune globulin (RhoGAM) unless the fetal blood is also Rh negative.
- Ultrasound examination is usually performed the day after the procedure to confirm the adequacy of the amniotic fluid and to assess fetal viability.

PROCEDURE AND PATIENT CARE

Before

- Explain the procedure to the patient.
- Obtain the patient's informed consent for this procedure.
- Assess the fetal heart rate before the test to serve as a baseline value.
- Administer meperidine (Demerol), if it is ordered, before the test because it crosses the placenta and quiets the fetus. This prevents excessive fetal movement, which would make the procedure more difficult.

During

- Note the following procedural steps:
  1. The patient is placed in the supine position on an examining table.
  2. A local anaesthetic is injected in the skin of the patient's abdomen.
  3. Ultrasonography is performed to locate the fetus and the placenta and to identify a safe area in the uterus to insert the endoscope.

4. The endoscope is inserted.
5. Biopsy specimens and blood samples may be obtained.
This procedure is performed in 1 to 2 hours by a physician.

 Remind the patient that the only discomfort associated with this study is the injection of the local anaesthetic.

After

- Assess the fetal heart rate and compare it with the baseline value to detect any side effects related to the procedure.
- Monitor the patient and fetus carefully for alterations in blood pressure, pulse rate, uterine activity, and fetal activity; for vaginal bleeding; and for loss of amniotic fluid.
- Administer RhoGAM to the patient who is Rh negative unless the fetal blood is determined to be Rh negative.
- If antibiotics are ordered, administer them prophylactically after the test to prevent amnionitis.

Home Care Responsibilities

- Instruct the patient to avoid strenuous activity for 1 to 2 weeks after the procedure.
- Advise the patient to report any pain, bleeding, amniotic fluid loss, or fever.

TEST RESULTS AND CLINICAL SIGNIFICANCE

Developmental defects (e.g., neural tube defects): *These defects are visible on a fetus older than 20 weeks.*
Congenital blood disorders (e.g., hemophilia, sickle cell disease): *These congenital abnormalities are identified by evaluation of the fetal blood.*
Primary skin disorders: *These may be obvious at the time of fetoscopy. Skin biopsy can be performed.*

RELATED TESTS

Amniocentesis (p. 660). This procedure involves placing a needle through the abdominal and uterine walls into the amniotic cavity to withdraw fluid for analysis. Valuable information about fetal status is obtained.

Chorionic Villus Sampling (p. 1134). This is a test whereby the chorionic placental tissue (which has the same genetic material as the fetus) is tested for genetic analysis and karyotyping. This is a rapid and accurate method of determining genetic defects. Chorionic villus sampling can be performed earlier in pregnancy than can amniocentesis.

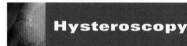

Hysteroscopy

NORMAL FINDINGS

Normal structure and function of the uterus

INDICATIONS

In this test, the endometrial cavity is visualized directly. Hysteroscopy is indicated for patients with abnormal results of a Papanicolaou (Pap) smear, dysfunctional uterine bleeding, or post-menopausal bleeding.

TEST EXPLANATION

Hysteroscopy is an endoscopic procedure by which the uterine cavity can be visualized directly by insertion of a hysteroscope (a thin, telescope-like instrument) through the vagina and cervix and into the uterus (Figure 4-12). Hysteroscopy can be used to identify the cause of abnormal uterine bleeding, infertility, and repeated miscarriages. It is also used to evaluate and diagnose uterine adhesions (Asherman syndrome), polyps, fibroids, and displaced intrauterine devices.

In addition to diagnosing and evaluating uterine problems, hysteroscopy can also be used to correct uterine problems. For example, uterine adhesions and small fibroids can be removed through the hysteroscope; thus open abdominal surgery is avoided. Hysteroscopy can also be used to perform endometrial ablation, which destroys the uterine lining to treat some cases of heavy uterine bleeding.

Hysteroscopy may confirm the results of other tests, such as hysterosalpingography (p. 1077). The level of anaesthesia used—general, spinal, or light sedative—depends on the amount of surgery and time associated with hysteroscopy. Simple hysteroscopy takes approximately 30 minutes. A gynecologist in the operating room usually performs this test. The patient receiving local anaesthesia or only light sedation may feel some cramping during the procedure. In general, it is not a painful procedure.

CONTRAINDICATIONS

- Pelvic inflammatory disease
- Vaginal discharge

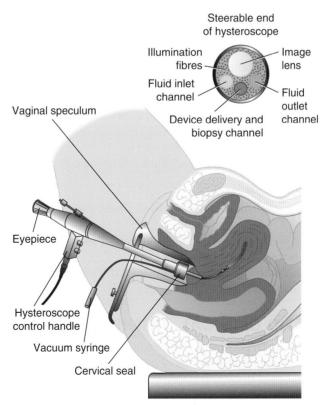

Figure 4-12 Illustration of hysteroscopy.

POTENTIAL COMPLICATIONS

- Uterine perforation
- Infection

PROCEDURE AND PATIENT CARE

Before

- Explain the procedure to the patient.
- Obtain the patient's informed consent for this procedure.
- Schedule the procedure for after menstrual bleeding has ceased and before ovulation. At this time, visualization of the inside of the uterus is better, and damage to a newly formed pregnancy is more easily avoided.
- Inform the patient that hysteroscopy may be performed with local, regional, or general anaesthesia. If general anaesthesia is needed, the patient should be on NPO status (nothing by mouth) for at least 8 hours before the test. This test may also be performed without the use of anaesthesia.
- Instruct the patient to void before the procedure because a distended bladder can be more easily perforated.

During

- Note the following procedural steps:
  1. Hysteroscopy may be performed in the operating room or in the physician's office. Local, regional, general, or no anaesthesia may be used. (The type of anaesthesia depends on other procedures that may be done at the same time.)
  2. The patient is placed in the lithotomy position. The vaginal area is cleansed with an antiseptic solution.
  3. The cervix may be dilated before this procedure.
  4. The hysteroscope is inserted through the vagina and cervix and into the uterus.
  5. A liquid (e.g., Ringer lactate) or gas (e.g., CO_2) is released through the hysteroscope to expand the uterus for better visualization.
  6. If minor surgery will be performed, small instruments will be inserted through the hysteroscope.
  7. For more detailed or complicated procedures, a laparoscope may be used (see following test) to concurrently view the outside of the uterus.
  8. After the desired procedure is performed, the hysteroscope is removed.

Aftercare

- Inform the patient that it is normal to have slight vaginal bleeding and cramps for a day or two after the procedure.
- Inform the patient that signs of fever, severe abdominal pain, or heavy vaginal discharge or bleeding should be reported to her physician.
- If the patient has any discomfort from the gas inserted during the hysteroscopy or laparoscopy, assure her that this usually lasts less than 24 hours.

TEST RESULTS AND CLINICAL SIGNIFICANCE

Endometrial cancer, polyps, or hyperplasia: *Cancer appears as thickened endometrium in one or multiple portions of the uterus. Hyperplasia looks similar but is not as isolated and seems more diffuse. Polyps appear as pedunculated mucosal tissue protruding from the endometrium.*

Uterine fibroids: *Small fibroids are easily seen because they distort the endometrium.*

Asherman syndrome: *Intrauterine adhesions may be associated with previous uterine infections and can be lysed through hysteroscopy.*

Septate uterus: *This and other developmental abnormalities can be visualized by hysteroscopy.*

Displaced intrauterine device: *A displaced intrauterine device is easily located.*

RELATED TEST

Dilation and Curettage. This is another procedure that enables clinicians to examine scrapings of the endometrium under a microscope. This test has nearly the same indications as hysteroscopy. However, sampling is random, and serious lesions may be missed.

 Laparoscopy (Pelvic Endoscopy, Gynecologic Video Laparoscopy, Peritoneoscopy)

NORMAL FINDINGS

Normal-appearing female reproductive organs

INDICATIONS

In laparoscopy, the abdominal and pelvic organs are visualized directly when a pathologic condition is suspected. Laparoscopy is used to evaluate patients with the following conditions:

- Acute abdominal or pelvic pain
- Chronic abdominal or pelvic pain
- Suspected advanced cancer
- Abdominal mass of uncertain cause
- Unexplained infertility

Operative procedures that can be performed with laparoscopic surgery include oophorectomy, appendectomy, cholecystectomy, colectomy, hernia repair, hiatal hernia repair, liver biopsy, nephrectomy, tubal ligation, and gastrectomy.

TEST EXPLANATION

During laparoscopy, the abdominal organs can be visualized by inserting a laparoscope through the abdominal wall and into the peritoneum (Figure 4-13). A television camera is attached to the laparoscope, and the camera's view is seen on colour monitors. This is particularly helpful in diagnosing abdominal and pelvic adhesions, tumours and cysts affecting any abdominal organ, and tubal and uterine causes of infertility. Endometriosis, ectopic pregnancy, ruptured ovarian cyst, and salpingitis can also be detected during a laparoscopic evaluation for pelvic pain. In addition, this procedure is used to stage cancers and determine their resectability. Surgical procedures, as described previously, can be performed with the laparoscope. As noted in Table 4-6, laparoscopy affords many advantages to the patient in comparison with an open laparotomy, which is the surgical opening of the abdomen.

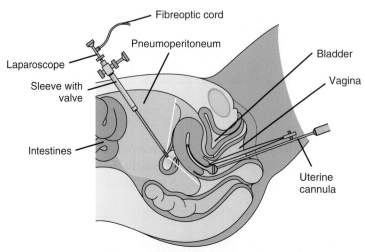

Figure 4-13 Illustration of gynecologic laparoscopy.

TABLE 4-6	Differences Between Laparotomy and Laparoscopy	
Characteristic	**Laparotomy**	**Laparoscopy**
Difficulty in technique	Moderate	High
Size of incision	One large	Multiple and small
Expense of equipment in the operating room	Moderate	High
Expense of postoperative care	High	Low
Postoperative mobility	Low	High
Postoperative pain	High	Minimal to moderate
Postoperative hospitalization	4–10 days	1–2 days
Duration of postoperative recovery	Weeks	Days
Return to work	6 weeks	1 week

Laparoscopy is performed by a surgeon. The patient is under general anaesthesia so that no pain or discomfort is experienced during the procedure. Most patients have mild to moderate incisional pain. However, the patient may complain of shoulder or subcostal discomfort from diaphragmatic irritation caused by pneumoperitoneum.

CONTRAINDICATIONS

- Multiple previous surgical procedures, because adhesions may have formed between the viscera and the abdominal wall, making safe access to the abdomen impossible; however, there are techniques that allow limited laparoscopy in these situations
- Suspected intra-abdominal hemorrhage, because visualization through the laparoscope will be obscured by the blood

POTENTIAL COMPLICATIONS

- Perforation of the bowel, with spilling of intestinal contents into the peritoneum
- Hemorrhage from the trocar site or surgical site
- Umbilical hernia, which results from inadequate repair of the hole in the fascia used to insert the laparoscope

INTERFERING FACTORS

- Adhesions may obstruct the field of vision.

 Clinical Priorities

- During the procedure, the peritoneal cavity is filled with 3 to 4 L of CO_2 to separate the abdominal wall from the intraabdominal viscera.
- After the procedure, patients may have shoulder or subcostal discomfort from pneumoperitoneum. This usually lasts only 24 hours.
- After the procedure, patients should be assessed for bleeding (increased pulse rate, decreased blood pressure) and perforated viscus (abdominal tenderness, guarding, decreased bowel sounds).

PROCEDURE AND PATIENT CARE

Before

- Explain the procedure to the patient.
- Obtain the patient's informed consent for this procedure. Because of the possibility of intra-abdominal injury, an open laparotomy may be required. Ensure that the patient is aware of that.
- If enemas are ordered to clear the bowel, assist the patient as needed, and record the results.
- Because the procedure is usually performed with the patient under general anaesthesia, follow the routine general anaesthesia precautions.
- Shave and prepare the patient's abdomen as ordered.
- Keep the patient on NPO status (nothing by mouth) after midnight on the day of the test. Intravenous fluids may be given.
- Instruct the patient to void before going to the operating room, because a distended bladder can be easily penetrated.

During

- After general anaesthesia is induced, a catheter and nasogastric tube are inserted to minimize the risk of penetrating a distended stomach or bladder with the initial needle placement.
- Note the following procedural steps:
  1. Laparoscopy is performed in the operating room. The patient is initially placed in supine position. Other positions may be used to maximize visibility.
  2. After the abdominal skin is cleansed, a blunt-tipped (Veress) needle is inserted through a small incision in the periumbilical area and into the peritoneal cavity. Alternatively, a slightly larger incision is placed in the skin, and the abdominal wall is separated from

the intra-abdominal viscera under direct vision. The peritoneal cavity is entered directly. Adhesions can be lysed under direct vision.

3. The peritoneal cavity is filled with approximately 2 to 3 L of CO_2 to separate the abdominal wall from the intra-abdominal viscera; this helps enhance visualization of pelvic and abdominal structures.

4. A laparoscope is inserted through a trocar to examine the abdomen (see Figure 4-13). Other trocars can be placed as conduits for other instrumentation.

5. After the desired procedure is completed, the laparoscope is removed, and the CO_2 is allowed to escape.

6. The incision is closed with a few skin stitches and covered with an adhesive bandage.

After

- Assess the patient frequently for signs of bleeding (increased pulse rate, decreased blood pressure) and perforated viscus (abdominal tenderness, guarding, decreased bowel sounds). Report any significant findings to the attending physician.
- If the patient has shoulder or subcostal discomfort from pneumoperitoneum, assure him or her that this usually lasts only 24 hours. Minor analgesics usually relieve this discomfort.
- If a surgical procedure has been performed laparoscopically, provide appropriate specific post-surgical care.

Home Care Responsibilities

- Instruct the patient to report increasing abdominal pain, which may indicate bowel perforation.
- Instruct the patient to report fever and chills, which may indicate a bowel perforation.
- Inform the patient that discomfort in the shoulder area or under the ribs may result from the carbon dioxide inserted into the peritoneal cavity during the procedure.

TEST RESULTS AND CLINICAL SIGNIFICANCE

Abdominal adhesions: *On occasion, these are the source of chronic abdominal pain.*

Ovarian tumour or cyst: *Tumours and cysts appear as obvious masses affecting the ovaries.*

Endometriosis: *The manifestation varies from small, white, wispy scars on the peritoneal surface to large inflammatory masses that distort normal anatomy.*

Ectopic pregnancy: *This usually appears as a large mass with or without a surrounding inflammation involving just one fallopian tube.*

Pelvic inflammatory disease (salpingitis): *The pelvic structures are red and inflamed.*

Uterine fibroids: *These appear as large, soft masses on and in the uterus.*

Abscess or infection: *This can have numerous abdominal or pelvic causes, including appendicitis, infection of fallopian tubes, diverticulitis, or acute cholecystitis.*

Cancer: *A large primary or metastatic cancer in the abdomen is usually obvious. The extent of tumour spread can be assessed.*

Ascites: *Fluid within the abdomen can be aspirated and tested to indicate its source, if that is not apparent at laparoscopy.*

Other abdominal pathologic conditions: *Nearly every significant abdominal pathologic process that affects the visceral or parietal peritoneal surface can usually be seen.*

Mediastinoscopy

NORMAL FINDINGS

No mediastinal tumours or abnormal lymph nodes

INDICATIONS

In this procedure, the mediastinum and the lymph nodes contained within can be visualized directly. Mediastinoscopy is used most commonly to determine the stage of a known lung cancer. It is also used to evaluate mediastinal masses of uncertain causes.

TEST EXPLANATION

In mediastinoscopy, a rigid mediastinoscope (a lighted instrument endoscope) is inserted through a small incision made at the suprasternal notch. The mediastinoscope is passed into the superior mediastinum to inspect the mediastinal lymph nodes and to remove biopsy specimens. Because these lymph nodes receive lymphatic drainage from the lungs, assessment of them can provide information on intrathoracic diseases such as carcinoma, granulomatous infections, and sarcoidosis; therefore, mediastinoscopy is used in establishing the diagnosis of various intrathoracic diseases. This procedure is also used to stage lung cancer and to assess whether the patient is a candidate for surgery. Evidence of metastasis to the mediastinal lymph nodes is usually a contraindication to thoracotomy because the tumour is considered inoperable. Biopsy of tumours in the mediastinum (e.g., thymoma or lymphoma) can also be performed through the mediastinoscope.

CONTRAINDICATIONS

- Superior vena cava obstruction, because of the tremendous venous collateralization in the mediastinum; mediastinoscopy in this situation can result in dangerous hemorrhage

POTENTIAL COMPLICATIONS

- Puncture of the esophagus, trachea, or great blood vessels
- Pneumothorax

PROCEDURE AND PATIENT CARE

Before

- Explain the procedure to the patient.
- Inform the patient that he or she will be asleep during the procedure.
- Obtain the patient's informed consent for this procedure.
- Check whether the patient's blood needs to be typed and crossmatched.
- Provide preoperative care as with any other surgical procedure.
- Keep the patient on NPO status (nothing by mouth) after midnight on the day of the test.
- Administer preprocedural medication approximately 1 hour before the test, as ordered.

During

- Note the following procedural steps:
  1. The patient is taken to the operating room for this surgical procedure.
  2. The patient is placed under general anaesthesia.
  3. An incision is made in the suprasternal notch.
  4. The mediastinoscope is passed through this neck incision and into the superior mediastinum.
  5. Biopsy samples of the lymph nodes are obtained.
  6. The mediastinoscope is withdrawn, and the incision is sutured closed.
- This procedure is performed in approximately 1 hour by a surgeon.

After

- Provide postoperative care as with any other surgical procedure.
- Note that subcutaneous emphysema may indicate a pneumothorax.
- Assess for mediastinal crepitus on auscultation, which may indicate mediastinal air from a pneumothorax or the bronchus or esophagus.
- Distended neck veins and pulsus paradoxus (abnormal decrease in systolic blood pressure and pulse wave amplitude during inspiration) may indicate lack of cardiac filling because of a large mediastinal hematoma.
- Observe for hypotension and tachycardia, which may indicate bleeding from the biopsy site or the great vessels.

Home Care Responsibilities

- Instruct the patient to report cough or shortness of breath, which may indicate a pneumothorax.
- Instruct the patient to report hoarseness, which may indicate injury to the recurrent laryngeal nerve.
- Instruct the patient to report fever and chills, which, with sepsis, may indicate mediastinitis from infection.

TEST RESULTS AND CLINICAL SIGNIFICANCE

Lung cancer, either primary into the mediastinum or metastatic to the lymph nodes: *It is routine to stage lung cancers with mediastinoscopy before thoracotomy.*

Thymoma: *Such a tumour of the anterior superior mediastinum can be easily seen in this technique.*

Tuberculosis or sarcoidosis: *Granulomatous inflammations can involve the mediastinal lymph nodes.*

Lymphoma or Hodgkin disease: *Lymphomas routinely involve the mediastinum. In a patient with previously established lymphoma, this procedure is not needed. However, mediastinoscopy may be the least invasive method of diagnosis if lymphoma has not yet been diagnosed.*

Infection (e.g., fungal, mycoplasmal): *Coccidioidomycosis, histoplasmosis, and* Pneumocystis jiroveci *infection can be diagnosed through this technique if the mediastinum is involved.*

RELATED TEST

Computed Tomography, Chest (p. 1068). This test can visualize the mediastinal structure but cannot identify a specific disease process.

Sigmoidoscopy (Proctoscopy, Anoscopy)

NORMAL FINDINGS

Normal anus, rectum, and sigmoid colon

INDICATIONS

In this test, the rectum and sigmoid colon can be visualized directly. Sigmoidoscopy is used to diagnose suspected pathologic conditions of these organs. It is recommended for patients who have had a change in bowel habits, have obvious or occult blood in the stool, or have abdominal pain. It is part of routine screening for colorectal cancer in individuals older than 50 years.

TEST EXPLANATION

Endoscopy of the lower gastrointestinal (GI) tract enables clinicians to visualize and obtain biopsy specimens of tumours, polyps, hemorrhoids, or ulcers of the anus, rectum, and sigmoid colon. *Anoscopy* refers to examination of the anus; *proctoscopy,* to examination of the anus and rectum; and *sigmoidoscopy* (the most frequent procedure), to examination of the anus, rectum, and sigmoid colon. Sigmoidoscopy can be performed with a rigid sigmoidoscopy (extending to 25 cm from the anus) or flexible sigmoidoscope (extending to 60 cm from the anus). Because the lower GI tract is difficult to visualize radiographically, direct visualization by sigmoidoscopy is diagnostically helpful.

Furthermore, sigmoidoscopy, like colonoscopy, can be used for therapeutic purposes. Reduction of sigmoid volvulus, removal of polyps, and obliteration of hemorrhoids can be performed through the sigmoidoscope.

A physician trained in GI endoscopy usually performs this procedure in the GI laboratory, operating room, or outpatient clinic or at the patient's bedside in approximately 15 to 20 minutes. Very little discomfort is associated with the test. An uncomfortable sense of having to defecate during the procedure is caused by the sigmoidoscope within the rectum.

CONTRAINDICATIONS

- Patient's inability to cooperate
- Diverticulitis, because the insufflation of air needed to distend the rectum and colon for passage of the scope may cause a perforation of the diverticula
- Painful anorectal conditions (e.g., fissures, fistulas, hemorrhoids), because of the anal pain associated with passage of the sigmoidoscope
- Severe bleeding, because blood clots obstruct the view of the sigmoidoscope
- Suspected perforation of colon lesions

POTENTIAL COMPLICATIONS

- Perforation of the colon
- Bleeding from biopsy sites

INTERFERING FACTORS

- Poor bowel preparation may obscure visualization of the bowel mucosa.
- Rectal bleeding may obstruct the lens system and preclude adequate visualization.

PROCEDURE AND PATIENT CARE

Before

- ⟨⟩ Explain the procedure to the patient.
- • Obtain the patient's informed consent for this procedure.
- ⟨⟩ Assist the patient with the bowel preparation. In most cases, two Fleet enemas are sufficient for examining the lower sigmoid colon and rectum. For examination extending as far as 60 cm, an oral cathartic is usually required.
- ⟨⟩ Instruct the patient to ingest only a light breakfast on the morning of the sigmoidoscopy.
- ⟨⟩ Assure the patient that he or she will be properly draped to avoid unnecessary embarrassment.

During

- • Note the following procedural steps:
  1. The patient is placed on the endoscopy table or bed in the left lateral decubitus position. Some physicians prefer the knee-chest position; many operating and examining tables are easily converted to make the knee-chest position more comfortable. This procedure also can be performed with the patient in the lithotomy position.
  2. Usually no sedation is required.
  3. The anus is mildly dilated with a well-lubricated finger.
  4. The rigid or flexible sigmoidoscope is placed into the rectum and advanced to its point of maximal penetration.
  5. Room air is insufflated during the procedure to more fully distend the lower intestinal tract.
  6. The sigmoid, rectum, and anus are visualized.
  7. Biopsy specimens can be obtained and polypectomy can be performed at the time of sigmoidoscopy.

After

- ⟨⟩ Remind the patient that because air has been insufflated into the bowel during the procedure, he or she may have flatulence or gas pains. Ambulation may help.
- • Observe the patient for signs of abdominal distension, increased tenderness, or rectal bleeding.
- ⟨⟩ If biopsy specimens have been taken, inform the patient that slight rectal bleeding may occur.

Home Care Responsibilities

- • Instruct the patient to report increasing abdominal pain, which may indicate bowel perforation.
- • Instruct the patient to report fever and chills, which may indicate a bowel perforation.
- • Inform the patient that frequent bloody bowel movements may indicate poor circulation of blood, if biopsy or polypectomy was performed.
- • Instruct the patient to report abdominal bloating and inability to pass flatus, which may indicate colon obstruction if a neoplasm was identified.

TEST RESULTS AND CLINICAL SIGNIFICANCE

Colorectal cancer: *This is seen as a red, friable, fleshy tumour concentrically involving the mucosa of the bowel.*

Colorectal polyp: *This tumour protrudes from only one part of the mucosa of the bowel. Some cancers and most polyps can be removed with the sigmoidoscope. Biopsy specimens can be obtained from neoplasms.*

Ulcerative proctitis: *Ulcerative colitis frequently involves the rectum, which results in ulcerative proctitis. This is one characteristic that distinguishes ulcerative colitis from Crohn's disease.*

Pseudomembranous colitis: *The rectum is the location that best facilitates the diagnosis of this disease. Usually this inflammation is the result of* Clostridium *overgrowth that results from prolonged use of clindamycin.*

Intestinal ischemia: *This usually is apparent as dark mucosa in the sigmoid colon. The sigmoid colon is the portion of colon most vulnerable if ischemia occurs. Ischemia always appears in the mucosa first.*

RELATED TESTS

Barium Enema (p. 1033). This is a radiographic contrast study of the colon and rectum. The rectum, however, is not well evaluated in this study.

Colonoscopy (p. 619). This is a direct visualization of the entire colon and rectum. It is more extensive and invasive than sigmoidoscopy. More complete preparation is required.

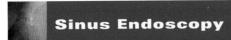

Sinus Endoscopy

NORMAL FINDINGS

Normal sinuses

INDICATIONS

This procedure is used to evaluate and treat recurrent or resistant sinus infections.

TEST EXPLANATION

Traditionally, patients with recurrent or resistant sinus infections often required surgical drainage. However, with the advent of sinus endoscopy, the sinus cavities can be accessed and drained without surgery. Cultures can be obtained, and antibiotic therapy can be more appropriately provided. The treatment of sinusitis is important to prevent the development of complications, such as mucoceles, cysts, or sinus bone destruction. The most accessible sinuses include the anterior ethmoid, middle turbinate, and middle meatus areas.

This procedure can also be used to visualize suspected neoplasms involving the sinuses. The test is usually performed by a surgeon trained in ear, nose, and throat diseases. Little postoperative pain is usually associated with this procedure.

POTENTIAL COMPLICATIONS

- Bleeding
- Cerebrospinal fluid leak (occurs only with ethmoid sinus endoscopy)

PROCEDURE AND PATIENT CARE

Before

- Explain the procedure to the patient.
- Obtain the patient's informed consent for this procedure.

Endoscopic Studies

4

If the procedure is to be performed with the patient under general anaesthesia, keep the patient on NPO status (nothing by mouth) after midnight on the day of the test. Intravenous fluids may be given. This procedure can also be performed with the use of local anaesthesia, depending on the amount of endoscopic surgery that is required.

During

- Note the following procedural steps:
    1. Sinus endoscopy is performed in the operating room if general anaesthesia is required; otherwise it can be performed in the office. The patient is initially placed in the supine position.
    2. After the skin near the nose and mouth is cleansed, the nose is sprayed with a lidocaine/epinephrine solution to diminish any bleeding.
    3. The sinuses are viewed with an endoscope preformed at various angles to enable optimal viewing.
    4. Sinus contents are examined and aspirated for culture testing.

After

- Place a 4 × 4 inch gauze pad under the nose to collect any fluid or blood that may further drain from the nose.
- If a cerebrospinal fluid leak is suspected, the fluid can be checked for glucose with a Dextrostix. Cerebrospinal fluid contains glucose.
- Assess the patient frequently for signs of bleeding. Report any significant findings to the attending physician.
- Allow the patient to have oral fluids.

TEST RESULTS AND CLINICAL SIGNIFICANCE

Chronic or resistant sinusitis: *These diseases usually result from inadequate drainage of the sinuses. Endoscopy should hasten cure.*

Sinus tumours: *These can be visualized and cells obtained to assist in the diagnosis of these tumours.*

Sinus cysts,

Sinus mucoceles: *These usually occur after years of chronic sinus infections.*

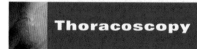

Thoracoscopy

NORMAL FINDINGS

Normal pleura and lungs

INDICATIONS

In this procedure, the pleura, lung, and mediastinum are visualized directly. Tissue can be obtained for testing. Thoracoscopy also assists in the staging and dissection of lung cancers.

TEST EXPLANATION

The use of thoracoscopy has been renewed as a result of the development of instrumentation for operative laparoscopy. With this technique, the parietal pleura, visceral pleura, and mediastinum can be directly visualized. Tumours involving the chest cavity can be staged through direct visualization. A biopsy for any abnormality can be performed. Collections of fluid can be drained and aspirated for testing. Dissection for lung resection can be carried out with the thoracoscope (video-assisted thoracotomy), which thereby minimizes the extent of a thoracotomy incision. Video-assisted thoracotomy is especially helpful for lung biopsy in patients with pulmonary nodules of uncertain cause or in immunocompromised patients with suspected *Pneumocystis* infections.

The patient must be aware of the possibility that an open thoracotomy is required if the procedure cannot be performed thoracoscopically or if bleeding occurs that cannot be controlled any other way. An open thoracotomy is a surgical incision into the chest wall. Any patient who can have an open thoracotomy can have a thoracoscopy.

CONTRAINDICATIONS

- Previous lung surgery, because it is difficult to obtain access to the free pleural space

POTENTIAL COMPLICATIONS

- Bleeding
- Infection or empyema
- Prolonged pneumothorax

PROCEDURE AND PATIENT CARE

Before

- Explain the procedure to the patient.
- Obtain the patient's informed consent for this procedure. Because of the possibility of intrathoracic injury, an open thoracotomy may be required. Ensure that the patient is aware of that.
- Because the procedure is usually performed with the patient under general anaesthesia, follow the routine general anaesthesia precautions.
- Shave and prepare the patient's chest as ordered.
- Keep the patient on NPO status (nothing by mouth) after midnight on the day of the test. Intravenous fluids may be given.

During

- Note the following procedural steps:
  1. Thoracoscopy is performed in the operating room. The patient is initially placed in the lateral decubitus position.
  2. After the thorax is cleansed, a blunt-tipped (Veress) needle is inserted through a small incision, and the lung is collapsed.
  3. A thoracoscope is inserted through a trocar to examine the chest cavity. Other trocars can be placed as conduits for other instrumentation.
  4. After the desired procedure is completed, the thoracoscope and trocars are removed.
  5. Usually a small chest tube is placed to ensure full re-expansion of the lung.
  6. The incision is closed with a few skin stitches and covered with an adhesive bandage.

After

- Assess the patient frequently for signs of bleeding (increased pulse rate, decreased blood pressure). Report any significant findings to the attending physician.

- Provide analgesics to relieve the minor to moderate pain that the patient may experience.
- If a surgical procedure has been performed thoracoscopically, provide appropriate specific postsurgical care.
- Note that a chest radiographic examination is performed after the procedure to ensure complete re-expansion of the lung.

TEST RESULTS AND CLINICAL SIGNIFICANCE

Primary lung cancer,

Metastatic cancer to the lung or pleura: *Often these tumours can be easily seen and biopsy performed, or the tumours can be removed through or with the help of thoracoscopy.*

Empyema: *The infected fluid can be drained directly, and good specimens obtained for cultures.*

Pleural diseases such as tumour, infection, or inflammation: *Biopsy of either the parietal or visceral pleura can be performed during this procedure.*

Pulmonary infection: *Thoracoscopy is particularly helpful in obtaining lung tissue for suspected infections such as tuberculosis,* Pneumocystis jiroveci *infection, coccidioidomycosis, or histoplasmosis.*

RELATED TEST

Laparoscopy (p. 645). This test is an examination of the abdomen in the same way that thoracoscopy is an examination of the chest. Most of the instruments are the same.

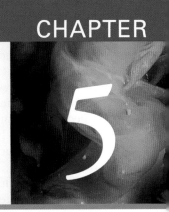
Fluid Analysis Studies

NOTE: *Throughout this chapter, SI units are presented in* **boldface colour,** *followed by conventional units in parentheses.*

OVERVIEW

TESTS

OVERVIEW

REASONS FOR PERFORMING FLUID ANALYSIS

Body fluid analysis can provide a significant amount of information concerning diseases that affect a patient. Normal body fluids can provide information concerning the body's hormonal status (cervical mucus test) and fertility (semen analysis, Sims-Huhner test). Analysis of cerebrospinal fluid (obtained by lumbar puncture) can provide significant data concerning diseases involving the central nervous system (brain and spinal cord). The normal collection of fluid that surrounds a fetus during pregnancy can be aspirated to gain information about the current and future health of the child and mother.

Abnormal accumulations of fluid (*effusions*) can be aspirated from the body to gain information about the disease process that caused the fluid to accumulate. Effusions can occur nearly anywhere in the body. Their presence is abnormal. In this chapter, effusions within the pericardium, pleura, peritoneum, and joints are discussed. An effusion is classified as a *transudate* or an *exudate*. The purpose of this classification is to categorize possible diagnoses. In general, exudates are caused by inflammatory, infectious, or neoplastic diseases. Transudates are generally caused by venous engorgement, hypoproteinemia, or fluid overload.

Other body fluids are analyzed to indicate specific disease such as cystic fibrosis (sweat electrolytes or pancreatic enzymes). The secretion of these body fluids is stimulated to obtain enough fluid for analysis.

Most body fluids are not easily obtained. Usually a cavity of the body must be invaded to obtain the fluids for analysis. A needle is used for aspiration of fluid from the subarachnoid space of the central nervous system (lumbar puncture), uterus (amniocentesis), pericardium (pericardiocentesis), pleura (thoracentesis), peritoneum (paracentesis), or joint (arthrocentesis). The aspiration technique must be completely sterile to avoid the introduction of infection to the body cavity. The quantity aspirated can vary from 20 mL to 5 L, depending on the location and original volume of the fluid. Testing of the fluid should be performed immediately to prevent cellular or chemical deterioration, which can cause inaccurate results. If the fluid cannot be tested immediately, guidelines for preservation should be closely followed. Usually the fluid is evaluated for gross appearance, colour, odour, red and white blood cell counts and differential, albumin and protein content, glucose and lactate dehydrogenase levels, cytologic features, fungi, tuberculosis, and bacteria (culture or Gram stain). Other tests may be performed, depending on the specifics of the fluid or the suspected disease.

The aspiration of fluid is helpful not only diagnostically but also often therapeutically. The aspiration of fluid from the pleura often improves ventilation and oxygenation. Aspiration of fluid from the peritoneum often relieves pressure and allows the patient to breathe more easily and eat more comfortably. Joint fluid aspiration may improve joint function. Pericardial fluid aspiration improves diastolic filling and cardiac output. Furthermore, therapeutic drugs (steroids or antibiotics) or diagnostic contrast materials (for radiographic evaluation) can be injected through the aspirating needle.

Although some other body fluids do not require aspiration, care must still be applied to obtaining and transporting the fluid properly (semen analysis, cervical mucus, sweat electrolytes, and pancreatic enzymes). The evaluation of some body fluids may be very important as criminal legal evidence (e.g., for the Sims-Huhner test in rape cases).

PROCEDURAL CARE FOR FLUID ANALYSIS
Before
- Explain the procedure to the patient.
- Obtain the patient's informed consent for this procedure.
- Inform the patient that no fasting is necessary unless heavy sedation is needed or an operative procedure is used to obtain the fluid.
- Have the patient urinate or empty the bladder before the test to avoid inadvertent puncture of the bladder during paracentesis or hip joint aspiration.
- Measure the patient's weight.
- Obtain baseline measurements of vital signs.

During

- The patient is positioned in a manner designed to make the fluid most accessible to the aspirating needle.
- Aspirating techniques are always performed in sterile conditions.
- When semen or cervical mucus is obtained, penile or vaginal preparation is contraindicated.
- With aspiration techniques, a variable amount of fluid is aspirated. Small volumes are aspirated into a syringe. For larger volumes, the aspirating needle is attached to a plastic tubing. The other end of the tubing is placed in the collection receptacle (usually a container with a pressurized vacuum).
- If medications are to be administered, a syringe containing the preparation is attached to the needle, and the drug is injected.
- To compare fluid levels with blood levels and to calculate ratios, blood samples are collected simultaneously for glucose, albumin, total protein, lactate dehydrogenase, and other measurements.

After

- All fluid samples should be analyzed immediately to avoid chemical or cellular deterioration, which could lead to false results.
- Place a small bandage over the needle site after aspiration is performed.
- Label the specimen with the patient's name, date, source of fluid, and diagnosis.
- Send the specimen promptly to the laboratory.
- Observe the puncture site for bleeding, continued drainage, or signs of infection if aspiration is performed.
- Monitor vital signs for evidence of hemodynamic changes if large volumes of fluid are withdrawn.
- On the microbiology laboratory requisition slip, write any recent antibiotic therapy that the patient has received.
- Place the patient in a position designed to minimize further leakage of fluid from an aspiration site.
- Monitor the patient and educate the patient about signs of potential complications.

POTENTIAL COMPLICATIONS OF FLUID ANALYSIS TESTING

The complications associated with fluid analysis are those of aspirating fluid for analysis. In general, they include the following:
- Injury to an organ by penetration with the aspirating needle
- Bleeding into the fluid space as a result of blood vessel penetration during aspiration
- Reflex bradycardia and hypotension because of the patient's anxiety about the procedure
- Infection of the soft tissue around the site of the needle aspiration
- Infection of the remaining fluid within the fluid space
- Seeding of the aspirating needle tract with tumour when malignant effusion is present
- Persistent leakage of effusion fluid after withdrawal of the aspirating needle
  Other specific complications are discussed with each test.

REPORTING RESULTS

In most instances, fluid is obtained by a physician. The laboratory tests are performed by technologists, and results are usually reported the same day. Cytologic study results are interpreted by a pathologist and are reported after several days. Culture and sensitivity reports also take several days.

Amniocentesis (Amniotic Fluid Analysis)

NORMAL FINDINGS

Length of Gestation	Amniotic Fluid Volume (mL)
15 weeks	450
25 weeks	750
30–35 weeks	1500
Full term	>1500

Amniotic fluid appearance: clear; pale to straw yellow
Lecithin/sphingomyelin (L/S) ratio: 2:1
Bilirubin level at 40 weeks' gestation: ≤**0.4 Mcmol/L** (≤0.024 mg/dL)
No chromosomal or genetic abnormalities
Phosphatidylglycerol level: positive
Lamellar body count: >30000/μL
Alpha-fetoprotein level: dependent on gestational age and laboratory technique
Fetal lung maturity (FLM) test
   Mature: >55 mg/g
   Borderline: >40 mg/g or <50 mg/g
   Immature: <40 mg/g

INDICATIONS

Amniocentesis is performed in pregnant women to gather information about the fetus. Fetal maturity, fetal distress, and risk for respiratory distress syndrome can be assessed. Genetic and chromosomal abnormalities can be identified. Maternal-fetal Rh incompatibility can be diagnosed. The sex of the child can be ascertained; this is important for a woman who carries a gene for a sex-linked disorder. Neural tube defects can also be recognized. The test is performed when a pregnancy is considered to be at high risk for complications. Affected patients include diabetic women; very obese women; women older than 35 years, especially if there is a family history of trisomy 21; women with repeated spontaneous abortions; women whose prior children have genetic defects; and women in a partnership in which either the woman or the man is a carrier for genetic defects. This test is also done on women in whom obstetric ultrasonography yields abnormal results.

TEST EXPLANATION

In amniocentesis, a needle is inserted through the patient's abdominal and uterine walls into the amniotic cavity to withdraw fluid for analysis. Studying amniotic fluid is vitally important in assessing the following:

1. Fetal maturity status, especially pulmonary maturity (when early delivery is preferred). Fetal maturity is determined by analysis of the amniotic fluid in the following manner:

   a. *Lecithin and sphingomyelin (L/S) ratio.* The measurement of the L/S ratio has emerged as the standard criterion test to evaluate fetal lung maturity. Lecithin is the major constituent of surfactant, an important substance required for alveolar ventilation. If surfactant is insufficient, the alveoli collapse during expiration. This results in atelectasis and respiratory distress syndrome (RDS), which is a major cause of death in immature infants. In the immature fetal lungs, the sphingomyelin concentration in amniotic fluid is higher than the lecithin concentration. At 35 weeks of gestation, the concentration of lecithin rapidly increases, whereas the sphingomyelin concentration decreases. An L/S ratio of 2:1 or greater ($\geq$3:1 in women with diabetes) is a highly reliable indication that the fetal lungs, and therefore the fetus, are mature. In such a case, the infant would be unlikely to develop RDS after birth. As the L/S ratio decreases, the risk of RDS increases.

b. Unfortunately, the L/S ratio assay involves a long and labour-intensive thin-layer chromatographic separation of the lipids. An alternative test is an assay based on fluorescence polarization, implemented on the fluorescence polarimeter and is called the *fetal lung maturity (FLM)* test. This test, which yields the ratio of surfactant (expressed in milligrams) to albumin (expressed in grams) in amniotic fluid samples, is quite sensitive. The mean expected weekly increment in FLM test results is $14.4 \pm 9.9\,\text{mg/g}$.

c. FLM results are affected less by other factors such as contaminated blood or meconium. A fluorescent phospholipid analogue (C_6-NBD-PC) is added to amniotic fluid and its fluorescence polarization is measured with a fluorescence polarimeter. Polarization values decrease during gestation in parallel with maturation of the pulmonary surfactant system. Polarization value can be used to predict the probability that a fetus will develop RDS after birth. Infrared spectroscopy is an alternative method of detecting and quantifying the key surfactants. The infrared spectrum of amniotic fluid shows strong absorptions from protein such as albumin in comparison with the surfactant lipids, which contribute subtle absorption differences to the overall profile.

d. *Phosphatidylglycerol.* This is a minor component (~10%) of lung surfactant phospholipids. However, because phosphatidylglycerol is synthesized almost entirely by mature lung alveolar cells, it is a good indicator of lung maturity. Because phosphatidylglycerol appears late in gestation, a positive finding in this test indicates a more mature surfactant than that found in the L/S ratio described previously. In healthy pregnant women, phosphatidylglycerol appears in amniotic fluid after 35 weeks of pregnancy, and levels gradually increase until term. An advantage of the phosphatidylglycerol assay is that it is not affected by contamination of amniotic fluid by blood or meconium. These two contaminants cause false-positive and false-negative results for the L/S ratio evaluation. In addition, the presence of phosphatidylglycerol in the amniotic fluid in the vagina after the membranes are ruptured indicates a low risk for RDS of the newborn. The simultaneous determination of the L/S ratio and the presence of phosphatidylglycerol is an excellent method of assessing fetal maturity on the basis of pulmonary surfactant.

e. *Lamellar body count.* This test to determine fetal maturity is also based on the presence of surfactant. Lamellar bodies are concentrically layered structures produced by type II pneumocytes. In cross-section, these small (~3 μm) structures look like onion layers. Lamellar bodies represent the storage form of pulmonary surfactant. Because cell counters cannot distinguish lamellar bodies from platelets, the lamellar body count is obtained through analysis of the amniotic fluid with a cell counter and recording the platelet count. Lamellar body results are calculated in units of particle density per microlitre of amniotic fluid. Some researchers have recommended cutoffs of $30\,000/\mu L$ and $10\,000/\mu L$ to predict low and high risk for RDS, respectively. If the count is greater than $30\,000/\mu L$, the negative predictive value for RDS is 100% (i.e., there is a 100% chance that the infant's lungs are mature enough to preclude RDS). If the lamellar body count is less than $10\,000/\mu L$, the probability of RDS is high (67%). Values between $10\,000/\mu L$ and $30\,000/\mu L$ represent intermediate risk for RDS. Not enough information is available on lamellar body count in diabetic patients to advocate its use in this population at high risk. There are several advantages of lamellar body counts. First, counts are faster, more precise, and more objective, and they require less amniotic fluid than does phospholipid analysis. Second, test results are not invalidated by the presence of blood or meconium. Third, the instrumentation required for this test is readily available, which thus allows it to be performed in all laboratories.

    f. *Microviscosity.* Microviscosity in lipid aggregates is dependent on the L/S ratio and the degree of saturation of fatty acid side chains. The pattern of change in amniotic fluid microviscosity during gestation parallels the expected development of the surfactant system. Amniotic fluid microviscosity is high during early gestation and abruptly and sequentially decreases between the twenty-eighth and thirty-sixth weeks of gestation. The measurements are an accurate reflection of the development of the surfactant system and thereby fetal lung maturity. With the development of more accurate testing such as FLM, this testing is no longer routinely performed; it is mentioned here more for recent historical value.

2. Sex of the fetus. Sons of women who are known to be carriers of X-linked recessive traits have a 50:50 risk of inheritance. Of importance is that amniocentesis is not performed to determine the sex of the child just out of interest.

3. Genetic and chromosomal aberrations, such as hemophilia, Down syndrome, and galactosemia. Genetic and chromosomal studies performed on cells aspirated within the amniotic fluid can indicate the gender of the fetus (important in sex-linked diseases such as hemophilia) or any of the described genetic and chromosomal aberrations (e.g., trisomy 21).

4. Fetal status affected by Rh isoimmunization. Women with Rh isoimmunization have a series of amniocentesis procedures during the second half of pregnancy to assess the level of bilirubin pigment in the amniotic fluid. The quantity of bilirubin is used to assess the severity of hemolytic anemia in Rh-sensitized fetuses. The higher the amount of bilirubin, the lower is the amount of fetal hemoglobin. Amniocentesis is usually initiated at 24 to 25 weeks. This allows assessment of the severity of the disease and the status of the fetus. Early delivery or blood transfusion may be indicated. It is important to take into consideration the volume of amniotic fluid because bilirubin concentration will be affected by total fluid volume.

5. Hereditary metabolic disorders, such as cystic fibrosis.

6. Anatomic abnormalities, such as neural tube closure defects (myelomeningocele, anencephaly, spina bifida). Increased levels of alpha-fetoprotein in the amniotic fluid may indicate a neural crest abnormality (p. 60). Decreased levels of alpha-fetoprotein may be associated with increased risk of trisomy 21.

7. Fetal distress, detected by meconium staining of the amniotic fluid. This is caused by relaxation of the anal sphincter. In this case, the amniotic fluid, which is normally colourless or straw-coloured and pale, may be tinged with green. Other colour changes may also indicate fetal distress. For example, yellow discoloration may indicate a blood incompatibility. A yellow-brown opaque appearance may indicate intrauterine death. A red colour indicates blood contamination from either the mother or the fetus.

Amniocentesis may be performed on the premise that elective abortion could be performed if the fetus is severely defective. Chorionic villus sampling (CVS) may be even better than amniocentesis for karyotyping and genetic analysis. CVS can be performed earlier in the pregnancy than can amniocentesis. (The earliest that amniotic fluid can be aspirated safely is at approximately 12 to 14 weeks' gestation.) Thus CVS enables a decision about abortion much earlier in the pregnancy than does amniocentesis.

The timing of the amniocentesis varies according to the clinical circumstances. With advanced maternal age and if chromosomal or genetic aberrations are suspected, the test should be performed early enough to allow a safe abortion. If information on fetal maturity is sought, performing the study during or after the thirty-fifth week of gestation yields the most information. Placental localization by ultrasonography (see p. 617) should be performed before amniocentesis to avoid passing the needle into the placenta, possibly interrupting the placenta, and inducing bleeding or miscarriage.

CONTRAINDICATIONS

- Abruptio placentae (a premature detachment of the placenta)
- Placenta previa (the placenta is implanted in the lower segment of the uterus)
- History of premature labour (before 34 weeks' gestation, unless the patient is receiving antilabour medication)
- Incompetent cervix

POTENTIAL COMPLICATIONS

- Miscarriage
- Fetal injury
- Leak of amniotic fluid
- Infection (amnionitis)
- Abortion
- Premature labour
- Maternal hemorrhage with possible maternal Rh isoimmunization
- Amniotic fluid embolism
- Abruptio placentae
- Inadvertent damage to the bladder or intestines

INTERFERING FACTORS

- Fetal blood contamination can cause artificial elevations in alpha-fetoprotein levels.
- Hemolysis of the specimen can alter results.
- Contamination of the specimen with meconium or blood may result in inaccurate L/S ratios.

✔ Clinical Priorities

- Instructions regarding emptying the bladder vary according to gestational age. Before 20 weeks of gestation, the bladder should be kept full during the test to support the uterus. After 20 weeks, the bladder must be emptied to minimize the chance of puncture.
- Before this procedure, the placenta should be located on ultrasonography in order to select a site to avoid placental puncture.
- Women who have Rh-negative blood should receive Rho(D) immune globulin (RhoGAM) because of the risk of immunization from fetal blood.

PROCEDURE AND PATIENT CARE

Before

 Explain the procedure to the patient. Allow the patient to verbalize her concerns, and allay any fears.

▷ Inform the patient that the discomfort associated with amniocentesis is usually described as a mild uterine cramping that occurs when the needle contacts the uterus. Some women may complain of a "pulling" sensation as the amniotic fluid is withdrawn.

• Obtain informed consent from the patient and her partner.

▷ Inform the patient that no food or fluid is restricted.

• Evaluate the patient's blood pressure and the fetal heart rate.

▷ Give the patient instructions regarding emptying the bladder, which depend on gestational age. Before 20 weeks of gestation, the bladder should be kept full to support the uterus. After 20 weeks, the bladder should be emptied to minimize the chance of puncture.

• Locate the placenta by ultrasound examination before the study so as to select a site that will avoid placental puncture.

During

• Place the patient in the supine position.
• Note the following procedural steps:
  1. The skin overlying the chosen site (often determined by obstetric ultrasonography) is prepared and usually anaesthetized locally.
  2. A needle with a stylet is inserted through the midabdominal wall and directed at an angle toward the middle of the uterine cavity (Figure 5-1).
  3. The stylet is then removed, and a sterile plastic syringe is attached.
  4. After 5 to 10 mL of amniotic fluid is withdrawn, the needle is removed. (This fluid volume is replaced by newly formed amniotic fluid within 3 to 4 hours after the procedure.)
  5. The specimen is placed in a light-resistant container to prevent breakdown of bilirubin.
  6. The site on the patient's abdomen is covered with an adhesive bandage.

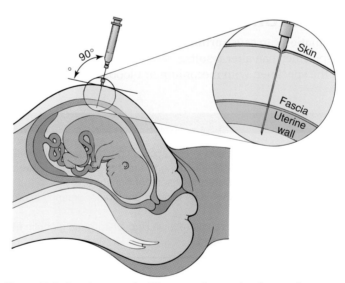

Figure 5-1 Amniocentesis. Ultrasound scanning is usually used to determine the placental site and to locate a pocket of amniotic fluid. The needle is then inserted. Three levels of resistance are felt as the needle penetrates the skin, fascia, and uterine wall. When the needle is placed within the uterine cavity, amniotic fluid is withdrawn.

7. If the amniotic fluid is bloody, the physician must determine whether the blood is maternal or fetal in origin. Kleihauer-Betke stain will turn fetal cells pink. If the amniotic fluid is stained dark brown it may indicate that meconium is present in the fluid (the earliest stools of an infant that are usually stored in the bowel until after birth). Meconium in the amniotic fluid is usually associated with compromise of the fetus.

- Amniotic fluid volume is calculated by injecting a known concentration of solute (such as para-aminohippuric acid [PAH]) into the amniotic fluid to distribute throughout the amniotic fluid. Amniotic fluid is then withdrawn, and the PAH concentration is determined.
- Note that this procedure takes approximately 20 to 30 minutes.
- Remember that many women are extremely anxious during this procedure. Provide emotional support.

After

- Place amniotic fluid in a sterile, siliconized glass container, and transport it to a special chemistry laboratory for analysis. Sometimes the specimen may be sent by air mail to another commercial laboratory for genetic and other testing.
- Inform the patient that the results of this study are usually not available for over 1 week.
- For women who have Rh-negative blood, administer Rho(D) immune globulin (RhoGAM) because of the risk of immunization against Rh-positive antibody from the fetal blood.
- Assess the fetal heart rate after the test to detect any ill effects related to the procedure. Compare this value with the preprocedural baseline value.
- If the patient felt dizzy or nauseated during the procedure, instruct her to lie on her left side for several minutes before leaving the examining room.
- Observe the puncture site for bleeding or other drainage.
- Instruct the patient to call her physician if she has any amniotic fluid loss, bleeding, temperature elevation, abdominal pain or cramping, fetal hyperactivity, or unusual fetal lethargy.

Home Care Responsibilities

- Inform the patient that the puncture site should be checked for bleeding and amniotic fluid loss.
- Instruct the patient to call her physician if she has any fluid loss, bleeding, temperature elevation, or abdominal cramping, or if she feels unusual fetal movement or fetal lethargy.

TEST RESULTS AND CLINICAL SIGNIFICANCE

Hemolytic disease of the newborn: *This may be apparent as increased bilirubin in the amniotic fluid. The fetal hemolysis causes free heme to form. This heme is then catabolized to bilirubin.*

Rh isoimmunization: *A rising anti-Rh antibody titre in an Rh-negative woman would indicate potential for erythroblastosis fetalis (Rh-positive fetus). The higher the bilirubin level in the amniotic fluid, the greater the risk to the fetus is.*

Neural tube defects (e.g., myelomeningocele, anencephaly, spina bifida),

Abdominal wall defects (e.g., gastroschisis, omphalocele),

Sacrococcygeal teratoma: *An elevated alpha-fetoprotein level most commonly indicates neural tube defects. However, other closing defects (e.g., in the abdominal wall) may be present. Neoplasms associated with neural tube defects may also be associated with increases in alpha-fetoprotein levels. Blood levels of alpha-fetoprotein are also increased with these abnormalities.*

Meconium staining: *This is evidence of fetal distress and is noted as greenish staining of the amniotic fluid.*

Immature fetal lungs: *This may occur with premature labour, maternal hypertension, or placental injuries. The risk of RDS increases as evidence of fetal lung immaturity increases. Fetal lung maturity is diminished in diabetic women and is also noted in hydrops fetalis.*

Hereditary metabolic disorders (e.g., cystic fibrosis, Tay-Sachs disease, galactosemia),

Genetic or chromosomal aberrations (e.g., sickle cell disease, thalassemia, Down syndrome),

Sex-linked disorders (e.g., hemophilia): *The genetic defects of many diseases can be recognized through gene recognition and karyotyping. Other genetic defects causing metabolic disorders can be recognized from the results of protein analysis of the amniotic fluid.*

Polyhydramnios: *This occurs in patients who have diabetes. When polyhydramnios (amniotic fluid level >2 000 mL) is present, the risk of congenital aberrations is significantly higher.*

Oligohydramnios: *This is recognized as less than 300 mL of amniotic fluid at 25 weeks' gestation. It is associated with fetal renal diseases. Near term, it is associated with early membrane rupture, intrauterine growth restriction, or significant post-term gestation.*

RELATED TESTS

Chorionic Villus Sampling (p. 1134). This is a test whereby the chorionic placental tissue (which has the same genetic material as the fetus) is tested for genetic analysis and karyotyping. This is a rapid and accurate method of determining genetic defects. CVS can be performed earlier in pregnancy than can amniocentesis.

Maternal Screen Testing (p. 369). This is a series of screening tests that can reveal fetal distress and chromosomal abnormalities.

Fetoscopy (p. 640). This is another method of obtaining fetal tissue for genetic and maturity testing.

Pelvic Ultrasonography (p. 917). Significant fetal disease and evidence of fetal distress can be detected on obstetric ultrasound examination. If findings are abnormal, amniocentesis is indicated.

Amyloid Beta Protein Precursor, Soluble (SBPP)

NORMAL FINDINGS

Ranges vary among laboratories. The testing laboratory should be consulted in order to interpret the results.

INDICATIONS

This test is performed on patients who increasingly show signs of dementia and confusion. It is a test used to help diagnose Alzheimer's disease and other forms of senile dementia.

TEST EXPLANATION

Amyloid protein is a 42–amino-acid peptide that is broken off of a larger amyloid precursor protein (amyloid beta precursor protein). These amyloid beta proteins have been shown to be neurotrophic and neuroprotective. In Alzheimer's disease, for some unknown reason, amyloid beta is deposited on the brain in the form of plaques. It has been discovered that these plaques contain damaged nerve cells in a compacted core of amyloid beta protein. As a result of this deposition, levels of amyloid beta are decreased in the cerebrospinal fluid of patients with Alzheimer's disease and other forms of dementia. Research has demonstrated the diagnostic potential of this biochemical marker for Alzheimer's disease.

Ongoing research has also focused on using cerebrospinal fluid levels of tau protein as another biochemical marker for Alzheimer's disease. Neurofibrillary tangles, also noted in the brains of patients with Alzheimer's disease, are composed primarily of hyperphosphorylated tau protein. There is a general consensus that cerebrospinal fluid levels of tau protein are significantly increased in patients with Alzheimer's disease in comparison with healthy control subjects and in patients with non–Alzheimer's neurologic disease. For these tests, a cerebrospinal fluid sample should be obtained through lumbar puncture (p. 676).

At present, there is little or no consensus on the use of screening tests for diagnosing early Alzheimer's disease. This is because of a lack of sensitivity and specificity and sufficient normative data. However, there is consensus that using a combination of early neuropsychologic changes and biomarkers will facilitate diagnosis of prodromal Alzheimer's disease earlier than current criteria for probable diagnosis allow.

Positron emission tomography (PET) with amyloid imaging has shown promise for the diagnosis of Alzheimer's disease. Pittsburgh agent B appears to reliably reveal brain amyloid deposits caused by the accumulation of the isoform amyloid beta$_{42}$ within plaques. Studies so far have revealed high levels of amyloid retention in the brain at prodromal stages of Alzheimer's disease, and scanning with Pittsburgh agent B thus may have potential for discriminating Alzheimer's disease from other dementia disorders. The PET scans with Pittsburgh agent B as the imaging agent have shown that the amyloid deposition pattern in Alzheimer's disease is dramatically different from appearance of normal brains. Because amyloid accumulation is one of the earliest signs of Alzheimer's disease, early diagnosis may be facilitated by identifying amyloid deposition early in the disease progression, perhaps before symptoms emerge.

With the use of multiparameter immunoassay, the plasma form of soluble amyloid beta protein precursor can be measured with the INNO-BIA AlzBio3 assay in a manner different from a simple blood sample. This could—in the long term and after further investigation—lead to improved and accelerated development of drugs to treat Alzheimer's disease and possibly to earlier diagnosis of the condition.

PROCEDURE AND PATIENT CARE

Before
- Explain the procedure to the patient.
- Refer to the instructions for a lumbar puncture and cerebrospinal fluid examination (see p. 676).

During
- Collect a cerebrospinal fluid specimen as indicated in the discussion of lumbar puncture (p. 676).

After
- Follow the postprocedure guidelines for lumbar puncture.

TEST RESULTS AND CLINICAL SIGNIFICANCE
▼ Decreased Levels
Alzheimer's disease,

Other senile dementia: *Amyloid beta levels in the cerebrospinal fluid are low, possibly because of its deposition in the brain. How these plaques of amyloid beta exert the neurologic damage is unknown.*

RELATED TEST
Lumbar Puncture and Cerebrospinal Fluid Examination (p. 676). In this diagnostic procedure, the cerebrospinal fluid is obtained to be studied for the presence of amyloid beta proteins.

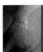

Arthrocentesis With Synovial Fluid Analysis (Synovial Fluid Analysis, Joint Aspiration)

NORMAL FINDINGS
Synovial fluid: clear and straw-coloured with few white blood cells (WBCs), no crystals, and a good mucin clot

Chemical test values (e.g., glucose determination): approximating those found in the bloodstream

INDICATIONS
Arthrocentesis is performed to establish the diagnosis of joint infection, arthritis, crystal-induced arthritis (gout and pseudogout), synovitis, or neoplasms involving the joint. This procedure is also used to identify the cause of joint inflammation or effusion, to monitor chronic arthritic diseases, and to inject anti-inflammatory medications (usually corticosteroids) into a joint space.

TEST EXPLANATION
Arthrocentesis is performed by inserting a sterile needle into the joint space of the involved joint to obtain synovial fluid for analysis. Synovial fluid is a liquid found in small amounts within the joints. Aspiration (withdrawal of the fluid) may be performed on any major joint, such as the knee, shoulder, hip, elbow, wrist, or ankle.

The fluid sample is examined microscopically and chemically. A culture of the fluid is usually performed. Normal joint fluid is clear, straw-coloured, and quite viscous because of the hyaluronic acid, which acts as a lubricant. Viscosity is reduced in patients with inflammatory arthritis. Viscosity can be estimated by forcing some synovial fluid from a syringe. Fluid of high viscosity forms a "string" several centimetres long; fluid of low viscosity drips in a manner similar to water.

The result of the *mucin clot test* is correlated with the viscosity. This test is performed by adding acetic acid to joint fluid. The formation of a tight, ropy clot indicates qualitatively good mucin and the presence of adequate molecules of intact hyaluronic acid. The mucin clot is poor in quality and quantity in the presence of an inflammatory joint disease, such as rheumatoid arthritis. By itself, synovial fluid should not spontaneously form a fibrin clot (clot without the addition of acetic acid) because normal joint fluid does not contain fibrinogen. If, however, bleeding into the joint (from trauma or injury) has occurred, the synovial fluid does clot.

The synovial fluid glucose value is usually within **0.6 mmol/L** (10 mL/dL) of the serum glucose value. For proper interpretation, the synovial fluid glucose and serum glucose samples should be collected simultaneously after the patient has fasted for 6 hours. The synovial fluid glucose level falls with increasing severity of inflammation. Although this level is lowest in septic arthritis (the synovial fluid glucose value may be less than 50% of the serum glucose value), the synovial glucose level may also be low in patients with rheumatoid arthritis. The synovial fluid is also tested for protein, uric acid, and lactate levels. Increased uric acid levels indicate gout. Increased protein and lactate levels indicate bacterial infection.

Cell counts are also performed on the synovial fluid. Normally the joint fluid contains less than 0.2×10^9/L (<200 WBCs/mm^3) and no red blood cells. An increased WBC count with a high percentage of neutrophils (>75%) supports the diagnosis of acute bacterial infectious arthritis. The WBC count can also be high in other conditions, such as acute gouty arthritis and rheumatoid arthritis. The differential WBC count, however, reveals monocytosis or lymphocytosis with these later-mentioned diseases.

Bacterial and fungal cultures are usually requested and performed when infection is suspected. Administering antibiotics before arthrocentesis may diminish the growth of bacteria in synovial fluid cultures and can confound the results. Smears with acid-fast stains for tubercle bacilli are also performed on the synovial fluid. In addition, synovial fluid is examined under polarized light for the presence of crystals, which enables differentiating between gout and pseudogout: The calcium pyrophosphate dihydrate crystals of pseudogout are birefringent (blue on red background) when examined with a polarized light microscope.

The synovial fluid is also analyzed for complement levels (p. 185). Complement levels are decreased in patients with systemic lupus erythematosus, rheumatoid arthritis, or other immunologic arthritis. Decreases in these joint complement levels are caused by consumption of the complement induced by the antigen-antibody immune complexes within the joint cavity.

One of the most important tests routinely performed on synovial fluid is the microscopic examination for crystals. For example, the presence of urate crystals indicates gouty arthritis. Calcium pyrophosphate crystals are present in pseudogout. Cholesterol crystals are present in rheumatoid arthritis.

A physician performs this procedure in approximately 10 minutes in an office or at the patient's bedside. The only discomfort associated with this test is from the injection of the local anaesthetic. The joint-space pain may worsen after fluid aspiration, especially in patients with acute arthritis. The administration of steroids is also associated with pain for as long as 2 days after the injection.

CONTRAINDICATIONS

- Skin or wound infections in the area of the needle puncture, because of the risk for sepsis

POTENTIAL COMPLICATIONS

- Joint infection
- Hemorrhage in the joint area

PROCEDURE AND PATIENT CARE

Before

- Explain the procedure to the patient.
- Obtain the patient's informed consent if this is the institution's policy.
- Keep the patient on NPO status (nothing by mouth) after midnight on the day of the test. Fasting prevents alterations of the chemical determinations (e.g., glucose) that may be performed with

the study. However, this study may be done more conveniently in a physician's office without the patient's fasting.

During

- Have the patient lie on his or her back with the joint fully extended.
- Note the following procedural steps:
  1. The skin is locally anaesthetized to minimize pain.
  2. The area is aseptically cleansed, and a needle is inserted through the skin and into the joint space.
  3. Fluid is obtained for analysis. The joint area sometimes may be wrapped with an elastic bandage to compress free fluid within a certain area, thereby maximizing collection of fluid.
  4. If a corticosteroid or other medications (e.g., antibiotics) are to be administered, a syringe containing the steroid preparation is attached to the needle, and the drug is injected.
  5. The needle is removed, and a pressure dressing may be applied to the site.
  6. Sometimes a peripheral venous blood sample is taken to compare results of chemical tests on the blood with those of chemical studies on the synovial fluid.

After

- Assess the joint for any pain, fever, or swelling, which may indicate infection.
- Apply ice to decrease pain and swelling.
- Keep a pressure dressing on the joint to avoid buildup of joint fluid or development of a hematoma.
- Advise the patient to avoid strenuous use of the joint for the next several days.

TEST RESULTS AND CLINICAL SIGNIFICANCE

Infection,

Septic arthritis: *This can be the result of penetrating trauma or bloodborne infection resulting from bacteremia. The affected joint is usually red, warm, swollen, and painful. The joint fluid usually has a reduced level of glucose and increased levels of WBCs, protein, and lactate (because of the lactate produced by the bacteria). The offending organism is expected to be visible with Gram stains and to grow in cultures (p. 733).*

Degenerative arthritis (osteoarthritis): *Excess nongouty crystals within the joint space and cartilage may cause degenerative changes involving the joint space. The course is usually chronic and without acute flare-up. Nonsteroidal anti-inflammatory drugs are usually helpful.*

Synovitis: *This can be inflammatory or infectious. The synovial membrane is the tissue surrounding the joint space.*

Neoplasm: *Synovial, cartilaginous, and bony tumours (benign and malignant) can begin in the joint. Protein levels can be expected to be elevated. Microscopy may reveal malignant cells.*

Joint effusion: *Joint effusion (fluid in the joint) causes the joint to be swollen. The fluid is obtained to determine the source of the effusion.*

Systemic lupus erythematosus,

Rheumatoid arthritis: *Autoimmune or collagen-vascular diseases can be associated with immunogenic arthritis. Levels of complement are reduced, and levels of WBCs and protein are increased.*

Gout,

Pseudogout: *Crystal-induced arthritis occurs when urate (gout) or calcium pyrophosphate (pseudogout) is deposited into the joint-surrounding structures and joint surface cartilage. Inflammation follows, and arthritis occurs. In time, cartilage is destroyed.*

Trauma: *When a joint is injured, a joint effusion may develop. This is usually a transudate. However, if a ligament or cartilage is torn, bleeding may occur within the joint.*

RELATED TEST

Arthroscopy (p. 610). This is an endoscopic procedure designed to view the joint space directly and to provide access to the joint for surgical treatment of disease and injury.

Breast Cyst and Nipple Discharge Fluid Analysis

NORMAL FINDINGS

No evidence of atypical or neoplastic (cancer) cells

INDICATIONS

These two tests are used to attempt to make the diagnosis of cancer within breast cysts or to exclude the diagnosis of breast cancer as a cause of persistent nipple discharge.

TEST EXPLANATION

Fluid from breast cysts or nipple discharge can be examined cytologically for evidence of cancer cells. Most simple cysts (cysts that contain fluid and no tissue, as recognized on ultrasonography, p. 901) are benign. The exceptions are those in which the aspirated fluid is bloody, those that repeatedly recur after aspirations, or those that do not completely collapse after aspiration. The contents of these simple cysts should be sent for cytologic examination. A complex cyst (cyst that contains some tissue) can be cancerous (cystic adenocarcinoma of the breast), and its contents should also be aspirated and examined microscopically. The cyst aspiration can be directed by palpation of the physician or by ultrasonography.

Cytologic examination of nipple discharge is not terribly reliable in the identification of cancer. Nearly all nonbloody nipple discharge results from benign pathologic processes. Only 10% to 12% of bloody discharges are related to breast cancer. Of that small percentage, fewer than 50% can be detected in cytologic examination of the nipple discharge. Cellular deterioration can be misinterpreted as atypical or suspect cytologic changes. This misinterpretation may lead to an unnecessary breast biopsy.

POTENTIAL COMPLICATIONS

- Infection in the breast as a result of the needle aspiration
- Pneumothorax as a result of the needle's penetrating a thin chest wall in the attempt to aspirate a cyst in the posterior portion of the breast
- Hematoma in the breast as a result of intraglandular bleeding from a blood vessel penetrated by the aspirating needle

PROCEDURE AND PATIENT CARE

Before

- Because cyst aspiration may cause intraglandular bleeding that may temporarily distort findings on the mammogram, bilateral mammography may be performed before cyst aspiration.
- Inform the patient of the proposed procedure.

5 Fluid Analysis Studies

⚖ Allow patient to verbalize concern about anticipated pain related to cyst aspiration, and allay those concerns. Mention that a needle with only a very small bore is used. If a larger bore needle is required, local anaesthetic is administered first.

During

Nipple Discharge.
- Note the following procedural steps:
  1. Express the nipple discharge from the breast.
  2. Smear the discharge onto a clean microscope slide as for a Papanicolaou (Pap) smear.
  3. The cells must be fixed immediately, either by immersion of the slide in equal parts of 95% alcohol and ether or by application of a commercial hair spray before drying, because drying will distort the cells and make interpretation difficult. In addition, this fixing process kills any infectious organisms so that the specimen is less infectious to the personnel who handle the specimen.
  4. The slide is labelled with the patient's name, date of birth, date of test, and site of the lesion.

Cyst Aspiration.
- Note the following procedural steps:
  1. While the patient is in the supine position, the cyst is identified by palpation or through ultrasound guidance.
  2. The skin overlying the cyst is prepared in a sterile manner.
  3. If a 25-gauge needle is to be used for aspiration, no local anaesthetic is required. If, however, the fluid is suspected to be thick, a 20-gauge needle is used. In this circumstance, local anaesthetic is infiltrated into the skin.
  4. The aspirating needle is inserted through the skin and into the cyst. Fluid is aspirated until the cyst is completely collapsed.
  5. The fluid is injected into a fixative solution (Carbowax) and appropriately labelled as described previously.

After

- Pressure is applied to the aspiration site. An adhesive bandage is applied.
- ⚖ The patient should be informed that it is not uncommon to develop an ecchymosis in the area of the breast where the aspiration was performed.
- ⚖ Allow the patient to verbalize concerns, and allay those concerns. Mention that if the cyst fluid is clear, the lesion is most certainly benign.

TEST RESULTS AND CLINICAL SIGNIFICANCE

Cancer,

Benign cyst: *As indicated previously, cystic adenocarcinoma of the breast is very rare. If the fluid is clear and the cyst collapses completely, the cyst is considered benign.*

Intraductal papilloma: *This is a common cause of breast discharge. Intraductal papillomas are benign, and no treatment is required unless the discharge is copious.*

RELATED TESTS

Breast Ultrasonography (p. 901). This method of cyst visualization can be used to direct cyst aspiration.

Mammography (p. 1086). Cysts are apparent as soft tissue densities within the breast tissue.

Breast Ductal Lavage

NORMAL FINDINGS
No atypical cells in the effluent

Possible Critical Values
Cancer cells in the effluent

INDICATIONS
The cytologic evaluation of breast ductal lavage specimens is a low-yield tool for assessing or identifying in situ or invasive breast cancer. A number of long-term follow-up studies have confirmed that the presence of atypical ductal cells does constitute a risk factor for breast cancer.

This test is performed on women who are at increased risk for developing breast cancer and who would make a decision to accept treatment designed to diminish that risk if atypical (premalignant) cells were found in their ducts.

TEST EXPLANATION
The theory behind ductal lavage is that study of exfoliated cells washed out from a few breast ducts enables clinicians to assess the patient's risk of developing breast cancer in the near future. If atypical cells are identified, the risk of developing breast cancer in the next decade may be as high as 4 to 10 times normal. Once that risk is identified, the patient may choose to attempt to alter that risk by using chemopreventive medications (such as selective estrogen receptor modulators) or surgery.

Initially, it was hoped that ductal lavage would identify ductal carcinoma of the breast at its earliest stages. The results of several large studies did not support that hope. Its use has now been limited to women who, in *breast cancer risk models,* have been found to be at a statistically higher personal risk for breast cancer. These statistical models are based on age at menarche, age at first pregnancy, prior breast surgery, family history, and history of atypical changes in previous breast biopsy specimens. Many women found to be at increased risk prefer more data before they decide to take a medication designed to reduce those risks. If atypical cells are found in the lavage, most patients would choose to take the medication. If no atypical cells were found, they may choose just close observation.

There are still no data to confirm that the findings do accurately reflect a true risk for breast cancer. Furthermore, there are no data to indicate what a negative finding of lavage means.

CONTRAINDICATIONS
- Prior breast cancer surgery, because the risks for such patients are known to be high

POTENTIAL COMPLICATIONS
- Infection

PROCEDURE AND PATIENT CARE

Before

- Explain the procedure to the patient. Many such patients have already received extensive counselling regarding their risks for breast cancer.
- Ensure that the findings of the breast examination and mammogram are normal.
- Apply a topical anaesthetic to the nipple area approximately 30 minutes before the test.

During

- Note the following procedural steps:
  1. Before suction, the breast is massaged for a few minutes.
  2. A suction apparatus is applied to the nipple area. Ducts that reveal fluid with the suction are then chosen for cannulation.
  3. A tiny catheter is gently placed into the nipple, and lavage is performed on the duct with 5 to 10 mL of saline.
  4. The effluent is then collected in a small tube and sent for cytologic study.
  5. The procedure is then repeated for other ducts that produced fluid with nipple suction. A separate catheter is used for each duct.
  6. The sites for each cannulated duct are recorded on a grid representing the nipple for future reference.
- This procedure is performed by a surgeon in approximately 30 minutes in the office. Minimal to moderate discomfort is associated with the nipple suction, duct cannulation, and lavage.

TEST RESULTS AND CLINICAL SIGNIFICANCE

Atypical cells: *Atypical cells indicate that the patient is at an increased risk for developing breast cancer and should consider cancer-preventive therapy.*

Ductal cancer cells: *Identification of cancer cells presents a very perplexing problem because the location of the cancer often cannot be determined; therefore, conservative simple excision cannot be performed as treatment. It is prudent to confirm the presence of malignant cells through a second cytopathologic opinion.*

RELATED TESTS

Mammography (p. 1086). This is a radiographic study of the breast that has proved to be a very accurate method of screening and diagnosing breast cancer.

Ductoscopy (p. 630). This test provides an endoscopic view of the breast ducts.

Magnetic Resonance Imaging (p. 1148). This is a very sensitive method of breast imaging.

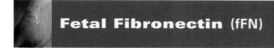

Fetal Fibronectin (fFN)

NORMAL FINDINGS

Negative (<0.05 Mcg/mL)

INDICATIONS

To help predict preterm delivery, women with symptoms of preterm labour can be screened for the presence of fetal fibronectin (fFN). The presence of fFN in the cervicovaginal secretions of symptomatic women during weeks 22 through 34 of pregnancy indicates an increased risk of preterm delivery. However, the absence of fFN is a more reliable predictor that the pregnancy will continue for at least another 2 weeks.

TEST EXPLANATION

Fibronectin may help with implantation of the fertilized egg into the uterine lining. Normally, fibronectin cannot be identified in vaginal secretions after 22 weeks of pregnancy. However, concentrations are very high in the amniotic fluid. If fibronectin is identified in vaginal secretions after 24 weeks, the patient is at high risk for preterm (premature) delivery within the next 2 weeks. Its use is limited to women whose membranes are intact and to women with signs and symptoms of labour in whom cervix dilatation is less than 3 cm.

A negative fFN test result is a highly reliable predictor that preterm delivery will not occur within the next 2 weeks. A positive result is a less reliable predictor of preterm labour: There is still a fair chance that the pregnancy will continue for at least another 2 weeks. The greatest value of the fFN test is the high level of reliability of a negative test result. A negative test result reassures medical providers and expectant parents that the risk of preterm delivery is currently low, and it helps reduce the need for medical interventions. A positive fFN result, although less reliable, allows physicians and patients to take preventive measures to delay labour for as long as possible, by hospitalization or administration of labour-suppressing (tocolytic) medications, or both.

This test has the best predictive screening capacity for determining whether pregnancy will continue for at least 7 days and beyond 34 weeks' gestation. The test has been shown to be very useful in Canadian women presenting with symptoms of preterm labour between 24 and 34 weeks' gestation. The American College of Obstetricians and Gynecologists (ACOG) currently recommends this test in women with signs of preterm labour.

This test can be performed at the patient's bedside in a few minutes. Results of this quick assay have been shown to be highly concordant with those of the original enzyme-linked immunosorbent assay (ELISA), which requires 48 hours to yield a result.

PROCEDURE AND PATIENT CARE

Before

- Explain the procedure to the patient.
- Inform the patient that no fasting is required.
- Determine whether the patient has had a recent cervical examination. The result may be inaccurate if a cervical examination has been performed within 24 hours.

During

- Note the following procedural steps:
  1. The patient is placed in the lithotomy position
  2. A vaginal speculum is inserted to expose the cervix.
  3. Vaginal secretions are collected from the posterior vagina and paracervical area with a polyester (Dacron) swab that comes with the fibronectin laboratory kit.
  4. The slide is labelled with the patient's name, age, and estimated date of confinement.
- Inform the patient that no discomfort, except at insertion of the speculum, is associated with this procedure.
- Note that this procedure is performed in several minutes by a physician or other licensed health care provider.

After

 Inform the patient that the result is usually available the next day.

 Educate the patient of the signs of preterm labour: cramps, uterine contractions, pelvic pressure, or the rupture of membranes.

 Encourage the patient to express concerns regarding the plans for preterm delivery.

TEST RESULTS AND CLINICAL SIGNIFICANCE

▲ Increased Levels

High risk for preterm premature delivery: *Fetal fibronectin, a component of the extracellular matrix of fetal membranes, leaks into the cervix when the interaction between the fetal membranes and the uterine wall weakens.*

Lumbar Puncture and Cerebrospinal Fluid Examination (LP and CSF Examination, Spinal Tap, Spinal Puncture, Cerebrospinal Fluid Analysis)

NORMAL FINDINGS

Cerebrospinal fluid (CSF) pressure: 100–200 mm Hg H_2O

Colour: crystal clear and colourless

Blood: none

Cells

Red blood cells (RBCs): 0

White blood cell (WBC) total:

- Neonate: **0–30 × 10⁶ WBCs/L** (0–30 cells/µL)
- Child 1–5 years: **0–20 × 106 WBCs/L** (0–20 cells/µL)
- Child 6–18 years: **0–10 × 106 WBCs/L** (0–10 cells/µL)
- Adult: **0–5 × 106 WBCs/L** (0–5 cells/µL)

WBC differential:

- Neutrophils: 0%–6%
- Lymphocytes: 40%–80%
- Monocytes: 15%–45%

Culture and sensitivity testing: no organisms present

Protein: **0.15–0.45 g/L of CSF** (15–45 mg/dL of CSF); up to **0.7 g/L** (70 mg/dL) in older adults and children

Protein electrophoresis

Prealbumin: 2%–7%

Albumin: 56%–76%

Alpha₁-globulin: 2%–7%

Alpha₂-globulin: 4%–12%

Beta-globulin: 8%–18%

Gamma-globulin: 3%–12%

Oligoclonal bands: none

Immunoglobulin G (IgG): **0–45 mg/L** (0.0–4.5 mg/dL)

Glucose: **2.8–4.2 mmol/L of CSF** (50–75 mg/dL of CSF) or 60%–70% of blood glucose level

Chloride: **116–122 mmol/L of CSF** (116–122 mEq/L of CSF)

Lactate dehydrogenase (LDH): <40 U/L for adults, <70 U/L for neonates
Lactic acid: **1.0–2.5 mmol/L of CSF** (10–25 mg/dL of CSF)
Cytologic findings: no malignant cells
Serologic finding for syphilis: negative
Glutamine: **0.4–1.2 mmol/L of CSF** (8–18 mg/dL of CSF)

INDICATIONS

This examination may assist in the diagnosis of primary or metastatic brain or spinal cord neoplasm, cerebral hemorrhage, meningitis, encephalitis, degenerative brain disease, autoimmune diseases involving the central nervous system, neurosyphilis, and demyelinating disorders (e.g., multiple sclerosis, acute demyelinating polyneuropathy).

TEST EXPLANATION

By placing a needle in the subarachnoid space of the spinal column (Figure 5-2), it is possible to measure the pressure of that space and obtain CSF for examination and diagnosis. Lumbar puncture may also be used to inject therapeutic or diagnostic agents and to administer spinal anaesthetics. Furthermore, lumbar puncture may be used to reduce intracranial pressure (ICP) in patients who have normal-pressure hydrocephalus with pseudotumour cerebri.

CSF is made by selective secretion from the plasma by the choroid plexus (a group of small blood vessels) in the ventricles of the brain. Three membranes surround the brain and spinal cord. From inner to outer, they are the pia mater, arachnoid, and dura mater. The CSF exists within the space between the pia mater and the arachnoid (the *subarachnoid space*). This fluid (~150 to 200 mL) bathes and protects the brain and spinal cord. The fluid acts as a shock absorber when head or back trauma occurs or when position suddenly changes. The CSF transports nutrients and clears metabolic wastes. Because the CSF is made from plasma, its constituents are approximately the same as plasma. Chloride levels are higher, however. Blood constituents of larger molecular size cannot be secreted by the choroid plexus (as a result of the blood-brain barrier).

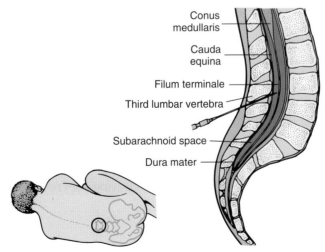

Conus medullaris
Cauda equina
Filum terminale
Third lumbar vertebra
Subarachnoid space
Dura mater

Figure 5-2 Patient position for a lumbar puncture.

Fluid Analysis Studies

5

Examination of the CSF includes evaluation for the presence of blood, bacteria, and malignant cells, as well as quantification of the amounts of glucose and protein present. Colour is noted, and various other tests, such as a serologic test for syphilis (p. 487), are performed.

On occasion, lumbar puncture is contraindicated because of nearby infection or suspected CSF blockage in the spinal canal.

Pressure

To measure the CSF pressure, a sterile manometer is attached to the needle used for lumbar puncture. The pressure exerted because of CSF, plus the total volume of the brain tissue and the total volume of the blood, is the ICP. To measure ICP, an external pressure transducer is attached to a catheter inserted into the lateral ventricle of the brain. The normal ICP ranges from 0 to 15 mm Hg. A pressure higher than 15 mm Hg is considered abnormal and indicative of increased ICP. Because the subarachnoid space surrounding the brain is connected to the subarachnoid space of the spinal cord, any increase in ICP is reflected directly as an increase at the lumbar site. Tumours, infection, hydrocephalus, and intracranial bleeding can cause increases in ICP and spinal pressure. If it is suspected that tumour or postinfection scarring obstructs this normal connection, a Queckenstedt-Stookey test is performed (see "Procedure and Patient Care" section) to document it. ICP is related to the volume of CSF fluid, which is determined by the homeostatic balance between production and resorption of CSF. Also, because the cranial venous sinuses are connected to the jugular veins, obstruction of those veins or of the superior vena cava increases ICP.

Decreased ICP is noted in hypovolemia (dehydration or shock). Chronic leakage of CSF through a previous lumbar puncture site, or through a nasal sinus fracture with a dura tear, is associated with reduced pressures.

Pressures are routinely measured at the beginning and the end of a lumbar puncture procedure. If these values differ significantly, a spinal cord obstruction (tumour) is suspected. In these instances, a small amount of CSF is present below the tumour. Removal of a large percentage of that fluid reduces the pressure drastically. Large differences in opening and closing pressures are also present in patients with hydrocephalus. If opening pressures are high, normal volumes of CSF should not be removed, to prevent the risk of cerebellar herniation. If, during the procedure, a child is crying and holding the breath, the pressure may elevate transiently and then reduce as the child relaxes.

Colour

Normal CSF is clear and colourless. The term *xanthochromia* (usually refers to a yellow tinge) is commonly used when the CSF is an abnormal colour. Colour differences can occur with hyperbilirubinemia, hypercarotenemia, melanoma, or elevated protein levels.

A cloudy appearance may indicate an increase in the WBC count or protein level. Normally, CSF contains no blood. A red tinge to the CSF indicates the presence of blood. Blood may be present because of bleeding into the subarachnoid space or because the needle used in the lumbar puncture has inadvertently penetrated a blood vessel on the way into the subarachnoid space. These causes of bleeding must be differentiated because it is important to identify and document subarachnoid bleeding (Table 5-1).

With a traumatic puncture, the blood within the CSF will clot. No clotting occurs with subarachnoid hemorrhage. Also, with a traumatic tap, the fluid clears toward the end of the procedure when successive CSF samples are obtained. This clearing does not occur with a subarachnoid hemorrhage.

Blood

Blood within the CSF indicates cerebral hemorrhage into the subarachnoid space or a traumatic puncture, as just described.

TABLE 5-1	Causes of Blood in the Cerebrospinal Fluid	
Characteristic	**Traumatic Puncture**	**Subarachnoid Bleeding**
CSF pressure	Low	High
Duration of bleeding	Decreases when CSF is withdrawn	No change in colour when CSF is withdrawn
Clotting	Present	Absent
Sample for repeat lumbar puncture	Not bloody	Bloody
Appearance after centrifugation	Clear fluid	Xanthochromia

CSF, Cerebrospinal fluid.

TABLE 5-2	Causes of Leukocytes in the Cerebrospinal Fluid	
Cell Type	**Infection**	**Other Diseases**
Neutrophils	Bacterial meningitis Tubercular meningitis Cerebral abscess	Subarachnoid bleeding Tumour
Lymphocytes or plasma cells	Viral, tubercular, fungal, syphilitic meningitis	Multiple sclerosis Guillain-Barré syndrome
Eosinophils	Parasitic meningitis	Allergic reaction to radiopaque dyes
Macrophages	Tubercular, fungal meningitis	Hemorrhage, brain infarction

Cells

The number of red blood cells (RBCs) is merely an indication of the amount of blood present within the CSF. Except for a few lymphocytes, the presence of WBCs in the CSF is abnormal (Table 5-2). The presence of polymorphonuclear leukocytes (neutrophils) is indicative of bacterial meningitis or cerebral abscess.

When mononuclear leukocytes are present, viral or tubercular meningitis or encephalitis is suspected. Leukemia or other primary or metastatic malignant tumours may cause elevations in WBC numbers. *Pleocytosis* is a term used to indicate turbidity of CSF because of an increased number of cells within the fluid. WBCs can be present in the CSF as a result of a traumatic puncture, in which the spinal needle hits a blood vessel while the spinal tap is being performed. However, the presence of more than 1 WBC per 500 RBCs is considered pathologic and can indicate infection such as meningitis.

Culture and Sensitivity

The organisms that cause meningitis or brain abscess can be cultured from the CSF. Other organisms that may be found include atypical bacteria, fungi, or *Mycobacterium tuberculosis*. A Gram stain (p. 733) of the CSF may yield preliminary information about the causative infectious agent. This may allow appropriate antibiotic therapy to be initiated before the 24 to 72 hours necessary to complete the culture and sensitivity report.

The most common causes of meningitis include *Haemophilus influenzae* (in children) and *Neisseria* or *Streptococcus* organisms (in adults).

Fluid Analysis Studies

5

Protein

Normally, very little protein is found in CSF because protein is a large molecule that does not cross the blood-brain barrier. The proportion of albumin to globulin is normally higher in CSF than in blood plasma (p. 440) because albumin is smaller than globulin and therefore can pass more easily through the blood-brain barrier. The amount of protein is usually lower in CSF obtained from the cisternal puncture, and even lower still with a ventricular puncture, than in the CSF obtained from a lumbar puncture. Disease processes, however, can alter the permeability of the blood-brain barrier, allowing protein to leak into the CSF. Examples of diseases that may be associated with a more permeable blood-brain barrier include infectious or inflammatory processes such as meningitis, encephalitis, or myelitis. Furthermore, tumours of the central nervous system (CNS) may produce and secrete protein into the CSF. Obstruction of CSF flow in the spinal canal caused by tumours or a herniated disc is also associated with high protein counts because normal CSF circulation and resorption are impaired by the obstruction.

CSF protein electrophoresis is very important in the diagnosis of CNS diseases. In patients with multiple sclerosis, neurosyphilis, or other immunogenic degenerative CNS disease, immunoglobulin levels in the CSF are elevated. Normally, less than 12% of the total protein consists of gamma-globulin. An increase in the CSF level of immunoglobulin G (IgG), an increase in the ratio of IgG to other proteins (e.g., albumin), and the detection of oligoclonal gamma-globulin bands are highly suggestive of inflammatory and autoimmune diseases of the CNS, especially multiple sclerosis. Levels of myelin basic protein, a component of myelin (the substance that surrounds normal nerve tissue), can be elevated when demyelinating diseases (such as multiple sclerosis or amyotrophic lateral sclerosis) occur. This protein, detected by radioimmunoassay of the CSF, can be monitored to assess the course of these deteriorating diseases.

Because albumin and prealbumin are not made in the CNS, increased levels of these specific proteins indicate increased permeability of the blood-brain barrier (as discussed previously).

Glucose

The glucose level is decreased when bacteria, inflammatory cells, or tumour cells are present. A blood sample for glucose (p. 269) is usually collected before the spinal tap is performed. A CSF glucose level less than 60% of the blood glucose level may indicate meningitis or neoplasm.

Chloride

The chloride concentration in CSF may be decreased in patients with meningeal infections, tubercular meningitis, and conditions of low blood chloride levels. An increase in the chloride level in CSF is not significant neurologically; it correlates with the blood levels of chloride (p. 167). CSF is not routinely evaluated for chloride; this test is done only if specifically requested.

Lactate Dehydrogenase

Quantification of lactate dehydrogenase (LDH)—specifically, fractions 4 and 5 (p. 339)—is helpful in diagnosing bacterial meningitis. The source of LDH is the neutrophils that fight the invading bacteria. When the LDH level is elevated, infection or inflammation is suspected. The elevated WBC count associated with CNS leukemia is also associated with elevated LDH levels. The nerve tissue in the CNS is also high in LDH (isoenzymes 1 and 2). Therefore, disease directly affecting the brain or spinal cord (e.g., stroke) is associated with elevated LDH levels.

Lactic Acid

Elevated levels indicate anaerobic metabolism associated with decreased oxygenation of the brain. The lactic acid level in CSF is increased in both bacterial and fungal meningitis but not in viral meningitis. The lactic acid level is also increased when the glucose level in CSF is very low or the WBC count in CSF is elevated. Because lactic acid does not readily pass through the blood-brain barrier, elevated blood lactate levels are not reflected in the CSF. Chronic cerebral hypoxemia or cerebral ischemia (hypoxic encephalopathy) is associated with elevated lactic acid levels in CSF. Lactic acid levels can also be increased in patients with some forms of mitochondrial diseases that affect the CNS.

Cytologic Study

Examination of cells found in the CSF can help determine whether they are malignant. Tumours in the CNS may shed cells from their surface. These cells can float freely in CSF. Their presence suggests neoplasm as the cause of any neurologic symptoms.

Tumour Markers

Increased levels of tumour markers such as carcinoembryonic antigen, alpha-fetoprotein, or human chorionic gonadotropin may indicate metastatic tumour.

Serologic Study for Syphilis

Latent syphilis is diagnosed by performing one of many available serologic tests on CSF. These include the following:
- The Wassermann test
- The Venereal Disease Research Laboratory (VDRL) test (p. 487)
- The fluorescent treponemal antibody test (p. 487): This test is considered to be the most sensitive and specific. When test results are positive, the diagnosis of neurosyphilis is established, and appropriate antibiotic therapy is initiated.

Glutamine

The CSF can be evaluated for the presence of glutamine. Elevated glutamine levels are helpful in the detection and evaluation of hepatic encephalopathy and hepatic coma. The glutamine is made by increased levels of ammonia, which are commonly associated with liver failure. (See discussion of serum ammonia on p. 65.) Levels of glutamine are also often increased in patients with Reye syndrome.

C-Reactive Protein

As noted on p. 199, C-reactive protein (CRP) is a nonspecific, acute-phase reactant present in bacterial infections and inflammatory disorders. Elevated CSF levels of CRP have been useful in the diagnosis of bacterial meningitis. Failure to find elevated CSF levels of CRP appears to be strong evidence against bacterial meningitis. Some research studies have shown that CSF levels of CRP have been valuable in distinguishing bacterial meningitis from viral meningitis, tuberculosis meningitis, febrile convulsions, and other central nervous system disorders. Serum levels of CRP (see p. 199) are more frequently studied for the diagnosis of bacterial meningitis.

Lumbar puncture is performed by a physician in approximately 20 minutes. This procedure is described as uncomfortable or painful by most patients. Some patients complain of feeling pressure from the needle. Some patients complain of a shooting pain in their legs.

CONTRAINDICATIONS

- Increased ICP, because the lumbar puncture may induce cerebral or cerebellar herniation through the foramen magnum
- Severe degenerative vertebral joint disease, because it is very difficult to pass the needle through the degenerated arthritic interspinal space

Fluid Analysis Studies

5

- Infection near the lumbar puncture site, because meningitis can result from contamination of CSF with infected material
- Anticoagulation drug regimen, because of the risk for epidural hematoma

POTENTIAL COMPLICATIONS

- Persistent CSF leak, causing severe headache
- Introduction of bacteria into CSF, causing suppurative meningitis
- Herniation of the brain through the tentorium cerebelli or herniation of the cerebellum through the foramen magnum: In patients with increased ICP, the quick reduction of pressure in the spinal column by release through the lumbar puncture may induce herniation of the brain. This can cause compression of the brain stem, which may result in deterioration of neurologic status and in death. In adults, especially, most clinicians obtain a computed tomographic scan of the head before performing lumbar puncture, so as to identify intracranial abnormalities and thus avoid the risk of brain herniation.
- Inadvertent puncture of the spinal cord, caused by inappropriately high puncture of the spinal canal
- Puncture of the aorta or vena cava, causing serious retroperitoneal hemorrhage
- Transient back pain and pain or paraesthesia in the legs
- Transient postural headache (worse when standing)

PROCEDURE AND PATIENT CARE

Before

- Explain the procedure to the patient. Many patients have misconceptions regarding lumbar puncture. Allow the patient to verbalize concerns, and allay any fears.
- Obtain the patient's informed consent if it is required by the institution.
- Perform a baseline neurologic assessment of the legs by assessing the patient's strength, sensation, and movement.
- Inform the patient that no fasting or sedation is required.
- Instruct the patient to empty the bladder and bowels before the procedure.
- Explain to the patient that he or she must lie very still throughout this procedure. Movement may cause traumatic injury. Encourage the patient to relax and take deep, slow breaths with the mouth open.

Clinical Priorities

- Lumbar puncture is contraindicated in patients with increased ICP because the lumbar puncture may induce cerebral or cerebellar herniation.
- A basic neurologic assessment should be done before this test, especially to evaluate the patient's legs for strength, sensation, and movement.
- If a blockage in CSF circulation is suspected in the subarachnoid space, a Queckenstedt-Stookey test (described in the next section) may be performed.

During

- Note the following procedural steps:
  1. This study is a sterile procedure that can be easily performed at the patient's bedside. The patient is usually placed in the lateral decubitus (fetal) position (see Figure 5-2).
  2. The patient is instructed to clasp the hands on the knees to maintain this position. Someone usually helps the patient maintain this position. (A sitting position also may be used.)
  3. A local anaesthetic is injected into the skin and subcutaneous tissues after the site has been aseptically cleaned.
  4. A spinal needle containing an inner obturator is placed through the skin and into the spinal canal.
  5. The subarachnoid space is entered.
  6. The insert (obturator) is removed, and CSF can be seen slowly dripping from the needle.
  7. The needle is attached to a sterile manometer, and the pressure (opening pressure) is recorded.
  8. Before the pressure reading is taken, the patient is asked to relax and straighten the legs to reduce the intra-abdominal pressure, which causes an increase in CSF pressure.
  9. Three sterile test tubes are filled with 5 to 10 mL of CSF. Usually the first tube is sent for chemical and immunologic testing because these results are not affected by any blood if a traumatic puncture occurs. The second may be sent for culture, and the third is used for microscopic examination.
  10. The pressure (closing pressure) is measured.
- Note that if blockage in CSF circulation in the spinal subarachnoid space is suspected, a *Queckenstedt-Stookey test* may be performed. For this test, the jugular vein is occluded either manually by digital pressure or by a medium-sized blood pressure cuff inflated to approximately 20 mm Hg. Within 10 seconds after jugular occlusion, CSF pressure should increase 15 to 40 mm Hg; within 10 seconds after release, the pressure should promptly return to normal. A sluggish rise or fall of CSF pressure is suggestive of partial blockage of CSF circulation. No rise after 10 seconds is suggestive of complete obstruction within the spinal canal.

After

- Apply digital pressure and an adhesive dressing to the puncture site.
- Place the patient in the prone position with a pillow under the abdomen to increase the intra-abdominal pressure, which will indirectly increase the pressure in the tissues surrounding the spinal cord. This retards continued CSF flow from the spinal canal.
- All testing of the CSF is ordered stat to diminish the false results that may occur (e.g., because of cellular deterioration).
- Encourage the patient to drink increased amounts of fluid with a straw to replace the CSF removed during the lumbar puncture. Drinking with a straw will enable the patient to keep the head flat.
- Usually keep the patient in a reclining position for up to 12 hours to avoid the discomfort of potential postpuncture spinal headache. Allow the patient to turn from side to side as long as the head is not raised.
- Label and number the specimen jars appropriately and deliver them to the laboratory immediately after the test. Refrigeration will alter test results. A delay between collection time and testing can invalidate results especially cell counts.
- Assess the patient for numbness, tingling, and decreased movement of the extremities; pain at the injection site; drainage of blood or CSF at the injection site; and the ability to void. Notify the physician of any unusual findings.

- The patient should be kept flat in bed for up to 12 hours to avoid a postprocedure spinal headache.
- Encourage the patient to drink increased amounts of fluid to replace CSF removed during the lumbar puncture.
- Instruct the patient to report any abnormalities, such as numbness and tingling in the legs, to the physician.

TEST RESULTS AND CLINICAL SIGNIFICANCE

Brain neoplasm,
Spinal cord neoplasm,
Metastatic tumour: *The CSF can be expected to be turbid, to contain malignant cells, and to have elevated protein and LDH levels.*
Degenerative brain disease,
Autoimmune disorder,
Multiple sclerosis and other demyelinating diseases: *The CSF of these patients may be turbid; it may contain increased protein levels (including myelin basic protein) and oligoclonal bands of proteins; and it may be associated with elevated LDH levels.*
Neurosyphilis: *Not only do affected patients have elevated protein levels, increased turbidity, and increased LDH levels in their CSF, but immunologic test results are also positive.*
Subarachnoid bleeding,
Cerebral hemorrhage,
Traumatic lumbar puncture: *The CSF in these patients has high protein levels, is turbid, has xanthochromia, and contains RBCs.*
Encephalitis,
Myelitis,
Hepatic encephalopathy or coma: *Elevated glutamine levels are noted in affected patients.*
Meningitis,
Encephalitis,
Cerebral abscess: *Elevated WBC and protein levels support the culture findings of infection.*

RELATED TESTS

Glucose, Blood (p. 269). This test is concomitantly performed with the lumbar puncture to assess the CSF glucose level in comparison with the blood glucose level.

Protein Electrophoresis (p. 440). Along with the lumbar puncture, measurement of serum protein levels is helpful in the calculation of many formulas involved in the evaluation of CSF.

Amyloid Beta Protein Precursor, Soluble (p. 666). This test is performed on CSF to diagnose Alzheimer's disease.

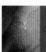

Paracentesis (Peritoneal Fluid Analysis, Abdominal Paracentesis, Ascitic Fluid Cytologic Study, Peritoneal Tap)

NORMAL FINDINGS

Gross appearance: clear, serous, light yellow
Red blood cells (RBCs): none

White blood cells (WBCs): **<100 × 10^9/L** (<100/mm^3)
Protein: **<41 g/L** (<4.1 g/dL)
Glucose: **3.3–6.1 mmol/L** (60–110 mg/dL)
Amylase: 138–404 U/L
Ammonia: <50 *Mcg*/dL
Alkaline phosphatase
Adult male: 90–240 U/L
Female <45 years: 76–196 U/L
Female >45 years: 87–250 U/L
Lactate dehydrogenase (LDH): similar to serum LDH
Cytologic findings: no malignant cells
Bacteria: none
Fungi: none
Carcinoembryonic antigen (CEA): **<5 *Mcg*/L** (<5 ng/mL)

INDICATIONS

Paracentesis is performed to determine the cause of unexplained ascites. It is an important part of evaluating the patient with multiple trauma to confirm or rule out abdominal trauma. Paracentesis is also performed to relieve the intra-abdominal pressure that accumulates with large-volume ascites.

TEST EXPLANATION

Paracentesis is an invasive procedure entailing the insertion of a needle into the peritoneal cavity to remove ascitic fluid. The peritoneum is defined as the space between the visceral peritoneum (thin membrane covering all the abdominal organs) and the parietal peritoneum (thin membrane covering the inside of the abdominal wall). Within the peritoneal membrane is an intricate network of capillary and lymphatic vessels. Fluid is constantly being secreted by the peritoneal membranes and constantly being reabsorbed by those same membranes. If secretion is increased or reabsorption blocked, buildup of peritoneal fluid (ascites) develops.

Paracentesis is performed in less than 30 minutes by a physician at the patient's bedside, in a procedure room, or in the physician's office. Usually the volume removed is limited to approximately 4 L at any one time to avoid hypovolemia if the fluid is rapidly reaccumulated. Although local anaesthetics eliminate pain at the insertion site, the patient may feel a pressure-like pain as the needle is inserted.

Peritoneal fluid is removed for diagnostic and therapeutic purposes. For diagnostic purposes, paracentesis is performed to obtain and analyze fluid to determine the cause of the peritoneal effusion. Peritoneal fluid is classified as transudate or exudate (Table 5-3). This is an important differentiation and is very helpful in determining the cause of the effusion. Transudates are most frequently caused by heart failure, cirrhosis, nephrotic syndrome, myxedema, peritoneal dialysis, hypoproteinemia, and acute glomerulonephritis. Exudates are most often found in infectious or neoplastic conditions. However, collagen-vascular disease, pulmonary infarction, gastrointestinal diseases, trauma, and drug hypersensitivity also may cause an exudative effusion.

For therapeutic purposes, this procedure is performed to remove large amounts of ascitic fluid from the abdominal cavity. Affected patients usually experience transient relief of symptoms (shortness of breath, distension, and early satiety) because of the fluid within the abdominal cavity.

TABLE 5-3	Differentiation Between Transudate and Exudate	
Characteristic	**Transudate**	**Exudate**
Total protein fluid/serum ratio	<0.5	>0.5
Total protein level	**<30 g/L** (<3 g/dL)	**>30 g/L** (>3 g/dL)
LDH fluid/serum ratio	<0.6	>0.6
Albumin gradient	<1.1	>1.1
Serum − Fluid = Albumin gradient		
Specific gravity	>1.015	>1.015
Clotting	None	Present
WBC count	<100 × 10⁹/L	>1 000 × 10⁹/L
Differential	Mononuclear	Neutrophils
Glucose level	Equal to that of serum	**<3.3 mmol/L** (<60 mg/dL)
Serum glucose − Cerebrospinal fluid glucose = Glucose difference	**<1.7 mmol/L** (<30 mg/dL)	**>1.7 mmol/L** (>30 mg/dL)
Appearance	Clear, thin fluid	Cloudy, viscous
Cause	Cirrhosis, nephrosis, heart failure, low protein level	Infection, inflammation, malignancy, collagen-vascular diseases

LDH, Lactate dehydrogenase; *WBC,* white blood cell.

The peritoneal fluid is usually evaluated for gross appearance; for levels of RBCs, WBCs, protein, glucose, amylase, ammonia, alkaline phosphatase, and LDH; for cytologic study; for bacteria and fungi; and for other entities such as CEA levels. Each is discussed separately as follows. Urea and creatinine levels may be measured if there is a possibility that the fluid may represent urine from a perforated bladder.

Gross Appearance

Transudative peritoneal fluid may be clear, serous, or light yellow, especially in patients with hepatic cirrhosis. Milk-coloured peritoneal fluid may result from the escape of chyle from blocked abdominal or thoracic lymphatic ducts. Conditions that may cause lymphatic blockage include lymphoma, carcinoma, and tuberculosis involving the abdominal or thoracic lymph nodes. The triglyceride value in a chylous effusion exceeds **1.24 mmol/L** (>110 mg/dL).

Cloudy or turbid fluid may result from inflammatory or infectious conditions such as peritonitis, pancreatitis, and appendicitis. Blood in the fluid may be the result of a traumatic puncture (the aspirating needle penetrates a blood vessel), intra-abdominal bleeding, tumour, or hemorrhagic pancreatitis. The fluid may be bile-stained and green as a result of a ruptured gallbladder, acute pancreatitis, or perforated intestines.

Cell Counts

Normally, no RBCs are present. The presence of RBCs may indicate neoplasms, tuberculosis, or intra-abdominal bleeding. WBC counts may be increased with peritonitis, cirrhosis, and tuberculosis.

Protein Count

Total protein levels greater than **30 g/L** (>3 g/dL) are characteristic of exudates, whereas transudates usually have a protein content of less than **30 g/L** (<3 g/dL). It is now thought that the albumin gradient between serum and ascitic fluid can differentiate better between the transudate and exudate nature of ascites than can the total protein content. This gradient is obtained by subtracting the ascitic albumin value from the serum albumin value. Values of **11 g/L** ($\geq$1.1 g/dL) or greater are suggestive of a transudate, which is usually caused by portal hypertension due to cirrhosis. Values less than **11 g/L** (<1.1 g/dL) are suggestive of an exudate but do not specify the potential cause of the exudate (malignancy from infection or inflammation).

Because protein values that differentiate transudate from exudate overlap significantly, the total protein ratio (fluid/serum) has been considered to be a more accurate criterion. A fluid/serum total protein ratio higher than 0.5 is considered to indicate an exudate.

Glucose

Usually peritoneal glucose levels approximate serum glucose levels. Decreased levels may indicate tuberculous or bacterial peritonitis or peritoneal carcinomatosis.

Amylase

Amylase levels may be increased in patients with pancreatic trauma, pancreatic pseudocyst, acute pancreatitis, and intestinal necrosis, pancreatic perforation, or pancreatic strangulation. In these diseases, the fluid amylase level is usually less than 1.5 times higher than serum levels.

Ammonia

Ammonia levels are high with ruptured or strangulated intestines and also with a ruptured appendix or ulcer.

Alkaline Phosphatase

Levels of alkaline phosphatase are greatly increased with infarcted or strangulated intestines.

Lactate Dehydrogenase

A peritoneal fluid/serum LDH ratio higher than 0.6 is typical of an exudate. An exudate is identified with a higher degree of accuracy if the peritoneal fluid/serum protein ratio is greater than 0.5 and the peritoneal fluid/serum LDH ratio is greater than 0.6.

Cytologic Findings

A cytologic study is performed to detect tumours. The tumours most often observed are ovarian, pancreatic, colon, and gastric. To interpret cytologic changes, the pathologist must have considerable experience in cytology. It can be difficult to differentiate malignancy from severely inflammatory mesothelial cells. In general, malignant cells tend to clump together and to have a high nucleus/cytoplasm ratio, prominent and multiple nucleoli, and unevenly distributed chromatin.

Cytologic examination of the fluid is improved by centrifugation of a large volume of fluid and examination of the sediment. A large number of cells can be seen and compared with each other.

Bacteria

Usually the fluid is cultured and the antibiotic sensitivities are determined. Gram stains (p. 733) are often performed.

Gram Stain and Bacteriologic Culture

The presence of bacteria may indicate a ruptured intestine, primary peritonitis, or infections such as appendicitis, pancreatitis, or tuberculosis. Culture and Gram stains help identify the

Fluid Analysis Studies

5

organisms involved in the infection and also provide information concerning antibiotic sensitivity. (See p. 733 for a more thorough discussion of Gram stains, cultures, and sensitivity testing.) These tests are routinely performed to diagnose bacterial peritonitis. If possible, these tests should be performed before initiation of antibiotic therapy.

Fungi

Fungi that are present may include *Histoplasma, Candida,* or *Coccidioides* species.

Carcinoembryonic Antigen

Elevated peritoneal fluid levels for CEA are associated with abdominal malignancy, usually arising from the gastrointestinal tract.

CONTRAINDICATIONS

- Coagulation abnormalities or bleeding tendencies
- The presence of only a small amount of fluid and a history of extensive previous abdominal surgery

POTENTIAL COMPLICATIONS

- Hypovolemia if a large volume of peritoneal fluid was removed and the fluid reaccumulates, with the fluid coming from the intravascular volume
- Hepatic coma in a patient with chronic liver disease
- Peritonitis
- Seeding of the needle tract with tumour cells when malignant ascites is present

Clinical Priorities

- The classification of peritoneal fluid as either a transudate or an exudate helps differentiate the cause of the effusion.
- Usually the volume of peritoneal fluid removed is limited to 4 L to avoid hypovolemia in case the fluid rapidly reaccumulates.
- The patient should empty the bladder before this test to avoid inadvertent puncture by the aspirating needle during the procedure.
- After this test, the patient should be frequently monitored for hemodynamic changes, especially hypotension, if a large volume of fluid was removed.

PROCEDURE AND PATIENT CARE

Before

 Explain the procedure to the patient.
- Obtain the patient's informed consent for this procedure.

 Inform the patient that no fasting or sedation is necessary.

 Instruct the patient to urinate or empty the bladder before the test to avoid inadvertent puncture of the bladder with the aspirating needle.
- Measure the patient's abdominal girth.
- Measure the patient's weight.
- Measure baseline vital signs.

During

- Paracentesis is performed under strict sterile technique. A paracentesis tray usually contains all necessary supplies.
- Note the following procedural steps:
  1. The patient is positioned in a high Fowler position in bed.
  2. The needle insertion site is aseptically cleansed and anaesthetized locally.
  3. A scalpel may be used to make a stab wound into the peritoneal cavity approximately 1 to 5 cm below the umbilicus.
  4. A trocar, cannula, or needle is threaded through the incision.
  5. A piece of plastic tubing is attached to the cannula. The other end of the tubing is placed in the collection receptacle (usually a container with a pressurized vacuum).

After

- Place a small bandage over the needle site.
- On occasion, ascitic fluid continues to leak out of the puncture site after removal of the needle. A suture can stop that leakage. If this is unsuccessful, a collection bag should be applied to the skin to allow for measurement of the volume of fluid loss.
- Label the specimen with the patient's name, date, source of fluid, and diagnosis.
- For all tests performed on peritoneal fluid, the fluid should be analyzed immediately to avoid false results related to chemical or cellular deterioration. Send the specimen to the laboratory promptly.
- Observe the puncture site for bleeding, continued drainage, or signs of inflammation.
- Measure the abdominal girth and weight of the patient; compare measurements with baseline values.
- Monitor vital signs frequently for evidence of hemodynamic changes. Watch for signs of hypotension if a large volume of fluid was removed.
- On the laboratory requisition slip, note whether the patient has received any recent antibiotic therapy.
- Because of the high protein content of ascitic fluid, albumin infusions may be ordered after paracentesis to compensate for protein loss. Monitor serum protein and electrolyte (especially sodium) levels.

TEST RESULTS AND CLINICAL SIGNIFICANCE

Exudate,

Lymphoma: *These tumours can involve the lymph nodes of the chest and abdomen. Fluid cannot be reabsorbed, and chylous effusion develops.*

Carcinoma: *When cancer involves the peritoneal membranes, reabsorption of fluid is diminished. Furthermore, the tumours (especially ovarian) can secrete large volumes of fluid. Ascites develops.*

Tuberculosis,

Peritonitis,

Pancreatitis,

Ruptured viscus:

Infections tend to increase peritoneal capillary permeability, and fluid is secreted into the abdominal cavity.

Transudate

Hepatic cirrhosis,

Portal hypertension: *The capillary vessels experience an increased portal venous drainage pressure. Reabsorption is diminished, and fluid accumulates.*

Nephrotic syndrome,

Hypoproteinemia: *The nephrotic syndrome is characterized by renal albumin wasting. This and other forms of hypoproteinemia are associated with decreased intravascular oncotic pressure. The fluid tends to leak out of the intravascular space into the peritoneum.*

Heart failure: *The venous drainage of peritoneum is diminished by right-sided heart failure and causes increased venous pressures. Peritoneal fluid accumulates.*

Abdominal trauma,

Peritoneal bleeding: *Intra-abdominal bleeding or ruptured viscus can be determined by means of identifying a bloody effusion (hemoperitoneum) or aspirating bowel contents from the free abdominal cavity.*

RELATED TESTS

Glucose, Blood (p. 269), Lactate Dehydrogenase (p. 339), Protein Electrophoresis (p. 440), and Amylase, Blood (p. 67). These blood tests are performed concomitantly to assist in the evaluation of the peritoneal fluid.

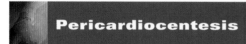

Pericardiocentesis

NORMAL FINDINGS

<50 mL of clear, straw-coloured fluid with no evidence of any bacteria, blood, or malignant cells

INDICATIONS

Pericardiocentesis is performed to determine the cause of an unexplained pericardial effusion. It is also performed to relieve the intrapericardial pressure that accumulates with a large volume of fluid and inhibits diastolic filling.

TEST EXPLANATION

Pericardiocentesis, which involves the aspiration of fluid from the pericardial sac with a needle, may be performed for therapeutic and diagnostic purposes. For therapeutic purposes, the test is performed to relieve cardiac tamponade by removing blood or fluid to improve diastolic filling. For diagnostic purposes, pericardiocentesis is performed to remove a sample of pericardial fluid for laboratory examination to determine the cause of the fluid accumulation. This is similar to the evaluation described for pleural fluid on p. 705.

A physician usually performs this procedure in approximately 10 to 20 minutes in the cardiac catheterization laboratory, operating room, or emergency room. This procedure is associated with very little discomfort. Most patients feel pressure when the needle is inserted into the pericardial sac.

CONTRAINDICATIONS

- Patients' inability to cooperate, because of the risk of lacerations to the epicardium or coronary artery
- A bleeding disorder, because inadvertent puncture of the myocardium may create uncontrollable bleeding into the pericardial sac, leading to tamponade

POTENTIAL COMPLICATIONS

- Laceration of the coronary artery or myocardium
- Needle-induced ventricular arrhythmias (dysrhythmias)
- Myocardial infarction
- Pneumothorax caused by inadvertent puncture of the lung
- Liver laceration caused by inadvertent puncture of that organ
- Pleural or pericardial infection caused by the aspirating needle
- Vasovagal hypotension or arrest

Clinical Priorities

- For therapeutic purposes, this test can be performed to relieve cardiac tamponade by removing blood or fluid to improve diastolic filling. For diagnostic purposes, it is performed to determine the cause of a fluid accumulation.
- Atropine may be given before the procedure to prevent the vasovagal reflex of bradycardia and hypotension.
- After this test, the vital signs are carefully monitored. Pericardial bleeding may be indicated by hypotension and pulsus paradoxus. Temperature elevations may indicate infection.

PROCEDURE AND PATIENT CARE

Before

 Explain the procedure to the patient.
- Obtain the patient's informed consent for this procedure.
- Restrict fluid and food intake for at least 4 to 6 hours (if this is an elective procedure).
- Obtain intravenous access for infusion of fluids and cardiac medications if they are required.
- Administer pretest medication. Atropine is frequently given to prevent the vasovagal reflex of bradycardia and hypotension.

During

- Note the following procedural steps:
  1. The patient is placed in the supine position.
  2. An area in the fifth to sixth intercostal space at the left sternal margin (or subxyphoid space) is prepared and draped. Alternatively, the subxyphoid space is used for access to the pericardium.
  3. After a local anaesthetic is administered, a pericardiocentesis needle is placed on a 50-mL syringe and introduced into the pericardial sac (Figure 5-3).
  4. An electrocardiographic lead is often attached by a clip to the needle to identify any ST segment elevations, which may indicate penetration into the epicardium. Echocardiography may be used to help guide the needle.
  5. Pericardial fluid is aspirated and placed in multiple specimen containers.
  6. Some patients who have recurring cardiac tamponade may require placement of an indwelling pericardial catheter for continuous draining for 1 to 3 days. On occasion, a surgical pericardial window (excision of a small portion of the pericardium) is necessary to prevent recurrent effusions.
  7. With certain types of pericarditis, medications (e.g., antibiotics, antineoplastic drugs, corticosteroids) may be instilled during pericardiocentesis to diminish the risk of recurrent effusions.

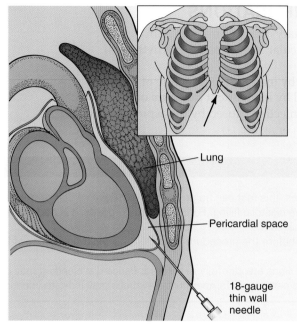

Lung

Pericardial space

18-gauge
thin wall
needle

Figure 5-3 Illustration of pericardiocentesis in which the subxyphoid route is used for aspiration of pericardial fluid. The 18-gauge needle is introduced at 30- to 40-degree angle.

After

- Closely monitor the patient's vital signs. An increase in temperature may indicate infection. Hypotension or pulsus paradoxus (abnormal decrease in systolic blood pressure during inspiration) is an indicator of pericardial bleeding.
- Label and number the specimen tubes that contain the pericardial fluid and deliver them to the appropriate laboratories for examination:
  1. Usually the fluid is taken to the chemistry laboratory, where the colour and turbidity are noted and the glucose, albumin, protein, and lactate dehydrogenase levels are measured. (See the discussion of thoracentesis on p. 705.)
  2. A tube of blood often goes to the hematology laboratory, where the quantities of red and white blood cells are recorded. (See the discussion of thoracentesis on p. 705.)
  3. The bacteriology laboratory performs routine cultures, Gram stains, fungal studies, acid-fast bacilli smears, and cultures.
  4. When malignancy is suspected, the fluid should be sent for cytologic examination.
- All tests performed on pericardial fluid should be performed immediately to avoid false results caused by chemical or cellular deterioration.
- Apply a sterile dressing to the catheter if one has been left for continuing pericardial drainage.
- Establish a closed system if continued pericardial drainage is required. This is usually performed by means of the straight drainage method.
- To minimize infection, pericardial catheters, if used, are usually removed after 2 days, although there are exceptions (e.g., to relieve cardiac tamponade). After the sutures are cut and the catheter is removed, apply a sterile dressing to the puncture site.

Home Care Responsibilities

- Instruct the patient to check the dressing frequently for drainage.
- Instruct the patient to report an increase in temperature, which may indicate infection.
- Instruct the patient to report any symptoms of hypotension, such as lightheadedness, fatigue, shortness of breath, or chest pain. Hypotension may be a sign of pericardial bleeding.

TEST RESULTS AND CLINICAL SIGNIFICANCE

Pericarditis: *Pericarditis can occur as a sequela to myocardial infarction; myocarditis; viral, bacterial, or tuberculous infections; or collagen-vascular diseases. The fluid is usually an exudate. (See the discussion of thoracentesis on p. 705.)*

Nephrotic syndrome: *The nephrotic syndrome is characterized by renal albumin wasting. This and other forms of hypoproteinemia are associated with decreased intravascular oncotic pressure. The fluid tends to leak out of the intravascular space into the peritoneum. This fluid is usually a transudate.*

Heart failure: *Normally, a small amount of fluid is present within the pericardial space. Fluid is constantly secreted and reabsorbed by the pericardium. If venous pressure of the pericardium is increased as a result of passive congestion of the pericardium associated with heart failure, fluid accumulates.*

Metastatic cancer: *Neoplasms affecting the pericardium primarily (mesothelioma) or secondarily (breast, lung, ovarian, lymphoma) secrete excess volume of fluid into the pleural space. This fluid is an exudate.*

Blunt or penetrating cardiac trauma,

Rupture of ventricular aneurysm: *These events cause sudden accumulation of blood within the closed pericardial space. As a result, diastolic filling is diminished, and cardiac output diminishes. The patient will die if immediate treatment is not given.*

Collagen-vascular disease: *In these autoimmune diseases, an inflammatory pericardial effusion can develop. Usually the effusion develops slowly, allowing enough time for anatomic and functional compensatory changes. Sometimes, however, the effusion is acute enough or large enough to necessitate pericardiocentesis.*

RELATED TESTS

Glucose, Blood (p. 269), Lactate Dehydrogenase (p. 339), Protein Electrophoresis (p. 440), and Amylase, Blood (p. 67). These blood tests are performed concomitantly to assist in the evaluation of the peritoneal fluid.

Chest Radiography (p. 1053). This is an important part of identifying a pericardial effusion. Furthermore, a chest radiograph should be routinely obtained on completion of pericardiocentesis to ensure that a pneumothorax has not iatrogenically occurred.

Electrocardiography (p. 568). This test is performed simultaneously with pericardiocentesis to indicate location of the aspirating needle.

Computed Tomography, Chest (p. 1068). This test can accurately assess the volume of fluid in the pericardium.

Secretin-Pancreozymin (Pancreatic Enzymes)

NORMAL FINDINGS

Volume: 2–4 mL/kg body weight
HCO_3^- (bicarbonate): **<80 mmol/L** (<80 mEq/L)
Amylase: 6.6–35.2 IU/kg

INDICATIONS

This is a corroborative test used in the evaluation of cystic fibrosis. This test is indicated in children with recurrent respiratory tract infections, malabsorption syndromes, or failure to thrive.

TEST EXPLANATION

Cystic fibrosis is an inherited disease characterized by abnormal secretion by exocrine glands within the bronchi, small intestines, pancreatic ducts, bile ducts, and skin (sweat glands). Because of this abnormal exocrine secretion, children with cystic fibrosis develop mucus plugs that obstruct their pancreatic ducts. The pancreatic enzymes (e.g., amylase, lipase, trypsin, chymotrypsin) cannot be expelled into the duodenum and therefore are either completely absent or present only in diminished quantities within the duodenal aspirate. For the same reasons, bicarbonate and other neutralizing fluids cannot be secreted from the pancreas. In the secretin-pancreozymin test, secretin and pancreozymin are used to stimulate pancreatic secretion of these enzymes and bicarbonate into the duodenum. The duodenal contents are then aspirated and examined for pH, bicarbonate, and enzyme levels; amylase is the most frequently measured enzyme. Diminished values are suggestive of cystic fibrosis.

A physician performs this test in approximately 2 hours in the laboratory or at the patient's bedside. Discomfort and gagging may occur during placement of the Dreiling tube.

PROCEDURE AND PATIENT CARE

Before

- Explain the procedure to the patient or parents, or both.
- Instruct the adult patient to fast for 12 hours before testing.
- Determine pediatric fasting times according to the patient's age.

During

- Note the following procedural steps:
    1. With the use of fluoroscopy, a Dreiling tube is passed through the patient's nose and into the stomach.
    2. The distal lumen of the tube is placed within the duodenum.
    3. The proximal lumen of the tube is placed within the stomach.
    4. Both lumens are aspirated. The gastric lumen is continually aspirated to avoid contamination of the gastric contents in the duodenum aspirate.
    5. A control specimen of the duodenal juices is collected for 20 minutes.
    6. The patient is tested for sensitivity to secretin and pancreozymin by low-dose intradermal injection.
    7. If no sensitivity is present, these hormones are administered intravenously. Secretin can be expected to stimulate pancreatic water and bicarbonate secretion. Pancreozymin can be expected to stimulate pancreatic enzyme (lipase, amylase, trypsin, chymotrypsin) secretion.
    8. Four duodenal aspirates are collected at 20-minute intervals and placed in four separate specimen containers.
    9. Each specimen is analyzed for pH, volume, bicarbonate, and amylase levels.

After

- Place the aspirated specimens in a container of water and crushed ice. Send them to the chemistry laboratory as soon as the test is completed.

- Remove the Dreiling tube after completion of the test. Give the patient appropriate nose and mouth care.
- 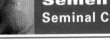 Allow the patient to resume a normal diet.

TEST RESULTS AND CLINICAL SIGNIFICANCE

Cystic fibrosis: *Affected patients do not have adequate levels of exocrinic pancreatic enzymes or bicarbonates because of mucus plugging of the small pancreatic duct tributaries.*

Celiac disease: *The pathophysiologic mechanism underlying this observation is not definitely known. It is thought that in patients with celiac disease, the intestinal mucosa is damaged. As a result, they do not have a normal stimulatory response to secrete secretin and pancreozymin. Therefore, the pancreas is chronically understimulated. When these hormones are administered, the pancreas can respond to a slight degree, but not as much as normal because of the previous prolonged periods of absence of stimulation.*

RELATED TESTS

Sweat Electrolytes (p. 702). This is the definitive test used in the diagnosis of cystic fibrosis. Skin sweat is analyzed for sodium and chloride content.

Genetic Testing (p. 1139). This is another confirmatory test for cystic fibrosis.

Semen Analysis (Sperm Count, Sperm Examination, Seminal Cytologic Study, Semen Examination)

NORMAL FINDINGS

Volume: 1.5–5 mL
Liquefaction time: 20 to 30 minutes after collection
pH: 7.12–8.00
Sperm count (density): **≥20 × 10^6/ejaculate** (>20 million/mL)
Sperm motility: ≥50% at 1 hour
Sperm structure: >30% (Kruger criteria, >14%) normally shaped

INDICATIONS

Semen analysis is used to evaluate the quality of sperm, to evaluate infertility, and to document the adequacy of operative vasectomy.

TEST EXPLANATION

Semen production depends on the function of the testicles; semen analysis is a measure of testicular function. Gonadotropin-releasing hormone (GnRH) is secreted by the hypothalamus in response to decreased levels of testosterone. GnRH stimulates the pituitary to produce follicle-stimulating hormone (FSH) and luteinizing hormone (also called *interstitial cell–stimulating hormone*). FSH stimulates the Sertoli cell growth within the seminiferous tubules (location of sperm production). Luteinizing hormone stimulates the Leydig cells to produce testosterone, which in turn stimulates the seminiferous tubules to produce sperm. Inadequate sperm production can be the result of primary gonadal failure (because of age, genetic cause [Klinefelter's syndrome], infection, irradiation, or surgical orchiectomy) or secondary gonadal failure (because of pituitary diseases). Measuring luteinizing hormone and FSH levels can differentiate these forms of gonadal failure. In primary gonadal failure, these levels are increased. In secondary gonadal failure, they are decreased. Stimulation tests with GnRH agonists such as leuprolide acetate clomiphene or human chorionic gonadotropin are also used in the differentiation. Men with *aspermia* (no sperm) or *oligospermia* ($<20 \times 10^6$/ejaculate [<20 million/mL]) should undergo endocrinologic evaluation for pituitary, thyroid, or testicular aberrations.

Semen analysis is one of the most important aspects of the fertility workup because the cause of a couple's inability to conceive often lies with the man. After 2 to 3 days of sexual abstinence, semen is collected and examined for volume, sperm count, motility, and structure.

The freshly collected semen is first measured for volume. After liquefaction of the white, gelatinous ejaculate, a sperm count is performed. Men with very low or very high counts are probably infertile. The motility of the sperm is then evaluated; at least 50% should show progressive motility. To study structure, a semen preparation is stained, and the numbers of normal versus abnormal sperm forms are calculated.

More exhaustive semen analysis for male infertility may include a *sperm penetration assay,* a multistep laboratory test that offers a biologic assessment of several aspects of human sperm fertilizing ability. Hyaluronan-binding assay is a qualitative assay used to determine the maturity of sperm in a fresh semen sample. The assay is based on the ability of mature, but not immature, sperm to bind to hyaluronan, the main mucopolysaccharide of the egg matrix and a component of human follicular fluid. Hyaluronan-binding capacity is acquired late in the sperm maturation process; immature sperm lack this capacity. Therefore, if the number of sperm binding to hyaluronan is low, the proportion of mature sperm in the sample is low. As with the sperm penetration assay, it has been suggested that the hyaluronan-binding assay may be used to determine the need for an intracytoplasmic sperm injection procedure as part of an assisted reproductive technique.

Aside from the conventional parameters of sperm quality such as concentration, motility, and structure, *sperm DNA integrity* is a potential cause of idiopathic male infertility. Although sperm with fragmented DNA may be able to fertilize oocytes, subsequent embryo and fetal development may be impaired. DNA fragmentation in sperm increases with age. Therefore, impaired DNA integrity may be an increasing infertility factor among older men. Available flow cytometry tests of DNA integrity include the *sperm chromatin structure assay test* and the *sperm DNA fragmentation assay test.* The sperm specimen is considered abnormal if more than 70% of the sperm have abnormal forms.

A single sperm analysis, especially if it indicates infertility, is inconclusive because sperm count varies from day to day. A semen analysis should be performed at least twice and possibly a third time, 3 weeks apart. A normal semen analysis alone does not accurately assess the male factor unless the effect of the partner's cervical secretion on sperm survival is also determined (see the discussion of the Sims-Huhner test on p. 701). In addition to its value in infertility workups, semen analysis is also helpful in documenting adequate sterilization after a vasectomy. It is usually performed 6 weeks after the surgery. If any sperm are seen, the adequacy of the vasectomy must be suspect.

INTERFERING FACTORS

Drugs that may cause *decreases* in sperm counts include antineoplastic agents (e.g., nitrogen mustard, procarbazine, vincristine, methotrexate), cimetidine, estrogens, and methyltestosterone.

Clinical Priorities

- It is best to collect the semen for this test after 2 to 3 days of sexual abstinence.
- For best results, the man should produce the semen specimen in the physician's office by masturbation.
- A single sperm analysis is inconclusive because the sperm count varies from day to day. A semen analysis should be performed two or three times for best results.

PROCEDURE AND PATIENT CARE

Before

✗ Explain the procedure to the patient.

✗ Instruct the patient to abstain from sexual activity for 2 to 3 days before the specimen is collected. Prolonged abstinence before the collection should be discouraged, because the quality of the sperm cells, and especially their motility, may diminish.

- Give the patient the proper container for the semen collection.

✗ Instruct the patient to avoid alcoholic beverages for several days before the collection.

✗ For evaluation of the adequacy of vasectomy, the patient should ejaculate once or twice before the day of examination to clear the distal portion of the vas deferens.

During

- Note that semen is best collected by ejaculation into a clean container. For best results, the man should produce the specimen in the physician's office or laboratory by masturbation.
- Less satisfactory specimens can be obtained in the patient's home through coitus interruptus or masturbation. Note the following procedural steps:
  1. Instruct the patient to deliver these home specimens to the laboratory within 1 hour after collection.
  2. Instruct the patient to avoid excessive heat and cold during transportation of the specimen.

After

- Record the date of the previous semen emission, along with the collection time and date of the fresh specimen.

✗ Inform the patient when and how to obtain the test results. Remember that abnormal results may have a devastating psychologic effect on the man.

TEST RESULTS AND CLINICAL SIGNIFICANCE

Infertility: *One of the most common causes of infertility is inadequate sperm production.*

Vasectomy (obstruction of vas deferens): *Semen analysis is necessary before vasectomy can be considered to be adequate.*

Orchitis: *This is usually caused by a virus (varicella) or, in rare cases, by a bacterium.*

Testicular failure: *This can be congenital (Klinefelter's syndrome) or acquired (e.g., infection). Usually, with acquired forms of testicular failure, sperm are present but in low quantities. With congenital forms of testicular failure, no sperm are seen.*

Hyperpyrexia,

Varicocele: *A common finding in sperm analysis is called "stress pattern." This is said to exist when more than 20% of the sperm have an abnormal appearance and sperm counts are low. The stress pattern indicates presence of a varicocele or recent febrile illness.*

Pituitary pathologic condition (adenoma, infarction): *This causes hypospermia because of reduced levels of luteinizing hormone and FSH or their absence. As a result, spermatogenesis does not occur.*

RELATED TESTS

Antispermatozoal Antibody (p. 106). These antibodies can exist in the blood of men and destroy sperm quality. Furthermore, these antibodies can be produced by women and exist in the cervical mucus, thereby undermining fertility.

Sims-Huhner (p. 701). The Sims-Huhner test consists of a postcoital examination of the cervical mucus to measure the ability of the sperm to penetrate the mucus and maintain motility. It is used in the diagnostic workup of infertility. This analysis is also helpful in documenting cases of suspected rape by testing the vaginal and cervical secretions for sperm.

Luteinizing Hormone and Follicle-Stimulating Hormone (p. 361). Measurements of these hormones are useful in determining the pituitary effect on gonadal function and spermatogenesis.

Sexual Assault Testing

NORMAL FINDINGS

No physical evidence of sexual assault

INDICATIONS

This testing is used to obtain evidence of a recent sexual assault and to obtain specimens to identify sexually transmitted infection.

TEST EXPLANATION

Victims of sexual assault need psychologic-emotional support, treatment of any physical injuries, and accurate and reliable evidentiary testing. Nearly all acute care centres have protocols in place to provide that care to victims of sexual assault. Furthermore, in most circumstances, nurses specifically trained in obtaining the appropriate specimens are employed. These nurses know the importance of following the chain-of-evidence protocols to ensure that evidence is admissible in court. Sexual Assault Nurse Examiner programs, now available in both Canada and the United States, provide round-the-clock, first-response care to victims of rape in a variety of health care settings, including hospitals and clinics. These programs also have highly trained nurses who specialize in forensic specimen collection and provide patients with comprehensive postrape care and counselling. Sexual Assault Nurse Examiner programs are effective in promoting the psychologic recovery of survivors, ensuring accurate and complete collection of forensic evidence, and improving the prosecution of sexual assault cases.

While being provided with emotional support and assistance, the patient is first interviewed in a nonjudgemental manner. A thorough gynecologic history is obtained. A brief summary of the assault (documenting whether vaginal, oral, or anal penetration occurred) and timing of the assault is important. After 48 hours, very little evidence persists. It is important to ascertain whether the victim changed clothing, showered, or used a douche before coming to the hospital. These actions affect the presence of evidence. The general demeanour of the patient, status of the clothing, and physical maturation assessment are documented.

The patient's clothes are removed and each garment is placed in a separate paper bag to assess for possible DNA from the victim's or assailant's body parts. Plastic bags are not used because bacteria may grow in them and can destroy DNA. All injuries should be photographed,

BOX 5-1	DNA Evidence Collection: Special Precautions

To avoid contamination of evidence that may contain DNA, the Sexual Assault Evidence Collection Kit (SAECK) should be used and the following precautions taken:
- Wear gloves, and change them often.
- Use disposable instruments, or clean instruments thoroughly before and after handling each sample.
- Avoid touching any area where you believe DNA may be present.
- Avoid talking, sneezing, or coughing over evidence.
- Avoid touching your face, nose, and mouth when collecting and packaging evidence.
- Keep evidence dry, and transport it at room temperature.
- Ensure that the chain of custody of evidence is maintained at all times.

if possible. The patient is then examined for signs of external and internal injuries. A pelvic examination is then performed. A "sexual assault evidence collection kit" (SAECK) is now most commonly used to obtain all the needed specimens. The directions must be followed carefully to ensure that any and all evidence is obtained and is useful toward identification and conviction of any perpetrator (Box 5-1).

Vaginal secretions are obtained for sperm (see p. 695) or other cells from the assailant. Acid phosphatase (see p. 30) and prostate-specific antigen (see p. 434) are also obtained from this specimen. Cervical secretions are obtained to test for sexually transmitted infection (p. 787). These anatomic areas, along with the anorectal area, are swabbed per directions in the kit. In the male victim, penile and anorectal areas are swabbed. Pubic hair is obtained by combing or plucking. Testing for sexually transmitted infections includes tests for syphilis (p. 487), trichomoniasis (p. 774), gonorrhea (p. 787), and chlamydia (p. 751). Later, blood testing for human immunodeficiency virus (HIV) infection (p. 310) and pregnancy (p. 426) is performed.

Next, blood specimens are obtained for DNA testing per the testing kit directions—usually an ethylenediamine tetra-acetic acid (EDTA)–containing tube (lavender top). More blood or urine may also be collected for evidence of mind-altering drugs/alcohol or for serologic evidence of sexually transmitted infections. After this testing, a more detailed examination of the vagina, cervix, and rectum is performed with a Wood lamp to more easily identify saliva or sperm from the assailant. These areas are examined for subtle injuries from forced penetration. Two methods used to identify these injuries are the toluidine blue dye test and use of a colposcope (see p. 623). The *toluidine blue dye test* can also be used to identify recent or healed genital or anorectal injuries. A 1% aqueous solution is applied to the area of concern and washed off with a lubricant (e.g., K-Y Jelly) or a 1% acetic acid solution. Injured mucosa retains the dye, and the injury becomes more apparent to the examiner's naked eye. Finally, the patient's fingernails are scraped underneath because they may contain tissue from the assailant. On completion of the examination, the victim is usually interviewed by the police for further investigation.

Unless antimicrobial therapy is medically contraindicated, all victims should be offered this medication to prevent sexually transmitted infections. The following combination of drugs is used in many hospitals: ciprofloxacin, 250 mg PO stat dose; doxycycline, 100 mg bid for 7 days; and metronidazole, 2 g stat. The use of antiretroviral drugs in the prevention of HIV transmission may be recommended, and the current guideline for postexposure prophylaxis after needlestick injuries should be used. It may also be advisable to offer victims a hepatitis B vaccination or hepatitis B immunoglobulin, inasmuch as these diseases may be fatal. Victims who are at risk for HIV infection should also be given counselling about HIV/acquired immune deficiency syndrome (AIDS).

A pregnancy test should be performed before any treatment or drugs are prescribed. If there is a risk of pregnancy, the victim should be offered postcoital contraception if the rape occurred less than 72 hours before examination by the health care provider. If it occurred more than 72 hours but less than 7 days before the examination, an intrauterine contraceptive device may be used to prevent pregnancy. Pregnancy testing may be repeated in the week after the rape.

CONTRAINDICATIONS

- The patient's emotional inability to undergo the examination

INTERFERING FACTORS

- Delays in examination after the alleged attack diminish the possibilities of identifying meaningful evidence.

PROCEDURE AND PATIENT CARE

Before

- Explain the procedure to the patient, and provide emotional support.
- Obtain the patient's or family's consent to treat the patient.
- Notify any family members the patient wants present during the examination.
- Assess the patient's emotional condition and determine whether the patient is able to undergo sexual assault testing.

During

- Obtain a thorough history, as described previously.
- Use the SAECK or a similar test kit exactly as instructed to maintain the chain of evidence (see Box 5-1).
- Properly handle the kit specimens to maintain the chain of custody.
- Refrigerate all samples containing biologic evidentiary material such as DNA to prevent putrefaction (decomposition).
- It is important to carefully examine all area of the patient's body to help corroborate the patient's version of the alleged events.

After

- Notify police of the alleged assault.
- Assess the patient's need for urgent counselling support, and make arrangements as needed.
- If additional or ongoing counselling is required, the patient should be referred to a counsellor trained in victim support.

TEST RESULTS AND CLINICAL SIGNIFICANCE

Rape,

Sexual assault: *The psychologic effect of a sexual assault in either sex is overwhelming. Such patients do best if referred for psychologic support. Often the legal conviction of the offender lessens the fear of the victim. Furthermore, observing just punishment of the offender may hasten healing. It is important to obtain accurate evidence so that all data is admissible and useful to law enforcement agencies.*

Sims-Huhner (Postcoital Testing, Postcoital Cervical Mucus, Cervical Mucus Sperm Penetration)

NORMAL FINDINGS

Cervical mucus adequate for sperm transmission, survival, and penetration; 6 to 20 active sperm per high-power field

INDICATIONS

The Sims-Huhner test consists of a postcoital examination of the cervical mucus to measure the ability of the sperm to penetrate the mucus and maintain motility. This test is invaluable in the evaluation of infertility.

TEST EXPLANATION

This study enables the clinician to evaluate interaction between the sperm and the cervical mucus. The quality of the cervical mucus can also be measured. This test can help determine the effect of vaginal and cervical secretions on the activity of the sperm. This procedure is performed only after previous semen analysis has yielded normal results.

This test is performed during the middle of the ovulatory cycle because at that time, the secretions should be optimal for sperm penetration and survival. During ovulation, the quantity of cervical mucus is maximal, whereas the viscosity is minimal, thus facilitating sperm penetration. The endocervical mucus sample is examined for colour, viscosity, and tenacity (spinnbarkeit). The fresh specimen is then spread on a clean glass slide and examined for the presence of sperm. Estimates of the total number and of the number of motile sperm per high-power field are reported. Normally, 6 to 20 active sperm cells should be seen in each microscopic high-power field; if the sperm are present but not active, the cervical environment is unsuitable for their survival (e.g., the pH is abnormal). After the specimen has dried on the glass slide, the mucus can be examined for ferning to demonstrate estrogen effect. The Sims-Huhner study is invaluable in fertility examinations; however, it is not a substitute for the semen analysis. If the results of the Sims-Huhner test are less than optimal, the test is usually repeated during the same or the next ovulatory cycle.

This analysis is also helpful in documenting cases of suspected rape by testing the vaginal and cervical secretions for sperm. A physician performs this procedure in approximately 5 minutes. The only discomfort associated with this study, in the absence of injury, is insertion of the speculum.

Clinical Priorities

- This test is performed during the middle of the ovulation cycle, when the secretions should be optimal for sperm penetration and survival.
- Instruct the female patient to remain in bed for 10 to 15 minutes after coitus to ensure cervical exposure to the semen. She should then report to the physician within 2 hours of coitus.

PROCEDURE AND PATIENT CARE

Before

- Explain the procedure to the patient.
- Instruct the patient to use basal body temperature recordings to estimate the time of ovulation.

Fluid Analysis Studies

5

X Inform the patient that no vaginal lubrication, douching, or bathing is permitted until after the vaginal cervical examination, because these actions will alter the cervical mucus.

X Inform the patient that this study should be performed after 3 days of male sexual abstinence.

X Instruct the patient to remain in bed for 10 to 15 minutes after coitus to ensure cervical exposure to the semen. After this rest period but within 2 hours after coitus, the patient should report to her physician for examination of her cervical mucus.

During

- Note that the patient is in the lithotomy position; the cervix is then exposed by an unlubricated speculum.
- The specimen is aspirated from the endocervix and delivered to the laboratory for analysis.

After

X Inform the patient how and when she may obtain the test results.

TEST RESULTS AND CLINICAL SIGNIFICANCE

Infertility: *This test determines the capability of the sperm to function and exist in an environment outside the male urethra. It is the final determinant of the adequacy of sperm. Semen analysis may indicate adequacy of sperm count, motility, and structure; however, if the sperm cannot function within the vaginal or cervical environment, fertility is improbable.*

Suspected rape: *The demonstration of sperm within vaginal secretions indicates that intercourse has occurred.*

RELATED TESTS

Semen Analysis (p. 695). Semen analysis is used to evaluate the quality of sperm, to evaluate infertility, and to document the adequacy of operative vasectomy.

Antispermatozoal Antibody (p. 106). These antibodies can exist in the blood of men and destroy sperm quality. Furthermore, these antibodies can be produced by women and exist in the cervical mucus, thereby undermining fertility.

Luteinizing Hormone and Follicle-Stimulating Hormone (p. 361). Measurements of these hormones are useful in determining the pituitary effect on gonadal function and spermatogenesis.

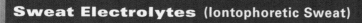

Sweat Electrolytes (Iontophoretic Sweat)

NORMAL FINDINGS

Sodium values in children
   Normal: **<70 mmol/L** (<70 mEq/L)
   Abnormal: **>90 mmol/L** (>90 mEq/L)
   Equivocal: **70–90 mmol/L** (70–90 mEq/L)
Chloride values in children
   Normal: **<50 mmol/L** (<50 mEq/L)
   Abnormal: **>60 mmol/L** (>60 mEq/L)
   Equivocal: **50–60 mmol/L** (50–60 mEq/L)

INDICATIONS

This test is used to diagnose cystic fibrosis. The sweat electrolytes test is indicated in children with recurrent respiratory tract infections, chronic cough, early-onset asthma, malabsorption syndromes, late passage of meconium stool, or failure to thrive. This test is also used to screen for the disease in children or siblings of patients with cystic fibrosis.

TEST EXPLANATION

In cystic fibrosis, the sodium and chloride contents are increased in sweat. That forms the basis of this test, which is both sensitive and specific for cystic fibrosis. Cystic fibrosis is an inherited (autosomal recessive) disease characterized by abnormal secretion by exocrine glands within the bronchi, small intestine, pancreatic ducts, bile ducts, and skin (sweat glands). Sweat, induced by electrical current (pilocarpine iontophoresis), is collected, and its sodium and chloride contents are measured. The degree of abnormality is no indication of the severity of cystic fibrosis; any abnormality merely indicates that the patient has the disease.

Patients with cystic fibrosis have a mutation in the cystic fibrosis transmembrane conductance regulator (*CFTR*) gene. This gene encodes the synthesis of a protein that serves as a channel through which chloride enters and leaves the cells. A mutation in this gene alters the cell's capability to regulate the transport of chloride (and, as a result, of sodium). Normally, at the base of a sweat gland, sodium and chloride concentrations are very high. As the sweat moves closer to the skin surface, chloride is transported through the lining cells out of the sweat. Sodium follows. By the time the sweat comes to the surface, nearly all of the chloride and sodium has been removed. In patients with cystic fibrosis, the transport of these ions does not occur. The sweat, therefore, has high concentrations of sodium and chloride. In almost all patients with cystic fibrosis, the sweat sodium and chloride contents are two to five times higher than normal values. In patients with suspect clinical manifestations, these levels are diagnostic of cystic fibrosis.

Abnormal sweat test results can also occur in patients with glycogen storage diseases, adrenal hypofunction, and glucose-6-phosphate dehydrogenase (G6PD) deficiency.

The sweat test is not reliable during the first few weeks of life. Measurement of serum concentrations of immunoreactive trypsin may be a better test for this age group. An experienced technologist performs the sweat test in approximately 90 minutes in the laboratory or at the patient's bedside. A small electrical current is experienced during the test, but this is not painful. In general, no discomfort or pain is associated with this test.

INTERFERING FACTORS

- In a cold room, sweating is inhibited. The room should be warmed or the child covered to maintain body heat.
- Dehydration is associated with reduced volume of sweat and increased concentration of sodium and chloride. The test results are not accurate.
- Sodium and chloride values in pubertal adolescents may vary significantly and are not accurate.

PROCEDURE AND PATIENT CARE

Before

✗ Explain the procedure to the patient or parents, or both.
✗ Inform the patient or parents, or both, that no fasting is required.

During

- Note the following procedural steps:
  1. For iontophoresis, a low-level electrical current is applied to the test area (the thigh in infants, the forearm in older children) (Figure 5-4).
  2. The positive electrode is covered by gauze and saturated with pilocarpine hydrochloride, a stimulating drug that induces sweating.
  3. The negative electrode is covered by gauze saturated with a bicarbonate solution.
  4. The electrical current is allowed to flow for 5 to 12 minutes.
  5. The electrodes are removed, and the arm is washed with distilled water.
  6. Paper discs are placed over the test site with the use of clean, dry forceps.
  7. These discs are covered with paraffin to create an airtight seal, preventing evaporation of sweat.
  8. After 1 hour, the paraffin is removed. The paper discs are transferred immediately by forceps to a weighing jar and sent for sodium and chloride analysis.

A screening test may be done to detect sweat chloride levels. For screening, a test paper containing silver nitrate is pressed against the child's hand for several seconds. The test is positive when the excess chloride combines with the silver nitrate to form a white powder (silver chloride) on the paper. That is, the child with cystic fibrosis will leave a "heavy" handprint on the paper. A positive screening test is usually validated by iontophoresis.

After

- Initiate extensive education, emotional support, and counselling for the patient or parents, or both, if the results indicate cystic fibrosis.

TEST RESULTS AND CLINICAL SIGNIFICANCE

Cystic fibrosis: *Normally, the sweat produced at the bottom of a sweat duct is rich in chloride and sodium. As the fluid traverses the duct leading to the outer skin level, the chloride (followed by sodium) escapes the lumen through the epithelial cells, leaving only water behind. In patients with cystic fibrosis, the epithelial lining cells of the ducts of sweat glands fail to take up the electrolytes efficiently from the lumen. The sweat at the skin level is therefore high in sodium and chloride.*

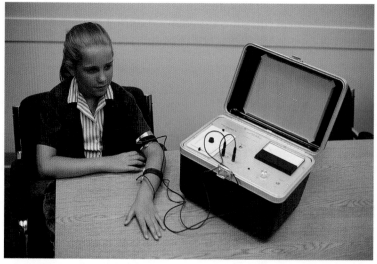

Figure 5-4 Child undergoing sweat test for cystic fibrosis.

RELATED TESTS

Secretin-Pancreozymin (p. 693). In this test, pancreatic efflux is measured for amylase and other components. It is a corroborative test for cystic fibrosis.

Genetic Testing (p. 1139). Identification of the cystic fibrosis transmembrane conductance regulator (*CFTR*) gene is another confirmatory test for the disease. It is more commonly used to identify carriers of the gene that causes cystic fibrosis.

Thoracentesis and Pleural Fluid Analysis

NORMAL FINDINGS

Gross appearance: clear, serous, light yellow, 50 mL
Red blood cells (RBCs): none
White blood cells (WBCs): **<100 × 10⁹/L** (<100/mm³)
Protein: **<41 g/L** (<4.1 g/dL)
Glucose: **3.3–6.1 mmol/L** (60–110 mg/dL)
Amylase: 138–404 U/L
Alkaline phosphatase
    Adult male: 90–240 U/L
    Female <45 years: 76–196 U/L
    Female >45 years: 87–250 U/L
Lactate dehydrogenase (LDH): similar to serum LDH
Cytologic findings: no malignant cells
Bacteria: none
Fungi: none
Carcinoembryonic antigen (CEA): **<5 Mcg/L** (<5 ng/mL)

INDICATIONS

Thoracentesis is performed to determine the cause of an unexplained pleural effusion. It is also performed to relieve the intrathoracic pressure that accumulates with a large volume of fluid and inhibits respiration.

TEST EXPLANATION

Thoracentesis is an invasive procedure in which a needle is inserted into the pleural space to remove fluid or, in rare cases, air (Figure 5-5). The *pleural space* is defined as the space between the visceral pleura (thin membrane covering the lungs) and the parietal pleura (thin membrane covering the inside of the thoracic cavity). Within the peritoneal membrane is an intricate network of capillary and lymphatic vessels. Fluid is constantly being secreted by the pleural membranes and constantly being reabsorbed by those same membranes. If secretion is increased or reabsorption blocked, pleural fluid accumulates.

Pleural fluid is removed for diagnostic and therapeutic purposes. For therapeutic purposes, it is performed to relieve pain, dyspnea, and other symptoms of pleural pressure. Removal of this fluid also enables better radiographic visualization of the lung.

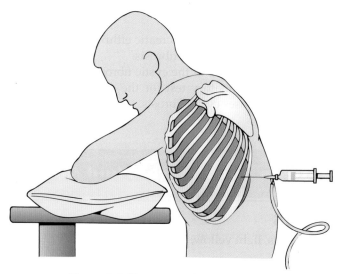

Figure 5-5 Illustration of thoracentesis.

For diagnostic purposes, thoracentesis is performed to obtain and analyze fluid to determine the cause of the pleural effusion. Pleural fluid is classified as a transudate or an exudate. This is an important distinction and is very helpful in determining the cause of the effusion. See Table 5-3 (p. 686) for differentiation between transudate and exudate. Transudates are most frequently caused by heart failure, cirrhosis, nephrotic syndrome, and hypoproteinemia. Exudates most often occur in inflammatory, infectious, or neoplastic conditions. However, collagen-vascular disease, pulmonary infarction, trauma, and drug hypersensitivity also may cause an exudative effusion.

A decubitus chest radiograph (p. 1053) is obtained before thoracentesis to ensure that the pleural fluid is mobile and accessible to a needle placed within the pleural space.

Pleural fluid is usually evaluated for gross appearance; cell counts; protein, LDH, glucose, and amylase levels; Gram stain and bacteriologic cultures; the presence of *Mycobacterium tuberculosis* and fungus; cytologic study; CEA levels; and sometimes other specific tests. Each is discussed separately as follows.

Gross Appearance

The colour, optical density, and viscosity are noted as the pleural fluid appears in the aspirating syringe. Transudative pleural fluid may be clear, serous, and light yellow, especially in patients with hepatic cirrhosis. Milk-coloured pleural fluid may result from the escape of chyle from blocked thoracic lymphatic ducts. An opalescent, pearly appearance is characteristic of chylothorax (chyle in the pleural cavity). Conditions that may cause lymphatic blockage include lymphoma, carcinoma, and tuberculosis involving the thoracic lymph nodes. The triglyceride value in a chylous effusion exceeds **1.24 mmol/L** (>110 mg/dL).

Fluid may be cloudy or turbid as a result of inflammatory or infectious conditions such as empyema. Empyema is characterized by the presence of a foul odour, and the fluid is thick and pus-like. Blood in the fluid may be the result of a traumatic puncture (the aspirating needle penetrates a blood vessel), intrathoracic bleeding, or tumour.

Cell Counts

The WBC count and differential are determined. A WBC count higher than $1\,000 \times 10^9$/L (>1 000/mm^3) is suggestive of an exudate. The predominance of polymorphonuclear leukocytes usually is an indication of an acute inflammatory condition (e.g., pneumonia, pulmonary infarction, early tuberculosis effusion). When more than 50% of the WBCs are small lymphocytes, the effusion is usually caused by tuberculosis or tumour. Normally, no RBCs are present. The presence of RBCs may indicate neoplasms, tuberculosis, or intrathoracic bleeding.

Protein Content

Total protein levels higher than **30 g/L** (>3 g/dL) are characteristic of exudates, whereas transudates usually have a protein content of less than **30 g/L** (<3 g/dL). It is now thought that the albumin gradient between serum and pleural fluid can differentiate better between the transudate and exudate nature of pleural fluid than can the total protein content. To obtain this gradient, the pleural albumin value is subtracted from the serum albumin value. Values of **11 g/L** ($\geq$1.1 g/dL) or greater are suggestive of a transudate. Values of less than **11 g/L** (<1.1 g/dL) are suggestive of an exudate but do not specify the potential cause of the exudate (malignancy from infection or inflammation).

Because protein values that differentiate transudate from exudate overlap significantly, the total protein ratio (fluid/serum) has been considered to be a more accurate criterion. A fluid/serum total protein ratio higher than 0.5 is considered to indicate an exudate.

Lactate Dehydrogenase

A pleural fluid/serum lactate dehydrogenase (LDH) ratio higher than 0.6 is typical of an exudate. An exudate is identified with a high degree of accuracy if the pleural fluid/serum protein ratio is greater than 0.5 and the pleural fluid/serum LDH ratio is greater than 0.6.

Glucose

Usually pleural glucose levels approximate serum levels. Low values appear to be a combination of glycolysis by the extra cells within an exudate and impairment of glucose diffusion because of damage to the pleural membrane. Values of less than **3.3 mmol/L** (<60 mg/dL) also indicate exudate.

Amylase

In a malignant effusion, the amylase concentration is slightly elevated. Amylase levels are above the normal range for serum or two times the serum level when the effusion is caused by pancreatitis or rupture of the esophagus associated with leakage of salivary amylase into the chest cavity.

Triglyceride

Measurement of triglyceride levels is an important part of identifying chylous effusions. These effusions are usually produced by obstruction or transection of the lymphatic system caused by lymphoma, neoplasm, trauma, or recent surgery. The triglyceride value in a chylous effusion exceeds **1.24 mmol/L** (>110 mg/dL).

Gram Stain and Bacteriologic Culture

Culture and Gram stains are routinely performed when bacterial pneumonia or empyema is a possible cause of the effusion. These tests identify the organisms involved in the infection and also provide information concerning antibiotic sensitivity. (See p. 733 for a more thorough discussion of Gram stains, cultures, and sensitivity.) If possible, these tests should be performed before antibiotic therapy is initiated.

Cultures for *Mycobacterium Tuberculosis* and Fungus

Tuberculosis is less often a cause for pleural effusion in Canada today than it was in the past (although its incidence is now on the rise, especially among immunosuppressed patients). Fungus may be a cause of pulmonary effusion in patients with compromised immunologic defences. (See p. 798 for more information about tuberculosis culture techniques.)

Cytologic Study

A cytologic study is performed to detect tumours. The findings are positive in approximately 50% to 60% of patients with malignant effusions. Breast and lung are the two most frequent tumours; lymphoma is the third. To interpret cytologic changes, the pathologist must have considerable experience in cytology. It can be difficult to differentiate malignancy from severe inflammatory mesothelial cells. In general, malignant cells tend to clump together and have a high nucleus/cytoplasm ratio, prominent and multiple nucleoli, and unevenly distributed chromatin.

Cytologic examination of the fluid is improved by centrifugation of a large volume of fluid and examination of the sediment. A large number of cells can be seen and compared with each other.

Carcinoembryonic Antigen

Pleural fluid CEA levels are elevated in various malignant (gastrointestinal, breast) conditions.

Special Tests

The pH of pleural fluid is usually 7.4 or greater. The pH is typically less than 7.2 when empyema is present. The pH may be 7.2 to 7.4 in tuberculosis or malignancy. In some instances, the rheumatoid factor (p. 467) and the complement levels (p. 185) are also measured in pleural fluid. Pleural fluid antinuclear antibody (ANA) levels and the pleural fluid/serum ratio for antinuclear antibody are often used to evaluate pleural effusion secondary to systemic lupus erythematosus.

Thoracentesis is performed in less than 30 minutes by a physician at the patient's bedside, in a procedure room, or in the physician's office. Although local anaesthetics eliminate pain at the insertion site, the patient may feel a pressure-like pain when the pleura is entered and the fluid is removed.

CONTRAINDICATIONS

- Significant thrombocytopenia, because the aspirating needle may initiate bleeding

POTENTIAL COMPLICATIONS

- Pneumothorax caused by puncture of the lung or entry of air into the pleural space through the aspirating needle
- Intrapleural bleeding because of puncture of a blood vessel
- Hemoptysis caused by needle puncture of a pulmonary vessel
- Reflex bradycardia and hypotension
- Pulmonary edema
- Seeding of the needle track with tumour when malignant pleural effusion is present
- Empyema caused by infection delivered by the aspirating needle

Clinical Priorities

- To prevent needle damage to the lung or pleura, the patient should remain still during this procedure. A cough suppressant may be needed if the patient has a troublesome cough.
- A radiograph, an ultrasound scan, or a fluoroscopic view is used to assist in localizing the pleural fluid and in determining the needle insertion site.
- Chest radiographic examinations are done after this procedure to check for pneumothorax. The lungs are carefully assessed for decreased breath sounds, which could be a sign of pneumothorax.

PROCEDURE AND PATIENT CARE

Before

- Explain the procedure to the patient.
- Obtain the patient's informed consent for this procedure.
- Inform the patient that no fasting or sedation is necessary.
- Inform the patient that movement or coughing should be minimized to avoid inadvertent needle damage to the lung or pleura during the procedure.
- Administer a cough suppressant before the procedure if the patient has a troublesome cough.
- Note that a radiograph, an ultrasound scan, or fluoroscopic examination is often used to assist in location of the fluid.

During

- Note the following procedural steps:
  1. The patient is usually placed in an upright position with the arms and shoulders raised and supported on a padded overhead table. This position spreads the ribs and enlarges the intercostal space for insertion of the needle.
  2. Patients who cannot sit upright are placed in a side-lying position on the unaffected side; the side to be tapped is uppermost.
  3. The thoracentesis is performed under strict sterile technique.
  4. The needle insertion site, which is determined by percussion, auscultation, and examination of a chest radiograph, ultrasound scan, or fluoroscopy, is aseptically cleansed and anaesthetized locally.
  5. The needle is positioned in the pleural space, and the fluid is withdrawn with a syringe and a three-way stopcock. In most thoracentesis kits, a blunt-tip soft catheter is over the needle. The needle is withdrawn, and the soft Silastic catheter is left in place. The fluid is aspirated. The use of these soft catheters has greatly diminished the incidence of pneumothorax as a complication of this procedure.
  6. Various mechanisms to stabilize the pleural needle or catheter are available to secure the needle depth during the fluid collection.
  7. A short polyethylene catheter may be inserted into the pleural space for fluid aspiration; this decreases the risk of puncturing the visceral pleura and inducing a pneumothorax.
  8. Also, connecting the catheter to a gravity-drainage system may collect large volumes of fluid.
  9. Monitor the patient's pulse for reflex bradycardia, and evaluate the patient for diaphoresis and the feeling of faintness during the procedure.

After

- Place a small bandage over the needle site. In most cases, turn the patient on the unaffected side for 1 hour to allow the pleural puncture site to heal.

Fluid Analysis Studies

5

- Label the specimen with the patient's name, date, source of fluid, and diagnosis. Send the specimen promptly to the laboratory.
- All pleural fluid should be analyzed immediately to avoid false results caused by chemical or cellular deterioration.
- Obtain a chest radiographic study as indicated to check for pneumothorax.
- Monitor the patient's vital signs.
- Observe the patient for coughing or expectoration of blood (hemoptysis), which may indicate trauma to the lung.
- Evaluate the patient for signs and symptoms of pneumothorax, tension pneumothorax, sub-cutaneous emphysema, and pyogenic infection (e.g., tachypnea, dyspnea, diminished breath sounds, anxiety, restlessness, fever).
- Assess the patient's lung sounds for diminished breath sounds, which could be a sign of pneumothorax.
- ⚠ If the patient has no complaints of dyspnea, normal activity usually can be resumed 1 hour after the procedure.

TEST RESULTS AND CLINICAL SIGNIFICANCE

Exudate

Empyema,

Pneumonia: *Empyema is most often the result of pneumonia. On occasion, however, it can follow surgery, pleuritis, or trauma.*

Tuberculosis effusion: *This is usually a bloody effusion that is the result of the primary tuberculous infection of the lung and pleura.*

Pancreatitis: *This pleural effusion is most often a "sympathetic" effusion in response to the inflammatory process below the diaphragm.*

Ruptured esophagus: *The pleural fluid can appear as a result of a free communication of the ruptured esophagus with the pleural cavity. The pleura covering the mediastinum usually prevents this free communication, and the fluid is a "sympathetic" reaction to the mediastinal infection. The fluid, however, subsequently becomes infected and acts as an empyema.*

Tumours: *Neoplasms affecting the pleura primarily (mesothelioma) or secondarily (breast, lung, ovarian) secrete excess volumes of fluid into the pleural space.*

Lymphoma: *The tumour infiltrates the lymph nodes through which the thoracic lymphatic ducts flow. As a result, the lymph fluid is not reabsorbed and accumulates as a chylous effusion within the pleural space (chylothorax).*

Pulmonary infarction: *This bloody effusion is also a "sympathetic" effusion in response to the necrosis of lung tissue following a pulmonary embolus.*

Collagen-vascular disease,

Rheumatoid arthritis,

Systemic lupus erythematosus,

Drug hypersensitivity: *An immunogenic pleuritis and subsequent effusion may be the sequelae of autoimmune diseases or drug hypersensitivities, as indicated previously.*

Transudate,

Cirrhosis,

Heart failure: *With increased venous pressure that results from either portal vein hypertension or passive congestion from heart failure, pleural fluid is not absorbed. As a result, pleural fluid accumulates.*

Nephrotic syndrome,

Hypoproteinemia: *The nephrotic syndrome is characterized by renal albumin wasting. This and other forms of hypoproteinemia are associated with decreased intravascular oncotic pressure. The fluid tends to leak out of the intravascular space into the pleural space.*

Trauma: *Injury to the thorax, lungs, or great blood vessels can cause bleeding into the pleural space (hemothorax).*

RELATED TESTS

Glucose, Blood (p. 269), Lactate Dehydrogenase (p. 339), Protein Electrophoresis (p. 440), and Amylase, Blood (p. 67). These blood tests are performed concomitantly to assist in the evaluation of the peritoneal fluid.

Chest Radiography (p. 1053). This is an important part of identifying a pleural effusion. Furthermore, a chest radiograph should be routinely obtained on completion of thoracentesis to ensure that a pneumothorax has not iatrogenically occurred.

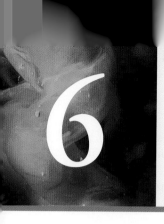

6 Manometric Studies

NOTE: *Throughout this chapter, SI units are presented in* **boldface colour,** *followed by conventional units in parentheses.*

OVERVIEW

TESTS

OVERVIEW

In manometric studies, certain areas of the body are evaluated with a manometric device to measure and record pressures. These devices can be as familiar to the patient as a blood pressure instrument or as unusual as the one used in oculoplethysmography to record eye pressures. Table 6-1 lists the uses of manometry.

PROCEDURAL CARE FOR MANOMETRIC STUDIES
Before

- Explain the purpose and procedure to the patient. The patient's cooperation is essential in these studies.
- Obtain informed consent per agency polices.
- Fasting requirements vary according to the specific study performed. For example, no fasting is required for cystometry. The patient must fast for esophageal function studies.

TABLE 6-1	Manometric Studies and Areas of Evaluation
Test	**Area Evaluated**
Cystometry	Bladder
Esophageal function studies	Esophagus
Oculoplethysmography	Ophthalmic artery
Plethysmography	Arterial pressures
Tilt-table testing	Blood pressure
Urethral pressure profile	Urethra
Urine flow studies	Urine flow

During

- Patient positioning depends on the procedure indicated.
- A particular type of manometer is applied to the patient. For example, for arterial plethysmography, blood pressure cuffs are applied to the extremities; for cystometry, a catheter is inserted into the bladder and attached to a pressure monitor.
- The patient must remain very still during the procedure. Movement can affect the pressure readings.

After

- Postprocedure care varies with each particular test. For example, some tests (e.g., tourniquet test) necessitate no special aftercare. Oculoplethysmography necessitates some specific eye precautions.

POTENTIAL COMPLICATIONS OF MANOMETRIC STUDIES

Few complications are associated with these tests. The few that do occur vary markedly from test to test. For example, gastric aspiration is a potential complication of esophageal function studies. Conjunctival hemorrhage is a potential complication of oculoplethysmography.

REPORTING OF RESULTS

Most tests are performed by a technician. The physician reviews the test results and explains them to the patient.

Cystometry (Cystometrography [CMG])

NORMAL FINDINGS

Normal sensations of fullness and temperature
Normal pressures and volumes
Maximal cystometric capacity
    Male: 350–750 mL
    Female: 250–550 mL
Intravesical pressure when bladder is empty: usually <40 cm H_2O
Detrusor pressure: <10 cm H_2O
Residual urine: <30 mL

Maximal Urethral Pressures in Normal Patients (cm H$_2$O)

Age (Years)	Male	Female
<25	37–126	55–103
25–44	35–113	31–115
45–64	40–123	40–100
>64	35–105	35–75

INDICATIONS

This test is used to measure pressures within the bladder to diagnose bladder dysfunction. It is used in patients with bladder outlet obstruction, urinary incontinence, and a suspected neurogenic disorder of the bladder. It is also used to document progress in treatment of these abnormalities.

TEST EXPLANATION

The purpose of cystometry is to evaluate the motor and sensory function of the bladder when incontinence is present or neurologic bladder dysfunction is suspected. A graphic recording of pressure exerted at varying phases of the filling of the urinary bladder is produced, and a pressure/volume relationship of the bladder is determined. This urodynamic study assesses the neuromuscular function of the bladder by measuring the efficiency of the detrusor muscle, intravesical pressure and capacity, and the bladder's response to thermal stimulation.

Cystometry can determine whether a bladder function abnormality is caused by neurologic, infectious, or obstructive diseases. Cystometry is indicated to elucidate the causes of bladder outlet obstruction or frequency and urgency, especially before surgery on the urologic outflow tract. Cystometry is also part of the evaluation for incontinence, persistent residual urine, vesicoureteral reflux, motor and sensory disorders affecting the bladder, and the effect of certain drugs on bladder function.

This test is performed in approximately 45 minutes by a urologist and is often performed at the same time as cystoscopy. The only discomfort is that associated with the urethral catheterization. Nocturnal examinations can be performed to evaluate nocturnal incontinence.

CONTRAINDICATIONS

- Urinary tract infections, because of the possibility of false results and the potential for the spread of infection

 Clinical Priorities

- This is an important test for diagnosing bladder dysfunction. It can also document response to therapy.
- Certain medications can be administered during cystometry to distinguish between underactivity of the bladder that is related to muscle failure and underactivity caused by denervation.
- This test can be performed at the same time as cystoscopy.
- Patients should be carefully evaluated for infection after this test.

PROCEDURE AND PATIENT CARE

Before

- Explain the purpose and the procedure to the patient.
- Inform the patient that no fluid or food restrictions are required.
- Assure the patient that he or she will be draped to prevent unnecessary exposure.
- Assess the patient for signs and symptoms of urinary tract infection.
- Instruct the patient not to strain while voiding because the results can be skewed.
- If the patient has a spinal cord injury, transport him or her on a stretcher. The test will then be performed with the patient on the stretcher.

During

- Note the following procedural steps:
  1. The patient is first asked to void.
  2. The amount of time required to initiate voiding and the size, force, and continuity of the urinary stream are recorded. The amount of urine, the time of voiding, and the presence of any straining, hesitancy, or terminal urine dribbling are also recorded. (See the discussion of urine flow studies, p. 729.)
  3. The patient is then placed in a lithotomy or supine position.
  4. A retention catheter is inserted through the urethra and into the bladder.
  5. Residual urine volume is measured and recorded.
  6. Thermal sensation is evaluated by the instillation of approximately 30 mL of room-temperature saline solution into the bladder, followed by an equal amount of warm water. The patient reports any sensations such as pain, flushing, sweating, or an urgency to void.
  7. This fluid is then withdrawn from the bladder.
  8. The urethral catheter is connected to a cystometer (a machine used to monitor bladder pressure).
  9. Sterile water, normal saline solution, or carbon dioxide gas is slowly introduced into the bladder at a controlled rate, usually with the patient in a sitting position. While the bladder is slowly filled, pressures are simultaneously recorded. This procedure is called *cystometrography.*
  10. Patients are asked to indicate when they first feel the urge to void and then when they have the feeling that they must void. The bladder is full at this time.
  11. The pressures and volumes are plotted on a graph.
  12. The patient is asked to void around the catheter, and the maximal intravesical voiding pressure is recorded.
  13. The bladder is drained for any residual fluid or gas.
  14. If no additional studies are to be done, the urethral catheter is removed.
  15. For urethral pressures, fluid or gas is instilled through the catheter, which is withdrawn while pressures along the urethral wall are obtained. (See the discussion of the urethral pressure profile, p. 728.)
- Throughout the study, ask the patient to report any sensations, such as pain, flushing, sweating, nausea, bladder filling, and an urgency to void.
- Note that certain drugs may be administered during the cystometric examination to distinguish between underactivity of the bladder caused by muscle failure and underactivity caused by denervation. Cholinergic drugs (e.g., bethanechol [Duvoid]) may be given to enhance the tone of a flaccid bladder. Anticholinergic drugs (e.g., atropine) may be given to promote relaxation of a hyperactive bladder. If these drugs are to be administered, the catheter is left in place.

After these drugs are administered, the examination is repeated 20 to 30 minutes later; the first test result is used as a control value. The information obtained with the drugs assists in the decision of whether drugs will be effective treatment.

After

- Observe the patient for any manifestations of infection (e.g., elevated temperature, chills, or dysuria).
- Examine the urine for hematuria. If the hematuria persists after several voidings, notify the physician.
- Provide a warm sitz bath or tub bath for comfort if the patient desires.
- Note that pelvic floor sphincter electromyography (p. 602) can be performed to evaluate the urethral sphincter in incontinent patients.

TEST RESULTS AND CLINICAL SIGNIFICANCE

Neurogenic disorder of the bladder: *With loss of motor function of the bladder, filling pressures and detrusor pressures are reduced, and residual volume of urine is increased. Sensation of fullness and temperature is often diminished or absent. There are several different classifications of neurogenic disorders of the bladder, some of which are based on the cystometric findings. Spina bifida, cord injury, compression, or demyelinating diseases can cause a neurogenic disorder of the bladder. Diabetic neuropathy, anticholinergic agents, and alpha-adrenergic antagonists also diminish bladder muscle tone. Extensive pelvic surgery can interrupt the peripheral nerve fibres to the bladder, thereby creating a neurogenic disorder of the bladder.*

Bladder obstruction: *Bladder outlet obstruction is evidenced by reduced urine flow, increased intravesicular pressures during voiding, and residual urine volume. Although bladder outlet obstruction can have congenital causes (e.g., urethral valves, phimosis, meatal stenosis), the most common cause of bladder outlet obstruction is a prostatic pathologic condition (cancer or hypertrophy). In women, the most common cause of outlet obstruction is a neoplasm (usually of the cervix) or a neurogenic disorder of the bladder (see previous discussion of neurogenic disorder of the bladder).*

Bladder infection: *Urgency and reduced bladder capacity are noted. Discomfort associated with bladder distension may be enhanced.*

Bladder hypertonicity: *Increased pressures are noted with filling. Capacity is reduced. This occurs with some forms of spastic paralysis. This is most common with upper motor neuron disease or injury.*

Diminished bladder capacity: *This may be the result of fibrosis that occurs after radiation therapy or the result of compression of the bladder by an extrinsic tumour. A fibrotic and inflamed bladder cannot distend adequately. Likewise, when a tumour compresses the bladder, the bladder cannot distend. Capacity is thereby reduced.*

RELATED TESTS

Urine Flow Studies (p. 729). In these studies, urine flow is measured per unit of time, and the values are used to diagnose bladder outlet obstruction.

Pelvic Floor Sphincter Electromyography (p. 602). This study is a measurement of the electrical activity of the periurethral sphincter function.

Cystography (p. 1075). This is a radiographic contrast study of the bladder. Outlet obstruction is evident on this study.

Esophageal Function Studies (Esophageal Manometry, Esophageal Motility Studies)

NORMAL FINDINGS

Lower esophageal sphincter pressure: 10–20 mm Hg
Swallowing pattern: normal peristaltic waves
Acid reflux: none
Acid clearing: <10 swallows
Bernstein test: negative result

INDICATIONS

This test is used to identify and document the severity of diseases affecting the swallowing function of the esophagus. It is also used to document and quantify gastroesophageal reflux. A wide variety of motor disturbances can be identified. It is commonly used in patients with heartburn, chest pain, or difficulty swallowing.

TEST EXPLANATION

Esophageal function studies include the following:
1. Determination of the lower esophageal sphincter (LES) pressure (manometry)
2. Graphic recording of esophageal swallowing waves, or swallowing pattern (manometry)
3. Detection of reflux of gastric acid back into the esophagus (acid reflux)
4. Detection of the ability of the esophagus to clear acid (acid clearing)
5. An attempt to reproduce symptoms of heartburn (Bernstein test)

Manometric Studies

Two manometric studies are used in assessing esophageal function: (1) measurement of LES pressure and (2) graphic recording of swallowing waves (motility). The LES is a sphincter muscle that acts as a valve to prevent reflux of gastric acid into the esophagus. Free reflux of gastric acid occurs when the sphincter pressures are low. An example of such a disorder in adults is gastroesophageal reflux; an example in children is chalasia (incompetent or relaxed LES).

With increased sphincter pressure, as found in patients with achalasia (failure of the LES to relax normally with swallowing) and with diffuse esophageal spasms, food cannot pass from the esophagus into the stomach. Increased LES pressures are noted on manometry. In achalasia, few if any swallowing waves are detected. In contrast, diffuse esophageal spasm is characterized by strong, frequent, asynchronous, and nonpropulsive waves.

Acid Reflux With pH Probe

Acid reflux is the primary component of gastroesophageal reflux. Patients with an incompetent LES regurgitate gastric acid into the esophagus. This then causes a drop in the esophageal pH during esophageal pH monitoring. With the newer and smaller catheters, 24-hour pH monitoring can be performed. Episodes of acid reflux are evident during this monitoring. If they coincide with the patient's symptoms of chest pain, esophagitis may be the cause. Transnasal pH catheters can cause discomfort in patients, sometimes causing them to avoid pH testing, which is the "gold standard" for measuring pH levels in the esophagus. Such avoidance limits the clinician's ability to definitively diagnose and ultimately treat gastroesophageal reflux disease.

6   Manometric Studies

With wireless pH probes, patients can eat and drink normally, as well as engage in their usual activities, while having their pH levels tested. A small, wireless pH-probe capsule is now being used with increasing frequency. It collects pH data in the esophagus and transmits it via radiofrequency telemetry to an external pager-sized receiver worn by the patient. This allows patients to maintain regular diet and activities during the monitoring period (24 to 48 hours). The pH capsule is attached to the wall of the esophagus by esophagoscopy (p. 636). Within days, the capsule spontaneously sloughs off the wall of the esophagus and passes through the patient's gastrointestinal tract. After the study is completed, the patient returns the receiver, and the data is downloaded to a computer for analysis.

Acid Clearing

Patients with normal esophageal function can completely clear hydrochloric acid from the esophagus in fewer than 10 swallows. Patients with decreased esophageal motility (frequently caused by severe esophagitis) require a greater number of swallows to clear the acid.

Bernstein Test (Acid Perfusion)

The Bernstein test is simply an attempt to reproduce the symptoms of gastroesophageal reflux. If the patient suffers pain with the instillation of hydrochloric acid into the esophagus, the test result is positive and is proof that the patient's symptoms are caused by reflux esophagitis. If the patient has no discomfort, a cause other than esophageal reflux must be sought to explain the patient's discomfort.

CONTRAINDICATIONS

- Patient's inability to cooperate
- Medical instability

POTENTIAL COMPLICATIONS

- Aspiration of gastric contents

INTERFERING FACTORS

- Eating shortly before the test may affect results.
- Drugs such as sedatives can alter test results. Other drugs that can reduce the LES include nitroglycerine, anticholinergics, beta-adrenergic agonists, and benzodiazepines.

PROCEDURE AND PATIENT CARE

Before

- Explain the procedure to the patient.
- Instruct the patient not to eat or drink anything for at least 8 hours before the test.
- Allow the patient to verbalize concerns, and allay those concerns. Be sensitive to the patient's fears about choking during the procedure.

During

- Note the following procedural steps:
  1. Esophageal studies are usually performed in the endoscopy laboratory.
  2. The fasting, unsedated patient is asked to swallow two or three very tiny tubes. The tubes are equipped so that pressure measurements can be taken at 5-cm intervals (Figure 6-1).

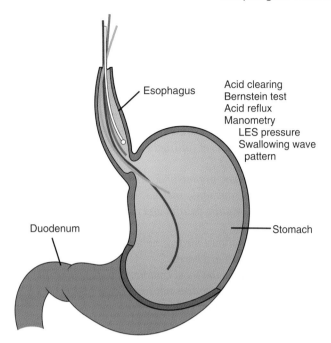

Esophagus

Acid clearing
Bernstein test
Acid reflux
Manometry
LES pressure
Swallowing wave
pattern

Duodenum

Stomach

Figure 6-1 Illustration of esophageal function studies, demonstrating placement of manometry tubes and a pH probe within the esophagus. LES, lower esophageal sphincter.

3. The outer ends of the tubes are attached to a pressure transducer.
4. All tubes are passed into the stomach; then three tubes are slowly pulled back into the esophagus. A rapid and extreme increase in the pressure readings indicates the high-pressure zone of the LES.
5. The LES pressure is recorded.
6. With all tubes in the esophagus, the patient is asked to swallow. Motility wave patterns are recorded.
7. The pH indicator probe is placed in the esophagus.
8. The patient's stomach is filled with approximately 100 mL of hydrochloric acid at a concentration of **0.1 mol/L** (commonly written as "0.1-N"). A decrease in the pH of the esophageal pH probe indicates gastroesophageal reflux.
9. Hydrochloric acid is instilled into the esophagus, and the patient is asked to swallow. The number of swallows is counted to determine acid clearing. More than 10 swallows to clear the acid (as determined by the pH probe) indicate decreased esophageal motility.
10. Finally, 0.1-N hydrochloric acid and saline solution are alternately instilled into the esophagus for the Bernstein test. The patient is not informed which solution is being infused. If the patient volunteers symptoms of discomfort while the acid is running, the test result is considered positive. If no discomfort is recognized, the test result is negative.

• Note that these tests are performed in approximately 30 minutes by an esophageal technician.
- Inform the patient that the test results are interpreted by a physician and are available in several hours.
- Inform the patient that, except for some initial gagging when he or she swallows the tubes, these tests are not uncomfortable.

After

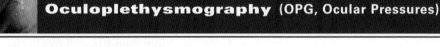 Inform the patient that it is not unusual to have a mildly sore throat after placement of the tubes.

TEST RESULTS AND CLINICAL SIGNIFICANCE

Presbyesophagus: *This is a common motility pattern noted in older adults. It is evident as synchronous esophageal contractions. As a result, the food is not propelled down the esophagus but, rather, becomes temporarily lodged between the two areas of contraction. This can be quite painful and can cause a functional obstruction to the passage of food.*

Diffuse esophageal spasm: *Spastic synchronously occurring contractions of the esophagus do not allow the food to be propelled down the esophagus; instead, it becomes lodged temporarily between the two areas of contraction. This, too, can be quite painful and can cause a functional obstruction to the passage of food.*

Chalasia: *Absence of tone in the LES allows for free reflux of food and gastric juices into the esophagus. This is a common cause of vomiting in newborns.*

Achalasia: *This is the opposite of chalasia and most commonly occurs in young adults. The tone of the LES is significantly increased, and the sphincter does not relax. As a result, the LES acts as an obstruction to the passage of food through the esophagus.*

Gastroesophageal reflux,

Reflux esophagitis: *The presence of gastric contents in the esophagus causes esophagitis. The pathophysiologic mechanism underlying gastroesophageal reflux is not completely understood. It is known that the LES tone is reduced, which allows reflux of acid into the esophagus. This is evident during pH monitoring. Esophagitis follows, and acid clearing is prolonged because the swallowing function of the inflamed esophagus is reduced.*

RELATED TESTS

Esophagogastroduodenoscopy (p. 636). Esophagoscopy is an endoscopic test of the esophagus. The processes of reflux esophagitis, esophageal obstruction, achalasia, and other diseases can be observed.

Barium Swallow (p. 1038). This is a radiographic study of the esophagus. Evidence of diseases of the esophagus (reflux esophagitis, esophageal obstruction, achalasia) can be visualized.

Oculoplethysmography (OPG, Ocular Pressures)

NORMAL FINDINGS

Normal and equal blood flow in both carotid arteries

INDICATIONS

Oculoplethysmography is a method of indirectly determining the flow within the internal carotid artery. It is used to identify carotid arterial atherosclerotic occlusive disease.

Oculoplethysmography is indicated in patients who have symptoms of carotid occlusive disease (e.g., transient ischemic attacks, carotid bruits, neurologic symptoms such as dizziness and fainting). This test is often performed to monitor the success of carotid endarterectomy.

TEST EXPLANATION

Oculoplethysmography is a noninvasive study used to indirectly measure blood flow in the ophthalmic artery. Because the ophthalmic artery is the first major branch of the internal carotid artery, its blood flow reflects the carotid blood flow and the alternative blood flow to the brain.

   For this study, eye pressures are measured through suction cups placed on the eyes for the recording. If the pressures measured are reduced (in comparison with normal pressure or in comparison with pressure in the other eye), carotid atherosclerotic occlusive disease is suspected. This procedure may be followed by cerebral angiography, if indicated. Carotid Doppler flow studies (p. 903) are more easily performed and less invasive and are therefore being used more frequently.

CONTRAINDICATIONS

- Eye surgery within the past 2 to 6 months
- A lens implant
- History of retinal detachment
- Cataracts
- Eye infection
- Allergy to local anaesthetics

POTENTIAL COMPLICATIONS

- Conjunctival hemorrhage
- Corneal abrasions: If corneal abrasions occur, a lubricant (e.g., Dacriose solution) is applied to the patient's eye, and then the eye is covered with a patch.
- Transient photophobia

PROCEDURE AND PATIENT CARE

Before

- Explain the procedure to the patient.
- Instruct the patient to arrange for transportation after the test if necessary.
- Inform the patient that eyes usually burn slightly when the ophthalmic drops are applied.
- Inform the patient that when suction is applied, he or she may feel a pulling sensation and vision may temporarily be lost.
- If the patient is wearing contact lenses, instruct the patient to remove the lenses.
- If the patient has glaucoma, advise the patient to take the usual medications and eye drops.
- Inform the patient that no fasting or sedation is necessary.

During

- Note the following procedural steps:
  1. The patient is asked to lie on his or her back on a table or bed.
  2. Blood pressure in both arms is taken before the test.
  3. Electrocardiographic electrodes are applied to the patient's extremities to detect abnormal cardiac rhythms.
  4. Anaesthetic eye drops are instilled in both eyes to minimize discomfort.
  5. Small detectors are attached to the earlobes to detect blood flow to the ear through the external carotid artery.

6. Tracings of blood flow in both ears are taken and compared.
7. Suction cups resembling contact lenses are applied directly to the eyeballs.
8. Tracings of the pulsations within each eye are recorded.
9. A vacuum source is applied to the suction cup. This increased pressure causes the pulse in both eyes to disappear temporarily, because all blood flow to the eye is stopped.
10. When the suction source is stopped, the blood flow returns to the eyes. Both pulses should return simultaneously.
11. The time difference in the pulse rate from one eye to the other, one ear to the other, and one ear to the eye on the other side is measured in milliseconds. If internal carotid stenosis is present, blood flow to the eye, on the affected side, is delayed.

- Note that a trained technologist performs this test in approximately 20 to 30 minutes.

After

✗ Inform the patient that the eye anaesthetic usually wears off in approximately 30 minutes.
✗ Instruct the patient not to rub his or her eyes for at least 2 hours. If tears appear, the eye should be blotted dry.
✗ Inform the patient that contact lenses should not be inserted for at least 2 hours after oculoplethysmography.

Home Care Responsibilities

- Inform the patient that the eyes may appear bloodshot for several hours after the test.
- Artificial tears may be instilled to soothe any irritation in the eyes.
- Advise the patient to wear sunglasses if photophobia is present.
- Instruct the patient to report pain or severe burning sensation in the eyes.

TEST RESULTS AND CLINICAL SIGNIFICANCE

Carotid atherosclerotic stenosis: *Carotid arterial occlusive plaques can significantly reduce carotid artery blood flow, as determined on oculoplethysmography.*

RELATED TESTS

Carotid Artery Duplex Scan (p. 903). Doppler flow study of the carotid artery is an accurate and more easily performed method of identifying and monitoring carotid arterial occlusive disease.

Arteriography (p. 1026). Cerebral angiography is a radiographic examination of the carotid artery and its branches. This is an invasive method to more clearly delineate carotid anatomy and pathologic conditions.

Plethysmography, Arterial

NORMAL FINDINGS

<20 mm Hg difference in systolic blood pressure between the lower extremity and the upper extremity

Normal pulse wave amplitude showing a steep upswing; an acute, narrow peak; and a gentler
   downward slope containing a dicrotic notch (normal arterial pulse wave)
Ankle/brachial ratio: 0.9–1.3.

INDICATIONS

This is a noninvasive method of identifying and monitoring treatment of arterial occlusive
disease.

TEST EXPLANATION

Plethysmography is usually performed to rule out occlusive disease of the lower extremities; however, it also can identify arteriosclerotic disease in the upper extremities. For this
test, one extremity must be normal, so as to compare normal findings with those in the other
extremities.

This test usually is performed in approximately 30 minutes in the noninvasive vascular laboratory or at the patient's bedside by a noninvasive vascular technologist. In arterial plethysmography, three blood pressure cuffs are applied to the proximal, middle, and distal parts of an
extremity. Pressure readings are also taken in the upper arm (brachial) artery. The blood pressure
cuffs are then attached to a pulse volume recorder (plethysmograph) that enables each pulse
wave to be displayed. A reduction in amplitude of a pulse wave in any of the three cuffs indicates
arterial occlusion immediately proximal to the area where the decreased amplitude is noted. Also,
arterial pressures are measured at each cuff site. A difference in pressure of more than 20 mm
Hg indicates a degree of arterial occlusion in the extremity. A positive result is reliable evidence
of arteriosclerotic peripheral vascular occlusion. However, a negative result does not definitely
exclude this diagnosis, because extensive vascular collateralization can compensate for even a
complete arterial occlusion.

An *ankle/brachial ratio* of less than 0.9 indicates peripheral vascular disease in the lower
extremity. Arterial plethysmography can also be performed immediately after exercise to
determine whether symptoms of claudication are caused by peripheral vascular occlusive
disease.

Although it is not as accurate as arteriography (see p. 1026), plethysmography entails no serious complications and can be performed in extremely ill patients who cannot be transported to
the arteriography laboratory.

INTERFERING FACTORS

• Arterial occlusion proximal to the extremity
• Cigarette smoking, because nicotine can cause transient arterial constriction

Clinical Priorities

• A positive result is reliable evidence of arteriosclerotic peripheral vascular occlusion.
• Patients should not smoke before this test because nicotine causes constriction of the peripheral
  arteries and thereby alters test results.
• This test is usually performed in approximately 30 minutes by a technologist in the noninvasive
  vascular laboratory or at the patient's bedside.

**Manometric
Studies**

6

PROCEDURE AND PATIENT CARE

Before

✗ Explain the procedure to the patient.
✗ Inform the patient that this test is painless.
✗ Inform the patient that he or she must lie still during the testing procedure.
✗ Instruct the patient to avoid smoking for at least 30 minutes before the test. Nicotine creates constriction of the peripheral arteries and alters the test results.
✗ Inform the patient that no fasting is required.
• Remove all clothing from the patient's extremities.

During

• Note the following procedural steps:
  1. The patient is placed in the semirecumbent position.
  2. The cuffs are applied to the extremities and then inflated to 65 mm Hg to increase their sensitivity to pulse waves.
  3. The pulse waves are recorded on the plethysmographic paper.
  4. The amplitudes and form of the pulse wave of each cuff are measured and compared. A marked reduction in wave amplitude indicates arterial occlusive disease.
✗ Inform the patient that results are usually interpreted by a physician and are available in several hours.
✗ Remind the patient that no discomfort is associated with this test.

After

✗ Encourage the patient to verbalize any concerns regarding the test results, and allay those concerns.

TEST RESULTS AND CLINICAL SIGNIFICANCE

Arterial atherosclerotic occlusive disease,
Arterial trauma,
Arterial embolization: *A decreased pressure in the cuff immediately distal to the occlusion notes arterial occlusion.*
Small vessel diabetic changes: *Little or no change may be noted in this disease. Vascular insufficiency in small vessels is usually observed in diabetic patients.*
Vascular diseases (e.g., Raynaud's phenomenon): *Arterial occlusion that is episodic is classic for Raynaud's phenomenon. This is difficult to identify on plethysmography unless larger vessels of the wrist or hand are involved. Often this diagnosis requires that pressure-sensitive cuffs be placed on the fingers.*

RELATED TESTS

Arteriography (p. 1026). This is a radiographic examination of the arteries of the extremities. Although more invasive and associated with greater complications, arteriography is more accurate than plethysmography.

Carotid Artery Duplex Scan (p. 903). Doppler arterial flow study is an ultrasound examination to determine blood flow within the artery suspected to be stenotic. This is a very accurate test of arterial patency.

Tilt-Table Testing

NORMAL FINDINGS

<20 mm Hg decrease in systolic blood pressure and <10 mm Hg increase in diastolic blood pressure
Heart rate increase <10 beats/minute

INDICATIONS

The tilt-table test is a test used to diagnose vasopressor syncope. It can help to understand the effect of posture and medications on blood pressure.

TEST EXPLANATION

Patients with this vasomotor syncope syndrome usually demonstrate symptomatic hypotension and syncope within a few to 30 minutes of being tilted upright by approximately 60 to 90 degrees. This test is usually performed along with an electrophysiologic study (p. 587). Tilt-table testing is often used to assess the efficacy of prophylactic pacing in some patients with vasopressor syncope. It is also used to evaluate the effect of posture on some forms of tachyarrhythmias. Normally, in the tilted position, systolic blood pressure drops minimally, diastolic blood pressure rises, and heart rate increases. In patients with vasopressor syncope, these changes are exaggerated, and they become lightheaded and dizzy on assuming the tilted position.

INTERFERING FACTORS

- Patients with dehydration or hypovolemia demonstrate comparable changes in blood pressure and heart rate. This is especially true in older adult patients.
- Patients taking antihypertensive medications or diuretics also may demonstrate similar changes when placed in the tilted position.

PROCEDURE AND PATIENT CARE

Before

- Explain the procedure to the patient.
- Patient should fast after midnight.
- Obtain intravenous access in the event that emergency drugs are required.
- Note that an arterial line may be placed to accurately monitor blood pressure, or cardiac monitoring may be initiated.
- Ask whether the patient has had excessive fluid loss (diarrhea or vomiting) in the previous 24 hours.
- Record any medications the patient is taking, including antihypertensive or diuretic medicines.

During

- Position the patient supine on a horizontal tilt table.
- Obtain the patient's blood pressure and pulse as baseline values before tilting is carried out.
- Monitor these vital signs during the procedure.

⇡ Question the patient about the presence of symptoms of dizziness and lightheadedness.
- Note that the table is progressively tilted to 60 to 80 degrees while the patient is being monitored. Alternatively, the patient is asked to sit or stand.

After
- Monitor the arterial intravenous site for bleeding after removal of the vascular access.
- Firmly secure a pressure dressing to both sites (arterial and venous).
- Monitor the vital signs as the patient adjusts to positioning changes.

TEST RESULTS AND CLINICAL SIGNIFICANCE

Vasomotor syncope: *Tachyarrhythmias, overmedication for hypertension or heart disease, hyperreactive vagal activity, and various forms of vasomotor instability can cause a positive result on a tilt-table test.*

RELATED TEST

Electrophysiologic Study (p. 587). This is a method of studying evoked potentials within the heart. It is used to evaluate patients with syncope, palpitations, or arrhythmias.

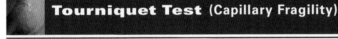

Tourniquet Test (Capillary Fragility)

NORMAL FINDINGS
<2 Petechiae

INDICATIONS

This test evaluates capillary integrity and platelet number and function. It is part of the new WHO case definition for dengue fever and can be used as a triage tool to help differentiate between dengue fever and other conditions such as acute gastroenteritis.

TEST EXPLANATION

Petechiae are small, round nonraised red spots in the skin. They occur as a result of increased capillary fragility (microvessels easily rupture, and a small amount of bleeding occurs just under the skin) or as a result of thrombocytopenia (causing spontaneous bleeding under the skin).

Production of petechiae can be induced in patients who have increased capillary fragility or thrombocytopenia. There are two methods of inducing petechiae. The most common method is with positive pressure; a blood pressure cuff is applied to an extremity and inflated above venous pressure. The second method is with negative pressure; a suction cup is applied to an area of skin for a specific period of time. Patients with thrombocytopenia, poor platelet function, purpura, or dengue develop petechiae. The number of petechiae are counted per 6 cm^2 (per square inch) and is graded as follows:

1+: Few petechiae present
2+: Many petechiae present
3+: Multiple petechiae present over a broader area
4+: Confluent petechiae present

The number of petechiae is generally proportional to the severity of the disease. A positive test is more than approximately 10 petechaie per 6 cm^2 (per square inch). The size of petechiae, if uniform, may indicate the source of the positive result. Large petechiae are associated with thrombocytopenia. Pinpoint petechiae are more likely to be related to increased capillary fragility.

INTERFERING FACTORS

- Premenstrual women experience transient episodes of increased capillary fragility.
- Postmenopausal women who do not use hormones experience increased capillary fragility.
- Women, especially those with sun-damaged skin, can have increased capillary fragility.
- Prolonged use of steroids increases capillary fragility.

PROCEDURE AND PATIENT CARE

Before

- Explain the procedure to the patient.
- Obtain informed consent from the patient, if it is required by the institution.
- Inform the patient that no fasting is required.
- Examine the extremity for pre-existing petechiae or ecchymoses.

During

Positive Pressure Test

- Take the patient's blood pressure and record.
- Place a blood pressure cuff on the upper arm and inflate it to midway between systolic plus diastolic blood pressure and maintain for 5 minutes (e.g., systolic (100) + diastolic (80) ÷ 2 = 90, so inflate cuff to 90 and maintain for 5 minutes).
- Relieve the cuff pressure and wait 2 minutes.
- Inspect the distal extremity for petechiae. Count the petichiae below the anticubital fossa.

Negative Pressure Test

- Place a lubricated suction cup (2 cm in diameter) on the skin of the upper arm.
- Remove the suction cup after 1 minute.
- Examine the site for petechiae.

After

- Explain the results to the patient.
- If the result is positive, explain to the patient that appropriate precautions should be taken to avoid injury to soft tissues.

TEST RESULTS AND CLINICAL SIGNIFICANCE

Positive: Fewer Than Two Petechiae

Immunologic thrombocytopenia (e.g., idiopathic thrombocytopenic purpura),
Drug-induced thrombocytopenia,
Thromboasthenia (poor platelet function): *Reduced platelets cause spontaneous microbleeding. Nonimmunologic thrombocytopenia is rarely associated with a positive result of the tourniquet test.*
Hereditary telangiectasia,
Vascular purpura (autoimmune diseases),

Senile purpura,
Allergic purpura,
Scurvy: *Increased capillary permeability causes petechiae.*
Hemophilia: *Spontaneous bleeding causes petechiae.*

RELATED TESTS

Platelet Count (p. 416). This is a direct measurement of platelet number.
   Platelet Volume, Mean (p. 419). This is a direct measurement of platelet volume.
   Platelet Aggregation (p. 409). This is a direct measurement of platelet function.
   Platelet Antibody (p. 411). This test identifies platelet antibodies that destroy platelets.

 Urethral Pressure Profile (UPP, Urethral Pressure Measurements)

NORMAL FINDINGS

Maximal Urethral Pressures in Normal Patients (cm H_2O)

Age (Years)	Male	Female
<25	37–126	55–103
25–44	35–113	31–115
45–64	40–123	40–100
>64	35–105	35–75

INDICATIONS

This test is often a part of cystometry (p. 713). It is used to document reduced urethral pressures in incontinent patients (e.g., women with stress incontinence or men after prostatectomy). It is also used to indicate the degree of compression applied to the urethra from an abnormally enlarged prostate (which will increase urethral pressure profile value).

TEST EXPLANATION

The urethral pressure profile indicates the intraluminal pressure along the length of the urethra with the bladder at rest. Indications for this urodynamic investigation include the following:
1. Assessment of prostatic obstruction
2. Assessment of stress incontinence in women
3. Assessment of the postprostatectomy sequela of incontinence
4. Assessment of the adequacy of external sphincterotomy
5. Analysis of the effects of drugs on the urethra
6. Analysis of the effects of stimulation on urethral flow
7. Assessment of the adequacy of implanted artificial urethral sphincter devices

This test is usually performed in less than 15 minutes by a urologist. This test is only slightly more uncomfortable than urethral catheterization.

CONTRAINDICATIONS

• Urinary tract infections, because catheterization may induce bacteremia

PROCEDURE AND PATIENT CARE

Before

 Explain the procedure to the patient.

Because many patients are embarrassed by this procedure, assure the patient that he or she will be draped to ensure privacy.

Inform the patient that no fasting or sedation is required.

During

- Note the following procedural steps:
  1. A catheter is placed into the bladder and attached to a pressure monitor machine.
  2. Fluids (or gas) are instilled through the catheter, which is withdrawn while the pressures along the urethral wall are measured.
  3. A motorized syringe pump maintains a constant infusion of the fluids or gas.
  4. The catheter is removed.

After

- The patient may take a sitz bath, if desired.

TEST RESULTS AND CLINICAL SIGNIFICANCE

Prostatic obstruction secondary to benign prostatic hypertrophy or cancer: *Increased urethral pressures are noted because of the extrinsic compression applied by the enlarged prostate.*

Urinary incontinence: *Reduced urethral pressures are noted because of the reduced tone of the urethral sphincter.*

RELATED TEST

Cystometry (p. 713). This test often includes the urethral pressure profile. Cystometry, which can identify bladder neuromuscular pathologic conditions, is a measure of bladder pressures.

Urine Flow Studies (Uroflowmetry, Urodynamic Studies)

NORMAL FINDINGS

Depend on the patient's age, gender, and volume voided

INDICATIONS

This test is a measurement of the urine flow rate during micturition. If the rate is reduced, outflow obstruction can be documented and measured. The test is used to monitor micturition for decisions concerning timing and adequacy of treatment. It is indicated to investigate dysfunctional voiding or suspected outflow tract obstruction. It is also performed before and after any procedure designed to modify the function of the urologic outflow tract.

Manometric Studies

6

TEST EXPLANATION

Uroflowmetry is the simplest of the urodynamic techniques, being noninvasive and requiring uncomplicated and relatively inexpensive equipment. The volume of urine expelled from the bladder is measured per second.

The urine flow depends greatly on the volume of urine voided. Normally, on initiation of urination, flow is slow. However, almost immediately, flow rate rapidly rises until bladder volume quickly decreases. Then the flow decreases rapidly. In patients with outlet obstruction—for example, secondary to an enlarged prostate—the flow slowly rises to a level lower than normal. The flow plateaus for a longer time until the bladder volume decreases, and then flow diminishes slowly. The flow rates are highest and most predictable in the urine volume range of 200 to 400 mL. When the bladder contains more than 400 mL of urine, the efficiency of the bladder muscle is greatly decreased. Nomograms of maximal flow versus voided volume may be used for accurate test result interpretation; these guidelines must take into account the patient's gender and age. If the flow rates are abnormally low, the test should be repeated to check for accuracy.

Modern urine flowmeters provide a permanent graphic recording. If flowmeters are not available, the patient can time the urinary stream with a stopwatch and record the voided volume; in this way, the average flow is calculated.

In some cases, it is more valuable to analyze several voided volumes and flow rates rather than a single flow rate. If this is to be done, the patient is taught to use a flowmeter. A graph of flow versus volume can be plotted. Together with clinical observation, this provides valuable information on the severity of outflow obstruction, the likelihood of urinary retention, and the state of compensation or decompensation of the detrusor muscle.

This test is often performed in conjunction with cystometry (p. 713).

PROCEDURE AND PATIENT CARE

Before

- Explain the procedure to the patient.
- Instruct the patient to arrive for the test with a full bladder.
- Instruct the patient how to void into the urine flowmeter.
- Determine the number of flow rates that will be needed.

During

- Note that this test should be performed when the patient has a normal desire to void and in conditions suitable for privacy. The bladder should be adequately full. Essentially, all the patient must do is urinate into the flowmeter. Several different types of flowmeters are available.
- Inform the patient that no discomfort is associated with this test.
- Note that the duration of this test is several seconds.

After

- Record the position of the patient, the method of filling the bladder (it should be natural), and whether this study was part of another evaluation.

TEST RESULTS AND CLINICAL SIGNIFICANCE

Dysfunctional voiding: *Flow rates may be normal but intermittent or delayed.*

Outflow tract obstruction: *Flow rates are diminished significantly, which indicates obstruction caused by urethral stricture, prostatic cancer, or hypertrophy. The flow rate curve plateaus at a lower rate and stays there longer than normal.*

RELATED TEST

Cystometry (p. 713). This is a measurement of the pressures within the bladder during filling and micturition. Uroflowmetry may be part of that study.

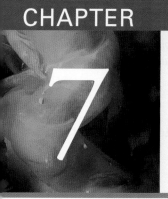

Microscopic Examinations

NOTE: *Throughout this chapter, SI units are presented in* boldface colour, *followed by conventional units in parentheses.*

OVERVIEW

TESTS

OVERVIEW
REASONS FOR PERFORMING MICROSCOPIC STUDIES

Microscopic examinations are essential for the diagnosis and treatment of numerous diseases and infectious processes. Included in this chapter are descriptions of microbiologic studies and studies that require a microscopic review of tissue. Microbiologic specimens can be collected from many sources, such as tissue and organ biopsy samples, blood, urine, wound drainage, cervical secretions, and sputum. This testing usually takes place in the microbiology or bacteriology section of the laboratory. Microscopic examination is used in a wide variety of clinical situations, some of which include the following:

1. To evaluate hematologic disorders (bone marrow biopsy)
2. To detect sexually transmitted infections (sexually transmitted infection culture)
3. To evaluate dysfunctional uterine bleeding (endometrial biopsy)
4. To determine pathologic liver conditions (liver biopsy)
5. To detect lung cancer (lung biopsy)
6. To screen for cancer of the vagina, cervix, and uterus (Papanicolaou smear)
7. To determine the sensitivity of breast cancer to hormonal therapy (estrogen and progesterone receptor assays)
8. To detect renal disease, such as malignancy, glomerulonephritis, and transplant rejection (renal biopsy)
9. To detect tuberculosis (tuberculosis culture)
10. To evaluate and treat infections (wound and soft tissue culture and sensitivity)

Microscopic examinations are used to evaluate histologic and cytologic specimens and to identify bacteria (and other infecting organisms). Determination of hormone receptor assay results along with chromatin identification also requires microscopic examination of various types.

Included in microscopic studies are culture and sensitivity testing. Microscopic examination is an important part of identifying an infecting organism. A *Gram stain* is just one of the microscopic examinations performed with microbiologic testing. A Gram stain is a method by which all bacteria are classified. All forms of bacteria are grossly classified as Gram-positive (turning blue with staining) or Gram-negative (turning red with staining). Furthermore, knowledge of the shape of the organism (e.g., spherical, rod-shaped) also may be very helpful in the tentative identification of the infecting organism. For example, if the Gram stain indicates the presence of Gram-negative rods, the infecting organism may be *Escherichia coli.* With knowledge of the Gram stain results, the physician can institute reasonable antibiotic treatment on the basis of past experiences regarding the organism's possible identity. The Gram stain can yield results less than 10 minutes after the specimen is smeared on a microscopic slide. Treatment can then be altered on the basis of the final results of culture and sensitivity testing.

The usual culture is obtained from a smear of an infected area (e.g., a wound culture). However, body fluids or tissue samples can be subjected to culture techniques. When smeared on the appropriate culture medium, an infecting organism can be expected to grow. It is important that several different kinds of culture media are used in the culture process to maximize the chances of growing the infecting organism. Some bacteria or fungi grow better in one medium than in another.

In most cases, the infecting organism is identified from a culture plate on which the organism is growing. In rare situations, the infecting organism is found by microscopic review of a tissue specimen. In still other situations, the only evidence of infection is derived from serologic testing (e.g., antistreptolysin O titre; see Chapter 2).

Although no potential complications are associated with culture testing, the risks involved in obtaining tissue for microscopic examination may be considerable. They are well outlined in the discussion of each specific study.

PROCEDURAL CARE FOR MICROSCOPIC STUDIES
Before
- Explain the procedure to the patient.
- Inform the patient of any special preprocedure requirements. For example, patients should not use douches or take a tub bath before cervical cultures for herpes. Men should not void for 1 hour before collection of urethral specimens.
- Inform the patient about the collection technique. These techniques vary from being noninvasive (throat culture) to invasive (liver biopsy).
- Invasive studies require an informed consent. Coagulation profile studies are often performed before invasive studies because of the risk of bleeding.
- If an invasive procedure is to be performed to obtain tissue, the patient should be prepared as if surgery were a possibility, because if bleeding or organ injury occurs, the patient may need immediate surgery.

During
- Follow universal precautions in handling all specimens because of the risk of transmitting infection.
- Specific protocols for collection are described with each test in this chapter.
- Instruct the patient to remain still during specimen collection. The quality of the specimen depends in part on the cooperation of the patient.

After
- The specimen should be carefully labelled with the patient's name, the source, and any other pertinent information, such as whether the patient is receiving antibiotic therapy.
- The specimen should be transported promptly to the laboratory or pathology department.
- Antibiotic therapy should be initiated after the specimen is collected.
- Vital signs should be carefully evaluated to detect bleeding, infection, or other potential complications of an invasive procedure.
- If the test results indicate a sexually transmitted infection, sexual partners should be notified, evaluated, and treated. In Canada, three STIs must be reported, according to national law: *Chlamydia* infection, gonorrhea, and infectious syphilis.

LABORATORY HANDLING OF SPECIMENS
The laboratory has protocols to minimize factors that may interfere with test results. Certain specimens must be processed immediately (such as cerebrospinal fluid cultures). Some specimens (such as urine) may be refrigerated if analysis will be delayed. Stained smears of medically urgent specimens should be evaluated and reported immediately. Cultures should be plated immediately; this is essential to avoid bacterial deterioration. All efforts must be made to avoid the contamination of a culture so as to decrease the likelihood of incorrect results.

In addition to protocols concerning timeliness in handling of the specimen, the laboratory must also have strict guidelines for rejecting a specimen. Improper identification is the main reason for rejection of a specimen: It is obvious that labelling the wrong patient with a diagnosis such as gonorrhea or other sexually transmitted infection can have devastating consequences. Desiccated or poorly preserved specimens would also be considered unsatisfactory.

REPORTING OF RESULTS
Most microbiologic examinations require several days before results are available. The specimens often must go through a staining process that takes at least 24 hours. Some tissue for microscopic

examination needs to be sent to reference laboratories for evaluation. In such cases, results take much longer to obtain. Preliminary culture reports and Gram stain results, however, are available within a few hours. The quality of microscopic study results depends on how efficaciously the specimen is obtained, transported, and handled in the laboratory. The experience of the physician reporting the results is also a key component in the process. Microscopic studies are invaluable in making a diagnosis. Not only is communication among the various health care providers imperative but also reporting must be timely, concise, and accurate.

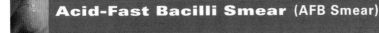

Acid-Fast Bacilli Smear (AFB Smear)

NORMAL FINDINGS

No bacilli seen

INDICATIONS

This smear (usually of sputum) is used to support the diagnosis of tuberculosis. The diagnosis of tuberculosis cannot be made with positive results of an acid-fast bacilli (AFB) smear alone; tuberculosis cultures are required. AFB smears are also used to monitor the patient's response to treatment of tuberculosis. The test is indicated in any patient with a persistent productive cough, night sweats, anorexia, weight loss, fever, hemoptysis, or an abnormal chest radiograph. This smear should especially be considered in patients at high risk for tuberculosis, such as those who are immunocompromised, have a history of alcohol abuse, or have had a recent exposure to tuberculosis.

TEST EXPLANATION

The most clinically significant AFB is *Mycobacterium tuberculosis.* This is the causative agent in the disease. After taking up a dye such as fuchsin, *M. tuberculosis* is not decolorized by acid alcohol (i.e., it is acid-fast). It is seen under the microscope as a red, rod-shaped organism. If this bacillus is seen, the patient may have active tuberculosis. However, other species of *Mycobacterium, Nocardia,* and some fungi are acid-fast. The AFB smear is performed most commonly on sputum. At least 5000 organisms must be present in each millilitre of specimen to be seen on a microscope smear. Specimens from other body secretions—such as cerebrospinal fluid, tissue, and synovial fluid—may be used. Smears may be negative as much as 50% of the time even with positive cultures. The diagnosis of tuberculosis cannot be based solely on a positive smear for AFB. Cultures (p. 798) must be positive for a definitive diagnosis. Also, cultures are the only way to determine drug sensitivities for treatment.

AFB is also used to monitor treatment for tuberculosis. If after adequate therapy (2 months) the sputum still contains AFB (even though the culture may be negative because of antituberculosis drugs), treatment should be considered a failure. Cavitary disease may cause this same scenario (positive smear, negative cultures).

INTERFERING FACTORS

- False-negative results can occur because of faulty laboratory techniques.
- False-positive results can occur when the water used to suspend the smear on the slide contains a non–tuberculosis-causing organism.

Clinical Priorities

- The AFB smear is used to support the diagnosis of tuberculosis. A definitive diagnosis requires a sputum culture and sensitivity.
- Inform the patient that sputum must be coughed up from the lungs. The first morning specimen is usually the best.
- Withhold antibiotic treatment until after the sputum has been collected.
- If the patient is suspected of having tuberculosis, health care providers should wear an N95 respirator mask when in contact with the patient. Ideally, the patient should be in a negative-pressure room.

PROCEDURE AND PATIENT CARE

Before

𝕏 Explain the procedure for sputum collection.

𝕏 Remind the patient that the sputum must be coughed up from the lungs and that saliva is not sputum. The first morning specimen is usually best.

- Withhold antibiotic treatment until after the sputum has been collected.
- Give the patient a sterile sputum container the night before the sputum is to be collected so that the patient can produce the morning specimen upon awakening.

𝕏 Instruct the patient to rinse out his or her mouth with water before the sputum collection to decrease contamination by particles in the oropharynx. Remind the patient not to use antiseptic mouthwash before sputum collection.

During

- For best results, obtain sputum collection when the patient awakens in the morning.
- Collect at least 5 mL (1 teaspoon) of sputum in a sterile sputum container.
- To produce sputum, the patient should take several deep breaths and then cough.
- If the patient is unable to produce a sputum specimen, stimulate coughing by lowering the head of the patient's bed or by giving the patient an aerosol administration of a warm hypertonic solution.
- Note that other methods to collect sputum—such as endotracheal aspiration, fibreoptic bronchoscopy, and transtracheal aspiration—may be used if necessary.
- For AFB determinations, collect sputum on three separate occasions.

After

- Avoid personal contamination, and wear gloves when handling all patient secretions.

𝕏 Instruct the patient to notify the nurse as soon as the specimen is collected.

- Label the specimen and send it to the laboratory as soon as possible.

𝕏 Inform the patient that culture results may take 3 weeks or longer.

TEST RESULTS AND CLINICAL SIGNIFICANCE

Tuberculosis: *Although tuberculosis is highly suspected when AFB is identified on a sputum smear, other organisms can cause positive AFB smears. Such organisms include atypical mycobacteria and some fungi.*

RELATED TESTS

Tuberculosis Culture (p. 798). This is the only manner in which the diagnosis of tuberculosis can be made with certainty. When tuberculosis is grown from the culture of a specimen, the diagnosis of tuberculosis can be established and treatment started on the basis of drug sensitivities.

Tuberculin Skin Testing (p. 1168). Purified protein derivative is administered intradermally to test for prior exposure to tuberculosis. Skin testing cannot indicate active or dormant tuberculosis. Positive results indicate nothing more than previous exposure.

Chest Radiography (p. 1053). Tuberculosis usually infects the lungs because of inhalation of airborne infectious material; therefore, the chest radiographic examination often demonstrates the results (Ghon complex) of the acute granulomatous infection.

Blood Culture and Sensitivity (Blood C&S)

NORMAL FINDINGS
Negative

INDICATIONS
Blood cultures are obtained to detect the presence of bacteria in the blood.

TEST EXPLANATION
Bacteremia (the presence of bacteria in the blood) can be intermittent and transient, except in endocarditis or suppurative thrombophlebitis. Chills and fever usually accompany the episode of bacteremia; thus the blood sample should be obtained when the patient manifests these signs in order to increase the chances that bacteria will grow in the cultures. It is important that at least two culture specimens be obtained from two different sites. Some agencies may require multiple specimens within a specific time frame. If bacteria are found in blood from one site and not from the other, it is safe to assume that the bacteria in the first culture may be a contaminant and not the infecting agent. When the infecting agent grows in both cultures, bacteremia is present and is caused by the organism that is growing in the culture. If the patient is receiving antibiotics during the time that the cultures are collected, the laboratory should be notified. Resin can be added to the culture medium to negate the antibiotic effect in inhibiting growth of the offending bacteria in the culture. If cultures are to be performed while the patient is receiving antibiotics, the blood culture specimen should be taken shortly before the next dose of the antibiotic is administered. All cultures preferably should be performed before antibiotic therapy is initiated.

Culture specimens collected through an intravenous catheter are frequently contaminated, and tests should not be performed on such specimens unless catheter sepsis is suspected. In these situations, blood culture specimens collected through the catheter help identify the causative agent more accurately than does a culture specimen from the catheter tip.

Most organisms require approximately 24 hours to grow in the laboratory, and preliminary findings can be reported at that time. Often, 48 to 72 hours are required for growth and identification of the organism. Anaerobic organisms may take longer to grow. Cultures may be repeated after antibiotic therapy to assess resolution of the infection.

INTERFERING FACTORS
- Contamination of the blood specimen, especially by skin bacteria, may occur.
- Drugs that may *alter* test results include antibiotics.

PROCEDURE AND PATIENT CARE

Before

- Explain the procedure to the patient.
- Inform the patient that no fasting is required.

During

- Carefully prepare the proposed venipuncture site with povidone-iodine (Betadine). Allow the skin to dry.
- Clean the tops of the sterile Vacutainer tubes or culture bottles with povidone-iodine, and allow them to dry. Some laboratories suggest cleaning with 70% alcohol after cleaning with povidone-iodine and air drying.
- Collect 10 to 15 mL of venous blood by venipuncture from each site in a 20-mL syringe.
- Discard the needle on the syringe and replace with a second, sterile needle before injecting the blood sample into the culture bottle.
- Inoculate the anaerobic bottle first if both anaerobic and aerobic cultures are needed.
- Mix gently after inoculation.
- Label the specimen with the patient's name, date, time, and tentative diagnosis.
- On the laboratory slip, list any medications that the patient is taking that could affect test results.

After

- Transport the culture bottles to the laboratory immediately (within 30 minutes).
- Notify the physician of any positive results so that appropriate antibiotic therapy can be initiated.

TEST RESULTS AND CLINICAL SIGNIFICANCE

Bacteremia: *The bacteria growing in the blood can often be grown in the culture medium within the microbiology laboratory. When bacteremia exists, the patient must be considered gravely ill, and antibiotics should be started immediately after blood cultures are obtained.*

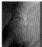

Blood Smear (Peripheral Blood Smear, Red Blood Cell Morphology, RBC Smear)

NORMAL FINDINGS

Normal quantity of red blood cells (RBCs), white blood cells (WBCs), and platelets
Normal size, shape, and colour of RBCs
Normal WBC differential count

INDICATIONS

The peripheral blood smear can provide a significant amount of information concerning drugs and diseases that affect the RBCs and the WBCs. Furthermore, other congenital and acquired diseases can be diagnosed by an examination of the peripheral blood smear. When special stains are applied to the blood smear, infection, infestation, leukemia, and other diseases can be identified.

TEST EXPLANATION

When adequately prepared and examined microscopically by an experienced technologist and pathologist, a smear of peripheral blood is the most informative of all hematologic tests. All three hematologic cell lines—erythrocytes (RBCs), platelets, and leukocytes (WBCs)—can be examined. In the peripheral blood, five different types of leukocytes can routinely be identified: neutrophils, eosinophils, basophils, lymphocytes, and monocytes. The first three are also referred to as *granulocytes.* (See discussion of bone marrow biopsy on p. 740 for more information concerning the various elements of blood.)

Microscopic examination of the RBCs can reveal variations in RBC size (anisocytosis), shape (poikilocytosis), colour, or intracellular content. Classification of RBCs according to these variables is most helpful in identifying the causes of anemia and the presence of other diseases.

RBC Size Abnormalities

Microcytes (small RBCs)
   Iron deficiency
   Thalassemia
   Hemoglobinopathies
Macrocytes (larger size)
   Vitamin B_{12} or folic acid deficiency
   Reticulocytosis secondary to increased erythropoiesis (RBC production)
   Liver disorder

RBC Shape Abnormalities

Spherocytes (small and round)
   Hereditary spherocytosis
   Acquired immunohemolytic anemia
Elliptocytes (crescent)
   Hereditary elliptocytosis
Codocytes, or target cells (thin cells with less hemoglobin)
   Hemoglobinopathies
   Thalassemia
Echinocytes (Burr cells)
   Uremia
   Liver disease

RBC Colour Abnormalities

Hypochromic (pale)
   Iron deficiency
   Thalassemia
Hyperchromasia (intense coloration)
   Concentrated hemoglobin, usually caused by dehydration

RBC Intracellular Structure Abnormalities

Nucleated (normoblasts; usually RBCs do not have a nucleus, but immature RBCs do, and higher
   numbers of immature nucleated cells indicate increased RBC synthesis.)
   Anemia
   Chronic hypoxemia
   "Normal" for an infant
   Marrow-occupying neoplasm or fibrotic tissue

Basophilic stippling (refers to bodies enclosed or included in the cytoplasm of the RBCs)
   Lead poisoning
   Reticulocytosis
Howell-Jolly bodies (small, round remnants of nuclear material remaining within the RBC)
   After a surgical splenectomy
   Hemolytic anemia
   Megaloblastic anemia
   Functional asplenia (after splenic infarction)
   The WBCs are examined for total quantity, differential count, and degree of maturity. An increased number of immature WBCs can indicate leukemia or infection. A decreased WBC count indicates a failure of marrow to produce WBCs (as a result of drugs, chronic disease, neoplasia, or fibrosis), peripheral destruction, or sequestration.
   Finally, an experienced pathologist also can estimate platelet number.

PROCEDURE AND PATIENT CARE

Before
- Explain the procedure to the patient.
- Inform the patient that no fasting is required.

During
- Collect a drop of blood from a fingerstick or (in an infant) heelstick, and place it on a slide.
- If necessary, perform a venipuncture and collect the blood in a lavender-top tube.
- Note that there are two methods for conducting a blood smear: the slide method and the covered glass method. Once the blood has been "smeared" on the slide or covered glass, it is then stained and placed under a microscope, and the cells are counted and examined for abnormal blood cell shapes and other irregularities. The most accurate smear requires review by a pathologist.

After
- Apply pressure or a pressure dressing to the venipuncture site.
- Assess the venipuncture site for bleeding.

TEST RESULTS AND CLINICAL SIGNIFICANCE

See the list of abnormalities in the "Test Explanation" section.

RELATED TESTS

Complete Blood Cell Count and Differential Count (p. 187). This is a battery of tests performed on the peripheral blood to measure the quantity of each blood component.
   Bone Marrow Biopsy (see following test). This is an examination of the bone marrow, which forms the components of the peripheral blood.

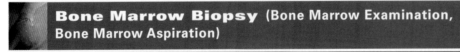

Bone Marrow Biopsy (Bone Marrow Examination, Bone Marrow Aspiration)

NORMAL FINDINGS

Active erythroid cell line, myeloid and lymphoid cell lines, and megakaryocyte (platelet) production: Normal iron content demonstrated by staining with Prussian blue

Cell Type	Range (%)
Neutrophilic Series	49.2–65.0
Myeloblasts	0.2–1.5
Promyelocytes	2.1–4.1
Myelocytes	8.2–15.7
Eosinophilic Series	1.2–5.3
Myelocytes	0.2–1.3
Metamyelocytes	0.4–2.2
Bands	0.2–2.4
Segmented	0–1.3
Basophilic and Mast Cells	0–0.2
Erythrocyte Series	18.4–33.8
Pronormoblasts	0.2–1.3
Basophilic	0.5–2.4
Polychromatophilic	17.9–29.2
Orthochromatic	0.4–4.6
Monocytes	0–0.8
Lymphocytes	11.1–23.2
Plasma Cells	0.4–3.9
Megakaryocytes	0–0.4
Reticulum Cells	0–0.9
Monocyte to Erythrocyte Ratio	1.5–3.3

 Critical Values

A physician should be notified when there is a new diagnosis of leukemia, lymphoma, metastatic malignancy, infection, or hemolytic anemia. The interpreting pathologist usually performs this notification.

INDICATIONS

Bone marrow examination is an important part of the evaluation of patients with hematologic diseases. Indications for bone marrow examination include the following:
1. To evaluate anemias
2. To diagnose leukemia, myeloma, or lymphoma
3. To determine whether a marrow disorder is the cause of reduced numbers of blood cells in the peripheral bloodstream
4. To document deficiency of iron stores
5. To document bone marrow infiltrative diseases (neoplasm, infection, or fibrosis)
   Bone marrow examination is also used to stage lymphomas.

TEST EXPLANATION

All the cells circulating through the bloodstream—leukocytes (white blood cells) that fight infections, erythrocytes (red blood cells) that carry oxygen to the tissues, and platelets (clotting cells) that prevent bleeding—are made by precursor cells in a fatty matrix inside the hollow of our bones called bone marrow. At birth there is bone marrow in the hollow space inside all the bones of the body, as well as some bone marrow cells in the liver, spleen, and bloodstream. As the

Microscopic Examinations

7

human body grows, the bone marrow cells are confined to the hollow space of the flat bones of the body, specifically the skull, the sternum, the ribs, or the bones of the pelvis (the iliac bones). When a patient has unexplained abnormal blood counts, has abnormal cells circulating in the blood, or is diagnosed with a disease that can involve the bone marrow (lymphoma) or metastasize to the bone marrow (some carcinomas), a bone marrow biopsy is performed to examine the cells in the marrow space. Because the marrow in adults is in the flat bones, the standard location for sampling bone marrow is the iliac bones of the pelvis. Accepted practice is that the safest location to use for entering the iliac bone to obtain a sample is the posterior superior iliac spine of the pelvis (Figure 7.1). There, the blood-forming cells in the marrow produce the blood cells and release them into the circulation

By examining a bone marrow specimen, the hematologist can evaluate hematopoiesis fully. The hematologist can determine the number, size, and shape of the RBCs, WBCs, and megakaryocytes (platelet precursors) as these cells evolve through their various stages of development in the bone marrow. Samples of the bone marrow can be obtained by either aspiration or surgical removal; the latter samples reveal more information. Also, with aspiration, the sample may be uninformative because there is very little cellular activity or because the cells are too tightly packed to aspirate through a needle. Under those circumstances, bone marrow biopsy is necessary to obtain marrow tissue. Microscopic examination includes estimation of cellularity, determination of the presence of fibrotic tissue or neoplasms (both primary and metastatic), and estimation of iron storage.

For the estimation of cellularity, the relative quantity of each cell type in the specimen is determined. Such estimation is more accurately performed on a biopsy specimen than on an aspirate because the aspirate may not be truly representative of the entire marrow. Leukemias or leukemoid drug reactions are suspected when numbers of leukocyte precursors are increased. Physiologic marrow leukemoid compensation for infection is also recognized from the finding of an increased number of leukocyte precursors. Numbers of marrow leukocyte precursors are decreased in patients with myelofibrosis, metastatic neoplasia, or agranulocytosis; in older adult (>65 years) patients; and after radiation therapy or chemotherapy.

The numbers of marrow RBC precursors are increased with polycythemia vera or as physiologic compensation for hemorrhagic or hemolytic anemias. The numbers of marrow RBC precursors are decreased with erythroid hypoplasia after chemotherapy, radiation therapy, administration of other toxic drugs, iron administration, or marrow replacement by fibrotic tissue or neoplasms.

The numbers of platelet precursors (megakaryocytes) are increased in the marrow of patients who are compensating after an episode of acute hemorrhage. They are also increased in some forms of acute and chronic myeloid leukemias. This increase may be compensatory in patients with secondary hypersplenism associated with portal hypertension or other conditions. In these patients, the spleen prematurely extracts platelets from the circulation. Platelet counts decrease, and the marrow compensates by increasing production. The numbers of megakaryocytes are decreased in patients who have had radiation therapy, chemotherapy, or other drug therapy; in patients with neoplastic or fibrotic marrow infiltrative diseases; and in patients with aplastic anemia.

The numbers of lymphocyte precursors are increased in chronic, viral, or mycoplasmal infections (e.g., mononucleosis); in lymphocytic leukemia; and in lymphoma. Plasma cells (plasmocytes) are increased in number in patients with multiple myelomas, Hodgkin disease, hypersensitivity states, rheumatic fever, and other chronic inflammatory diseases.

Estimation of cellularity also can be expressed as a ratio of myeloid (WBC) to erythroid (RBC) cells (M/E ratio). The normal M/E ratio is approximately 3:1. The M/E ratio is higher than normal in the diseases mentioned previously in which increased leukocyte precursors are present or erythroid precursors are decreased. The M/E ratio is lower than normal when either numbers of leukocyte precursors are decreased or numbers of erythroid precursors are increased. A more detailed list of diseases affecting the M/E ratio can be found in most hematology textbooks.

Drug-induced or idiopathic myelofibrosis can be detected through examination of the bone marrow. With the use of special stains, it is possible to estimate iron stores with marrow biopsy. Although fibrosis or neoplasia is occasionally detected in aspiration studies, biopsy is the best method. Leukemias and multiple myelomas can easily be detected in biopsy specimens. Similarly, lymphomas and other metastatic tumours (e.g., cancers of the breast, kidney, lung) can be detected. Bone marrow biopsy is an important part of staging for lymphomas and Hodgkin disease.

A physician usually performs bone marrow aspiration and biopsy. The duration of each of these procedures is approximately 20 minutes. The patient may have some apprehension when pressure is applied to puncture the outer table of the bone during biopsy or aspiration. The patient probably will feel pain during lidocaine infiltration and pressure when the syringe plunger is withdrawn for aspiration.

CONTRAINDICATIONS

- Acute coagulation disorders, because of the risk of excessive bleeding
- Patients' inability to cooperate and remain still during the procedure

POTENTIAL COMPLICATIONS

- Hemorrhage, especially if the patient has a coagulopathy, or other bleeding disorder
- Infection, especially if the patient is leukopenic
- Sternal fracture as a result of overaggressive application of pressure to the sternum if a sternal biopsy is performed
- Inadvertent puncture of the heart or great vessels when the test is performed on the sternum

Clinical Priorities

- Assess the results of the coagulation studies before bone marrow biopsy. Patients with coagulation disorders cannot undergo this procedure because of the risk for excessive bleeding.
- It is essential that patients remain still and cooperate during this invasive procedure.
- During bone marrow aspiration, most patients feel pain during lidocaine infiltration and pressure when the syringe plunger is withdrawn for aspiration.

PROCEDURE AND PATIENT CARE

Before

 Explain the procedure to the patient.
- Obtain the patient's written informed consent for this procedure.

 Encourage the patient to verbalize fears, because many patients are anxious concerning this study.
- Assess the results of the coagulation studies. Report any evidence of coagulopathy to the physician.
- Obtain an order for sedatives if the patient appears extremely apprehensive.

 Remind the patient to remain very still throughout the procedure.

During

✗ Inform the patient that he or she may have some apprehension when pressure is applied to puncture the outer table of the bone during biopsy specimen removal or aspiration.

✗ Inform the patient that he or she probably will feel pain during lidocaine infiltration and discomfort when the syringe plunger is withdrawn for aspiration.

- Note the following procedural steps for bone marrow aspiration, which is performed on the iliac crest, anterior or posterior iliac crests, sternum, and (in children) the proximal tibia:
  1. The procedure is usually performed at the patient's bedside with the use of local anaesthesia.
  2. A preferred site is the posterior superior iliac crests (the part of the iliac crest that is closest to the surface), with the patient placed prone or on the side.
  3. The area overlying the bone is prepared with an antiseptic solution and draped in a sterile manner.
  4. The overlying skin and soft tissue, along with the periosteum, is infiltrated with lidocaine.
  5. A small (<1-mm) incision is made in the skin directly over the posterior superior iliac spine.
  6. A large-bore needle containing a stylus is slowly advanced through the soft tissue and into the outer table of the bone (Figure 7-1).
  7. Once the needle is inside the marrow, the stylus is removed and a syringe is attached.
  8. A 0.5- to 2-mL sample of bone marrow is aspirated, smeared on slides, and allowed to dry.
- Note the following procedural steps for bone marrow biopsy:
  1. The skin and soft tissues overlying the bone are incised.
  2. A core biopsy instrument is "screwed" into the bone.
  3. The biopsy specimen is obtained and sent to the pathology laboratory for analysis.

After

- Apply pressure to the puncture site to arrest minimal bleeding. Apply an adhesive bandage.
- Observe the puncture site for bleeding. Ice packs may be used to help control bleeding.
- Assess for tenderness and erythema, which may indicate infection. If either is present, report this to the physician.
- Evaluate the patient for signs of shock (increased pulse rate, decreased blood pressure).
- If there are no complications, place the patient on bed rest for 30 to 60 minutes after the test.
- Note that some patients complain of tenderness at the puncture site for several days after this study. Mild analgesics may be ordered.

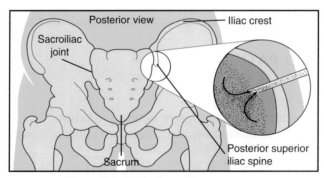

Figure 7-1 Aspiration of bone marrow.

Home Care Responsibilities

- Instruct the patient to observe the puncture site for bleeding.
- Inform the patient that tenderness and erythema may indicate infection. This should be reported to the physician.
- Mild analgesics may be needed for several days after this procedure for tenderness at the puncture site.

TEST RESULTS AND CLINICAL SIGNIFICANCE

Neoplasm,

Myelofibrosis: *Infiltrative diseases are evident histologically with regard to the specific cause; the evidence is hypocellularity within the marrow.*

Infection (viral, bacterial, fungal): *Bacterial infection is usually associated with increased amounts of neutrophilic elements. However, in overwhelming sepsis, these elements may be depressed. Viral and some fungal infections are characterized by increases in monocytic elements.*

Agranulocytosis: *The marrow has no myeloblast cells.*

Polycythemia vera: *Erythroid cellular elements are abundant.*

Multiple myelomas,

Hodgkin disease,

Lymphoma: *These cancers may be associated with overwhelming abundance of mononuclear elements within the marrow.*

Leukemia: *The myeloid precursor cells are significantly increased in number and crowd the marrow.*

Hypersensitivity states: *These states may be evident as an increase in eosinophilic and basophilic myeloblast elements.*

Acute hemorrhagic marrow hyperplasia: *After an acute hemorrhage, the erythroid (and to some extent, the myeloid) elements are greatly increased in number to compensate for the loss of cells in the peripheral blood.*

Anemia: *If the anemia is caused by marrow failure, erythroid precursors are deficient in number. Specifics about the appearance of the marrow cells (e.g., megaloblasts in B_{12} deficiency) may indicate the cause of the marrow failure. Special stains may reveal deficient iron storage and other disorders.*

Chronic inflammatory disease,

Rheumatic fever: *Mononuclear precursor elements may be increased in number.*

Acquired immune deficiency syndrome (AIDS): *Decreased numbers of leukocytic elements may be noted, especially as the disease progresses.*

RELATED TEST

Blood Smear (p. 738). These test results are usually reported in the bone marrow biopsy report so as to corroborate the findings and support the indications for the procedure.

Complete Blood Cell Count and Differential Count (p. 187). This is a measurement of the number and relative percentages of the myeloid, erythroid, and platelet elements in the peripheral bloodstream.

7   Microscopic Examinations

Breast Cancer Tumour Analysis (Breast Cancer Predictors, DNA Ploidy Status, S-Phase Fraction, Cathepsin D, HER2 [c-erbB2, neu] Protein, Ki67 Protein, p53 Protein)

NORMAL FINDINGS

DNA Ploidy

Diploid is favourable
(Aneuploid is unfavourable)

S-phase Fraction

<5.5% is favourable
(>5.5% is unfavourable)

Human Epidermal Growth Factor Receptor 2 (HER2) Protein

Immunohistochemistry method: 0 to 1+
Fluorescence in situ hybridization (FISH) method: <2 copies/cell
OncoType Dx method: <10.7 units

Cathepsin D

<10% is favourable
(>10% is unfavourable)

p53 Protein (TP53)

<10% is favourable
(>10% is unfavourable)

Ki67 Protein

<20% is favourable
(10%–20% is borderline; >20% is unfavourable)

INDICATIONS

This testing is performed on the breast cancer tissue and is used to predict the possibility of breast cancer relapse after curative primary surgery.

TEST EXPLANATION

The most important predictor of recurrent breast cancer is lymph node status. In patients with positive lymph node metastasis, recurrence is more likely. However, nearly 30% of the patients whose tumour has been completely removed and who have no evidence of lymph node metastasis also experience recurrence. It would be helpful to predict which patients are destined for recurrence so that they can be selected for systemic therapy, whereas patients who will not have a recurrence can be spared the morbidity of a treatment that is not needed. Conventional predictors such as tumour size, grade, histologic type, and hormone receptors have not proved to be reliable. As a result, there has been a marked increase in the efforts to identify newer markers that more accurately reflect cellular function and growth. Although estrogen and progesterone receptors are also breast cancer prognostic indicators, they are discussed separately on pp. 248 and 429. Furthermore, in addition to *HER2/neu* testing, there are more accurate prognosticators for breast cancer (e.g., breast cancer genomic testing, discussed on p. 1131).

Ploidy (DNA Index) and S-Phase Fraction

Measurement of the rapidity with which the cells in a breast cancer grow includes ploidy status and S-phase analysis. Normally, cells are diploid (each cell has one set of paired chromosomes), and a small number of cells are present in the S-phase of cell division. During the mitotic phase of cell division, the amount of DNA doubles (two sets of paired chromosomes) in preparation for cell division. Because the more aggressive cancer cells divide more rapidly, many cells are in various stages of the mitotic phase. These cells may have a variable number of chromosome sets (the state of aneuploidy).

The more aggressive cancer cells are more often in S-phase (a time of intracellular protein synthesis in preparation for division). This is usually reported as the *S-phase fraction:* that is, the number of cells in S-phase divided by the total number of cancer cells in the particular specimen. The laboratory methods have been automated by flow cytometry with laser-stimulated DNA fluorescence.

Cathepsin D

This protein is a lysosomal cysteine protease that is absent in resting breast tissue but markedly abundant in malignant tissue. It was thought that this protein on the cellular membrane contributed, in some way, to the malignant potential of the tumour, but there is insufficient evidence to support the routine use of this breast cancer tumour marker test in clinical practice. The exact cutoff point between a favourable prognosis and an unfavourable prognosis has yet to be standardized. As with most protein markers, monoclonal antibody immunohistochemical techniques are used to identify this protein.

HER2 (c-erbB2, neu) Protein

HER2 is a protein whose gene is associated with a higher aggressiveness in breast cancers. The *HER2/neu* oncogene encodes a transmembrane tyrosine kinase receptor with extensive similarity to other epidermal growth factor receptors. It is normally involved in the pathways leading to cell growth and survival. In approximately 15% to 20% of breast cancers, the *HER2/neu* oncogene is amplified, or its protein product is overexpressed. Overexpression of this receptor in breast cancer is associated with increased risk of disease recurrence and worse prognosis.

Two methods are commonly used to measure HER2/neu protein. *Fluorescence in situ hybridization* (FISH) has become the "standard criterion" method of measuring HER2/neu protein in tumour tissue. In this test method, fluorescent probes are used to determine the number of *HER2* gene copies in a tumour cell. If there are more than four copies of the *HER2* gene, the cancer is considered *HER2*-positive. *Immunohistochemical testing*, although the easier, can be less accurate than the FISH method. In this test, the production of the HER2 protein by the tumour is measured. The test results are ranked as 0, 1+, 2+, or 3+. If the results are 3+, the cancer is *HER2*-positive. Reverse-transcription polymerase chain reaction is a third method that is more accurate but more cumbersome and more costly.

HER2 testing is also helpful in making treatment decisions. Because tumours that overexpress the *HER2/neu* oncogene are more aggressive, more aggressive adjuvant chemotherapy is recommended to women with these tumours. It has been found that the *HER2* oncogene can act as a target for trastuzumab (Herceptin), an antineoplastic monoclonal antibody drug. Trastuzumab is effective only in breast cancer in which *HER2/neu* is overexpressed. One of the mechanisms of trastuzumab after it binds to the HER2 protein is to halt cell proliferation.

p53 Protein

The *p53* gene is a tumour suppressor gene that is overexpressed in more aggressive breast cancer cells. Mutation of the gene causes overexpression and a buildup of mutant proteins on the surface of the cancer cells. Overexpression of *p53* can be identified by studying the gene or by immunohistochemical staining of paraffin-embedded breast cancer tissue for the mutant proteins.

Ki67 Protein

The *Ki67* gene encodes the synthesis for Ki67 protein that is associated with a more aggressive breast cancer. This protein is identified by immunohistochemical staining of paraffin-embedded breast cancer tissue.

INTERFERING FACTORS

- Delay in tissue fixation may cause deterioration of marker proteins and produce lower values.
- Preoperative use of some chemotherapy agents can decrease levels of some marker proteins.

PROCEDURE AND PATIENT CARE

Before

- Inform the patient that an examination for these tumour predictor markers will be performed on their breast cancer tissue.
- Provide psychologic and emotional support to the patient with breast cancer.

During

- The surgeon obtains tumour tissue.
- This tissue should be placed on ice or in formalin.
- Part of the tissue is used for routine histologic examination. A portion of the paraffin block is sent to a reference laboratory.

After

- Explain to the patient that results are usually available in 1 week.

TEST RESULTS AND CLINICAL SIGNIFICANCE

Unfavourable: *In general, when these prognostic tumour markers are present in high quantities, the cancer acts more aggressively, and the risk of recurrence is higher.*

RELATED TESTS

Estrogen Receptor Assay (p. 759) and Progesterone Receptor Assay (p. 781). These tests are used to identify other prognostic markers for breast cancer.

   Breast Cancer Genomics (p. 1131). This test is used to predict the possibility of cancer susceptibility to chemotherapy. It is also a powerful indicator of the likelihood of breast cancer recurrence after primary breast cancer surgery.

Cervical Biopsy (Simple Cervical [Punch] Biopsy, Endocervical Biopsy [Endocervical Curettage], Loop Electrosurgical Excision Procedure [LEEP], Cone Biopsy [Conization])

NORMAL FINDINGS
Normal squamous cells

 Critical Values

Cancer cells

INDICATIONS
A biopsy of the cervix is performed to more accurately identify and treat premalignant and superficial malignant lesions of the cervix.

TEST EXPLANATION
When a Papanicolaou (Pap) smear reveals an "epithelial cell abnormality" or when a pelvic examination reveals a possible neoplastic abnormality in the cervix, a biopsy of that structure is indicated. The biopsy can be performed with several different methods, in which an increasing amount of tissue is obtained. Cervical biopsy procedures include the following:

- In a *simple cervical biopsy,* sometimes called a *punch biopsy,* a small piece of tissue is removed from the surface of the cervix. This is often performed during colposcopy (p. 623).
- In an *endocervical biopsy (endocervical curettage),* a sharp instrument is used to scrape tissue from high in the cervical canal.
- In *loop electrosurgical excision procedure* (LEEP), a thin, low-voltage electrified wire loop is used to cut out abnormal tissue on the cervix and high in the endocervical canal. This procedure is sometimes called a *large-loop excision of the transformation zone* (LLETZ).
- A *cone biopsy (conization)* is a more extensive form of a cervical biopsy in which a cone-shaped wedge of tissue is removed from the cervix. Both normal and abnormal cervical tissues are removed. This can be performed by means of LEEP, with a surgical knife (scalpel), or with a carbon dioxide laser.

After colposcopy or a cervical biopsy, LEEP may be used to treat abnormal, precancerous cells found in the biopsy sample. It can also be used to assess the extent of noninvasive superficial cervical cancers and, sometimes, to treat them.

CONTRAINDICATIONS
- Active menstrual bleeding
- Pregnancy

POTENTIAL COMPLICATIONS
- After the surgery, a small number of women (<10%) may have significant bleeding that necessitates vaginal packing or a blood transfusion.
- Infection of the cervix or uterus may occur. (This is rare.)
- Narrowing of the cervix (cervical stenosis) can occur and can cause infertility. (This is rare.)

Microscopic Examinations

7

PROCEDURE AND PATIENT CARE

Before

- ⟋ Explain the procedure to the patient.
- Obtain the patient's informed consent if it is required by the institution.
- ⟋ Instruct the patient to take a non–aspirin-containing analgesic 30 minutes before the procedure.

During

- Note the following procedural steps:
  1. The patient is placed in the lithotomy position, and a vaginal speculum is used to expose the vagina and cervix.
  2. The cervix is cleansed with a 3% acetic acid solution or iodine to remove excess mucus and cellular debris and to accentuate the difference between normal and abnormal epithelial tissues.
  3. Medication may be injected to numb the cervix (*cervical block*).
  4. The physician chooses the instrument to perform a simple cervical biopsy, an endocervical biopsy, LEEP, or cone biopsy.
- Note that a physician performs the procedure in approximately 5 to 10 minutes.
- Cone biopsy is performed in the operating room; the other procedures can be performed in the physician's office.
- ⟋ Inform the patient that some women complain of pressure pains from the vaginal speculum and that discomfort may be felt if biopsy specimens are obtained.
- Most women can return to normal activities immediately after a simple cervical biopsy or an endocervical biopsy.
- Most women are able to return to normal activities within 2 to 4 days after LEEP or cone biopsies. This length of time varies, depending on the amount of tissue removed during the procedure.

After

- ⟋ Inform the patient that it is normal to experience the following:
- Vaginal bleeding if biopsy specimens were taken (suggest that she wear a sanitary pad)
- Mild cramping for several hours after the procedure
- Brownish-black vaginal discharge during the first week
- Vaginal discharge or spotting for about 1 to 3 weeks
- ⟋ Instruct the patient that sanitary pads should be used instead of tampons for 1 to 3 weeks.
- ⟋ Inform the patient when and how to obtain the results of this study.

 Home Care Responsibilities

- Instruct the patient to avoid sexual intercourse for 3 to 4 weeks after the procedure.
- Advise the patient not to douche for 3 to 4 weeks.
- Instruct the patient to call the physician for any of the following symptoms:
  - Fever
  - Spotting or bleeding that lasts longer than 1 week
  - Bleeding that is heavier than a normal menstrual period and contains blood clots
  - Increasing pelvic pain
  - Foul-smelling, yellowish vaginal discharge, which may indicate an infection

TEST RESULTS AND CLINICAL SIGNIFICANCE

Cervical chronic infection,
Cervical intraepithelial neoplasia,
Cervical carcinoma in situ,
Invasive cervical carcinoma,
Endocervical adenocarcinomas: *Any of these lesions can lead to cellular changes on Pap smear that could appear to be cancerous and therefore necessitate biopsy. Visual observation of any abnormal lesion on the cervix would also necessitate biopsy.*

RELATED TESTS

Colposcopy (p. 623). This procedure is a more thorough evaluation of the cervix and is used to identify malignant and premalignant lesions of the vagina and cervix.

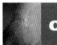

Chlamydia

NORMAL FINDINGS

Negative culture
Antibodies:
 Chlamydophila pneumoniae
 IgG: <1:64
 IgM: <1:10
 Chlamydophila psittaci
 IgG: <1:64
 IgM: <1:10
 Chlamydia trachomatis
 IgG: <1:64
 IgM: <1:10

INDICATIONS

Chlamydia testing is performed in patients with symptoms of the wide variety of diseases this organism can cause. This form of sexually transmitted infection (STI) commonly manifests as pelvic pain, vaginal discharge, or both. Cervical cultures or smears are performed in patients who report these symptoms.

TEST EXPLANATION

Chlamydia is the most commonly reported STI in Canada with 103 716 cases reported in 2012. Between 2003 and 2012, *chlamydia* rates in Canada increased by 57.6% from 189.6 to 298.7 per 100 000. A number of *Chlamydia* species cause various diseases within the human body. *Chlamydia psittaci* causes respiratory tract infections and occurs with close contact with infected birds. *Chlamydia pneumoniae*, another species, causes pneumonia. *C. trachomatis* infection is probably the most frequently occurring STI in developed countries. Infections of the genitalia are most common, followed by those of the conjunctiva, pharynx, urethra, and rectum. Lymphogranuloma venereum was the first form of venereal disease recognized as a *C. trachomatis* infection; this infection is very common in central Africa. The second serotype of *C. trachomatis* causes the eye disease trachoma, which is the most common form of preventable blindness. A third serotype produces genital and urethral infections different from lymphogranuloma. This third type is transmitted to newborns by direct contact with the mother's cervix during vaginal delivery and to sexually active persons by direct contact during sexual activity.

C. trachomatis infection is thought to be the most widespread STI in developed countries, including Canada and the United States. Sexually active youth and young adults are overrepresented in the case reports of *C. trachomatis* in Canada; the reported rate is highest in young adults 15 to 24 years of age. This disease is also prevalent in nulliparous women and in users of nonbarrier contraceptive methods. Also, in persons with multiple or recent new sexual partners, *Chlamydia* infection is frequently associated with gonorrhea.

Chlamydia is underdiagnosed because most women colonized with *Chlamydia* are asymptomatic. *Chlamydia* may be associated with pelvic inflammatory disease, particularly in adolescents. Also, screening is underperformed in men at high risk, who represent a forgotten reservoir for *Chlamydia* and the source of reinfections in female partners.

The *Chlamydia* organism can be detected in many different ways. It is, in most cases, accurately demonstrated by tissue culture. Although these tests require a special cell culture line, which takes several days to develop, they are used as the standard criterion against which other methods of detection of *Chlamydia* are measured. It is now possible to detect the *Chlamydia* antigen by direct fluorescent antibody slide staining, enzyme-linked immunosorbent assay (ELISA) technique, and DNA probes. These techniques are less expensive and more widely available than culture techniques; however, their sensitivity and specificity are lesser.

Invasive infection with *C. trachomatis* does not produce an immunogenic response. Therefore, *Chlamydia* antibodies can be measured with complement fixation, microimmunofluorescence, and ELISA techniques. When a fourfold rise in immunoglobulin G titre or the presence of specific immunoglobulin M antibodies is documented, *Chlamydia* disease may be diagnosed.

With the increasing use of ThinPrep Cervical cytologic test (see Papanicolaou Smear, p. 774), increasing numbers of *Chlamydia* infections are being diagnosed. Transcription-mediated amplification can be used to amplify *Chlamydial* ribosomal RNA on a ThinPrep sample. This same technology can even detect *Chlamydia* from a urine swab sample.

INTERFERING FACTORS

- Presence of routine menses
- Antibiotic therapy

✓ Clinical Priorities

- In Canada, *Chlamydia* infection is a reportable STI.
- Because of the rapidly increasing prevalence of *Chlamydia* infection, screening should take place in all at-risk groups, particularly sexually active adolescents and individuals with other STIs.
- Female patients are evaluated for *Chlamydia* with cervical cultures, and male patients are evaluated with urethral cultures.
- All affected patients should be treated with antibiotics. Sexual partners should be evaluated.
- High-risk groups also include sexually active men and women younger than 25 years, individuals with a history of *Chlamydia* infection, and men and women practising unprotected sexual intercourse.
- In female patients, signs and symptoms include vaginal discharge, cervicitis, lower abdominal pain, abnormal vaginal bleeding, conjunctivitis, and proctitis.
- In male patients, signs and symptoms include urethral discharge, urethritis, urethral itch, dysuria, testicular pain, conjunctivitis, and proctitis.
- Potential specimen sites for culture include the cervix and vagina in pubertal or older female patients, the urethra in male patients, the conjunctivae, the nasopharynx, the oropharynx, and the rectum.

Age-Related Concerns

- Neonates with *Chlamydia* infection can present with conjunctivitis.
- Infants younger than 6 months with *Chlamydia* infection can present with pneumonia.
- Infants younger than 6 months may need a culture of nasopharyngeal aspirate to diagnose *Chlamydia* infection.
- All pregnant women should be screened for *Chlamydia* infection during their first prenatal visit. For those who are positive or at high risk for reinfection, rescreening during the third trimester is recommended.

PROCEDURE AND PATIENT CARE

Before
- Explain the procedure to the patient.
- Note that many different methods are used to perform *Chlamydia* tests.
- Inform the patient that minimal discomfort is associated with these procedures.

During
- Collect a venous blood sample in a red-top tube.
- Acute and convalescent samples of serum should be collected 2 to 3 weeks apart.
- A conjunctival smear is obtained by swabbing the eye lesion with a cotton-tipped applicator or scraping with a sterile ophthalmic spatula and smearing on a clean glass slide.
- Sputum cultures (p. 791) are used to check for *C. psittaci* respiratory infections.
- Note the following procedural steps for cervical culture:
  1. The female patient should refrain from using douches and taking tub baths before the cervical culture is performed.
  2. The patient is placed in the lithotomy position.
  3. A nonlubricated vaginal speculum is inserted to expose the cervix.
  4. The mucus is removed from the squamocolumnar junction of the cervix.
  5. A sterile, cotton-tipped swab is inserted into the endocervical canal and moved from side to side for 30 seconds to obtain the culture.
- Note the following procedural steps for urethral culture:
  1. It is preferable that the male patient not void for at least 2 hours before urethral testing; however, having voided within 2 hours does not preclude testing.
  2. A culture is taken by gently inserting a sterile thin swab 3 to 4 cm into the urethra.
- Note that a physician or nurse performs these tests in several minutes.

After
- For patients who have positive smears, administer antibiotics.
- Advise affected patients to recommend that their sexual partners be examined.

TEST RESULTS AND CLINICAL SIGNIFICANCE

Chlamydia infections: *This organism causes many different diseases, as indicated in the "Test Explanation" section. In developing countries, this is the most significant STI.*

RELATED TEST

Sexually Transmitted Infection Culture (p. 787). This is a general test for the presence of STIs and their causative agents.

Colon Cancer Tumour Analysis (Microsatellite Instability [MSI] Testing, DNA Mismatch Repair [MMR] Genetic Testing, BRAF Mutation Analysis, Oncotype DX Colon Cancer Assay)

NORMAL FINDINGS

Recurrence score <10 (on a scale of 0 to 100)
No mismatch repair gene
No microsatellite instability

INDICATIONS

This test is used to indicate the prognosis of a patient recently surgically treated for colon cancer to determine if additional chemotherapy will improve survival. Furthermore this test can be used to indicate the possibility that the colon cancer was hereditary, thereby encouraging other members of the patient's family to undergo testing.

TEST EXPLANATION

Patients with stage 1 colon cancer have a high cure rate with surgery alone. Patients with stage 3 colon cancer benefit from the use of adjuvant chemotherapy. However, patients with stage 2 colon cancer may or may not benefit from adjuvant chemotherapy. Colon cancer tumour analysis can help differentiate stage 2 patients who may benefit from adjuvant chemotherapy. This test is used to indicate the risk of recurrence colon cancer in the years succeeding surgical treatment.

Deficiencies in *DNA mismatch repair (MMR) gene* function, either because of decreased gene expression or mutation, result in the accumulation of DNA alterations that can manifest as abnormal shortening or lengthening of microsatellite DNA sequences in the colon cancer cell. This causes *microsatellite instability (MSI)*. Patients with MMR deficient (MMR-D) colon tumours have high MSI and have been shown to have significantly lower colon cancer recurrence risk. Therefore, testing the colon tumour for MMR and MSI can assist in determining the likelihood of recurrence after surgery and quantify any benefit from adjuvant chemotherapy.

Furthermore, hereditary colon cancers frequently are positive for MSI as compared with sporadic colon cancers. Lynch syndrome (a hereditary form of colon cancer) can be suspected if the tumour is MSI positive. MSI is performed by immunohistochemical identification of specific nucleic acid. MMR genetic testing is most frequently performed by PCR testing.

BRAF is another important gene that is used to indicate the likelihood that a colon tumour is hereditary. *BRAF* is a kinase-encoding gene in the RAS/RAF/MAPK pathway. The presence of a *BRAF* V600E mutation in a microsatellite unstable tumour indicates that the tumour is probably sporadic and not associated with hereditary non-polyposis colorectal cancer (HNPCC). The lack of this mutation indicates that a tumour may either be sporadic or HNPCC associated.

The *Oncotype DX Colon Cancer Assay* evaluates 12 genes and provides an individualized score reflective of the risk of colon cancer recurrence for individual patients with stage 2 colon cancer. The assay uses a RT-PCR platform to quantitate the level of expression of each of the 12 genes in the panel using the patient's colon tumour. For each patient, the assay produces a recurrence score that is closely associated with the patient's risk of recurrent colon cancer 3 years after surgery (the peak time of recurrence). MMR and MSI testing can complement the information provided by the Oncotype DX Colon Cancer Assay.

PROCEDURE AND PATIENT CARE

Before

 Inform the patient that an examination for these tumour predictor markers may be performed on his or her colon cancer tissue.

- Provide psychological and emotional support to the colon cancer patient.

During

- The surgeon obtains tumour tissue.
- This tissue should be placed on ice or in formalin.
- Part of the tissue is used for routine histology. A portion of the paraffin block is sent to a reference laboratory.

After

Explain to the patient that results are usually available in 1 week.

TEST RESULTS AND CLINICAL SIGNIFICANCE

Colon cancer with unfavourable prognosis: *This helps determine patients who by the genomic make up of their colon cancer and other prognostic factors will benefit from the use of adjuvant chemotherapy. Patients whose prognosis is very good by genomic testing will not benefit from the addition of preventive chemotherapy.*

Hereditary colon cancer: *Patients with a BRAF genetic mutation or whose colon cancer has microsatellite instability have an increased risk that their cancer was hereditary. After genetic counselling, other family members may want to consider being tested for genetic predisposition to colon cancer and have early screening testing such as colonoscopy (p. 619) if they are positive.*

RELATED TEST

Genetic Testing (p. 1139). This discussion included genetic testing for other forms of familial colon cancer, including Lynch syndrome and familial polyposis.

Cutaneous Immunofluorescence Biopsy
(Immunofluorescence Skin Biopsy, Skin Biopsy Antibodies, Skin Immunohistopathology)

NORMAL FINDINGS

Normal skin histologic appearance

INDICATIONS

This test of inflamed skin is performed to evaluate and diagnose immunologically mediated dermatitis. It is indicated when an immunologic source for a skin rash is suspected.

TEST EXPLANATION

For this study, a skin biopsy is obtained and evaluated by immunofluorescence methods. Deposition of human immunoglobulins or complement components is determined by immunofluorescent patterns. This test is useful in detecting immune complexes, complement, and immunoglobulin skin deposition in systemic and discoid lupus erythematosus, pemphigus, bullous pemphigoid, and dermatitis herpetiformis. This test is also used to confirm the histopathologic features of skin lesions and to monitor the results of treatment.

PROCEDURE AND PATIENT CARE

Before
✗ Explain the procedure to the patient.
• Obtain the patient's informed consent for the procedure.

During
• The skin area used for biopsy is anaesthetized locally to minimize discomfort.
• A 4-mm punch biopsy or elliptical tissue excision is obtained.

After
• Apply a dry, sterile dressing over the biopsy site.
✗ Inform the patient that results may not be available for several days.
• Deliver the specimen on ice to the laboratory immediately after the biopsy is taken.

TEST RESULTS AND CLINICAL SIGNIFICANCE

Systemic lupus erythematosus (SLE),
Discoid lupus erythematosus: *Lupus erythematosus is associated with acute, subacute, and chronic skin lesions. All are associated with deposits of immunoglobulins and complement in the epidermal basement membrane zone. The acute changes are represented by the butterfly rash of SLE. Subacute changes of SLE are represented by photosensitive ulcers. The chronic changes of discoid lupus are scalelike areas about the neck and face. Once the scale is removed, an ulcer remains until healing and scarring occur.*
Pemphigus,
Bullous pemphigoid: *These immunologic dermatitis diseases are highlighted clinically as subepidermal blistering of skin, usually in older adults.*
Dermatitis herpetiformis: *This urticarial immunologic dermatitis is often associated with gluten-sensitive enteropathy.*

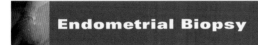
Endometrial Biopsy

NORMAL FINDINGS

No pathologic conditions
Presence of a "secretory-type" endometrium 3 to 5 days before normal menses

INDICATIONS

Endometrial biopsy had been used to determine whether the patient has adequate ovarian estrogen and progesterone levels. This is indicated in women with suspected ovarian dysfunction (such as women who are nearing menopause, are not menstruating, or are infertile). It is most often used to diagnose and evaluate women who have dysfunctional uterine bleeding and uterine cancer.

TEST EXPLANATION

An endometrial biopsy can determine whether ovulation has occurred. A biopsy specimen taken 3 to 5 days before normal menses should demonstrate a "secretory-type" endometrium on histologic examination if ovulation and corpus luteum formation have occurred. If not, the specimen should demonstrate only a preovulatory "proliferative-type" endometrium.

Two other major uses of endometrial biopsy are to diagnose endometrial cancer, polyps, or inflammatory conditions and to evaluate uterine bleeding.

This procedure is performed in approximately 10 to 15 minutes by an obstetrician/gynecologist. Minor discomfort (menstrual-type cramping) may be felt. It is important to recognize that an endometrial biopsy is not a substitute for dilation and curettage, which is much more extensive and tests all surfaces of the endometrium.

CONTRAINDICATIONS

- Infections (e.g., trichomonal, candidal, suspected gonococcal) of the cervix or vagina, because the infection may spread to the uterus
- Inability to visualize the cervix (e.g., because of abnormal position or previous surgery), because the cervix is the access to the uterus

POTENTIAL COMPLICATIONS

- Perforation of the uterus
- Uterine bleeding
- Interference with early pregnancy
- Infection

PROCEDURE AND PATIENT CARE

Before

- Explain the procedure to the patient.
- Obtain the patient's written informed consent for this procedure.
- Inform the patient that no fasting or sedation is usually required unless ordered by the physician. Menstrual-type cramping may be experienced.

During

- Note the following procedural steps:
  1. The patient is placed in the lithotomy position, and a pelvic examination is performed to determine the position of the uterus.
  2. The cervix is exposed and cleansed.
  3. A biopsy instrument is inserted into the uterus, and specimens are obtained from the anterior, posterior, and lateral walls. The biopsy can be performed with a curette or forceps or through the use of endometrial uterine lavage and a suction device to collect the specimen (Figure 7-2). Suction endometrial biopsy is most commonly performed because it is the least painful and can be performed in the physician's office.
  4. The specimens are placed in a solution containing 10% formalin and sent to the pathologist for histologic examination.

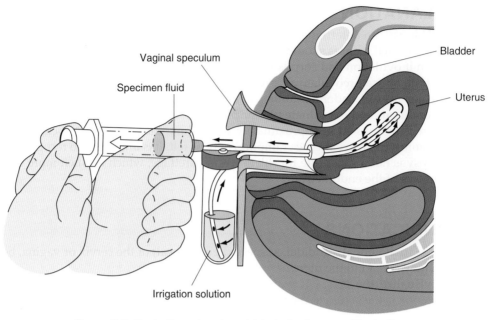

Figure 7-2 Illustration of endometrial uterine lavage with sterile normal saline and negative pressure. Arrows indicate the flow of the irrigating solution and collection of the specimen. Fluid does not enter the fallopian tubes. A plug at the cervical os helps maintain negative pressure within the uterus.

After

- Any temperature elevation should be reported to the physician because this procedure may activate pelvic inflammatory disease.
- Advise the patient to wear a sanitary pad because some vaginal bleeding is to be expected.
- Instruct the patient to call her primary care or family physician if excessive bleeding (necessitating more than one pad per hour) occurs.
- Instruct the patient to avoid douching and intercourse for 72 hours after the biopsy procedure.
- Instruct the patient to rest during the next 24 hours and to avoid heavy lifting, to prevent increased intra-abdominal pressure and uterine hemorrhage.

 Home Care Responsibilities

- Instruct the patient to report any temperature elevation to her physician because this procedure may activate pelvic inflammatory disease.
- Advise the patient to wear a sanitary pad after this procedure because some vaginal bleeding is expected. Instruct the patient to call her primary care or family physician for excessive bleeding (more than one pad per hour).
- Instruct the patient to avoid heavy lifting after this procedure to prevent increased intra-abdominal pressure and possible uterine bleeding.

TEST RESULTS AND CLINICAL SIGNIFICANCE

Anovulation: *Without ovulation, the endometrium is persistently in the proliferative stage. No secretory changes are noted.*

Tumour,

Polyps: *Endometrial adenocarcinoma with or without squamous carcinoma components is the most common uterine cancer. Hyperplastic proliferative polyps are a common cause of dysfunctional uterine bleeding.*

Inflammatory condition: *Endometrial infections, although rare, do occur. Ascending sexually transmitted infections are the most common type of primary infection not associated with prior surgical instrumentation.*

Estrogen Receptor Assay (ER Assay, ERA, Estradiol Receptor)

NORMAL FINDINGS

Negative: fewer than 1% of the cells take up stain for receptors

INDICATIONS

Estrogen receptor assay is performed on breast cancer tissue to indicate sensitivity to hormonal manipulative therapy and to indicate prognosis of breast cancer.

TEST EXPLANATION

The estrogen receptor assay is useful in determining the prognosis and treatment of breast cancer and to determine whether a tumour is likely to respond to endocrine therapy. Tumours for which the estrogen receptor assay yields positive results are more than twice as likely to respond to endocrine therapy as are estrogen receptor–negative tumours. Hormone receptor assays should be performed on all breast cancers. Breast tumours tend to be positive more often in postmenopausal women than in premenopausal women. In general, estrogen receptor–positive tumours have a better prognosis than estrogen receptor–negative tumours.

Slightly more than half of patients with breast carcinoma who are estrogen receptor–positive respond to endocrine therapy (e.g., tamoxifen, estrogens, aromatase inhibitors, oophorectomy). The response is greater when the results of the progesterone receptor assay (see p. 781) are also positive. Patients whose breast cancers lack these hormone receptors (i.e., are estrogen receptor–negative) have a much lower chance of tumour response to hormone therapy and may not be candidates for this form of treatment.

A pathologist obtains assay specimens from surgical specimens. Estrogen receptor assays are performed most commonly with immunohistochemical methods on fixed, paraffin-embedded tissue. Positive immunohistochemical reactivity is observed in the nuclei of the tumour cells. This method of measuring estrogen receptors is considered very accurate. Results are usually available in less than 1 week.

INTERFERING FACTORS

- Delay in tissue fixation may cause deterioration of receptor proteins and may lead to lower values.
- Hormone therapy should be discontinued before breast biopsy is performed. Ingestion of antiestrogen preparations (e.g., tamoxifen [Nolvadex]) during the previous 2 months may cause false-negative results of estrogen receptor assays.
- Exogenous hormones that are taken for contraceptive purposes or menopausal estrogens may lead to lower receptor values.

PROCEDURE AND PATIENT CARE

Before

- Explain the biopsy procedure to the patient.
- Instruct the patient to discontinue taking hormones as per physician's orders, usually 2 months before breast biopsy is performed.
- Before biopsy, obtain the patient's gynecologic history, including menopausal status and exogenous hormone use.

During

- The surgeon obtains tumour tissue.
- This tissue should be placed on ice or in formalin.
- Part of the tissue is used for routine histologic examination. A portion of the paraffin block is sent to a reference laboratory.

After

- Explain to the patient that results are usually available in 1 week.

TEST RESULTS AND CLINICAL SIGNIFICANCE

Estrogen receptor–positive: *The treatment of this cancer is more likely to be successful with hormone manipulation in a therapeutic or adjuvant clinical setting.*

RELATED TESTS

Progesterone Receptor Assay (p. 781). Like estrogen receptor assay, this test helps predict the likelihood of tumour response to endocrine manipulative therapy.

Breast Cancer Genomics (p. 1131). This test is used as a prognosticator indicating the risk of recurrent breast cancer. It is a powerful predictor of benefit from hormone therapy or chemotherapy.

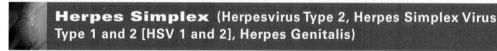

Herpes Simplex (Herpesvirus Type 2, Herpes Simplex Virus Type 1 and 2 [HSV 1 and 2], Herpes Genitalis)

NORMAL FINDINGS

No virus present
No herpes simplex virus (HSV) antigens or antibodies present

INDICATIONS

Herpes testing is performed to diagnose acute initial herpes infections. It is used in patients with suspected initial genital infection. It is also used in immunocompromised patients who have aggressive oral mucosal or genital eruptions characteristic of the infection. Furthermore, it is used on patients (especially immunocompromised patients) who have a fever of unknown origin.

Herpes cultures are used to identify active genital herpes infection in women who are expecting to deliver a baby vaginally in the next 6 to 8 weeks.

TEST EXPLANATION

HSV can be classified as either herpes simplex virus type 1 (HSV-1) or herpes simplex virus type 2 (HSV-2). HSV-1 is responsible primarily for oral lesions (blisters on the lips, or "cold sores") or even corneal lesions. At present, HSV-1 is treatable, but about half of the patients with HSV-1 develop recurrent infections. Recurrences of the HSV-1 symptoms can be triggered by excess sunlight, fever, stress, acute illness, and medications or conditions that weaken the immune system (such as cancer, human immunodeficiency virus [HIV] infection/acquired immune deficiency syndrome [AIDS], or the use of corticosteroids). HSV-2 is a sexually transmitted viral infection of the urogenital tract, also known as *genital herpes*. At present, HSV-2 is treatable but incurable and is usually acquired through genital-genital contact, but also by exposure to HSV-1, usually through oral-genital contact.

Vesicular lesions may occur on the penis, scrotum, vulva, perineum, perianal region, vagina, or cervix. Initial infections are often associated with generalized symptoms of fever and malaise.

Because most infants become infected if they pass through a birth canal containing HSV, its presence at delivery must be determined. Congenital infections may result in problems such as microcephaly, chorioretinitis, and mental retardation in the newborn. Disseminated neonatal HSV infections carry a high incidence of infant mortality. A vaginal delivery is possible if no virus is present, but birth by Caesarean section is necessary if HSV is present. Viral testing can be performed on male or female patients to determine the risk for sexual transmission.

Culture is still the standard criterion for HSV detection and can identify HSV in 90% of infected patients. Serologic tests are more easily and conveniently available for detection of HSV-1 and HSV-2 antigen. Unfortunately, the accuracy is not high; only about 85% of patients who have positive culture results also have positive serologic results. The advantage of antigen tests is that results can be available in a day. Serologic tests for antibodies are cumbersome because they necessitate repeated blood tests during the acute and convalescent phases of an acute viral outbreak (about 2 weeks apart). A fourfold rise in titre is expected for the diagnosis of acute initial herpes infection. Recurrent infections are far less likely to demonstrate titre elevations. Despite the high psychosexual and physical consequences of infection, there is almost no information on the epidemiologic features of genital herpes infection in Canada; however, HSV-1 now accounts for approximately 40% of first genital episodes in Canadian patients.

The antigen tests are performed with fluorescent immunoassay or latex agglutination. The antibody tests involve immunofluorescent immunoassay or enzyme-linked immunosorbent assay (ELISA) methods. Antibody testing cannot diagnose active recurrent genital herpes; culture testing is required for this diagnosis.

7   Microscopic Examinations

Clinical Priorities

- Neonatal HSV infections carry a high incidence of infant mortality. A Caesarean delivery may be needed if HSV is present in the pregnant woman.
- Women should refrain from using douches and from taking tub baths for 24 hours before the cervical culture.
- Men should not urinate within 1 hour before a urethral culture because voiding washes secretions out of the urethra.
- If herpes is diagnosed, it should be treated, and patients' sexual partners should be evaluated. Although acute outbreaks of genital herpes are treatable, this disease is not curable.

PROCEDURE AND PATIENT CARE

Before

✗ Explain the procedure to the patient.

✗ Instruct the female patient to refrain from using douches and from taking tub baths for 24 hours before the cervical culture is performed.

- Obtain the urethral specimen from the male patient as he voids.
- Note that blood study results can be diagnostic in both male and female patients.

During

Urethral Culture

1. A culture is taken by inserting a sterile swab gently into the anterior urethra or genital skin lesion of the male patient (see Figure 7-8, p. 790).
2. It is advisable to place the male patient in the supine position to prevent his falling if vasovagal syncope occurs during introduction of the cotton swab or wire loop into the urethra.
3. The patient is observed for hypotension, bradycardia, pallor, sweating, nausea, and weakness.

Cervical Culture

1. The female patient is placed in the lithotomy position, and a vaginal speculum is inserted.
2. Cervical mucus is removed with a cotton ball.
3. A sterile cotton-tipped swab is inserted gently into the endocervical canal and moved from side to side to obtain the culture. If a genital lesion is present, swabs from that area will be more sensitive in indicating infection.
4. For pregnant women with genital herpes, note that the cervix is cultured weekly for HSV beginning 4 to 6 weeks before the due date. Vaginal delivery is possible if the following criteria are met:
   1. The two most recent cultures are negative.
   2. The woman is not experiencing any symptoms.
   3. No lesions are visible on inspection of the vagina and vulva.
   4. Throughout pregnancy the woman has not had more than one positive culture, during which she was free of symptoms.

Blood for Serologic Study

- Obtain a venous blood sample in a red-top tube.

Molecular PCR Tissue and Other Fluids
- Obtain CSF (p. 676) or other fluids by sterile technique as described elsewhere in this book.
- Obtain tissue by appropriate biopsy techniques.
- Place specimen in an appropriate container designated by the reference laboratory.

After
- Apply pressure or a pressure dressing to the venipuncture site.
- Observe the venipuncture site for bleeding.
- Inform the patient how to obtain the test results.

TEST RESULTS AND CLINICAL SIGNIFICANCE

Herpes virus infection: *Like other sexually transmitted infections (STIs), this disease can significantly affect patients, their children, and their sexual partners. If herpes or other STIs have been diagnosed, treatment should begin immediately and active sexual partners should be evaluated. Although acute outbreaks of genital herpes are treatable, the disease is not curable.*

RELATED TESTS

Sexually Transmitted Infection Culture (p. 787). This is a general test for the presence of STIs and their causative agents.

Chlamydia (p. 751), Syphilis Detection (p. 487), Hepatitis Virus Studies (p. 304), and HIV Serology (p. 310). These are tests for other STIs.

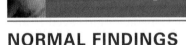

Human Papillomavirus (HPV Test, HPV DNA Testing)

NORMAL FINDINGS

No human papillomavirus (HPV) present

INDICATIONS

An HPV test is performed to identify genital HPV infection in a woman with abnormal results of a Papanicolaou (Pap) smear.

TEST EXPLANATION

HPV is a small, nonenveloped, double-stranded, circular DNA tumour virus, classified in the genus *Papillomavirus* of the Papovaviridae family of viruses. More than 100 distinct types of HPV have been identified, and approximately 50 of these infect the epithelial membranes of the ano-genital tract of women. HPV DNA incorporates itself into the cervical cell genome, promoting its effects through activation of oncogenes and suppression of host cell immune response. HPV protein products prevent DNA repair and programmed cell death, which can lead to instability and unchecked cell growth.

HPV infects the genital epithelium and is spread through skin-to-skin contact. Some strains of HPV cause genital warts, but HPV infections often produce no signs or symptoms. As a result,

Microscopic Examinations

7

infected individuals are frequently unaware that they are carriers, and they unknowingly transmit the virus to other people.

Genital HPV strains are divided into two groups (low and high risk) on the basis of their oncogenic potential and ability to induce the development of virus-associated tumours. Low-risk strains (HPV-6, -11, -42, -43, and -44) are associated with condylomata genital warts and low-grade cervical changes, such as mild dysplasia. Lesions caused by low-risk HPV infection have a high likelihood of regression and little potential for progression and are considered of no or low oncogenic risk. High-risk strains (HPV-16, -18, -31, -33, -35, -39, -45, -51, -52, -56, -58, -59, and -68) are associated with intraepithelial neoplasia and are more likely to progress to severe lesions and cervical cancer.

A clear causal relationship has been established between HPV infection and cervical cancer (70% of cervical cancers are related particularly to HPV-6, -11, -16, and -18). HPV is found in almost all cases of cervical malignancies worldwide. Of the high-risk HPV strains, HPV-16 and HPV-18 are the most carcinogenic and most prevalent. HPV-16 is the predominant strain in almost all regions of the world, with the exception of Southeast Asia, where HPV-18 has the highest prevalence. High-grade cervical intraepithelial lesions are most commonly associated with HPV-16 and HPV-18, and yet these strains are also frequently found to be the causative factor in minor lesions and mild dysplasia. The latency period between initial HPV exposure and development of cervical cancer may be months or years. It is estimated that more than 70% of sexually active Canadian men and women will have HPV infection in their lifetime. Although progression may be rapid, average time from initial infection to manifestation of invasive cervical cancer is estimated at approximately 15 years. Women who have normal Pap smear results and no HPV infection are at very low risk (0.2%) for developing cervical cancer. Women who have an abnormal Pap smear result and a positive result of the HPV test are at higher risk (6% to 7% or greater) for developing cervical cancer.

Two HPV vaccines are now authorized for use in Canada: Gardasil and Cervarix. Gardasil provides protection against four HPV types (HPV-6, -11, -16, and -18): two that cause 70% of all cervical cancers and two that cause 90% of all genital and anal warts. It is approved for use in all individuals aged 9 to 26 years. Cervarix, a vaccine that protects against the two HPV types that cause 70% of all cervical cancers, has been approved for use in Canada for girls aged 10 and up and women up to age 25 years. Gardasil is given as an intramuscular injection in a series of three shots. Second and third boosters are provided at 2 months and 6 months after the first. Both the National Advisory Committee on Immunization (NACI) and the Canadian Immunization Committee (CIC) recommend the use of these vaccines in these populations.

The HPV test is now performed routinely on most women but particularly those who have an abnormal Pap smear result. Pap smear results such as "atypical squamous cells of undetermined significance" or "low-grade squamous intraepithelial lesion" often prompt a routine HPV test. The most commonly used test is the Hybrid Capture II DNA assay. In this test, RNA probes are used in a modified enzyme-linked immunosorbent assay (ELISA) platform to identify the presence or absence of 13 strains of "high-risk" HPV DNA. In another commonly performed method of HPV testing, nucleic acid probe/polymerase chain reaction is used.

Numerous sources indicate that more than 60% of women with an abnormal Pap smear test positive for high-risk HPV infection. If the HPV test result is positive, a woman should undergo colposcopy to detect a more serious cervical lesion such as cancer. It is well known that HPV infection in younger women is more prevalent and often spontaneously regresses, particularly in those younger than 30 years. In contrast, persistent high-risk infection peaks in women older than 30 years. As a result, some physicians recommend that HPV testing be reserved for clinical use in the evaluation of women older than 30 to 35 years or for younger women with high-grade squamous intraepithelial lesions. Most recent studies have suggested that HPV testing is more sensitive than the Pap smear in the detection of serious cervical disease.

INTERFERING FACTORS

- HPV testing may be affected by the number of cells in the specimen. Cervical specimens with few cells may not provide an adequate number for DNA testing.

PROCEDURE AND PATIENT CARE

Before

🖊 Explain the procedure for Pap smear (p. 774).

🖊 Instruct the patient not to use a douche or take a tub bath during the 24 hours before the Pap smear. (Some health care providers prefer that patients refrain from sexual intercourse for 24 to 48 hours before the test.)

🖊 Instruct the patient to empty her bladder before the examination.

🖊 Instruct the patient to reschedule testing if she is menstruating.

🖊 Inform the patient that no fasting or sedation is required.

During

- Note the following procedural steps:
  1. The patient is placed in the lithotomy position as for a Pap smear.
  2. With the use of either a cytology brush or a wooden spatula, a cervical mucus specimen is obtained by placing the instrument into the cervical os and rotating 3 to 5 times in clockwise and counterclockwise directions.
  3. After specimen collection, rotate the broomlike device or spatula and cytobrush several times in the collection vial to remove the specimen. Firmly cap the vial, and discard the collection devices.
  4. Affix a patient identification label to the vial.
  5. Seal the vial and place in a plastic specimen bag along with a properly filled-out cytology requisition form, and send to the laboratory.
- Specimens for the Hybrid Capture II assay can be obtained in two ways. Reflex testing entails the use of the residual cell suspension from liquid-based cytologic study of the original Pap smear. A second sample can also be obtained at the time of the original Pap smear or during a second procedure. The cervical specimen is then placed into a transport medium in a separate tube for HPV testing.
- Note that a nurse or a physician obtains a Pap smear in approximately 10 minutes.

🖊 Inform the patient that no discomfort, except for insertion of the speculum, is associated with this procedure.

After

🖊 Inform the patient that usually she will not be notified unless further evaluation is necessary.

🖊 Inform the patient that HPV is a sexually transmitted infection. All proper precautions should be taken to prevent infecting sexual partners.

TEST RESULTS AND CLINICAL SIGNIFICANCE

HPV infection: *Infected women should consider more aggressive cervical cancer screening.*

RELATED TEST

Papanicolaou Smear (p. 774). This is a commonly performed screening test for cervical/uterine cancer that is performed at the same time the specimen is obtained for HPV testing.

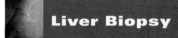

Liver Biopsy

NORMAL FINDINGS

Normal liver histologic features

INDICATIONS

Liver biopsy is a safe, simple, and valuable method of diagnosing pathologic liver conditions.

TEST EXPLANATION

For this study, a specially designed needle is inserted through the abdominal wall and into the liver (Figure 7-3). A piece of liver tissue is removed for microscopic examination. Percutaneous liver biopsy is used in the diagnosis of various liver disorders, such as cirrhosis, hepatitis, drug reaction, granuloma, and tumour. Biopsy is indicated for patients with the following conditions:

1. Unexplained hepatomegaly
2. Persistently elevated liver enzyme levels
3. Suspected primary or metastatic tumour, as determined by other studies
4. Unexplained jaundice
5. Suspected hepatitis
6. Suspected infiltrative diseases (e.g., sarcoidosis, amyloidosis)

The biopsy may be performed by a "blind stick" method or may be directed with the use of computed tomography, magnetic resonance imaging, ultrasonography, or laparoscopy. Directed biopsy is used if there is a specific focal area of the liver that is suspect and from which tissue must be obtained (e.g., a metastatic tumour). The "blind stick" method is used if the liver is diffusely involved.

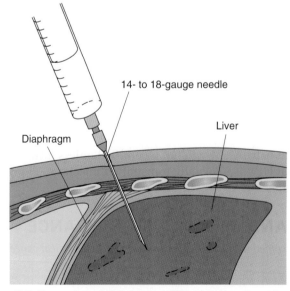

Figure 7-3 Illustration of liver biopsy. Percutaneous liver biopsy requires the patient's cooperation. The patient must be able to lie quietly and hold his or her breath after exhaling.

A physician performs this test in approximately 15 minutes. Minor discomfort may be experienced during injection of the local anaesthetic and during needle insertion and biopsy. In the past, blind biopsy was performed with small aspiration or small tissue-sampling needles. With guided biopsies, larger-core needles can obtain a significant amount of tissue for histologic review. This has reduced sampling errors both in placing the needle in the suspect area and in obtaining enough tissue for histologic study.

CONTRAINDICATIONS

- Inability of patients to remain still and hold their breath after sustained exhalation
- Impaired hemostasis
- Anemia with inability to tolerate major blood loss associated with inadvertent puncture of an intrahepatic blood vessel
- Infections in the right pleural space or right upper quadrant, because the biopsy may spread the infection
- Obstructive jaundice, in which bile within the ducts is under pressure and may subsequently leak into the abdominal cavity after needle penetration
- Hemangioma, because this is a very vascular tumour, and bleeding after a biopsy may be severe
- Ascites, because persistent leak of fluid may occur (further bile leaks will not seal off)

POTENTIAL COMPLICATIONS

- Hemorrhage caused by inadvertent puncture of a blood vessel within the liver
- Chemical peritonitis caused by inadvertent puncture of a bile duct, with subsequent leakage of bile into the abdominal cavity
- Pneumothorax (collapsed lung) caused by improper placement of the biopsy needle into the adjacent chest cavity

 Clinical Priorities

- Assess the coagulation profile before performing a liver biopsy because of the possibility of bleeding.
- After the liver biopsy, instruct the patient to remain on the right side for about 1 to 2 hours. This position decreases the risk of hemorrhage by compressing the liver capsule against the chest wall.
- Carefully evaluate the patient after this test for evidence of hemorrhage (increased pulse rate, decreased blood pressure) and peritonitis (increased temperature).

PROCEDURE AND PATIENT CARE

Before

- Explain the procedure to the patient. Allow the patient to verbalize concerns, and allay any fears.
- Obtain the patient's informed consent for this procedure.
- Ensure that all coagulation test results are normal.
- Instruct the patient to keep on NPO status (nothing by mouth) after midnight on the day of the test. Surgery may be necessary if a complication occurs. The patient must be prepared for the possibility of surgery.
- Administer any sedative medications as ordered.

During

- Note the following procedural steps:
  1. The patient is placed in the supine or left lateral position.
  2. The skin area used for puncture is locally anaesthetized.
  3. The patient is asked to exhale and hold the exhalation. This causes the liver to descend and reduces the possibility of a pneumothorax. Frequently, the patient practises exhalation two or three times before insertion of the needle.
  4. During the patient's sustained exhalation, the physician rapidly introduces the biopsy needle into the liver and obtains liver tissue. Several types of needles are available. Often the biopsy needle is inserted under computed tomographic guidance. This is especially useful when tissue from a specific area of the liver is needed.
  5. The needle is withdrawn from the liver.
- If laparoscopy is used to obtain the biopsy, follow the procedure outlined for laparoscopy (p. 645).

After

- Place the tissue sample into a specimen bottle containing formalin and send it to the pathology department.
- Apply a small dressing over the needle insertion site.
- Place the patient on his or her right side for approximately 1 to 2 hours. In this position, the liver capsule is compressed against the chest wall, which decreases the risk for hemorrhage or bile leak.
- Assess the patient's vital signs frequently for evidence of hemorrhage (increased pulse rate, decreased blood pressure) and peritonitis (increased temperature).
- If laparoscopy was performed, provide routine postoperative care.
- Evaluate the rate, rhythm, and depth of respirations. Assess breath sounds. Report chest pain and signs of dyspnea, cyanosis, and restlessness—which may be indicative of pneumothorax—to the physician performing the procedure.

 Clinical Priorities

- Instruct the patient to report signs of bleeding (increased pulse and decreased blood pressure) or peritonitis (increased temperature).
- Advise the patient to avoid coughing and straining that may cause increased intra-abdominal pressure. Strenuous activities and heavy lifting should be avoided for 1 to 2 weeks.

TEST RESULTS AND CLINICAL SIGNIFICANCE

Benign tumour (adenoma),

Malignant tumour (primary [hepatoma, cholangiocarcinoma] and metastatic [e.g., bowel, breast, lung]): *Biopsy of these focal lesions can be performed and specimens obtained for histologic study. Usually these biopsies are guided by imaging studies.*

Abscess,

Cyst: *These fluid lesions can be aspirated and catheters left for drainage.*

Hepatitis,

Infiltrative diseases (e.g., amyloidosis, hemochromatosis, cirrhosis, fat): *Diffuse liver abnormality is much more easily obtainable by the liver biopsy needle because more tissue contains the pathologic condition.*

RELATED TESTS

Computed Tomography, Abdomen (p. 1059). This radiographic study provides excellent visualization of the liver for guided biopsy.

Magnetic Resonance Imaging (p. 1148). In MRI of the liver, variations in electromagnetic characteristics are used to provide an accurate image of the liver. Technology has advanced to allow the guidance of a biopsy needle to the suspect area within the liver.

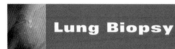
Lung Biopsy

NORMAL FINDINGS

No evidence of pathologic conditions

INDICATIONS

Lung biopsy is indicated to determine the nature of a pulmonary parenchymal nodule that has been identified on plain chest radiograph or chest computed tomography. Carcinomas, granulomas, infections, and sarcoidosis can be diagnosed with this procedure. This procedure is also useful in detecting environmental exposures, infections, or familial disease, which may lead to better prevention and treatment.

TEST EXPLANATION

This invasive procedure is used to obtain a specimen of pulmonary tissue for a histologic examination through either an open or a closed technique. The open method involves a limited thoracotomy. The closed technique includes methods such as transbronchial lung biopsy, transbronchial needle aspiration biopsy, transcatheter bronchial brushing, percutaneous needle aspiration biopsy, and video-assisted thoracostomy surgery.

This procedure is performed in 30 to 60 minutes by a radiologist, surgeon, or pulmonologist. Most patients describe the percutaneous biopsy procedure as painful. Postoperative incisional pain can be expected if the open technique or video-assisted thoracostomy surgery is used.

CONTRAINDICATIONS

- Bullae or cysts of the lung, because the risk of pneumothorax is greater with needle lung biopsy
- Suspected vascular anomalies of the lung, because bleeding may occur
- Bleeding abnormalities, because bleeding may occur
- Pulmonary hypertension, because bleeding is more likely to occur
- Respiratory insufficiency, because if a pneumothorax occurs, the patient is not likely to survive

POTENTIAL COMPLICATIONS

- Pneumothorax
- Pulmonary hemorrhage
- Empyema

Clinical Priorities

- Assess the results of the coagulation studies before lung biopsy because postprocedure bleeding can occur.
- The patient is usually kept on NPO status (nothing by mouth) after midnight before this test.
- After the procedure, carefully assess the patient for signs of bleeding (increased pulse rate, decreased blood pressure) and shortness of breath.
- A chest radiograph is usually ordered after the procedure to check for complications (such as pneumothorax).

PROCEDURE AND PATIENT CARE

Before

- Explain the procedure to the patient.
- Obtain the patient's signed informed consent for this procedure.
- Explain to the patient that fasting is usually ordered. The patient may be kept on NPO status after midnight on the day of the test.
- Administer the preprocedural medications 30 to 60 minutes before the test as ordered. Medications are usually given to decrease bronchial secretions and sedate anxious patients.
- Instruct the patient to remain still during the lung biopsy. Any movement or coughing could cause laceration of the lung by the biopsy needle.

During

- Note that the patient's position depends on the method used and that the histologic lung specimen may be obtained by several different methods:

Transbronchial Lung Biopsy

See discussion of bronchoscopy on p. 613.
1. This technique is performed with flexible fibreoptic bronchoscopy with cutting forceps.
2. Fluoroscopy is used to ensure proper opening and positioning of the forceps on the lesions.
3. Fluoroscopy also enables visualization of the "tug" of the lung as the specimen is removed.

Transbronchial Needle Aspiration

See discussion of bronchoscopy on p. 613.
1. The specimen is obtained through a fibreoptic bronchoscope with a needle (Figure 7-4).
2. The bronchoscope is inserted, and the target site is identified through fluoroscopy.
3. The needle is inserted through the bronchoscope and into the tumour or desired area, where aspiration is performed with the attached syringe.
4. The needle is retracted within its sheath, and the entire catheter is withdrawn from the fibreoptic bronchoscope.

Transcatheter Bronchial Brushing

1. This is also performed through a fibreoptic bronchoscope (see discussion of bronchoscopy, p. 613).
2. During bronchoscopy, a small brush is moved back and forth over the suspect area in the bronchus or its branches.
3. The cells adhere to the brush, which is then removed and used to make microscopic slides.

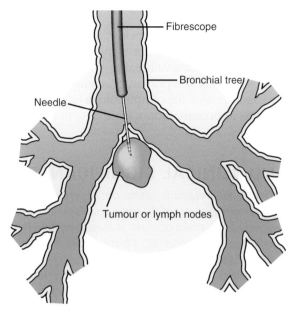

Figure 7-4 Illustration of transbronchial needle biopsy. The transbronchial needle penetrates the bronchial wall and enters a mass of subcarinal lymph nodes or tumour.

Percutaneous Needle Biopsy

1. In this method for obtaining a closed specimen, the biopsy is obtained after fluoroscopic radiography or computed tomography is used for localization of the desired site.
2. The procedure is carried out with a cutting needle or by aspiration with a spinal type of needle to obtain a specimen.
3. The main problem with this procedure is potential damage to major blood vessels.
4. During the lung biopsy procedure, assess the patient carefully for signs of respiratory distress (e.g., shortness of breath, rapid pulse rate, cyanosis).

Open Lung Biopsy

1. The patient is taken to the operating room, and general anaesthesia is induced.
2. The patient is placed in the supine or lateral position, and an incision is made into the chest wall.
3. After a piece of lung tissue is removed, the lung is sutured.
4. Chest tube drainage is used for approximately 24 hours after an open lung biopsy.
5. This procedure can be performed by thoracoscopy, as described in the following section.

Thoracoscopic Biopsy

1. The lung is collapsed with a double-lumen endotracheal tube placed during induction of general anaesthesia.
2. A thoracoscope (similar to a laparoscope [p. 645]) is used to grasp the lung, and a cutting/stapling device is used to cut off a piece. Large-wedge lung resections can be obtained.
3. The bronchoscope and trocars are removed, and a small chest tube is left in place.
4. The tiny incisions are closed.

After

- Place biopsy specimens in appropriate containers for histologic and microbiologic examination.
- Observe the patient's vital signs frequently for signs of bleeding (increased pulse rate, decreased blood pressure) and for shortness of breath.
- Assess the patient's breath sounds, and report any decrease on the biopsy side.
- A chest radiograph is ordered to check for complications (e.g., pneumothorax).
- Observe the patient for signs of pneumothorax (e.g., dyspnea, tachypnea, decrease in breath sounds, anxiety, restlessness).

TEST RESULTS AND CLINICAL SIGNIFICANCE

Carcinoma: *Biopsy of both primary and metastatic lesions can be performed with this technique. The lesion must be peripheral enough to ensure that one of the great vessels is not punctured.*

Granuloma: *If the lesion is observed to contain calcium, it may be an old granuloma from previous granulomatous infection. If calcification is not observed, a biopsy of the lesion must be performed to rule out cancer, active fungal infection, or tuberculosis.*

Exposure lung diseases (e.g., black lung, asbestosis): *It is important to recognize and document the presence of exposure lung disease for medical reasons (prognosis and treatment) and legal reasons (workers' compensation or disability).*

Sarcoidosis: *Sarcoidosis of the lung is an interstitial disease highlighted by chronic inflammation and fibrosis. This is obvious on lung biopsy.*

Infection: *For unusual infections (such as that caused by* Pneumocystis jiroveci) *and unusual fungal diseases, tissue is required for culture and microscopic identification.*

RELATED TESTS

Bronchoscopy (p. 613). This endoscopic test is the access through which transbronchial biopsy and aspirations are performed.

Lung Scan (p. 838). This scan is a computed tomographic method of localizing a lung lesion for biopsy.

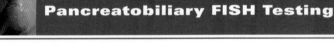

Pancreatobiliary FISH Testing

NORMAL FINDINGS

No chromosomal ploidy abnormalities

INDICATIONS

This test is used to assist in the diagnosis of pancreatic/biliary cancer.

TEST EXPLANATION

It is sometimes difficult to differentiate benign bile duct strictures from early pancreatobiliary cancer. When a stricture is identified on an endoscopic retrograde cholangiopancreatography (ERCP, p. 632), cancer must be considered as a possible cause. If an obvious cancer is not seen at the time of ERCP, a brush is repeatedly swept along the bile duct to obtain duct surface cells for conventional cytology to identify cancer cells. In conventional cytology, the brushing specimens are placed on a slide and stained with a PAP stain. Slides are then interpreted by a cytopathologist to determine whether they show features that are positive for malignancy, suspicious for malignancy, atypical (meaning there are cells that are not normal but cannot be definitely ascribed to a neoplastic process), or negative for malignancy.

With the use of fluorescence in situ hybridization (FISH) testing, three chromosome enumeration probes and a gene-specific probe to P16 tumour suppressor gene are able to determine if more than one pair of chromosomes or P16 genes exists in the cells obtained from the brushings of the bile duct during ERCP. If extra copies of two or more of the chromosomes or P16 genes are evident, the cells are considered to be *polysomic*, which indicates a high chance of malignancy. Based on conventional cytology, FISH testing, and other clinical data, the likelihood of cancer can be calculated.

CONTRAINDICATIONS
- See ERCP (p. 632).

POTENTIAL COMPLICATIONS
- See ERCP (p. 632).

INTERFERING FACTORS
- Errors in obtaining a good specimen can influence results.
- Cytologic examination is always affected by physician interpretation.

PROCEDURE AND PATIENT CARE

Before
- Explain the procedure to the patient.
- Obtain informed consent from the patient.
- Keep the patient NPO as of midnight the day of the test.
- Follow the procedure for ERCP (p. 632).

During
- During ERCP, a rounded brush is placed through the accessory lumen of the endoscope and passed repeatedly through the stricture.
- The brush is then swished in a cytology solution for FISH or directly smeared on a slide and preserved for conventional cytology.

After
- Follow the procedure for ERCP.

TEST RESULTS AND CLINICAL SIGNIFICANCE
Sclerosing cholangitis,
Biliary sclerosis,

Strictures of the pancreatobiliary duct: *These benign abnormalities will not be associated with any P16 gene abnormalities.*

Pancreatobiliary cancer: *If P16 genetic abnormalities are noted, the likelihood of cancer is very high.*

RELATED TESTS

ERCP (p. 632). With upper GI endoscopic techniques, the pancreatobiliary tree can be accessed for pancreatic biliary FISH testing.

Papanicolaou Smear (p. 774). Pap smears are the mainstay of screening for cancer of the vagina, cervix, and uterus.

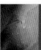

Papanicolaou Smear (Pap Smear, Pap Test, Cytologic Test for Cancer, Liquid-Based Cervical Cytology [LBCC])

NORMAL FINDINGS

No abnormal or atypical cells

INDICATIONS

Papanicolaou (Pap) smears are the mainstay of screening for cancer of the vagina, cervix, and uterus. They are routinely performed on women older than 21 years and on women younger than 21 years who are sexually active. Approaches to cervical cancer screening vary across Canada. Each province or territory has its own recommendations for how often women should be screened for cervical cancer, the type of test used, and human papillomavirus (HPV) vaccine. Refer to provincial recommendations for guidance on screening.

TEST EXPLANATION

A Pap smear is taken to detect neoplastic cells in cervical and vaginal secretions. This test is based on the fact that normal cells and abnormal cervical and endometrial neoplastic cells are shed into the cervical and vaginal secretions. Microscopic examination of these secretions enables detection of early cellular changes associated with premalignant conditions or an existing malignant condition. The Pap smear is 95% accurate in detecting cervical carcinoma; however, its accuracy in the detection of endometrial carcinoma is only approximately 40%.

The Bethesda System for reporting cervical and vaginal cytologic diagnoses was developed and revised by the National Cancer Institute to minimize discrepancy in result reporting and create a standardized framework for reporting results that were clinically useful. This system was updated in 2001 and includes evaluation of the following five components (see Box 7-1):

1. Adequacy of specimen: The specimen either has enough cells that can be evaluated or does not.
2. General categorization (optional): This is a quick summary of the cellular findings that allows the clinician to triage results readily.
3. Interpretation/result: This is a report of the cytopathologist's interpretation of the cells examined. It is not a diagnosis because other diagnostic data may be required in order to make a diagnosis.

BOX 7-1   Bethesda System for Reporting Cervical and Vaginal Cytologic Diagnoses

Adequacy of Specimen
- Satisfactory for evaluation
- Unsatisfactory for evaluation
  - Specimen rejected/not processed
  - Specimen processed and examined but unsatisfactory for evaluation

General Categorization
- Negative for intraepithelial lesion or malignancy
- Epithelial cell abnormality
- Other

Interpretation/Results
- Negative for intraepithelial lesion or malignancy
  - Organism causing infection
  - Other nonneoplastic findings
- Epithelial cell abnormalities
- Squamous
  - Atypical squamous cells
  - Low-grade squamous intraepithelial lesions
  - High-grade squamous intraepithelial lesions
  - Squamous cell carcinoma
- Glandular cell
  - Atypical glandular cells
  - Atypical glandular cells, favour neoplastic
  - Endocervical adenocarcinoma in situ
  - Adenocarcinoma

Automated Review and Ancillary Testing

Educational Notes/Suggestions

Nayar, R., and Wilbur, D. (2015). The Pap test and Bethesda 2014. *Acta Cytological, 59*, 121–132. DOI: 10.1159/000381842.

Microscopic Examinations

7

    a. Negative for intraepithelial lesion or malignancy: This report includes the possibility of infections such as those caused by *Trichomonas* or *Candida* organisms and of reactive changes from an intrauterine device or radiation therapy.

    b. Epithelial cell abnormalities: These range from atypical to cancer for both the squamous and glandular cancer lines.

4. Automated review and ancillary testing (where appropriate): These are reported if slides are scanned by automated computer systems (described later). Also, the use of any ancillary molecular tests such as HPV (described later) should be specified in this report.

5. Educational notes (optional): Here comments are written regarding the significance of the cytology results, or recommendations for further diagnosis are provided.

    A more common method of Pap smear specimen collection is *liquid-based cervical cytology* (LBCC). With this technique, the specimen obtained from the cervix is placed into a preservative solution instead of being smeared onto a slide, as is done during conventional Pap smear testing. Any blood cells and debris are then isolated by centrifuge, which leaves only cervical cells. A thin film of the residuum is then placed on a slide to be evaluated. The specimen can be split into two parts. The first is evaluated for cytopathologic features. If cytologic abnormalities of undetermined significance are found that could be better elucidated with further testing, the cells in the second part of the split specimen are used for that testing (to avoid having to obtain another cervical sample). For example, if cellular changes are found that may be related to HPV, the second part of the specimen is tested by real-time polymerase chain reaction for HPV DNA (see p. 763). HPV has been implicated as the cause of more than 95% of cervical cancers.

In comparison with conventional Pap smear testing, LBCC yields a significantly greater percentage of satisfactory specimens for Pap testing. A significantly greater percentage of low-grade and high-grade squamous intraepithelial lesions were reported with LBCC than with conventional Pap smear testing. The predictive value of a positive result of LBCC (93.9%) was similar to that for a positive result of conventional Pap smear testing (87.8%) in comparison with histology results.

Automated Pap smear readings are increasingly being used because the volume of screening Pap smears exceeds the ability of the cytopathologists to spend enough time to accurately interpret the slides. Automation is especially accurate when performed on LBCC specimens. The ThinPrep Imaging System, for example, integrates automated imaging with screening by cytotechnologists to identify fields that contain potentially relevant cellular abnormalities. If the cytotechnologist identifies significant abnormalities, the slide is examined by the cytopathologist. LBCC may eventually replace Pap testing because with LBCC, the application of cells to the glass slide is standardized; cells are distributed evenly on the slide; the amounts of mucus, blood, and inflammatory cells are reduced; fixation is effective and even; higher rates of serious cervical pathologic conditions are detected; and the material is less often considered inadequate for interpretation. In a slightly different and less expensive technique called the *PapSpin,* a special brush is placed in a collection device and centrifuged to provide a cellular concentrate.

❧ According to the Canadian Task Force on the Periodic Health Examination, general guidelines for screening include the following:
- Cervical cancer screening should begin at 18 years of age if the woman has not been sexually active.
- Regardless of age, screening should be initiated once the patient is sexually active.
- After the initial screening test, women should then have the test every 3 years after two normal results.
- Screening can cease at 70 years of age.
- Women with certain risk factors such as human immunodeficiency virus (HIV) infection, a weak immune system, in utero diethylstilbestrol exposure, or a previous diagnosis of cervical cancer may need more frequent screening.
- Among women who have had a total hysterectomy (removal of the uterus and cervix) for benign conditions, those who do not have a history of cervical dysplasia and have a negative and adequate screening history do not require screening after their hysterectomy.

CONTRAINDICATIONS
- Presence of routine, normal menses, because this can alter test interpretation
- Vaginal infections, because the infections can create cellular changes that may be misinterpreted as precancerous

INTERFERING FACTORS

- A delay in fixing a specimen allows the cells to dry, destroys effectiveness of the stain, and makes cytologic interpretation difficult.
- Using lubricating jelly on the speculum can alter the specimen.
- Using douches and taking tub baths before testing may wash away cellular deposits and interfere with the test results.
- Menstrual flow may alter test results. The best time to perform a Pap test is 2 weeks after the start of the last menses.
- Infections may interfere with hormonal cytologic study.
- Drugs such as digitalis and tetracycline may *alter* the test results by affecting the squamous epithelium.

Clinical Priorities

- Pap smears should not be collected during menstruation because results may be altered.
- A maturation index can be determined to detect endocrine abnormalities (such as estrogen-progesterone imbalance).
- Usually patients are not notified of Pap smear results unless further evaluation is needed.

PROCEDURE AND PATIENT CARE

Before

- Explain the procedure to the patient.
- Instruct the patient not to use douches or take tub baths during the 24 hours before the Pap smear. (Some health care providers prefer that the patients refrain from sexual intercourse for 24 to 48 hours before the test.)
- Instruct the patient to empty her bladder before the examination. A full bladder inhibits complete palpation of pelvic structures.
- Inform the patient that no fasting or sedation is required.

During

- Note the following procedural steps:
  1. The patient is placed in the lithotomy position.
  2. A vaginal speculum is inserted to expose the cervix.
  3. Material is collected from the cervical canal by rotating a cotton swab moistened with saline or a wooden (plastic for LBCC) spatula within the cervical canal and in the squamocolumnar junction (Figure 7-5). If a maturation index is requested for hormonal information, the smear is taken off the vaginal wall. Care is taken to exclude the cervix.
  4. The cells are immediately wiped across a clean glass slide and fixed either by immersing the slide in equal parts of 95% alcohol and ether or by using a commercial spray (e.g., hairspray). The secretions must be fixed before drying because drying will distort the cells and make interpretation difficult. Furthermore, this fixing process kills any infectious organisms so that the specimen is less infectious to the personnel who handle the specimen.
  5. The slide is labelled with the patient's name, unique patient identifier number, age, parity, and date of her most recent menstrual period. If this is not done, the specimen is considered unsatisfactory for interpretation.

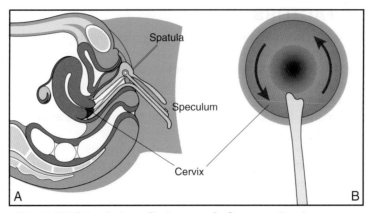

Figure 7-5 Papanicolaou (Pap) smear. **A**, Cross-sectional illustration of the process of obtaining a cervical specimen. **B**, The cervix is scraped with the bifid end of a spatula to obtain a specimen for Pap smear.

6. If LBCC is performed, the cervical specimen is placed in the fixative preservative solution. Once placed in this solution, cells can be evaluated anytime within the next 3 weeks (if kept frozen).
7. The patient's medication history (e.g., oral contraceptives) and the reason for the examination should be written on the laboratory request form.

After

- If the Pap smear has induced some bleeding, provide the patient with a perineal napkin.
- Note that once in the laboratory, the Pap smear slide is stained and reviewed microscopically by the pathologist. Several computer programs are now able to recognize abnormal cells and classify them. These programs are used to assist the pathologist in screening, particularly cellular smears.
- Inform the patient that her primary care physician will notify her of the test results.

TEST RESULTS AND CLINICAL SIGNIFICANCE

Cancer: *The diagnosis of malignancy can be made only on biopsy of the tumour. All patients with suspect Pap smear results must be more thoroughly examined with colposcopy, cone biopsy, or dilation and curettage.*

Sexually transmitted infections,

Fungal infection,

Parasite infection,

Herpes infection: *Many of these infectious diseases cause cellular changes on Pap smears. Culture of these organisms, however, is required in order to establish the diagnosis.*

Infertility: *Lack of estrogenic effect noted on vaginal Pap smears may indicate ovarian failure in a woman of usual menstrual age.*

RELATED TESTS

Cervical Biopsy (p. 749). This procedure is performed to accurately identify and treat premalignant and superficial malignant lesions of the cervix.

Colposcopy (p. 623). This is one of the follow-up tests performed when the results of a Papanicolaou smear are abnormal.

Pleural Biopsy

NORMAL FINDINGS
No evidence of pathologic conditions

INDICATIONS
This test is indicated when the pleural fluid obtained by thoracentesis (p. 705) is exudative, which suggests infection, neoplasm, or tuberculosis. The pleural biopsy is indicated to distinguish among these disease processes. It is also performed when chest imaging indicates a pleural-based tumour, reaction, or thickening.

TEST EXPLANATION
Pleural biopsy is the removal of pleural tissue for histologic examination. Pleural biopsy is usually performed as a percutaneous needle biopsy. It also can be performed through thoracoscopy, which is done by inserting a thoracoscope into the pleural space for inspection and biopsy of the pleura (see Thoracoscopy, p. 654). Pleural tissue also may be obtained by an open pleural biopsy, which involves a limited thoracotomy and requires that the patient be under general anaesthesia. For this procedure, a small intercostal incision is made, and the biopsy of the pleura is performed under direct observation. The advantage of these open procedures is that a larger piece of pleura can be obtained.

Percutaneous needle biopsy is usually performed in approximately 30 minutes by a physician at the patient's bedside, in a special procedure room, or in the physician's office. Because of the local anaesthetic, little discomfort is associated with this procedure. Open biopsy is performed in the operating room.

CONTRAINDICATIONS
• Prolonged bleeding or clotting times

POTENTIAL COMPLICATIONS
• Bleeding or injury to the lung
• Pneumothorax

PROCEDURE AND PATIENT CARE
Before
𝄪 Explain the procedure to the patient.
• Obtain the patient's informed consent for this procedure.
𝄪 Inform the patient that no fasting or sedation is required.
𝄪 Instruct the patient to remain very still during the procedure. Any movement may lead to inadvertent damage by the needle.

During
• Note the following procedural steps for percutaneous needle biopsy:
  1. This procedure is usually performed with the patient in a sitting position with his or her shoulders and arms elevated and supported by a padded overhead table.

2. After the presence of the fluid has been determined by the thoracentesis technique, the skin overlying the biopsy site is anaesthetized and pierced with a scalpel blade.
3. A needle is inserted with a cannula until most fluid is removed. (Some fluid is left in the pleural space after the thoracentesis to make the biopsy easier.)
4. The inner needle is removed, and a blunt-tipped, hooked biopsy trocar, attached to a three-way stopcock, is inserted into the cannula.
5. The patient is instructed to exhale all air and then perform the Valsalva manoeuvre to prevent air from entering the pleural space.
6. The cannula and biopsy trocar are withdrawn while the hook catches the parietal wall and takes a specimen with its cutting edge.
7. Usually three biopsy specimens are taken from different sites at the same session.
8. The specimens are placed in a fixative solution and sent to the laboratory immediately.
9. After the specimens are taken, additional parietal fluid can be removed.

After

- Apply an adhesive bandage to the biopsy site.
- Note that a chest radiograph is usually taken to detect the potential complication of pneumothorax.
- Observe the patient for signs of respiratory distress (e.g., shortness of breath, diminished breath sounds) on the side of the biopsy.
- Observe the patient's vital signs frequently for evidence of bleeding (increased pulse rate, decreased blood pressure).
- Ensure that the biopsy specimen is sent to the laboratory immediately.

 Home Care Responsibilities

- Instruct the patient to report any signs of shortness of breath.
- Instruct the patient to report any signs of bleeding, such as decreasing blood pressure or increasing pulse rate.

TEST RESULTS AND CLINICAL SIGNIFICANCE

Neoplasm: *Pleural tumours can be primary (mesothelioma) or metastatic (e.g., breast, lung, ovarian, gastrointestinal). These tumours are often associated with a pleural effusion.*

Infection: *Lung and pleural space infections can cause thickening of the pleura and pleural effusions (empyema). Most infections can be identified on Gram stains or cultures of the pleural fluid. However, some infections cannot be identified without tissue for culture or tissue for other forms of identification. This is especially true for the unusual infections occurring in immunocompromised patients* (Pneumocystis jiroveci).

RELATED TESTS

Thoracentesis and Pleural Fluid Analysis (p. 705). In this procedure, pleural fluid is aspirated from the pleural space for analysis.

Chest Radiography (p. 1053) and Lung Scan (p. 838). These radiographic studies visualize most surfaces of the pleura.

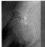

Progesterone Receptor Assay (PR Assay, PRA, PgR)

NORMAL FINDINGS

Immunochemistry
Negative: <5% of the cells stain for receptors
Positive: >5% of the cells stain for receptors

Reverse-Transcriptase Polymerase Chain Reaction (RT-PCR)
Negative: <5.5 units
Positive: >5.5 units

INDICATIONS

Progesterone receptor assay is performed on breast cancer tissue to indicate sensitivity to hormone manipulative therapy and to indicate prognosis of breast cancer.

TEST EXPLANATION

The progesterone receptor assay is used in determining the prognosis and treatment of breast cancer and, to a lesser degree, other cancers. These assays help determine whether a tumour is likely to respond to endocrine medical or surgical therapy. The test is conducted on breast cancer specimens when a primary or recurrent cancer is identified; it is usually performed in conjunction with estrogen receptor assay (see p. 759) to increase the predictability of a tumour response to hormone therapy. Breast tumours tend to be progesterone receptor–positive more often in postmenopausal women than in premenopausal women. Progesterone receptor–positive tumours are suspected to be associated with a better prognosis than are progesterone receptor–negative tumours. Tumour response rates to medical or surgical hormonal manipulation are found to be potentiated if the result of the estrogen receptor assay is positive.

The two most common ways to report estrogen receptor and progesterone receptor test results are the proportion score (Table 7-1) and the intensity score. Both scores are based on immunohistochemical staining of tumour cells. The proportion score is the percentage of tumour cells with positive nuclear staining. The intensity score is the average intensity of all positive tumour cells

TABLE 7-1	Estrogen Receptor and Progesterone Receptor Proportion Score
Score	**Proportion of Tumour Cells With Positive Nuclear Staining**
0	None
1	>0 to <1%
2	1% to <10%
3	10% to <33%
4	33% to 66%
5	>66%

Microscopic Examinations 7

on a scale from pale to dark, with results of 0 (none), 1 (weak), 2 (intermediate), and 3 (strong). In some cases, the proportion and intensity scores are combined for a total score. If the total scores are 0 (none + none) or 2 (<1% + weak), the test result is considered negative, but any total score of 3 to 8 is considered a positive result.

The most commonly used laboratory method provides accurate information on paraffin-embedded tissue with immunohistochemical staining for progesterone receptor proteins. Positive reactivity to immunohistochemical staining is observed in the nuclei of the tumour cells. Only a small portion of the paraffin-embedded tissue is required for testing. Results are usually available in less than 1 week. Only the cancerous tissue is evaluated for progesterone receptor receptors.

Other tumours (such as ovarian, melanoma, uterine, or pancreatic) are occasionally sampled for estrogen receptor and progesterone receptor assay. This is mostly performed within clinical trials.

INTERFERING FACTORS

▮ Use of exogenous hormones such as progesterone or estrogen may cause false-negative results.

PROCEDURE AND PATIENT CARE

Before

- Prepare the patient for breast biopsy according to routine protocol.
- Record the menstrual status of the patient.
- Record any exogenous hormone the patient may have used during the previous 2 months.
- Instruct the patient to discontinue exogenous hormone therapy before breast biopsy. This is done in consultation with the attending physician.

During

- The surgeon obtains tissue.
- This tissue should be placed on ice or in formalin.
- Part of the tissue is used for routine histologic examination. A portion of the paraffin block is sent to a reference laboratory.

After

- Provide routine postoperative care.
- Inform the patient that results are usually available in 1 week.

TEST RESULTS AND CLINICAL SIGNIFICANCE

Progesterone receptor–positive: *This cancer is more likely to be successfully treated with hormone manipulation in a therapeutic or adjuvant clinical setting.*

RELATED TESTS

Estrogen Receptor Assay (p. 759). Like the progesterone receptor assay, this test helps predict the likelihood of tumour response to endocrine manipulative therapy.

Breast Cancer Genomics (p. 1131). This test helps predict the risk of recurrent breast cancer. It is also a powerful predictor of benefit from hormone therapy or chemotherapy.

Renal Biopsy (Kidney Biopsy)

NORMAL FINDINGS
No pathologic conditions

INDICATIONS
Renal biopsy is performed for the following purposes:
1. To diagnose the cause of renal disease (e.g., poststreptococcal glomerulonephritis, Goodpasture's syndrome, lupus nephritis)
2. To detect primary and metastatic malignancy of the kidney in patients who may not be candidates for surgery
3. To evaluate rejection of kidney transplant, which enables the physician to determine the appropriate dose of immunosuppressive drugs

TEST EXPLANATION
Biopsy of the kidney affords microscopic examination of renal tissue. Renal biopsy is most often obtained percutaneously (Figure 7-6). During this procedure, a needle is inserted through the skin and into the kidney to obtain a sample of kidney tissue. The biopsy needle is more accurately

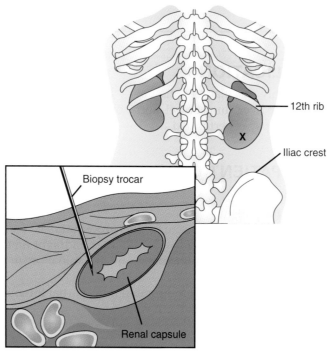

Figure 7-6 Illustration of renal biopsy. The renal biopsy trocar is inserted into the renal capsule, which is located below the twelfth rib and above the iliac crest and identified in the figure by the area marked with an "X."

placed when computed tomography, ultrasonography, or fluoroscopy is used for guidance. These visualization techniques allow more precise localization of the desired kidney tissue. A physician performs this procedure in approximately 10 to 30 minutes. The biopsy is uncomfortable, but only minimally if enough lidocaine is used.

On occasion, renal biopsy is an open procedure. This involves an incision through the flank and dissection to expose the kidney surgically.

CONTRAINDICATIONS

- Coagulation disorders, because of the risk of excessive bleeding
- Operable kidney tumours, because tumour cells may be disseminated during the procedure
- Hydronephrosis, because the enlarged renal pelvis can be easily entered and cause a persistent urine leak, necessitating surgical repair
- Urinary tract infections, because the needle insertion may disseminate the active infection throughout the retroperitoneum

Clinical Priorities

- Assess the coagulation profile before performing a kidney biopsy because of the possibility of bleeding. Often, hemoglobin and hematocrit values are obtained after the procedure to check for bleeding.
- After a renal biopsy, the patient is usually kept in bed on his or her back for about 24 hours.
- After this test, carefully evaluate the vital signs for evidence of bleeding. Inspect the urine for gross hematuria.

POTENTIAL COMPLICATIONS

- Hemorrhage from the highly vascular renal tissue
- Inadvertent puncture of the liver, lung, bowel, aorta, or inferior vena cava
- Infection when an open biopsy is performed

PROCEDURE AND PATIENT CARE

Before

- Explain the procedure to the patient.
- Obtain the patient's written informed consent for this procedure.
- Keep the patient on NPO status (nothing by mouth) after midnight on the day of the test in the event that bleeding or inadvertent puncture of an abdominal organ necessitates surgical intervention.
- Assess the patient's coagulation profile (prothrombin time, partial thromboplastin time).
- Check the patient's hemoglobin and hematocrit values.
- Note that the patient's blood may need to be typed and crossmatched in case of severe hemorrhage that necessitates transfusions.
- Inform the patient that no sedative is required.
- Note that the needle biopsy may be performed at the patient's bedside.
- If computed tomographic or ultrasound guidance is to be used, note that the needle biopsy is performed in the radiology or ultrasonography department.

During

- Note the following procedural steps:
  1. The patient is placed in a prone position with a sandbag or pillow under the abdomen to straighten the spine.
  2. Under sterile conditions, the skin overlying the kidney is infiltrated with a local anaesthetic (lidocaine).
  3. While the patient holds his or her breath to stop kidney motion, the physician inserts the biopsy needle into the kidney and takes a specimen.
  4. After this procedure is completed, the needle is removed, and pressure is applied to the site for approximately 20 minutes.

After

- Apply a pressure dressing.
- Turn the patient on his or her back, and have the patient stay in bed for approximately 24 hours.
- Check the patient's vital signs; puncture site, and hematocrit values frequently during the 24-hour period.
- Instruct the patient to avoid any activity that increases abdominal venous pressure (e.g., coughing).
- Assess the patient for signs and symptoms of hemorrhage (e.g., decrease in blood pressure, increase in pulse rate, pallor, backache, flank pain, shoulder pain, light-headedness).
- Evaluate the patient's abdomen for signs of bowel or liver penetration (e.g., abdominal pain and tenderness, abdominal muscle guarding and rigidity, decreased bowel sounds).
- Inspect all urine specimens for gross hematuria. In most cases, the patient's urine contains blood initially, but this generally does not continue after the first 24 hours. Urine samples may be placed in consecutive chronologic order to facilitate comparison for evaluation of hematuria. This is referred to as *rack, or serial, urine samples.*
- Encourage the patient to drink large amounts of fluid to prevent clot formation and urine retention.
- To assess for active bleeding, obtain blood to determine hemoglobin and hematocrit level after the biopsy. One lavender-top tube of blood is needed.
- Instruct the patient to avoid strenuous exercise (e.g., heavy lifting, contact sports, horseback riding) or any activity that could cause jolting of the kidney for at least 2 weeks.
- Teach the patient the signs and symptoms of renal hemorrhage, and instruct him or her to call the physician if any of these symptoms occur.
- Instruct the patient to report burning sensation on urination or any temperature elevations. These could indicate a urinary tract infection.

TEST RESULTS AND CLINICAL SIGNIFICANCE

Renal disease (e.g., poststreptococcal conditions, Goodpasture's syndrome, lupus nephritis): *These primary diseases of the kidney have classical histologic appearances. The type of renal disease must be documented to ensure proper therapy. Immunofluorescent stains are often applied to the tissue to identify renal disease of immunologic origin (e.g., Goodpasture's disease).*

Primary and metastatic malignancy of the kidney: *The most common cancers of the kidney are primary renal cell carcinomas. It is dangerous to perform a biopsy of this tumour because it is quite vascular. Furthermore, the biopsy could cause tumour studding along the needle tract. However, in cases of metastatic disease, or if medical conditions preclude surgery, tissue can be obtained by kidney biopsy.*

Rejection of kidney transplant: *Renal biopsy is the definitive manner in which rejection is diagnosed. If the problem is caught early enough, the immunosuppressive medication regimen can be altered to stop the rejection process.*

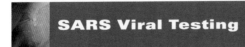

SARS Viral Testing

NORMAL FINDINGS

No severe acute respiratory syndrome (SARS) virus

INDICATIONS

This test is used to diagnose SARS.

TEST EXPLANATION

According to the World Health Organization (WHO), from November 2002 to July 2003, SARS caused 774 deaths worldwide and resulted in 8096 cases of confirmed infection in 29 countries. During that same time period, there were 27 confirmed cases but no deaths in the United States and 251 confirmed cases and 43 deaths in Canada. Since 2003, the WHO has declared SARS to be contained, and active global surveillance for SARS has not detected any person-to-person transmissions.

A coronavirus causes SARS. China's southern Guangdong province, which includes Hong Kong, is believed to be the source of the virus, which has about an 8- to 10-day incubation period. Symptoms are similar to those of any pneumonia (fever, chills, and cough). The diagnosis should be suspected in a symptomatic patient who lives in or has travelled to an area where transmission of the illness has been documented. Routine testing for the SARS virus is not conducted unless a cluster of cases develops and health officials are able to rule out all other infectious agents.

Three tests are currently available:

1. *Enzyme-linked immunosorbent assay (ELISA):* This test detects antibodies to coronavirus. The test identifies antibodies 20 days after the start of symptoms. That means it cannot be used to detect cases in the early stage of illness.
2. *Immunofluorescence assay (IFA):* With this method, SARS antibodies are detected as early as 10 days after infection, but it is a complex and relatively slow test that requires growing the virus in the laboratory.
3. *Reverse-transcription polymerase chain reaction (RT PCR):* This molecular test detects the SARS virus by amplifying RNA genetic information from a cultured sample. It is good at detecting early stages of the infection, and results can be available in 2 days.

The diagnosis can be made only with positive test results in the following situations:

- With one specimen tested on two occasions; thus, the original clinical specimen is used on each occasion
- With two clinical specimens from different sources (e.g., nasopharyngeal and stool)
- With two clinical specimens collected from the same source on two different days (e.g., two nasopharyngeal aspirates).

The following types of respiratory specimens may be collected for viral or bacterial diagnostic tests, or both: (1) nasopharyngeal wash/aspirates, (2) nasopharyngeal swabs, (3) oropharyngeal swabs, (4) bronchioalveolar lavage, (5) tracheal aspirate, (6) pleural fluid tap, (7) sputum, and (8) postmortem tissue. Nasopharyngeal wash/aspirates are the specimen of choice for detection of most respiratory viruses.

Serum and blood (plasma) should be collected early in the illness for RT PCR testing. The reliability of RT PCR testing performed on blood specimens decreases as the illness progresses. Both acute- and convalescent-stage serum specimens should be collected for antibody testing. To confirm or rule out SARS-coronavirus infection, it is important to collect convalescent-stage serum specimens more than 28 days after the onset of illness.

A virus culture to isolate SARS coronavirus is available but takes a few days for results. The capability to isolate and cultivate the virus is particularly important for epidemiologists and researchers.

PROCEDURE AND PATIENT CARE

Before
- Explain the procedure to the patient.
- Observe standard precautions and transmission-based precautions.
- Observe strict isolation technique. This disease is contagious and dangerous.

During
- To obtain a *nasopharyngeal wash/aspirate,* have the patient sit with the head tilted slightly backward. Instill 1 to 1.5 mL of nonbacteriostatic saline (pH, 7.0) into one nostril. Flush a plastic catheter or tubing with 2 mL to 3 mL of saline. Insert the tubing into the nostril. Aspirate nasopharyngeal secretions. Repeat this procedure for the other nostril. Collect the specimens in sterile vials.
- To obtain a *nasopharyngeal* or *oropharyngeal swab,* use only sterile polyester (Dacron) or rayon swabs with plastic shafts. Do not use a cotton swab or swabs with wooden sticks, because they may contain substances that inactivate some viruses and inhibit RT PCR testing. Insert the swab into the nostril. Leave the swab in place for a few seconds to absorb secretions. Swab both nostrils. (For *oropharyngeal culture,* swab the posterior pharynx and tonsillar areas, avoiding the tongue.)
- To collect *sputum,* educate the patient about the difference between sputum and oral secretions. Have the patient rinse the mouth with water and then expectorate deep-cough sputum directly into a sterile screw-cap sputum collection cup or sterile dry container.
- To collect *blood,* collect 5 to 10 mL of whole blood in a serum separator tube for serum RT PCR testing or for ELISA antibody testing. Collect 5 to 10 mL of blood in a purple-top tube for plasma testing.

After
- Provide acute care for respiratory illness.
- If the specimen is to be shipped domestically, use cold packs to keep the sample at 4°C. If shipping is international, pack the sample in dry ice.

TEST RESULTS AND CLINICAL SIGNIFICANCE

SARS: *Initial diagnostic testing for suspected SARS should include chest radiograph, oximetry, blood cultures, sputum for Gram stain and culture, and testing for influenza A and B.*

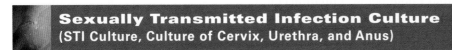

Sexually Transmitted Infection Culture
(STI Culture, Culture of Cervix, Urethra, and Anus)

NORMAL FINDINGS

No evidence of sexually transmitted infection (STI), such as gonorrhea, *Chlamydia* infection (p. 751), or *Trichomonas* infection

INDICATIONS

These cultures and smears are performed for patients who have a vaginal discharge, pelvic pain, urethritis, or penile discharge and are at risk for STIs.

TEST EXPLANATION

Sexually transmitted infections (STIs) are a significant public health concern in Canada, with reported cases of *Chlamydia*, gonorrhea, and infectious syphilis rising since the late 1990s. In Canada in 2012 there were 103 716 cases of *Chlamydia*, 12 561 cases of gonorrhea, and 2 003 cases of infectious syphilis reported. When these three STIs are detected, the law requires that they be reported to the Public Health Agency of Canada. The organisms can cause urethritis, vaginitis, endometritis, pelvic inflammatory disease, pharyngitis, proctitis, epididymitis, prostatitis, and salpingitis. Children born to infected mothers may develop conjunctivitis, pneumonia, neonatal blindness, and neonatal neurologic injury and may even die.

Cultures for STI infections are performed on men and women with suggestive symptoms. If the culture result is positive, sexual partners should be evaluated and treated. Cervical cultures are usually performed for women; urethral cultures are performed for men. Rectal and throat cultures are performed in individuals who have engaged in anal and oral intercourse. Because rectal gonorrhea accompanies genital gonorrhea in a high percentage of women, rectal cultures may be recommended in all women with suspected gonorrhea. Performing a culture for gonorrhea is also part of the prenatal workup. If the STI culture result is positive, treatment during pregnancy can prevent possible fetal complications (e.g., ophthalmia neonatorum) and maternal complications. Rectal and orogastric cultures should be performed on the neonates of infected mothers.

Gram stains of smears or bacterial cultures should be taken before a patient begins antibiotic therapy. For bacterial cultures for gonorrhea, a special medium is used, such as Thayer-Martin, designed for the cultivation of *Neisseria gonorrhoeae*.

The culture or smear of a genital lesion, tissue biopsy, serologic testing, and observation of classic clinical lesions identifies other STIs. DNA probes tagged with chemiluminescent dye are also used for identification of some of these STI organisms. Testing for each suspected organism must be specifically requested. Some laboratories do routine "genital cultures" that include testing for gonorrhea, beta-hemolytic streptococci, and *Gardnerella* infection.

A physician or nurse obtains STI cultures and smears in several minutes. Very little discomfort is associated with these procedures.

INTERFERING FACTORS

- *N. gonorrhoeae* is very sensitive to lubricants and disinfectants.
- Menses may alter test results.
- Female douching within 24 hours before a cervical culture makes fewer organisms available for culture.
- Male voiding within 1 hour before a urethral culture washes secretions out of the urethra.
- Fecal material may contaminate an anal culture.

Clinical Priorities

- If cultures for STIs yield positive results, sexual partners should be evaluated and treated.
- Women should not douche within 24 hours before cervical cultures because douching may decrease the number of organisms available for culture.
- Men should not urinate within 1 hour before a urethral culture because voiding washes secretions out of the urethra.

PROCEDURE AND PATIENT CARE

Before

𝒳 Explain the purpose and procedure to the patient. Use a matter-of-fact, nonjudgemental approach.

𝒳 Inform the patient that no fasting or sedation is required.

During

Cervical Culture

𝒳 The female patient is told to refrain from using douches and taking tub baths for 24 hours before the cervical culture.

• The patient is placed in the lithotomy position, and a moistened, unlubricated vaginal speculum is inserted to expose the cervix (see Figure 7-5*A*, p. 778).

• Cervical mucus is removed with a cotton ball held in a ring forceps.

• A sterile cotton-tipped swab is inserted into the endocervical canal and moved from side to side to obtain the culture.

• The swab is placed in sterile saline or a transporting fluid obtained from the laboratory. The specimen should be plated as soon as possible. The specimen should not be refrigerated.

Anal Canal Culture

• An anal culture of the female or male patient is taken by inserting a sterile, cotton-tipped swab approximately 2.5 cm into the anal canal (Figure 7-7).

• If stool contaminates the swab, swabbing is repeated.

Oropharyngeal Culture

• This culture should be obtained in male and female patients who have engaged in oral intercourse.

• A throat culture is best obtained by depressing the patient's tongue with a wooden tongue blade and touching the posterior wall of the throat with a sterile cotton-tipped swab.

**Microscopic
Examinations**

7

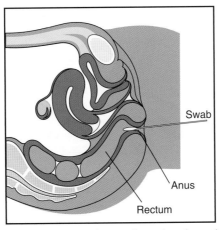

Figure 7-7 Obtaining a specimen of exudate from the rectum.

Urethral Culture

X Instruct the male patient to refrain from urinating for the hour before the test. Voiding within 1 hour before collection washes secretions out of the urethra, making fewer organisms available for culture. The best time to obtain the specimen is before the first morning void.

- A culture is taken by inserting a sterile swab gently into the anterior urethra (Figure 7-8).
- It is advisable to place the male patient in the supine position to prevent his falling if vasovagal syncope occurs during introduction of the cotton swab or wire loop into the urethra.
- The patient is observed for hypotension, bradycardia, pallor, sweating, nausea, and weakness.
- In the male, prostatic massage may increase the chances of obtaining positive cultures.

After

- Place the swabs for gonorrhea in a Thayer-Martin medium, and roll them from side to side.
- Label and send the culture bottle to the microbiology laboratory.
- Transport the specimen to the laboratory as soon as possible.
- Handle all specimens as though they were capable of transmitting disease.
- Do not refrigerate the specimen.
- On the laboratory slip, note the collection time, date, source of specimen, patient's age, current antibiotic therapy, and clinical diagnosis.

X Advise the patient to avoid sexual intercourse and all sexual contact until test results are available.

X If the culture results are positive, advise the patient to receive treatment and to recommend to their sexual partners that they be evaluated.

- Note that repeat cultures should be obtained after completion of treatment to evaluate therapy.

TEST RESULTS AND CLINICAL SIGNIFICANCE

Gonorrhea,

Chlamydia infection (p. 751),

Trichomonas infection: *These and other STIs can be identified by these and other diagnostic tests (Table 7-2).*

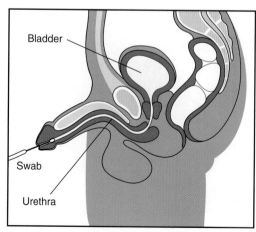

Figure 7-8 Obtaining a urethral specimen.

TABLE 7-2	Sexually Transmitted Infections and Methods of Diagnosis

Disease	Methods of Diagnosis
Gonorrhea	Cervical, urethral, anal, oropharyngeal cultures
Chlamydia infection	Cervical, urethral culture; serologic study
Lymphogranuloma venereum	DNA probe testing
Chlamydia trachomatis infection	
Herpes genitalis	Culture from lesion, serologic study
Syphilis	Serologic study, fluid cultures (central nervous system), darkfield slide
Hepatitis	Serologic study
Acquired immune deficiency syndrome (AIDS)	Serologic study
Granuloma inguinale	Tissue biopsy
Trichomoniasis	Cervical, urethral, vaginal smear on a wet mount
Scabies	Characteristic scabies lesion, skin scraping from lesion
Molluscum contagiosum (molluscum virus)	Characteristic wartlike lesion
Condylomata acuminata (papillomavirus infection)	Characteristic wartlike lesion
Chancroid (*Haemophilus* infection)	Culture of the chancre, smear of the chancre, DNA probe
Candida (*Monilia*) infection	Wet mount, Gram stain, fungal culture
Pediculosis pubis (lice)	Characteristic appearance of louse
Gardnerella vaginalis	Cervical, urethral, anal cultures

Microscopic Examinations

7

RELATED TESTS

Chlamydia (p. 751), Herpes Simplex (p. 760), Syphilis Detection (p. 487), Hepatitis Virus Studies (p. 304), and AIDS Serology (p. 310). These are tests for other STIs.

Sputum Culture and Sensitivity (Sputum C&S, Sputum Culture, and Gram Stain)

NORMAL FINDINGS

Normal upper respiratory tract flora

INDICATIONS

Sputum culture is indicated in any patient with a persistent productive cough, fever, hemoptysis, or a chest radiographic picture characteristic of pulmonary infection. This test is used to diagnose pneumonia, bronchiectasis, bronchitis, or pulmonary abscess. Bacterium, fungus, or virus can be cultured.

TEST EXPLANATION

Sputum cultures are obtained to determine the presence of pathogenic bacteria in patients with respiratory infections, such as pneumonia. A *Gram stain* is the first step in the microbiologic analysis of sputum. Through sputum staining, bacteria are classified as Gram-positive or Gram-negative. This finding may be used to guide drug therapy until the culture and sensitivity report is complete. The sputum sample is then applied to a series of bacterial culture plates. The bacteria that grow on those plates in the next 1 to 3 days are then identified. To identify the most appropriate antimicrobial drug therapy, bacterial sensitivity to various antibiotics (also called *drug sensitivity testing*) is determined by observing a ring of growth inhibition around an antibiotic plug in the culture medium.

Sputum for culture and sensitivity should be collected before antimicrobial therapy is initiated, unless the test is being performed to evaluate the effectiveness of medications already being given. Preliminary reports are usually available in 24 hours. Cultures require at least 48 hours for completion. Sputum cultures for fungus and *Mycobacterium tuberculosis* may take 6 to 8 weeks.

PROCEDURE AND PATIENT CARE

Before

- Explain the procedure for sputum collection to the patient.
- Remind the patient that sputum must be coughed up from the lungs and that saliva is not sputum (Figure 7-9).
- Withhold antibiotics until after the sputum has been collected.
- If an elective specimen is to be obtained, give the patient a sterile sputum container on the night before the sputum is to be collected so that the morning specimen may be obtained when the patient awakens.

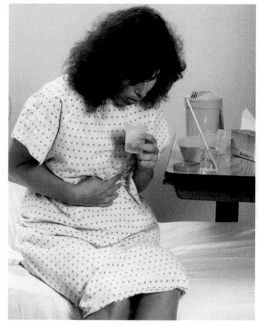

Figure 7-9 Collection of sputum specimen. The specimen should be representative of pulmonary secretions, not saliva.

Instruct the patient to rinse out his or her mouth with water—but not antiseptic mouthwash—before the sputum collection, to decrease contamination of the sputum by particles in the oropharynx.

During

- Note that sputum specimens are best taken when the patient awakens in the morning before eating or drinking.
- Collect at least 5 mL (1 teaspoon) of sputum in a sterile sputum container.
- Usually obtain sputum by having the patient cough after taking several deep breaths.
- If the patient is unable to produce a sputum specimen, stimulate coughing by lowering the head of the patient's bed or giving the patient an aerosol administration of a warm, hypertonic solution.
- Note that other methods to collect sputum include endotracheal aspiration, fibreoptic bronchoscopy, and transtracheal aspiration.

After

Instruct the patient to notify the nurse as soon as the sputum is collected.
- Label the sputum, and send it to the laboratory as soon as possible.
- On the laboratory slip, note whether the patient is receiving any current antibiotic therapy.

TEST RESULTS AND CLINICAL SIGNIFICANCE

Bacterial infection (e.g., pneumonia),
Viral infection,
Atypical bacterial infection (e.g., tuberculosis),
Fungal infection: *Sputum that is obtained for these types of organisms is plated on several types of culture media to grow the organisms that could grow in the pulmonary tree. Some of these organisms are quite difficult to grow in the laboratory, and great attention to detail is necessary to grow these pathogens effectively and demonstrate disease.*

RELATED TEST

Tuberculosis Culture (p. 798). This is the only method by which tuberculosis can be diagnosed with certainty. When tuberculosis-causing organisms are grown from the culture of a specimen, the diagnosis of tuberculosis can be made and treatment based on drug sensitivities can be started.

Sputum Cytologic Study

NORMAL FINDINGS

Normal epithelial cells

INDICATIONS

Sputum for cytologic examination is indicated whenever the diagnosis of cancer of the lung is considered. Bronchoscopy and percutaneous lung biopsy have supplanted the need for sputum cytologic study to a great degree. Now its greatest use is in patients who have productive cough, abnormal findings on chest radiograph, but nothing visible on bronchoscopic study. It is also used to monitor smokers in whom some atypical changes have been noted on prior examination of the lower respiratory tract.

TEST EXPLANATION

Tumours within the pulmonary system frequently slough cells into the sputum. When the sputum is gathered, the cells are examined. If the cytologic examination indicates malignant cells, a lung tumour exists within the mucosa of the trachea, bronchi, and lungs. If only normal epithelial cells are observed, either no malignancy exists or any existing tumour is not shedding cells at that time. Therefore, a positive sputum cytology test result indicates malignancy; a negative result means nothing. The test result is more likely to be positive in smokers who have a chronic productive cough, hemoptysis, or both. Furthermore, the more specimens obtained, the more accurate the test result is. This test is now rarely performed because tissue for biopsy can be easily obtained by bronchoscopic biopsy (p. 613).

Bronchial brushings can obtain excellent specimens for cytologic examination. A brush is placed through the bronchoscope and wiped on the bronchial mucosa. It is then withdrawn back into its sheath and wiped on a dry slide, which is immediately fixed.

INTERFERING FACTORS

- Findings can be falsely negative as a result of poor cytologic preparation or inadequate specimen acquisition. Interpretation of cytologic changes is difficult, but most pathologists who have had cytologic experience maintain good accuracy. This is usually monitored by quality assurance studies within the pathology department.

PROCEDURE AND PATIENT CARE

Before

- Explain the procedure for sputum collection to the patient.
- Remind the patient that sputum must be coughed up from the lungs and that saliva is not sputum.
- Give the patient a sterile sputum container the night before the sputum is to be collected so that the morning specimen may be obtained on arising.
- Instruct the patient to rinse out his or her mouth with water—but not antiseptic mouthwash—to decrease contamination of the sputum by particles in the oropharynx.

During

- Note that sputum specimens are best collected when the patient awakens in the morning.
- Collect at least 5 mL (1 teaspoon) of sputum in the sterile sputum container. The container may or may not contain alcohol as an immediate fixative; this varies according to the laboratory. If a 24-hour specimen is requested, the alcohol fixative must be within the container to diminish cellular deterioration during the collection period.
- Usually, obtain sputum by having the patient cough after taking several deep breaths.
- If the patient is unable to produce a sputum specimen, stimulate coughing by lowering the head of the patient's bed or with aerosol administration of a warm hypertonic solution.
- Note that other methods to collect sputum include endotracheal aspiration, fibreoptic bronchoscopy, and transtracheal aspiration.
- Usually, collect sputum for cytologic examination once daily on 3 successive days. The first morning specimen is the best.

After

✍ Instruct the patient to notify the nurse as soon as the sputum is collected.

• Label the specimen, and send it to the laboratory as soon as possible.

TEST RESULTS AND CLINICAL SIGNIFICANCE

Malignancies: *Malignancies of the trachea, bronchus, and lung can be detected. Marked changes in the nuclear/cytoplasmic ratio, size of the cell, and differentiation of the cell indicate suspect changes. It is now thought that cellular changes progress from benign, normal appearance to metaplastic features, atypical appearance, and finally frankly cancerous status. The cytologic report may indicate what part of that spectrum the cells appear to reflect. The cells may be labelled* benign, abnormal, suspect, *or* definitely cancer. *In smokers, the epithelial cells of the lower respiratory system seem to make those progressive changes the longer the person smokes.*

Benign cellular changes: *This is most commonly related to infection (bronchiectasis), exposure (asbestosis), or viral pneumonitis.*

Asthma: *The sputum of affected patients often has an increased number of eosinophils.*

RELATED TEST

Bronchoscopy (p. 613). This is an endoscopic test through which pulmonary lavage can be performed and specimens for cytologic examination can be obtained.

Throat and Nose Cultures

NORMAL FINDINGS

Normal oral and respiratory flora

INDICATIONS

A throat or nose culture is obtained to diagnose bacterial, viral, gonococcal, or candidal pharyngitis. It is indicated for patients who complain of a sore throat, have a fever of unknown cause, or may be chronic carriers of recurrent infection. Nose cultures are used to identify acute nasal or sinus infections and to identify carriers of pathogenic bacteria.

TEST EXPLANATION

Because the throat is normally colonized by many organisms, culture of this area serves only to isolate and identify a few particular pathogens (e.g., streptococci, meningococci, gonococci, *Bordetella pertussis, Corynebacterium diphtheriae*). Recognition of these organisms necessitates treatment. Streptococci are most often sought, because a group A beta-hemolytic streptococcal pharyngitis (Figure 7-10) may be followed by rheumatic fever or glomerulonephritis. This type of streptococcal infection most frequently affects children between 3 and 15 years of age. Therefore, for all children with a sore throat and fever, a throat culture should be performed to attempt to identify streptococcal infections. In adults, however, fewer than 5% of patients with pharyngitis have a streptococcal infection. Therefore, throat cultures in adults are indicated only when sore

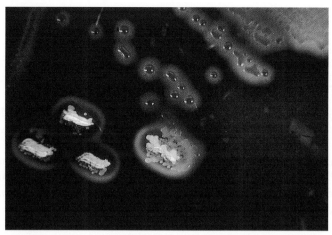

Figure 7-10 Blood agar plate showing colonies (clear zone around colony) of group A beta-hemolytic streptococci, the organism that causes bacterial pharyngitis.

throat is severe or recurrent, often in association with fever and palpable lymphadenopathy. Such adults often have a history of previous streptococcal infections.

Rapid immunologic tests ("strep screen") with antiserum against group A beta-hemolytic *Streptococcus* antigen are now available and are very accurate for the identification of the organism without culture. With these newer kits, the streptococcal organism can be identified directly from the swab specimen. With this method, the organism is chemically or enzymatically extracted from the swab specimen. It is then tested with the antisera containing the antibodies to group A beta-hemolytic streptococci. Agglutination on the slide indicates that group A beta-hemolytic streptococci are present. If no agglutination occurs, the specimen is still cultured for streptococci. If that culture is negative, no streptococcal infection exists. The rapid serologic tests can be performed in about 15 minutes. The final results of the culture take at least 2 days, and the normal values for the "strep screen" would be negative for streptococci.

In a routine throat culture, several different types of culture media (chocolate, streptococcus-specific, and other agar) are used to grow various bacteria. When a specific *Streptococcus* culture is requested or if the "strep screen" is negative, the specimen is plated on *Streptococcus*-specific agar only. All cultures should be performed before antibiotic therapy is initiated; otherwise, the antibiotic may interrupt the growth of the organism in the laboratory. In cases of acute infection, antibiotic therapy may need to be initiated before the culture yields results. In these instances, a Gram stain of the specimen smeared on a slide is most helpful and can yield results in less than 10 minutes. All forms of bacteria are grossly classified as Gram-positive (blue staining) or Gram-negative (red staining). Knowledge of the shape of the organism—for example, spherical (typical of cocci) or rod-shaped (typical of bacilli)—also can be very helpful in the tentative identification of the infecting organism. With knowledge of the Gram stain results, the physician can initiate a reasonable antibiotic regimen on the basis of past experience regarding the organism's possible identity and sensitivity. Most organisms take approximately 24 hours to grow in the laboratory, and preliminary findings can be reported at that time. On occasion, a period of 48 to 72 hours is required for growth and identification of the organism. Cultures may be repeated on completion of appropriate antibiotic therapy to identify resolution of the infection.

Nasal and pharyngeal cultures are often performed to screen for infections and carrier states caused by various other organisms such as *Staphylococcus aureus, Haemophilus influenzae,* and *Neisseria meningitidis* and viruses such as respiratory syncytial virus and viruses that cause rhinitis. Health care providers in the operating room and neonatal nursery may have these cultures performed to screen potential sources of spread once an outbreak occurs in a hospital setting. These cultures are also used to detect infection in older adult and debilitated patients.

INTERFERING FACTORS

Drugs that may *affect* test results include antibiotics and antiseptic mouthwashes.

PROCEDURE AND PATIENT CARE

Before

Explain the procedure to the patient.

During

- Obtain a *throat culture* with the following steps:
  1. Depress the patient's tongue with a wooden tongue blade, and use a sterile cotton swab to touch the posterior wall of the throat (Figure 7-11) and areas of inflammation, exudation, or ulceration.
  2. Two swabs are preferred. Growth of streptococci from both swabs is more confirmatory of infection, and the second swab can also be used in the "strep screen."
  3. Avoid touching any other part of the patient's mouth. Place the swabs in a sterile container.

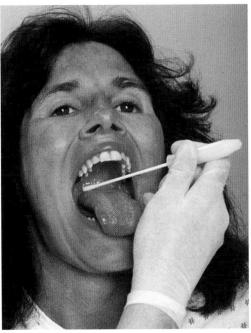

Figure 7-11 Collection of specimen from posterior pharynx.

- Obtain a *nasal culture* with the following steps:
  1. Gently raise the tip of the patient's nose, and insert a flexible swab into the nares.
  2. Rotate the swab against the side of the nares.
  3. Remove the swab, and place it in an appropriate culture tube.
- Obtain a *pharyngeal culture* with the following steps:
  1. Gently raise the tip of the patient's nose, and insert a flexible swab along the bottom of the nares.
  2. Guide this swab until it reaches the posterior pharynx. Rotate the swab to obtain secretions.
  3. Remove the swab, and place it in an appropriate culture tube.
- Wear gloves, and handle the specimen as if it were capable of transmitting disease.
- Place the swab in a sterile container and send it to the microbiology laboratory within 30 minutes.
- On the laboratory slip, list any medications that the patient is taking that could affect test results.

After

- Notify the physician of any positive results so that appropriate antibiotic therapy can be initiated.

 Age-Related Concerns

- When throat and nose cultures are collected in young children, an adult should hold the child on his or her lap; the person obtaining the specimen should then place one hand on the child's forehead to stabilize the head. The specimen is then obtained in a manner similar to that for adults.

TEST RESULTS AND CLINICAL SIGNIFICANCE

Acute pharyngitis: *Throat cultures are used to identify pathogenic bacteria such as streptococci,* Corynebacterium diphtheriae, *gonococci,* Bordetella pertussis, Neisseria *organisms, and staphylococci.* Candida *and other* Bordetella *infections can also be identified.*

Tonsillar infections: *These infections can be identified and their source determined if the swab is applied adequately to the tonsillar areas.*

Chronic nasal carriers of bacteria: *Some people are chronic carriers of bacteria that can initiate an infection when transmitted to other people. Such bacteria include staphylococci, streptococci, influenza, or respiratory syncytial virus.*

RELATED TEST

Anti–Streptolysin O Titre (p. 109). This serologic test verifies a recent *Streptococcus* infection.

 Tuberculosis Culture (TB Culture, BACTEC Method, Polymerase Chain Reaction)

NORMAL FINDINGS

Negative for tuberculosis

INDICATIONS

Tuberculosis culture is indicated in any patient with a persistent productive cough, night sweats, anorexia, weight loss, fever, and hemoptysis. This diagnosis should be especially considered in patients at high risk for such infection, such as those who are immunocompromised, patients with a history of alcohol abuse, or those who have been exposed recently to tuberculosis.

TEST EXPLANATION

The diagnosis of tuberculosis can be made only by identification and culture of *Mycobacterium tuberculosis* in the specimen. (See p. 1168 for other tuberculosis testing.) Conventional culture techniques for growth, identification, and susceptibility testing of acid-fast mycobacteria take 4 to 6 weeks. Because a patient who actually has tuberculosis cannot be isolated from society for that duration, the disease may spread to many other people during that time. With the resurgence and increasing incidence of tuberculosis in the U.S. and Canadian populations (especially among Indigenous people and immunocompromised patients with acquired immune deficiency syndrome [AIDS]), newer, more rapid culture techniques have been developed and are now being used.

The BACTEC blood culture system is a radiometric technique in which the growth medium for culturing mycobacteria is supplanted with a substrate labelled with radioactive carbon (^{14}C). This substrate is used by mycobacteria, and during metabolism, radioactive carbon dioxide ($^{14}CO_2$) is produced from the substrate. The examiner detects $^{14}CO_2$ quantitatively by counting the radioactivity with the Becton Dickinson Diagnostic Instrument System. The rate and amount of $^{14}CO_2$ produced is directly proportional to the rate and amount of growth occurring on the medium. With this technique, very small quantities of $^{14}CO_2$ can be detected. This enables quick identification of mycobacterial growth. This technique is used not only to isolate mycobacteria from clinical specimens but also to differentiate *M. tuberculosis* complex from other mycobacteria and for antimicrobial susceptibility testing.

Polymerase chain reaction culture methods also have been developed. With the addition of a DNA polymerase, genetic chromosomal parts can be multiplied. This allows amplification of genomes, which then can be detected by genetic DNA probes. With the newer techniques already described, *M. tuberculosis* can be identified in as little as 36 to 48 hours. Because of this reduction in diagnostic time, treatment can be started earlier. It is anticipated that the spread of tuberculosis will therefore be greatly reduced. The average detection time, however, is longer for extrapulmonary specimens than for sputum specimens. The time for identification is greatly reduced when numerous mycobacteria are present. In general, organisms in specimens from patients already receiving antituberculosis treatment take longer to grow.

After identification and growth of mycobacteria, antibiotic susceptibility testing is performed to identify the most effective antimycobacterial drugs. The culture can be performed on sputum, body fluids, cerebrospinal fluid, and even biopsy tissue specimens.

INTERFERING FACTORS

Antituberculosis drugs that have been started before culture could interfere with the growth of tuberculosis.

Cultural Considerations

- In Canada, the incidence of tuberculosis is considerably higher among Indigenous people (27.5 per 100 000) than among the general population (5.0 per 100 000).

PROCEDURE AND PATIENT CARE

Before

Explain the procedure to the patient.
Inform the patient that no fasting is required.

During

- For sputum, obtain an early morning specimen. It is best to induce sputum production with an ultrasonic or nebulizing device.
- Collect three to five early-morning specimens. All specimens must contain mycobacteria in order to establish the diagnosis of tuberculosis.
- For urine collection, obtain three to five single, clean-voided specimens early in the morning.
- Note that swabs, intestinal washings, and biopsy specimens should be transported to the laboratory immediately for preparation.
- Follow the institution's policy for universal specimen handling. Staff should wear an N95 respirator mask when in contact with the patient. Ideally, the patient should be placed in a negative-pressure room.
- Note the following procedural steps:
  1. Once the laboratory receives the specimen, a decontamination process is applied to it to kill all nonmycobacterial organisms. The specimen is then cultured in the appropriate medium.
  2. With the rapid growth techniques, the specimen is evaluated every 24 hours.
  3. When cultural growth is considered adequate, the organisms are stained for acid-fast bacilli and identified (p. 735).
  4. With DNA genetic probes, the *Mycobacterium* species is identified.
  5. At this point, if *M. tuberculosis* is present, the report will read "culture more positive for mycobacteria." If the species has been identified, the report will also contain this information.
  6. Drug-susceptibility testing then will be carried out and the results subsequently reported.

After

Instruct the patient in appropriate isolation about sputum and other body fluids to avoid potential spread of suspected tuberculosis.

TEST RESULTS AND CLINICAL SIGNIFICANCE

Tuberculosis,

Atypical mycobacterial nontuberculous disease: *These organisms require special medium plates to grow. Any fluid or tissue can be used as a culture specimen. If the lungs are thought to be the site of infection, sputum or pleural fluid is used. If the kidneys are suspected to be involved, urine should be tested. Other specimens include abdominal fluid, stomach aspirate, and bone tissue.*

RELATED TESTS

Acid-Fast Bacilli Smear (p. 735). This smear is used to support the diagnosis of tuberculosis; by itself, it cannot confirm this diagnosis. The smear (usually of sputum) is also used to monitor treatment for tuberculosis.

Tuberculin Skin Testing (p. 1168). Purified protein derivative is administered intradermally to test for prior exposure to tuberculosis. Results of skin testing cannot indicate active or dormant tuberculosis. Positive results imply nothing more than previous exposure.

Chest Radiography (p. 1053). Because tuberculosis usually infects the lungs through inhalation of airborne infectious material, the chest radiograph often demonstrates the results (Ghon complex) of the acute granulomatous infection.

QuantiFERON-TB Gold (p. 450). This assay is a whole-blood test for use as an aid in diagnosing *M. tuberculosis* infection. It is a diagnostic aid that measures a component of cell-mediated immune reactivity to *M. tuberculosis*.

Viral Cultures

NORMAL FINDINGS
No virus isolated

INDICATIONS
This test is used to diagnose viral disease by culturing the virus.

TEST EXPLANATION
It is now recognized that viral infections are the most common infections affecting children and adults. Viruses are subdivided by the nuclear material they contain (RNA or DNA). Infections from viruses are often indistinguishable from bacterial infections. Definitive diagnosis of viral disease is made by culture of the virus (discussed here). Other methods used to identify viral disease include the following:
1. Serologic methods of identifying antibodies to a specific virus
2. Serologic methods of identifying antigen parts of a virus
3. Direct detection by electron microscopy
4. Indirect detection by nucleic acid probes

    Ability to isolate a viral culture depends on many aspects of the culture process. The first is determining the correct specimen for culture. That depends on the organ involved and the type of virus suspected (Table 7-3). Timing is important. Viral load is always greatest in the early

TABLE 7-3	Specimen Culture for Common Viruses and Diseases	
Common Virus	**Specimens**	**Disease**
Adenovirus	Throat culture	Influenza
Influenza	Bronchoscopic aspiration	Pneumonia
Respiratory syncytial rhinovirus	Throat and nose culture	Pharyngitis
Rubella virus	Throat culture	Skin rash
Rubeola	Skin vesicle	Zoster
Coxsackievirus		
Varicella		
Arbovirus	Throat culture	Meningitis
Enterovirus	Cerebrospinal fluid	Encephalitis
Herpesvirus	Blood	Herpes simplex
Cytomegalovirus		
Parvovirus	Stool	Skin rash
Adenovirus	Blood	Arthropathy
	Sputum	Upper respiratory infection
Influenza A virus	Throat culture	Flu syndrome
Epstein-Barr virus	Blood	Mononucleosis
West Nile virus	Blood	Skin rash, lymphadenopathy, polyarthropathy
	Cerebrospinal fluid	

stages of the disease. Cultures obtained in the first few days after symptoms appear to offer the best chance of identifying the infective organism. Using the correct culture medium is essential. In general, the culture medium used to grow the viral culture is a tissue/cell culture. Different viruses vary greatly in their ability to grow in specific cell cultures. Viral cultures take 3 to 7 days to yield results.

INTERFERING FACTORS

- Inadequate specimen, inadequate timing, or inappropriate choice of culture medium will cause false-negative test results.
- The use of a cotton swab or wooden applicator for specimen collection may destroy the virus.

PROCEDURE AND PATIENT CARE

Before

☒ Explain the method of collection of the specimen to the patient.
- Obtain a history regarding the timing of symptoms.
- Accurately record the source of the specimen.

During

- If blood is the specimen, obtain a venous blood sample in a lavender-top or blue-top tube.

After

- Use a closed-specimen system to obtain and transport the specimen to the laboratory.
- Transport the specimen immediately to the laboratory. Viruses in specimens quickly lose their vitality.
- Place samples on ice if delivery to the laboratory is not immediate.
- Small-volume specimens such as tissue aspirates are often best transported in a liquid medium. If bacterial cultures are to be performed, use sterile saline solution for transfer.
☒ Explain to the patient that he or she may still be infectious and should minimize exposure to other people.

TEST RESULTS AND CLINICAL SIGNIFICANCE

Viral infectious disease; see Table 7-3.

RELATED TESTS

Blood Culture and Sensitivity (p. 737). Blood tests are used to detect bacteria in the blood.

Sputum Culture and Sensitivity (p. 791). This test is used in patients who have signs and symptoms of a pulmonary infection.

Throat and Nose Cultures (p. 795). This test is obtained to diagnose bacterial, viral, gonococcal, or candidal pharyngitis.

West Nile Virus Testing (p. 547). This series of tests is used to detect and confirm the presence of the antibody to West Nile virus.

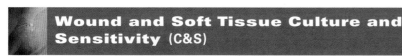

Wound and Soft Tissue Culture and Sensitivity (C&S)

NORMAL FINDINGS
Negative

INDICATIONS
A wound or soft tissue culture is indicated when a wound or soft tissue has signs of infection (redness, warmth, swelling, purulent exudate, foul odour, or pain). In a postoperative patient with a persistent fever of unknown origin, a wound may be probed and cultured even if the signs of infection are not present. Any spontaneous drainage from a wound or soft tissue should be cultured to document infection for treatment and drug sensitivities and to document the appropriateness of skin and wound isolation precautions.

TEST EXPLANATION
Wound cultures are obtained to determine the presence of pathogens in patients with suspected wound infections. Pus-forming organisms most often cause wound infections. All cultures should be performed before antibiotic therapy is initiated; otherwise, the antibiotic may interrupt the growth of the organism in the laboratory. More often than not, however, physicians initiate antibiotic therapy after the wound is cultured but before the culture results are reported. In these instances, a Gram stain of the specimen smeared on a slide is most helpful and can yield results in less than 10 minutes. All forms of bacteria are grossly classified as Gram-positive (blue staining) or Gram-negative (red staining). Knowledge of the shape of the organism (e.g., spherical, rod shaped) also may be very helpful in the tentative identification of the infecting organism. With knowledge of the Gram stain results, the physician can initiate a reasonable antibiotic regimen on the basis of past experience regarding the organism's possible identity. Most organisms require approximately 24 hours to grow in the laboratory, and preliminary findings can be reported at that time. On occasion, 48 to 72 hours is required for growth and identification of the organism. Cultures may be repeated after appropriate antibiotic therapy to assess for complete resolution of the infection.

It is important to recognize that many wound infections contain more than one organism. Multiple organisms may grow on culture. Deep-space wounds, wounds containing necrotic debris or gas, and postoperative wounds commonly contain aerobic and anaerobic bacteria.

INTERFERING FACTORS
■ Drugs that may *alter* test results include antibiotics.

PROCEDURE AND PATIENT CARE
Before
✍ Explain the procedure to the patient.
• Assemble all equipment (Figure 7-12).

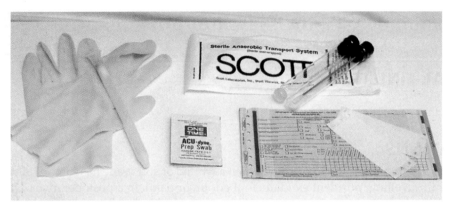

Figure 7-12 Equipment for collection of specimens from wounds and decubitus ulcers.

During

- Prior to taking the culture, cleanse the wound with sterile or normal saline, or sterile water.
- Aseptically place a sterile cotton swab into the pus of the patient's wound, and then place the swab into a sterile, covered test tube. (Cultures of specimens from the skin edge yield much less accurate results than do cultures of the suppurative material.)
- If an anaerobic organism is suspected, obtain an anaerobic culture tube from the microbiology laboratory. The specimen is best obtained by aspirating a closed wound and directly transferring the pus to the anaerobic culture tube.
- If the patient is to undergo wound irrigation, obtain the culture before the wound is irrigated.
- If any antibiotic ointment or solution has been previously applied, remove it with sterile water or saline, wait several hours, and then obtain the culture.
- Handle all specimens carefully. These specimens are capable of transmitting disease.
- On the laboratory slip, list any medications that the patient is taking that could affect test results.

After

- Transport the specimen to the laboratory immediately after testing (within no more than 30 minutes).
- Notify the physician of any positive results so that appropriate antibiotic therapy can be initiated.
- Note that if pus was observed in the wound or soft tissue, skin and wound isolative precautions should be instituted for that patient immediately. The culture report documenting the infection does not need to be received before appropriate protective precautions are instituted.

TEST RESULTS AND CLINICAL SIGNIFICANCE

Wound infection: *The best treatment of a wound infection is incision (widely opening the infection) and providing good drainage. Antibiotic treatment is secondary.*

CHAPTER 8

Nuclear Scanning

NOTE: *Throughout this chapter, SI units are presented in* **boldface colour,** *followed by conventional units in parentheses.*

OVERVIEW

TESTS

OVERVIEW
REASONS FOR PERFORMING NUCLEAR MEDICINE STUDIES

With the administration of a radiopharmaceutical and subsequent detection of the photons emitted from a particular organ, anatomic and functional abnormalities of various body areas can be detected. Nuclear medicine studies do not identify the specific cause (disease) of the abnormality. They do provide supportive information to be used in conjunction with other diagnostic modalities. The many indications for nuclear scanning include the following:

1. To stage cancer by detecting metastasis (positron emission tomography [PET]) or to test specific organs such as bone (bone scan), the liver (liver scan), or the brain (brain scan)
2. To diagnose acute and chronic cholecystitis (gallbladder scan)
3. To detect cerebral pathologic conditions (brain scan)
4. To evaluate gastric emptying (gastric emptying scan)
5. To localize sites of gastrointestinal bleeding (gastrointestinal bleeding scan)
6. To diagnose pulmonary embolism (lung scan)
7. To determine perfusion, structure, and function of the kidneys (renal scanning) or heart (cardiac nuclear scanning)
8. To evaluate thyroid nodules (thyroid scan)
9. To evaluate testicular swelling and pain (scrotal nuclear imaging)
10. To evaluate cardiac function and coronary artery patency

The radionuclides used in diagnostic medicine are artificially produced by either a nuclear reactor or a charged particle accelerator (cyclotron) by irradiating the nuclei and causing them to be unstable. Because of this instability, the nucleus of the radionuclide atom emits radioactive particles (photons in the gamma radiation range). The radionuclides used in nuclear scanning have short half-lives, which refers to the time required for 50% of the radioactive atoms to undergo decay. Technetium-99m (^{99m}Tc) is used extensively in nuclear scanning because its half-life is 6.01 hours and it emits low levels of gamma rays. ^{99m}Tc is used in approximately 80% of nuclear medical scans in Canada. Other commonly used radionuclides include gallium-67, thallium-201, and iodine-123.

To get to the desired organ, radionuclides are combined with a transport molecule. This combination of radionuclide and transport molecule is called a *radiopharmaceutical*. A *radiopharmaceutical* is labelled with the radionuclide that is administered to the patient and localized in the organ to be studied. For most nuclear scans, radiopharmaceuticals are administered intravenously. Less commonly used methods of administration include the oral and inhalation routes. Radiopharmaceuticals concentrate in target organs by various mechanisms. For example, some labelled compounds, such as iodohippurate sodium iodine-131 (Hippuran ^{131}I), are cleared from the blood and excreted by the kidneys. Some phosphate compounds concentrate in the bone and infarcted tissue. Lung function can be studied by imaging the distribution of inhaled gases and aerosols. Other radiopharmaceuticals (such as fluorodeoxyglucose) are selectively taken up by cancer cells.

After the radioisotope concentrates in the desired area, it emits gamma rays. The area is scanned with a gamma camera or a scintillation scanner that detects and records the emission of gamma rays. With each gamma ray detected, a light particle is emitted from the scintillation scanner. A computer translates these light readings into a two-dimensional image or scan (scintigram) that is printed in various shades of grey. Through the use of multiple scanners, a three-dimensional image can be obtained through single-photon emission computed tomography (SPECT). Scintigrams can also be produced in colour. The shades of grey or colour show the distribution of the radionuclide in the organ. When a scintigram is superimposed on a baseline-computed tomogram, an image of accurate anatomy can be created. "Hot" spots are areas of increased uptake of the radionuclide, and "cold" spots are areas with decreased uptake. Normally, the uptake of the radionuclide in an organ is diffuse and homogeneous. Hot and cold spots may mean different things on different scans. For example, a cold spot identified in the liver, spleen, or brain indicates tumour, abscess, or some other space-occupying lesion. A cold spot detected on a thallium scan of the heart would not be suggestive of tumour; rather, it indicates an area of ischemia or infarction. On bone scan, hot spots may indicate areas of osteoblastic activity surrounding tumour. Arthritis or fracture may also be evident as hot spots. The scanning usually takes place in the nuclear medicine department. A large part of nuclear medicine includes blood studies and in vitro staining of microscopic slides through radioimmunoassay techniques. These studies are discussed in Chapter 2; in vivo nuclear scanning is discussed in this chapter.

Scanning can be *static,* which means that the patient and the camera are held in one position until an image is completed. After one image is completed, the patient is often rotated into another position for a static image of another view of the same organ. *Dynamic* scanning enables the examiner to evaluate the blood flow to a certain organ, such as the brain or the liver. SPECT is a technique in which a gamma camera is serially placed at multiple angles around the entire circumference of the patient. This method is used to obtain three-dimensional images of the organ to be studied; in addition, sensitivity is increased. PET can demonstrate anatomic, functional, and biochemical abnormalities in an organ.

Although nuclear scanning includes a risk of radiation for the patient, the risk associated with most radionuclides is much lower than that associated with a radiographic study. The half-lives of the radioisotopes are short; thus, radiation contamination by way of fecal and urine wastes is minimal. Unless the benefit outweighs the risk, nuclear scanning is contraindicated in pregnant women and nursing mothers because of the risk of injury to the fetus or infant. To help protect patients and others, patients should take some precautions for 12 hours after injection of radionuclides. Whenever possible, a toilet should be used, rather than a urinal. The toilet should be flushed several times after each use. Spilled urine should be cleaned up completely. After each time voiding or fecal elimination, patients should thoroughly wash their hands. All clothes soiled with urine or feces should be washed separately.

PROCEDURE AND PATIENT CARE FOR NUCLEAR SCANNING
Before

- Explain the procedure to the patient. Assure the patient that radiation exposure is limited and minimal.
- Assess the patient for an allergy to the radiopharmaceutical (especially when iodine is used).
- Note whether the patient has had any recent exposure to radionuclides. The previous study could interfere with the interpretation of the results of the current study.
- Record the patient's age and current weight. This information is used to calculate the amount of radioactive substance needed.
- Many of the scanning procedures do not require any preparation. However, a few do have special requirements. For example, in bone scanning, the patient is encouraged to drink several glasses of water between the time of the injection of the isotope and the actual scanning.
- For some studies, blocking agents may need to be given to prevent other organs from taking up the isotope. For example, Lugol iodine solution may be needed to protect the thyroid gland from iodine-tagged radioisotopes. Potassium chloride may be used during a brain scan to prevent an inordinate amount of ^{99m}Tc uptake by the choroid plexus, which would simulate a pathologic condition.

During
- Take the patient to the nuclear medicine department.
- Most radionuclides are injected intravenously. Patients are often encouraged to drink water between administration of the radioisotope and the scanning. Radionuclides can also be administered orally (for a gastric emptying scan) or by inhalation (for a ventilation scan).
- The area is scanned at the designated time. The delay between administration of the radionuclide and scanning depends on the length of time required for the specific organ or tissue to take up the radionuclide and concentrate it. The patient must lie still during the scanning. Scans are usually repeated over a period that may extend from 1 hour to 3 days. The patient returns to the nuclear medicine department for each scanning.

After
- Reassure the patient that only tracer doses of radioisotopes have been used and that no precautions against radioactive exposure to the patient or others are necessary.
- Although the amount of radionuclide excreted in the urine is very low, rubber gloves are sometimes recommended if the urine must be handled. Some physicians may advise the patient to flush the toilet several times after voiding.
- Encourage the patient to drink extra fluids to aid in excretion of the isotope from the body.
- If the isotope was injected intravenously, inspect the site for signs of infection, bruising, or hematoma.
- Most agencies have specific protocols and guidelines, so refer to your agency's policies regarding the care of patients before, during, and after nuclear studies.

REPORTING OF RESULTS
A nuclear medicine technologist in the nuclear medicine department performs most tests. A physician trained in diagnostic nuclear medicine interprets the test results.

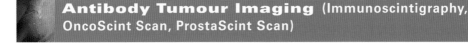

Antibody Tumour Imaging (Immunoscintigraphy, OncoScint Scan, ProstaScint Scan)

NORMAL FINDINGS
No increased uptake of radionuclide in the body

INDICATIONS
This scan is used to identify recurrent prostate, ovarian, or colorectal cancer. It is indicated in patients in whom recurrence is suspected on the basis of elevated levels of blood tumour markers (prostate-specific antigen, CA-125, or carcinoembryonic antigen [CEA], respectively).

TEST EXPLANATION
Immunoscintigraphy is an additional nuclear medicine technique for tumour imaging that is based on the ability of a radiolabelled monoclonal antibody to attach to tumour markers overproduced by certain cancers. At present, it is used to detect recurrent or metastatic prostate, colorectal, or ovarian cancer. The radionuclide indium chloride-111 or indium-111 satumomab

pendetide is attached to a monoclonal antibody. When injected, this radionuclide-antibody conjugate attaches to the protein tumour markers on the cancer cell surface. With the use of a scintillation camera, whole-body images are obtained and the anatomic location of tumour recurrence can be identified. Positron emission tomography (PET; p. 849) has largely replaced this type of scanning, but immunoscintigraphy still has a role in oncology. This scan can be incorrectly negative up to 30% of the time. When positive, however, its information is helpful. In OncoScint scanning, anti-CEA antibody is used; in ProstaScint scanning, an antibody to anti–prostate-specific antigen is used.

PROCEDURE AND PATIENT CARE

Before
- Explain the procedure to the patient.
- Explain that no fasting is required before the test.
- Because the radionuclide can be concentrated in areas of degenerative joint disease, abdominal aortic aneurysms, abdominal inflammatory processes, or inflammatory bowel disease, a thorough history should be obtained before the scanning. Usually a computed tomogram of the abdomen (p. 1059) is performed before this test. The diseases just listed would have been identified in the computed tomogram.

During
- Take the patient to the nuclear medicine department.
- The radiolabelled monoclonal antibody is injected into the patient.
- Initial images are obtained 48 to 72 hours after intravenous infusion.
- The patient is asked to lie on a padded table.
- A scintigraphy camera is placed over the anterior or posterior surface of the chest, abdomen, and pelvis. Approximately 10 minutes is required for each view.
- The patient may be asked to return the following day or the day after that for repeated images.
- Little or no discomfort is associated with this procedure.
- The procedure takes approximately 1 hour each day over a period of 1 to 4 days.
- If an amount of radionuclide occurs in the bowel sufficient to obscure the rest of the abdomen, a cathartic or enema can be administered.

After
- Reassure the patient that because only tracer doses of radioisotopes are used, other people do not need to take precautions against radiation exposure.

TEST RESULTS AND CLINICAL SIGNIFICANCE
Recurrent prostate, colorectal, or ovarian cancer

RELATED TESTS
Prostate-Specific Antigen (p. 434). This is a screening test for prostate cancer.

CA-125 Tumour Marker (p. 148). This tumour marker is measured to detect ovarian cancer.

Carcinoembryonic Antigen (p. 159). This tumour marker is measured to determine the extent of cancer and its prognosis.

Nuclear Scanning

8

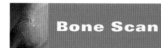

Bone Scan

NORMAL FINDINGS
No evidence of abnormality

INDICATIONS
The bone scan is used to identify metastatic cancer involving the bone. It is often performed on patients with cancer as a routine part of staging before and after treatment. To a lesser degree, bone scanning is used to identify pathologic bone conditions that cannot be identified on plain radiographs of the bone (e.g., osteomyelitis, hairline fractures).

TEST EXPLANATION
The bone scan enables examination of the skeleton by a scanning camera after intravenous injection of a radionuclide material. Usually technetium-99m (^{99m}Tc) is the radionuclide used. After injection of the ^{99m}Tc, the bone takes up the radiopharmaceutical. Gamma rays are emitted through the body from the ^{99m}Tc in the bone and are detected by a scintillation scanner. The scintillation scanner emits light with each photon it receives from the gamma ray. When these light patterns are arranged in a spatial order, a realistic image of the bones is produced.

The degree of radionuclide uptake is related to the metabolism of the bone. Normally, the concentration should be uniform throughout the bones of the body. Distribution of the radionuclide activity is symmetric throughout the skeletal system in healthy adults. Radionuclide activity in the urinary bladder, the kidneys (faint), and soft tissues (minimal) is also normally visible. An increased uptake of isotope is abnormal and may represent tumour, arthritis, fracture, degenerative bone and joint changes, osteomyelitis, bone necrosis, osteodystrophy, or Paget's disease (Figure 8-1). These areas of concentrated radionuclide uptake are often called "hot" spots and are detectable months

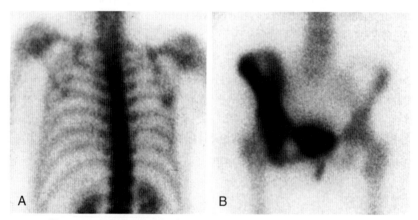

Figure 8-1 Bone scans. **A,** Upper body. Uptake of radionuclide is normal in the bones of the upper body. **B,** Lower body. Uptake of radionuclide is increased diffusely in the right iliac bones, ischium, and pubic bones, which is consistent with Paget's disease.

before an ordinary radiograph can reveal the pathologic condition. Hot spots occur because new bone growth is usually stimulated around areas of abnormality. If a pathologic condition exists but no new bone forms around the lesion, the scan does not pick up the abnormality. Uptake of radionuclide is also increased in the normal physiologic active epiphyses of children (growth plates).

The major reason a bone scan is performed is to detect cancer metastatic to the bone. All malignancies capable of metastasis may involve the bone, especially cancers of the prostate, breast, lung, kidney, urinary bladder, and thyroid gland. Bone scans are also useful in staging primary bone tumours such as osteogenic sarcomas and Ewing sarcoma. Bone scans may be repeated serially to monitor tumour response to antineoplastic therapy.

Bone scans also provide valuable information for the evaluation of patients with trauma or unexplained pain. Bone scanning is much more sensitive than routine radiographs in detecting small and difficult-to-find fractures, especially in the spine, ribs, face, and small bones of the extremities. Bone scans are used to determine the age of a fracture as well. If a fracture line is seen on a plain radiograph and the uptake around that fracture is not increased on a bone scan, the injury is said to be an "old" fracture, having occurred more than several months earlier.

Although the bone scan is extremely sensitive, it is, unfortunately, not very specific. Fractures, infections, tumours, and arthritic changes all appear similar in this scan. When plain radiographs fail to identify the classic findings of bone infection (osteomyelitis), bone scans are helpful.

A three-phase bone scan may be performed if inflammation (arthritis) or infection (osteomyelitis, septic arthritis) is suspected. In a three-phase bone scan, imaging is performed at three different times after injection of the radionuclide. Early uptake of the radionuclide indicates infection or inflammation rather than neoplasm. Uptake of the radionuclide visible on delayed images that had not been visible on early images indicates neoplasm.

When the metastasis process is diffuse, virtually all of the radiotracer is concentrated in the skeleton, with little or no activity in the soft tissues or urinary tract. The resulting pattern, which is characterized by excellent bone detail, is frequently referred to as a *superscan*. A superscan may also be associated with metabolic bone diseases such as Paget's disease, renal osteodystrophy, and osteomalacia. Unlike the pattern of uptake in metastatic disease, however, the uptake in metabolic bone disease is more uniform in appearance and extends into the distal appendicular skeleton. Intense calvarial uptake disproportionate to that in the remainder of the skeleton is another feature of a metabolic superscan.

The bone scan is performed in 30 to 60 minutes by a nuclear medicine technician. A physician trained in nuclear medicine imaging interprets the image. The injection of the radioisotope causes slight discomfort. Lying on the hard scanning table for an hour may cause pain. In many circumstances, magnetic resonance imaging (MRI) is used in place of bone scans. It is more specific in indicating disease.

CONTRAINDICATIONS

- Pregnancy, unless the benefits of the procedure outweigh the risk of injury to the fetus
- Lactation, because of the risk of contaminating maternal milk

Clinical Priorities

- Bone scans are performed primarily to detect metastatic cancer to the bone.
- Bone scans are often repeated to monitor tumour response to antineoplastic therapy.
- Bone scans should not be performed on pregnant or lactating women.

PROCEDURE AND PATIENT CARE

Before

☒ Explain the procedure to the patient.

☒ Assure the patient that he or she will not be exposed to large amounts of radioactivity because only tracer doses of the isotope are used.

☒ Inform the patient that no fasting or sedation is required.

☒ Inform the patient that the injection of the radioisotope may cause slight discomfort, nausea, vomiting, a metallic taste in the mouth, or a flushing sensation in the face.

During

• Take the patient to the nuclear medicine department.

• Note the following procedural steps:

1. The patient receives an intravenous injection of an isotope, usually ^{99m}Tc in a peripheral vein.

2. The patient is encouraged to drink several glasses of water between the time of radioisotope injection and the scanning. This facilitates renal clearance of any circulating tracer not picked up by the bone. The waiting period before scanning is approximately 1 to 3 hours.

3. The patient is instructed to urinate to eliminate any tracer that is in the bladder because it may block the view of the underlying pelvic bones.

4. The patient is positioned supine on the scanning table in the nuclear medicine department (Figure 8-2).

5. A scintillation camera is placed over the patient's body and records the radiation emitted by the skeleton.

6. This information is translated into a two- or three-dimensional view of the skeleton, which is then visualized on radiographs.

7. The patient is moved into the prone and lateral positions during the test.

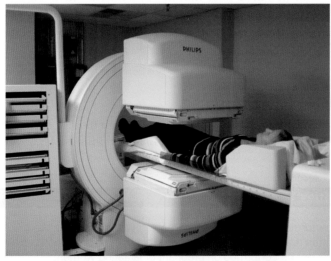

Figure 8-2 Preparation of a patient for a bone scan.

After

 Because only tracer doses of radioisotope are used, reassure the patient that no precautions need to be taken to prevent radioactive exposure to other personnel or family present.

 Assure the patient that the radioactive substance is usually excreted from the body within 6 to 24 hours.

Home Care Responsibilities

- Instruct the patient to observe the injection site and to report any redness or swelling.
- Encourage the patient to drink fluids to aid the excretion of the radioactive substance.

TEST RESULTS AND CLINICAL SIGNIFICANCE

Primary or metastatic tumours of the bone: *These can be singular or multiple. It is difficult to diagnose the specific tumour. Serial scans may help.*

Fracture: *Increased uptake in the bone of a patient with anatomic pain is very suggestive of a fracture missed on routine plain radiographs.*

Degenerative arthritis,

Rheumatoid arthritis: *Increased uptake involving the joints (especially multiple joints) is a hallmark of arthritis.*

Osteomyelitis: *Within the bone of a patient with a compatible clinical history, small "islands" of increased uptake indicate infection.*

Bone necrosis: *Uptake may be decreased ("cold" spot) if there is no new bone growth surrounding the area of bone necrosis.*

Renal osteodystrophy,

Paget's disease: *These two diseases are usually evident as multiple or diffuse uptake of the tracer in the bones.*

RELATED TESTS

Bone (Long) Radiography (p. 1045). The routine bone radiograph often provides information that is additional to or supportive of findings of the bone scan.

Magnetic Resonance Imaging (p. 1148). This test is sometimes more reliable than bone scan in detecting disease or traumatic injury to the bone.

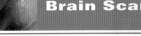

Brain Scan (Cisternal Scan, Cerebral Blood Flow)

NORMAL FINDINGS

No areas of increased radionuclide uptake within the brain

INDICATIONS

In the past, the brain scan was the only test available to study the brain directly. Since the advent of computed tomography of the brain (p. 1065) and magnetic resonance imaging (MRI) (p. 1148), the usefulness of the nuclear brain scan has diminished. This test is used to identify pathologic

8   Nuclear Scanning

conditions (tumour, infarction, infection) involving the cortex. It is used for patients with ongoing headaches, epilepsy, and other neurologic symptoms.

The nuclear brain scan for cerebral blood flow is still commonly used to support the diagnosis of brain death.

TEST EXPLANATION

The brain scan enables examination of the brain by a scanning camera after intravenous injection of a radionuclide material (Figure 8-3). Usually technetium-99m (^{99m}Tc) is the radionuclide used. After injection of the ^{99m}Tc, the radiopharmaceutical is deposited anywhere in the brain in which the blood-brain barrier has been disrupted by disease. Gamma rays are emitted through the skull from the ^{99m}Tc and are detected by a scintillation scanner. The scintillation scanner emits light with each photon it receives from the gamma ray. When these light patterns are arranged in a spatial order, a realistic image of the blood vessels, grey matter, and meninges of the brain and pathologic deposits is produced. This study is performed in patients with frequent and severe headaches, stroke (cerebrovascular accident syndrome), seizure complaints, or other neurologic complaints.

Normally, the blood-brain barrier does not allow blood (containing the radionuclide) to come in direct contact with brain tissue. Frequently used isotopes (e.g., ^{99m}Tc) are unable to cross the blood-brain barrier. However, in localized pathologic conditions, this normal barrier is disrupted. The isotopes are then preferentially localized or concentrated in abnormal regions of the brain.

Various pathologic processes can disrupt the blood-brain barrier. Unfortunately, the brain scan is not a precise indicator of the specific pathologic process. Study of the location, size, and shape of the abnormality, as well as the timing of the scan, may help specify the pathologic process.

The timing of brain scanning in relation to the onset of symptoms of a cerebrovascular accident is usually significant. For example, in cerebral infarction, scanning may yield normal findings when performed soon after the onset of symptoms and then yield abnormal findings 2 weeks later; this combination is virtually pathognomonic of infarction. Brain scans in patients with

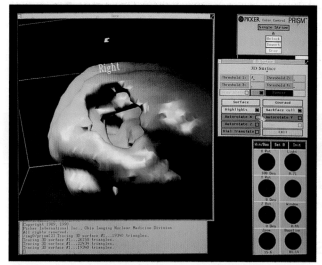

Figure 8-3 Image produced by radionuclide brain scan. This particular image demonstrates a deficit in cerebral blood flow as a result of an arteriovenous malformation.

cerebral thrombosis without infarction may never reveal abnormalities. Tumours and abscesses manifest abnormalities on the initial scan.

Clinicians may inject isotopes and then perform immediate scanning to detect changes in the dynamics of cerebral blood flow by comparing one side of the brain with the other. For example, cerebrovascular occlusive disease is characterized by decreased flow, in contrast to an arteriovenous malformation, which is associated with an increased flow rate. ^{99m}Tc may be used for cerebral perfusion studies. A *cerebral blood flow scan* can demonstrate lack of blood flow to the brain and concurrent blood flow to the scalp and is thereby used to support the findings of "brain death."

Cisternal scans may be performed by injecting radioactive material into the subarachnoid space and then taking serial scans of the head. These scans are useful in evaluating ventricular size and patency of the cerebrospinal fluid (CSF) pathways and reabsorption. Because only a small amount of CSF enters the ventricles, their uptake of radioactive material is normally minimal. Blocks in the CSF pathways may prevent this reabsorption, however, and thus large amounts of isotopes may appear in the ventricles. Cisternal scans also may be used to evaluate CSF leakage (e.g., into the nasal sinuses) in patients with recurrent meningitis and to evaluate hydrocephalus.

The technique of single-photon emission computed tomography (SPECT) has significantly improved the quality of brain scanning. With SPECT scanning, the radionuclide is injected and the scintillation cameras are placed to receive images from multiple angles (around the circumference of the head). This technique greatly increases the usefulness of nuclear brain scanning. In general, computed tomography, MRI, and carotid duplex scans have replaced the brain scan in diagnostic neurology.

CONTRAINDICATIONS

- Pregnancy, unless the benefits of the procedure outweigh the risk of injury to the fetus
- Inability of patients to cooperate during the testing

Clinical Priorities

- Pathologic conditions disrupt the normal blood-brain barrier and allow isotopes to concentrate in abnormal regions of the brain.
- The brain scan is not specific for indicating the cause of a pathologic process. Study of the location, shape, and size of the abnormality, along with the timing of the scan, may help delineate the problem.
- The SPECT technique has greatly improved the quality of brain scanning.

PROCEDURE AND PATIENT CARE

Before

✍ Explain the procedure to the patient.
- Administer blocking agents as ordered before the scanning. For example, potassium chloride prevents an inordinate amount of ^{99m}Tc uptake by the choroid plexus, which would simulate a pathologic cerebral condition. Similar solutions (e.g., potassium iodine, Lugol iodine solution) may be administered orally to block radioisotope uptake by the thyroid.
- Check the patient for allergy to iodine if an iodinated solution will be used.
- For agitated patients, consider having a sedative ordered.
✍ Inform the patient that no discomfort is associated with this study other than the peripheral intravenous puncture required for injection of the radioisotope.

During

- Take the patient to the nuclear medicine department.
- Note the following procedural steps:
    1. After administration of the radioisotope, the patient is placed in the supine, lateral, and prone positions while a counter is placed over the patient's head (Figure 8-4).
    2. The radioisotope counts are anatomically displayed and photographed while the patient remains very still.
    3. When cerebral flow studies are performed, the counter is immediately placed over the patient's head.
    4. The counts are anatomically recorded in timed sequence to follow the isotope during its first flow through the brain.
    5. Another scan is obtained 30 minutes to 2 hours later for identification of pathologic tissues.
- Note that this study is performed in approximately 35 to 45 minutes by a technician in the nuclear medicine department.

After

- Assure the patient that the radioactive material is usually excreted from the body within 6 to 24 hours.
- Because only tracer doses of radioisotopes are used, remember that no precautions need to be taken to prevent radioactive exposure to other personnel or family present.
- Encourage the patient to drink fluids to aid in the excretion of the isotope from the body.
- Observe the injection site for redness and swelling.

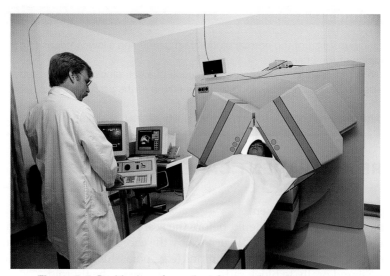

Figure 8-4 Positioning of a patient for a radionuclide scan of the brain. In this diagnostic study, a small amount of radioactive material crosses the blood-brain barrier to produce an image. This study is known as *single-photon emission computed tomography (SPECT)*.

TEST RESULTS AND CLINICAL SIGNIFICANCE

Cerebral neoplasm,

Brain abscess,

Cerebral hemorrhage,

Cancer metastasis to the brain: *These pathologic conditions are associated with disruption in the blood-brain barrier, which results in increased uptake of radionuclide in the cerebral cortex.*

Acute cerebral infarction: *In the first few days to weeks after a stroke, the scan may appear normal. After a few weeks, however, the blood-brain barrier has been disrupted, and cortical uptake occurs. This appearance is pathognomonic of stroke.*

Subdural hematoma: *The cortex/subcortical tissue and meninges may become distorted and lateralized.*

Cerebral thrombosis,

Cerebrovascular occlusive disease,

Hematoma,

Arteriovenous malformation,

Aneurysm: *These vascular abnormalities are evident in cerebral flow studies.*

CSF leakage: *The most common site of leakage of CSF is into the nasal cavity. This can be the result of tumour or infection.*

Hydrocephalus: *This is evident on cisternal scans.*

RELATED TESTS

Computed Tomography, Brain (p. 1065). This test is very accurate in identifying pathologic conditions of the brain. X-ray beams are directed to the brain from multiple circumferential angles and then gathered to produce multiple images of the brain.

Magnetic Resonance Imaging (p. 1148). MRI of the brain does not involve radiation; rather, it detects electromagnetic differences among the brain tissues. The brain is visualized from similar angles as in computed tomography, and an accurate image is produced.

Cardiac Nuclear Scanning (Myocardial Scan, Cardiac Scan, Nuclear Cardiac Scanning, Heart Scan, Thallium Scan, Multigated Acquisition [MUGA] Scan, Isonitrile Scan, Sestamibi Cardiac Scan, Cardiac Flow Studies)

NORMAL FINDINGS

Heterogeneous uptake radionuclide throughout the myocardium of the left ventricle

Left ventricular end diastolic volume ≤70 mL

Left ventricular end systolic volume ≤25 mL

Left ventricular ejection fraction >50%

Right ventricular ejection fraction >40%

Normal cardiac wall motion

No muscle wall thickening

INDICATIONS

Cardiac nuclear scanning is used to detect myocardial ischemia, infarction, wall dysfunction, and decreased ejection fraction. It is commonly used as the imaging method portion of cardiac stress testing. Specific indications for cardiac nuclear scanning include the following:

1. Evaluation of ventricular function in patients with myocardial disease or in patients receiving cardiotoxic drugs (e.g., doxorubicin [Adriamycin] chemotherapy)
2. Screening of adults for past and recent infarction
3. Evaluation of patients with chest pain and uninterpretable or equivocal electrocardiographic changes caused by drugs, bundle branch block, or left ventricular hypertrophy
4. Evaluation of myocardial perfusion before and after therapy (e.g., coronary artery bypass surgery)

TEST EXPLANATION

Cardiac radionuclear scanning is a noninvasive and safe method of recognizing alterations of left ventricular muscle function and coronary artery blood distribution. In this test, radionuclide is injected intravenously into the patient. Myocardial perfusion images are then obtained while the patient is lying down under a single-photon emission computed tomography (SPECT) camera that generates a picture of the radioactivity coming from the heart. Perfusion images, ventricular function, and gated-pool ejection fractions can all be obtained with a single injection (a *myocardial perfusion scan*). Furthermore, with the use of ^{99m}Tc isonitrile, an ischemic area will remain visible several hours after an ischemic event. This scan can be performed at rest or with exercise such as treadmill or bicycling (*myocardial nuclear stress testing*). Medications may be administered that duplicate exercise stress testing. Vasodilators (dipyridamole, adenosine, and Regadenoson) or chronotropic agents (dobutamine) are commonly used. Regadenoson is the most recent A_{2A} adenosine receptor agonist that instigates coronary vasodilatation. It is associated with fewer side effects (e.g., heart block, bronchospasm) and can be injected more quickly. See Table 8-1 for an overview of cardiac nuclear scanning.

Many different radiocompound materials can be used; in Canada, however, the isotope used most often in these compounds is technetium-99m (^{99m}Tc). When these compounds are injected intravenously and a radiation detector is placed over the heart, an image of the heart can be recorded and photographed. In the evaluation of the patency of the coronary arteries, the characteristic abnormality varies according to the type of radiocompound used. When thallium-201 is used, all normal myocardial cells take up the substance and appear on the photoscan. Ischemic or infarcted cells do not take up the substance and appear as "cold" spots, devoid of nuclear material and surrounded by normal cells (Figure 8-5).

^{99m}Tc sestamibi (isonitrile) produces a similar appearance and is an even better cardiac imaging agent. Higher quality images can be obtained on the first pass, providing information similar to that of angiocardiography. ^{99m}Tc pyrophosphate is a radionuclide that binds with calcium. When ischemia or early infarction has occurred, intracellular calcium leaks out of the cardiac muscle cells. The calcium level in the area of injury is very high. The ^{99m}Tc pyrophosphate binds to that calcium and creates an area of increased radionuclide uptake ("hot" spot). This is often called a *myocardial infarction scan*. Cardiac scanning with ^{99m}Tc pyrophosphate is particularly useful when ischemia is difficult to diagnose. For example, in a patient with ventricular hypertrophy or left bundle branch block, the electrocardiogram is unreliable. If such a patient has chest pain and the ^{99m}Tc pyrophosphate scan is positive, muscle injury has indeed occurred. This type of scan is also especially helpful if the patient has had ongoing chest pain for 5 to 10 days before seeing a physician. Because the ^{99m}Tc pyrophosphate scan stays positive for that long, the delayed diagnosis of a myocardial infarction can be made.

With the radionuclides discussed, cardiac nuclear scanning is used to indicate myocardial ischemia or myocardial infarction. It can be used in acute events of chest pain. Ischemia or infarction would be evident as described previously. Cardiac scanning also can be used to assess myocardial ischemia during stress testing (p. 563). In some cases, no evidence of diminished blood supply to

TABLE 8-1	**Overview of Cardiac Nuclear Scanning**			
Scan	**Radionuclide**	**Use**	**Positive Results**	**Comments**
Myocardial perfusion	99mTc isonitrile (sestamibi) Thallium-201	To identify ischemic or infarcted heart muscle	Cold spots are areas of ischemia	Commonly performed with nuclear ventriculography
Myocardial infarction scan	99mTc pyrophosphate	To identify ischemic or infarcted heart muscle	Hot spots are areas of ischemia	Rarely performed
Myocardial function (MUGA)	99mTc-labelled albumin or RBCs	To calculate the cardiac ejection fraction	Reduced cardiac ejection fraction	The most accurate method for determining cardiac ejection fraction
Cardiac flow	99mTc alone or labelled RBCs	To determine the direction of cardiac flow	Abnormal cardiac blood flow patterns	Performed most commonly in children with suspected cardiac anomalies
Nuclear ventriculography	Thallium-201 99mTc	To evaluate muscle wall activity	Poor wall contractility in ischemia or infarction	Commonly performed with a perfusion scan
Exercise stress testing	Thallium-201 99mTc Isontrile	To evaluate muscle wall activity during stress (physical or chemical)	Poor wall contractility in ischemia or infarction	Commonly includes a perfusion scan and ventriculography

MUGA, Multigated acquisition; *RBCs,* red blood cells; *99mTc,* technetium-99m.

8   Nuclear Scanning

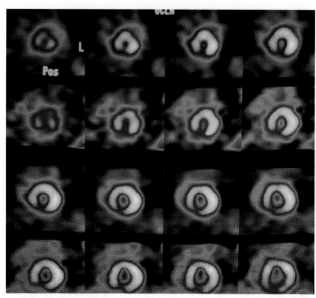

Figure 8-5 Thallium-201 scintigraphy produces a series of images of blood flow and tissue perfusion.

the myocardium is evident during the resting state. When the heart is stressed, however, evidence of myocardial ischemia can become quite obvious and is easily detected by nuclear stress testing. In this form of nuclear cardiac scanning, the radionuclide is injected intravenously at the point of maximal cardiac stress. The radionuclide accumulates in the myocardium in direct proportion to the regional myocardial blood flow. A normal myocardium has much greater radionuclide activity than does an ischemic myocardium. In comparing results of this stress testing with a resting cardiac nuclear scan, the examiner can detect exercise-induced ischemia. In this form of stress testing, cardiac nuclear scanning is the method of cardiac imaging or monitoring. This test is not only beneficial in detecting coronary occlusive disease but also successful in assessing postoperative patency of a coronary artery bypass graft. Another method for detecting myocardial ischemia is to obtain delayed images to show clearance of the radionuclide from the myocardium. Hot spots on the delayed images indicate poor wash-out in areas of decreased coronary perfusion.

For an evaluation of myocardial function, ^{99m}Tc pertechnetate or ^{99m}Tc-labelled albumin is used to measure the portion of blood ejected from the ventricle during one cardiac cycle (ejection fraction). Normally, more than 65% of the blood is ejected from the ventricle during systole. Values lower than 65% indicate decreased contractility of the heart as a result of ischemia, infarction, or cardiomyopathy. Computers can be synchronized with the electrocardiogram during scanning; this is called *gating*. The amount of blood ejected during systole also can be calculated on the basis of the size of the heart at the end of systole and at the end of diastole (Figure 8-6). This form of determination of ventricular function is called *gated pool imaging,* and the measurement is the *gated pool ejection fraction. Multigated acquisition (MUGA) scanning* is another name for this test, derived from the name of the computer machinery originally required for this determination. Because the MUGA scan is three-dimensional, it is the most accurate means of determining cardiac function and ejection fraction.

This type of computer-assisted gated (synchronized) cardiac scanning can also allow the myocardial wall to be photographed while in motion. This enables visualization of the myocardium during several cardiac cycles, and contractility of the myocardium can be determined. This imaging

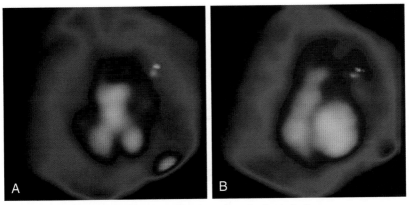

Figure 8-6 Blood pooling imaging. **A,** Systolic frame. **B,** Diastolic frame.

technique is called *nuclear ventriculography* and can provide the same information as radiographic ventriculography, which is performed during cardiac catheterization (p. 1047); however, nuclear scanning is noninvasive and much safer. Ischemic areas appear hypokinetic on scans, whereas infarcted areas appear akinetic on scans. This is also evident after stress during a cardiac stress test.

Cardiac flow studies can be performed by the rapid injection of the radionuclide into a vein (jugular or antecubital) and obtaining images immediately to follow the "first pass" of the radionuclide through the heart and great vessels. This provides excellent information about the direction of blood flow to and from the ventricles. It is particularly helpful in the evaluation of children with suspected congenital heart disorders. Ventricular septal defects that cause abnormal direction of blood flow are apparent. Transposition of great vessels is easily demonstrated. Valvular regurgitation is also obvious. This test also allows the physician to quantify the amount of blood flow affected by those disorders.

In single-photon emission computed tomography (SPECT), the radionuclear materials discussed emit single photons. SPECT has been used to visualize the heart from many different angles. These images are then reconstructed with the use of techniques similar to computed tomography, and three-dimensional images of the physiologic cardiac processes are obtained. Areas of myocardial ischemia can be seen with far greater resolution and can be more accurately quantified.

CONTRAINDICATIONS

- Patients who are uncooperative or medically unstable
- Patients with severe cardiac arrhythmia
- Pregnancy, unless the benefits of the procedure outweigh the risk to the fetus from exposure to radionuclide material
- See contraindications to cardiac stress testing (p. 563)

INTERFERING FACTORS

- Myocardial trauma
- Cardiac flow studies can be altered by excessive alterations in chest pressure, such as that caused by excessive crying in pediatric patients
- Recent nuclear scanning (e.g., thyroid or bone scan)
- Drugs such as long-acting nitrates may only temporarily improve coronary perfusion and cardiac function.

Nuclear Scanning

8

Clinical Priorities

- Nuclear scanning is commonly used as the imaging portion of cardiac stress testing to assess myocardial ischemia.
- This test can be used to evaluate myocardial function by measuring the ejection fraction.
- ^{99m}Tc isonitrile produces a better cardiac image than does thallium-201. It is often used to replace thallium-201.

PROCEDURE AND PATIENT CARE

Before

✗ Explain the procedure to the patient.
✗ Instruct the patient that a short fasting period may be required.
✗ Inform the patient that the only discomfort associated with this test is the venipuncture required for injection of the radioisotope.

During

- Take the patient to the nuclear medicine department. Depending on the type of nuclear myocardial scan, each scanning protocol is different.
- Note the following procedural steps:
    1. An intravenous injection of radionuclide material is performed.
    2. Depending on the radionuclide used, scanning is performed 15 minutes to 4 hours later.
    3. Gamma ray detectors are placed over the precordium.
    4. The patient is placed in the supine position (Figure 8-7), then in the lateral position, and then in both the right and left oblique positions. In some departments, the detector can be rotated around the patient, who remains in the supine position.

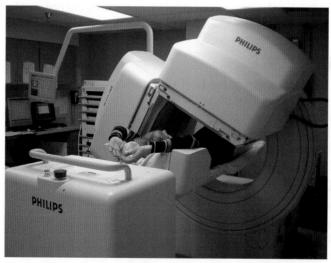
Figure 8-7 Positioning of a patient for cardiac nuclear scanning.

5. The gamma ray scanner records the image of the heart, and an image is immediately produced.
6. For a *thallium exercise stress test,* radioactive thallium is injected during exercise when the patient reaches a maximum heart rate. The patient then lies on a table, and scanning is done. A repeat scan may be performed 3 to 4 hours later.
7. If a ^{99m}Tc *isonitrile stress test* is needed, the radionuclide material is injected and a scan performed 30 to 60 minutes later for the resting phase. Four hours later, cardiac stress testing is performed. After a second injection, scanning is repeated. After each ^{99m}Tc isonitrile injection, a carbohydrate snack such as milk and a muffin is usually given to facilitate clearing of the radionuclide from the hepatobiliary system.

- Note that myocardial scans are usually performed in less than 30 minutes by a nuclear medicine technician.

After

- Apply pressure or a pressure dressing to the venipuncture site.
- Assess the venipuncture site for bleeding.
- Because only tracer doses of radioisotopes are used, note that no precautions need to be taken against radioactive exposure to personnel or family.
- Encourage the patient to drink fluids to aid in the excretion of the radioactive substance.
- If stress testing was performed, evaluate the patient's vital signs at frequent intervals (as indicated).

TEST RESULTS AND CLINICAL SIGNIFICANCE

Coronary artery occlusive disease: *This diagnosis can be made during a resting scan or during cardiac stress nuclear scanning. The appearance of this abnormality depends on the radionuclide used.*

Decreased myocardial function in association with ischemia, myocarditis, cardiomyopathy, or heart failure: *These myocardial diseases are evident as hypokinesia of the cardiac wall. Infarcted areas, in comparison, have no wall motion.*

Decreased cardiac output: *A number of coronary, myocardial, and valvular diseases are associated with reduced cardiac output. A reduced ejection fraction is an indirect measurement of cardiac output. A reduced ejection fraction is often the first sign of those diseases.*

RELATED TESTS

Cardiac Stress Testing (p. 563). In this test, the patient receives a stressor (such as exercise) to maximize cardiac function. The heart is then often imaged with nuclear scanning to measure the effect of the stress.

Cardiac Catheterization (p. 1047). This test provides similar images through the use of radio-opaque dyes injected through catheters placed in and around the heart.

Echocardiography (p. 906). This is an ultrasound directed image of the cardiac muscle and chambers.

Gallbladder Nuclear Scanning (Hepatobiliary Scintigraphy, Hepatobiliary Imaging, Biliary Tract Radionuclide Scan, Cholescintigraphy, Diisopropyl Iminodiacetic Acid [DISIDA] Scanning, Hepatobiliary Iminodiacetic Acid [HIDA] Scanning, Iminodiacetic Acid [IDA] Gallbladder Scanning)

NORMAL FINDINGS

Gallbladder, common bile duct, and duodenum visualized within 60 minutes after radionuclide injection (confirmation of patency of the cystic and common bile ducts)

INDICATIONS

Cholescintigraphy is valuable in evaluating patients for suspected gallbladder disease. The primary use of this study is to diagnose acute cholecystitis in patients who have acute right upper quadrant abdominal pain. When the gallbladder ejection fraction is calculated, chronic cholecystitis can be diagnosed. This study is also used to assist in the diagnosis of extrahepatic biliary obstruction.

TEST EXPLANATION

Through the use of iminodiacetic acid analogues (IDAs) labelled with technetium-99m (^{99m}Tc), the biliary tract can be evaluated in a safe, accurate, and noninvasive manner. These radionuclide compounds are extracted by the liver and excreted into the bile. Gamma rays are emitted through the body from the ^{99m}Tc in the bile and are detected by a scintillation camera. The scintillation camera emits light with each photon it receives from the gamma ray. When these light patterns are arranged in a spatial order, a realistic image of the biliary tree is produced.

Failure to visualize the gallbladder 60 to 120 minutes after injection of the radionuclide dye is virtually diagnostic of an obstruction of the cystic duct, which instigates the pathophysiologic process of acute cholecystitis. Delayed filling of the gallbladder is associated with chronic or acalculous cholecystitis. This procedure is also helpful in diagnosing biliary duct obstructions. The identification of the radionuclide in the biliary tree but not in the bowel is diagnostic of common bile duct obstruction.

This procedure is superior to oral cholecystography, intravenous cholangiography, ultrasonography, and computed tomography of the gallbladder in the detection of cholecystitis (Table 8-2). Also, with cholescintigraphy, it is possible to determine gallbladder function numerically by calculating the capability of the gallbladder to eject its contents. It is believed that an ejection fraction of less than 35% indicates primary gallbladder disease. Digital ultrasonography (p. 896) has largely replaced this test in the diagnosis of acute cholecystitis.

On occasion, morphine sulphate is administered intravenously during nuclear scanning. The morphine causes increased ampullary contraction. This not only can reproduce the patient's symptoms of biliary colic but also serves to force the bile containing the radionuclide into the gallbladder. If no radionuclide is seen in the gallbladder with the use of morphine within 15 to 60 minutes, the diagnosis of acute cholecystitis is nearly certain. This greatly decreases the scanning time because without morphine, obtaining a definitive diagnosis of acute cholecystitis takes 4 hours.

A nuclear medicine technologist performs this study in 1 to 4 hours in the nuclear medicine department. A physician trained in interpretation of diagnostic nuclear medicine interprets the

TABLE 8-2	Comparison of Methods of Visualizing the Gallbladder and Biliary System	
Test	**Advantages**	**Disadvantages**
Cholecystography	Easily performed, inexpensive	Visualization is not possible with acute cholecystitis or if other inflammatory processes are in the abdomen
		Visualization is not possible if bilirubin level **54.2 Mcmol/L** (>2 mg/dL)
		Visualization is not possible if patient vomits or has diarrhea
Intravenous cholangiography	Easily performed, inexpensive	Visualization is not possible if bilirubin level **54.2 Mcmol/L** (>2 mg/dL)
Intravenous cholangiography	Easily performed, inexpensive	Visualization is not possible if bilirubin level **54.2 Mcmol/L** (>2 mg/dL)
Endoscopic retrograde cholangiopancreatography (ERCP)	Good visualization of the bile duct Stones can be extracted Stents can be placed to drain bile	Technically difficult The gallbladder might not be visualized Invasive procedure
Percutaneous transhepatic cholangiography (PTC)	Good visualization of the biliary tree Stents can be placed to drain bile	Invasive procedure The gallbladder might not be visualized
Ultrasonography	Easily performed, accurate, inexpensive	May not accurately help visualize pathologic conditions of the common bile duct
Scintigraphy (nuclear scanning)	Can help diagnose acute cholecystitis The biliary tree can be visualized even if bilirubin level >2 mg/dL	Not accurate for chronic cholecystitis More complicated to perform Identifying pathologic condition takes several hours May yield false-positive results if other inflammatory processes are occurring within the abdomen

test in several minutes. The only discomfort associated with this procedure is the intravenous injection of radionuclide.

CONTRAINDICATIONS

- Pregnancy, unless the benefits of the procedure outweigh the risk of injury to the fetus

INTERFERING FACTORS

- If the patient has not eaten for more than 24 hours, the radionuclide may not fill the gallbladder. This would produce a false-positive result.

PROCEDURE AND PATIENT CARE

Before

- Explain the procedure to the patient.
- Assure the patient that he or she will not be exposed to large amounts of radioactivity.
- Instruct the patient to fast for at least 2 hours before the test. This fasting is preferable but not mandatory.

Clinical Priorities

- Gallbladder scanning is used primarily to diagnose acute cholecystitis in patients who have acute right upper quadrant pain.
- This procedure is superior to oral cholecystography, intravenous cholangiography, ultrasonography, and computed tomography of the gallbladder in the diagnosis of cholecystitis.
- This procedure can also help determine the ejection fraction of the gallbladder.
- Morphine sulphate can be administered intravenously during scanning to markedly reduce the scanning time from 4 hours to less than 1 hour; however, careful monitoring is required because one of the adverse effects of morphine is biliary tract spasm, which can be very painful for the patient.

During

- Take the patient to the nuclear medicine department.
- Note the following procedural steps:
  1. After intravenous administration of a ^{99m}Tc-labelled iminodiacetic acid (IDA) analogue, the right upper quadrant of the abdomen is scanned.
  2. Serial images are obtained over a period of 1 hour.
  3. Subsequent images can be obtained at 15- to 30-minute intervals.
  4. If the gallbladder, common bile duct, or duodenum is not visualized within 60 minutes after injection, delayed images are obtained up to 4 hours later.
  5. Images are recorded.
  6. When an ejection fraction is to be determined, either the patient is given a fatty meal or cholecystokinin is administered to evaluate emptying of the gallbladder. The gallbladder is continually scanned to measure the percentage of isotope ejected.

After

- Obtain a meal for the patient, if it is indicated.

TEST RESULTS AND CLINICAL SIGNIFICANCE

Acute cholecystitis: *The gallbladder cannot be visualized because a gallstone is stuck in the cystic duct, causing acute cholecystitis. The rest of the biliary tree is visualized.*

Chronic cholecystitis,

Acalculous cholecystitis,

Cystic duct syndrome: *Visualization of the gallbladder is delayed after several hours. The gallbladder ejection fraction is less than 35%. The pathophysiologic mechanism of cystic duct syndrome is not well known.*

Obstruction of the common bile duct secondary to gallstones, tumour, or stricture: *This is evident when the radionuclide is seen in a large bile duct but not in the bowel. The bile duct is obstructed.*

RELATED TESTS

See Table 8-2, p. 825.

Abdominal Ultrasonography (p. 896). With the use of ultrasonography, gallstones can be identified within the gallbladder. The diagnosis of acute cholecystitis, however, cannot be made with the same degree of certainty as it can with biliary scintigraphy.

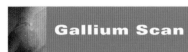

Gallium Scan

NORMAL FINDINGS

Diffuse, low level of gallium uptake, especially in the liver and spleen
No increased gallium uptake within the body

INDICATIONS

Gallium-67 becomes concentrated in areas of the body where white blood cells (WBCs) tend to congregate (areas of tumour, infection, and inflammation). It is used to stage gallium-avid tumours (those that attract high concentrations of gallium; e.g., Hodgkin disease, lymphomas, lung cancer). It is used to locate infection or inflammation in patients with fever of unknown origin. In addition, it is used to monitor response to treatment of infection, inflammation, or tumour.

TEST EXPLANATION

A gallium scan of the total body is usually performed 24, 48, and 72 hours after an intravenous injection of radioactive gallium-67. Most commonly, however, a single scan is performed 2 to 4 days after injection of the gallium. Gallium-67 is a radionuclide that is taken up in areas of inflammation and infection, by abscesses, and by benign and malignant tumours. Not all types of tumours, however, take up gallium. Lymphomas are particularly gallium avid. Other tumours that can be detected by a gallium scan include sarcomas, hepatomas, and carcinomas of the gastrointestinal tract, kidney, uterus, stomach, and testicle.

This test is useful in detecting metastatic tumour, specifically Hodgkin disease and lymphoma, even when results of other diagnostic imaging tests are normal. Positron emission tomography (PET; p. 849) has largely replaced gallium scans for the identification of malignancy. Gallium scans are also useful in demonstrating a source of infection in patients with a fever of unknown origin. Gallium can be used to identify noninfectious inflammation within the body in patients who have an elevated sedimentation rate. Unfortunately, this test is not specific enough to differentiate among tumour, infection, inflammation, and abscess. Although a gallium scan is better able to detect sites of chronic inflammation, PET is more commonly used to identify areas of acute infection.

Some organs (liver, spleen, bone, colon) normally retain gallium. Therefore, a normal total-body gallium scan study would demonstrate some uptake in these organs, but this uptake is much less concentrated than in diseased areas (e.g., tumour, inflammation).

Another common method of scanning is single-photon emission computed tomography (SPECT). For SPECT, the patient lies supine on the table surrounded by a doughnut-like gantry.

The photon detection camera rotates around the patient to obtain proton counts from 360 degrees. This provides a more detailed image.

A nuclear medicine technologist performs each separate scan in approximately 30 to 60 minutes. Repeated scanning is required. Repeated injections are not necessary. The test results are interpreted by a physician trained in nuclear medicine and are usually available 72 hours after the injection. No pain or discomfort is associated with this procedure other than the intravenous injection. However, lying still on a hard table for the duration required is occasionally uncomfortable for the patient.

CONTRAINDICATIONS

• Pregnancy, unless the benefits of the procedure outweigh the risk of injury to the fetus

INTERFERING FACTORS

• Recent barium studies interfere with the visualization of the gallium within the abdomen.

Clinical Priorities

• Gallium scans are useful in detecting metastatic tumour, even when results of other diagnostic imaging tests are normal.
• Gallium-67 is normally retained in the liver, colon, spleen, and bone. Therefore, small amounts of uptake in these organs are normal during scanning.
• Scanning can be repeated without additional injections of the radionuclide.

PROCEDURE AND PATIENT CARE

Before

✗ Explain the procedure to the patient.
• Usually administer a cathartic or enema as ordered by the physician, to minimize increased gallium uptake within the bowel.

During

• Take the patient to the nuclear medicine department.
• Note the following procedural steps:
  1. Gallium is injected into the unsedated patient.
  2. A total-body scan may be performed 4 to 6 hours later by slowly passing a scintillation camera over the body.
  3. The images provided by the scintillation camera are recorded.
  4. Additional scans are usually performed 24, 48, and 72 hours later.
  5. During the scanning process, the patient is positioned in the supine, prone, and lateral positions.

After

✗ Reassure the patient that because only tracer doses of radioisotopes have been used, other people do not need to take precautions against radioactive exposure.

TEST RESULTS AND CLINICAL SIGNIFICANCE

Tumour,

Noninfectious inflammation (sarcoidosis, rheumatoid arthritis),

Infection,

Abscess: *These processes can take up gallium, but visualization is not 100% accurate. These pathologic conditions may exist in patients in whom results of the gallium scan are normal.*

 Gastric Emptying Scan

NORMAL FINDINGS

Normal values are determined by type and quantity of radiolabelled ingested food.

Time	Lower Normal Limits	Upper Normal Limits
0 minutes		
30 minutes	70%	
1 hour	30%	90%
2 hours		60%
3 hours		30%
4 hours		10%

Values lower than normal represent abnormally fast gastric emptying. Values higher than upper limits represent delayed gastric emptying.

INDICATIONS

This scan is used to determine the rate of gastric emptying. It is used to diagnose gastroparesis or gastric obstruction in patients who have postcibal nausea, vomiting, bloating, early satiety, belching, or abdominal pain.

TEST EXPLANATION

In this study, the patient ingests a solid or liquid "test meal" containing a radionuclide such as technetium-99m (^{99m}Tc). The stomach is then scanned until gastric emptying is complete. This study is used to assess the stomach's ability to empty solids or liquids and to evaluate disorders that may cause a delay in gastric emptying, such as obstruction (caused by peptic ulcers or gastric malignancies) and gastroparesis. This scan is also useful in determining the patency of a gastrointestinal surgical anastomosis.

This procedure lasts approximately 4 hours, depending on the gastric emptying time. The test result is interpreted by a nuclear medicine physician. Results are available the same day. No discomfort is associated with the test.

CONTRAINDICATIONS

- Pregnancy or lactation, unless the benefits of the procedure outweigh the risk of injury to the fetus or infant

Nuclear Scanning

8

INTERFERING FACTORS

▌ Drugs that *increase* gastric emptying time include anticholinergics, opiates, and sedatives/hypnotics. These medications should be withheld for 2 days before the test.

PROCEDURE AND PATIENT CARE

Before

✗ Explain the procedure to the patient. Assure the patient that no pain is associated with this study.
✗ Inform the patient that only a small dose of nuclear material is ingested. Reassure the patient that this is a safe dose.
✗ Instruct the patient to keep on NPO status (nothing by mouth) after midnight on the day of the test.
✗ Instruct the diabetic patient not to take insulin or oral medications before testing because he or she will be fasting until the next meal.
✗ Inform the patient that smoking is prohibited on the day of examination because exposure to tobacco can inhibit gastric emptying.

During

• Take the patient to the nuclear medicine department.
• Note the following procedural steps:
  1. In the nuclear medicine department, the patient is asked to ingest a test meal. In the solid-emptying study, the patient usually eats scrambled egg whites containing ^{99m}Tc, unless contraindicated. In the liquid-emptying study, the patient drinks orange juice or water containing ^{99m}Tc.
  2. After ingestion of the test meal, the patient lies supine under a gamma camera that records gastric images. Images are obtained for 2 minutes every 30 to 60 minutes until gastric emptying is complete. This may take several hours, although each particular timed scan takes only a few minutes.
• With the use of computer calculations of timed images, the rate of gastric emptying can be determined.

After

✗ Assure the patient that he or she has ingested only a small amount of nuclear material. No radiation precautions need to be taken against the patient or his or her body secretions.

TEST RESULTS AND CLINICAL SIGNIFICANCE

Gastric obstruction caused by gastric ulcer or cancer: *Tumours located at the gastric outlet can obstruct or delay gastric emptying. Ulcers, particularly those in the duodenum, can cause edema and scarring, which also can cause delay in gastric emptying. The scan, although not specific about the cause of the obstruction, demonstrates prolonged gastric emptying.*
Nonfunctioning gastrointestinal anastomosis: *Postoperative edema is suspected to be the cause of delayed gastric emptying after gastric surgery. Gastroparesis also may play a role.*
Gastroparesis: *The muscle function required for gastric emptying can be affected by nerve damage caused by diabetes or other neuropathies. Endocrine factors (gastrin related) may also affect gastric emptying. This process is not uncommon after prolonged periods of gastric obstruction. In this case, again, the gastric emptying scan is prolonged.*

RELATED TEST

Gastroesophageal Reflux Scan (see following test). This is very similar to gastric emptying scan, but the patient is evaluated for reflux of the gastric contents into the esophagus.

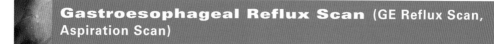

Gastroesophageal Reflux Scan (GE Reflux Scan, Aspiration Scan)

NORMAL FINDINGS

No evidence of gastroesophageal reflux

INDICATIONS

This scan is performed on patients who report symptoms of heartburn, reflux of food, water brash (sour taste in the mouth), aspiration, or paroxysmal nocturnal dyspnea (from nocturnal aspiration). It can detect gastroesophageal reflux and aspiration.

TEST EXPLANATION

Gastroesophageal reflux scans are used to evaluate patients with symptoms of heartburn, regurgitation, vomiting, and dysphagia. These scans are also used to evaluate the response to medical or surgical treatment in patients with gastroesophageal reflux. In addition, aspiration scans may be used to detect aspiration of gastric contents into the lungs and to evaluate swallowing function.

This procedure is performed in approximately 30 minutes in the nuclear medicine department. No discomfort is associated with this test.

CONTRAINDICATIONS

- Intolerance of abdominal compression
- Pregnancy or lactation, unless the benefits of the procedure outweigh the risk of injury to the fetus or infant

 Age-Related Concerns

- Aspiration scans can be used to evaluate infants for chalasia.
- The tracer is added to the infant's formula or feeding. Images are taken over the next hour, with delayed images taken as needed.
- Older adults (>65 years) are at high risk for gastroesophageal reflux because of a decline in the motility of esophagus, which can result in dysphagia, heartburn, or vomiting of undigested food.
- Older adults may also experience a decrease in the resting pressure of the lower esophageal sphincter, which can result in symptoms of dysphagia, feelings of fullness, heartburn, and sternal pain.

PROCEDURE AND PATIENT CARE

Before

✗ Explain the procedure to the patient.
✗ Assure the patient that no pain is associated with this test.
✗ Instruct the patient to eat a full meal just before the study.

During

Gastroesophageal Reflux Scan

- Take the patient to the nuclear medicine department.
- Note the following procedural steps:

1. The patient is placed in the supine position and asked to swallow 100 to 150 mL of a tracer "cocktail" (e.g., orange juice, diluted hydrochloric acid, and technetium-99m [^{99m}Tc]–labelled colloid).
2. Images of the patient's esophageal area are immediately taken.
3. The patient is asked to assume other positions to determine whether gastroesophageal reflux occurs and, if so, in what position.
4. A large abdominal binder that contains an air-inflatable cuff is placed on the patient's abdomen. This is insufflated to increase abdominal pressure.
5. Images are again taken over the esophageal area to determine whether any gastroesophageal reflux occurs.

Aspiration Scan
- Take the patient to the nuclear medicine department.
- Note the following procedural steps:
  1. This scan may be performed by adding a radionuclide to the patient's evening meal and keeping the patient in the supine position until the next morning.
  2. Images are made over the lung fields to detect esophagotracheal aspiration of the tracer.
  3. In infants being evaluated for chalasia, the tracer is added to the feeding or formula. Nuclear tracer images are then taken over the next hour, with delayed images as needed.

After
- With the use of computer calculations based on the images of the scans, the severity and percentage of reflux can be calculated.
- Assure the patient that he or she has ingested only a small dose of nuclear material. No radiation precautions need to be taken against the patient or his or her body secretions.

TEST RESULTS AND CLINICAL SIGNIFICANCE

Gastroesophageal reflux: *The radionuclide can be seen to flow backwards from the stomach into the esophagus. This should diminish or disappear with successful medical or surgical treatment.*

Pulmonary aspiration: *This can be the result of severe gastroesophageal reflux or the result of faulty swallowing function.*

RELATED TEST

Gastric Emptying Scan (p. 829). This is similar to gastroesophageal reflux scan, but it is used to identify delayed gastric emptying, which can contribute to gastroesophageal reflux.

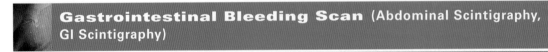

Gastrointestinal Bleeding Scan (Abdominal Scintigraphy, GI Scintigraphy)

NORMAL FINDINGS

No collection of radionuclide in gastrointestinal tract

INDICATIONS

This study is mainly used to localize sites of gastrointestinal bleeding.

TEST EXPLANATION

The gastrointestinal (GI) bleeding scan is a test used to localize the site of bleeding in patients who are having active GI hemorrhage. The scan also can be used in patients who have suspected intra-abdominal (non-GI) hemorrhage from an unknown source. Localization of the source of GI or other bleeding can be quite difficult. When surgery is required under these circumstances, it is difficult, cumbersome, and prolonged. The surgeon, too, may have extreme difficulty finding the source of bleeding. The bleeding scan helps localize the bleeding for the surgeon.

Box 8-1 provides an overview of the diagnostic procedures used in evaluating GI bleeding. The limitations of many of these studies warrant the use of the GI bleeding scan. For example, endoscopy has proved to be extremely useful in determining the source of intestinal bleeding; however, endoscopy is not helpful if the source is within the small intestine or the colon. Although colonoscopy allows excellent visualization of the colon when the colon is cleared out, it is extremely difficult to see when acute, active intestinal bleeding is occurring. Arteriography has three limitations in the evaluation of GI bleeding: First, arteriography can determine the site of bleeding, but the rate of bleeding must exceed 0.5 mL/minute for detection. Second, if GI bleeding is intermittent, the results of the arteriogram can be artificially negative. Third, arteriography visualizes only the blood vessels to the small bowel, right colon, and transverse colon through a superior mesenteric angiogram. If the left colon and sigmoid vessels are to be visualized (most bleeding comes from these areas), inferior mesenteric angiography must be undertaken. This is more difficult to perform.

The GI bleeding scan has several advantages over arteriography. The GI bleeding scan can detect bleeding if the rate is in excess of 0.05 mL/min. Also, with the use of technetium-99m (^{99m}Tc)–labelled red blood cells (RBCs), imaging can be delayed (as long as 24 hours) to indicate the site of an intermittent or extremely slow intestinal bleed.

A GI scintigram is much more sensitive in locating the site of GI bleeding; however, it is not very specific in pinpointing the site or the cause of bleeding. Usually, when the results of a GI scintigram are positive, the exact source of bleeding cannot be localized any more precisely than the affected quadrant of the abdomen (e.g., right upper, left lower). This test is usually performed with the injection of sulphur colloid labelled with ^{99m}Tc or of ^{99m}Tc-labelled RBCs into the patient. If the bleeding is at a rate in excess of 0.05 mL/minute, the radionuclide will ultimately pool in the abnormal segment of the intestine. False-positive results are rare. Again, it is important to recognize that the test only localizes the bleeding; it does not indicate the exact pathologic

Nuclear Scanning

8

BOX 8-1	**Diagnostic Procedures for Gastrointestinal Bleeding**

Upper Gastrointestinal Bleeding (Hematemesis or Blood in the Nasogastric Tube)
- Esophagogastroduodenoscopy
- Celiac angiography
- Aortography (to rule out aortoduodenal fistula)

Lower Gastrointestinal Bleeding (Hematochezia or Melena)
- Passage of nasogastric tube to eliminate upper gastrointestinal bleeding
- Proctoscopy to eliminate hemorrhoids
- Colonoscopy if patient is stable and bowel is relatively free of stool
- Arteriography if bleeding is fast enough
- Gastrointestinal scintigraphy if bleeding is slow but persistent
- Barium enema if other tests cannot localize bleeding and bleeding is persistent

cause of the bleeding. With this test result, if surgery is required, the surgeon is directed to the abnormal area and, it is hoped, can detect and resect the pathologic bleeding source.

It is important to realize that this test can take at least 1 to 4 hours to obtain useful information. Unstable patients should not leave the intensive care environment for that long. Furthermore, the unstable patient may need to go to surgery within minutes, and the surgeon may not have the luxury of taking several hours to determine the region of active bleeding.

CONTRAINDICATIONS

- Pregnancy or lactation, unless the benefits of the procedure outweigh the risk of injury to the fetus or infant
- Medical instability, in which case a stay in the nuclear medicine department may be risky

INTERFERING FACTORS

- Barium within the GI tract may mask a small source of bleeding.

Clinical Priorities

- GI bleeding scans can localize the bleeding. They cannot indicate the cause of the bleeding.
- Because this test requires several hours, unstable patients may not be candidates for it. They may be unable to leave the intensive care unit for that long.
- Imaging may be delayed up to 24 hours to detect slow, intermittent, or chronic bleeding.

PROCEDURE AND PATIENT CARE

Before

- Explain the procedure to the patient.
- Assess the patient's vital signs to ensure that the patient is stable enough for transfer to and from the nuclear medicine department.
- Accompany the patient to the nuclear medicine department if the stability of vital signs is in question.
- Assure the patient that only a small amount of nuclear material will be administered.
- Instruct the patient to notify the nuclear medicine technologist if he or she has a bowel movement during the test. Blood in the GI tract can act as a cathartic.
- Inform the patient that no pretest preparation is required.
- Instruct the nuclear medicine technologist to notify the nurse of all bloody bowel movements that occur while the patient is in the nuclear medicine department.
- Inform the patient that the only discomfort associated with this study is the injection of the radioisotope.

During

- Take the patient to the nuclear medicine department.
- Note the following procedural steps:
  1. Ten millicuries of freshly prepared ^{99m}Tc-labelled sulphur colloid is administered to the patient intravenously. If ^{99m}Tc-labelled RBCs are to be used, 3 to 5 mL of the patient's own blood is combined with the ^{99m}Tc and reinjected into the patient.
  2. Immediately after administration of the radionuclide, the patient is placed under a scintillation camera.

3. Multiple images of the abdomen are obtained at short intervals (5 to 15 minutes). Imaging may be delayed as late as 6 to 24 hours to detect slow, intermittent, or chronic bleeding. The scintigrams are recorded.

4. Pooling of radionuclide in the abdomen indicates the site of bleeding. If no bleeding sites are noted in the first hour, the scan is repeated at hourly intervals for as long as 24 hours.

• Note that areas of the bowel hidden by the liver or spleen may not be adequately evaluated by this procedure. Also, the rectum cannot be easily evaluated because other pelvic structures (e.g., the bladder) obstruct the view. If the initial study is negative and subsequent images show evidence of active bleeding, a repeat scan may be performed.

• Note that each scan is usually performed in approximately 20 to 30 minutes by a technologist in the nuclear medicine department.

After

• Reevaluate the patient's vital signs on return to the nursing unit.

• Reassure the patient that because only tracer doses of radioisotopes have been used, other people do not need to take precautions against radioactive exposure.

TEST RESULTS AND CLINICAL SIGNIFICANCE

Ulcers,

Tumours,

Angiodysplasia and other vascular malformations,

Polyps,

Diverticulosis,

Inflammatory bowel disease: *The mucosa and submucosa in the areas of these diseases are quite friable and can bleed profusely.*

Aortoduodenal fistulas: *These usually manifest as rapid exsanguinating and recurrent upper GI bleeding episodes in a patient who has had prior aortic aneurysm surgery or prior radiation therapy to the area of the midabdomen to upper abdomen.*

RELATED TESTS

Arteriography (p. 1026). This is a radiographic study used to evaluate the patient with GI bleeding at a rate faster than 1 mL/minute.

Esophagogastroduodenoscopy (p. 636) and Colonoscopy (p. 619). These endoscopic tests can be very helpful in identifying the source of GI bleeding. In some cases, endoscopic therapies can be used to stop the bleeding.

Liver/Spleen Scan (Liver Scanning)

NORMAL FINDINGS

Normal size, shape, and position of the liver and spleen with no filling defects

INDICATIONS

This test allows for visualization of the liver and spleen. It is indicated in patients with cancer to rule out tumour metastases to the liver. It is a routine part of tumour staging. It is also indicated

∞ **Nuclear Scanning**

in patients with primary tumours (hepatomas) or in patients with cirrhosis who are at high risk for the development of primary hepatomas. Patients with abnormal liver enzyme values also have their liver visualized. Liver scanning is used to monitor hepatic diseases and response to therapy.

TEST EXPLANATION

This radionuclide procedure is used to outline and detect structural changes of the liver and spleen. A radionuclide, usually technetium-99m (^{99m}Tc)–labelled sulphur colloid, is administered intravenously. Later, a scintillation camera is placed over the right upper and left upper quadrants of the patient's abdomen. This camera records the distribution of the radioactive particles emitted from the liver and spleen. The gamma ray emissions are collected to form an image, which is recorded.

Because the scan can demonstrate only filling defects larger than 2 cm in diameter, results may be artificially negative in patients with space-occupying lesions (e.g., tumours, cysts, granulomas, abscesses) smaller than 2 cm. The scan may be incorrectly interpreted as positive for filling defects in patients with cirrhosis because of the distortion of the patient's liver parenchyma. The liver scan can detect tumours, cysts, granulomas, abscesses, and diffuse infiltrative processes affecting the liver (e.g., amyloidosis, sarcoidosis).

When a hepatic filling defect is observed, the most common cause is a benign hemangioma. This can be differentiated from tumour with the use of ^{99m}Tc-labelled red blood cells (RBCs). The patient's own RBCs are labelled with ^{99m}Tc and reinjected into the patient. Immediate uptake of the radionuclide by the filling defect is suggestive of a hemangioma, for which no therapy is usually required.

In general, computed tomography and magnetic resonance imaging (MRI) have replaced the liver scan in diagnostics. Single-photon emission computed tomography (SPECT) has significantly improved the quality and accuracy of liver scanning. With SPECT, the radionuclide is injected and the scintillation camera is placed to receive images from multiple angles (around the circumference of the liver). Positron emission tomography (PET; p. 849) has also greatly increased the usefulness of nuclear liver scanning. With PET, radioactive carbon, nitrogen, fluorine, or oxygen is used to visualize anatomic and biochemical changes within the liver.

The liver scan can also identify portal hypertension. Normally, most of the radionuclide administered during a liver scan is taken up by the liver (the normal liver/spleen ratio >1). Reversal of the liver/spleen ratio (i.e., the spleen takes up more of the radionuclide) indicates reversal of hepatic blood flow, as a result of portal hypertension.

Splenic hematoma, abscess, cyst, tumour, infarction, and infiltrate processes such as granulomas can be detected. SPECT can also be used to improve visualization of the spleen.

CONTRAINDICATIONS

- Pregnancy or lactation, unless the benefits of the procedure outweigh the risk of injury to the fetus or infant

INTERFERING FACTORS

- Barium in the gastrointestinal tract overlying the liver or spleen produces the appearance of defects on the scan that may be mistaken for masses.

Clinical Priorities

- This test is a routine part of tumour staging. It is used to rule out metastasis to the liver in patients with cancer.
- Results can be artificially negative in patients with lesions smaller than 2 cm in diameter.
- A combination lung-liver scan can be performed to identify subpulmonic or subdiaphragmatic abscesses.

PROCEDURE AND PATIENT CARE

Before

✗ Explain the procedure to the patient.
✗ Inform the patient that no fasting or premedication is required.
✗ Assure the patient that he or she will not be exposed to large amounts of radiation because only tracer doses of isotopes are used.
✗ Inform the patient that the only discomfort associated with this procedure is the intravenous injection of the radionuclide.

During

- Take the patient to the nuclear medicine department.
- Note the following procedural steps:
  1. The patient is taken to the nuclear medicine department, where the radionuclide is administered intravenously. (For inpatients, a nuclear medicine technologist may administer the radionuclide at the patient's bedside.)
  2. Thirty minutes after injection, a gamma ray detector is placed over the right upper quadrant of the patient's abdomen.
  3. The patient is placed in supine, lateral, and prone positions so that all surfaces of the liver can be visualized.
  4. The radionuclide images are recorded.
- Note that this procedure is performed in approximately 1 hour by a trained technologist. A physician trained in nuclear medicine interprets the results.

After

✗ Reassure the patient that because only tracer doses of radioisotopes are used, other people do not need to take precautions against radiation exposure.

TEST RESULTS AND CLINICAL SIGNIFICANCE

Primary or metastatic tumour of the liver or spleen,
Abscess of the liver or spleen,
Hematoma of the liver or spleen,
Hepatic or splenic cyst,
Hemangioma: *These diseases are evident as filling defects localized within the liver-spleen parenchyma.*
Lacerations of the liver or spleen: *The organ can be seen to be lacerated, with a hematoma within the laceration.*
Infiltrative processes (e.g., sarcoidosis, amyloidosis, tuberculosis, or granuloma of the liver or spleen),
Cirrhosis: *These diseases are apparent as diffuse irregularity in the uptake of the radionuclide within the liver or spleen.*

Nuclear Scanning

8

Portal hypertension: *The liver/spleen ratio of uptake of the radionuclide is reversed. Usually the liver takes up most of the radionuclide. In portal hypertension, with reversal of hepatic portal blood flow, the spleen takes up more of the radionuclide.*

Accessory spleen: *The radionuclide aggregates in extrasplenic sites. This is very helpful to the surgeon who is planning a splenectomy and removal of all spleen tissue for patients with autoimmune thrombocytopenia or hemolytic anemia.*

Splenic infarction: *This is evident as a space-filling defect localized within the spleen in a patient with sudden onset of left upper quadrant pain.*

RELATED TESTS

Computed Tomography, Abdomen (p. 1059). Computed tomography of the liver and spleen is probably a more accurate test for the evaluation of these organs than is nuclear scanning. However, to establish the diagnosis of hemangioma, liver scanning with autologous RBCs labelled with ^{99m}Tc is superior in accuracy to computed tomography.

Magnetic Resonance Imaging (p. 1148). MRI of the liver and spleen is considered to be more accurate than nuclear scanning; however, it is more difficult to obtain and more expensive.

Lung Scan (Ventilation/Perfusion Scanning [VPS], Pulmonary Scintiphotography, V/Q Scan)

NORMAL FINDINGS

Diffuse and homogeneous uptake of nuclear material by the lungs

INDICATIONS

The lung scan is very helpful in making the diagnosis of pulmonary embolism. It is easily and rapidly performed on patients who have sudden onset of noncardiac chest pain or shortness of breath. It is often performed on patients who have unexplained tachycardia or hypoxemia (Box 8-2).

TEST EXPLANATION

This nuclear medicine procedure is used to identify defects in blood perfusion of the lung in patients with suspected pulmonary embolism. To evaluate blood flow to the lungs, macroaggregated albumin tagged with technetium-99m (^{99m}Tc) is injected into the patient's peripheral vein. Because the diameter of the radionuclide aggregates is larger than that of the pulmonary capillaries, the aggregates become temporarily lodged in the pulmonary vasculature. A scintillation camera detects the gamma rays from within the lung microvasculature. With the use of light conversion, a realistic image of the lung is obtained.

A homogeneous uptake of particles that fills the entire pulmonary vasculature conclusively rules out pulmonary embolism. The appearance of a defect in an otherwise smooth and diffusely homogeneous pattern indicates a perfusion abnormality (Figure 8-8). This can indicate pulmonary embolism. Unfortunately, many other serious pulmonary parenchymal lesions (e.g., pneumonia, pleural fluid, emphysematous bullae) also cause a defect in pulmonary blood perfusion. Therefore, although the scan may be sensitive, it is not specific because many different pathologic conditions can cause the same abnormal results.

BOX 8-2   Diagnosis of Pulmonary Embolism

Symptoms
Chest pain
Shortness of breath
Feelings of impending doom
Pleurodynia (pleuritic pain with deep inspiration)

Signs
Tachycardia
Hypoxemia
S_4 gallop

Tests	Results
Chest radiograph	Normal, although if the pulmonary embolism progresses to pulmonary infarction, a wedge-shaped abnormality can be identified.
Electrocardiography	Normal, although if the pulmonary embolism is large enough, right-sided heart strain may be evident (i.e., S wave in lead I, Q wave in lead III, and inverted T wave in lead III).
Arterial blood gases	Po_2 is reduced. O_2 saturation is reduced. Pco_2 may be slightly increased.
Lung scan	Poor perfusion to an isolated segment of lung is observed.
V/Q scan	Mismatch of ventilation and perfusion is evident.
Pulmonary angiography	Cutoff of blood flow to one or more segments of the lung and filling defects in the pulmonary arteries or arterioles are observed.
Computed tomography of the chest	Embolism is visible in a branch of the pulmonary artery.

Pco_2, Partial pressure of carbon dioxide; Po_2, partial pressure of oxygen.

Nuclear Scanning

8

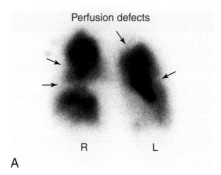
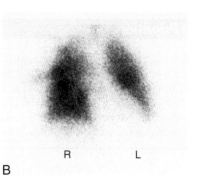

Perfusion defects

A   B

R   L   R   L

Figure 8-8 Lung scan. **A,** Perfusion. **B,** Ventilation. Multiple perfusion defects are noted on the perfusion lung scan. However, the uptake of radionuclide on the ventilation scan is normal. This combination of findings is indicative of pulmonary emboli.

The chest radiograph aids in the interpretation of the perfusion scan because a defect on the perfusion scan seen in the same area as a pulmonary parenchymal abnormality on the chest radiograph does not indicate pulmonary embolism. Rather, the defect may represent pneumonia, atelectasis, effusion, and other pathologic processes. When a perfusion defect is visible in an area of the lung that is normal on a chest radiographic study, however, pulmonary embolism is very likely to be the cause.

Specificity of a perfusion scan also can be enhanced by the concomitant performance of a *ventilation lung scan*, which detects parenchymal abnormalities in ventilation (e.g., pneumonia, pleural fluid, emphysematous bullae). The ventilation scan reflects the patency of the pulmonary airways, whereby krypton gas or ^{99m}Tc diethylenetriamine pentaacetic acid (DTPA) is used as an aerosol. When vascular obstruction (embolism) is present on a perfusion scan, ventilation scans demonstrate normal wash-in and normal wash-out of radioactivity from the embolized lung area. If parenchymal disease (e.g., pneumonia) is responsible for the perfusion abnormality, however, wash-in or wash-out is abnormal. Therefore, the "mismatch" of perfusion and ventilation is characteristic of embolic disorders, whereas the "match" is indicative of parenchymal disease. Synchronously performed ventilation and perfusion scans are known collectively as a *ventilation/perfusion (V/Q) scan*.

Most nuclear physicians classify the lung scan results in one of several categories: negative for pulmonary embolism, low probability of pulmonary embolism, high probability of pulmonary embolism, or positive for pulmonary embolism.

With the increased availability of rapid-access spatial computed tomography of the chest (see p. 1068), the diagnosis of pulmonary embolism is now more easily made with computed tomographic angiography. This procedure is faster and more accurate than ventilation/perfusion lung scans and is less invasive than pulmonary angiography.

CONTRAINDICATIONS

- Pregnancy, unless the benefits of the procedure outweigh the risk of injury to the fetus

INTERFERING FACTORS

- Known pulmonary parenchymal or pleural problems (e.g., pneumonia, emphysema, pleural effusion, tumours), which will have the appearance of a perfusion defect and simulate pulmonary embolism

Clinical Priorities

- This nuclear medicine procedure is used mainly to detect pulmonary embolism.
- Because lung scans are sensitive but not specific, several types of pulmonary problems (other than pulmonary embolism) can cause a defect in pulmonary blood perfusion.
- The specificity of a perfusion scan can be improved by the performance of a ventilation scan. The performance of both together is called a *ventilation/perfusion (V/Q) scan*.
- The chest radiographic study aids in the interpretation of the lung scan.

Age-Related Concerns

- In older adults, approximately two of three lung scans are inconclusive for diagnosing pulmonary embolism.

PROCEDURE AND PATIENT CARE

Before

- Explain the procedure to the patient.
- Obtain the patient's informed consent for the procedure, if this is required by the institution.
- Assure the patient that he or she will not be exposed to large amounts of radioactivity because only tracer doses of isotopes are used.
- If iodine-123 will be administered (this is rarely done), give the patient 10 drops of Lugol iodine solution several hours before the test as a blocking agent for the thyroid gland. This will prevent iodine uptake by the thyroid gland.
- Inform the patient that no fasting is required.
- Note that a chest radiograph should be obtained within 24 to 48 hours before the test.
- Instruct the patient to remove jewellery around the chest area.
- Inform the patient that no discomfort is associated with this test other than the peripheral venipuncture.

During

- The unsedated, nonfasting patient with suspected pulmonary embolism is taken to the nuclear medicine department (Figure 8-9).
- Note that this test is usually performed in approximately 30 minutes by a physician.

Perfusion Scan

- Note the following procedural steps:
  1. The patient is given a peripheral intravenous injection of macroaggregated albumin tagged with ^{99m}Tc.
  2. While the patient lies in the appropriate position, a gamma ray detector is passed over the patient and records radionuclide uptake.

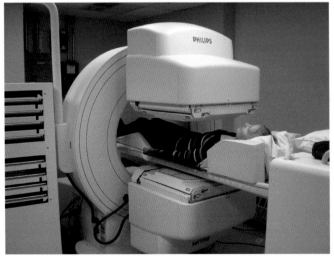

Figure 8-9 Positioning of a patient for a lung scan.

3. The patient is placed in the supine, prone, and various lateral positions, which allows for anterior, posterior, and lateral and oblique views, respectively.
4. The results are interpreted by a physician trained in diagnostic nuclear medicine.

Ventilation Scan
- Note the following procedural steps:
  1. During the ventilation scan, the patient inhales radioactive gas through a mask while sitting or lying on a table under the scanner arm.
  2. Patient cooperation is less of an issue with a krypton tracer. Ventilation scans can be performed with krypton even on comatose patients. Krypton images can be obtained before, during, or after perfusion images.
  3. In contrast, ^{99m}Tc DTPA images are usually obtained before perfusion images and require patient cooperation with deep breathing and appropriate use of breathing equipment to prevent contamination.

After
✗ Inform the patient that no radiation precautions are necessary.

TEST RESULTS AND CLINICAL SIGNIFICANCE

Pulmonary embolism: *This is evident as a perfusion defect on a perfusion lung scan. It is also apparent as a "mismatch" of ventilation and perfusion on a V/Q scan. Positive results are definitive, but negative results can be false.*

Pneumonia,

Tuberculosis,

Asthma,

Chronic obstructive pulmonary disease,

Tumour,

Atelectasis,

Bronchitis: *These parenchymal abnormalities can cause perfusion defects. When a defect is apparent on the plain chest radiograph or a ventilation lung scan, a ventilation/perfusion "match" is identified. Matched defects are caused not by pulmonary emboli but rather by the parenchymal diseases listed.*

RELATED TESTS

Computed Tomography, Chest (p. 1068). Computed tomography of the lung has now become the preferred test for diagnosing pulmonary embolism.

Arterial Blood Gases (p. 121). These measurements are used to detect hypoxemia, which is the hallmark of pulmonary embolism.

Electrocardiography (p. 568). Although the electrocardiogram is usually normal with pulmonary embolism, right-sided heart strain can be identified with large acute pulmonary embolism.

Chest Radiography (p. 1053). Although pulmonary embolisms are not evident on the plain chest radiograph, this test can help identify parenchymal abnormalities, which is important for accurately interpreting the perfusion lung scan.

NORMAL FINDINGS

No increased uptake of radionuclide in the right lower quadrant of the abdomen

INDICATIONS

This scan is designed to identify a Meckel diverticulum that contains ectopic gastric mucosa. The test is indicated in patients who have recurrent lower abdominal pain or in pediatric or young adult patients who have occult gastrointestinal bleeding.

TEST EXPLANATION

Meckel diverticulum is the most common congenital abnormality of the intestinal tract. It is a persistent remnant of the omphalomesenteric tract. The diverticulum usually occurs in the ileum, approximately 2 feet (60 cm) proximal to the ileocecal valve. Approximately 20% to 25% of Meckel diverticula are lined internally by ectopic gastric mucosa. This gastric mucosa can secrete acid and cause ulceration of the intestinal mucosa nearby. Bleeding, inflammation, and intussusception are other potential complications of this congenital abnormality. The majority of these complications occur by the age of 2 years.

Both normal gastric mucosa within the stomach and ectopic gastric mucosa in Meckel diverticulum take up technetium-99m (^{99m}Tc) pertechnetate. When this radionuclide is injected intravenously, it is concentrated in the ectopic gastric mucosa of Meckel diverticulum. A "hot" spot is usually visible in the right lower quadrant of the abdomen at approximately the same time that the normal stomach mucosa is visualized. This is a very sensitive and specific test for this congenital abnormality.

It is possible that a Meckel diverticulum is present but contains no ectopic gastric mucosa within. In most such cases, this is not symptomatic. Radionuclide is not taken up within the diverticulum. Therefore, this test is not helpful in these cases.

Other conditions can simulate a hot spot like that of a Meckel diverticulum containing ectopic gastric mucosa. Usually these findings are associated with inflammatory processes within the abdomen (e.g., appendicitis, Crohn's disease, or ectopic pregnancy).

PROCEDURE AND PATIENT CARE

Before

- Explain the procedure to the patient.
- Advise the patient to refrain from eating or drinking anything for 6 to 12 hours before the examination.
- A histamine H_2-receptor antagonist is usually given for 1 to 2 days before the scan. This blocks secretion of the radionuclide from the ectopic gastric mucosa and improves visualization of a Meckel diverticulum.
- Inform the patient that no pain is associated with this test.

Nuclear Scanning

8

During

- Take the patient to the nuclear medicine department.
- The patient lies in a supine position, and a large-view nuclear detector camera is placed over the patient's abdomen to identify concentration of nuclear material after intravenous injection.
- Images are taken at 5-minute intervals for 1 hour.
- The patient may be asked to lie on the left side to minimize the excretion of the radionuclide from the normal stomach because that would flood the intestine with radionuclide and preclude visualization of a Meckel diverticulum.
- On occasion, glucagon is administered to prolong intestinal transit time and avoid downstream contamination with the radionuclide.
- On occasion, gastrin is administered to increase the uptake of the radionuclide by the ectopic gastric mucosa.

After

- The patient is asked to void, and a repeat image is obtained. This is to ensure that a distended bladder has not hidden a Meckel diverticulum.
- Reassure the patient that because only tracer doses of radioisotopes are used, other people do not need to take precautions against radiation exposure.

TEST RESULTS AND CLINICAL SIGNIFICANCE

Increased uptake in the right lower quadrant: *This is characteristic of a Meckel diverticulum containing ectopic gastric mucosa. As indicated previously, if the diverticulum does not contain ectopic gastric mucosa, the test result is not positive. Furthermore, other inflammatory diseases can cause false-positive results.*

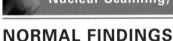

Octreotide Scan (Carcinoid Nuclear Scanning, Neuroendocrine Nuclear Scanning)

NORMAL FINDINGS

No evidence of increased uptake of radionuclide throughout the body

INDICATIONS

Octreotide scans are used to identify and localize neuroendocrine primary and metastatic tumours. This scan is indicated in patients with known neuroendocrine tumours (e.g., carcinoid tumours and gastrinomas). It is used preoperatively to direct the surgeon to primary and metastatic tumours. This scan is also used to monitor the patient's response to therapy for these tumours.

TEST EXPLANATION

Octreotide scan is a specific example of *nuclear peptide scanning* that is increasingly being used to identify neoplasms by their altered physiologic state. The use of peptides for which tumours have an increased uptake—because of cellular membrane receptors or idiosyncratic physiologic processes (glycolysis, proliferation, angiogenesis, or oxidation)—allows anatomic localization of many previously hidden tumours. These molecular imaging techniques can also provide information regarding the effect of anticancer therapy on tumour growth and survival.

Most neuroendocrine cells have a somatostatin receptor on the cellular membrane. Neuroendocrine tumours retain these receptors. Octreotide is an analogue of somatostatin. When combined with a radiopharmaceutical (such as iodine-123), octreotide attaches to the somatostatin receptors of the neuroendocrine tumour cells. With the use of a scintillation camera, the uptake can be observed and localized. In pediatric imaging, metaiodobenzylguanidine (MIBG) is used more frequently than octreotide as the radioisotope for identification of neuroendocrine tumours. Lanreotide is another peptide used in this imaging.

In patients with known neuroendocrine tumours, this test is used to direct the surgeon to the primary and metastatic sites within the body (especially the abdomen). This test is also used in the surveillance of patients who have been or are being treated for these neuroendocrine tumours. When this test is used as a monitor of disease, recurrence or progression can be identified quite easily and accurately. The liver, however, is more difficult to evaluate with octreotide scans. The use of single-photon emission computed tomography (SPECT) improves the sensitivity of this test. Many different types of hormone-producing tumours—most notably, carcinoid, gastrinoma, insulinoma, glucagonoma, pheochromocytoma, and small cell lung cancer—can be detected with SPECT. Other abnormalities that can take up octreotide include granulomatous infections (such as sarcoidosis or tuberculosis), rheumatoid arthritis, and nonhormonal cancers (breast, lymphoma, and non–small cell lung cancers).

The imaging procedure is performed in approximately 30 minutes by a trained technologist. A physician trained in nuclear medicine interprets the results. The only discomfort associated with this procedure is the intravenous injection of the radionuclide.

CONTRAINDICATIONS

- Pregnancy or lactation, unless the benefits of the procedure outweigh the risk of injury to the fetus or infant

INTERFERING FACTORS

- Barium in the gastrointestinal tract overlying the liver or spleen produces the appearance of defects on the scan that may be mistaken for masses.

PROCEDURE AND PATIENT CARE

Before

- Explain the procedure to the patient.
- Inform the patient that no fasting or premedication is required.
- Assure the patient that he or she will not be exposed to large amounts of radiation because only tracer doses of isotopes are used.
- If an iodinated radionuclide is to be used, ensure that the patient does not have an allergy to iodine.
- If an iodinated dye is to be used, administer 5 drops of Lugol iodine solution daily for 3 days. This will block uptake of the radionuclide by the thyroid gland.
- If the patient has been receiving octreotide as a form of antineoplastic treatment, this must be discontinued for 2 weeks before scanning.

Nuclear Scanning

8

During

- Take the patient to the nuclear medicine department.
- Note the following procedural steps:
  1. The patient is taken to the nuclear medicine department, where the radionuclide is administered intravenously. (For inpatients, a nuclear medicine technologist may administer the radionuclide at the patient's bedside.)
  2. One hour after injection, a gamma camera is positioned over the entire body.
  3. The patient is placed in supine, lateral, and prone positions so that all surfaces can be visualized.
  4. The radionuclide image is recorded. SPECT may also be performed.
  5. Usually the patient is given a fatty meal 2 hours after octreotide injection to clear the radiopharmaceutical from the gallbladder.
  6. After 4 hours, the patient is given a strong laxative to clear the octreotide from the bowel.
  7. Repeat scanning is again performed 2, 4, 24, and 48 hours after administration of the octreotide.

After

Reassure the patient that because only tracer doses of radioisotopes are used, other people do not need to take precautions against radiation exposure.

TEST RESULTS AND CLINICAL SIGNIFICANCE

Carcinoid tumours: *These tumours consist of neuroendocrine argentaffin cells that have somatostatin receptors. They usually arise from the appendix, small bowel, or colon. However, any organ can be the primary site of a carcinoid tumour.*

Neuroendocrine tumours: *Neuroendocrine tumours and many different types of hormone-producing tumours as listed previously can take up octreotide.*

Granulomatous infections such as sarcoidosis and tuberculosis: *The pathophysiologic mechanism underlying this observation is not well understood.*

Parathyroid Scan (Parathyroid Scintigraphy)

NORMAL FINDINGS

No increased uptake by the parathyroid glands

INDICATIONS

This test is used to locate the parathyroid glands before surgery. It also indicates the cause of hyperparathyroidism.

TEST EXPLANATION

Hypercalcemia can be caused by hyperparathyroidism. Parathyroid hyperplasia, adenoma, or cancer, in turn, can cause hyperparathyroidism. It is important for the surgeon planning resection of the parathyroid abnormality to know how many parathyroid glands are involved and their location. Preoperative parathyroid scanning is the most accurate method of providing this information. Parathyroid hyperplasia causes enlargement of all four parathyroid glands. A parathyroid adenoma or cancer, however, causes enlargement of only one parathyroid gland and suppression (decrease in size) of the other three glands. On the basis of the parathyroid scan, the surgeon will know whether the abnormality is hyperplasia or adenoma/cancer.

Parathyroid glands are located most commonly on the lateral borders of the thyroid lobes, two on each side. However, parathyroid anatomic location varies considerably and they may be located anywhere from the upper neck to the lower mediastinum. They can even be located in the centre of the thyroid lobe. Parathyroid scanning demonstrates the location of the pathologic parathyroid glands with high degrees of resolution and accuracy. Single-photon emission computed tomography (SPECT) is even more accurate than routine nuclear imaging.

Scanning is now performed more frequently in patients with newly diagnosed hyperparathyroidism. In some centres, scanning is reserved for patients in whom an initial neck exploration failed to identify all four parathyroid glands and the hypercalcemia persisted after the operation.

There are two methods of parathyroid scanning. The first is the single-tracer double-phase (STDP) test with technetium-99m (^{99m}Tc) sestamibi. In this method, the ^{99m}Tc sestamibi tracer is injected into the patient. Images are obtained at 15 minutes and 3 hours. The tracer initially illuminates both the thyroid and the parathyroid glands. At 3 hours, however, the tracer is washed out of all normal endocrine tissue and remains only in the pathologic parathyroid tissue.

The second method is the double-tracer subtraction test (DTST), in which ^{99m}Tc pertechnetate or iodine-123 (^{123}I) is administered. Only the thyroid gland takes up either of these two latter tracers. Scanning is performed, and the ^{99m}Tc sestamibi is then administered and is taken up by both the thyroid and the parathyroid glands. Scanning is repeated, and the earlier image is then "subtracted" from the repeated image, leaving an image of only the parathyroid glands.

Parathyroid scanning is also performed immediately before surgery to help the surgeon identify the parathyroid glands, particularly the pathologic glands. In this test, a scan is performed in the parathyroid glands as described previously. Once in the operating room, the surgeon scans the entire anterior portion of the patient's neck with a gamma ray detector. Increased counts are noted in the regions where the parathyroid glands are located. The surgeon can then direct dissection to that particular area.

CONTRAINDICATIONS

- Allergy to iodine if radioactive iodine is to be used
- Pregnancy, unless the benefits of the procedure outweigh the risk of injury to the fetus

INTERFERING FACTORS

- Patient movement can inhibit the quality of imaging, especially when subtraction scanning is performed.
- Recent administration of radiographic contrast agents can alter test results.
- Ingestion of iodine-containing foods or drugs (including cough medicines) can affect test results.

8 **Nuclear Scanning**

PROCEDURE AND PATIENT CARE

Before

- Explain the procedure to the patient.
- Inform the patient that fasting is usually not required. Check first with the laboratory.
- Check the patient for allergies to iodine.
- Instruct the patient about medications and food that need to be restricted for weeks before the test (e.g., thyroid drugs, medications or food containing iodine).
- Obtain a history concerning recent contrast radiographic studies, nuclear scanning, or intake of any thyroid-suppressive or antithyroid drugs.
- Inform the patient that no discomfort is associated with this study.

During

- Take the patient to the nuclear medicine department.

STDP Method
- Note the following procedural steps:
  1. ^{99m}Tc sestamibi is injected intravenously.
  2. At 15 minutes and 3 hours, the patient is positioned supine, a detector is passed over the neck and upper chest area, and the radioactive counts are recorded and displayed. At some centres, images are acquired as rapidly as every 5 minutes for 90 to 120 minutes.

DTST Method
- Note the following procedural steps:
  1. ^{99m}Tc pertechnetate or ^{123}I is injected intravenously.
  2. At 15 minutes, the patient is positioned supine, a detector is passed over the neck and upper chest area, and the radioactive counts are recorded and displayed.
  3. ^{99m}Tc sestamibi is then injected intravenously, and imaging is repeated.
  4. With the computer, images are "subtracted," only the parathyroid gland appears on the final images.
- A radiologic technologist or a physician in the nuclear medicine department performs this procedure. The duration of the test is approximately 30 minutes. Scanning can be repeated several hours later for the STDP method.

After

- Assure the patient that the dose of radioactive ^{99m}Tc used in this test is minute and therefore harmless. No isolation and no special urine precautions are needed.

TEST RESULTS AND CLINICAL SIGNIFICANCE

Parathyroid adenoma, carcinoma, or hyperplasia: *Adenomas and cancers of the parathyroid gland usually involve only one gland. Hyperplasia usually involves all four parathyroid glands. All must be found at the time of surgery. Parathyroid scanning specifies the location of those glands for the surgeon.*

Aberrantly located parathyroid tissue in the upper neck, thyroid gland, or mediastinum: *The information provided by this scan can identify abnormally malpositioned parathyroid tissue. This information is invaluable before surgery.*

Positron Emission Tomography (PET)

NORMAL FINDINGS
No abnormal areas of increased or decreased uptake

INDICATIONS
Positron emission tomography (PET) is used in many areas of medicine, most commonly for evaluation of the heart and brain. It is also commonly used in many aspects of oncology.

TEST EXPLANATION
In PET, radioactive chemicals are administered to the patient. These chemicals are used in the normal metabolic process of the cells of the particular organ being imaged. Positrons emitted from the radioactive chemicals in the organ are sensed by a series of detectors positioned around the patient. These detectors receive positron counts and—with the combination of computed tomography—the positron emissions are recorded into a high-resolution three-dimensional image that depicts a particular metabolic process in a specific anatomic site (Figure 8-10). Therefore, PET provides images representing not only anatomy but also physiology. Like computed tomography, magnetic resonance imaging (MRI) merely produces images of the body's anatomy or structure,

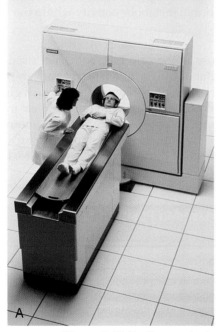
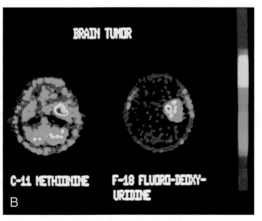

Figure 8-10 Positron emission tomography (PET). **A,** Clinical setting for PET. Shown are the Siemens ECAT scanner gantry and patient bed. **B,** Images received from PET scan with different radioisotopes such as carbon-11 and fluorine-18. The study positively identified a brain tumour.

8 Nuclear Scanning

not its metabolism. In most disease states, physiologic changes precede anatomic changes. In still other disease states, such as Alzheimer's disease, no anatomic changes occur, but PET can identify classic physiologic changes that are diagnostic of the disease. Depending on the particular radionuclide used, PET can demonstrate the glucose metabolism, oxygenation, blood flow, and tissue perfusion of any specific area. Pathologic conditions are recognized and diagnosed by alterations in the normal metabolic process.

Certain radioactive chemical compounds provide specific information, depending on the information required and the organ being evaluated. A cyclotron is used to create the radioactive chemical. Radioactive fluorine is applied to a glucose analogue; the combination is called *fluorodeoxyglucose* (FDG). Because most cells use glucose as an energy source, FDG is particularly useful because it is concentrated in regions of high metabolic activity of a particular organ. Radioactive carbon-labelled glucose is also useful for this purpose. Radioactive nitrogen is used in radioactive ammonia, which can be used in evaluating the liver. Other applications of radionuclides approved in Canada are listed in Table 8-3. PET is becoming more widely applied and more commonly used as research continues. Thus far, its use has been most extensive in the fields of neurology, cardiology, and oncology.

In many centres, PET images can be superimposed with computed tomography (CT) or MRI to produce an anatomically accurate image that shows the physiology or metabolism of the organ imaged with newer units. PET/CT can be performed in the same unit (Figure 8-11). This is called *PET/CT image fusion* or *PET/CT co-registration*. These composite views allow the information from two different studies to be digitally correlated and superimposed onto one image, which provides more precise information and accurate diagnoses. The computed tomographic images are acquired with the use of iodine contrast. In less than 60 minutes after the FDG is administered, PET is performed in the same unit. The images are imposed on each other. The combined PET/CT provides images that pinpoint the location of abnormal metabolic activity within the body.

Neurology

Most brain imaging is performed with FDG. Glucose is the sole metabolic fuel used by the brain. Pathologic areas of the brain that are more metabolically active (such as cancers) take up FDG more avidly than do normal areas. Because of the high physiologic rate at which glucose is metabolized by normal brain tissue, it is difficult to detect tumours with only modest increases in glucose metabolism (such as low-grade tumours and, in some cases, recurrent tumours) with FDG. Alzheimer's disease is classically recognized as hypometabolism in multiple areas of the brain (temporal and parietal lobe) as scanning is performed during cognitive exercises. PET can

TABLE 8-3	Canadian Approved Isotopes Used in Positron Emission Tomography
Radionuclide	**Application**
^{18}F FDG	Approved for some cancer scans
^{18}F Sodium fluoride	Bone scanning through clinical trials
Nitrogen-13 ammonia	Heart procedures and at the request of a physician or through clinical trials
Rubidium-82	Can be made available through Health Canada to replace a small number of heart studies at the request of a physician or through clinical trials

^{18}F, Fluorine-18; *FDG*, fluorodeoxyglucose.

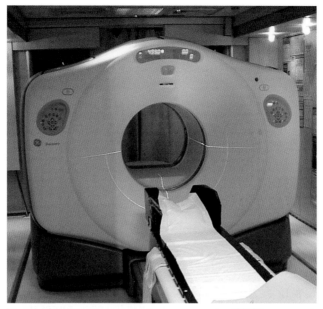

Figure 8-11 Positron emission tomography (PET)/computed tomography (CT) is performed on this unit.

identify these changes several years before other imaging modalities can, thereby providing an opportunity for earlier treatment. Epilepsy, Parkinson's disease, and Huntington's disease are identified as localized areas of increased metabolic activity indicating rapid nerve firing. Brain trauma resulting in a hematoma or bleeding is evident as decreased metabolic activity in the area of trauma. Stroke can also be identified and its extent determined. With the use of radioactive water ($H_2{}^{15}O$), brain blood flow can be determined. Areas of decreased blood flow will take up less $H_2{}^{15}O$ than normal areas and represent areas at risk for stroke.

Cardiology

Matching of flow studies (e.g., thallium-201 scan) with scans obtained with PET allows visualization of areas of decreased blood flow, indicating coronary artery occlusive disease. PET is also used when cardiac muscle function is reduced. PET can indicate whether the dysfunction arises from reversible ischemic muscle that would benefit from revascularization or from muscle tissue that is no longer viable. In the former case, surgical revascularization should be considered. In the latter case, revascularization would not be beneficial.

Oncology

The agent most commonly used in oncology is FDG because increased glucose metabolism is so prevalent in malignant tumours in comparison with normal or benign pathologic tissue. PET can be used to visualize rapidly growing tumours and indicate their anatomic location. It is used to determine tumour response to therapy, identify recurrence of tumour after surgical removal, and differentiate tumour from other pathologic conditions (e.g., infection). PET is particularly helpful in identifying regional and metastatic spread for a particular tumour (Figures 8-12 [head and neck] and 8-13 [chest]). PET is more accurate in oncologic staging than is CT. Its sensitivity exceeds 95%, and its specificity exceeds 80%. In lung cancer, for example, if the FDG fails to concentrate in any area other than the primary tumour, no spread is suspected, and the patient is

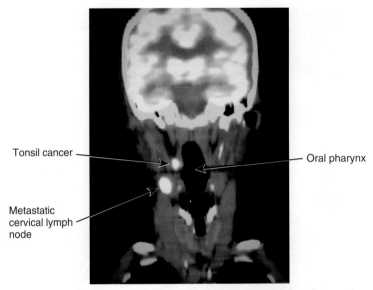

Tonsil cancer

Oral pharynx

Metastatic
cervical lymph
node

Figure 8-12 PET scan of the head and neck. Avid uptake of normal brain is noted. See two hotspots noted in the neck, representing primary tonsil cancer and metastatic cervical lymph node.

considered an ideal candidate for surgery. PET has also been particularly useful for identifying metastasis from melanoma, from lymphoma, and from lung, breast, pancreas, colon, and brain cancers. (See Figure 8-13.)

Rapidly growing tumours have a high metabolic rate and therefore concentrate FDG particularly well. The amount of uptake of FDG is measured by the standardized uptake value: the amount of FDG uptake by the tumour in comparison with the normal tissue in the same area. The standardized uptake value helps distinguish between benign and malignant lesions; the higher the standardized uptake value, the more likely the tumour is to be malignant.

When the standardized uptake value (SUV) is greater than the "cutoff value" (as determined by each institution), cancer rather than a benign pathologic condition is suspected. PET is particularly helpful in the evaluation of solitary pulmonary nodules. CT and chest radiographs are inadequate in distinguishing benign from malignant lesions. PET can accurately provide that information in more than 75% of cases.

Bone

A PET/CT scan with a sodium fluoride F18 injection (^{18}F NaF) scans the entire skeletal system and produces high-resolution images of the bones. These images are used to detect areas of abnormal bone growth associated with tumours. This test is more accurate than conventional nuclear bone scans. The PET/CT scan of the bone is particularly helpful for patients with prostate or breast cancer. The uptake of ^{18}F NaF in the skeleton reflects sites of increased blood flow and bone remodelling associated with bone injury or metastatic disease. A bone PET/CT scan's high-resolution images and its ability to scan the entire skeleton make it very helpful in detecting bone disease.

PET for small body parts is being used with increasing frequency for inflammatory pathologic processes of the foot. *PET mammography* or *positron emission mammography* (PEM) is being used increasingly as a tool for diagnostic breast imaging. PEM holds the promise of improving sensitivity and specificity of routine mammography (see p. 1086).

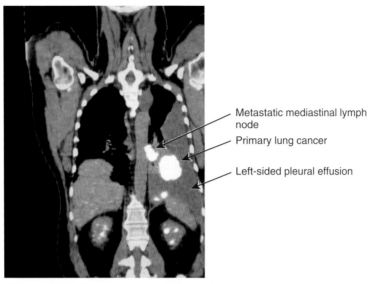

Metastatic mediastinal lymph node

Primary lung cancer

Left-sided pleural effusion

Figure 8-13 PET scan of the chest. Note two hot spots representing a primary lung cancer and multiple mediastinal lymph node metastases. A large pleural effusion is noted.

INTERFERING FACTORS

- Use of caffeine, alcohol, or tobacco within 24 hours of the test may affect test results.
- The liver and spleen avidly take up FDG. Therefore, those organs are difficult to evaluate on PET.
- FDG is excreted by the urinary system. As a result, the bladder may obscure areas of increased uptake in the pelvis.
- Vigorous exercise within a day of the study can markedly increase muscular metabolism and thereby cause a shift of the FDG to the muscles, thus "stealing" FDG from any pathologic region that may have concentrated FDG.
- Anxiety can cause increased uptake in multiple areas (e.g., neck, upper mediastinum) of the body. If the patient is anxious, sedatives, as per the physician's orders, could be administered 30 minutes before testing.
- Uptake of FDG can occur in the lymph node basin into which the injected FDG is drained. If PET is being performed to stage tumours that could metastasize to those lymph nodes, the FDG should be injected on the contralateral side.

Nuclear Scanning

8

Clinical Priorities

- Test results can be affected by recent use of caffeine, alcohol, or tobacco.
- Tests results can be affected by vigorous exercise within 24 hours of the study.
- Instruct patients that no sedatives or tranquillizers should be taken, because patients may need to perform mental activities during the test.
- After the test, patients should be encouraged to drink fluids and urinate frequently to aid in washing out the radioisotope from the bladder.

PROCEDURE AND PATIENT CARE

Before

- Explain the procedure to the patient. Because most patients have not heard of this study, they are often anxious and require emotional support.
- Explain that while lying in the bed, the patient will be moved into the scanner and may have feelings of being in a small space. Encourage him or her to discuss feelings with the health care provider to allay worries and answer questions. If the patient is anxious, sedatives should be administered, per the physician's orders, 30 minutes before testing.
- Obtain the patient's informed consent for the procedure if it is required by the institution.
- Inform the patient that he or she may have an intravenous line inserted.
- Inform the patient that he or she may need to restrict food or fluids for 4 hours on the day of the test. The patient should refrain from alcohol, caffeine, and tobacco for 24 hours.
- Instruct diabetic patients to take their pretest dose of insulin at a meal 3 to 4 hours before the test.
- Inform the patient that no sedatives or tranquillizers should be taken because he or she may need to perform certain mental activities during brain PET.
- Instruct the patient to empty the bladder before the test for comfort. A Foley catheter may be inserted for scanning of the pelvic region.
- Inform the patient that the only discomfort associated with this study is insertion of the intravenous line.
- Depending on the organ being evaluated, specific protocols are followed for the examination.

During

- Take the patient to the nuclear medicine department.
- Note the following procedural steps:
  1. The patient is positioned on a bed that is moved into the scanner.
  2. The radioactive material can be infused through an intravenous line or inhaled as a radioactive gas.
  3. The gamma rays that penetrate the tissues are recorded outside the body by a circular array of detectors, and the recordings are displayed by a computer.
  4. If the brain is being scanned, the patient may be asked to perform different cognitive activities (e.g., reciting the alphabet) to measure changes in brain activity during reasoning or remembering.
  5. Assess patient for anxiety (e.g., hyperventilating) and intervene as appropriate with relaxation techniques such as talking with the patient in a calm and reassuring manner.
  6. Extraneous auditory and visual stimuli are minimized by a blindfold and ear plugs.
  7. If the chest is being scanned, instruct the patient to breathe in a shallow manner until the middle of the chest is reached. Then ask the patient to hold the breath after expiration until the middle of the abdomen is reached. This will improve visibility of the chest anatomy.
- Note that a physician performs this procedure with a trained technologist in approximately 40 to 90 minutes.

After

- Instruct the patient to change position slowly from lying to standing to avoid postural hypotension.
- Encourage the patient to drink fluids and urinate frequently to aid in washing out the radioisotope from the bladder.

TEST RESULTS AND CLINICAL SIGNIFICANCE

Myocardial infarction,

Coronary artery disease: *Areas of ischemia or infarction are associated with decreased flow and decreased glucose metabolism. This is indicated by hypoconcentration of FDG.*

Cerebrovascular accident (stroke): *These areas are evident as decreased blood flow and metabolism.*

Epilepsy,

Parkinson's disease,

Huntington's disease: *Focal areas of increased metabolism are evident during seizure or repetitive activity.*

Dementia,

Alzheimer's disease: *Specific areas of decreased metabolism are noted in typical regions of the brain (temporal and parietal lobes).*

Malignant tumour: *Malignancy is associated with increased glucose metabolism in rapidly dividing cells. This is indicated by concentration of FDG in levels exceeding cutoff points for the standardized uptake value.*

RELATED TESTS

Computed Tomography, Abdomen (p. 1059), Computed Tomography, Brain (p. 1065), Computed Tomography, Chest (p. 1068), and Computed Tomography, Heart (p. 1072). In CT, differences in density coefficients are used to visualize different organs and tissues. Unlike PET, CT cannot provide information concerning metabolism or function.

Single-Photon Emission Computed Tomography. This is another form of radionuclear imaging that can provide three-dimensional anatomic and perfusion images but lacks the capability to indicate metabolism.

Magnetic Resonance Imaging (p. 1148). This provides a picture of normal and pathologic anatomy by temporarily altering the magnetic field of the cells in the area to be evaluated.

Renal Scanning (Kidney Scan, Radiorenography, Renography, Radionuclide Renal Imaging, Nuclear Imaging of the Kidney, Disodium Monomethane Arsenate [DSMA] Renal Scanning, Diethylenetriamine Pentaacetic Acid [DTPA] Renal Scanning, Captopril Renal Scanning)

NORMAL FINDINGS

Normal size, shape, and function of the kidneys

INDICATIONS

Renal scanning is used to indicate the perfusion, function, and structure of the kidneys. It is also used to indicate the presence of obstruction or renovascular hypertension. Because no iodinated dyes are used in this study (except when iodohippurate is used), it is safe to perform on patients who have iodine allergies or compromised renal function. Renal scanning is used to monitor renal function in patients with known renal disease. This scan also plays a large part of the diagnosis of renal transplant rejection.

TEST EXPLANATION

This nuclear medicine procedure provides visualization of the urinary tract after intravenous administration of a radioisotope. The radioactive material is detected by a scintillation camera, which can detect the gamma rays emitted by the radionuclide in the kidneys. The scintillation camera information can be translated into light and thereby produce a realistic image of the renal structure. A computer collates that information, and the amount of gamma ray emission per unit of time is calculated to determine renal function, vascular insufficiency, or renal obstruction. Scans do not interfere with the normal physiologic process of the kidneys. The resultant image (scan) indicates distribution of the radionuclide within the kidney and ureters.

There are several types of renal scanning, depending on which information is needed (Table 8-4). Different isotopes may be more suitable for different scans, according to how the kidney handles the radioisotope.

Renal Blood Flow (Perfusion) Scan

This type of renal scanning is used to evaluate the blood flow to each kidney. It is used to detect renal artery stenosis, renovascular hypertension, and rejection of renal transplant. It is also used to demonstrate hypervascular lesions (renal cell carcinoma) in the kidney.

In the basic test, the radionuclide—usually technetium-99m (^{99m}Tc), diethylenetriamine pentaacetic acid (DTPA), ^{99m}Tc disodium monomethane arsenate (DSMA), or iodohippurate sodium (^{131}I)—is injected while the patient is positioned under the scintigraphy camera. Computers collate the data obtained by the camera and create a curve of gamma activity per unit of time. Each kidney is compared with the opposite kidney and with the aorta. Decreased gamma activity is noted in the kidney with arterial stenosis or renovascular hypertension. Decreased activity in relation to the aorta is noted in a transplanted kidney that is being rejected. Increased gamma activity is noted in a kidney that contains a hypervascular tumour (cancer).

TABLE 8-4	Renal Scanning	
Types	**Purpose**	**Examples of Findings**
Blood flow (perfusion)	Evaluation of blood flow to each kidney	Renal artery stenosis, renovascular hypertension, transplant rejection, hypervascular tumours
Structural	Identification of structural abnormalities	Tumour, cyst, abscess, congenital disorders, malposition or absence, horseshoe-shaped kidney
Function (renogram)	Evaluation of function by uptake and excretion of radioisotopes	Glomerulonephritis, decreased blood supply, transplant rejection, renal failure
Hypertension	Detection of presence and source of renal hypertension	Renal artery stenosis, vascular obstruction
Obstruction	Identification of outflow obstruction	Renal pelvis obstruction, ureter obstruction, bladder outlet obstruction

Renal Structural Scan

This type of renal scanning is performed to outline the structure of the kidney to identify a pathologic condition that may alter normal anatomic structure (e.g., tumour, cyst, abscess). Congenital disorders (e.g., hypoplasia or aplasia of the kidney, malposition of the kidney) can also be detected. Also, information after renal transplantation can be obtained with this scan. A filling defect in the renal parenchyma may indicate a tumour, cyst, abscess, or infarction. Horseshoe-shaped kidney, pelvic kidney, or absence of a kidney may be evident. Anatomic alterations in the parenchymal distribution of tracer may indicate transplant rejection.

^{99m}Tc DTPA or ^{99m}Tc DSMA can be used for this scan. ^{99m}Tc DSMA is particularly good because it is rapidly taken up by the kidney but excreted very slowly, allowing good visualization of the renal structure.

Renal Function Scan (Renogram)

Renal function can be determined by documenting the capability of the kidney to take up a particular radioisotope and excrete it. A well-functioning kidney can be expected to rapidly assimilate the isotope and then excrete the same isotope. A poorly functioning kidney is not able to take up the isotope rapidly or excrete it in a timely manner. Each radioactive tracer is handled by the kidney in a different manner. Different renal functions can be tested according to which isotope is used:

^{99m}Tc DTPA helps measures glomerular filtration.

^{99m}Tc DSMA helps measures tubular cell secretion.

Iodohippurate sodium (^{131}I) or iodohippurate sodium (^{133}I) helps measure both glomerular filtration and tubular cell secretion.

In this study, the dose of radionuclide is calculated on the basis of body weight or surface area. The patient is placed under the scintigraphy camera. The radioisotope is injected, and a computer analyzes the data obtained from the camera. Activity per unit of time equals the function of the kidney, which is plotted on a graph. This plot is called a *renogram curve* (and the study is *isotope renography*). The function tested depends on the radioisotope being used. Disappearance of the isotope is also plotted as part of that same curve and is a measurement of excretory function of the kidney. The curves are plotted, and their shapes can be compared with those of expected normal values and those of the opposite kidney. Furthermore, renal function can be monitored by serially repeating this test and comparing results. Renal function can be noted to be improved or deteriorating, depending on serial comparisons of the curves.

The kidney with diminished renal function (e.g., from glomerulonephritis) or decreased blood supply can be expected to have slower uptake activity and slower disappearance (excretion) of the radionuclide. The curve is much flatter. This pattern can also appear in rejection after transplantation. In addition, impending renal failure can be identified with this scan.

Renal Hypertension Scan

This scan is used to determine the presence and the source of renovascular hypertension. This scan usually entails the use of an angiotensin-converting enzyme inhibitor (such as captopril).

The captopril scan (captopril renography/scintigraphy) helps determine the functional significance of a renal artery or arteriole stenosis. After the administration of captopril, the glomerular filtration rate in a kidney with a partial vascular obstruction is reduced despite the preservation of renal plasma flow. The glomerular filtration rate in the contralateral kidney is maintained. This is demonstrated as delayed radioactivity in the affected kidney after injection of a radionuclide. These scans may help predict the response of the blood pressure to medical treatment, angioplasty, or surgery.

8 Nuclear Scanning

Renal Obstruction Scan

This scan is performed to identify obstruction of the outflow tract of the kidney because of obstruction of the renal pelvis, ureter, or bladder outlet. In this study, the radionuclide is rapidly injected while the patient is under the scintigraphy camera. Activity is measured and plotted per unit of time. After approximately 10 minutes, a diuretic (Lasix) is administered. The radionuclide in the unobstructed kidney washes out (is excreted) rapidly from the kidney. A slow excretion without wash-out is visible in an obstructed but still functioning kidney. Furthermore, when the collecting system does become visible, it is observed to be dilated.

Often, several of these types of scans are combined to obtain the maximum amount of information about the renal system. In a *triple renal study,* all of these techniques may be used to evaluate renal blood perfusion, structure, and excretion.

Renal scanning is superior to other testing in determining renal function, identifying renal infarction, monitoring renovascular hypertension, and identifying primary renal diseases and transplant rejection. This type of radionuclear scanning is also helpful in the evaluation of the following:

- Arterial atherosclerosis or trauma; the uptake of the radionuclear material by the kidneys is delayed or absent on the affected side or sides
- Pathologic renal or ureteral conditions in patients who cannot undergo intravenous pyelography (p. 1080) because of dye allergies or poor renal function
- Renal tumours, abscesses, or cysts in patients who may have an allergy to iodine; these appear as "cold" spots (areas without radionuclide uptake) because of the nonfunctioning tissue
- Renal or ureteral disease in patients whose renal function is already poor and who would be at risk for further reduction in function if iodinated dye were to be administered

For anatomic abnormalities, tumours, or cysts, ultrasonography (p. 917), computed tomography (p. 1059), and magnetic resonance imaging (p. 1148) are preferable and more accurate.

 Clinical Priorities

- Numerous types of renal scanning (such as blood flow, structure, function, hypertension, obstruction) can be performed, depending on which information is needed. Various isotopes are used, depending on how the kidney handles the radioisotopes.
- Renal scanning should not be scheduled within 24 hours after intravenous pyelography because the iodinated dye may diminish renal function.
- Renal scanning can be used to evaluate rejection of a transplanted kidney.

CONTRAINDICATIONS

- Pregnancy, unless the benefits of the procedure outweigh the risk of injury to the fetus
- Inability of patient to lie still during the study

PROCEDURE AND PATIENT CARE

Before

- Explain the procedure to the patient.
- Do not schedule renal scanning within 24 hours after intravenous pyelography. The iodinated dye may temporarily diminish renal function.

- Assure the patient that he or she will not be exposed to large amounts of radioactivity because only tracer doses of isotopes are used.
- Note that Lugol iodine solution (10 drops) may be ordered if ^{131}I will be used. This minimizes radioisotope uptake by the thyroid.
- Remind the patient to void before the scan.
- Inform the patient that no sedation or fasting is required but that good hydration is essential.
- Instruct the patient to drink two to three glasses of water before the scan.
- Inform the patient that no pain or discomfort is associated with this procedure.
- Inform the patient that he or she must lie still during this study.

During

- Take the patient to the nuclear medicine department.
- Note the following procedural steps:
  1. The unsedated, nonfasting patient is taken to the nuclear medicine department.
  2. A peripheral intravenous injection of radionuclide is given. It takes only minutes for the radioisotope to become concentrated in the kidneys.
  3. While the patient assumes a prone or sitting position, a gamma ray scintigraphy camera is passed over the kidney area and records the radioactive uptake.
  4. For *Lasix renal scanning* or *diuretic renal scanning,* ^{99m}Tc DTPA is injected. Images are obtained for 10 to 20 minutes; then 40 mg of Lasix is administered intravenously, and images are obtained for another 20 minutes.
  5. For *captopril renal scanning,* scanning is performed after the administration of an angiotensin-converting enzyme inhibitor, such as captopril.
  6. Scans may be repeated at different intervals after the initial isotope injection. For the renal blood flow and the renal function scans, scanning is started immediately after the injection.
  7. For *structural renal scanning,* the patient is asked to lie still for the entire time of the scan (30 minutes).
- Note that the duration of this test varies from 1 to 4 hours, depending on the specific information required. Perfusion scans are performed in approximately 20 minutes and functional scans in less than 1 hour. Static structure scans require 20 minutes to 4 hours for completion.
- Note that a nuclear medicine technologist or physician performs this study.

After

- Inform the patient that because only tracer doses of radioisotopes are used, no precautions need to be taken against radioactive exposure.
- Inform the patient that the radioactive substance is usually excreted from the body within 6 to 24 hours. Encourage the patient to drink fluids.

TEST RESULTS AND CLINICAL SIGNIFICANCE

Urinary obstruction: *This is obvious on a renal obstruction scan. After diuresis, the obstructed kidney fails to demonstrate wash-out (excretion) of the radionuclide. Prolonged obstruction ultimately leads to total loss of function of the obstructed kidney. That kidney is not illuminated after injection of a radionuclide.*

Renovascular hypertension: *The renal hypertension scan is performed after administration of captopril. The time for the affected kidney to become illuminated by the radionuclide is significantly prolonged.*

Renal infarction: *This can be visible as a wedge-shaped defect on the structural scan and perhaps as decreased blood flow on the perfusion scan.*

Renal arterial atherosclerosis: *This is evident as delayed illumination on the perfusion scan. The plotted curve is flatter than normal.*

Glomerulonephritis,

Pyelonephritis,

Acute tubular necrosis,

Absence of kidney function: *If significant enough to affect renal function, these diseases are evident on the renal function scans. The affected kidney is not illuminated as quickly as normal. The plotted curves of function per unit of time are flatter than normal. No uptake is seen with absence of renal function.*

Renal tumour,

Renal abscess,

Renal cyst: *These abnormalities are apparent as filling defects on the renal structural scan.*

Congenital abnormalities such as renal aplasia, hypoplasia, and malposition: *These abnormalities are evident on the renal structural scan.*

Renal trauma: *With arterial injury, the renal blood flow scan demonstrates prolonged filling or no visualization of the affected kidney. The renal structural scan may demonstrate a laceration of the kidney with extravasation of radionuclide out of the renal capsule.*

Transplant rejection: *This is apparent with many of the scans described in this section. With rejection of a transplanted kidney, blood flow to the transplanted kidney may be reduced, function of the transplanted kidney may be reduced, or renal structure of the transplanted kidney may be altered.*

RELATED TESTS

Intravenous Pyelography (p. 1080). This is a radiographic examination of the kidneys and lower urologic tract. With the use of iodinated intravenous contrast medium, this test can also provide information about renal function, blood flow, and structure. In addition, this test can demonstrate renal obstruction.

Computed Tomography, Abdomen (p. 1059), Computed Tomography, Brain (p. 1065), Computed Tomography, Chest (p. 1068), and Computed Tomography, Heart (p. 1072). Computed tomography is another radiographic study that can provide information about renal function, blood flow, and structure and can also demonstrate renal obstruction.

Salivary Gland Nuclear Imaging (Parotid Gland Nuclear Imaging)

NORMAL FINDINGS

Normal function of the salivary gland

No tumour or duct obstruction

INDICATIONS

This test is used to evaluate xerostomia (dry mouth), salivary gland pain, tumours, or possible parotid duct obstruction.

TEST EXPLANATION

The ability of the epithelial cells of the salivary glands to transport pertechnetate, a large anion, from the blood and to secrete it into the saliva is the principle on which imaging the salivary glands is based. The functional capabilities, structural integrity, and location of the glands can be assessed. Usually, the parotid gland alone is visualized. On occasion, the submandibular glands can be seen.

In this type of imaging, the radionuclide is injected, and its course is followed; thus, blood flow can be evaluated. Because this blood flow comes from the cerebral arteries, this test is a measure of the patency of those vessels. Tumours have increased blood flow that can be identified during this part of the study. Patients with acute inflammation also have increased blood flow during the early stages of the test.

Approximately 10 to 20 minutes after the injection, gland function becomes obvious by uptake of the nuclide into the gland. This uptake is usually compared with that of the thyroid, which is visualized at the same time. Function is diminished in patients with severe inflammation or auto-immune diseases, such as Sjögren syndrome. Five to 10 minutes later, nuclear material is seen being secreted into the mouth. Salivary calculi impede excretion and wash-out of the radionuclide because of obstruction of the excretory duct.

Wash-out demonstrates complete salivary gland excretion. Usually the patient is asked to suck on a lemon to encourage rapid wash-out. Static lateral pictures of the salivary glands can demonstrate tumours or cysts. The parotid gland is affected most commonly by tumours, and usually tumours are benign. In neoplasm of the salivary glands, wash-out is slow (i.e., the tumour may remain "hot" [retain radionuclide]) for longer periods of time. Nearly 50% of the benign tumours are hot. A "cold" appearance (which does not take up radionuclide as well as "cold" surrounding tissue) is common in malignant tumours.

CONTRAINDICATIONS

- Pregnancy, unless the benefits of the procedure outweigh the risk of injury to the fetus

INTERFERING FACTORS

- Rinsing the mouth before the study may reduce excretion.

PROCEDURE AND PATIENT CARE

Before

- Explain the procedure to the patient.
- Instruct the patient not to rinse the mouth before scan because this may reduce the effectiveness of the test.
- Inform the patient that no specific preparation is necessary.
- Ensure that the patient does not receive any thyroid-blocking agents within 48 hours of testing.

During

- Take the patient to the nuclear medicine department.
- Note the following procedure steps:
  1. Technetium-99m (^{99m}Tc) pertechnetate is injected into the antecubital vein.
  2. Dynamic images are obtained immediately when the detector is placed over the facial area. Radioactive counts are recorded and displayed.
  3. Repeat images are obtained every 3 to 5 minutes for total of 15 to 20 minutes.
  4. A salivary gland stimulant is administered after completion of static images. Either lemon juice or a lemon slice should be swished in the mouth and then expectorated.

TABLE 8-5 Salivary Gland Nuclear Imaging

Pathologic Process	Early Blood Flow	Static Images/ Function Phase	Wash-Out	Excretion
Sjögren syndrome	Normal	Poor uptake	Normal	Normal
Benign tumour	Increased or decreased	Local/hot or local/cold	Poor	Normal
Malignant tumour	Increased	Local/cold	Very slow	Normal
Acute inflammation	Increased	Diffuse/increased early then decreased	Slow	Normal
Chronic inflammation	Normal	Diffuse/decreased	Slow	Normal
Duct obstruction	Decreased	Diffuse/decreased	Slow	Slow or none

5. Wash-out images are obtained 5 to 10 minutes after the salivary gland stimulant. The thyroid gland is included in the images for reference or comparison.

• This procedure is performed in approximately 35 to 45 minutes by a nuclear medicine technologist or a physician in the nuclear medicine department.

After

 Assure the patient that the dose of radioactive ^{99m}Tc used in this test is minute and therefore harmless. No isolation and no special urine precautions are needed.

TEST RESULTS AND CLINICAL SIGNIFICANCE

Table 8-5 lists findings of salivary gland nuclear imaging.

Schilling Test (Vitamin B$_{12}$ Absorption Test)

NORMAL FINDINGS

Excretion of 8% to 40% of radioactive vitamin B_{12} within 24 hours

INDICATIONS

This test is performed on patients who have been found to have vitamin B_{12} deficiency and are thought to have pernicious anemia. It is useful to determine the cause of that deficiency. Abnormal results of the Schilling test indicate a defect in absorption of vitamin B_{12}.

TEST EXPLANATION

The Schilling test is performed to detect vitamin B_{12} absorption. Normally, ingested vitamin B_{12} combines with intrinsic factor, which is produced by the gastric mucosa, and is absorbed in the distal part of the ileum. Pernicious anemia results when absorption of vitamin B_{12} is inadequate. This may be caused by a primary malabsorption problem of the intestinal tract or by lack of intrinsic factor.

The two-stage Schilling test can help detect a defect in vitamin B_{12} absorption. When absorption is normal, the ileum absorbs more vitamin B_{12} than the body needs and excretes the excess into the urine. When absorption is impaired, however, little or no vitamin B_{12} is excreted into the urine.

In the Schilling test, urinary B_{12} levels are measured after the ingestion of radioactive vitamin B_{12}. The test can be performed in one stage (without intrinsic factor) or two stages (with intrinsic factor). When pernicious anemia results from lack of intrinsic factor, results are abnormal for the first stage and normal for the second stage of the Schilling test. When malabsorption results from an intestinal source, results are abnormal for both the first and second stages of the Schilling test. When malabsorption is related to a treatable condition such as Crohn's disease, small intestinal lymphoma, or bacterial intestinal overgrowth, the test may be repeated after appropriate treatment.

A combined one-stage and two-stage test is now commonly used. All bone marrow and hematologic studies, along with determination of serum vitamin B_{12} levels, must be performed before the Schilling test. Any vitamin B_{12} that is administered during this test can significantly alter Schilling test results.

The Schilling test has fallen out of favour because it is expensive and complicated to perform, because obtaining the radiolabelled vitamin B_{12} is difficult, and because interpretation of test results can be problematic in patients with renal insufficiency. Direct measurement of vitamin B_{12} levels in the serum and serologic studies—such as anti–parietal cell antibodies (see p. 102) and anti–intrinsic factor (see p. 332)—are easy to perform and available; thus, the diagnosis of pernicious anemia can be confirmed rapidly. The sooner the diagnosis is made, the sooner effective therapy can be initiated.

CONTRAINDICATIONS

- Pregnancy or lactation, unless the benefits of the procedure outweigh the risk of injury to the fetus or infant

INTERFERING FACTORS

- Radioactive nuclear material received up to 10 days before testing may affect results.
- Renal insufficiency may cause a reduction in excretion of radioactive vitamin B_{12}.
- In older adults, patients who have diabetes, or patients who have hypothyroidism, excretion of vitamin B_{12} may be reduced.
- Inadequate collection of urine can artificially reduce the vitamin B_{12} in the urine.
- Stool in the urine specimen alters test results.
- Drugs that may affect test results include laxatives because they could decrease the rate of vitamin B_{12} absorption.

PROCEDURE AND PATIENT CARE

Before

- Explain the procedure to the patient.
- Instruct the patient to remain on NPO status (nothing by mouth) except for water for 8 to 12 hours before the test. Food should not be given until after the patient receives the injections.
- Instruct the patient not to take laxatives during the test period.

During

- Take the patient to the nuclear medicine department.

First-Stage Schilling Test (Without Intrinsic Factor)

- Note the following procedural steps:
    1. Radioactive vitamin B_{12} is administered orally to the patient.
    2. Shortly thereafter, nonradioactive vitamin B_{12} is administered to the patient intramuscularly to saturate tissue-binding sites and to enable some excretion of radioactive vitamin B_{12} in the urine if it is absorbed.
    3. For vitamin B_{12} measurement, urine is collected for 24 to 48 hours.
    4. For the *second-stage Schilling test (with intrinsic factor)*, radioactive vitamin B_{12}, combined with human intrinsic factor, is administered orally, and the test is repeated.

Combined One-Stage and Two-Stage Schilling Test

- Note the following procedural steps:
    1. The fasting patient receives a capsule of vitamin B_{12} labelled with cobalt-57 (^{57}Co) plus intrinsic factor.
    2. A second capsule of vitamin B_{12} labelled with cobalt-58 (^{58}Co) is also administered.
    3. One hour later, nonradioactive vitamin B_{12} is injected intramuscularly.
    4. The urine is collected for 24 to 48 hours.
    5. Percentages of ^{57}Co and ^{58}Co are calculated. ^{57}Co-labelled vitamin B_{12} is present only in patients with pernicious anemia secondary to lack of intrinsic factor. No vitamin B_{12} will be present in the urine of patients in whom pernicious anemia is caused by primary bowel malabsorption.

After

- Ensure that the urine specimens are transported promptly to the laboratory.

TEST RESULTS AND CLINICAL SIGNIFICANCE

▼ Decreased Levels

Pernicious anemia: *Pernicious anemia is a type of megaloblastic anemia that results from vitamin B_{12} deficiency. This may result from lack of intestinal absorption of vitamin B_{12} because of a deficiency of intrinsic factor.*

Intestinal malabsorption (regional enteritis [Crohn's disease], blind-loop syndrome, small bowel lymphoma): *These diseases are associated with decrease in absorption of vitamin B_{12} as a result of thickening of the bowel, which precludes the passage of nutrients. When vitamin B_{12} absorption is poor, little or no vitamin B_{12} is present in the urine.*

Hypothyroidism,

Liver disease: *These diseases are also associated with abnormal vitamin B_{12} absorption and metabolism.*

RELATED TESTS

Vitamin B_{12} (p. 541). This is a direct measurement of vitamin B_{12} levels in the blood.

Anti–Parietal Cell Antibodies (p. 102). This test helps detect antibodies to the gastric parietal cells, and the result is positive in most patients with pernicious anemia.

Intrinsic Factor Antibody (p. 332). This test helps detect antibodies to intrinsic factor, and the result is positive in more than half of the patients with pernicious anemia.

> **Scrotal Nuclear Imaging** (Scrotal Scanning, Testicular Imaging)

NORMAL FINDINGS

Symmetric and prompt blood flow to both testicles

INDICATIONS

Scrotal imaging is helpful in the diagnosis of patients with a sudden onset of unilateral testicular swelling and pain. Scrotal imaging can differentiate unilateral testicular torsion from other causes of testicular pain (e.g., acute epididymitis, torsion of the testicular appendage, orchitis, strangulated hernia, testicular hemorrhage). This test is not used frequently because scrotal ultrasonography can reliably provide the same information more rapidly and less expensively.

TEST EXPLANATION

Testicular torsion is a medical emergency necessitating prompt surgical exploration to salvage the involved testicle. To provide immediate surgical care, the surgeon must differentiate the condition from other causes of painful testicular swelling that do not necessitate surgery. Use of radionuclide scrotal imaging enables the surgeon to diagnose testicular torsion. This study is usually performed on an emergency basis and in the nuclear medicine department.

The patient is positioned under the gamma camera with the scrotum supported between the abducted thighs. Technetium-99m (^{99m}Tc) pertechnetate is administered, and a dynamic radionuclide nuclear angiogram is obtained. Static images are obtained immediately afterward. An area of decreased perfusion corresponding to the involved testis is highly indicative of torsion of the testicle. If the clinically involved testis has normal perfusion or is hypervascular, a disease other than torsion of the testicle (as described earlier) is responsible for the symptoms.

PROCEDURE AND PATIENT CARE

Before

- Explain the procedure to the patient.
- Inform the patient that no fasting or premedication is required.
- Assure the patient that he will not be exposed to large amounts of radiation because only tracer doses of isotope are used.
- If the patient is a child, encourage one or both parents, or the caregiver, to be present during the test.

During

- Take the patient to the nuclear medicine department.
- The patient is placed on a padded table in the supine position.
- The patient's legs are placed in abduction, and the testicles are supported with tape or a lead shield. The penis is taped to the lower abdomen.
- A small dose of ^{99m}Tc pertechnetate is injected intravenously.
- Radionuclide imaging is then immediately performed over both testicles. Both dynamic and static images are obtained.

Nuclear Scanning

8

After

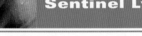 Reassure the patient that because only tracer doses of radioisotopes are used, other people do not need to take precautions against radiation exposure.

• If torsion of the testicle is identified, prepare the patient for immediate surgery.

TEST RESULTS AND CLINICAL SIGNIFICANCE

▲ Increased Testicular Blood Flow

Epididymitis,

Torsion of the testicular appendage,

Orchitis,

Trauma: *These abnormalities may be associated with increased blood flow to the testicle.*

▼ Decreased Testicular Blood Flow

Testicular torsion of the spermatic cord: *Torsion of the testicle inhibits blood flow to the testicle. This ultimately leads to infarction of the testicle if it is not treated immediately.*

RELATED TEST

Scrotal Ultrasonography (p. 923). This is now the preferred test for detecting torsion of the testicle. It is more rapidly performed and more accurate than scrotal imaging.

Sentinel Lymph Node Biopsy (SLNB, Lymphoscintigraphy)

NORMAL FINDINGS

Uptake noted in one or more lymph nodes

INDICATIONS

Lymphoscintigraphy is used to identify the "sentinel" lymph node: the one most likely to contain metastasis from a nearby primary tumour. It is used to map the lymphatic drainage of a primary cancer so that surgery can be directed for diagnostic and possibly therapeutic resection of lymph nodes. It is used primarily in the treatment of breast cancer and melanoma.

TEST EXPLANATION

In this procedure, the first (sentinel) lymph node in line to catch metastatic cells from a primary tumour is identified, and a biopsy sample is taken. To stage most breast or melanoma cancers, a lymph node draining the primary site must be evaluated microscopically. With the use of sentinel lymph node biopsy, the first lymph node in the chain of lymph nodes can be identified, and a biopsy sample can be obtained. If results are negative, as is the case in most patients with small tumours, the rest of the axillary lymph contents can be safely assumed to be free of tumour and are not removed. This saves women from the potential complications—including arm-swelling, cellulitis, postoperative pain, and reduced range of motion—associated with a full lymph node dissection. Furthermore, this test can identify unusual locations for lymph node metastasis that would not normally be identified by the surgeon.

In this procedure, a tracer (isosulfan or methylene blue dye or technetium-99m [^{99m}Tc]) is injected into the skin or tissue near the tumour. If ^{99m}Tc is used, a scan is performed approximately 1 to 2 hours after the injections. Lymph nodes that take up the radionuclide are the sentinel lymph nodes that the surgeon identifies and removes. In the operating room, the surgeon is able to identify the region of maximal radioactivity by using a handheld gamma detector. Nodes in this region are removed and sent to the pathology laboratory for immediate evaluation. If isosulfan or methylene blue dye is injected, a stained lymphatic vessel is identified by the surgeon in the subcutaneous tissue, and its course is followed to the first blue-coloured node. The sentinel lymph nodes are the blue, or "hot," nodes closest to the primary tumour.

If the sentinel lymph node is found not to contain tumour cells on frozen section or on touch preparation pathologic study, the lymph node dissection procedure is not required. If the sentinel lymph node does contain tumour cells, a full lymph node dissection is carried out. In some instances, light microscopy findings may be negative, but subsequent immunohistochemical staining may indicate the presence of cancer in the node.

This test is quickly becoming an important part of the standard treatment for breast and melanoma cancer surgery. The only discomfort associated with the test is the preoperative injections required around the tumour. The ^{99m}Tc injection and subsequent scanning are usually performed in the nuclear medicine department. When isosulfan or methylene blue dye is used as the lymph node tracer, the injection is administered in the operating room after anaesthesia induction.

CONTRAINDICATIONS
- Patients who have a large tumour from which lymph node metastasis is very likely to occur
- Early pregnancy, unless the benefits of the procedure outweigh the risk of injury to the fetus

POTENTIAL COMPLICATIONS
- Anaphylaxis has been reported with injection of isosulfan blue dye.

PROCEDURE AND PATIENT CARE
Before
- Explain the procedure to the patient.
- Because this is an operative procedure, routine preoperative nursing processes should be carried out, including obtaining operative consent, keeping the patient on NPO status (nothing by mouth), and surgical site preparation as ordered.

During
- Take the patient to the nuclear medicine department.

Technetium-99m (^{99m}Tc)
- Note the following procedural steps:
  1. The patient is taken to the nuclear medicine department, where the radionuclide is injected around the tumour.
  2. The site of lymph node drainage is then scanned immediately and 1 to 24 hours later.
  3. Lymph node uptake is reported to the surgeon.

4. In the operating room, a handheld gamma detector locates "hot" areas of radionuclide uptake in the area of the lymph nodes. The most proximal "hot" node is excised as the sentinel node.

Isosulfan and Methylene Blue

- Note the following procedural steps:
  1. In the operating room, 4 to 5 mL of isosulfan or methylene blue dye is injected around the tumour.
  2. After 5 to 9 minutes, a small incision is made overlying the lymph node–bearing area and the proximal blue lymph node is removed as the sentinel lymph node.
- If the sentinel lymph node does not contain tumour cells, the lymph node dissection procedure is discontinued. If the sentinel lymph node does contain tumour cells, a complete lymph node dissection is performed.

After

 If ^{99m}Tc is used, reassure the patient that because the radionuclide dose is minimal, other people do not need to take precautions against radiation exposure.
- If isosulfan or methylene blue dye is used, the patient's skin may develop a transient blue hue (looking almost like severe cyanosis). This appearance dissipates over the next 6 hours.
- If isosulfan blue dye is used, warn the patient that the urine will have a blue tinge as a result.
- Observe the patient for signs of allergy (rare) caused by the blue dye injection.

TEST RESULTS AND CLINICAL SIGNIFICANCE

Metastasis of tumour to lymph node,

Normal lymph node: *It is important to note that uptake of dye or radionuclide does not indicate whether a lymph node contains metastatic tumour cells. It only locates the lymph node that is most likely to contain tumour cells if metastasis occurred.*

Thyroid Scan (Thyroid Scintiscan)

NORMAL FINDINGS

Normal size, shape, position, and function of the thyroid gland
No areas of decreased or increased uptake

INDICATIONS

This test is used to visualize the thyroid gland when disease of the thyroid is suspected. It is particularly useful in the evaluation of patients with a suspected thyroid nodule. With thyroid nuclear scanning, the nodule can be classified and appropriately treated.

TEST EXPLANATION

Radionuclear thyroid scanning enables the examiner to determine the size, shape, position, and physiologic function of the thyroid gland. A radioactive substance such as technetium-99m (^{99m}Tc) is administered to the patient to visualize the thyroid gland. A scintigraphy camera is passed over the neck area, and an image is recorded.

Thyroid nodules are easily detected by this technique. Nodules are classified as functioning ("warm"/"hot") or nonfunctioning ("cold") according to the amount of radionuclide taken up by the nodule (Figure 8-14). A functioning nodule could represent a benign adenoma or a localized toxic goitre. A nonfunctioning nodule may represent a cyst, carcinoma, nonfunctioning adenoma or goitre, lymphoma, or localized area of thyroiditis.

Scanning is useful in patients with the following clinical conditions:

1. Neck or substernal mass.
2. Thyroid nodule. Thyroid cancers are usually nonfunctioning (cold) nodules.
3. Hyperthyroidism. Scanning assists in differentiating Graves' disease (diffusely enlarged hyperfunctioning thyroid gland) from Plummer disease (nodular hyperfunctioning gland).
4. Metastatic tumours without a known primary site. Normal findings on the scan rule out the thyroid gland as a possible primary site.
5. Well-differentiated form of thyroid cancer.

Another form of thyroid scanning is called *whole-body thyroid scanning*. This scan is performed on patients who have previously undergone treatment for thyroid cancer. Iodine-123 (^{123}I) is injected intravenously, and the entire body is scanned to detect metastatic thyroid tissue. A hot spot would indicate recurrent tumour. Before this test can be performed, all of the thyroid tissue in the neck must be either surgically excised or ablated with radioactive iodine-131 (^{131}I). If the patient is receiving thyroid replacement therapy, the thyroid medicine must be discontinued at least 6 weeks before the test. Any metastatic thyroid tissue will thus become particularly iodine avid. A high blood level of thyroid-stimulating hormone ensures that any thyroid cancer tissue will take up the administered radioactive iodine. This test is performed routinely (every 1 to 2 years) on

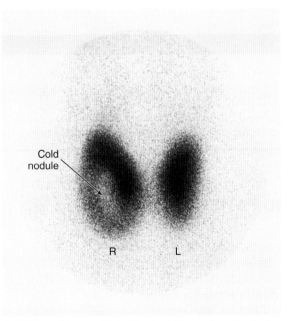

Figure 8-14 Thyroid scan. Note the "cold" (nonfunctioning) nodule in the right (larger) lobe of the thyroid gland. This finding is consistent with cyst, carcinoma, nonfunctioning adenoma or goitre, lymphoma, or localized area of thyroiditis.

Nuclear Scanning

8

patients who have had a thyroid cancer larger than 1 cm in diameter. Smaller cancers are unlikely to metastasize. Much of the procedure is similar to thyroid scanning.

CONTRAINDICATIONS

- Allergy to iodine or shellfish, because sometimes ^{123}I is used as the radionuclide
- Pregnancy, unless the benefits of the procedure outweigh the risk of injury to the fetus

POTENTIAL COMPLICATIONS

- Radiation-induced oncogenesis: This complication is eliminated if ^{99m}Tc or low-radioactive iodine isomers are used instead of ^{131}I.

INTERFERING FACTORS

- Iodine-containing foods affect results because the iodine may saturate all of the iodine-binding sites and the thyroid will take up very little iodine tracer. Also, if large quantities of iodine are ingested, the thyroid may shut down and will not take up even small amounts of the ^{99m}Tc tracer.
- The recent administration of radiographic contrast agents affects results because these agents contain large quantities of iodine. For the reasons described previously, contrast agents should be avoided before thyroid scanning.
- Drugs that may affect test results include cough medicines, multiple vitamins, some oral contraceptives, and thyroid drugs.

Clinical Priorities

- Thyroid nodules are classified as hot (greater area of intensity with more chemical activity) or cold (lesser intense area with less chemical activity), depending on the amount of radionuclide taken up by the nodule.
- Whole-body thyroid scanning can be used to detect metastatic thyroid tissue.
- Iodine in foods or radiographic contrast agents should be avoided before thyroid scanning.

PROCEDURE AND PATIENT CARE

Before

- Explain the procedure to the patient.
- Check the patient for allergies to iodine.
- Instruct the patient about medications that need to be restricted for 6 weeks before the test (e.g., thyroid drugs, medications containing iodine).
- Document the patient's history concerning previous contrast radiographic studies, nuclear scanning, or intake of any thyroid-suppressive or antithyroid drugs.
- Inform the patient that fasting is usually not required. Check first with the laboratory.
- Inform the patient that no discomfort is associated with this study.

During

- Take the patient to the nuclear medicine department.
- Note the following procedural steps:
  1. A standard dose of radioactive ^{99m}Tc or ^{123}I is usually given to the patient by mouth. The capsule is tasteless.
  2. Scanning is usually performed 24 hours later. If ^{99m}Tc is used, scanning may be performed 2 hours after administration of the capsule.
  3. At the designated time, the patient is positioned supine, and a scintigraphy camera is placed over the thyroid area.
  4. The radioactive counts are recorded and displayed.
- Note that this study is performed in less than 30 minutes by a radiologic technologist.

After

Reassure the patient that the dose of radioactive ^{99m}Tc used in this test is minute and therefore harmless. No isolation and no special urine precautions are needed.

TEST RESULTS AND CLINICAL SIGNIFICANCE

Adenoma: *This may be evident as a hot nodule if the lymph node is functioning or as a cold nodule if the node is not functioning.*

Toxic and nontoxic goitre: *The toxic goitre is apparent as a hot nodule. The nontoxic goitre is apparent as a cold nodule.*

Cyst,
Carcinoma,
Lymphoma,
Thyroiditis,
Metastasis: *These diseases usually appear as cold nodules or filling defects in normal thyroid tissue.*

Graves' disease: *This disease is evident as diffuse increased uptake of radionuclide involving the entire thyroid gland.*

Plummer disease: *This disease produces a single or multiple nodular areas of increased uptake.*

Hyperthyroidism,
Hypothyroidism: *In general, uptake of radionuclide is increased in hyperthyroidism and reduced in hypothyroidism.*

Hashimoto disease: *In this disease, uptake of radionuclide often has a mottled appearance.*

RELATED TESTS

Thyroid Ultrasonography (p. 925). This is an important part of evaluation of the thyroid gland. In general, all solid nodules demonstrated on ultrasonography that are cold on thyroid scan should be considered suggestive of cancer.

Triiodothyronine (p. 525), Thyroxine, Total (p. 516), and Thyroid-Stimulating Hormone (p. 500). These tests are the most common methods by which thyroid function is measured. They are more accurate than radioactive iodine uptake testing and thyroid scanning. No radioactive material needs to be administered to the patient. These tests should be a part of every thyroid evaluation.

Computed Tomography, Chest (p. 1068). With computed tomographic scan of the chest, the thyroid nodule can be more accurately located and its characteristics evaluated for malignancy.

Nuclear Scanning

8

Total Blood Volume (TBV, Red Blood Cell [RBC] Volume)

NORMAL FINDINGS

No deviation from normal

INDICATIONS

Total blood volume measurement may be useful in the following clinical circumstances:
1. Heart failure: The actual amount of fluid overload can be calculated and diuresis can be more appropriately determined.
2. Presurgery: The patient's fluid status can be accurately determined, as can RBC status.
3. Acutely ill patients: There are often large fluid shifts in these patients and TBV may help in guiding IV fluid replacement.
4. Azotemia: Measurement of TBV will indicate if azotemia is prerenal (hypovolemia) or primary renal.
5. Hypertension: TBV may indicate plasma volume overload versus vascular constriction.
6. Anemia: TBV and RBC volumes can indicate accurately the extent of anemia that otherwise could be affected by such things as fluid status.

TEST EXPLANATION

Measurement of total blood volume is an accurate indicator of true plasma (liquid components of blood) measurement. Based on the patient's height, weight, gender, and body composition, a TBV can determine whether the measured volumes are normal, high, or low compared with what would be ideal for the particular patient. The report indicates actual volumes for TBV and RBCs that deviate from normal.

To maintain blood volume within a normal range, the kidneys regulate the amount of water and sodium lost into the urine. For example, if excessive water and sodium are ingested, the kidneys normally respond by excreting more water and sodium into the urine. This auto adjustment is mediated through the renin-angiotensin-aldosterone system. Both angiotensin and aldosterone, although by different mechanisms, stimulate distal tubular sodium reabsorption and decrease sodium and water loss by the kidney and thereby adjust blood volume. Another important hormone in regulating blood volume is vasopressin (antidiuretic hormone [ADH]). The posterior pituitary releases this hormone. One of its actions is to stimulate water reabsorption in the collecting duct of the kidney, thereby decreasing water loss and increasing blood volume. Blood volume affects cardiac output and blood pressure.

Radioiodine labelled albumin is injected intravenously. Blood is withdrawn every 5 minutes for five samples. The radioactivity is counted and compared with what would be considered normal. A lower amount of the radioactivity in the sample indicates a higher plasma volume. The hematocrit is then used to derive the red cell volume. The total blood volume is obtained by adding the plasma volume and the red cell volume.

Before

✍ Explain the procedure and tell the patient that no fasting is required.

During

• Obtain venous access
• Fifteen minutes after radionuclide injection, the first venous blood specimen is collected in a red-top tube.
• Similar venous blood specimens are obtained every 5 minutes for a total of five samples.

After
- Apply pressure to the intravenous site upon removal after the extracting the last sample.

TEST RESULTS AND CLINICAL SIGNIFICANCE

▲ Increased Levels

Hypervolemia,
Hypertension,
Heart failure,
Primary renal disease,
Polycythemia vera: *These conditions are associated with increased total blood volume because of too much intravascular fluid or too many RBCs.*

▼ Decreased Levels

Dehydration,
Hypovolemia,
Acute bleeding,
Anemia: *These conditions are associated with decreased total blood volume because of too little intravascular fluid and/or too few RBCs.*

RELATED TEST

Hematocrit (p. 295). This is a measure of the volume of RBCs in the blood. This measurement is inversely related to the amount of intravascular fluid, given that the RBCs are normal in size.

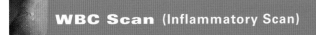

WBC Scan (Inflammatory Scan)

NORMAL FINDINGS

No signs of white blood cell (WBC) localization outside the liver or spleen

INDICATIONS

This scan is used to identify and localize occult inflammation or infection. It is used for patients who have a fever of unknown origin, suspected osteomyelitis, or inflammatory bowel disease. It is used to indicate whether an abnormal mass (e.g., a pancreatic pseudocyst) represents an infection.

TEST EXPLANATION

This test is based on the fact that WBCs are attracted to areas of infection or inflammation. When the patient has a suspected infection or inflammation but the site cannot be localized, the injection of radiolabelled WBCs may help identify and localize that area of inflammation or infection. Appropriate treatment can then be administered. This is especially helpful in patients who have a fever of unknown origin, in whom occult intra-abdominal infection is suspected, or in whom osteomyelitis is suspected (but radiographically unapparent). The scan can differentiate infectious from noninfectious processes. Areas of noninfectious inflammation (e.g., inflammatory bowel disease) also take up the radiolabelled WBCs.

This scan requires drawing a small amount of blood from the patient, separating out the WBCs, labelling the WBCs with technetium-99m (^{99m}Tc), and reinjecting them into the patient. Four to 24 hours later, imaging of the whole body may show an area of increased radioactivity, which suggests that radiolabelled WBCs have accumulated in an area of infection or inflammation.

In leukopenia, the WBC count is so low that separating them out from the other blood cellular components would be very difficult. In these instances, donor WBCs are used instead of autologous WBCs. Donor WBCs are also used for patients infected with the human immunodeficiency virus (HIV), to minimize the risk to laboratory workers.

The imaging procedure is performed in approximately 30 minutes by a trained technologist. A physician trained in nuclear medicine interprets the results. The only discomfort associated with this procedure is the intravenous injection of the radionuclide.

INTERFERING FACTORS

- These radiolabelled cells normally tend to accumulate in the reticuloendothelial system (liver, spleen, and bone marrow).

PROCEDURE AND PATIENT CARE

Before
- Explain the procedure to the patient.
- Assure the patient that he or she will not be exposed to large amounts of radioactivity because only tracer doses of the isotope are used.
- Inform the patient that no preparation or sedation is required.

During
- Take the patient to the nuclear medicine department.
- Note the following procedural steps:
  1. A small amount of blood is withdrawn from the patient, and the WBCs are extracted from the rest of the blood cells. This is usually accomplished by centrifugation.
  2. The WBCs are suspended in saline and tagged with ^{99m}Tc lipid-soluble product.
  3. The tagged WBCs are reinjected into the patient.
  4. In 4, 24, and 48 hours after injection, a gamma camera is placed over the body.
  5. The patient is placed in supine, lateral, and prone positions so that all surfaces of the body can be visualized.
  6. The radionuclide image is recorded.

After
- Inform the patient that because only tracer doses of radioisotopes are used, no precautions need to be taken against radioactive exposure.

TEST RESULTS AND CLINICAL SIGNIFICANCE

Infection (abscess, osteomyelitis, or poststernotomy infections): *The WBCs are localized to the area of infection, and their appearance is of increased radionuclear uptake (hot spot).*

Inflammation (e.g., inflammatory bowel disease, arthritis): *Like areas of infection, areas of noninfectious inflammation attract the radiolabelled WBCs.*

Stool Tests

NOTE: *Throughout this chapter, SI units are presented in* **boldface colour,** *followed by conventional units in parentheses.*

OVERVIEW

TESTS

OVERVIEW

REASONS FOR PERFORMING STOOL STUDIES

Stool represents the waste products of digested food. It also includes bile, mucus, shed epithelial cells, bacteria, and other inorganic salts. Food is normally passed through the stomach, into the duodenum, and into the small bowel. In the small bowel, most of the nutrient and electrolyte absorption occurs. The liquid stool is then passed into the colon, where most of the water is reabsorbed.

Stool studies are used to evaluate the function and integrity of the bowel. These studies are performed to evaluate intestinal bleeding, infections, infestations, inflammation, malabsorption, and diarrhea.

Some stool studies that are commonly performed are described in this chapter. Other testing can be done on the stool but is more often performed on other specimens. In those situations, the study is listed in the appropriate chapter for the specimen that is more commonly used.

Information obtained from stool studies is invaluable for proper care of the patient with gastrointestinal diseases.

PROCEDURAL CARE FOR STOOL STUDIES

Before

🖎 Explain the method of stool collection to the patient. Reassure the patient of the reasons for the test, and answer any questions as necessary.

🖎 Instruct the patient not to mix urine or toilet paper with the stool specimen.

- Instruct the patient to use an appropriate collection container.
- Instruct the patient not to undergo any diagnostic tests that require barium and to avoid laxatives and mineral oil.
- Observe universal or standard precautions/routine practices when handling stool specimens.

During

- Ask the patient to defecate into a clean bedpan.
- Place a small amount of stool in the appropriate container (e.g., a sterile collection container, developing card).
- If a rectal swab is needed, wear gloves and insert the cotton-tipped swab at least 2.5 cm (1 inch) into the patient's anal canal. Then rotate the swab for 30 seconds and place it in the clean container.

After

- Handle the stool specimen per standard precautions/routine practices.
- Promptly send the stool specimen to the laboratory. Delays in transfer of the specimen may affect test results.
- If there will be a delay in laboratory handling of the stool specimen, follow laboratory procedures or guidelines concerning storage. Stools for ova and parasites should be kept warm. Stools for enteric pathogens and *Clostridium difficile* should be refrigerated.
- Another option is to add a preservative to the stool. For example, for stool culture, a buffered glycerol-saline solution may be combined with the stool as a preservative.

REPORTING OF RESULTS

It may take several days or even weeks to obtain results of some stool specimens. However, most stool study results are available within 24 hours.

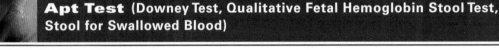

Apt Test (Downey Test, Qualitative Fetal Hemoglobin Stool Test, Stool for Swallowed Blood)

NORMAL FINDINGS

No fetal blood present
Maternal blood present

INDICATIONS

This is a screening test to indicate whether blood present in the stool or amniotic fluid of a newborn is fetal blood or swallowed maternal blood.

TEST EXPLANATION

Blood in the stool of a newborn must be rapidly evaluated. Although an adult can lose hundreds of millilitres of blood, that volume may represent the entire blood volume of a newborn. Newborns may have a serious disease causing the blood in the stool, or they may simply be defecating maternal blood that was swallowed during birth or breast-feeding. It is important to tell the difference rapidly. The Apt test is performed on the stool specimen to differentiate the source of the blood. Fetal hemoglobin is resistant to alkali denaturization; adult hemoglobin

(hemoglobin A) is not. When sodium hydroxide is added to the blood, maternal blood dissolves, leaving only a brown hematin stain. Fetal blood (containing hydroxide-resistant hemoglobin) does not dissolve, and blood will remain red in the specimen. This test can be performed on stool, a stool-stained diaper, amniotic fluid, or vomitus.

PROCEDURE AND PATIENT CARE

Before

 Explain the procedure to the newborn's parents.
- It is always important to assess vital signs of a newborn who develops possible intestinal bleeding.

During

- Obtain an adequate stool or vomitus specimen. Only a small amount is required.
- In the laboratory, 1% sodium hydroxide is added to the specimen. Vomitus is diluted and centrifuged first. Maternal blood turns brown; fetal blood stays red or pink.

After

- If maternal blood is present, reassure the parents, and examine the mother for nipple erosion and cracking.
- If fetal blood is present, begin close observation of the newborn, and provide emotional support to the parents during further diagnostic procedures.

TEST RESULTS AND CLINICAL SIGNIFICANCE

Maternal blood: *A newborn's defecation of maternal blood usually occurs in the first 3 to 5 days of life. If maternal nipple disease exists, the blood in the stool of a newborn can persist.*

Fetal blood: *This is an indication of disease within the gastrointestinal tract of the newborn and must be evaluated immediately.*

RELATED TEST

Stool for Occult Blood (p. 885). This is a method of identifying occult blood or substantiating the presence of blood in an adult's stool.

Clostridial Toxin Assay (*Clostridium difficile, Antibiotic-Associated Colitis Assay; Pseudomembranous Colitis Toxic Assay, C. diff.*)

NORMAL FINDINGS

Negative (no *Clostridium* toxin identified)

INDICATIONS

This test is indicated in patients with diarrhea who have been taking antibiotics for more than 5 days. It can also be performed on immunosuppressed patients with diarrhea even if they are not receiving antibiotics.

Stool Tests

9

TEST EXPLANATION

Clostridium difficile–associated diarrhea (CDAD) bacterial infections usually affect the intestine (colitis) and occur in patients who are immunocompromised or taking broad-spectrum antibiotics (e.g., clindamycin, ampicillin, and cephalosporins). The disease severity can range from mild nuisance diarrhea to severe pseudomembranous colitis and bowel perforation. The overwhelming predisposing factor is ongoing antibiotic therapy. Patient age, length of hospital stay, acuity of illness, and comorbidities are risk factors.

The infection possibly results from depression of the normal flora of the bowel caused by the administration of antibiotics. The clostridial bacterium produces two toxins (A and B) that cause inflammation and necrosis of the colonic epithelium. The standard for laboratory detection of *Clostridium difficile* toxins is the cytotoxicity assay in cell cultures. The specificity of the reaction is determined by the neutralization of the toxins with antisera directed to the toxin in the stool. However, the cytotoxin assay is labour intensive and may take up to 48 hours to obtain a result. Toxin detection by enzyme immunoassay (EIA) is insensitive. *C. difficile* can also be diagnosed by obtaining colonic-rectal tissue for this toxin. Stool cultures (p. 883) for *C. difficile* can be performed but are also labour intensive and take longer to get results.

A PCR assay for the qualitative in vitro rapid detection of *C. difficile* toxin B gene (tcdB) in human liquid or soft stool specimens is available. This method rapidly provides a definitive diagnosis of *C. difficile*. Quickly reaching a definitive diagnosis allows CDAD patients to get the proper treatment without delay and reduce hospital stays for inpatients with CDAD. At the same time they can be placed in isolation sooner to reduce transmission and prevent outbreaks. Definitive results can reduce inappropriate antimicrobial use in negative patients.

A positive PCR result for the presence of the gene-regulating toxin production (tcdC) indicates the presence of *C. difficile* and toxin A and/or B. A negative result indicates the absence of detectable *C. difficile* (tcdC) DNA in the specimen, but does not rule out *C. difficile* infection. False-negative results may occur because of inhibition of PCR, sequence variability underlying the primers and/or probes, or the presence of *C. difficile* in quantities less than the limit of detection of the assay.

Treatment of CDAD typically involves withdrawal of the associated antimicrobial(s) and, if symptoms persist, orally administered and intraluminally active metronidazole, vancomycin, or fidaxomicin. Intravenous metronidazole may be used if an oral agent cannot be administered. In recent years, a more severe form of CDAD with increased morbidity and mortality has been recognized as being caused by an epidemic toxin-hyperproducing strain of *C. difficile* (NAP1 strain). Many toxin-hyperproducing isolates also contain the binary toxin gene and are resistant quinolones.

PROCEDURE AND PATIENT CARE

Before

- Explain the method of stool collection to the patient. To avoid embarrassing the patient, be matter-of-fact in your demeanour.
- Instruct the patient not to mix urine or toilet paper with the stool specimen.
- Handle the specimen carefully, as though it were capable of causing infection. If someone is assisting with the specimen collection, that person should wear gloves.

During

- Instruct the patient to defecate into a clean container. A rectal swab cannot be used because it collects inadequate amounts of stool. The stool must not be retrieved from the toilet.
- Stool can be obtained from incontinence pads.
- A stool specimen also can be collected by proctoscopy or colonoscopy.

- Place the specimen in a closed container and then transport it to the laboratory immediately, to prevent deterioration of the toxin.
- If the specimen cannot be processed immediately, refrigerate it (depending on laboratory protocol).
- Submission of more than one specimen for testing is not recommended.

After

- Maintain enteric isolation precautions for all patients until appropriate therapy is completed.

TEST RESULTS AND CLINICAL SIGNIFICANCE

Antibiotic-related pseudomembranous colitis,

C. difficile colitis: *A number of names exist for the same clinical entity. This infection can progress to toxic megacolon and even death. In the extreme cases of this disease, medical therapy may not be adequate, and a total colectomy may be required.*

Age-Related Concerns

- Age-related changes in gastrointestinal physiology and function occur in adults older than 65 years. These changes are often accompanied by an increase in the incidence of gastrointestinal infections.
- *C. difficile* is isolated in the stools of older patients more often than in younger patients; therefore, older patients are at high risk for contracting *C. difficile* as a health care–associated infection.
- *C. difficile*–associated diarrhea is a persistent disease in older hospitalized patients that can result in a prolonged hospital stay and high medical costs.

RELATED TESTS

Sigmoidoscopy (p. 651). This endoscopic test is used to support the diagnosis of pseudomembranous colitis. Also, through this test, good specimens can be obtained for clostridial toxin testing.

Stool Culture (p. 883). This study is performed to identify pathogenic bacteria growing within the bowel.

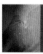
Fecal Fat (Fat Absorption, Quantitative Stool Fat Determination)

NORMAL FINDINGS

Timed Collection:
Fat: ≥ 18 years **7–21 mmol/day** (2–6 g/24 hr)
Reference values have not been established for patients who are <18 years of age.
Random collection:
All ages: 0%–19% fat

INDICATIONS

This test is performed to confirm the diagnosis of steatorrhea. Steatorrhea is suspected when stool is large, greasy, and foul smelling. The finding of an abnormally high fecal fat content confirms the diagnosis.

Stool Tests

9

TEST EXPLANATION

The fecal fat test measures the fat content in the stool. This qualitative or quantitative test is performed to confirm the diagnosis of steatorrhea. Steatorrhea occurs when fat content in the stool is high. Short-gut syndrome and any condition that may cause malabsorption (e.g., sprue, Crohn's disease, Whipple's disease) or maldigestion (e.g., bile duct obstruction, pancreatic duct obstruction secondary to tumour or gallstones) are also associated with increased fecal fat.

Neutral fats include the monoglycerides, diglycerides, and triglycerides, whereas split fats are the free fatty acids that are liberated from them. Maldigestion (impaired synthesis or secretion of pancreatic enzymes or bile) may cause an increase in neutral fats, whereas an increase in split fats suggests malabsorption.

The total output of fecal fat can be tested on a random stool specimen but is more accurate when total 24-, 48-, or 72-hour collection is carried out. Abnormal results from a random specimen should be confirmed by submission of a timed collection. Test values for random fecal fat collections are reported in terms of percentage of fat.

INTERFERING FACTORS

▮ Drugs that may *increase* levels of fecal fat include enemas and laxatives, especially mineral oil, and diaper rash ointments.

▮ Drugs that may *decrease* levels of fecal fat include barium and fibre laxatives or supplements.

Age-Related Concerns

- Children with cystic fibrosis have mucus plugs that obstruct the pancreatic ducts. This prevents fat absorption (malabsorption).
- A fat-retention coefficient (described in the "Procedure and Patient Care" section) is used in infants and children to determine the difference between ingested fat and fecal fat.
- The fat-retention coefficient should be at least 95%. A low value indicates steatorrhea.
- Age-related changes in the small intestine of adults older than 65 years may include atrophy of the intestinal muscle and thinning of villi. This may result in a decrease of the absorption of fats, which contributes to the increase in the secretion of fecal fats.

PROCEDURE AND PATIENT CARE

Before

✗ Explain the procedure to the patient.

✗ Give the patient instructions regarding the appropriate diet (a diet diary may be requested by the laboratory):

1. For adults (>18 years), usually 100 g of fat per day is suggested for 3 days before and throughout the collection period.

2. Children (<18 years), and especially infants (<1 year), cannot ingest 100 g of fat. Therefore, a *fat-retention coefficient* is determined by measuring the difference between ingested fat and fecal fat and then expressing that difference (the amount of fat retained) as a percentage of the ingested fat:

$$\left[(\text{Ingested fat} - \text{Fecal fat}) \div \text{Ingested fat}\right] \times 100\% = \text{Fat-retention coefficient}$$

- Note that the fat-retention coefficient in normal children and adults is 95% or greater. A low value indicates steatorrhea.
- Instruct the patient to defecate into a dry, clean container. On occasion, a tongue blade is required to transfer the stool to the specimen container.
- Instruct the patient not to urinate into the stool container.
- Inform the patient that even diarrheal stools should be collected.
- Instruct the patient not to mix urine or toilet paper with the stool specimen.
- Instruct the patient not to take any laxatives or enemas during this test because they will interfere with intestinal motility and alter test results.

During

- Collect each stool specimen and send it immediately to the laboratory during the 24- to 72-hour testing period.
- Label each specimen and include the time and date of collection.
- If the specimen is collected at home, give the patient a large stool container to keep in the freezer.

After

- Inform the patient that a normal diet can be resumed.

TEST RESULTS AND CLINICAL SIGNIFICANCE

▲ Increased Levels

Cystic fibrosis: *Affected patients experience maldigestion of fat because their pancreatic function is poor. They cannot absorb fat from the gut. As a result, they have steatorrhea.*

Malabsorption secondary to sprue, celiac disease, Whipple's disease, Crohn's disease (regional enteritis), or radiation enteritis: *The absorptive capability of the stool is markedly reduced. Transit time is markedly decreased. As a result of these changes, fat is not absorbed. Steatorrhea results.*

Maldigestion secondary to obstruction of the pancreatobiliary tree (e.g., cancer, stricture, gallstones): *Exocrine secretion of the pancreatobiliary tree is necessary for digestion of dietary fat. When disease affects these organs, steatorrhea results.*

Short-gut syndrome secondary to surgical resection, surgical bypass, or congenital anomaly: *The transit time in these patients is markedly diminished. The time available for digestion and absorption of fat is inadequate. Steatorrhea results.*

RELATED TEST

D-Xylose Absorption (p. 555). This test is used to evaluate the absorptive capability of the intestines. It is used in the evaluation of patients with suspected malabsorption.

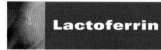

Lactoferrin

NORMAL FINDINGS

None detected

INDICATIONS

Lactoferrin is used to diagnose inflammatory bowel diseases such as ulcerative colitis or Crohn's disease. It is also used as a screening test to determine the possibility of bacterial colitis.

Stool Tests

9

TEST EXPLANATION

Lactoferrin is a glycoprotein expressed by activated neutrophils. The detection of lactoferrin in a fecal sample therefore serves as a surrogate marker for inflammatory white blood cells (WBCs) in the intestinal tract. WBCs in the stool are not stable and may be easily destroyed by temperature changes, delays in testing, and toxins within the stool. As a result, WBCs may not be detected by common microscopic methods. Lactoferrin assay has allowed the identification of inflammatory cells in the stool without the use of microscopy.

Detection of fecal lactoferrin allows for the differentiation of inflammatory and noninflammatory intestinal disorders in patients with diarrhea. Usually the test is used as a diagnostic aid to help identify patients with active inflammatory bowel disease (such as Crohn's disease or ulcerative colitis) and rule out those with active irritable bowel syndrome, which is noninflammatory. Lactoferrin is also present in patients with bacterial enteritis such as *Shigella, Salmonella, Campylobacter jejuni,* and *Clostridium difficile*. Diarrhea caused by viruses and most parasites is not associated with elevated lactoferrin levels. Lactoferrin testing is often used as a screening test for patients who may have bacterial enteritis. If the stool is negative for lactoferrin, it is unlikely that a stool culture will be positive.

The lactoferrin analyte may be qualitatively detected by two distinct methods: (1) a latex agglutination procedure (the most commonly used) and (2) a microwell enzyme immunoassay procedure. The former method has been used primarily in the evaluation of patients with diagnoses of bacterial infectious gastroenteritis, while the latter method has been developed primarily as a diagnostic aid to distinguish between active inflammatory bowel disease and active noninflammatory irritable bowel syndrome.

INTERFERING FACTORS

- Delays in testing can interfere with test results: The stool specimen should be examined immediately. In some instances a specific stool preservative–enteric transport media (Cary-Blair) can be used.
- Breast-feeding can affect test results: Because lactoferrin is a component of human breast milk, the test will be positive in breast-fed children and should not be used to evaluate neonates receiving breast milk. However, the test uses a human lactoferrin–specific antibody that does not cross-react with lactoferrin in cow's milk.

PROCEDURE AND PATIENT CARE

Before
- Explain the procedure to the patient.
- Instruct the patient not to mix urine or toilet paper with the specimen.

During
- Stool is collected in a clean bedpan.
- Place at least 5 g of stool in a clean specimen container.

After
- Observe appropriate contamination precautions.
- Transfer the specimen to the laboratory immediately.
- Inform the patient that results are available in less than half an hour.

TEST RESULTS AND CLINICAL SIGNIFICANCE

Bacterial enteritis,

Acute Crohn's disease,

Acute ulcerative colitis: *Each of these diseases is associated with an inflammatory immune response of WBCs causing positive lactoferrin results.*

RELATED TESTS

Stool Culture (p. 883). This test is used to identify the cause of bacterial enteritis.

Colonoscopy (p. 619). This is a commonly performed test to identify inflammatory bowel diseases such as ulcerative colitis and Crohn's disease.

Stool Culture (Stool for Culture and Sensitivity [Stool C&S], Stool for Ova and Parasites [O&P])

NORMAL FINDINGS

Normal intestinal flora

No ova or parasite infestation

INDICATIONS

Stool cultures are indicated in patients who have unrelenting diarrhea, fever, and abdominal bloating. The index of suspicion is especially high if the patient has been drinking well water, has been receiving a prolonged course of antibiotics, or has travelled to underdeveloped countries where clean and safe drinking water may not be accessible.

TEST EXPLANATION

Normally, stool contains many bacteria and fungi. The more common bacteria include *Enterococcus* organisms, *Escherichia coli*, *Proteus* organisms, *Pseudomonas* organisms, *Staphylococcus aureus*, *Candida albicans*, *Bacteroides* organisms, and *Clostridium* organisms. Bacteria are indigenous to the bowel; however, several bacteria act as pathogens within the bowel. These include pathogenic *E. coli* and *Salmonella, Shigella, Campylobacter, Yersinia, Clostridium,* and *Staphylococcus* species.

Parasites also may affect the stool. Common parasites are *Ascaris* (hookworm), *Strongyloides* (tapeworm), *Giardia* (protozoans), and *Cryptosporidium* (especially in patients with acquired immune deficiency syndrome [AIDS]). Identification of any of these pathogens in the stool incriminates that organism as the cause of the infectious enteritis.

Sometimes the normal stool flora can become pathogenic if overgrowth of the bacteria occurs as a result of antibiotic use (e.g., *C. difficile* as the source of toxin in pseudomembranous colitis), immunosuppression, or overaggressive catharsis. *Helicobacter pylori* can be found in the stool but indicates an increased risk for peptic ulcer disease and gastritis. Usually, however, this is better cultured from the stomach or determined by a serologic test on the blood.

Infections of the bowel from bacteria, virus, or parasites usually manifest with acute diarrhea, excessive flatus, abdominal discomfort, and fever. This situation may progress to toxic megacolon.

INTERFERING FACTORS

- Urine may inhibit the growth of bacteria. Therefore, urine should not be mixed with the feces during collection of a stool sample.
- Recent barium studies may obscure the detection of parasites.
- Drugs that may affect test results include antibiotics, bismuth, and mineral oil.

PROCEDURE AND PATIENT CARE

Before

 Explain the method of stool collection to the patient. Reassure the patient of the reasons for the test, and answer any questions as necessary.

 Instruct the patient not to mix urine or toilet paper with the stool specimen.

 Instruct the patient to use an appropriate collection container.

> ✓ **Clinical Priorities**
>
> - Stool cultures are usually performed for patients with unrelenting diarrhea, fever, and abdominal bloating.
> - The normal stool flora can become pathogenic if bacterial overgrowth occurs as a result of antibiotics, immunosuppression, or excessive catharsis.
> - Observe universal or standard precautions/routine practices when handling stool specimens.

During

 Instruct the patient to defecate into a clean bedpan.

- Place a small amount of stool in a sterile collection container.
- Send mucus and blood streaks with the specimen.
- If a rectal swab is to be used, observe universal or standard precautions/routine practices and insert the cotton-tipped swab at least 2.5 cm (1 inch) into the anal canal. Then rotate the swab for 30 seconds and place it in the clean container.

Tape Test

- Use this test when pinworms (*Enterobius*) are suspected.
- Place a strip of clear tape in the patient's perianal region. (This is especially helpful in children.)
- Because the female worm lays her eggs at night around the perianal area, apply the tape before bedtime and remove it in the morning before the patient gets out of bed.
- Press the sticky surface of the tape directly to a glass slide and examine it microscopically for pinworm ova.

After

- Observe universal or standard precautions/routine practices when handling stool specimens.
- Promptly send the stool specimen to the laboratory. Delays in transfer of the specimen may affect viability of the organism. If long delays are necessary, obtain a buffered glycerol-saline solution to be combined with the stool and used as a preservative.
- Note that some enteric pathogens may take as long as 6 weeks to isolate.
- When pathogens are detected, maintain isolation of the patient's stool until therapy is completed. Other individuals who have had close contact with the patient should be tested and treated to prevent spread of the infection.

TEST RESULTS AND CLINICAL SIGNIFICANCE

Bacterial enterocolitis,

Protozoan enterocolitis,

Parasitic enterocolitis: *These organisms can be grown on special culture plates. The parasites can also be detected on smear of the stool. Treatment of these infections must be prompt, especially in children, who can dehydrate rapidly and become septic.*

RELATED TEST

Clostridial Toxin Assay (p. 877). This test confirms the diagnosis of pseudomembranous colitis on basis of the presence of *C. difficile.*

 Stool for Occult Blood (Stool for OB, Fecal Occult Blood Test [FOBT], Fecal Immunotest [FIT], DNA Stool Sample)

NORMAL FINDINGS

No occult blood within stool

INDICATIONS

This test is used for colorectal cancer screening of asymptomatic individuals. It can also detect occult blood from other causes (e.g., ulcers, hemorrhoids, diverticulosis).

TEST EXPLANATION

Normally, only minimal quantities (2 to 2.5 mL) of blood are passed into the gastrointestinal tract. This bleeding is usually not significant enough to cause a positive result in stool for occult blood testing. This test can detect occult blood when as little as 5 mL of blood is lost per day.

Tumours of the intestine grow into the lumen and are subjected to repeated trauma by the fecal stream. Eventually, the friable neovascular tumour ulcerates, and bleeding occurs. Most often, bleeding is so slight that gross blood is not seen in the stool. The blood can be detected by chemical assay or by immunohistochemistry. Guaiac is the most commonly performed chemical assay. The peroxidase-like activity of hemoglobin catalyzes the reaction of peroxide and a chromogen called *orthotoluidine* to form blue-stained oxidized orthotoluidine.

Occult blood can also be detected by immunochemical methods that detect the human globin portion of hemoglobin using monoclonal antibodies. These tests are called the *fecal immunochemical test* or *immunochemical fecal occult blood test* (FOBT). These methods are as sensitive as guaiac testing but are not affected by red meats or plant oxidizers as described in the "Interfering Factors" section. Immunochemical methods may fail to recognize occult blood from the upper gastrointestinal tract because the globin is digested by the time it gets in the stool.

The *DNA stool sample* test is more sensitive than guaiac testing in the detection of significant colorectal precancerous, benign, and malignant tumours. Because most precancerous polyps do not bleed, they can be missed by FOBT. In contrast, all precancerous polyps shed cells that contain abnormal DNA. Thus, a stool-based DNA test designed to detect this DNA holds promise of being more accurate in the detection of precancerous polyps—which, when detected, can be removed before they turn into cancer.

Stool Tests

9

TABLE 9-1	Testing Options for Colorectal Cancer*
Test	**Frequency**
Fecal occult blood test (FOBT or FIT)	Every year
Flexible sigmoidoscopy	Every 5 years
Double-contrast barium enema	Every 5 years
Colonoscopy†	Every 10 years
Virtual colonoscopy	Every 10 years

*(See Table 4-3, p. 620, colonoscopy, p. 619). People at higher risk of developing colorectal cancer should begin screening at a younger age, and may need to be tested more frequently.
†Colonoscopy can be used as a follow-up diagnostic tool when the results of another screening test are positive.

Benign and malignant gastrointestinal tumours, ulcers, inflammatory bowel disease, arteriovenous malformations, diverticulosis, and hematobilia (hemobilia) can all cause occult blood within the stool. Other more common abnormalities (e.g., hemorrhoids, swallowed blood from oral or nasopharyngeal bleeding) may also cause occult blood within the stool.

When occult blood testing is properly performed, multiple specimens are collected on successive days; a positive result warrants a thorough gastrointestinal evaluation—usually esophagogastroduodenoscopy (see p. 636) and colonoscopy (see p. 619). Regular screening, beginning at age 50, can reduce the number of people who die from colorectal cancer by as much as 60%. There are several tests used for colorectal cancer screening (Table 9-1). Yet despite the availability of such screening tools, more than half of Canadian adults have never undergone colorectal cancer screening. This fact highlights the need for more user-friendly testing methods such as stool DNA testing.

♣ The Canadian Cancer Society recommends that all men and women older than 50 years have a FOBT or a fecal immunochemical test at least every 2 years. Routine screening, beginning at 50 years of age, can significantly reduce the number of deaths from colorectal cancer. Several other tests are used for colorectal cancer screening once a positive FOBT result, a positive fecal immunochemical test result, or both are established (see Table 4-3, p. 620).

INTERFERING FACTORS

- Reducing or oxidizing agents (such as iron, radish, cantaloupe or cauliflower, and vitamin C) can affect the results of guaiac or fecal immunochemical test (FIT).
- Vigorous exercise.
- Bleeding gums following a dental procedure or disease may affect results.
- The animal hemoglobin of ingested animal meat may instigate the guaiac peroxidation process and cause false-positive results. In most cases, even with the ingestion of 8 oz (227 g) of cooked red meat per day, guaiac reactions remain negative.
- Ingestion of peroxidase-rich vegetables (turnips, horseradish, artichokes, mushrooms, radishes, broccoli, bean sprouts, cauliflower, oranges, bananas, cantaloupes, and grapes) may affect results.
- Drugs that may cause gastrointestinal bleeding include anticoagulants, aspirin, colchicine, iron preparations (large doses), nonsteroidal antiarthritics, and steroids. Although these drugs do not interfere with the performance of the test, they can cause GI bleeding not associated with pathology.
- Drugs that may instigate the peroxidation reaction and cause false-positive results include boric acid, bromides, colchicine, iodine, iron, and *Rauwolfia* derivatives.
- Vitamin C may cause false-negative results by inhibiting the peroxidation reaction.

Clinical Priorities

- This test is part of the routine colorectal cancer screening performed in individuals older than 50 years.
- Patients must avoid red meats for 3 days before the test. Otherwise, false-positive results could be obtained because red meats contain animal hemoglobin.
- Positive test results for occult blood indicate the need for a thorough gastrointestinal evaluation.

PROCEDURE AND PATIENT CARE

Before

✗ Explain the procedure to the patient.

✗ Instruct the patient to refrain from eating any red meat for at least 3 days before the test.

✗ Instruct the patient to refrain from taking drugs known to interfere with occult blood testing.

✗ Instruct the patient to collect a sample of stool by placing a sheet of plastic wrap loosely across the toilet bowl to catch the stool, or use a dry container to collect the stool.

✗ Instruct the patient in the method of obtaining appropriate stool specimens. Many procedures are available (e.g., specimen cards, tissue wipes, test paper). Specimens may be obtained at home with specimen cards (e.g., Heme-Screen, Hemoccult) and mailed to a local testing laboratory or physician's office when collected (Figure 9-1).

✗ Instruct the patient not to let the stool specimen mix with urine or toilet paper.

✗ Instruct the patient that multiple specimens must be obtained on separate days to increase the test's accuracy.

- Note that in some centres, a high-residue diet is recommended to increase the abrasive effect of the stool.
- Be gentle in obtaining stool by digital rectal examination. Traumatic digital examination can cause a false-positive result, especially in patients with prior anorectal disease such as hemorrhoids.

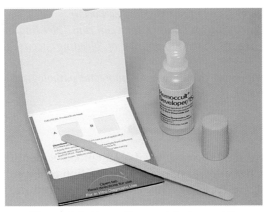

Figure 9-1 Heme-Screen take-home kit.

Stool Tests

9

During

Hemoccult Slide Test

1. Place stool samples on one side of guaiac paper. Stool samples should be from two different areas of the specimen.
2. Place two drops of developer on the other side.
3. Note that a bluish discoloration indicates occult blood in the stool.

Tablet Test

1. Place a stool sample on the test paper.
2. Place a tablet on top of the stool specimen.
3. Put two or three drops of tap water on the tablet and allow to flow onto the paper.
4. Note that a bluish discoloration indicates occult blood in the stool.

After

⚕ Inform the patient of the results.

⚕ If the test results are positive, inquire whether the patient violated any of the preparation recommendations.

TEST RESULTS AND CLINICAL SIGNIFICANCE

Gastrointestinal tumour (cancers and polyps): *The mucosa overlying neoplasm is friable. Bleeding occurs when stool passes by.*

Gastrointestinal bleeding: *With lower gastrointestinal hemorrhage, occult blood can be present in the stool. The presence of blood in the stool is a concern because in the gastrointestinal tract, blood is broken down into ammonia. Elevations in blood ammonia levels can result in manifestations of hepatic encephalopathy, which are primarily neurologic and range from mild confusion to deep coma.*

Peptic diseases (esophagitis, gastritis, and ulceration): *In peptic disease, the mucosa becomes inflamed, thickened, and friable. Bleeding easily occurs. Ulcers can erode into blood vessels within the wall of the gut.*

Varices: *Caused by portal hypertension, these large venous complexes are covered by a thin lining of mucosa. With increased intra-abdominal pressure, varices can rupture and bleed.*

Inflammatory bowel disease (ulcerative colitis, Crohn's disease): *The inflammatory reaction causes the mucosa to become thickened and friable, which causes bleeding.*

Ischemic bowel disease: *The mucosa of the bowel is the first layer to be affected by diminished blood supply. This mucosa easily sloughs, and minor bleeding can occur.*

Gastrointestinal trauma: *Penetrating or blunt trauma can cause bleeding into the gut.*

Recent gastrointestinal surgery: *Small amounts of bleeding occur at the new gastrointestinal anastomosis.*

Hemorrhoids and other anorectal problems: *An anorectal pathologic condition is the most common nonneoplastic cause of blood in the stool.*

RELATED TESTS

The following tests are performed successively if occult blood is identified on multiple specimens:

Colonoscopy (p. 619). This test allows endoscopic evaluation of the entire colon.

Esophagogastroduodenoscopy (p. 636). This endoscopic procedure visualizes the esophagus, stomach, and duodenum.

Barium Enema (p. 1033). In this test, barium is used to provide radiographic visualization of the colon.

Upper Gastrointestinal Tract Radiography (p. 1117). In this test, barium is used to provide radiographic visualization of the upper gastrointestinal tract.

Small Bowel Follow-Through (p. 1109). In this test, barium is used to provide radiographic visualization of the small intestines.

Stool Tests

9

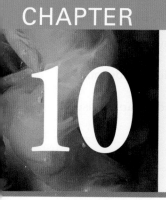

CHAPTER 10

Ultrasound Studies

NOTE: *Throughout this chapter, SI units are presented in* **boldface colour,** *followed by conventional units in parentheses.*

OVERVIEW

TESTS

OVERVIEW

Ultrasonography is a diagnostic technique in which high-frequency sound waves (ultrasonic waves) are directed at internal body structures, and a record is made of the wave pulses as they are reflected back (echoed) through the tissues. Solid and cystic structures have different acoustic densities, which thereby form an "image" of the organ being studied.

REASONS FOR PERFORMING ULTRASOUND STUDIES

Ultrasonography is performed for the following reasons:
1. To determine whether a lump or other abnormality is a fluid-filled cyst or a solid tumour (e.g., kidney, thyroid, breast lesions)
2. To guide needle-directed biopsy of a suspected tumour site to establish a diagnosis (e.g., prostate or breast cancer)
3. To stage a tumour (e.g., esophageal, rectal, or breast cancer)
4. To evaluate pregnancy and placental status
5. To detect ectopic pregnancy
6. To determine fetal status, size, and growth
7. To evaluate disorders of arteries (e.g., aneurysm) and veins (e.g., deep-vein thrombosis)

PRINCIPLES OF ULTRASONOGRAPHY

Tissues of different composition reflect sound waves differently, which enables differentiation of normal and diseased tissue. Sound waves are transmitted well through fluid but not through air, bone, or contrast media (e.g., barium).

The advantages of ultrasonography are that it is noninvasive and requires no ionizing radiation. Therefore, repeated studies can be performed and multiple images obtained with no risk. Because no radiation exposure occurs, ultrasonography can be performed in a physician's office, in a laboratory, or at the patient's bedside. Ultrasonography is less expensive than either computed tomography or magnetic resonance imaging.

Ultrasonography is painless. The skin overlying the body area to be evaluated (e.g., heart, gallbladder) is covered with a lubricating gel to provide an air-free barrier between the skin and the ultrasonographic probe, which contains a transducer. The probe is passed over the specific body area, and ultrasonic waves, with frequencies in a range above human hearing, are transmitted through the tissues. The transducer converts the echoes to electric impulses and transforms them into visual images, or sonograms, which can be viewed singly (like a photograph) or in rapid sequence (like a movie) to evaluate the data obtained. Light (hyperechoic) or dark (hypoechoic) areas seen on a sonogram are a result of the manner in which various tissues reflect ultrasonic waves.

In some types of ultrasonography, the probe (transducer) is placed within the body. For example, in transesophageal echocardiography, the transducer is incorporated in the tip of a fibreoptic endoscope, which is placed in the esophagus, behind the heart; in rectal or prostate ultrasonography, the transducer is introduced through the anus into the rectum; and during surgery, the transducer can be held directly on the organ to be evaluated (e.g., the liver).

Various scans and techniques can be used to display the ultrasonic echoes. Some of these are as follows:
1. *B-scan:* A B-scan image is made up of a series of dots, each indicating a single ultrasonic echo. The position of a dot corresponds to the time elapsed, and the brightness of a dot corresponds to the strength of the echo. Movement of the transducer over the skin yields a two-dimensional cross-sectional image (Figure 10-1).
2. *M-mode scan:* An image obtained with M-mode echocardiography shows the motion (M) of the heart over time.
3. *Real-time imaging:* Multiple transducers are used to display a rapid sequence of data that can be instantaneously converted into accurate anatomic images of the organ being evaluated.
4. *Doppler ultrasonography:* As opposed to static ultrasonography, in which the sound wave returning to the transducer is the same frequency as that which was emitted, Doppler ultrasonography is a different technique. In Doppler ultrasonography of blood vessels, the red blood

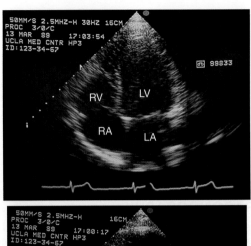

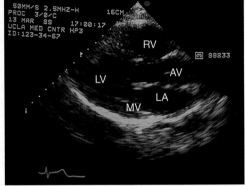

Figure 10-1 Two-dimensional echocardiogram. *AV,* aortic valve; *LA,* left atrium; *LV,* left ventricle; *MV,* mitral valve; *RA,* right atrium; *RV,* right ventricle.

cells (RBCs) within the vessel distort the frequency of the ultrasound waves. The change in frequency of the ultrasound wave is proportional to the velocity of the RBCs. The better the blood flow, the faster the RBCs move by the stationary ultrasound beam and the greater the frequency distortion (or Doppler shift). With this technique, sound waves are transformed into audible sounds or linear graphic recordings. This is important for assessing blood flow through arteries and veins. It is also used in pregnant women to assess the fetal heart rate and with increasing frequency to determine blood flow to organs (e.g., kidneys, testicles).

5. *Colour flow Doppler imaging:* This imaging technique is used to determine direction (recorded as colours) and velocity (shades) of blood flow in the chambers of the heart (Figure 10-2). This technique is important in evaluating heart valve regurgitation and blood shunting in patients with heart defects.

6. *Duplex scanning:* This technique is a combination of real-time imaging and colour flow Doppler imaging to demonstrate how the arteries and veins are functioning and velocity and turbulence within the vessels. Duplex scanning is useful in detecting plaque within arteries, demonstrating aneurysms, and assessing renal or liver transplants for rejection.

7. *Three-dimensional (3D) ultrasound:* This imaging technique is often used during pregnancy to provide 3D images of the fetus. The common obstetric mode is 2D. In 3D fetal scanning, a computer program can construct a 3D image of the fetus that is more realistic than 2D imaging (Figure 10-3). Four-dimensional (4D) shows a 3D picture in real time (e.g., can see fetus moving).

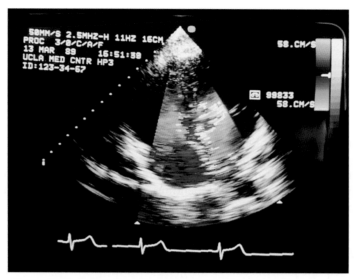

Figure 10-2 Colour flow Doppler echocardiography. Flow, or signals, moving toward the transducer are recorded in shades of yellow and red, and those moving away from the transducer are recorded as blue.

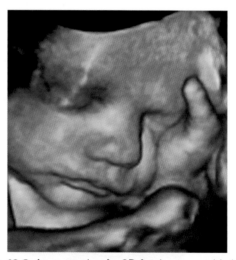

Figure 10-3 An example of a 3D fetal sonographic image.

Ultrasonography is often used in conjunction with other diagnostic testing. For example, if a computed tomographic scan of the kidney demonstrates a filling defect, an ultrasound scan can indicate whether that defect is a benign fluid-filled cyst or a malignant solid tumour.

PROCEDURAL CARE FOR ULTRASONOGRAPHY
Before

- Refer to agency guidelines and protocols for specific ultrasound tests.
- Most ultrasound procedures require little or no preparation. However, patients undergoing pelvic scanning must have a full bladder, which may become uncomfortable. Patients

10 Ultrasound Studies

undergoing ultrasound examination of the gallbladder should be fasting to avoid the gallbladder contraction that usually follows ingestion of a meal. A contracted gallbladder is difficult to identify with ultrasonography.
- The patient's informed consent is needed if the transducer will be inserted into a body cavity or if an ultrasonography-directed biopsy is planned.

During
- Ultrasound examinations are usually performed in an ultrasonography suite (Figure 10-4) but can be performed on the patient's unit or in a physician's office.
- A gel lubricant is applied to the tissue overlying the organ to be studied. Air impedes transmission of sound waves, and this lubricant ensures good contact between the skin and the transducer. Different probes are used depending on the area being evaluated (Figure 10-5). Thus sound transmission and reception are enhanced.

After
- Because ultrasonography is noninvasive, no special nursing measures are needed after the study except to help the patient remove the gel lubricant.
- Ultrasound examinations can be repeated as often as necessary without harm to the patient. No cumulative effects have been noted.

INTERFERING FACTORS
- Air impedes transmission of ultrasonic waves into the body. The use of a lubricant is essential to ensure good transmission of sound waves to and from the body.

ESSENTIAL CONSIDERATIONS FOR AN ULTRASOUND ROOM

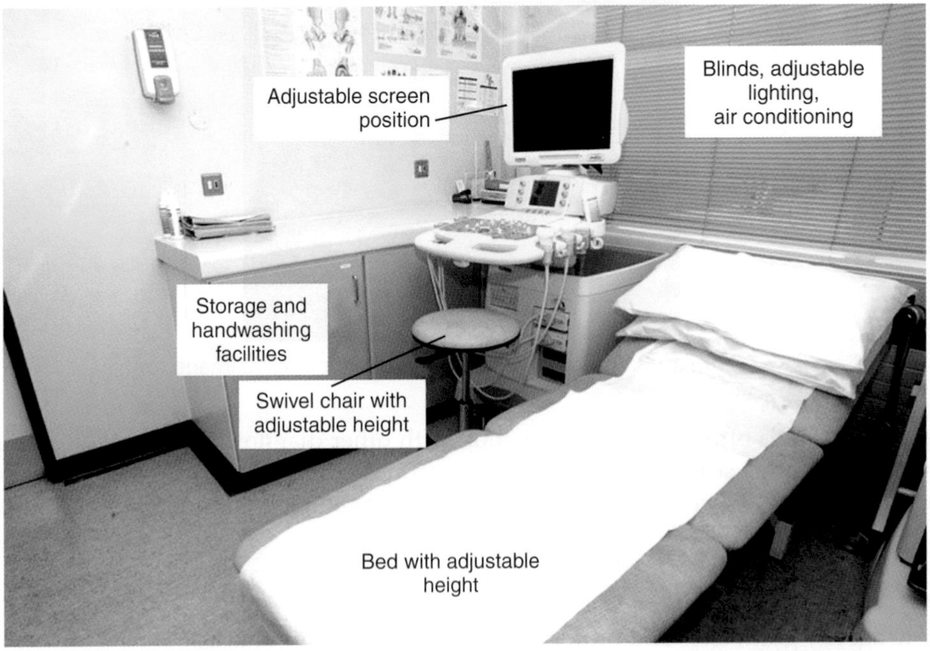

Adjustable screen position

Blinds, adjustable lighting, air conditioning

Storage and handwashing facilities

Swivel chair with adjustable height

Bed with adjustable height

Figure 10-4 Ultrasonography room.

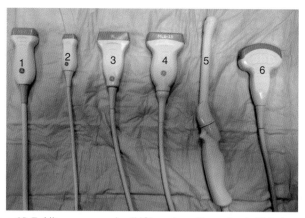

Figure 10-5 Ultrasonography (US) probes (from the left) 1, low frequency sector probe used for abdominal US; 2, high-frequency sector probe used for infant US and intraoperative brain surgery US; 3, linear probe used for vascular US; 4, high-frequency linear probe used for superficial structures such as thyroid, scrotum, or breast; 5, intracavitary probe used for vaginal/rectal US; 6, general low-frequency probe used for abdominal US.

- Barium blocks transmission of ultrasonic waves. For this reason, ultrasonography of the abdomen should be performed before any barium contrast studies.
- Large amounts of gas in the bowel distort visualization of abdominal organs, because bowel gas reflects sound. Likewise, ultrasonic evaluation of the lungs yields poor results.
- Obesity may affect the results of the study because sound waves are altered by fatty tissue. For this reason, it may be difficult to obtain an accurate scan in an obese patient.
- Movement causes artifacts. Some patients may need to be sedated to remain still. Uncooperative patients (especially children) may not be candidates for ultrasonography.
- Because ultrasonography requires direct contact between the transducer and the skin, it may not be possible to perform this study in postoperative patients with dressings.
- The quality of the ultrasound image and the sufficiency of the study depend to a large extent on the abilities of the ultrasound technician performing the study.

POTENTIAL COMPLICATIONS

No potential complications have been directly related to ultrasonography at the intensities used for medical diagnosis. However, in some procedures (e.g., transesophageal echocardiography), complications may occur as a result of the invasive method used to place the ultrasound probe inside the body. These complications are described for individual tests.

REPORTING OF RESULTS

The patient can usually observe the scan on a monitor in the room. The technician may point out some aspects of the scan, however; the physician reviews the scan and explains the results to the patient. Printouts of the ultrasound image can be obtained if requested.

Abdominal Ultrasonography (Abdominal Sonography; Echography; Ultrasonography of the Kidney, Liver, Pancreatobiliary System, Gallbladder, Pancreas, Biliary Tree)

NORMAL FINDINGS

Normal abdominal aorta, liver, gallbladder, bile ducts, pancreas, kidney, and bladder

INDICATIONS

This technique is used to visualize the abdomen and the organs within it. It has a number of uses, as described in Table 10-1.

TEST EXPLANATION

Through use of reflected sound waves, ultrasonography provides accurate visualization of the abdominal aorta, liver, gallbladder, pancreas, bile ducts, spleen, kidneys, and bladder. In ultrasonography, high-frequency sound waves are emitted from the transducer to penetrate the organ being studied. The sound waves are bounced back to the transducer and electronically converted to a pictorial image that is recorded. Real-time ultrasonography provides an accurate picture of the organ being studied. Doppler ultrasonography provides information about blood flow to those organs.

The *kidney* (Figure 10-6) is evaluated ultrasonographically for the following reasons:
1. Diagnose and locate renal cysts
2. Differentiate renal cysts from solid renal tumours
3. Demonstrate renal and pelvic calculi
4. Document hydronephrosis
5. Guide a percutaneously inserted needle for cyst aspiration, biopsy, or nephrostomy placement

Ultrasonography of the urologic tract is used to detect malformed or ectopic kidneys and perinephric abscesses. Renal transplantation surveillance is possible with ultrasonography. One advantage of kidney ultrasonography over intravenous pyelography (p. 1080) is that it can be performed in patients with impaired renal function, because no intravenous contrast medium is required.

Endourethral urologic ultrasonography can also be performed through a stent that has a transducer at its end. The stent probe is placed into the urethra to examine that segment for diverticula. The stent probe can then be advanced into the bladder, where the depth of a tumour into

TABLE 10-1	Overview of Abdominal Ultrasonography
Area Visualized	**Possible Findings**
Kidney	Cysts, tumours, calculi, hydronephrosis, malformations, abscess, transplant rejection
Aorta	Aneurysm
Liver	Cysts, abscess, dilated hepatic ducts, tumours
Gallbladder, extrahepatic ducts	Gallstones, polyps, dilation secondary to strictures or tumours
Pancreas	Tumours, pseudocysts, inflammation, abscess

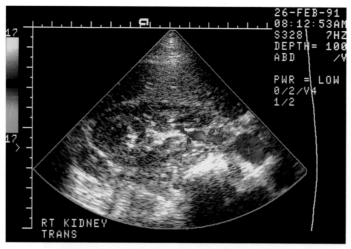

Figure 10-6 Ultrasonogram of the kidney.

the bladder wall can be measured. With the use of wire lead guidance, the stent probe can be passed into the ureter, where stones (especially those embedded in the submucosa), tumours, or extraurethral compression can be identified and localized. Finally, as the probe is advanced in the proximal ureter, renal tumours or cysts can be better delineated.

The *testes* (p. 923) can be evaluated for neoplasm, abscess, infection, inflammation, or torsion. The *prostate gland* (p. 921) can be examined for neoplasm, hypertrophy, or infection. Ultrasonography is used to guide biopsy of the prostate gland.

The abdominal aorta can be assessed for aneurysmal dilation. Sonographic evidence of an aortic aneurysm larger than 5 cm in greatest dimension, or of any aneurysm that is documented to be significantly enlarging, is an indication for resection of the abdominal aortic aneurysm. Ultrasonography is also an ideal way to monitor aneurysms before and after surgery.

Ultrasonography is used to detect cystic structures of the *liver* (e.g., benign cysts, hepatic abscesses, dilated hepatic ducts) and solid intrahepatic tumours (primary and metastatic). Hepatic ultrasonography can also be performed intraoperatively with a sterile probe. This technique allows accurate location of small, nonpalpable hepatic tumours or abscesses. The *gallbladder* and *extrahepatic ducts* can be visualized for evidence of gallstones (Figure 10-7), polyps, or dilation secondary to obstructive strictures or tumours. The *pancreas* is examined for evidence of tumour, pseudocysts, acute or chronic inflammation, or pancreatic abscess. Ultrasound scans of the pancreas are frequently repeated to document resolution of acute pancreatic inflammatory processes. Often, the pancreas is better visualized if the stomach and duodenum are filled with water.

Because ultrasonography requires no contrast material or radiation, it is especially useful in patients who are allergic to contrast media or are pregnant. Fasting is desirable but not mandatory. (See discussion of pelvic ultrasonography [p. 917] for evaluation of pelvic organs.)

INTERFERING FACTORS

- Barium and gas distort the sound waves and alter test results. This test should be performed before any radiographic testing with barium contrast.
- The quality of the results of ultrasound studies depends on the skills of the sonographer.

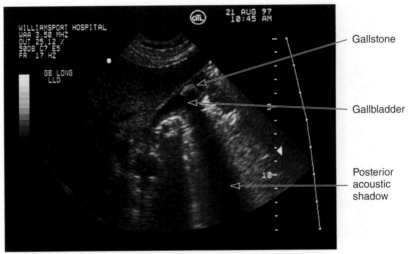

Figure 10-7 Ultrasonogram of the gallbladder. Long-axis view of the gallbladder demonstrates a gallstone. Note the posterior acoustic shadowing, typical for gallstones.

 Clinical Priorities

- Because this study requires no contrast material and no radiation, it is especially useful in patients allergic to dyes and in pregnant patients.
- The need for preprocedure fasting depends on the organ to be examined.
- Ultrasonography of the kidney can be used to evaluate rejection of a kidney transplant.

PROCEDURE AND PATIENT CARE

Before

🖎 Explain the procedure to the patient.

🖎 Assure the patient that no discomfort is associated with the procedure.

🖎 Inform the patient that fasting may or may not be required, depending on the organ to be examined. No fasting is required for ultrasonography of the abdominal aorta, kidney, liver, spleen, or pancreas, but it is preferred before ultrasonography of the gallbladder and biliary tree.

During

- Procedure:
    1. The patient is placed on the ultrasonography table in the prone or supine position, depending on the organ to be examined.
    2. A gel lubricant is applied to the patient's skin to enhance sound wave transmission and reception.
    3. A transducer is placed on the skin (Figure 10-8).
- Images are made from the reflections from the organ being studied.
- For water distension of the stomach, the patient is asked to drink 8 to 10 oz (235 to 295 mL) of water while standing.
- The test is completed in approximately 20 minutes, usually by an ultrasound technologist, and the results are interpreted by a radiologist.

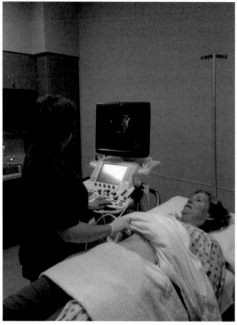

Figure 10-8 Technician performing abdominal ultrasonography.

After

- Remove the gel from the patient's skin.
- If a biopsy was performed, refer to the discussion of the specific organ (e.g., liver biopsy, kidney biopsy) for postprocedure care.

TEST RESULTS AND CLINICAL SIGNIFICANCE

Kidney

Renal cysts and polycystic kidney: *Renal cysts appear as dark (echo free, or hypoechoic) areas with smooth, well-defined walls. In polycystic kidneys, these cysts are of various sizes.*

Renal tumour: *Renal tumours appear as white (hyperechoic) areas.*

Renal calculi,

Hydronephrosis,

Ureteral obstruction: *Dilation of the collecting system is indicative of obstruction.*

Perinephric collection (e.g., perirenal abscess, perirenal hematoma): *Perirenal collections of pus or blood appear as a hypoechoic (dark) halo surrounding the kidney.*

Primary renal disease (e.g., glomerulonephritis, pyelonephritis): *Primary renal disease is evidenced by small, isoechoic kidneys, especially in end-stage disease.*

Pancreas

Tumour: *Pancreatic tumour is evident as an echogenic (solid) mass, usually in the head of the pancreas.*

Cysts or pseudocysts: *These appear as dark (hypoechoic) masses. Neoplastic cysts are difficult to differentiate from pseudocysts. Malignant cystic tumours cannot be differentiated from benign cysts.*

Abscess: *Hypoechoic (dark) areas in an inflamed pancreas could represent cysts or abscesses, which cannot be differentiated.*

Inflammation: *Acute inflammation of the pancreas has the appearance of an enlarged edematous pancreas. Chronic inflammation has the appearance of a small, contracted echogenic (dense) pancreas.*

Gallbladder

Polyps,

Tumour: *Neoplasms appear as echogenic (solid) masses in the gallbladder that do not move with changes in position.*

Gallstone: *Ultrasonography is accurate for detection of gallstones. An echogenic mass with "shadowing" behind it is the classical appearance of a gallstone.*

Liver

Tumour primary or metastatic: *The ultrasound appearance of liver metastasis is variable. In general, liver neoplasms are echogenic.*

Abscess,

Cysts: *Liver abscesses and cysts cannot be differentiated with certainty on ultrasonography.*

Bile Ducts

Gallstone,

Tumour: *Tumours and gallstones appear as echogenic masses with posterior acoustic "shadowing" within the bile duct.*

Dilation caused by stricture, stones, or tumour,

Intrahepatic dilated bile ducts: *The entire biliary tree has the appearance of a hypoechoic tube in the portal area or liver.*

Abdominal Aorta

Aneurysm: *The aorta appears as a hypoechoic tubular structure in the retroperitoneum. Aortic aneurysm is evident as a saccular dilation.*

Abdominal Cavity

Ascites: *Ultrasonography is sensitive for detection of fluid within the abdomen. As little as 10 mL of fluid can be detected.*

Abscess: *Abscesses secondary to appendicitis or diverticulitis are easily demonstrated. Phlegmon (inflammatory involvement of tissue) may surround an abscess.*

RELATED TESTS

Prostate and Rectal Ultrasonography (p. 921), Scrotal Ultrasonography (p. 923), and Pelvic Ultrasonography (p. 917). Ultrasound studies of the prostate gland, testes, uterus, and ovaries are discussed separately.

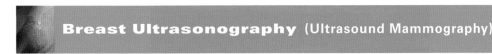

NORMAL FINDINGS
No evidence of cyst or tumour

INDICATIONS
Ultrasound examination of the breast is diagnostically performed to determine whether a mammographic abnormality or a palpable lump is a cyst (fluid-filled) or a solid tumour (benign or malignant). It is also used in screening for breast cancer for women whose breasts appear dense on mammography.

TEST EXPLANATION
In diagnostic real-time ultrasonography, harmless high-frequency sound waves penetrate the breast. The sound waves are reflected back to the sensor and arranged in a pictorial image by electronic conversion. Ultrasonography of the breast has the following uses:
1. Differentiating cystic from solid breast lesions
2. Identifying masses in women with breast tissue too dense for accurate mammography
3. Monitoring a cyst to determine whether it enlarges or disappears
4. Measuring the size of a tumour
5. Evaluating the axilla in women with newly diagnosed breast cancer

Ultrasonography is also useful for examining breasts with symptoms in women in whom the radiation of mammography is potentially harmful. Such patients include the following:
1. Pregnant women, because radiation may be harmful to the fetus
2. Women younger than 25 years, who may be at greater oncologic risk from the radiation of mammography
3. Women who refuse mammography because of fear of diagnostic radiation

With high-quality diagnostic ultrasonography, the characteristics of an abnormality can be evaluated, and a reasonable prediction can be made whether it is malignant. Characteristics of malignancy are indicated in Table 10-2. Diagnostic accuracy is improved when breast ultrasonography is combined with mammography (see p. 1086). Ultrasonography is especially useful in

TABLE 10-2	Characteristics of Ultrasound Findings: Benign Versus Malignant	
Characteristic	**Benign**	**Suspect for Malignancy**
Contents	Cystic	Solid
Effect on surrounding tissue	No interruption	Invasive
Dimensions	Wider than tall	Taller than wide
Homogeneity of contents	Homogeneous	Heterogeneous
Acoustic effects beyond the lesion	Good sound transmission (acoustic enhancement)	Poor sound transmission (acoustic attenuation)

Ultrasound Studies 10

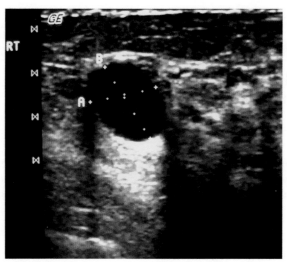

Figure 10-9 Ultrasonography of the breast, demonstrating a simple cyst of the breast measuring 1.14× 0.94 cm.

patients with an abnormal mass identified on a mammogram because the nature (cystic or solid) of the mass can be determined. Most cysts are benign (Figure 10-9).

Ultrasonography can be used to locate and accurately direct percutaneous biopsy probes to a nonpalpable breast abnormality for biopsy or aspiration. Ultrasonography is painless and harmless and has no radiation effects on the breast tissue.

PROCEDURE AND PATIENT CARE

Before

- Explain the procedure to the patient, and assure the patient that no discomfort is associated with the examination.
- Inform the patient that no fasting or sedation is required. Instruct the patient not to apply any lotions or powders to the breasts on the examination day.

During

- The patient is placed in the supine position, a gel lubricant is applied, and a handheld transducer is placed directly on the skin overlying the breast (Figure 10-10).
- The test is performed in approximately 15 minutes by an ultrasound technician.

After

- After the test is completed, the gel lubricant is removed.

TEST RESULTS AND CLINICAL SIGNIFICANCE

Cyst: *These are apparent as very dark (hypoechoic), well-circumscribed abnormalities with posterior acoustic enhancement. They are benign, and no intervention is required unless they are symptomatic.*
Hematoma,
Abscess,
Cancer: *These appear as hypoechoic (dark), poorly circumscribed masses with acoustic "shadowing" behind the back wall of the mass.*

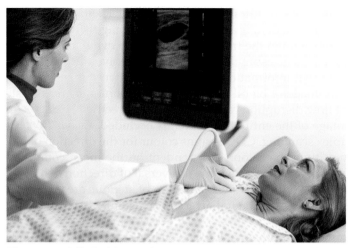

Figure 10-10 Technician performing ultrasonography of the breast.

Fibroadenoma: *These appear as hypoechoic (dark) well-circumscribed lesions within the breast acoustic "enhancement" behind the back wall.*

Fibrocystic disease: *This is evident as diffuse, echogenic, localized tissue within the breast.*

RELATED TESTS

Mammography (p. 1086). This radiographic study of the breast can detect breast abnormalities but cannot differentiate between cystic and solid masses as ultrasonography can.

Magnetic Resonance Imaging (p. 1148). MRI is very sensitive in detecting abnormalities in the breast.

Carotid Artery Duplex Scanning (Carotid Ultrasonography)

NORMAL FINDINGS

Carotid artery free of plaques and stenosis

INDICATIONS

This Doppler ultrasound test is performed to identify occlusive disease in the carotid artery or its branches. It is recommended in patients with peripheral vascular disease and neurologic symptoms such as transient ischemic attacks, hemiparesis, paraesthesia, dizziness, syncope, or acute speech or visual deficits. It is also used on patients who have no symptoms but are found to have a carotid bruit.

TEST EXPLANATION

Carotid duplex scanning is a noninvasive, ultrasound test used to directly detect occlusive disease of the vertebral and extracranial carotid artery. It is called *duplex* because it combines the benefits of two methods of ultrasonography: Doppler and B-mode techniques. With the use of the transducer, a B-mode ultrasound grey-scale image of the carotid vessel is obtained. A pulsed Doppler probe within the transducer is used to evaluate blood flow velocity and direction in the artery and to measure the amplitude and waveform of the carotid arterial pulse. A computer combines that information and provides a two-dimensional image of the carotid artery, along with an image of blood flow. With this technique, areas of stenotic or occluded arteries and arterial flow disruption can be visualized directly. The degree of occlusion is measured as the percentage of the entire lumen that is occluded. *Colour Doppler Ultrasound (CDU)* can be added to duplex scanning. CDU assigns colour for the direction of blood flow within the vessel, and the intensity of the colour is dependent on the mean computed velocity of blood travelling in the vessel. By showing slowing or reversal of direction of blood flow at a particular area of the artery, this method allows visualization of stenotic areas. Reversal of blood flow is sometimes associated with contralateral arterial occlusion, which can be easily demonstrated with this technique.

This test is performed in approximately 15 to 30 minutes by an ultrasound technologist in the ultrasonography or radiology department. Results are interpreted by a radiologist, usually the same day. No discomfort is associated with the test. The accuracy of this test is limited by the skill of the technologists.

Measurement of the thickness of the wall of the carotid artery (*carotid intimal–medial thickness [CIMT]*) is used as a measurement of cerebrovascular atherosclerosis specifically and is a predictor of coronary atherosclerosis in general. CIMT is also used to monitor progression of atherosclerosis (particularly in diabetic patients). It is also used to monitor atherosclerotic regression in patients who are undergoing treatment for atherosclerosis.

Many studies have documented the relation between the CIMT and the presence and severity of atherosclerosis. Because the carotid artery is elastic, most of its wall represents the intima (innermost part of the arterial wall). The wall of a muscular artery such as the femoral artery, in comparison, is made up mostly of the muscular media. Because atherosclerosis most affects the intima, the carotid artery is the best location for evaluation. Furthermore, because of its proximity to the skin in the neck, it is easily measured with external ultrasonography. The CIMT can also be measured by intravascular ultrasonography (see p. 914). Nonatherosclerotic diseases such as intimal hyperplasia and intimal fibrocellular hypertrophy can also cause increased CIMT. In more recent research, investigators have used the combined CIMT and femoral artery intimal–medial thickness measurements to more accurately determine the atherosclerotic burden of the coronary arteries.

CIMT measurements above thresholds (0.9 mm) almost certainly indicate atherosclerosis. For every 0.1 mm increase, the risk of a heart attack or stroke increases 15%. CIMT is able to identify and monitor subclinical atherosclerosis. B-mode ultrasonography is most commonly used. The intimal-medial thickness is measured and averaged over six sites in each carotid artery. A limitation of CIMT in the evaluation of coronary artery disease is that it does not accurately assess the total atherosclerotic burden and therefore cannot help predict the severity of coronary artery disease or distinguish patients with one-vessel, two-vessel, or more extensive coronary artery disease.

PROCEDURE AND PATIENT CARE

Before

- Explain the procedure to the patient.
- Inform the patient that no special preparation is required.
- Assure the patient that the study is painless.

During
- Place the patient supine with the head supported to prevent lateral motion.
- Note the following procedural steps:
  1. A gel lubricant is used to couple the sound from the transducer to the skin surface.
  2. Images of the carotid artery and pulse waveform are obtained.

After
- Remove the gel from the patient's skin.

TEST RESULTS AND CLINICAL SIGNIFICANCE

Carotid artery occlusive disease: *Narrowing of the lumen of the carotid artery or any of its branches can be accurately determined as a percentage of the vessel occluded (e.g., 90% occlusion). Most often, occlusion is a result of atherosclerotic disease.*

Carotid artery aneurysm: *The arterial flow disruption is easily visualized.*

RELATED TEST

Arteriography (p. 1026). Arteriography is a more accurate test of the carotid system and is performed if surgery is contemplated. The angiogram demonstrates where and how extensive occlusive plaques are.

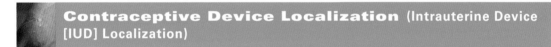

Contraceptive Device Localization (Intrauterine Device [IUD] Localization)

NORMAL FINDINGS

An intrauterine contraceptive device (IUD) is located in the endometrial cavity

INDICATIONS

This ultrasound test is performed to locate an IUD when its string cannot be palpated.

TEST EXPLANATION

When a woman is unable to visualize or palpate the string of an IUD, ultrasonography is indicated to determine whether the IUD has perforated the uterus, has been evacuated, or has been incorporated with an intrauterine pregnancy. IUDs have a particular type-specific structure and can be easily recognized on a sonogram. If an IUD can be seen on an abdominal radiograph but cannot be demonstrated in the endometrial cavity on a sonogram, the IUD has probably perforated the uterus.

IUD localization is performed in approximately 20 minutes. No discomfort is associated with this study other than that of having a full bladder and the urge to urinate.

INTERFERING FACTORS

- In patients who have recently undergone gastrointestinal contrast studies, barium severely distorts reflective sound waves.

- In patients with gas-filled bowel loops, the air does not transmit sound waves well.
- The bladder is often used as a reference point in pelvic sonography; failure to fill the bladder may render the image uninterpretable.

PROCEDURE AND PATIENT CARE

Before

- Explain the procedure to the patient.
- Give the patient three to four glasses (200 to 300 mL) of water or other liquid 1 hour before the examination, and instruct her not to void until after the procedure is completed. This allows the bladder to fill and to be used as a reference point.
- Inform the patient that no fasting or sedation is required.

During

- Note the following procedural steps:
    1. The patient is taken to the ultrasonography room and placed supine on the examination table.
    2. The ultrasonographer, usually a radiologist, applies a gel lubricant to the abdomen to enhance sound transmission and reception.
    3. A transducer is passed vertically and horizontally over the skin.
    4. Pictures are taken of the sound waves, and a real-time image is produced.

After

- Remove the lubricant from the patient's skin.
- Allow the patient to void.

TEST RESULTS AND CLINICAL SIGNIFICANCE

Perforation of the uterus: *If an IUD is seen on a plain radiograph of the abdomen but cannot be found in the uterus at ultrasonography, it can be suspected that the IUD has perforated and is outside the uterus.*

Expulsion of the IUD: *The IUD cannot be located in the uterus or on a plain radiograph of the abdomen.*

Incorporation of the IUD in an intrauterine pregnancy: *The IUD was in place when pregnancy began and has become incorporated in the uterus along with the placenta.*

Echocardiography (Cardiac Echography, Heart Sonography, Transesophageal Echocardiography [TEE], Transthoracic Echocardiography [TTE])

NORMAL FINDINGS

Normal position, size, and movement of the cardiac valves and heart muscle wall
Normal directional flow of blood within the heart chambers

INDICATIONS

Echocardiography is performed most commonly to evaluate heart wall motion (a measure of heart wall function), to detect valvular disease, to evaluate the heart during stress testing, and to identify and quantify pericardial fluid.

TEST EXPLANATION

Echocardiography is a noninvasive ultrasound procedure used to evaluate the structure and function of the heart. In diagnostic ultrasonography, harmless, high-frequency sound waves emitted from a transducer penetrate the heart and are reflected back to the transducer as a series of echoes (Figure 10-11). These echoes are amplified and displayed on a computer monitor. Tracings also can be recorded on moving graph paper or digitally recorded. The study usually includes M-mode recordings, two-dimensional recordings, a Doppler study, and real-time three-dimensional imaging.

M-mode echocardiography produces a one-dimensional recording of the amplitude and rate of motion (M) of the heart structures in real time. This allows the various cardiac structures to be located and studied with regard to their movement during a cardiac cycle.

In *two-dimensional echocardiography,* the ultrasonic beam is moved within one sector of the heart. Computer reconstruction produces a two-dimensional image of the spatial relationships within the heart. *Three-dimensional echocardiography* is routinely added to most new cardiac imaging procedures. This allows for improved images of the heart wall and valves. The addition of high temporal resolution improves images still further.

Colour flow Doppler imaging demonstrates the direction and velocity of blood flow within the heart and great vessels. These variations in blood flow and velocity alter the ultrasound frequency. Computerized weighted numbers are assigned to these altered frequencies; in this way, origins of velocity change and blood turbulence can be mapped. Altered direction and velocity of blood flow are coded as colours and shades, respectively (e.g., blue and red represent the direction of blood flow; various shades from dull to bright represent blood velocity). The most useful application of colour flow Doppler imaging is to determine the direction and turbulence of blood flow across regurgitant or narrowed valves. Colour flow Doppler imaging also may be helpful in assessing proper functioning of prosthetic valves.

Echocardiography is used to diagnose pericardial effusion, valvular heart disease (e.g., mitral valve prolapse, stenosis, regurgitation), subaortic stenosis, myocardial wall abnormalities (e.g., cardiomyopathy), infarction, aneurysm, and cardiac tumours (e.g., myxomas). Atrial and ventricular septal defects, other congenital heart diseases, and postinfarction mural thrombi are also recognized with this testing.

Echocardiography is one method of choice for cardiac stress testing. During an exercise or chemical cardiac stress test, ischemic muscle areas are evident as hypokinetic areas within the myocardium. Echocardiography can be used in an emergency evaluation of chest pain. If the myocardium is normal and without areas of hypokinesia, no coronary artery occlusive disease is suspected. A hypokinetic or akinetic area, however, indicates ischemia or infarction and that the chest pain is cardiac in origin.

Echocardiography can be performed via the esophagus with a transducer mounted on an endoscope. This procedure is referred to as *transesophageal echocardiography* (TEE; see discussion on p. 927). Fetal echocardiograms enable identification of significant congenital heart disease before birth.

Perflutren (DEFINITY or Optison) is an opacifying agent that highlights the endocardial borders during echocardiography by lowering acoustic impedance and enhancing the intrinsic backscatter of blood in the heart. This improves images of any abnormalities in heart wall activity.

Echocardiography usually takes approximately 45 minutes and is performed by an ultrasound technician in a darkened room in the cardiac laboratory or radiology department. Some slight discomfort may be associated with this study from minor pressure as the transducer is placed on the chest and from the gel lubricant, which is usually cooler than body temperature.

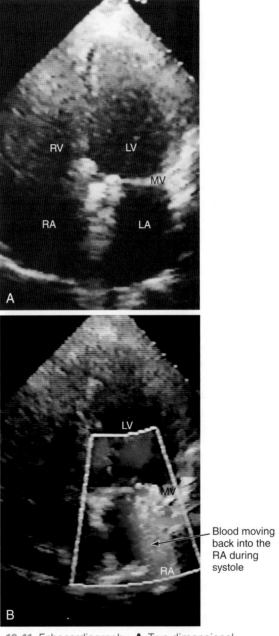

Figure 10-11 Echocardiography. **A,** Two-dimensional echocardiogram (black and white). **B,** Colour Doppler echocardiogram. The heart is oriented with the ventricles on the upper portion of the images and the atria on the lower portion. The four chambers of the heart are easily identified. The right side of the heart is seen on the left side of the figure. On the colour Doppler echocardiogram, *blue* indicates abnormal reversal of blood flowing from the left ventricle and into the left atrium during systole because of mitral valve regurgitation. *LA,* left atrium; *LV,* left ventricle; *MV,* mitral valve leaflets (white line) closed during systole; *RA,* right atrium; *RV,* Right ventricle.

CONTRAINDICATIONS
- Inability of patients to cooperate

INTERFERING FACTORS
- Patients with chronic obstructive pulmonary disease (COPD) have a substantial amount of air between the heart and the chest cavity. Air space does not conduct ultrasound waves well.
- In obese patients, the space between the heart and the transducer is greatly enlarged; therefore, accuracy of the test is decreased.

Clinical Priorities

- Echocardiography is an effective method of heart imaging for stress testing.
- This test is frequently used in the emergency evaluation of chest pain.
- Because of the large amount of air between the heart and the chest cavity, it is difficult to evaluate patients who have COPD with echocardiography. TEE is a better procedure in such patients.

Age-Related Concerns

- In adults older than 65 years who have no clinical heart disease, an echocardiogram may reveal a decrease in heart size caused by age-related cardiovascular changes.
- Cardiovascular changes in adults older than 65 years may also include a thickening in the left ventricular wall; the extent of this thickening may be as much as 25% by 80 years of age.
- Mitral and aortic heart valves in older adults may also be thicker and stiffer, as a result of lipid accumulation, degeneration in the collagen, and fibrosis. This can result in changes to the movement of the cardiac valves, as shown on the echocardiogram.

PROCEDURE AND PATIENT CARE

Before
- Assure the patient that the study is painless.
- Include pertinent patient history on the echocardiography request form.

During
- Note the following procedural steps:
  1. The patient is placed supine.
  2. Electrocardiographic leads are placed (p. 568).
  3. A gel lubricant, which allows better transmission of sound waves, is placed on the chest wall, over which the transducer is passed.
  4. Ultrasonic waves are directed at the heart, and appropriate tracings are obtained (Figures 10-12 and 10-13).

After
- Remove the gel from the patient's chest wall.
- Inform the patient that the physician must interpret the study and that the results will be available in a few hours.

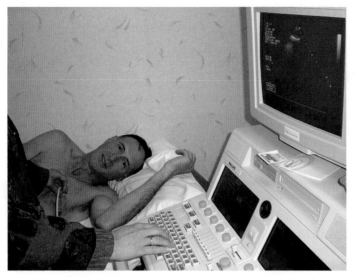

Figure 10-12 Echocardiography laboratory.

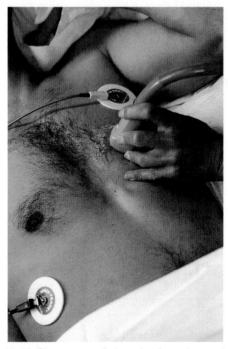

Figure 10-13 Placement of chest leads and transducer on precordium.

TEST RESULTS AND CLINICAL SIGNIFICANCE

Valvular heart disease (e.g., stenosis, regurgitation, mitral valve prolapse): *This is readily evident on echocardiograms. All valves can be easily seen with the linear mode. The circulatory effects of valvular disease are apparent on Doppler studies.*

Pericardial effusion: *Fluid around the heart is easily evident. Echocardiography can be used to guide a needle into the pericardial space for aspiration of fluid for analysis and treatment.*

Ventricular or atrial mural thrombi: *When these are evident, anticoagulation therapy is required. These thrombi may be the result of previous myocardial infarction, ventricular aneurysm, heart failure, or cardiomyopathy.*

Myxomas: *These tumours are often evident as a mass partially attached to the endocardium.*

Poor ventricular muscle motion: *Hypokinesia is evident in a portion of or in the entire myocardial wall in patients with myocardial ischemia, cardiomyopathy, and heart failure.*

Ventricular hypertrophy: *This chronic disease is evident as an unusually thickened myocardium.*

Endocarditis: *Vegetations are readily evident on the valves. Aggressive antibiotic or anticoagulation therapy, or both, is needed.*

Septal defects: *Left-to-right shunting is readily evident with colour flow Doppler imaging.*

RELATED TEST

Transesophageal Echocardiography (p. 927). This test provides information similar to that obtained with transthoracic echocardiography, but TEE allows better visualization of the posterior portion of the heart and thoracic vessels.

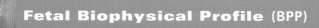

Fetal Biophysical Profile (BPP)

NORMAL FINDINGS

Score of 8 to 10 points (if amniotic fluid volume is adequate)

 Critical Values

Score of less than 4 indicates fetal distress, which may necessitate immediate delivery.

INDICATIONS

The premise of the biophysical profile (BPP) is that assessment of variable factors of fetal biophysical activity are more reliable than examination of a single parameter (e.g., fetal heart rate). Indications for BPP include postdate pregnancy, maternal hypertension, diabetes mellitus, vaginal bleeding, maternal Rh factor sensitization, maternal history of stillbirth, and premature rupture of membranes. The BPP is probably more useful in identifying a fetus that is in jeopardy than in predicting future fetal well-being. Testing usually begins at approximately 32 weeks but can be performed earlier if maternal complications are present.

TEST EXPLANATION

The BPP is a method of evaluating antepartal fetal status on the basis of five variables: fetal heart rate, fetal breathing movement, gross fetal movement, fetal muscle tone, and amniotic fluid volume. Fetal heart rate reactivity is measured with the nonstress test (p. 597); the other four parameters are measured with ultrasonography. Each variable is scored as either 2 or 0. Therefore, 10 is a perfect score, and 0 is the lowest score.

1. *Fetal heart rate reactivity:* This variable is measured and interpreted in the same way as in the nonstress test (p. 597). Fetal heart rate is considered reactive when there are movement-associated fetal heart rate accelerations of at least 15 beats/minute above baseline and 15 seconds in duration, over a 20-minute time period. A score of 2 indicates reactivity; a score of 0 indicates that the fetal heart rate is nonreactive.

2. *Fetal breathing movements:* This variable is assessed on the assumption that fetal breathing movements indicate fetal well-being, and their absence may indicate hypoxemia. Rate and uniformity of fetal breathing become increasingly regular after week 36 of gestation. At least one episode of fetal breathing lasting a minimum of 60 seconds within a 30-minute observation period is scored as 2; absence of this breathing pattern is scored as 0. Several factors can alter fetal breathing movements. For example, fetal breathing movements increase during the second and third hours after maternal meals and also at night during sleep. Fetal breathing movements may decrease in conditions such as hypoxemia and hypoglycemia and with nicotine use and alcohol ingestion.

3. *Fetal body movements:* Fetal activity is a reflection of neurologic integrity and function. The presence of at least three discrete episodes of fetal movement within a 30-minute observation period is scored as 2; that of two or fewer fetal movements in 30 minutes is scored as 0. Fetal activity is greatest 1 to 3 hours after the woman has consumed a meal. For this reason, it is often suggested that this test be scheduled in relation to mealtime.

4. *Fetal muscle tone:* In the uterus, the fetus is normally in a position of flexion but also stretches, rolls, and moves. The arms, legs, trunk, and neck may be flexed and extended. The occurrence of at least one episode of active extension with return to flexion (e.g., opening and closing of a hand) is scored as 2; slow extension with return to only partial flexion, fetal movement not followed by return to flexion, limbs or spine in extension, and a fetal hand remaining open are scored as 0.

5. *Amniotic fluid volume:* Measurement of amniotic fluid volume is an effective method of predicting fetal distress. Oligohydramnios (too little amniotic fluid) has been associated with fetal anomalies, intrauterine growth restriction, and postterm pregnancy. Immediate delivery is recommended in postterm pregnancy with oligohydramnios because of the high risk of associated problems, such as umbilical cord compromise. If there is at least one pocket of amniotic fluid that measures 1 cm in two perpendicular planes, the score is 2; if fluid is absent in most areas of the uterine cavity or else the largest pocket measures 1 cm or less in the vertical axis, the score is 0.

A score of 8 or 10 with an acceptable amount of amniotic fluid is normal. A score of 8 with oligohydramnios or a score of 4 to 6 is equivocal and is interpreted as possibly abnormal. Some clinicians recommend repeating the test within 24 hours; others advocate extending testing after any equivocal test result. A score of 0 or 2 is abnormal and indicates the need for assessment for immediate delivery.

Modifications can be made to the BPP. Some physicians omit the nonstress test if the ultrasound parameters are normal; some include placental grading as a sixth parameter. Information about fetal size, position, and location of the placenta can also be obtained.

Another measure of fetal well-being is the *amniotic fluid index.* This is determined with the use of ultrasonography to measure the largest collection of amniotic fluid in each of the four quadrants within the uterus. The sum represents a number that is plotted on a graph in which the age of gestation is also taken into account. If the amniotic fluid index is less than percentile 2.4, oligohydramnios is present. If amniotic fluid index exceeds the ninety-seventh percentile, polyhydramnios is present. An abnormal amniotic fluid index observed in antepartum testing is associated with an increased risk of intrauterine growth restriction and overall adverse perinatal outcome. Some authorities have suggested that borderline amniotic fluid index be calculated twice weekly, whereas other studies have shown amniotic fluid index to be so weak a predictor for poor neonatal outcome as to be useless. The percentile value seems to be a better indicator than an absolute fluid volume. Oligohydramnios is associated with placental failure or fetal renal problems. Polyhydramnios is associated with maternal diabetes or fetal upper gastrointestinal malformation/obstruction.

Additional information about fetal well-being can be gained from Doppler ultrasound evaluation of the placenta and the *umbilical artery flow velocity*. Changes in umbilical artery flow or direction may indicate fetal stress or illness.

INTERFERING FACTORS

- Maternal hyperglycemia may increase fetal biophysical activity.
- Hypoxemia and trauma may decrease fetal biophysical activity.
- Maternal or fetal infection affects fetal biophysical activity.
- On occasion, no movement is noted. If no eye movement or respiratory movement is noted, the fetus may be sleeping.
- Central nervous system stimulants, such as catecholamines, can increase fetal biophysical activity.
- Magnesium sulphate, analgesics, anaesthetics, sedatives, and nicotine can depress fetal biophysical activity.

Clinical Priorities

- The BPP is more useful in identifying a fetus in jeopardy than in predicting future fetal well-being.
- The BPP is usually indicated in women with high-risk pregnancies. Testing usually begins at approximately week 32 of gestation but can be performed earlier if maternal complications occur.
- Several BPP variables are affected by the maternal blood glucose level. For this reason, it is often recommended that this test be performed 1 to 3 hours after the woman has eaten.

PROCEDURE AND PATIENT CARE

Before

- Explain the procedure to the patient.
- Inform the patient that no fasting is required.

During

- Fetal heart rate reactivity is measured and interpreted from a nonstress test (p. 597).
- Fetal breathing movements, fetal body movements, fetal muscle tone, and amniotic fluid volume are determined by ultrasound imaging (see Obstetric Ultrasonography, p. 917).

After

- If test results are abnormal or equivocal, provide emotional support to the mother in the next phase of the fetal evaluation process.

TEST RESULTS AND CLINICAL SIGNIFICANCE

Fetal asphyxia,
Congenital anomalies,

10   **Ultrasound Studies**

Oligohydramnios,
Intrauterine growth restriction,
Postterm pregnancy,
Fetal distress or death

RELATED TESTS

Fetal Contraction Stress Test (p. 594) and Nonstress Test (p. 597). These tests are performed to monitor fetal heart rate and movement.

Pelvic Ultrasonography (p. 917). This test is used in the obstetric patient to identify a tubal or molar pregnancy, indicate the number of fetuses, and determine fetal age, rate of growth, position, and size.

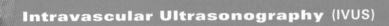

Intravascular Ultrasonography (IVUS)

NORMAL FINDINGS

Normal coronary arteries.

INDICATIONS

Intravascular ultrasonography (IVUS) is used to determine the patency of blood vessels, particularly the coronary arteries. IVUS is used to evaluate the need for or the effectiveness of coronary artery stents.

TEST EXPLANATION

Percutaneous IVUS imaging requires very small, specially made transducers that are mounted on the tip of an intravascular catheter. The ultrasound catheter tip is slid in over the guide wire and positioned with angiographic techniques, so that the tip is in the blood vessel to be studied. Sound waves are emitted from the catheter tip. The catheter receives and conducts the echo information from the blood vessel to the external digital ultrasound equipment. The equipment then constructs and displays a real-time ultrasound image of a thin section of the blood vessel currently surrounding the catheter tip.

Unlike arteriography, which shows a shadow of the arterial lumen, IVUS shows a tomographic, cross-sectional view of the vessel. This orientation enables direct measurements of lumen dimensions, which are considered to be more accurate than angiographic dimensions. The guide wire is kept stationary, and the ultrasound catheter tip is slid backward, usually under motorized control at a pullback speed of 0.5 mm/second. The motorized pullback tends to be smoother than the physician's hand movement. The data obtained can be restructured by the ultrasound machine software to create a longitudinal three-dimensional image of the particular segment of artery that is being studied.

IVUS is an important technology for studying the progression, stabilization, and potential regression of coronary atherosclerosis. IVUS enables imaging of the lumen size, vessel wall structure, and any atheroma that may be present. It allows characterization of atheroma size, plaque distribution, and lesion composition and enables accurate visualization of not only the lumen of the coronary arteries but also the atheroma that may be "hidden" within the vessel wall. In this way, IVUS has enabled advances in clinical research, providing a more thorough perspective and a better understanding of vascular disease. It is a reproducible, safe, and sensitive method for assessing the development and extent of atherosclerosis, particularly in the earlier, presymptomatic stages. This procedure is used predominantly in the coronary arteries.

Normal coronary arteries usually have a triple-layered appearance on IVUS imaging, which corresponds to the three histologic layers of the arterial wall. The innermost layer is the echogenic (brighter) intima, the middle layer is the echolucent (darker) media, and the outermost layer is the echogenic adventitia. The tomographic orientation of IVUS enables visualization of the full 360-degree circumference of the vessel wall, so that lumen dimensions can be measured directly on a cross-sectional image. This enables the examiner to assess precisely the extent of disease in vessels that are often difficult to assess with angiography. IVUS also allows excellent resolution of structures within the arterial wall that may represent other atheromatous disease.

IVUS is used in the following clinical situations:

1. Assessment of coronary stent placement and determination of minimum luminal diameter within the stent
2. Determination of the mechanism of stent restenosis (inadequate expansion vs. neointimal proliferation) and selection of appropriate therapy (plaque ablation vs. repeated balloon expansion)
3. Evaluation of coronary obstruction at a location difficult to image with angiography (such as the left main coronary artery, the ostia of the anterior descending artery, the left circumflex artery, and the right coronary artery)
4. Assessment of a suboptimal angiographic result after stent placement in cases in which the degree of stenosis of a coronary artery is unclear
5. Guidance and assessment for vascular atherectomy
6. Determination of plaque location and circumferential distribution for guidance of directional coronary atherectomy
7. Determination of the extent of atherosclerosis in patients with characteristic anginal symptoms and a positive functional study result with no focal stenoses or mild coronary artery disease on angiography (IVUS can directly quantify the percentage of stenosis and give insight into the anatomy of the plaque)
8. Preinterventional assessment of lesion characteristics and vessel dimensions as a means of selecting an optimal revascularization device
9. Assessment of the changes in plaque volume after lipid-lowering therapy

INTERFERING FACTORS

- The accuracy of ultrasonography depends on the skills of the sonographer (the technician who performs the study).

PROCEDURE AND PATIENT CARE

Before

- Explain the procedure to the patient.
- Inform the patient that fasting is required from midnight before the test.

During

- The IVUS probe is placed by coronary angiographic procedures. See p. 1026.
- The test is completed in approximately 1 hour, usually by a cardiologist.

After

- See the discussion of cardiac catheterization (p. 1047) for postprocedure care.

TEST RESULTS AND CLINICAL SIGNIFICANCE

Coronary occlusive disease: *With IVUS, the degree of disease of a coronary artery can be directly quantified by percentage of stenosis. IVUS can give insight into the anatomy of the plaque when the degree of stenosis of a coronary artery is unclear.*

RELATED TEST

Cardiac Catheterization (p. 1047). The anatomy and degree of stenosis of a coronary artery is most commonly determined by this method because it is less technically demanding and provides a better indication of anatomy if heart surgery is required.

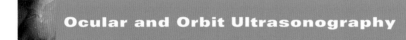

Ocular and Orbit Ultrasonography

NORMAL FINDINGS

Normal pattern of orbital and posterior orbital structures

INDICATIONS

Ocular ultrasonography is used to examine the eye when the extraocular and intraocular spaces cannot be adequately evaluated by other methods because of disease, scarring, or surgery. This test is also used to evaluate the posterior bulbar area for tumours and cysts.

TEST EXPLANATION

Ultrasonography of the eye is used to detect intraocular disease such as vitreous hemorrhage, retinal or choroidal detachment, and intraocular foreign bodies. It is also used to identify retro-ocular abnormalities such as tumour (e.g., glioma, meningioma), benign cysts (e.g., dermoid, mucocele), and cavernous hemangioma. Changes in corneal and ocular shape as a result of disease, surgery, or trauma can be identified. Computed tomography and magnetic resonance imaging are also excellent methods for evaluating the ocular and retrobulbar spaces. The orbital fossae and eyes can be evaluated in the fetus by ultrasonography if cranial or ocular abnormalities are suspected.

PROCEDURE AND PATIENT CARE

Before

- Explain the procedure to the patient.
- Topical anaesthetic drops are administered to the eyes 5 to 10 minutes before the study.

During

- The ultrasound probe is applied directly to the eye.
- Ultrasound images are obtained.

- Alternatively, ultrasound immersion technique can be performed (i.e., with this technique the probe tip does not come into direct contact with the cornea. A scleral shell, filled with fluid, is centred over the cornea, and the probe tip is placed in the fluid for the reading).

After

Inform the patient that the cornea is still anaesthetized and that because no discomfort can be appreciated, it is important to refrain from rubbing or otherwise touching the eye.

TEST RESULTS AND CLINICAL SIGNIFICANCE

Retinal or choroidal detachment: *This can result from senile deterioration, trauma, or posterior ocular bleeding.*

Thickened orbit: *The most common cause is hyperthyroidism (Graves' disease).*

Vitreous opacities: *These "floaters," or dark spots in vision, can be caused by foreign bodies, desquamated cells, or hemorrhage.*

Neoplasm: *Neoplasms include posterior ocular tumours (such as melanoma, hemangioma, or metastatic tumours), retrobulbar tumours (such as glioma, meningioma, or neurofibroma), or metastatic tumour.*

Pelvic Ultrasonography (Obstetric Echography, Pregnant Uterus Ultrasonography, Pelvic Ultrasonography in Pregnancy, Obstetric Ultrasonography, Vaginal Ultrasonography)

NORMAL FINDINGS

Normal fetal and placental size and position
Normal maternal genital tract

INDICATIONS

Pelvic ultrasonography is used in obstetric patients to evaluate the pregnancy and the fetus. It is especially important in high-risk pregnancies. In nonpregnant women, it is used to evaluate the genital tract for disease and to monitor known pelvic disease (e.g., benign ovarian cysts).

See the "Prostate and Rectal Ultrasonography" section (p. 921) for discussion of pelvic ultrasound examination in male patients.

TEST EXPLANATION

Ultrasound examination is a harmless, noninvasive method of evaluating the female genital tract and the fetus. In real-time diagnostic ultrasonography, high-frequency sound waves are emitted from the transducer and penetrate the structure to be studied (e.g., uterus, ovaries, parametria, placenta, fetus). These sound waves are reflected back to a sensor within the transducer and, by electronic conversion, are arranged into a pictorial image of the studied structure.

Pelvic ultrasonography can be performed with the transducer placed on the anterior abdomen or in the vagina with a specially designed vaginal probe, which provides the best view of the pelvic organs in a nonpregnant woman. The images obtained with both transducers are complementary. Vaginal ultrasonography provides significant accuracy in identifying paracervical, endometrial, and ovarian disease that may not be detected with the anterior abdominal probe.

On occasion, abdominal organs are displaced into the pelvis and preclude adequate pelvic visualization with the anterior abdominal probe. Vaginal ultrasonography provides better visualization under these circumstances. In obese patients, the thick abdominal wall inhibits transmission of ultrasonic waves, and vaginal ultrasonography is preferred. The anterior abdominal probe, however, provides better visualization of the upper pelvis than does the vaginal probe, especially in pregnant women.

Pelvic ultrasonography may be useful in *obstetric patients* in the following circumstances:

1. To make an early diagnosis of normal pregnancy or abnormal pregnancy (e.g., fetal malformations)
2. To identify multiple fetuses
3. To differentiate a tumour (e.g., hydatidiform mole) from a normal pregnancy
4. To determine the age of the fetus from the diameter of the head
5. To measure fetal growth rate
6. To identify placental abnormalities such as abruptio placentae and placenta previa
7. To determine the position of the placenta (ultrasound localization of the placenta is performed before amniocentesis)
8. To make differential diagnoses of various uterine and ovarian enlargements (e.g., polyhydramnios, neoplasms, cysts, abscesses)
9. To determine fetal position
10. To diagnose ectopic pregnancy
11. To provide a realistic image of the fetus using 3D and 4D imaging (see p. 892) for expectant parents

Ultrasonography is quickly becoming a very accurate and easily performed screening test to recognize risks of fetal abnormalities (see discussion of amniotic fluid index in the "Fetal Biophysical Profile" section, p. 911). *Fetal nuchal translucency (FNT)* is an ultrasound measurement of subcutaneous edema in the neck region of the fetus. It is performed at 10 to 14 weeks of gestation. Major heart defects, trisomy 21, and other genetic defects are associated with increased edema in this location at this gestational age. Screening for chromosomal defects by measurement of FNT identifies 80% of fetuses with trisomy 21; the false-positive rate is 5%. This is especially helpful for older pregnant women. With FNT, these abnormalities can be identified earlier in the pregnancy when abortion is still a safe option. Although there may be advantages in early detection of fetal anomalies, a specific disadvantage should be considered: Many pregnancies complicated by fetal abnormality—both aneuploidy and other anomalies—end in an early miscarriage. If these pregnancies are identified early, parents may be asked to make difficult decisions regarding termination of pregnancy. This imposes a potential psychologic burden that could be avoided if the pregnancy were lost spontaneously.

Pelvic ultrasonography is useful in *nonpregnant women* to monitor the endometrium in patients who take tamoxifen and to aid in the diagnosis of several conditions:

1. Ovarian cyst
2. Ovarian tumour
3. Tuboovarian abscess
4. Uterine fibroids
5. Uterine cancer
6. Pelvic inflammatory disease
7. Uterine stripe (endometrium)

The procedure is performed in approximately 20 minutes. No discomfort is associated with the study, other than that of having a full bladder and the urge to void. Some patients may be uncomfortable lying on a hard table.

CONTRAINDICATIONS

- Latex allergy could be a contraindication, because vaginal ultrasonography requires placement of the probe in a latex condom-like cover; however, a non-latex cover could be used with these patients.

INTERFERING FACTORS

- In patients who have recently undergone barium contrast studies, barium creates severe distortion of reflective sound waves.
- In patients with gas-filled bowels, air does not transmit sound waves well.
- In patients who are obese or who cannot fill the bladder, the image may be uninterpretable.

Clinical Priorities

- Pelvic ultrasonography can be performed with the transducer placed on the anterior abdomen or in the vagina.
- Vaginal ultrasonography is preferred in obese patients because a thick abdominal wall inhibits transmission of sound waves.
- A full bladder is essential in patients undergoing transabdominal ultrasonography, to provide a reference point for interpreting pelvic ultrasonograms.
- No discomfort is associated with the study other than that of having a full bladder and the urge to void.

PROCEDURE AND PATIENT CARE

Before

- Explain the procedure to the patient.
- Assure the patient that the study has no known deleterious effect on maternal or fetal tissues, even if repeated several times.
- Give the patient three to four glasses (200 to 350 mL) of water or other liquid 1 hour before the examination, and instruct her not to void until after the procedure is completed. This will enable visualization of the bladder, which is used as a reference point in pelvic anatomy. The full bladder also displaces the bowel from the pelvis and pushes the uterus and ovaries away from the pubis. The fluid in the bladder acts as a window to the pelvis for transmission of sound waves.
- No water is required if ultrasonography is to be performed vaginally only.
- If a transabdominal ultrasonography is required urgently and there is no time to fill the bladder by ingestion or administration of fluids, the bladder can be filled by means of a bladder catheter.
- Inform the patient that no fasting or sedation is required.

During

- Note the following procedural steps:
  1. The patient is taken to the ultrasonography room and placed supine on the examining table (Figure 10-14).
  2. The ultrasonographer, usually a radiologist, applies a greasy, conductive gel to the patient's abdomen to enhance sound wave transmission and reception.
  3. A transducer is passed vertically and horizontally over the skin.
  4. If a vaginal probe is used, a thin cover is applied to the probe; it is inserted in the vagina, and then angled to identify the various parts of the pelvis.

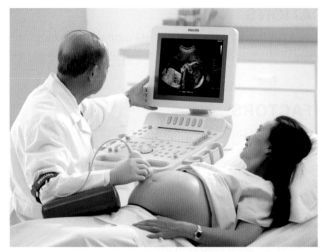

Figure 10-14 Pelvic ultrasonography. Ultrasonography is often used in pregnant women for obtaining diagnostic information.

5. The sound waves are reflected back by the transducer, and an image appears on the monitor.
6. During the examination, fetal structures are pointed out to the patient.

After

- Remove the lubricant from the patient's skin.
- Allow the patient to void.
- If vaginal ultrasonography is used, provide patient with a small sanitary pad.

TEST RESULTS AND CLINICAL SIGNIFICANCE

Abdominal or tubal pregnancy: *Extrauterine pregnancy is evident when the placental complex is outside the uterus.*

Hydatidiform mole: *Molar pregnancy can be diagnosed and monitored by ultrasonography.*

Intrauterine growth restriction,

Fetal hydrocephalus,

Multiple fetuses,

Fetal death,

Abnormal fetal position (e.g., breech, transverse),

Polyhydramnios: *Fetal characteristics are easily evaluated with ultrasonography (see Fetal Biophysical Profile, p. 911).*

Abnormal position of the placenta (e.g., placenta previa, abruptio placentae): *Placenta position and quality can be evaluated with ultrasonography. Doppler ultrasonography can be used to evaluate placental blood flow.*

Neoplasm of the ovaries, uterus, or fallopian tubes: *Ultrasonography is sensitive in detection of tumours of the female genital tract. The uterine stripe (endometrial lining of the uterus) is monitored in patients taking medications associated with hyperplasia or cancer (e.g., tamoxifen).*

Cysts: *Ultrasonography is the most accurate method for differentiating an ovarian cyst from a solid ovarian tumour. Pure cysts (well-defined hypoechoic mass with clean walls) are more likely to be benign than are complex cysts (containing echogenic material).*

Pelvic inflammatory disease and abscesses: *Abscesses (tuboovarian) appear similar to ovarian cysts but can be differentiated by means of their clinical features.*

Localization of an intrauterine device (IUD): *This test can locate an IUD.*

RELATED TESTS

Contraceptive Device Localization (p. 905). An IUD can be located with ultrasonography when its string cannot be palpated.

Prostate and Rectal Ultrasonography (see following test). Ultrasonography of the rectum is used in the staging of rectal tumours in men and women.

Prostate and Rectal Ultrasonography

NORMAL FINDINGS

Normal size, contour, and consistency of the prostate gland

Normal mucosa with no polyps, bleeding, cancer, or other perirectal disease

INDICATIONS

Prostate or rectal ultrasonography is helpful in the detection of prostate cancer in patients with an elevated prostate-specific antigen titre. This study can also be used to stage and monitor rectal cancer and to detect other perirectal diseases.

TEST EXPLANATION

Rectal ultrasonography of the prostate is a valuable tool in the early diagnosis of prostate cancer. When combined with rectal digital examination and prostate-specific antigen testing (p. 434), very small prostate cancers can be identified. Ultrasonography is also useful in evaluating the seminal vessels and other perirectal tissue and in guiding prostate biopsy (Figure 10-15), and it can be helpful in quantifying the volume of prostate cancer. When radiation therapy implantation is required for treatment, ultrasonography is used to map the exact location of the prostate cancer. Rectal ultrasonography is helpful in staging rectal cancers as well. The depth of transmural involvement and presence of extrarectal extension can be accurately assessed.

Real-time ultrasonography requires the emission of high-frequency sound waves from a special transducer placed in the rectum. The sound waves are reflected back to the transducer and electronically converted into a pictorial image. This test can be performed in the ultrasonography section of the radiology department and is now being performed routinely in most urologists' offices. Results are available almost immediately.

CONTRAINDICATIONS

- Latex allergy could be a contraindication, because rectal ultrasonography requires placement of the probe in a latex condom-like cover; however, a non-latex cover could be used with these patients.

INTERFERING FACTORS

- Stool in the rectum can prevent adequate visualization.

10 Ultrasound Studies

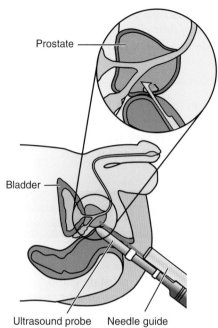

Figure 10-15 Rectal ultrasonography. Diagram demonstrating transrectal biopsy of the prostate.

Clinical Priorities

- By combining rectal or prostate ultrasonography with a digital rectal examination and prostate-specific antigen test, small prostate cancers can be identified.
- This test can be easily performed in the offices of most urologists.
- This test cannot be performed in patients with latex allergy.

Age-Related Concerns

- Prostatic hypertrophy is not considered a normal age-related change, but its prevalence is increased among older men.
- Enlargement of the prostate can interfere with normal voiding and bladder emptying.

PROCEDURE AND PATIENT CARE

Before

✗ Explain the procedure to the patient.
✗ Inform the patient that a small-volume enema must be administered approximately 1 hour before the ultrasound examination.

During

- The patient is placed in the left lateral decubitus position.
- A digital rectal examination may be performed to assess the prostate gland or rectal tumour.

- A draped and lubricated ultrasound probe is placed within the rectum.
- Scans are obtained in various spatial planes.

After
- Provide the patient with tissue material to cleanse the perianal area.

TEST RESULTS AND CLINICAL SIGNIFICANCE

Prostate cancer,

Benign prostatic hypertrophy: *An enlarged solid prostate mass anterior to the rectum is suggestive of prostate disease.*

Prostatitis: *An enlarged, bulging, echogenic gland indicates inflammation.*

Seminal vesicle tumour: *An echogenic mass in the region of the seminal vesicle may indicate tumour.*

Prostate abscess,

Perirectal abscess: *A hypoechoic fluid-filled mass that is well circumscribed indicates abscess, especially if surrounded by a phlegmonous reaction.*

Intrarectal or perirectal tumour: *Extent of tumour can be accurately assessed with ultrasonography. Lymph node metastasis, if present, is evident.*

RELATED TEST

Pelvic Ultrasonography (p. 917). This test is used to assess the female genital tract and the pregnant uterus.

Scrotal Ultrasonography (Ultrasonography of Testes)

NORMAL FINDINGS

Normal size, shape, and configuration of the testicles

INDICATIONS

Ultrasonography of the scrotum allows thorough evaluation of the testes and other scrotal structures for evidence of suspected disease.

TEST EXPLANATION

Scrotal ultrasonography is a noninvasive, nonionizing, rapid method for scrotal examination. Through the use of reflected sound waves, ultrasonography provides accurate visualization of the scrotum and its contents. Ultrasonography requires the emission of high-frequency sound waves from the transducer to penetrate the organ being studied. The sound waves are reflected back to the transducer and electronically converted into an accurate digital pictorial image.

Current uses for scrotal ultrasonography include the following:

1. Evaluation of scrotal masses
2. Measurement of testicular size
3. Evaluation of scrotal trauma
4. Evaluation of scrotal pain and identification of torsion of the testicle

10 Ultrasound Studies

5. Evaluation of occult testicular neoplasm
6. Surveillance in patients with previous primary or metastatic contralateral testicular neoplasms
7. Follow-up of testicular infections
8. Location of undescended testicles
9. Identification of microlithiasis

The scrotum is examined with real-time ultrasonography. The testes and extratesticular intrascrotal tissues are examined. The accuracy of scrotal ultrasound findings is 90% to 95%. Both benign and malignant tumours (primary and metastatic) can be identified with ultrasonography. Benign abnormalities (e.g., testicular abscess, orchitis, testicular infarction, testicular torsion) can be identified. Extratesticular lesions such as hydrocele (fluid in the scrotum), hematocele (blood in the scrotum), and pyocele (pus in the scrotum) can be identified. Scrotal and groin ultrasonography has been helpful in locating undescended testes.

Ultrasound of the scrotum is now the preferred method to identify torsion of the testicle. Ultrasound is a very accurate method of identifying microlithiasis in the testicles. When identified, microcalcifications in the testicle indicate marked increased risk for testicular cancer. Calcifications can also occur following orchitis or trauma. In most cases, both testicles are routinely imaged during the ultrasound exam.

The use of colour Doppler imaging is very helpful in determining blood flow to the testicle. With torsion of the testicle, colour Doppler imaging indicates markedly reduced blood flow to the testicle, and immediate surgical exploration is required. Scrotal ultrasonography has replaced scrotal nuclear imaging for the diagnosis of testicular torsion because results can be obtained immediately.

Very little discomfort is associated with testicular ultrasonography. The study is usually performed by an ultrasound technologist, and the results are interpreted by a physician.

PROCEDURE AND PATIENT CARE

Before
- Explain the procedure to the patient.
- Inform the patient that no fasting is required.

During
- Note the following procedural steps:
  1. Careful examination of the scrotum is performed by the physician. Usually, a short history is documented.
  2. The scrotum is supported by a towel or cradled by the examiner's gloved hand.
  3. A gel lubricant is applied to the scrotum before scanning. This gel enhances sound wave transmission and reception.
  4. Thorough scanning in the sagittal, transverse, and oblique projections is performed.
- The test takes approximately 20 to 30 minutes.

After
- Assist the patient in removing the gel from the scrotum.

TEST RESULTS AND CLINICAL SIGNIFICANCE

Benign testicular tumour,
Malignant testicular tumour: *Seminoma of the testicle is evident as a hypoechoic mass in the testicle. Other cancers may appear as hyperechoic dense masses in the testicle.*

Testicular infection (e.g., orchitis),

Hydrocele (fluid around the testicle),

Hematocele (blood around the testicle),

Pyocele (pus around the testicle),

Varicocele (venous varicosities in the spermatic cord, usually on the left side),

Spermatocele (cystic collection surrounding the spermatic cord or epididymis): *These abnormalities appear as hypoechoic (dark) areas surrounding the testicle or spermatic cord.*

Epididymitis: *This has the appearance of an enlarged epididymis. It is a painful infection involving the epididymis.*

Scrotal hernia: *Bowel contents can be seen in the scrotum and indicate hernia.*

Cryptorchidism: *Undescended testes can be located anywhere from the retroperitoneum to the inlet of the scrotum. It is important to locate these organs and evaluate their consistency, because undescended testes are at high risk of becoming malignant.*

Hematoma: *A testicular hematoma from trauma is seen as a hypoechoic mass in the parenchyma of the testicle.*

Testicular torsion: *Inadequate suspension of the testicle in the scrotum results in the testicle twisting around on its blood supply. The testicle appears to have an irregular texture, with echogenic areas that correspond to areas of intratesticular hemorrhage. Doppler ultrasonography can indicate reduced blood flow to the testicle.*

Thyroid Ultrasonography (Thyroid Echography, Thyroid Sonography)

NORMAL FINDINGS

Normal size, shape, and position of the thyroid gland

INDICATIONS

The primary purpose of thyroid ultrasonography is to indicate whether a thyroid nodule is a fluid-filled cyst (likely benign) or a solid tumour (possibly malignant). Ultrasonography is also used to monitor the medical treatment or observation of a thyroid nodule, and to monitor the contralateral thyroid lobe when one side was surgically removed because of cancer.

TEST EXPLANATION

Ultrasound examination of the thyroid gland is valuable for distinguishing cystic from solid thyroid nodules. If the nodule is found to be purely cystic (fluid-filled), the fluid can simply be aspirated (cysts are not cancerous), and surgery is avoided. If the nodule has a mixed or solid appearance, however, a tumour may be present, and surgery may be required for diagnosis and treatment.

This study may be repeated at intervals to determine the response of a thyroid mass to medical therapy. This test is the procedure of choice for studying the thyroid gland in pregnant women, because no radioactive material is used.

An ultrasound technologist usually performs this study in approximately 15 minutes; a radiologist interprets the results. No discomfort is associated with this study.

10 Ultrasound Studies

PROCEDURE AND PATIENT CARE

Before

- Explain the procedure to the patient.
- Assure the patient that breathing or swallowing will not be affected by the placement of a transducer on the neck.
- Inform the patient that a liberal amount of lubricant will be applied to the neck to ensure effective transmission and reception of sound waves.
- Inform the patient that no fasting or sedation is required.

During

- Note the following procedural steps:
  1. The patient is taken to the ultrasonography department (usually in the radiology department) and placed supine with the neck hyperextended.
  2. Gel is applied to the patient's neck.
  3. A transducer is passed over the gland (Figure 10-16).
  4. Photographs are taken of the image displayed.

After

- Assist the patient in removing the lubricant from the neck.

TEST RESULTS AND CLINICAL SIGNIFICANCE

Cyst: *A thyroid cyst is evident as a hypoechoic, well-circumscribed mass in the thyroid gland.*
Thyroid adenoma,
Thyroid carcinoma,
Goitre: *This is evident as a solid echogenic mass within the thyroid gland.*

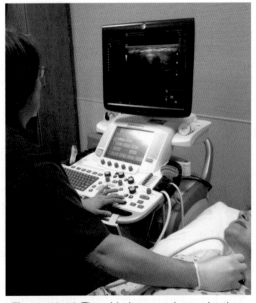

Figure 10-16 Thyroid ultrasound examination.

RELATED TEST

Thyroid Scan (p. 868). This nuclear medicine study allows visualization of the thyroid gland after intravenous administration of a radionuclide. Cysts, tumours, and goitres appear as space-occupying filling defects (cold nodule) within the thyroid gland. This study is often performed with ultrasonography of the thyroid. A cold nodule that appears solid on ultrasonography is the type of lesion with the greatest chance of being a cancer.

Transesophageal Echocardiography (TEE)

NORMAL FINDINGS

Normal position, size, and movement of the heart muscle, valves, and chambers

INDICATIONS

An ultrasonography probe, placed endoscopically in the distal esophagus or proximal stomach, provides accurate information about the heart muscle, heart valves, and heart function. It is also capable of providing accurate information about the thoracic aorta. Transesophageal echocardiography (TEE) is helpful in evaluation of structures that are inaccessible or poorly visualized by the transthoracic probe approach, especially in patients who are obese or have large lung-air spaces (e.g., as in chronic obstructive pulmonary disease).

TEE is performed for the following reasons:
1. To better visualize the mitral valve
2. To differentiate intracardiac from extracardiac masses and tumours
3. To better visualize the atrial septum (for atrial septal defects)
4. To diagnose thoracic aortic dissection
5. To better detect valvular vegetation indicative of endocarditis
6. To determine cardiac sources of arterial embolism
7. To detect coronary artery disease by identifying areas of muscle wall hypokinesia

TEST EXPLANATION

TEE provides ultrasonic imaging of the heart from a retrocardiac vantage point, avoiding interference by the interposed subcutaneous tissue, the bony areas of the thorax, and the lungs. A high-frequency ultrasound transducer placed in the esophagus at endoscopy provides better resolution than does routine transthoracic echocardiography (see "Echocardiography" section, p. 906). For TEE, the distal end of the endoscope is advanced into the esophagus, and the transducer is positioned behind the heart (Figure 10-17). Controls on the handle of the endoscope enable the sonographer to rotate and flex the transducer in the anteroposterior, right lateral, and left lateral planes. TEE images have better resolution than those obtained by routine transthoracic echocardiography because of the higher-frequency sound waves and closer proximity of the transducer to the cardiac structures.

TEE can be used intraoperatively to monitor patients at high risk for ischemia. Ischemic muscle movement is much different from normal muscle movement. Because TEE is a sensitive indicator of myocardial ischemia, it can be used to monitor patients undergoing major abdominal, peripheral vascular, and carotid artery procedures who are at high risk for intraoperative ischemia because of coronary artery disease.

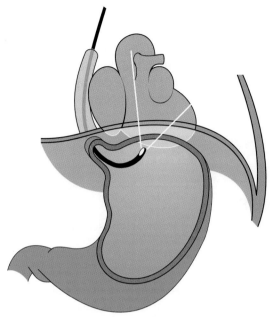

Figure 10-17 Transesophageal echocardiography. Diagram illustrating the location of the transesophageal endoscope in the esophagus.

TEE is more sensitive than electrocardiography for detecting ischemia. TEE is also used intraoperatively to evaluate surgical results of valvular or congenital heart disease and to detect air emboli, a serious complication of neurosurgery performed with the patient in the upright position (e.g., cervical laminectomy).

Perflutren (DEFINITY or Optison) is an opacifying agent that provides enhancement of the endocardial borders during echocardiography by lowering acoustic impedance and enhancing the intrinsic backscatter of blood in the heart. This improves images of any abnormalities in heart wall activity.

TEE is performed in approximately 20 minutes by a cardiologist or a gastrointestinal endoscopist in the endoscopy suite or at the patient's bedside. Little discomfort is associated with this test, and light sedation is induced.

CONTRAINDICATIONS

- Known upper esophageal disease
- Known esophageal varices
- Zenker diverticulum
- Esophageal abnormalities (e.g., stricture diverticula, scleroderma, esophagitis)
- Bleeding disorders
- Recent esophageal surgery
- Inability of patients to cooperate during the procedure

POTENTIAL COMPLICATIONS

- Esophageal perforation or bleeding
- Cardiac arrhythmias

Clinical Priorities

- TEE is especially useful in patients who are obese or have chronic obstructive pulmonary disease.
- TEE can be used intraoperatively to monitor patients at high risk for ischemia.
- TEE is the most sensitive technique for detecting air emboli, a serious complication of neurosurgery performed with the patient in the upright position (e.g., cervical laminectomy).

PROCEDURE AND PATIENT CARE

Before

- ☒ Explain the procedure to the patient.
- ☒ Instruct the patient to fast for 4 to 6 hours before the test.
- Remove all oral prostheses.
- Obtain intravenous access.

During

- Refer to and follow the agency's procedural sedation protocols.
- Intravenous sedation is commonly provided with a short-acting benzodiazepine. Other sedatives may be provided.
- Apply electrocardiographic leads, and monitor heart rhythm continually.
- Apply a blood pressure cuff, and monitor blood pressure periodically.
- On occasion, pulse oximetry is monitored to determine oxygen saturation in heavily sedated patients.
- Note the following procedural steps:
  1. The pharynx is anaesthetized with a locally applied topical agent to depress the gag reflex.
  2. The patient is placed in the left lateral decubitus position.
  3. The endoscope is inserted through the mouth and into the upper esophagus.
  4. The patient is asked to swallow, and the transducer is positioned behind the heart by manipulation through the endoscope.
  5. The room is darkened, and the ultrasound images are displayed on a monitor.

After

- Observe the patient closely for approximately 1 hour after the procedure, until the effects of sedation have worn off.

TEST RESULTS AND CLINICAL SIGNIFICANCE

Myocardial ischemia,

Myocardial infarction: *These are suspected from the presence of abnormal (hypokinetic) wall motion.*

Valvular heart disease: *Motion of heart valves is evaluated.*

Intracardiac thrombi: *These can be a cause of arterial emboli. Thrombi usually form in the area of akinetic muscle because of myocardial infarction or myocardial aneurysm.*

Cardiac valvular vegetation: *This is a result of endocarditis and is a cause of arterial emboli.*

Cardiomyopathy: *Heart muscle is hypokinetic, may or may not be thickened, and may or may not be dilated.*

Marked cardiac chamber dilatation: *This usually occurs as a result of chronic heart failure.*

Cardiac tumours: *The most common (although rare) cardiac tumour is a myxoma.*

Thoracic aortic aneurysm: *TEE is considered the standard for diagnosis of dissecting thoracic aortic aneurysm.*

10 **Ultrasound Studies**

Aortic plaque: *Arterial sclerotic plaques can easily be seen with TEE.*

Pulmonary hypertension: *When pulmonary arterial thrombosis (embolism) is the cause of acute or chronic pulmonary hypertension, TEE can demonstrate that clot.*

RELATED TEST

Echocardiography (p. 906). This test provides the same information as does TEE, but the posterior portion of the heart is not as well seen as with TEE.

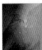

Vascular Ultrasound Studies (Venous/Arterial Doppler Ultrasonography, Venous/Arterial Duplex Scanning)

NORMAL FINDINGS

Venous

Normal Doppler venous signal
Normal venous system without evidence of occlusion

Arterial

Normal arterial Doppler signal with systolic and diastolic components
No reduction in blood pressure in excess of 20 mm Hg in comparison with the normal extremity
Normal ankle/brachial index (ABI) of 0.85 or greater
No evidence of arterial occlusion

 Critical Values

An ABI of less than 0.85 indicates a significant arterial occlusion in the arteries of the leg.

INDICATIONS

This ultrasound study provides information about arterial and venous patency without the use of invasive techniques. Arterial Doppler studies are used in patients with suspected arterial insufficiency (e.g., claudication, poorly healing skin ulcer, cold and pale leg, pulseless extremity, resting pain). Venous ultrasonography is used to evaluate the patency of the venous system in patients with a swollen painful leg, venous varicosities of the upper or lower extremities, or edematous extremities.

TEST EXPLANATION

Vascular ultrasound studies are used to identify occlusion or thrombosis of the veins or arteries of an extremity. Patency is demonstrated with *Doppler ultrasonography* by detecting moving red blood cells (RBCs) within the vein. The Doppler transducer directs an ultrasound beam at the vein. Moving RBCs scatter the beam. The change in frequency of the sound wave reflected back to the transducer is proportional to the velocity of the blood flow. The patency of the venous system can also be identified by evaluating the degree of venous reflux (backwards blood flow in the veins of the lower extremities in patients with venous valvular insufficiency). Venous Doppler studies are not accurate for detection of venous occlusive disease of the lower calf. *Vascular duplex scanning* combines the benefits of Doppler imaging with B-mode scanning. With the use of the transducer, a B-mode ultrasound grey-scale image of the vessel is obtained. A pulsed Doppler probe within the transducer is used to evaluate blood flow velocity and direction in the artery and to measure the amplitude and waveform of the carotid arterial pulse. A computer combines that information and provides a two-dimensional image of the vessel along with an image of blood flow. With this technique, areas of vascular narrowing or occlusion can be visualized directly. The degree of occlusion is measured as a percentage of the entire lumen that is occluded. Also, venous thrombosis is suspected when the vein is not easily compressible by the ultrasound probe.

Colour Doppler ultrasonography can be added to arterial duplex scanning. In colour Doppler ultrasonography, colours are assigned to represent direction of blood flow within the vessel, and the intensity of a particular colour depends on the mean computed velocity of blood travelling in the vessel. This allows visualization of stenotic areas on the basis of velocity or direction of blood flow in a particular area of the artery. With the use of duplex scanning, the vessel anatomy and patency can be represented accurately.

Duplex scanning is routinely used in patients suspected of having an extremity affected by deep-vein thrombosis. It is more rapidly performed, and the results are more rapidly interpreted, than is venography (p. 1026). In general, however, venous duplex scanning is less accurate than venography in identifying deep-vein thrombosis in the calf or in the iliac veins.

With a single-mode transducer, venous and arterial blood flow can be heard audibly and is augmented by an audio speaker as a swishing noise. If the vein or artery is occluded, no swishing sounds are detected. With single-mode arterial Doppler studies, peripheral arteriosclerotic occlusive disease of the extremities can be easily located. A Doppler ultrasound device can be used to detect the ABI, which is used to predict the severity of arterial disease within the arteries of the lower leg. By slowly deflating blood pressure cuffs placed on the arm and ankle, systolic pressure in the arteries of the extremities can be accurately measured by detecting the first evidence of blood flow with the Doppler transducer. The extremely sensitive Doppler ultrasound detector can detect the swishing sound of even the most minimal blood flow. Systolic blood pressure normally is slightly higher in the brachial arteries of the arms than in the arteries of the ankles. The ankle systolic pressure is divided by the brachial systolic pressure to determine the ABI. A decreased ABI is an indicator that disease is present. If the difference in blood pressure exceeds 20 mm Hg, occlusive disease is believed to exist immediately proximal to the area tested. The patency of an arterial bypass graft in the lower extremity can also be assessed with Doppler ultrasonography.

INTERFERING FACTORS

- Venous or arterial occlusive disease proximal to the site of testing can render this procedure unsafe.
- Nicotine ingested as a result of cigarette smoking can cause constriction of the peripheral arteries and alter the results.

Clinical Priorities

- Venous patency is demonstrated with Doppler ultrasonography, which detects moving RBCs within a vein.
- Flow velocity and direction within an artery can be evaluated with duplex Doppler scanning.
- Because nicotine can cause vasoconstriction, cigarette smoking is prohibited before and during this test.
- An ABI of less than 0.85 indicates significant arterial occlusive disease in the extremity.

Age-Related Concerns

- Low ABI is associated with increased risk of cardiovascular disease in adults older than 65 years.
- Among adults older than 80 years who are living in nursing homes, the prevalence of low ABI is high; however, results of research studies indicate that a low ABI (<0.90) in this population is not related to cardiovascular mortality.

PROCEDURE AND PATIENT CARE

Before

✗ Explain the procedure to the patient.
✗ Inform the patient that the procedure is painless.
✗ Instruct the patient to abstain from cigarette smoking for at least 30 minutes before the test.

During

Venous Doppler Studies

- Remove all clothing from the extremity to be examined.
- Note the following procedural steps:
  1. A gel lubricant is applied in multiple areas to the skin overlying the venous system of the extremity.
  2. In the lower extremity, the deep venous system is usually identified in the ankle, calf, thigh, and groin.
  3. The characteristic "swishing" sound indicates that the venous system is patent. Failure to detect this signal indicates venous occlusion.
  4. Usually, both the superficial and deep venous systems are evaluated.

Arterial Doppler Studies: Lower Extremities

- Note the following procedural steps:
  1. Blood pressure cuffs are placed around the thigh, calf, and ankle.
  2. A gel lubricant is applied to the skin overlying the artery distal to the cuffs.
  3. The proximal cuff is inflated to a level above systolic blood pressure in the normal extremity.
  4. The Doppler ultrasound transducer is placed immediately distal to the inflated cuff.
  5. The pressure in the cuff is slowly released.
  6. The highest pressure at which blood flow is detected by the characteristic swishing Doppler signal is recorded as the blood pressure of that artery.
  7. The test is repeated at each successive level.
- Venous and arterial Doppler studies are usually performed in the vascular laboratory or radiology department and take approximately 30 minutes.

Arterial Doppler Studies: Ankle/Brachial Index

- Note the following procedural steps:
  1. Blood pressure cuffs are placed around the arm (brachial artery) and calf area above the ankle.
  2. A conductive gel is applied to the skin overlying the artery distal to the cuffs.
  3. The arm cuff is inflated to a level above systolic blood pressure in the normal extremity.
  4. The Doppler ultrasound transducer is placed immediately distal to the inflated cuff.
  5. The pressure in the cuff is slowly released.

6. The highest pressure at which blood flow is detected by the characteristic swishing Doppler signal is recorded as the blood pressure of that artery.
7. The test is repeated at the calf area above the ankle level.
8. The ABI is determined by dividing the ankle systolic pressure by the brachial systolic pressure.

• These studies are usually performed in the vascular laboratory or radiology department and take approximately 30 minutes.

After

✗ Encourage the patient to verbalize fears regarding the test results. Provide emotional support.
• Remove the gel lubricant from the extremity.
✗ Inform the patient that the radiologist must interpret the studies and that results will be available in a few hours.

TEST RESULTS AND CLINICAL SIGNIFICANCE

Venous occlusion secondary to thrombosis or thrombophlebitis: *Complete or partial occlusion is apparent at any level above the upper calf. Results are not accurate below the upper calf.*

Venous varicosities: *Doppler ultrasonography can recognize flow reversal as a result of incompetent valves of varicose veins.*

Small or large vessel arterial occlusive disease,

Spastic arterial disease (e.g., Raynaud's phenomenon),

Small vessel arterial occlusive disease (as in diabetes),

Embolic arterial occlusion,

Arterial aneurysm: *These vascular diseases are most evident with duplex Doppler scanning. Colour flow Doppler imaging, in which designated colours demonstrate flow velocity and direction, can be performed. Partial or complete occlusion is readily visualized. Turbulence, as with an aneurysm, is obvious. Reversal of flow that may occur distal to an occluded artery is evident.*

RELATED TESTS

Venography, Lower Extremities (p. 1120). This is a radiographic study of the veins of an extremity. It is more accurate for detection of deep-vein thrombosis in the lower calf, but it is no more accurate than Doppler studies in the more proximal extremity. Intravenous iodinated contrast medium used for this test may precipitate an allergic reaction or renal failure.

Arteriography (p. 1026). This radiographic study of the arteries of an extremity can more accurately indicate the exact location and anatomy of the arterial occlusion.

Urine Studies

NOTE: *Throughout this chapter, SI units are presented in* **boldface colour,** *followed by conventional units in parentheses.*

OVERVIEW

TESTS

OVERVIEW

Urine is derived from filtration of the blood by the nephrons in the kidney. Blood enters the kidney through the renal artery and passes into small capillaries in the glomerulus. There, solute and water are filtered through the capillary and into the Bowman capsule. This fluid progressively passes through the capsule and into the renal tubule. More capillaries surround the tubule, and water and other solutes can pass through the tubule into and out of the capillaries according to the body's needs. Within the renal medulla, the collecting system collects all the urine from each nephron and transports it to the renal pelvis. The urine then passes through the ureters and into the bladder. At micturition (voiding), the urine passes through the urethra and out of the body.

Urine is nearly all water, with a small percentage of solutes. All end products of metabolism and all potentially harmful materials are excreted in the urine to maintain normal acid-base balance, fluid and electrolyte balance, and homeostasis.

In general, the urine reflects the blood level for any analyte. If the analyte level is elevated in the blood and the kidneys are working well, the urine level for that same product can be expected to be high. If the urine level is not high, the kidneys may be diseased, which results in high levels in the blood. In some instances, certain blood solute products are not filtered from the blood unless "threshold" levels of the solute are exceeded. For example, glucose is not excreted by the kidney unless blood levels exceed approximately 180 mg/dL.

REASONS FOR OBTAINING URINE SPECIMENS

The urine specimen has been referred to as a "fluid biopsy" of the urinary tract. It is usually obtained painlessly, and it provides a great deal of information quickly and economically. Like other specimen tests, urine tests must be carefully performed and properly controlled. Most urine tests are performed for one of the following reasons:

1. To diagnose renal or urinary tract disease (e.g., proteinuria may indicate glomerulonephritis)
2. To monitor renal or urinary tract disease (e.g., urine cultures may be used to monitor the effectiveness of antibiotic therapy for urinary tract infections)
3. To detect metabolic or systemic diseases not directly related to the kidneys (e.g., glucose in the urine may be indicative of diabetes mellitus or Cushing's syndrome)

Although blood tests provide valuable information about the body, urinalysis may be preferred for several reasons:

1. Identification of urinary tract infection requires a urine specimen.
2. A 24-hour urine collection reflects homeostasis and disease better than does a blood specimen obtained at a random moment of the day.
3. Some products (e.g., Bence-Jones protein) are rapidly cleared by the kidneys and may not be apparent in the blood. Results of a blood test may be normal, whereas urinalysis indicates the presence of these products.
4. The level of the serum product being tested (e.g., sodium) may be affected by renal clearance. Therefore, a urine specimen to measure the sodium concentration provides significant information in addition to a serum sodium level.
5. Urine testing is easily performed and does not require an invasive skin puncture.
6. Many urine tests are less expensive than blood tests. The urine test result may be less accurate or only qualitative, but that information may be all that is needed.

TYPES OF URINE SPECIMENS

The type of urine specimen collected and the collection procedure depend on the test ordered. There are five basic types of urine specimens, discussed in the following sections. In addition, other body fluids can be evaluated to determine whether they contain urine.

First Morning Specimen

To collect a first morning specimen, the patient voids before going to bed. Immediately on awakening, the patient collects a urine specimen. The benefits of a first morning specimen are many. First, the urine in the bladder overnight represents all the urine for the previous 6 to 8 hours. Unlike a random spot urine sample, it is a more accurate reflection of the patient's 24-hour urine accumulation. Second, postural changes that may affect the urine can be avoided by obtaining the urine specimen immediately on awakening. Third, diurnal variations may affect test results. Collecting the first morning specimen allows the examiner to factor in the timing of the testing. Finally, because the urine has been retained in the bladder during a relative overnight fast, it is concentrated, and pathologic conditions are more likely to be detected. This specimen is ideal for detecting substances such as proteins and nitrites, and it is often used to confirm a diagnosis of orthostatic proteinuria.

Although the first morning specimen is frequently the specimen of choice, it is not the most convenient to obtain. The patient must follow specific instructions and be given the urine container at least 1 day before the specimen is needed. In addition, the specimen must be preserved if it is not delivered to the laboratory within 2 hours of collection.

Random Urine Specimen

Random urine specimens are usually obtained during daytime hours and without any prior patient preparation. For ease and convenience, routine screening is most often performed on a random specimen. Random testing is usually performed when the substance to be tested does not have significant diurnal variation and its normal concentration is adequate to be detected in a small volume of urine. Random urine is also the specimen of choice in screening for the presence of illegal drugs. This prevents the patient from tampering with results or changing behaviour in anticipation of testing.

Timed Urine Collection

Because substances such as hormones, proteins, and electrolytes are excreted in variable amounts over 24 hours, and because of the effects of exercise, posture, hydration, and body metabolism on excretion rates, quantitative urine tests often require collection to be timed. These time periods may range anywhere from 2 to 24 hours. Timed collections are of two types. The first type includes urine specimens collected at a predetermined time. For example, glucose is often measured 2 hours after a meal (postprandial), because that is when the glucose level in the urine is expected to be maximal. A 2-hour postprandial specimen can be collected after any meal. The second type includes specimens collected at a specific time of day. For example, a specimen for urobilinogen testing is best collected between 2:00 PM and 4:00 PM, when the amount of urobilinogen excreted is maximal. Depending on the substance being measured and the type of collection, a preservative may be needed to ensure stability throughout the collection period. In addition, certain foods and drugs may need to be avoided during the collection period. Box 11-1 lists several sources of the more common errors made in collecting and analyzing timed urine specimens.

BOX 11-1   **Sources of Error in Timed Urine Specimens**

- Loss of specimen
- Inadequate preservative used
- Inclusion of two first morning specimens in a 24-hour collection
- Inaccurate total volume measurement
- Transcription error

To collect a timed specimen, the patient is instructed to void and discard the first specimen. This is noted as the starting time of the test. All subsequent urine is saved in a special container for the designated period of time. At the end of the specified time period, the patient voids and adds this urine to the specimen container, completing the collection process. (For example, see 24-Hour Urine Collection, p. 938.)

Double-Voided Specimen

This collection method is performed to obtain and evaluate fresh urine. To obtain this specimen, the patient first empties the bladder. Shortly thereafter, the patient voids again. The second specimen in the double-voided specimen is the freshest urine and is used for testing. It accurately reflects blood concentrations at that particular time.

Urine Specimen for Culture and Sensitivity

This specimen is collected for examination of bacteria. The specimen must be collected as aseptically as possible in a sterile container. This requires meticulous cleansing of the urinary meatus with an iodine preparation to reduce contamination of the specimen by external organisms. A midstream collection technique cleanses the urethral canal of contaminant bacteria. The specimen should be submitted for culture within 1 hour of collection.

Other Body Fluids

Body fluids can be tested for blood urea nitrogen (BUN) and creatinine to determine whether the fluid is urine. This testing is commonly performed after pelvic surgery. Abdominal fluid serous drainage can look like urine. If the BUN and creatinine concentrations in that fluid are the same as in serum, the fluid is considered to be serous drainage or ascites. If, however, the concentration of BUN and creatinine in the fluid is more than three times that in serum, the fluid is urine. This testing is also helpful in obstetrics to differentiate amniotic fluid from urine.

COLLECTION METHODS

Collection methods vary from those requiring no patient preparation to invasive-type procedures. The reason for the test and the clinical situation influence the appropriate choice of collection method.

Common Collection Methods

Routine Void Specimen. A routine void specimen requires no preparation; the patient voids into an appropriate nonsterile container. Random and first morning specimens are collected in this manner.

Midstream and Clean-Catch Specimens. If a culture and sensitivity study is required or if the specimen is likely to be contaminated by vaginal discharge or bleeding, a clean-catch or midstream specimen is collected. For a clean-catch specimen, meticulous cleansing of the urinary meatus with an antiseptic preparation is necessary to reduce contamination of the specimen by external organisms. In male patients, the foreskin is retracted before the meatus is cleansed. Then the cleansing agent must be carefully removed, because it may inhibit growth of any bacteria in the specimen, which would affect the culture and sensitivity determination. For a midstream collection, the patient begins to void into a bedpan, urinal, or toilet, then stops. This washes the urine out of the distal urethra. The patient voids 3 to 4 oz ($\sim$90 to 120 mL) of urine into a sterile container, which is then capped, and the patient is allowed to finish voiding.

Twenty-Four-Hour Urine Collection. The patient is instructed to void and discard the first specimen (e.g., at 8:00 AM on day 1). This is noted as the starting time of the 24-hour collection. The patient collects all urine voided up to and including that at 8:00 AM the following day (day 2). In the laboratory, the total volume of the collection is recorded. After the collection is thoroughly mixed, a measured sample is withdrawn for analysis. See Box 11-2.

If any urine is removed or discarded during a timed collection, the entire timed collection is invalid. Twenty-four-hour urine collections are more accurate than specimens collected over a shorter time. Some analytes are excreted at different rates throughout the day or night, and if random specimens are discarded, the time of maximal excretion may be missed. Also, because greater concentrations of an analyte are present in a 24-hour collection, the chance of a false-negative result is reduced.

Special Collection Methods

Special collection methods are indicated when a specimen cannot be obtained by the more common techniques. Examples of such methods are described as follows.

Urethral Catheterization. A urine specimen can be obtained by inserting a sterile catheter through the urethra into the bladder. Although catheterization may cause infection, this collection method is used when patients are unable to void at all or cannot void when the specimen is required (e.g., during trauma).

In patients with an indwelling urinary catheter in place, a specimen is obtained by attaching a syringe to the catheter at a point distal to the sleeve leading to the balloon. Many tubes have an access area (sampling port) for this type of collection technique. Urine is aspirated and placed in a sterile urine container. (Usually the catheter tubing distal to the puncture site needs to be clamped for 15 to 30 minutes before the aspiration of urine to allow urine to fill the tubing. After the specimen is withdrawn, the clamp is removed.) The urine that accumulates in a plastic reservoir bag should never be used for a urine test.

Suprapubic Aspiration. In suprapubic aspiration, urine is collected directly from the bladder by inserting a needle through the abdominal wall and into the bladder. The urine is aspirated into a syringe and sent for analysis. This method is mainly used to obtain urine for anaerobic culture, when specimen contamination is unavoidable, and in infants and young children. Complications are rare.

BOX 11-2   Guidelines for a 24-Hour Urine Collection

1. Begin the 24-hour collection by discarding the first specimen.
2. Collect all urine voided during the next 24 hours.
3. Show the patient where to store the urine.
4. Keep the urine on ice or refrigerated during the collection period. Foley bags are kept in a basin of ice. Some collections require a preservative. Check with the laboratory.
5. Post the hours for the urine collection in a prominent place to prevent accidentally discarding a specimen.
6. Instruct the patient to void before defecating so that urine in not contaminated by stool.
7. Remind the patient not to put toilet paper in the urine collection container.
8. Collect the last specimen as close as possible to the end of the 24-hour period. Add this urine to the collection.

Pediatric Collections. Urine specimens from infants and young children are often collected in a pediatric collection bag. This clear, pliable, polyethylene bag has a hypoallergenic skin-adhesive backing around the opening. The perineal skin is cleansed and dried before the specimen bag is applied to the skin. The bag is placed over the penis in a boy and around the vagina (excluding the rectum) in a girl. Once the bag is in place, the patient is checked every 15 minutes until the urine is collected. The specimen bag should be removed as soon as the urine is collected. Bags may be folded and self-sealed for transportation. If a 24-hour specimen is needed, a tube is attached to the bag and connected to a storage container. This avoids repeated skin preparation and reapplication of adhesive to the child's sensitive skin.

TRANSPORT, STORAGE, AND PRESERVATION

Disposable plastic containers (100- to 200-mL capacity) with lids are sufficient for most routine urine tests. Screw-top containers are preferred because they are less likely to leak during transportation. Wax-coated cardboard containers should not be used because of the possibility of contaminating the specimen with fatty material. Sterile kits are available for bacterial cultures. Kits usually contain a disposable plastic urine container and cleansing pads.

Rigid, brown, light-resistant plastic containers (~3000-mL capacity) are suitable for most 12- and 24-hour urine collections. These containers have a wide mouth and a leak-proof screw cap. Preservatives may be added to these containers.

Specimen containers must be correctly labelled. Labels should not be placed on the lid, because when the lid is removed, the specimen is unlabelled. The patient identification label should be placed directly on the container.

Specimens should be transported promptly to the laboratory. If this is not possible and specimen transportation will be delayed 2 hours or longer, precautions need to be taken to preserve the integrity of the specimen. A variety of changes can occur in an unpreserved specimen. The findings of physical, chemical, and microscopic examinations can all be affected by oxidation, precipitation, and overgrowth of bacteria. Therefore, appropriate handling and storage are necessary to ensure that changes do not occur and that accurate results are obtained. Laboratories have written criteria describing when to reject a urine specimen as unsuitable for testing. Box 11-3 lists common criteria for rejecting a urine specimen.

Many analytes require preservatives to maintain viability during the collection period. The proper preservative depends on the type of collection, the delay before analysis, and the tests to be performed. No single urine preservative suits all testing requirements. Some analytes remain stable in an acidic pH; others are stable in an alkaline pH. For example, acetic acid can be used as a preservative to maintain acidity. Sodium carbonate may be used to maintain alkalinity. Boric acid may be used to inhibit bacterial multiplication. Some analytes are best preserved by refrigeration, which is the easiest means of preserving many urine specimens. If possible, all timed urine specimens should be refrigerated or on ice throughout the collection period. Foley catheter bags can be placed in a basin of ice. Timed specimens may also require the addition of a chemical preservative.

BOX 11-3	Criteria for Rejection of a Urine Sample

- Improper sample identification
- Incorrect urine preservation
- Insufficient urine quantity
- Improper specimen collection
- Missing or incomplete request form
- Visible contamination (e.g., stool)

Urine Studies

11

For example, sodium fluoride is used to preserve glucose in a 24-hour urine collection. Some analytes need to be protected from light; a dark container can be used, or the container can be wrapped with foil. Urine for the evaluation of tumour cells may be collected into a container with alcohol. Fixatives (e.g., Saccomanno fluid) also can be used to preserve cytologic specimens.

Collection preservatives may differ among laboratories, depending on (1) testing methods, (2) units of measurement, (3) how often the test is performed, (4) time delays, or (5) transportation to reference laboratories.

URINE REAGENT STRIPS

The use of urine reagent strips has replaced many complicated individual chemical analyses for determination of various components in the urine. For example, glucose, albumin, hemoglobin, and bile concentrations—as well as urinary pH, specific gravity, protein levels, presence of ketone bodies, nitrite levels, and leukocyte esterase level—can be estimated easily with a dipstick. Dipsticks are small strips of paper impregnated with a chemical that reacts to products in the urine by changing colour. The colour is correlated with concentrations of the analyte in the urine. Many tests can be performed with one dipstick.

This method of testing involves dipping a reagent strip or dipstick into urine and observing the colour change on the strip (Figure 11-1). It is important to check the expiry date of the strip prior to use. The colour is compared with the colour chart on the bottle of reagent strips at the exact time indicated. Dipstick testing is accurate and somewhat quantitative. However, a large number of products in a urine specimen can cause false-positive or false-negative results. Dipstick test results are considered preliminary findings or for screening. More definitive and quantitative studies are often necessary to confirm the results.

REPORTING OF RESULTS

Accuracy of results depends on appropriate collection, transport, storage, and preservation of the urine specimen. To be clinically useful, test results must be promptly reported because delays can render the data useless. The report must also be delivered to the appropriate medical record keeper and must be presented in a manner that is clear and easily interpreted.

The report should include the test results, reporting units, and reference ranges. Reference ranges vary from institution to institution. Comments may be included to help interpret results. For example, the technologist may note that the urine specific gravity is too low for proper interpretation of results. Proper reporting of "critical" or "panic" values (well outside the usual range of normal) is essential because such results generally necessitate immediate intervention. If these results are called in to a physician or nurse, such notification must be properly documented.

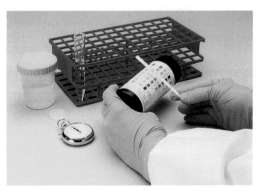

Figure 11-1 Dipstick urine testing.

Amylase, Urine

NORMAL FINDINGS

Urine amylase: **400–6 800 nkat/day*** (24–408 U/24 hr, Somogyi method)
Renal clearance ratio of amylase to creatinine: 1%–4%

INDICATIONS

The urine amylase concentration is used to assist in making the diagnosis of pancreatitis, although other nonpancreatic diseases can cause elevations in urine amylase levels. Urine amylase levels rise later than blood amylase levels. Several days after onset of the disease process, serum amylase levels may return to normal, whereas urine levels may be significantly elevated. Urine amylase concentration is particularly useful in detecting pancreatitis late in the disease course.

TEST EXPLANATION

Amylase is normally secreted from the pancreatic acinar cells into the pancreatic duct and then into the duodenum. Once in the intestine, it aids catabolism of carbohydrates to their component simple sugars. Destruction of acinar cells (as in pancreatitis) or obstruction to the pancreatic duct flow (as in pancreatic carcinoma) causes outpouring of this enzyme into the bloodstream.

Because the kidneys rapidly clear amylase, disorders that affect the pancreas cause elevations in urine amylase levels. Serum levels of amylase rise transiently but usually return to normal 1 to 2 days after resolution of the acute phase of disease. Levels of amylase in the urine, however, remain elevated 5 to 7 days after onset of disease. This is an important indicator of pancreatitis in patients who have had symptoms for 3 days or longer.

Like serum amylase levels (p. 67), urine amylase levels are sensitive but not specific for pancreatic disorders. Other diseases—such as parotiditis (mumps), cholecystitis, perforated bowel, penetrating peptic ulcer, ectopic pregnancy, and renal infarction—can cause elevations in urine levels; however, urine levels are usually highest with pancreatitis. The renal clearance ratio of amylase to creatinine provides more specific diagnostic information than either the urine amylase level or the serum amylase level alone. When the amylase/creatinine clearance ratio is 5% or higher, pancreatitis can be diagnosed with certainty. A ratio lower than 5% in a patient with elevated serum and urine amylase levels is indicative of a nonpancreatic pathologic conditions (e.g., perforated bowel, macroamylasemia).

INTERFERING FACTORS

- Intravenous dextrose solutions can cause a false-negative result.
- Drugs that may cause *increases* in amylase levels include salicylic acid, aspirin, azathioprine, corticosteroids, dexamethasone, ethyl alcohol, glucocorticoids, iodine-containing contrast media, loop diuretics (e.g., furosemide), methyldopa, narcotic analgesics, oral contraceptives, and prednisone.
- Drugs that may cause *decreases* in amylase levels include citrates, glucose, and oxalates.

---

* Values vary according to laboratory methods used. Check with your laboratory for values and units of measure.

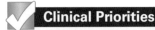

Clinical Priorities

- Urinary levels of amylase remain elevated for 5 to 7 days after disease onset. This is helpful in diagnosing pancreatitis after serum levels have returned to normal.
- When the amylase/creatinine clearance ratio is 5% or higher, pancreatitis can be diagnosed with certainty.

PROCEDURE AND PATIENT CARE

Before

✗ Explain the procedure to the patient.
✗ Inform the patient that no fasting is required.
- Record the exact time of the start of the urine collection.
✗ Show the patient where to store the urine specimen.

During

- Begin the 24-hour urine collection. Discard the initial specimen, and collect all urine voided during the next 24 hours.
- A 2-hour spot urine specimen can sometimes be used instead of the 24-hour urine collection.
- Keep the collection on ice or refrigerated during the entire 24 hours. Foley bags are kept in a basin of ice. No preservative is needed.
✗ Instruct the patient to post the times of the urine collection in a prominent location to prevent the patient from accidentally discarding a specimen.
✗ Instruct the patient to void before defecating so that the urine is not contaminated by feces.
✗ Instruct the patient not to put toilet paper in the urine container.
✗ Instruct the patient to collect the last specimen as close as possible to the end of the collection period. This specimen should be added to the urine container.

After

- Transmit the urine specimen to the laboratory promptly.

TEST RESULTS AND CLINICAL SIGNIFICANCE

▲ Increased Levels

Acute pancreatitis,
Chronic relapsing pancreatitis: *Damage to pancreatic acinar cells (as in pancreatitis) causes outpouring of amylase into the intrapancreatic lymph system and the free peritoneum. Blood vessels draining the free peritoneum and absorbing the lymph fluid pick up the excess amylase. The amylase is then cleared by the kidneys, and urine levels rise. Amylase/creatinine clearance ratio can be expected to be greater than 5.*
Penetrating peptic ulcer into the pancreas,
Gastrointestinal disease: *In patients with perforated peptic ulcer, necrotic bowel, perforated bowel, or duodenal obstruction, amylase leaks out of the gut and into the free peritoneal cavity. The amylase is picked up by the blood and lymphatic vessels of the peritoneum. The amylase is cleared by the kidneys, and urine levels rise. Amylase/creatinine clearance ratio is between 2 and 5.*
Acute cholecystitis,
Parotiditis (mumps),

Ruptured fallopian tube because of ectopic pregnancy: *Amylase is present in the salivary glands, gallbladder, and fallopian tubes. Diseases or other conditions that affect these organs are associated with elevated urine and blood levels of amylase. Amylase/creatinine clearance ratio is between 2 and 5.*
Diabetic ketoacidosis,
Pulmonary infarction,
Osteogenic sarcoma,
Cryoglobulinemia,
Rheumatoid diseases,
Postendoscopic retrograde pancreatography: *These clinical situations are sometimes associated with high urine amylase levels.*

RELATED TESTS

Amylase, Blood (p. 67). Amylase can be detected in the serum earlier than in the urine. This test is more easily performed and therefore used more frequently to monitor the course of disease.
Lipase (p. 353). Lipase is similar to amylase but is more specific for the pancreas.

Bence-Jones Protein (Free Kappa and Lambda Light Chains)

NORMAL FINDINGS

Kappa total light chain: <0.68 mg/dL
Lambda total light chain: <0.40 mg/dL
Kappa/lambda ratio: 0.7–6.2

INDICATIONS

The detection of Bence-Jones protein in the urine most commonly indicates multiple myeloma (especially when urine levels are high). The test is used to detect and monitor the treatment and clinical course of multiple myeloma and similar diseases.

TEST EXPLANATION

Bence-Jones protein consists of immunoglobulin light chains and is found in 75% of patients with multiple myeloma. This protein is most notably made by the plasma cells in these patients. It may also be associated with tumour metastases to bone, chronic lymphocytic leukemia, lymphoma, macroglobulinemia, and amyloidosis.

Normally, there is no protein in the urine because the glomerular spaces do not allow filtration of large molecules such as proteins. Bence-Jones protein, however, is very small and easily filtrated by the kidneys and excreted into the urine. Because Bence-Jones protein is rapidly cleared from the blood by the kidneys, it is difficult to detect in the blood; therefore, only urine is used for this study. Normally, urine contains no Bence-Jones protein.

Routine urine testing for proteins with reagent strips often does not reflect the type or amount of proteins in the urine. In fact, the strip may even show a negative result despite large amounts of Bence-Jones protein. Proteins in the urine are best identified by *protein electrophoresis* of the urine. With this method, the proteins are separated on the basis of size and electrical charge in an electric field when the urine specimen is applied to a gel plate. Once the various proteins are separated,

11 | Urine Studies

antisera to specific proteins can be added to the gel, and specific precipitin arcs can be identified and quantified (*immunofixation*). Monitoring the urine M-spike is especially useful in patients with light-chain multiple myeloma in whom the serum M-spike may be very small or absent, but in whom the urine M-spike is large.

INTERFERING FACTORS

- Dilute urine may yield a false-negative result.
- High doses of penicillin or aspirin can cause *false-positive* results.

PROCEDURE AND PATIENT CARE

Before

- Explain the procedure to the patient.
- Instruct the patient not to put toilet paper or stool in the urine container.

During

- Instruct the patient to collect an early morning specimen of at least 50 mL of uncontaminated urine in a container. If it would be helpful to know the amount of Bence-Jones protein excreted over 24 hours, a 24-hour collection is ordered.

After

- Immediately transport the specimen to the laboratory. If it cannot be taken to the laboratory immediately, refrigerate the specimen, because heat-coagulable proteins can decompose, causing false-positive test results.

TEST RESULTS AND CLINICAL SIGNIFICANCE

▲ Increased Levels

Multiple myeloma (plasmacytoma): *Approximately 2% of patients with myeloma do not produce Bence-Jones protein. Detection of Bence-Jones protein at high levels (>60 mg/L) is most common with this malignant disease.*

Chronic lymphocytic leukemia,

Lymphoma,

Metastatic colon, breast, lung, or prostate cancer: *Several neoplastic disorders are associated with monoclonal gammaglobulinopathies. Some can produce Bence-Jones protein.*

Amyloidosis: *Primary amyloidosis can produce immunoglobulin light chains similar to those of Bence-Jones protein.*

Waldenström macroglobulinemia: *This malignant lymphoproliferative disease is characterized by lymphadenopathy, hepatosplenomegaly, anemia, hyperviscosity, and Bence-Jones proteinuria (~20% of affected patients).*

RELATED TEST

Urinalysis (p. 991). Urinalysis includes determination of protein in the urine. If the result is positive, urine electrophoresis (similar to serum protein electrophoresis) can be performed (p. 440).

11 Beta-Prostaglandin F(2) Alpha, Urine

NORMAL FINDINGS
>1000 ng/24 hours

INDICATIONS
Measurement of 11 beta-prostaglandin F(2) alpha in urine is useful in the evaluation of patients suspected of having systemic mastocytosis (systemic mast-cell disease [SMCD]).

TEST EXPLANATION
SMCD is characterized by mast cell infiltration of extracutaneous organs (usually the bone marrow). Focal mast cell lesions in the bone marrow are found in approximately 90% of adult patients with systemic mastocytosis.

Prostaglandin D2 (PGD2) is generated by human mast cells, activated alveolar macrophages, and platelets. There are a large number of metabolic products of (PGD2); the most abundant is 11 beta-prostaglandin F2 alpha. Although the most definitive test for systemic mast cell disease is bone marrow biopsy (p. 740), measurement of mast cell mediators like beta prostaglandin in urine is advised for the initial evaluation of suspected cases. Elevated levels of 11 beta-prostaglandin F(2) alpha in urine are not specific for systemic mast cell disease and may be found in patients with angioedema, diffuse urticaria, or myeloproliferative diseases in the absence of diffuse mast cell proliferation.

Testing is most commonly performed using a commercially available alpha EIA kit.

PROCEDURE AND PATIENT CARE
Before
✍ Explain the procedure to the patient.

During
• See Box 11-2, Guidelines for a 24-Hour Urine Collection, p. 938.
✍ Encourage the patient to drink fluids during the 24 hours unless this is contraindicated for medical purposes.

After
• Send the urine to the chemistry laboratory as soon as the test is completed.

ABNORMAL FINDINGS
▲ Increased Levels
Systemic mast cell disease: *Proliferation of mast cells causes elevation of PGD2 that gets metabolized to 11 beta-prostaglandin F(2) alpha and is then excreted in urine.*
Angioedema,
Diffuse urticaria,

Urine Studies

11

Myeloproliferative diseases: *In the absence of diffuse mast cell proliferation associated with these diseases, PGD2 is abundant from a source other than mast cells, leading to increased 11 beta-prostaglandin F(2) alpha in urine.*

Bladder Cancer Markers (Bladder Tumour Antigen [BTA], Nuclear Matrix Protein 22 [NMP22])

NORMAL FINDINGS

Bladder tumour antigen (BTA): <14 U/mL
Nuclear matrix protein 22 (NMP22): <10 U/mL
Fluorescence in situ hybridization (FISH): No chromosomal amplification or deletions noted

INDICATIONS

This test is performed in patients who have had a transurethral resection of a superficial bladder cancer. The findings are used to predict or identify tumour recurrence.

TEST EXPLANATION

The rate of recurrence of superficial bladder cancers that have been resected by transurethral cystoscopy is high. Surveillance testing requires frequent urine testing for cytologic study and frequent cystoscopic evaluations. The use of bladder tumour markers may provide an easier and inexpensive method of diagnosing recurrent bladder cancer that also improves accuracy.

Bladder tumour antigen and NMP22 are proteins produced by bladder tumour cells and deposited into the urine. Normally, no or very low levels of these proteins are found in the urine. Elevated levels are associated with bladder cancer. When levels of bladder cancer tumour markers are normal, cystoscopy rarely yields positive results. When levels of these markers are elevated, bladder tumour recurrence is strongly suspected, and cystoscopy is indicated to confirm bladder cancer recurrence. As the stage (depth or grade) of the tumour increases, the likelihood that one of these markers will be positive also increases.

NMP22 may also be a good screening test for patients at increased risk for developing bladder cancer. These markers can be elevated in other circumstances (recent urologic surgery, urinary tract infection, or calculi). Cancers involving the ureters and renal pelvis may also be associated with increased levels of bladder tumour antigen and NMP22. These proteins can be quantified by immunoassay methods available in testing kits (Bard Diagnostics). At present, each is considered an adjunct to urinary cytologic study.

Bladder cancer cells have been found to exhibit aneuploidy (gene amplifications on chromosomes 3, 7, and 17, and the loss of the 9p21 locus on chromosome 9). With the use of DNA probes, through FISH, these chromosomal abnormalities can be identified with great accuracy. FISH can be performed on cells isolated in a fresh urine specimen or cells available on a ThinPrep slide (similar to Papanicolaou smears [see p. 774]). When these chromosomal abnormalities are present, fluorescent staining is obvious under a fluorescence microscope. In general, the test result may be considered positive when four or more cells show a gain of two or more chromosomes (3, 7, and 17) in the same cell or a loss of the 9p21 locus in 12 or more cells.

Although not actually a tumour marker, a specific cytologic test can be used in the early detection of bladder cancer recurrence. It is an immunocytofluorescence technique based on a patented cocktail of three monoclonal antibodies labelled with fluorescence markers. These antibodies bind to two antigens: a mucin glycoprotein and carcinoembryonic antigen (CEA). These antigens are expressed by tumour cells found in patients with bladder cancer and exfoliated in the urine.

INTERFERING FACTORS

- These proteins are very unstable. If the urine is not immediately stabilized, results may be falsely negative.
- Active infection (including sexually transmitted diseases) of the lower urologic tract can cause artificial elevations in levels of these bladder tumour markers.
- Kidney or bladder calculi can cause artificial elevations of levels of these tumour markers.

PROCEDURE AND PATIENT CARE

Before

- Explain the procedure to the patient.
- Inform the patient that no fasting is required.

During

- A single voided specimen should be collected before noon.
- The specimen should be transported to the laboratory immediately to avoid deterioration of the protein.
- If a time delay is required, the specimen should be refrigerated.

After

- Explain any other surveillance testing that may be required for bladder cancer follow-up.

TEST RESULTS AND CLINICAL SIGNIFICANCE

▲ Increased Levels

Bladder cancer: *The rapid cellular synthesis and destruction cause these proteins to be generated and washed into the urine.*

Bone Turnover Markers (N-Telopeptide [NTx], Osteocalcin [Bone G1a Protein, BGP, Osteocalc], Pyridinium [PYD] Crosslinks, Bone Alkaline Phosphatase [BAP], Procollagen Type I Intact N-Terminal Propeptide [PINP], C-Telopeptide [CTx])

NORMAL FINDINGS

N-telopeptide
  Urine
- Male: 21–66 nmol bone collagen equivalents (BCE)/mmol creatinine
- Female: 19–63 nmol BCE/mmol creatinine

  Serum
- Male: 5.4–24.2 nmol BCE
- Female: 6.2–19.0 nmol BCE

Urine Studies

11

C-telopeptide, serum
  Male:
  - 18–30 years: 155–873 pg/mL
  - 31–50 years: 93–630 pg/mL
  - 51–70 years: 35–836 pg/mL
  Female:
  - Premenopausal: 25–573 pg/mL
  - Postmenopausal: 104–1 008 pg/mL
Procollagen type I intact N-terminal propeptide (PINP), serum
  Male: 22–105 Mcg/L
  Female:
  - Premenopausal: 20–101 Mcg/L
  - Postmenopausal: 16–96 Mcg/L
Osteocalcin, serum
  ≤18 years: 9–42 ng/mL
Pyridinoline, urine
  Male: 20–61 nmol/mmol creatinine
  Female: 22–89 nmol/mmol creatinine
Bone-specific alkaline phosphatase, serum
  Male
  - <2 years: 25–221 Mcg/L
  - 2–9 years: 27–148 Mcg/L
  - 10–13 years: 35–169 Mcg/L
  - 14–17 years: 13–111 Mcg/L
  - Adults: ≤20 Mcg/L
  Female
  - <2 years: 28–187 Mcg/L
  - 2–9 years: 31–152 Mcg/L
  - 10–13 years: 29–177 Mcg/L
  - 14–17 years: 7–41 Mcg/L
  - Premenopausal: ≤14 Mcg/L
  - Postmenopausal: ≤22 Mcg/L

INDICATIONS

N-telopeptide, C-telopeptide, PINP, bone-specific alkaline phosphatase, pyridinoline, and osteocalcin are biochemical markers of bone turnover and are measured to monitor treatment for osteoporosis.

TEST EXPLANATION

With the increased use of bone density scans (see p. 1041), osteoporosis can now be diagnosed and treated more easily. This has prompted an interest in biochemical markers of bone metabolism. Bone is continuously being replaced: It is resorbed by osteoclasts and formed by osteoblasts. Osteoporosis is a common disease of postmenopausal women and is associated with increased bone resorption and decreased bone formation. The result is thin and weak bones that are prone to fracture. The same process is now becoming increasingly recognized in older adult men, as well. Early diagnosis enables therapeutic intervention to prevent bone fracture.

Bone mineral density studies are valuable tools in the identification of osteoporosis; however, they cannot recognize small changes in bone metabolism. Although bone density studies can be used to monitor the effectiveness of therapy, it takes years to detect measurable changes in bone density. Biochemical markers, however, can be measured to identify significant improvement in a few months after instituting successful therapy. Furthermore, the cost of bone density studies limits the feasibility of performing this test as frequently as may be necessary to monitor treatment.

Because the levels of bone turnover biochemical markers vary according to the time of day and bone volume, these studies are not helpful in screening for osteoporosis. Their use is in determining the effect of treatment as the posttreatment levels of these markers are compared with pretreatment levels. Levels decline with the use of antiresorption drugs (such as estrogen, alendronate, calcitonin, and raloxifene).

N- and C-telopeptides are protein fragments used in type 1 collagen that make up nearly 90% of the bone matrix. The C- and N-terminals of these proteins are crosslinked to provide tensile strength to the bone. When bone is broken down, C-telopeptide and N-telopeptide are released into the bloodstream and excreted in the urine. Serum levels of these fragments have been shown to be correlated strongly with urine measurements normalized to creatinine. Measurements of these fragments show early response to antiresorptive therapy (within 3 to 6 months). When used in conjunction with bone density scanning, the measurements provide a more complete picture of bone metabolism and status. Normal levels can vary with method of testing.

The concentration of PINP, like that of N-telopeptide, is directly proportional to the amount of new collagen produced by osteoblasts. Concentrations are increased in patients with various bone diseases and who are receiving therapies characterized by increased osteoblastic activity. PINP is the most effective marker of bone formation and is particularly useful for monitoring bone formation therapies and antiresorptive therapies.

Osteocalcin, or *bone G1a protein,* is a noncollagenous protein in the bone and is made by osteoblasts. It enters the circulation during both bone resorption and bone formation, and its level is a good indicator of bone metabolism. Serum levels of osteocalcin are correlated with rates of bone formation and destruction. Although osteocalcin is synthesized predominantly by osteoblasts, increased levels are associated with increased bone resorption. Osteocalcin is a vitamin K–dependent protein. Reduction in vitamin K intake is associated with reduced osteocalcin levels. This possibly explains the pathophysiologic process of vitamin K–deficiency osteoporosis.

Pyridinoline crosslinks are formed during maturation of the type I collagen during bone formation. During bone resorption, these pyridinoline crosslinks are released into the circulation.

These bone turnover biochemical markers cannot indicate the risk for bone fracture nearly as well as can a bone density scan. Besides osteoporosis, these markers can be used to monitor the activity and treatment of Paget's disease, hyperparathyroidism, and bone metastasis. After 3 months of antiresorptive therapy, levels of bone turnover markers are typically decreased by 30%.

Levels of biochemical markers are normally high in children because of increased bone resorption associated with growth and remodelling of the ends of the long bones. The levels reach a peak at 14 years of age and then gradually decline to adult values. Because estrogen is a strong inhibitor of osteoclastic (bone resorption) activity, loss of bone density begins soon after menopause begins. Marker levels therefore rise after menopause. Most urinary assays reflect creatinine excretion for normalization.

Bone-specific alkaline phosphatase is an isoenzyme of alkaline phosphate (p. 53) and is found in the cell membrane of the osteoblast. It is therefore an indicator of the metabolic status of osteoblasts and bone formation.

Urine Studies

11

INTERFERING FACTORS

- Measurements of these urinary markers can differ by as much as 30% in one person even on the same day. Collecting double-voided specimens in the morning can minimize variability.
- Osteocalcin production is dependent on the availability of vitamins D, C, and K.
- ⚖ Drugs taken for bodybuilding treatments, such as testosterone, can cause *reductions* in the levels of N-telopeptide.

PROCEDURE AND PATIENT CARE

Before

- 📖 Explain the procedure to the patient.
- It is important to obtain baseline levels before instituting therapy.
- Note that some laboratories require a 24-hour urine collection.

During

Urine

- A double-voided specimen is preferred.
  1. Obtain a urine specimen 30 to 40 minutes before the time the specimen is needed.
  2. Discard this first specimen.
  3. Give the patient a glass of water to drink.
  4. At the requested time, obtain a second specimen.

Blood

- Collect a venous blood sample in a red-top tube. Check with your laboratory for guidelines when collecting specimens for bone turnover markers.

After

- Apply pressure or a pressure dressing to the venipuncture site.
- Assess the venipuncture site for bleeding.
- Transmit the specimens to the laboratory for testing.

TEST RESULTS AND CLINICAL SIGNIFICANCE

▲ Increased Levels

Osteoporosis,
Paget's disease,
Advanced bone tumours (primary or metastatic),
Acromegaly,
Hyperparathyroidism,
Hyperthyroidism,
Osteodystrophy: *These diseases are associated with increased activity of osteoblasts and osteoclasts. Levels of these bone turnover markers are increased as a result of increased cellular function, increased bone matrix formation, or destruction.*

▼ Decreased Levels

- Hypoparathyroidism,
- Hypothyroidism,
- Cortisol therapy: *These situations are associated with decreased activity of osteoblasts and osteoclasts.*

RELATED TESTS

Bone Densitometry (p. 1041). This test is a measure of the density of central and peripheral bones. It is also a measure of bone mass.

Bone (Long) Radiography (p. 1045). Plain radiography can identify advanced bone demineralization and indicate severe osteoporosis.

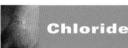
Chloride, Urine (Cl)

NORMAL FINDINGS

Adult/older adult: **110–250 mmol/day** (110–250 mEq/day)
Child: **15–40 mmol/day** (15–40 mEq/day)
Infant: **2–10 mmol/day** (2–10 mEq/day)

INDICATIONS

This test is performed with measurements of other urinary electrolytes to indicate the state of electrolyte or acid-base imbalance.

TEST EXPLANATION

Chloride is the major extracellular anion. Its main purpose is to maintain electrical neutrality, mostly as a salt with sodium. Chloride losses follow sodium (cation) losses, and chloride excesses accompany sodium excesses to maintain electrical neutrality. For example, when aldosterone prompts sodium reabsorption, chloride reabsorption follows to maintain electrical neutrality. Because water moves with sodium and chloride, chloride also affects water balance. Finally, chloride serves as a buffer to assist in acid-base balance. As levels of carbon dioxide (and hydrogen cation) increase, bicarbonate must move from the intracellular space to the extracellular space. To maintain electrical neutrality, chloride shifts back into the cell.

A 24-hour urine collection for chloride is useful for evaluating the electrolyte composition of urine and in helping determine acid-base imbalances. It is also useful in evaluating the patient's compliance with diets with restricted salt (sodium chloride). If sodium and chloride levels are high, the patient is not complying with the diet.

INTERFERING FACTORS

- Urine volume and perspiration can affect chloride levels.
- Dietary salt intake or saline infusion affects urinary levels.
- Drugs that may cause *increases* in chloride levels include bromides, diuretics, and steroids.

PROCEDURE AND PATIENT CARE

Before

- Explain the procedure to the patient.
- Inform the patient that no special diet is required.
- Show the patient where to store the urine container.

Urine Studies

11

During

- Begin the 24-hour urine collection. Discard the initial specimen, and collect all urine voided by the patient during the next 24 hours.
- Keep the collection on ice or refrigerated during the entire 24 hours.
- On the urine container and laboratory slip, note the starting time.
- Instruct the patient to post the times of the urine collection in a prominent location to prevent the patient from accidentally discarding a specimen.
- Instruct the patient to void before defecating so that the urine is not contaminated by feces.
- Instruct the patient not to put toilet paper in the urine container.
- Encourage the patient to drink fluids during the 24 hours unless drinking is contraindicated for medical reasons.
- Instruct the patient to collect the last specimen as close as possible to the end of the 24 hours. This specimen should be added to the urine container.

After

- Transport the urine specimen to the laboratory promptly.

TEST RESULTS AND CLINICAL SIGNIFICANCE

▲ Increased Levels

Dehydration,
Starvation,
Diuretic therapy,
Addison's disease: *Sodium (followed by chloride) reabsorption is decreased.*
Increased salt intake,
Intravenous saline infusion: *Output must equal input to maintain homeostasis. Therefore, urinary chloride increases with increased intake.*

▼ Decreased Levels

Cushing's syndrome,
Conn syndrome,
Steroid therapy,
Heart failure: *Sodium reabsorption (followed by chloride reabsorption) is increased.*
Malabsorption syndrome,
Prolonged gastric suction or vomiting,
Diarrhea,
Pyloric obstruction,
Diaphoresis,
Reduced salt intake: *Serum chloride levels are decreased. Therefore, urinary chloride levels are decreased.*

RELATED TESTS

Sodium, Urine (p. 980), and Potassium, Urine (p. 976). These are measurements of sodium and potassium electrolytes in the urine.

Chloride, Blood (p. 167). This is a measurement of serum chloride level.

Cortisol, Urine (Hydrocortisone, Urine Cortisol, Free Cortisol)

NORMAL FINDINGS
Adult/older adult: <276 nmol/day (<100 *Mcg*/24hr)
Adolescent: 14–152 nmol/day (5–55 *Mcg*/24hr)
Child: 5.5–74 nmol/day (2–27 *Mcg*/24hr)

INDICATIONS
This test, a measure of urinary cortisol, is performed in patients with suspected hyperfunction or hypofunction of the adrenal gland.

TEST EXPLANATION
An elaborate feedback mechanism for cortisol exists to coordinate the function of the hypothalamus, pituitary gland, and adrenal glands. Corticotropin-releasing hormone is made in the hypothalamus. This stimulates production of adrenocorticotropic hormone (ACTH) in the anterior pituitary gland. ACTH, in turn, stimulates the adrenal cortex to produce cortisol. The rising levels of cortisol act as a negative feedback and curtail further production of corticotropin-releasing hormone and ACTH. Free or unconjugated cortisol is filtered by the kidneys and excreted in the urine. Elevated urine cortisol levels reflect elevated serum cortisol levels.

Cortisol is a potent glucocorticoid released from the adrenal cortex. This hormone affects the metabolism of carbohydrates, proteins, and fats. It has an especially profound effect on glucose serum levels. Cortisol tends to increase glucose by stimulating gluconeogenesis from glucose stores. It also inhibits the effect of insulin and thereby inhibits glucose transport into the cells.

INTERFERING FACTORS
- Pregnancy causes increases in cortisol levels.
- Physical and emotional stress can cause elevations in cortisol levels.
- Stress stimulates the pituitary-cortical mechanism, which thereby stimulates cortisol production.
- Drugs that may cause *increases* in cortisol levels include danazol, hydrocortisone, oral contraceptives, and spironolactone (Aldactone).
- Drugs that may cause *decreases* in cortisol levels include dexamethasone, ethacrynic acid, ketoconazole, and thiazides.

PROCEDURE AND PATIENT CARE
Before
- Explain the procedure to the patient.
- Assess the patient for signs of physical stress (e.g., infection, acute illness) or emotional stress, and report these signs to the physician.

During

- Begin the 24-hour urine collection. Discard the initial specimen, and collect all urine passed by the patient during the next 24 hours.
- Ⓧ Instruct the patient to post the times of the urine collection in a prominent location to prevent the patient from accidentally discarding a specimen.
- Note that it is not necessary to measure each urine specimen.
- Ⓧ Instruct the patient to void before defecating so that the urine is not contaminated by feces.
- Ⓧ Instruct the patient not to put toilet paper in the urine container.
- Ⓧ Encourage the patient to drink fluids during the 24 hours, unless drinking is contraindicated for medical reasons.
- Ⓧ Instruct the patient to collect the last specimen as close as possible to the end of the 24 hours. This specimen should be added to the urine container.
- Place the 24-hour urine collection in a plastic container and keep on ice or refrigerated. Use a preservative.
- On the laboratory slip, note the dates and times that the specimen collection began and ended.
- On the laboratory slip, note whether the patient is taking any medications that may affect test results.

After

- Transmit the specimen to the laboratory promptly.

TEST RESULTS AND CLINICAL SIGNIFICANCE

▲ Increased Levels

Cushing's disease,

Ectopic ACTH-producing tumours,

Stress: *ACTH is overproduced as a result of neoplastic overproduction of ACTH in the pituitary gland or elsewhere in the body by an ACTH-producing cancer. Stress is a potent stimulus of ACTH production. Cortisol levels rise as a result.*

Cushing's syndrome (adrenal adenoma or carcinoma): *The neoplasm produces cortisol without regard to the normal feedback mechanism.*

Hyperthyroidism: *The metabolic rate is increased, and cortisol levels rise accordingly to maintain elevated glucose needs.*

Obesity: *All sterols are increased in obese patients, perhaps because fatty tissue may act as a depository or location of synthesis.*

▼ Decreased Levels

Adrenal hyperplasia: *Congenital absence of important enzymes in the synthesis of cortisol precludes adequate serum levels.*

Addison's disease: *As a result of hypofunctioning of the adrenal gland, cortisol levels drop.*

Hypopituitarism: *ACTH is not produced by a pituitary gland destroyed by disease, neoplasm, or ischemia. The adrenal gland is not stimulated to produce cortisol.*

Hypothyroidism: *Normal cortisol levels are not necessary to maintain the reduced metabolic rate in patients with hypothyroidism.*

RELATED TESTS

Adrenocorticotropic Hormone Stimulation (p. 37). This test is used to evaluate the differential diagnosis of Cushing's syndrome or Addison's disease.

Adrenocorticotropic Hormone (p. 34). The serum ACTH study is a test of anterior pituitary gland function that affords the greatest insight into the causes of Cushing's syndrome (overproduction of cortisol) and Addison's disease (underproduction of cortisol).

Cortisol, Blood (p. 192). This is a direct measurement of cortisol blood level.

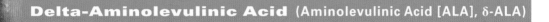

Delta-Aminolevulinic Acid (Aminolevulinic Acid [ALA], δ-ALA)

NORMAL FINDINGS

11–57 Mcmol/24 hr (1.5–7.5 mg/24 hr)

 Critical Values

>152.5 Mcmol/24 hr (>20 mg/24 hr)

INDICATIONS

This test is used to diagnose porphyria and in the evaluation of subclinical forms of lead poisoning in children.

TEST EXPLANATION

As the basic precursor for the porphyrins (p. 974), delta-aminolevulinic acid (δ-ALA) is needed for the normal production of porphobilinogen, which ultimately leads to heme synthesis in erythroid cells. Heme is used in the synthesis of hemoglobin. Genetic disorders (e.g., porphyria) are associated with lack of a particular enzyme that is vital for heme metabolism. These disorders are characterized by accumulation of porphyrin products in the liver or in red blood cells (RBCs). The liver porphyrias are most common. Symptoms of liver porphyrias include abdominal pain, neuromuscular signs and symptoms, constipation, and, on occasion, psychotic behaviour. This group of disorders results from enzymatic deficiency in synthesis of heme (a portion of hemoglobin). Acute intermittent porphyria is the most common form of liver porphyria and is caused by a deficiency in uroporphyrinogen-1-synthase (also called *porphobilinogen deaminase*).

Most patients with acute intermittent porphyria have no symptoms (latent phase) until the acute phase is precipitated by medication or some other factor (see Box 2-15, p. 540). The acute phase is characterized by abdominal and muscular pain, nausea, vomiting, hypertension, mental symptoms (e.g., anxiety, insomnia, hallucinations, paranoia), sensory loss, and urinary retention. Hemolytic anemia also may develop during the acute phase. These acute symptoms are associated with increased serum and urine levels of porphyrin precursors (δ-ALA, porphyrins, and porphobilinogens).

In lead intoxication, heme synthesis is similarly diminished by the inhibition of δ-ALA dehydrase. This enzyme assists in the conversion of δ-ALA to porphobilinogen. As a result of lead poisoning, δ-ALA accumulates in the blood and urine.

Urine Studies

11

INTERFERING FACTORS

Drugs that may cause *increases* in δ-ALA levels include barbiturates, and penicillin (see also Box 2-15, p. 540).

PROCEDURE AND PATIENT CARE

Before

Explain the procedure to the patient.

During

- Begin the 24-hour urine collection. Discard the initial specimen, and collect all urine passed by the patient during the next 24 hours.
- Show the patient where to store the urine container.
- Keep the collection on ice or refrigerated during the entire 24 hours.
- Keep the urine in a light-resistant container with a preservative.
- On the urine container and laboratory slip, note the starting time.
- Instruct the patient to post the times of the urine collection in a prominent location to prevent the patient from accidentally discarding a specimen.
- Instruct the patient to void before defecating so that the urine is not contaminated by feces.
- Instruct the patient not to put toilet paper in the urine container.
- Encourage the patient to drink fluids during the 24 hours, unless drinking is contraindicated for medical reasons.
- Instruct the patient to collect the last specimen as close as possible to the end of the 24 hours. This specimen should be added to the urine container.
- If the patient has a Foley catheter in place, cover the drainage bag to prevent exposure to light.
- On the laboratory slip, note whether the patient is taking any drugs that may affect test results.

After

- Transport the urine specimen promptly to the laboratory.

TEST RESULTS AND CLINICAL SIGNIFICANCE

▲ Increased Levels

Porphyria (acute intermittent, variegate, and coproporphyria): *During the acute phase, porphyrin precursors (including δ-ALA) accumulate in the blood and urine.*

Lead intoxication: *Chronic lead intoxication may be associated with increased levels of δ-ALA, which accumulates in the blood and urine.*

Chronic alcoholic liver disorders,

Diabetic ketoacidosis: *These diseases are associated with increased levels of δ-ALA. The pathophysiologic mechanism underlying these observations is complex and not well defined.*

RELATED TESTS

Uroporphyrinogen-1-Synthase (p. 539). This test is used to identify individuals at risk for development of porphyria and to diagnose porphyria in the acute and latent stages.

Porphyrins and Porphobilinogens (p. 974). This is a quantitative measurement of porphyrins and porphobilinogens in the urine. This test helps define a porphyrin pattern with which the type of porphyria can be classified.

Glucose, Urine (Urine Sugar)

NORMAL FINDINGS

Random specimen: Negative
24-hour specimen: **<2.78 mmol/day** (<0.5 g/day)

INDICATIONS

Testing for glucose in the urine is part of routine urinalysis. If glucose is present, it reflects the degree of glucose elevation in the blood. Urine glucose tests are also used to monitor the effectiveness of therapy for diabetes mellitus.

TEST EXPLANATION

A qualitative glucose test is part of routine urinalysis. This screening test for the presence of glucose within the urine may indicate the likelihood of diabetes mellitus or other causes of glucose intolerance (see Glucose, Blood, p. 269). This diagnosis must be confirmed by other tests (e.g., fasting glucose, glucose tolerance, glycosylated hemoglobin). Urine glucose tests may be used to monitor the effectiveness of diabetes therapy; however, this has largely been supplanted by fingerstick determinations of blood glucose levels.

In patients with diabetes that is not well controlled with hypoglycemic agents, blood glucose levels can become very high. Glucose is filtered from the blood by the glomeruli of the kidney. In the glomerular filtrate, the glucose concentration is the same as in the blood. Normally, all of the glucose is reabsorbed in the proximal renal tubules. When the blood glucose level exceeds the capability of the renal threshold to reabsorb the glucose (~10 mmol/L [~180 mg/dL]), the glucose begins to spill over into the urine (glycosuria). As the blood glucose level increases, the amount of glucose that spills into the urine also increases.

Glycosuria may occur immediately after a high-carbohydrate meal, in patients with otherwise normal glucose levels, or in prediabetic patients receiving dextrose-containing intravenous fluids. Furthermore, glycosuria does not always indicate diabetes; it can occur normally or in diseases that affect the renal tubule or in genetic defects in metabolism and excretion of glucose. In these diseases, the renal threshold for glucose is abnormally low. Despite a normal blood glucose concentration, the kidneys cannot reabsorb the normal glucose load. As a result, surplus glucose is spilled into the urine. In these patients, results of glucose tolerance tests are normal. In acute severe physical stress or injury, transient glycosuria can result from normal compensatory endocrine-mediated responses.

INTERFERING FACTORS

- Any substance that can reduce copper in the Clinitest can produce false-positive results. This may include other sugars (e.g., galactose, fructose, lactose).
- Drugs that may cause *false-positive* results with reagent tablets (e.g., in the Clinitest assay) but not with enzyme-impregnated strips (Clinistix, Tes-Tape) include acetylsalicylic acid, salicylic acid, ascorbic acid, cephalothin, chloral hydrate, nitrofurantoin, streptomycin, and sulphonamides.

Urine Studies

11

- Drugs that may cause *false-negative* results include ascorbic acid (Clinistix, Tes-Tape), levodopa (Clinistix), and phenazopyridine (Clinistix, Tes-Tape).
- Drugs that may cause *increases* in urine glucose levels include salicylic acid, cephalosporins, chloral hydrate, chloramphenicol, dextrothyroxine, diazoxide, diuretics (loop and thiazide), estrogen, glucose infusions, isoniazid, levodopa, lithium, nafcillin, nalidixic acid, and nicotinic acid (large doses).

PROCEDURE AND PATIENT CARE

Before

- Explain the procedure to the patient.
- Follow the directions on the bottle or container of reagent strips.
- Check the expiration date on the bottle before use.
- Inform the patient that urine tests for glucose may be performed at specified times during the day, generally before meals and at bedtime, and that test results may be used to help determine insulin requirements.

During

- Because accuracy is necessary, collect a "fresh" urine specimen. Stagnant urine that has been in the bladder for several hours does not accurately reflect the serum glucose level at the time of testing.
- Preferably, obtain a double-voided specimen by the following method:
  1. Instruct the patient to void 30 to 40 minutes before the time the urine specimen is actually needed.
  2. Discard this first specimen.
  3. Give the patient a glass of water to drink.
  4. At the required time, obtain a second specimen to be tested for glucose.
- Inform the patient that testing for glucose can be easily performed using enzyme tests such as Clinistix, Diastix, or Tes-Tape.
- If a 24-hour specimen is required, refrigerate the urine during the collection period.

After

- If bedside or office testing is performed, record the urine glucose level on the patient's chart.

TEST RESULTS AND CLINICAL SIGNIFICANCE

▲ Increased Levels

Diabetes mellitus and other causes of hyperglycemia,

Pregnancy: *Glycosuria is common in pregnant women. Persistently and significantly high levels may indicate gestational diabetes or other obstetric illness. Also, lactosuria is common in nursing women. Lactose is classified as a "reducing sugar" that may cause false-positive results for glucose, depending on the method of testing.*

Renal glycosuria: *This can occur normally or in patients with diseases that affect the renal tubule. It can also result from genetic defects in the metabolism and excretion of glucose. In these diseases, the renal threshold for glucose is abnormally low. Despite a normal blood glucose level, the kidneys cannot reabsorb the glucose that they should. As a result, the surplus glucose is spilled into the urine.*

Fanconi's syndrome: *This condition is associated with transport defects in the proximal renal tubules, causing glycosuria. This genetic defect can also affect the metabolism and excretion of amino acids and electrolytes.*

Hereditary defects in metabolism of other reducing substances (e.g., galactose, fructose, pentose): *These reducing substances may cause false-positive results of glucose tests, depending on the method of testing.*

Increased intracranial pressure (e.g., from tumours, hemorrhage): *The pathophysiologic mechanism underlying this observation is not well defined, although many theories exist.*

Nephrotoxic chemicals (e.g., carbon monoxide, mercury, lead): *These chemicals injure the kidneys and lower the renal threshold.*

RELATED TESTS

Glucose, Blood (p. 269). This is the main screening test for diagnosis of diabetes.

Glycosylated Hemoglobin (p. 281). This is an accurate method for indicating glucose tolerance in the recent past.

Glucose Tolerance (p. 276). This is a test of a patient's capability of handling a glucose load.

Glucose, Postprandial (p. 272). This is a timed glucose measurement after a carbohydrate meal.

Glucagon (p. 267). This is a direct measurement of glucagon, which acts to increase glucose in the blood.

Insulin Assay (p. 330). This is a direct measurement of insulin, which acts to decrease glucose in the blood.

17-Hydroxycorticosteroids (17-OCHS)

NORMAL FINDINGS

Adult
    Male: **8.3–27.6 Mcmol/24 hr** (3–10 mg/24 hr)
    Female: **5.2–22.1 Mcmol/24 hr** (2–8 mg/24 hr)
Older adult: values slightly lower than for adult
Child
    0–1 years: **1.4–2.8 Mcmol/24 hr** (0.5–1 mg/24 hr)
    <12 years: **2.8–12.4 Mcmol/24 hr** (1–4.5 mg/24 hr)

INDICATIONS

This urine study is used to assess adrenocortical function by measuring the cortisol metabolites (17-hydroxycorticosteroids [17-OCHS]) in a 24-hour urine collection.

TEST EXPLANATION

Levels of 17-OCHS are elevated in patients with adrenal hyperfunction (Cushing's syndrome), whether the condition is caused by a pituitary or adrenal tumour, bilateral adrenal hyperplasia, or ectopic tumours producing adrenocorticotropic hormone (ACTH). Levels of 17-OCHS are low in patients with adrenal hypofunction (Addison's disease) as a result of destruction of the adrenal glands (by hemorrhage, infarction, metastatic tumour, or autoimmunity), surgical removal of an adrenal gland without appropriate steroid replacement, congenital enzyme deficiency, hypopituitarism, or adrenal suppression after prolonged ingestion of exogenous steroid.

Testing the urine for this hormone metabolite is an indirect measure of adrenal function. Urine and plasma levels of cortisol (see p. 953 and p. 192, respectively) provide a much more accurate measurement of adrenal function. Because excretion of cortisol metabolites follows a diurnal variation, 24-hour urine collection is necessary.

INTERFERING FACTORS

- Emotional and physical stress (e.g., infection) and licorice ingestion may cause increased adrenal activity.
- Drugs that may cause *increases* in 17-OCHS levels include acetazolamide, chloral hydrate, chlorpromazine, colchicine, erythromycin, meprobamate, paraldehyde, quinidine, quinine, and spironolactone.
- Drugs that may cause *decreases* in 17-OCHS levels include estrogen, oral contraceptives, and phenothiazines.

PROCEDURE AND PATIENT CARE

Before

- Explain the procedure to the patient.
- Note that drugs are usually withheld for several days before urine collection. Check with the physician and laboratory for specific guidelines.
- Assess the patient for signs of stress, and report these signs to the physician.

During

- Do not administer any drugs that may interfere with test results.
- Begin the 24-hour urine collection. Discard the initial specimen, and collect all urine voided by the patient during the next 24 hours.
- Instruct the patient to post the times of the urine collection in a prominent location to prevent the patient from accidentally discarding a specimen.
- Note that it is not necessary to measure each urine specimen.
- Instruct the patient to void before defecating so that the urine is not contaminated by feces.
- Instruct the patient not to put toilet paper in the urine container.
- Encourage the patient to drink fluids during the 24 hours, unless drinking is contraindicated for medical reasons.
- Instruct the patient to collect the last specimen as close as possible to the end of the 24 hours. This specimen should be added to the urine container.
- Keep the collection refrigerated or on ice during the entire 24 hours.

After

- Transmit the urine to the chemistry laboratory as soon as the test is completed.

TEST RESULTS AND CLINICAL SIGNIFICANCE

▲ Increased Levels

Cushing's disease,
Ectopic ACTH-producing tumours: *Overproduction of ACTH results from ACTH-producing cancers in the pituitary gland or elsewhere in the body.*

Stress: *Stress is a potent stimulus of ACTH production. Cortisol and 17-OCHS levels rise as a result.*

Cushing's syndrome (adrenal adenoma or carcinoma): *The neoplasm produces cortisol without regard to the normal feedback mechanism, and 17-OCHS levels rise.*

Hyperthyroidism: *Metabolic rate is increased, and cortisol and 17-OCHS levels rise accordingly to maintain the elevated glucose needs.*

Obesity: *All sterols are increased in obese patients, perhaps because fatty tissue acts as a depository or location of synthesis.*

▼ Decreased Levels

Adrenal hyperplasia (adrenogenital syndrome): *Congenital absence of important enzymes in the cortisol synthesis process precludes adequate serum and urine levels.*

Addison's disease caused by adrenal infarction, adrenal hemorrhage, surgical removal of the adrenal glands, congenital enzyme deficiency, or adrenal suppression from steroid therapy: *As a result of hypofunctioning of the adrenal gland, cortisol and 17-OCHS levels are decreased.*

Hypopituitarism: *ACTH is not produced by a pituitary gland destroyed by disease, neoplasm, or ischemia. The adrenal glands are not stimulated to produce cortisol and 17-OCHS.*

Hypothyroidism: *Normal cortisol levels are not necessary to maintain the reduced metabolic rate in patients with hypothyroidism. Cortisol and 17-OCHS levels are decreased.*

RELATED TEST

Cortisol, Blood (p. 192). This test is a measure of serum cortisol and is performed in patients with suspected adrenal gland hyperfunction or hypofunction.

5-Hydroxyindoleacetic Acid (5-HIAA)

NORMAL FINDINGS

10–40 *Mc*mol/day (2–8 mg/24 hr)
   Concentrations are lower in female patients than in male patients.

INDICATIONS

This test is used to detect carcinoid tumour and to monitor affected patients' response to therapy.

TEST EXPLANATION

Quantitative analysis of 5-hydroxyindoleacetic acid (5-HIAA) in urine is performed to detect and monitor the clinical course of carcinoid tumours. Carcinoid tumours are serotonin-secreting tumours that may grow in the appendix, intestine, lung, or any tissue derived from the neuroectoderm. These tumours contain argentaffin-staining (enteroendocrine) cells, which produce serotonin and other powerful neurohormones that are metabolized by the liver to 5-HIAA and excreted in the urine. These powerful neurohormones are responsible for the clinical symptoms (e.g., bronchospasm, flushing, diarrhea) of carcinoid syndrome. This test is used not only to identify carcinoid tumours but also to reevaluate known tumours by means of serial levels of urinary 5-HIAA. Increasing levels of 5-HIAA indicate progression of the tumour; decreasing levels

11

Urine Studies

indicate a therapeutic response to antineoplastic therapy. To some extent, larger tumours are associated with higher urine levels than smaller tumours are.

INTERFERING FACTORS

- Bananas, plantains, pineapples, kiwis, walnuts, plums, pecans, and avocados can factitiously elevate 5-HIAA levels.
- Drugs that may cause *increases* in 5-HIAA levels include acetanilid, acetophenetidin, glyceryl guaiacolate, methocarbamol, and acetaminophen.
- Drugs that may cause *decreases* in 5-HIAA levels include aspirin, chlorpromazine, ethyl alcohol, heparin, imipramine, isoniazid, levodopa, methenamine, methyldopa, monoamine oxidase inhibitors, phenothiazines, promethazine, and tricyclic antidepressants.

PROCEDURE AND PATIENT CARE

Before

- Explain the procedure to the patient.
- Instruct the patient to refrain from eating foods containing serotonin (e.g., plums, pineapples, bananas, eggplants, tomatoes, avocados, walnuts) for several days (usually 3) before and during testing.

During

- Begin the 24-hour urine collection. Discard the initial specimen, and collect all urine voided by the patient during the next 24 hours.
- Show the patient where to store the urine specimen.
- Keep the collection on ice or in a refrigerator during the entire 24 hours. A preservative is needed to maintain an appropriate pH.
- Instruct the patient to post the times of the urine collection in a prominent location to prevent the patient from accidentally discarding a specimen.
- Instruct the patient to void before defecating so that the urine is not contaminated by feces.
- Instruct the patient not to put toilet paper in the urine container.
- Instruct the patient to collect the last specimen as close as possible to the end of the 24-hour collection period. This specimen should be added to the urine container.

After

- Transmit the urine specimen to the laboratory promptly.
- On the laboratory slip, note whether the patient is taking any medications that may affect the test results.

TEST RESULTS AND CLINICAL SIGNIFICANCE

▲ Increased Levels

Carcinoid tumour of the appendix, bowel, lung, breast, or ovary: *Serotonin is produced by the argentaffin-staining (enteroendocrine) cells within the tumour. The serotonin is metabolized by the liver to 5-HIAA, which is then excreted into the urine.*

Noncarcinoid illness,

Cystic fibrosis,

Intestinal malabsorption: *These conditions may be associated with elevated 5-HIAA levels. The pathophysiologic mechanism underlying these observations is not clear.*

▼ Decreased Levels

Depression,
Migraine: *Serotonin deficit has been noted in these conditions. The cause is unknown.*

17-Ketosteroid (17-KS)

NORMAL FINDINGS

Male: **20–70 M**c**mol/day** (6–20 mg/24 hr)
Female: **20–60 M**c**mol/day** (6–17 mg/24 hr)
Older adult (>60 years): **13–27 M**c**mol/day** (4–8 mg/24 hr)
Child/adolescent:
    <12 years: **<17 M**c**mol/day** (<5 mg/24 hr)
    12–15 years: **17–41 M**c**mol/day** (5–12 mg/24 hr)

INDICATIONS

This urine test is performed to assist in evaluation of adrenal cortex function, especially as it relates to androgenic function. It is especially useful for evaluation and monitoring of adrenal hyperplasia (adrenogenital syndrome) and adrenal tumours.

TEST EXPLANATION

This urine test is used to measure adrenocortical function by measuring 17-ketosteroids in the urine. 17-Ketosteroids are metabolites of testosterone and other androgenic sex hormones. The principal 17-ketosteroid is dehydroepiandrosterone (DHEA). In men, approximately one-third of the hormone metabolites are derived from testosterone, produced in the testes, and two-thirds are derived from other androgenic hormones, produced in the adrenal cortex. In women and children, almost all 17-ketosteroids are nontestosterone androgenic hormones, produced in the adrenal cortex. Therefore, this test is useful in diagnosing adrenocortical dysfunction. It is important to note that 17-ketosteroids are not metabolites of cortisol and do not reflect levels of cortisol production. 17-Ketosteroid levels are frequently elevated in congenital adrenal hyperplasia and androgenic tumours of the adrenal glands. In these diseases, excess steroid synthesis is of the "noncortisol" androgenic sterols. These diseases frequently cause virilization syndromes. Testicular tumours rarely cause elevations in 17-ketosteroid levels.

Low levels of 17-ketosteroids have little clinical significance because of the inaccuracy of determining low levels. The most common cause of low 17-ketosteroid levels is stress. During stress, the adrenal glands produce less androgen and more cortisol. In this regard, low 17-ketosteroid levels may reflect states of good health.

INTERFERING FACTORS

• Stress may decrease adrenal androgenic activity.

Urine Studies

11

🛠 Drugs that may cause *increases* in 17-ketosteroid levels include antibiotics, chloramphenicol, chlorpromazine, dexamethasone, meprobamate, phenothiazines, quinidine, secobarbital, and spironolactone.

🛠 Drugs that may cause *decreases* in 17-ketosteroid levels include estrogen, oral contraceptives, probenecid, promazine, salicylates (prolonged use), and thiazide diuretics.

PROCEDURE AND PATIENT CARE

Before

🗓 Explain the procedure to the patient.
- Withhold all drugs (with the physician's approval) for several days before the test.
- Assess the patient for signs of stress, and report these signs to the physician.

During

- Begin the 24-hour urine collection. Discard the initial specimen, and collect all urine voided by the patient during the next 24 hours.
🗓 Instruct the patient to post the times of the urine collection in a prominent location to prevent the patient from accidentally discarding a specimen.
- Note that it is not necessary to measure each urine specimen.
🗓 Instruct the patient to void before defecating so that the urine is not contaminated by feces.
🗓 Instruct the patient not to put toilet paper in the urine container.
🗓 Encourage the patient to drink fluids during the 24 hours, unless drinking is contraindicated for medical reasons.
- Remember that the urine collection needs a preservative.
🗓 Instruct the patient to keep the collection on ice or refrigerated during the entire 24 hours.
🗓 Instruct the patient to collect the last specimen as close as possible to the end of the 24 hours. This specimen should be added to the urine container.

After

- On the laboratory slip, note the starting and ending times of the specimen collection.
- Transmit the specimen to the laboratory as soon as the test is completed.

TEST RESULTS AND CLINICAL SIGNIFICANCE

▲ Increased Levels

Congenital adrenal hyperplasia: *In this condition, an enzyme defect results in underproduction of cortisol. In the normal feedback mechanism, ACTH is maximally produced. The result is maximal noncortisol adrenal (androgenic) sterol production. Levels of 17-ketosteroid are therefore elevated. This often causes masculinizing syndrome in female patients and precocious puberty in male patients. Congenital adrenal hyperplasia is the most common cause of elevations in 17-ketosteroid levels in children.*

Pregnancy: *Pregnancy is associated with slightly higher levels of androgens. 17-Ketosteroid levels are therefore elevated.*

ACTH administration,

ACTH-secreting ectopic tumours,

Hyperpituitarism: *ACTH stimulates adrenal cortisol and, to a lesser degree, androgenic sterol production. 17-Ketosteroid levels are therefore elevated in these three clinical situations.*

Testosterone-secreting or androgenic-secreting tumours of the adrenal glands, ovaries, or testes: *These tumours are most often associated with elevated 17-ketosteroid levels in adults and can elevate androgen levels to an extreme degree. 17-Ketosteroid levels also can be very high. Adrenal androgen (mostly DHEA)–producing cancers or adenomas also can elevate levels of 17-ketosteroid to an extreme degree.*

Cushing's syndrome: *17-Ketosteroid production varies, depending on the cause of adrenal overproduction.*

Stein-Leventhal syndrome: *This masculinizing syndrome is not well understood. Elevated 17-ketosteroid levels have been noted.*

▼ Decreased Levels

Severe debilitating disease,

Severe stress or infection,

Chronic disease: *In serious illness, the adrenal glands produce more cortisol and less androgenic hormone. 17-Ketosteroid levels are therefore low.*

Addison's disease: *With diminished adrenal function, production of androgenic hormones is reduced. 17-Ketosteroid levels are therefore low.*

Hypogonadism (Klinefelter's syndrome),

Castration: *With reduced testosterone production, 17-ketosteroid levels are low.*

Hypopituitarism: *Reduced production of ACTH reduces the activity of the adrenal cortex. 17-Ketosteroid levels are therefore low.*

RELATED TEST

17-Hydroxycorticosteroids (p. 959). This urine test measures the metabolites of cortisol and function of the adrenal cortex.

Microalbumin (MA)

NORMAL FINDINGS

Microalbumin: **0.03–0.08 g/24 hr** (30–80 *Mcg*/24 hr)
Microalbumin/creatinine ratio: 0–30 mg/g

INDICATIONS

This test is used as an indicator of complications (in the kidneys, heart, or small vessels) of diabetes. It is often the first indicator of renal disease.

TEST EXPLANATION

In microalbuminuria (MA), the albumin concentration in the urine is higher than normal, but this elevation is not detectable with routine protein testing. Normally, only small amounts of albumin are filtered through the renal glomeruli, and that small quantity can be reabsorbed by the renal tubules. However, when a disease causes glomerular permeability of albumin to exceed tubular reabsorption capability, albumin is spilled into the urine. Preceding this stage of a disease is a period in which only a very small amount of albumin (microalbuminuria) normally goes undetected by traditional urine protein tests (p. 991). Therefore, microalbuminuria is an early indication of renal disease.

For the diabetic patient, the amount of albumin in the urine is related to duration of the disease and the degree of glycemic control. Microalbuminuria is the earliest indicator for the development of diabetic complications (nephropathy, cardiovascular disease, and hypertension).

Urine Studies

11

The presence of MA can help identify diabetic nephropathy 5 years before routine protein urine tests reveal elevated levels of albumin. Diabetic patients with elevated MA levels have a five- to ten-fold increase in the occurrence of mortality from cardiovascular disease, retinopathy, and end-stage kidney disease.

It is recommended that all diabetic patients older than 12 years be screened annually for MA. This mass screening can be most inexpensively performed on a spot urine specimen with a semi-quantitative Micral Urine Test Strip. If MA is present, the test should be repeated two more times. If two of three MA urine test results are positive, a quantitative measurement with a 24-hour urine specimen should be performed.

The presence of MA in nondiabetic patients is an early indicator of shorter life expectancy because of cardiovascular disease and hypertension. Nondiabetic nephropathies may also be associated with microalbuminuria. Life insurance underwriters are increasingly using MA testing to estimate life expectancy. MA levels may be used as a predictor of outcome in critically ill patients.

Because MA levels may be affected by hydration status, the MA/creatinine ratio can be calculated. This is obtained by determining the ratio of urinary MA to urinary creatinine (an indicator of urine concentration). The ratio is calculated as follows:

$$\left\{ \frac{\text{Microalbumin (mg/dL)}}{\text{Creatinine (mg/dL)}} \right\} \times 1000\,\text{mg/g}$$

INTERFERING FACTORS

- Urinary tract infection, blood, or acid-base abnormalities can cause elevations in MA levels and falsely indicate a more serious prognosis.
- Vigorous exercise or febrile illnesses may temporarily cause MA to appear in the urine.
- Drugs that may *interfere* with test results include oxytetracycline.

PROCEDURE AND PATIENT CARE

Before

- Explain the procedure to the patient.
- Ensure that the patient does not have any acute infection or urinary bleeding that could cause a false-positive result.

During

- Collect a fresh urine specimen in a urine container.
- If the urine specimen contains vaginal discharge or bleeding, a clean-catch or midstream specimen is needed (see p. 937).
- Ensure that the urine sample is at room temperature for testing.
- If a Micral Urine Test Strip is used, follow these steps:
  1. Dip the test strip into the urine for 5 seconds.
  2. Allow the strip to dry for 1 minute.
  3. Compare the strip with the colour scale on the label. The concentration of the red colour is proportional to the amount of MA in the patient's sample.
- For quantification of MA, a 10-mL random sample or a portion of a 24-hour urine specimen is obtained. No preservative is used during the 24-hour collection.

After

- Transport the urine specimen to the laboratory promptly.
- If a 24-hour urine collection is requested, the specimen should be refrigerated. However, it will be warmed by the laboratory to room temperature before analysis.

 If the results are positive, inform the patient that the test should be repeated in 1 week.

TEST RESULTS AND CLINICAL SIGNIFICANCE

▲ Increased Levels

Diabetes mellitus,

Myoglobinuria,

Hemoglobinuria,

Bence-Jones proteinuria,

Nephrotoxic drugs,

Nephropathy: *These diseases are associated with renal glomerular injury that causes the permeability of albumin to exceed the reabsorption in the renal tubule.*

Atherosclerosis,

Lipid abnormalities,

Insulin resistance,

Hypertension,

Myocardial infarction: *These diseases also may be associated in some unknown way with increased renal glomerular permeability of albumin.*

Microglobulin (Beta-$_2$ Microglobulin [B$_2$M], Alpha 1 Microglobulin, and Retinol-Binding Protein)

NORMAL FINDINGS

Beta 2 microglobulin:
    Blood: 0.70–1.80 *Mcg*/mL
    Urine: ≤300 *Mcg*/L
    CSF: 0–2.4 mg/L

Alpha 1 microglobulin (urine):
    <50 years: <13 mg/g creatinine
    ≥50 years: <20 mg/g creatinine

Retinol-binding protein (RBP):
    Urine: <163 *Mcg*/24 hours

INDICATIONS

This test is used to evaluate patients with malignancies, chronic infections, inflammatory diseases, and renal diseases.

TEST EXPLANATION

Beta-$_2$ microglobulin (B$_2$M) is a protein found on the surface of all cells. It is a human leukocyte antigen (HLA) major histocompatibility antigen that exists in increased numbers on the cell surface and particularly on lymphatic cells. Production of this protein increases with cell turnover. B_2M is increased in patients with malignancies (especially B-cell lymphoma, leukemia, or multiple myeloma), chronic infections, and in patients with chronic severe inflammatory diseases. It is an accurate measurement of myeloma tumour disease activity, stage of disease, and prognosis and, as such, is an important tumour marker. This tumour marker is best determined in the blood.

B_2M, *alpha 1 microglobulin*, and *retinol-binding proteins* pass freely through glomerular membranes and are nearly completely reabsorbed by renal proximal tubules cells. Because of extensive tubular reabsorption, under normal conditions very little of these proteins appear in the final excreted urine. Therefore an increase in the urinary excretion of these proteins indicates proximal tubule disease or toxicity and/or impaired proximal tubular function. In patients with a urinary tract infection, these proteins indicate pyelonephritis. These proteins are helpful in differentiating glomerular from tubular renal disease. In patients with aminoglycoside toxicity, heavy metal nephrotoxicity, or tubular disease, protein urine levels are elevated. Excretion is increased 100 to 1 000 times normal levels in cadmium-exposed workers. This test is used to monitor these workers. Periodic testing is performed on these patients to detect kidney disease at its earliest stage. To date, there are no convincing studies to indicate that one protein has better clinical utility than the other.

B_2M is particularly helpful in the differential diagnosis of renal disease. If blood and urine levels are obtained simultaneously, one can differentiate glomerular from tubular disease. In glomerular disease, because of poor glomerular filtration, blood levels are high and urine levels are low. In tubular disease, because of poor tubular reabsorption, the blood levels are low and urine levels are high. Blood levels increase early in kidney transplant rejection.

Urinary excretion of these proteins can be determined from either a 24-hour collection or from a random urine collection. The 24-hour collection is traditionally considered the gold standard. For random or spot collections, the concentration of alpha 1 microglobulin is divided by the urinary creatinine concentration. This corrected value adjusts alpha 1 microglobulin for variabilities in urine concentration.

Increased CSF levels of B_2M indicate central nervous system involvement with leukemia, lymphoma, HIV, or multiple sclerosis.

Quantitative chemiluminescent immunoassay or nephelometry methods are used to identify these proteins in the urine/serum.

INTERFERING FACTORS

- Results could be affected by recent nuclear imaging when B_2M testing is performed by radioimmunoassay.
- B_2M is unstable in acid urine.

PROCEDURE AND PATIENT CARE

Before
⋈ Explain the procedure to the patient to minimize anxiety.

During
Blood
- Collect a venous blood sample in a red-top tube.

Urine. See Box 11-2, Guidelines for a 24-Hour Collection, p. 938.
⋈ Encourage the patient to drink fluids during the 24 hours unless this is contraindicated for medical purposes.

- If a single random urine collection is requested, collect specimen for protein and creatinine testing to adjust for urine concentration.

After
- Apply pressure to the venipuncture site.
- Send the urine collection to the laboratory

TEST RESULTS AND CLINICAL IMPLICATIONS

▲ Increased Urine Levels

Renal tubule disease,

Drug-induced renal toxicity,

Heavy metal–induced renal disease: *In primary renal tubular disease, these proteins cannot be reabsorbed by the renal tubule. Thus they are elevated in excreted urine.*

Lymphomas, leukemia, myeloma: *In patients with advanced disease, glomerular filtration of these proteins exceeds the ability of renal tubules to reabsorb them. Thus they are elevated in excreted urine.*

▲ Increased Serum Levels

Lymphomas, leukemia, myeloma,

Glomerular renal disease,

Renal transplant rejection: *Glomerular filtration of these proteins is diminished and serum levels rise.*

Viral infections, especially HIV and cytomegalovirus,

Chronic inflammatory processes: *Inflammation is associated with increased cell turnover. Thus shedding increases levels of these proteins into the serum.*

RELATED TESTS

Microalbumin (p. 965). Like the noted proteins, microalbumin is a marker for renal disease.

BUN (p. 534). This is a measure of renal function.

Creatinine (p. 205). This is a measure of renal function.

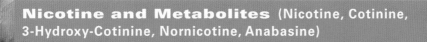

Nicotine and Metabolites (Nicotine, Cotinine, 3-Hydroxy-Cotinine, Nornicotine, Anabasine)

NORMAL FINDINGS
Urine

	Unexposed Non–Tobacco User (ng/mL)	Passive Exposure (Non–Tobacco User) (ng/mL)	Abstinent User for >2 Weeks (ng/mL)	Active Tobacco Product User (ng/mL)
Nicotine	<2	<20	<30	1 000–5 000
Cotinine	<5	<20	<50	1 000–8 000
3-OH-Cotinine	<50	<50	<120	3 000–25 000
Nornicotine	<2	<2	<2	30–900
Anabasine	<3	<3	<3	3–500

Urine Studies

11

Serum

	Unexposed Non–Tobacco User (ng/mL)	Passive Exposure (Non–Tobacco User) (ng/mL)	Abstinent User for >2 Weeks (ng/mL)	Active Tobacco Product User (ng/mL)
Nicotine	<2	<2	<2	30–50
Cotinine	<2	<8	<2	200–800
3-OH-Cotinine	<2	<2	<2	100–500

INDICATIONS

This test is used to document tobacco use. It is used to assess compliance with smoking cessation programs and qualify for surgical procedures. It is also used by insurance companies to determine if the applicant is a smoker.

TEST EXPLANATION

Nicotine is metabolized into cotinine and 3-hydroxy-cotinine which are measurable in urine and serum. The word *cotinine* is actually an anagram of *nicotine*—the eight letters are rearranged. In addition to nicotine and metabolites, tobacco products also contain other alkaloids (anabasine and nornicotine). The purpose of this testing is to differentiate patient tobacco use as the following:

• Active user
• Abstinent >2 weeks
• Passively exposed nonuser
• Unexposed nonuser

    Cotinine and 3-hydroxy-cotinine have an in vivo half-life of approximately 20 hours and are typically detectable from several days to up to 1 week after the use of tobacco. Because the level of these metabolites in the blood is proportionate to the amount of exposure to tobacco smoke, it is a valuable indicator of tobacco smoke exposure. Nicotine and its metabolites can be measured in the serum, urine, or other biofluids (most commonly the saliva). Cotinine is found in urine from 2 to 4 days after tobacco use. Serum/plasma testing is required when a valid urine specimen cannot be obtained (anuretic or dialysis patient) or to detect recent use (within the past 2 weeks). Blood cotinine will increase no matter how the tobacco is used (smoke, chew, dip, or snuff products). Nicotine levels have an in vivo half-life of approximately 2 hours, which is too short to be useful as a marker of smoking status.

    Anabasine (only measured in the urine) is present in tobacco products, but not nicotine replacement therapies. Nicotine, cotinine, 3-hydroxy-cotinine, and nornicotine will also be elevated by the use of any of the nicotine replacement gum, patch, or pill products. The presence of anabasine >10 ng/mL or nornicotine >30 ng/mL in urine indicates current tobacco use, irrespective of whether the subject is on nicotine replacement therapy. The presence of nornicotine without anabasine is consistent with use of nicotine replacement products. Heavy tobacco users who abstain from tobacco for 2 weeks exhibit urine nicotine values <30 ng/mL, cotinine <50 ng/mL, anabasine <3 ng/mL, and nornicotine <2 ng/mL. Passive exposure to tobacco smoke can cause accumulation of nicotine metabolites in non–tobacco users. Urine cotinine has been observed to accumulate up to 20 ng/mL from passive exposure. Neither anabasine nor nornicotine accumulates from passive exposure.

For smokers, another method of determining tobacco use is expired carbon monoxide. Again, a relatively short half-life (approximately 4 hours) limits the reliability and accuracy. Furthermore, carbon monoxide testing is unable to detect the use of smokeless tobacco.

Urine and salivary cotinine levels are less reliable. Nicotine and metabolite levels will vary by the amount of tobacco used, the use of a filter, the depth of the inhalation, and the size, gender, and weight of the person being tested. Because hydration status and renal function may affect urinary cotinine results, a spot urine cotinine test is always accompanied by a spot urine creatinine.

Quantification of urine nicotine and metabolites while a patient is actively using a tobacco product is useful to define the concentrations that a patient achieves through self-administration of tobacco. The nicotine replacement dose can then be tailored to achieve the same concentrations early in treatment to assure adequate nicotine replacement so the patient may avoid the strong craving he or she may experience early in the withdrawal phase.

Nicotine and metabolites can be accurately quantified with various laboratory methods, including high performance liquid chromatography, gas chromatography/mass spectroscopy, enzyme immunoassay (EIA), and enzyme-linked immunosorbent immunoassay (ELISA). Qualitative assays (including EIA and ELISA) are relatively easy to perform on urine and saliva but are less accurate than the blood measurement. Absolute laboratory normal values may vary depending on the method of testing.

INTERFERING FACTORS

- Menthol cigarettes may increase cotinine levels because the menthol retains cotinine in the blood for a longer period of time.
- Diluted/adulterated urine may alter results.

PROCEDURE AND PATIENT CARE

Before
- Explain the procedure to the patient and indicate the type of specimen needed.
- Obtain an accurate history of recent tobacco use.

During
Blood
- Collect venous blood in a red-top, lavender-top (EDTA), or pink-top (K_2 EDTA) tube.

Urine
- Obtain a random spot urine specimen of at least 5 mL.
- Immediately transport the specimen to the laboratory.

Saliva
- Ask the patient to spit at least 1 mL of saliva into a spit container.
- Alternatively, dental gauze rolls can be placed in the mouth for 15 minutes and then placed in a storage container for transport.

After
- Keep the specimens in a cool place if they cannot be transported to the laboratory immediately.

TEST RESULTS AND CLINICAL SIGNIFICANCE

Tobacco exposure: *With even minimal tobacco use, nicotine and metabolite levels will be elevated.*

Urine Studies

11

Osmolality, Urine

NORMAL FINDINGS

12- to 14-hour fluid restriction: **>850 mmol/kg H₂O** (>850 mOsm/kg H₂O)

Random specimen: **50–1200 mmol/kg H₂O** (50–1200 mOsm/kg H₂O), depending on fluid intake

INDICATIONS

This test is used to evaluate fluid and electrolyte abnormalities. It is an accurate determination of the kidney's concentrating capabilities. It is also used to investigate antidiuretic hormone (ADH) abnormalities (e.g., diabetes insipidus) and inappropriate ADH secretion.

TEST EXPLANATION

Urine osmolality is the measurement of the number of dissolved particles in the urine. It is a more exact measurement of urine concentration than specific gravity is, because specific gravity depends on the weight and density of the particles in the urine. Specific gravity also requires correction for the presence of glucose or protein, as well as for temperature; in contrast, osmolality depends only on the number of particles of solute in a unit of solution. Osmolality can be measured over a wider range, and with greater accuracy, than can specific gravity.

Osmolality is used in precise evaluation of the concentrating ability of the kidneys. This test is also used to monitor fluid and electrolyte balance. With normal fluid intake and normal diet, a patient will produce urine of about 500 to 850 mOsm/kg water. The normal kidney can concentrate urine to 800 to 1400 mOsm/kg. With excess fluid intake, a minimal osmolality of 40 to 80 mOsm/kg can be obtained. With dehydration, the urine osmolality should be three to four times the plasma osmolality.

Osmolality is used in the evaluation of kidney function and the ability to excrete ammonium salts. Osmolality may be used as part of the urinalysis when the patient has glycosuria or proteinuria or has had tests that use radiopaque substances. In these situations, the *urine osmolar gap* increases because of other organic osmolar particles. The urine osmolar gap is the sum of all the particles predicted or calculated to be in the urine (electrolytes, urea, and glucose) compared with the actual measurement of the osmolality. Urine levels of sodium, potassium, glucose, and urea nitrogen can then determine the predicted/calculated urine osmolality:

$$\text{Calculated urine osmolality} = 2 \times ([Na + K]) + [Urea\ nitrogen]/2.8 + [Glucose]/18$$

Normally, the osmolar gap is **80 to 100 mmol/kg H₂O** (80 to 100 mOsm/kg H₂O). The urine osmolality is more easily interpreted when the serum osmolality (see p. 391) is simultaneously performed. More information concerning the state of renal water handling or abnormalities of urine dilution or concentration can be obtained if urinary osmolality is compared with serum osmolality and urine electrolyte studies are performed. Normally the ratio of urine osmolality to serum osmolality is 1.0 to 3.0, reflecting a wide range of urine osmolality.

Clinical Priorities

- This test provides valuable information about fluid and electrolyte abnormalities.
- Urine osmolality is a more exact measure of urine concentration than is specific gravity.
- Urine osmolality is more easily interpreted when the serum osmolality is also measured.

PROCEDURE AND PATIENT CARE

Before
- Explain the procedure to the patient.
- Inform the patient that no special preparation is necessary for a random urine specimen.
- Inform the patient that preparation for a fasting urine specimen may require ingestion of a high-protein diet for 3 days before the test.
- Instruct the patient to eat a dry supper the evening before the test and to drink no fluids until the test is completed the next morning.

During
- Collect a first-voided urine specimen for a random sample.
- For a fasting specimen, instruct the patient to empty the bladder at approximately 6:00 AM and to discard the urine. Collect the test urine at 8:00 PM.
- On the laboratory slip, note the patient's fasting status.

After
- Transmit the specimen to the laboratory.
- Provide food and fluids for the patient.

TEST RESULTS AND CLINICAL SIGNIFICANCE

▲ Increased Levels

Syndrome of inappropriate antidiuretic hormone (SIADH) secretion: *Several illnesses can produce SIADH secretion. ADH is inappropriately secreted despite the presence of conditions that normally would inhibit its secretion. As a result, large quantities of water are reabsorbed by the kidneys. Less free water is excreted, and the urine osmolality rises.*

Paraneoplastic syndromes associated with carcinoma (e.g., lung, breast, colon): *These cancers act as an autonomous ectopic source for secretion of ADH. The pathophysiologic mechanism is the same as that described for SIADH.*

Shock: *The normal physiologic response to shock is to minimize the loss of free body water. The kidneys therefore absorb all the free water possible. Urine osmolality rises.*

Hepatic cirrhosis,

Heart failure: *These illnesses are associated with water retention because of reduced perfusion of the kidneys. Less free body water is excreted, and urine osmolality rises.*

▼ Decreased Levels

Diabetes insipidus: *Insufficient secretion of ADH despite physiologic stimulation by increased serum osmolality diminishes the kidneys' capability of concentrating urine. Urine osmolality decreases.*

Excess fluid intake: *Free water overload is excreted into the urine. Urine osmolality decreases.*

Renal tubular necrosis,

Severe pyelonephritis: *The concentrating capability of the kidneys is reduced. Excess free water is excreted. Urine osmolality decreases.*

RELATED TESTS

Osmolality, Blood (p. 391). This test is a measurement of osmolality of the serum. When it is combined with the test for urine osmolality, either test result can be interpreted more accurately.

Antidiuretic Hormone (p. 83). This provides a direct measurement of ADH in the blood.

Antidiuretic Hormone Suppression (p. 85). This test is helpful in the evaluation of ADH abnormalities.

Porphyrins and Porphobilinogens

NORMAL FINDINGS

Total porphyrins:
 Adult: **24–146 nmol/24 hr** (20–121 *Mcg*/24 hr)
Uroporphyrin:
 Male: **10–53 nmol/24 hr** (8–44 *Mcg*/24 hr)
 Female: **10–26 nmol/24 hr** (4–22 *Mcg*/24 hr)
Coproporphyrin:
 Male: **15–167 nmol/24 hr** (10–109 *Mcg*/24 hr)
 Female: **5–86 nmol/24 hr** (3–56 *Mcg*/24 hr)
Porphobilinogens: **0–6.6 mg/24 hr** (0–2 mg/24 hr)

INDICATIONS

This test is a quantitative measurement of porphyrins and porphobilinogen. It is used along with delta-aminolevulinic acid (ALA) to identify the various forms of porphyria.

TEST EXPLANATION

Porphyria is the name of any of a group of genetic disorders associated with enzyme deficiencies involved with porphyrin synthesis or metabolism. Porphyrins (e.g., uroporphyrin, coproporphyrin) and porphobilinogens are important building blocks in the synthesis of heme. Heme is incorporated into hemoglobin within the erythroid cells. Porphyrias are classified according to location of the accumulation of the porphyrin precursors. In most forms of porphyria, levels of porphyrins and porphobilinogen are increased in the urine.

Variable symptoms are associated with different types of porphyrias. Erythropoietic porphyria is associated with photosensitivity of the eyes and skin. Intermittent porphyria and, less often, variegate and hereditary coproporphyria are associated with abdominal pain and neurologic symptoms. Heavy-metal (e.g., lead) intoxication is also associated with increased levels of porphyrins in the urine. Certain drugs can induce porphyria and cause elevations in porphyrin levels in the urine (see Box 2-15, p. 540). This test is a quantitative analysis of urinary porphyrins and porphobilinogens. If porphyrins are present, the urine may be amber red or burgundy, or it may turn even darker after standing in the light.

Urine tests for porphyrins are not as accurate as plasma measurements and pattern identification for the various forms of porphyria, but they are accurate in screening for porphyria, especially the intermittent variety. Porphyrin fractionation of erythrocytes and of plasma provides specific assays for primary red blood cell (RBC) porphyrins such as protoporphyrin, uroporphyrin, and coproporphyrin. These assays are used predominantly to differentiate the various forms of congenital porphyrias. Plasma measurement of free erythrocyte protoporphyrin is helpful in the diagnosis of iron-deficiency anemia or lead intoxication. In these diseases, a small amount of excess porphyrin remains in the RBC after heme synthesis. This is measured as free erythrocyte protoporphyrin.

Although this test can also be done on a fresh stool specimen, random and 24-hour urine collections are more accurate. Colorimetric methods (or spectrophotometry) are used most often. *Porphyrin fractionation* of the various types of porphyrins within the urine enables identification of patterns commonly associated with the various porphyrias; this is accomplished with high-performance liquid chromatography. The diagnosis of porphyria and interpretation of test results are difficult. The Canadian Association for Porphyria/Association Canadienne de Porphyrie can provide evidence-based information and support for patients with porphyria, their families, health care providers, and the general public.

INTERFERING FACTORS

Drugs that may *alter* test results include salicylic acid, barbiturates, chloral hydrate, chlorpropamide, ethyl alcohol, morphine, oral contraceptives, phenazopyridine, procaine, and sulphonamides (see also Box 2-15, p. 540).

PROCEDURE AND PATIENT CARE

Before
- Explain the procedure to the patient.
- Inform the patient that no fasting is required.

During
Porphobilinogens
- Collect a freshly voided urine specimen.
- Protect the specimen from light.

Porphyrins
- Begin the 24-hour urine collection. Discard the initial specimen, and collect all urine voided by the patient during the next 24 hours.
- Instruct the patient to avoid alcohol use during the collection period.
- Show the patient where to store the urine container.
- Keep the collection on ice or refrigerated during the entire 24 hours.
- Keep the urine in a light-resistant specimen bottle with a preservative to prevent degradation of the light-sensitive porphyrin.
- On the urine container and laboratory slip, note the starting time.
- Instruct the patient to post the times of the urine collection in a prominent location to prevent the patient from accidentally discarding a specimen.
- Instruct the patient to void before defecating so that the urine is not contaminated by feces.
- Instruct the patient not to put toilet paper in the urine container.

✗ Encourage the patient to drink fluids during the 24 hours, unless drinking is contraindicated for medical reasons.

✗ Instruct the patient to collect the last specimen as close as possible to the end of the 24 hours. This specimen should be added to the urine container.

After
• Transport the urine specimen to the laboratory promptly.

TEST RESULTS AND CLINICAL SIGNIFICANCE
▲ Increased Levels

Porphyrias

Acute intermittent porphyria: *Porphobilinogen and, to a lesser degree, porphyrin levels are elevated during the acute phase. No real increase is noted during the latent phases.*

Congenital erythropoietic porphyria: *The porphobilinogen level is elevated.*

Hereditary coproporphyria: *Coproporphyrin and porphobilinogen levels are elevated.*

Variegate porphyria: *In acute episodes, porphobilinogen and delta-aminolevulinic acid (p. 955) levels are elevated.*

Lead poisoning: *The delta-aminolevulinic acid level is most significantly elevated; porphyrin levels are slightly elevated.*

RELATED TESTS

Uroporphyrinogen-1-Synthase (p. 539). This test is used to identify persons at risk for development of porphyria and to diagnose porphyria in the acute and latent stages.

Delta-Aminolevulinic Acid (p. 955). This test is used to diagnose porphyria and in the evaluation of children with subclinical forms of lead poisoning.

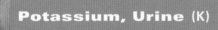

Potassium, Urine (K)

NORMAL FINDINGS
25–100 mmol/day (25–100 mEq/L/day)
  Values vary greatly with diet.

INDICATIONS

This test measures the amount of potassium in a spot or 24-hour urine collection to aid in determining electrolyte balance.

TEST EXPLANATION

Potassium is the major cation within the cell. The electrolyte balance of potassium can be measured in a spot specimen or a 24-hour urine collection. A 24-hour collection is essential for evaluating electrolyte (especially hypokalemia) balance, acid-base balance, and renal and adrenal diseases.

The serum potassium concentration depends on many factors. Aldosterone and, to a lesser extent, glucocorticosteroids tend to increase renal losses of potassium. If sodium blood levels are diminished, the renal tubules can reabsorb sodium in exchange for potassium, which is then excreted at increased rates. Acid-base balance depends to a small degree on potassium excretion. In alkalotic states, hydrogen can be reabsorbed in exchange for potassium. The kidneys cannot reabsorb potassium. Therefore, potassium intake is balanced by kidney excretion through the urine.

INTERFERING FACTORS

- Dietary intake affects potassium levels.
- Excessive intake of licorice may cause increases in urine levels of potassium because licorice acts like aldosterone and increases potassium excretion.
- Drugs that may cause *increases* in potassium levels include diuretics, glucocorticoids, and salicylates.

PROCEDURE AND PATIENT CARE

Before
- Explain the procedure to the patient.
- Inform the patient that no special diet is required.

During
- Begin the 24-hour urine collection. Discard the initial specimen, and collect all urine voided by the patient during the next 24 hours.
- Show the patient where to store the urine container.
- Keep the collection on ice or refrigerated during the entire 24 hours.
- On the urine container and laboratory slip, note the starting time.
- Instruct the patient to post the times of the urine collection in a prominent location to prevent the patient from accidentally discarding a specimen.
- Instruct the patient to void before defecating so that the urine is not contaminated by feces.
- Instruct the patient not to put toilet paper in the urine container.
- Encourage the patient to drink fluids during the 24 hours unless drinking is contraindicated for medical reasons.
- Instruct the patient to collect the last specimen as close as possible to the end of the 24 hours. This specimen should be added to the urine container.

After
- Transport the urine specimen promptly to the laboratory.

TEST RESULTS AND CLINICAL SIGNIFICANCE

▲ Increased Levels

Chronic renal failure: *Sodium loss is increased in some forms of renal failure because of loss of reabsorptive capabilities of the kidneys. Potassium loss follows sodium loss.*
Renal tubular acidosis: *Reductions in excretion of hydrogen lead to increases in excretion of potassium.*
Starvation: *To provide energy, protein- and fat-containing tissues are broken down. The cells in those tissues expel potassium into the bloodstream. The potassium is then excreted, at increased levels, into the urine.*
Cushing's syndrome,

Hyperaldosteronism: *Aldosterone increases potassium urinary excretion. Because glucocorticosteroids have an aldosterone-like effect, potassium excretion is also increased in Cushing's syndrome.*

Excessive intake of licorice: *Licorice has an aldosterone-like effect, as described previously.*

Alkalosis: *Hydrogen is reabsorbed in the renal tubules in exchange for potassium excretion.*

Diuretic therapy: *Most diuretics cause potassium wasting and increase potassium urinary excretion.*

▼ Decreased Levels

Dehydration: *Decreases in renal blood flow in association with dehydration cause decreases in urinary excretion of potassium.*

Addison's disease: *This disease is associated with diminished aldosterone effect on the kidneys. Because aldosterone increases urinary excretion of potassium, reduced levels of aldosterone are associated with reduced urinary potassium levels.*

Malnutrition,

Vomiting,

Diarrhea,

Malabsorption: *Diminished intake of potassium is matched by diminished urinary excretion of potassium.*

Acute renal failure: *Urinary excretion of potassium is diminished. This is the most common cause of hyperkalemia.*

RELATED TESTS

Sodium, Urine (p. 980). Sodium is often measured with potassium.

Potassium, Blood (p. 420). This is a direct measurement of potassium in serum.

Pregnanediol

NORMAL FINDINGS

Child: <0.312 *Mc*mol/day (<0.1 mg/day)

Adult male: 0–5.9 *Mc*mol/day (0–1.9 mg/day)

Adult female

　Follicular phase: <8.1 *Mc*mol/day (<2.6 mg/day)

　Luteal phase: 8.1–33.1 *Mc*mol/day (2.6–10.6 mg/day)

　Pregnancy

- First trimester: 31–109 *Mc*mol/day (10–35 mg/day)
- Second trimester: 109–218 *Mc*mol/day (35–70 mg/day)
- Third trimester: 218–312 *Mc*mol/day (70–100 mg/day)

INDICATIONS

This test measures pregnanediol, a metabolite of progesterone. It is used in the evaluation and decision making in women who are having difficulty becoming pregnant or maintaining a pregnancy. It is also used to monitor high-risk pregnancies.

TEST EXPLANATION

Urinary pregnanediol is measured to evaluate progesterone production by the ovaries and placenta. The main effect of progesterone is on the endometrium. It initiates the secretory phase of the endometrium in anticipation of implantation of a fertilized ovum. Normally, progesterone is secreted by the ovarian corpus luteum after ovulation. Both serum progesterone levels and urine concentration of progesterone metabolites (pregnanediol and others) are significantly increased during the second half of an ovulatory cycle. Pregnanediol is the most easily measured metabolite of progesterone. However, this test is difficult to standardize because it varies with sex, age, and the stage of pregnancy. The serum progesterone test (see Progesterone Assay, p. 429) is a more useful test of progesterone production.

Because pregnanediol levels rise rapidly after ovulation, this study is useful in documenting whether ovulation has occurred and, if so, exactly when. This is useful information for a woman who has difficulty becoming pregnant. During pregnancy, pregnanediol levels normally rise because of placental production of progesterone.

Repeated assays can be used to monitor the status of the placenta in high-risk pregnancy.

Hormone assays for urinary pregnanediol are used primarily to monitor progesterone supplementation in patients with an inadequate luteal phase to maintain an early pregnancy. Urinary assays may be supplemented by plasma assays (Progesterone Assay, p. 429), which are quicker and more accurate.

INTERFERING FACTORS

- Drugs that may cause *increases* in pregnanediol levels include adrenocorticotropic hormone (ACTH).
- Drugs that may cause *decreases* in pregnanediol levels include oral contraceptives and progesterone.

PROCEDURE AND PATIENT CARE

Before

- Explain the procedure to the patient.
- Inform the patient that usually no special diet is required, but he or she should consult with the physician to confirm the diet.
- Inform the patient that no sedation or fasting is necessary.

During

- Begin the 24-hour urine collection. Discard the initial specimen, and collect all urine voided by the patient during the next 24 hours.
- Show the patient where to store the urine collection.
- Keep the collection on ice or refrigerated during the entire 24 hours.
- Check with the laboratory to see whether a preservative is needed.
- On the urine container and laboratory slip, note the starting time.
- Instruct the patient to post the times of the urine collection in a prominent location to prevent the patient from accidentally discarding a specimen.
- Instruct the patient to void before defecating so that the urine is not contaminated by feces.
- Instruct the patient not to put toilet paper in the urine container.
- Encourage the patient to drink fluids during the 24 hours unless drinking is contraindicated for medical reasons.
- Instruct the patient to collect the last specimen as close as possible to the end of the 24 hours. This specimen should be added to the urine container.

After

- On the laboratory slip, record the date of the most recent menstrual period or the week of gestation during pregnancy.

Urine Studies

11

TEST RESULTS AND CLINICAL SIGNIFICANCE

▲ Increased Levels

Ovulation: *Ovulation occurs with development of a corpus luteum, which makes progesterone. Pregnanediol is a metabolite of progesterone.*

Pregnancy: *A healthy placenta produces progesterone. Pregnanediol is a metabolite of progesterone.*

Molar pregnancy: *Hydatidiform mole can produce progesterone, although at lower levels than during pregnancy.*

Luteal cysts of ovary: *The corpus luteum produces progesterone in the nonpregnant woman and in the early stages of pregnancy. Cysts can also produce progesterone for prolonged periods of time. Pregnanediol is a metabolite of progesterone.*

Arrhenoblastoma of ovary: *This tumour can secrete sex hormones or their metabolites (usually testosterone). 17-Hydroxyprogesterone is a precursor of sex hormones. Pregnanediol is a metabolite of progesterone.*

Hyperadrenocorticism,

Adrenocortical hyperplasia: *Adrenal cortical hormones are secreted at increased rates. 17-Hydroxyprogesterone is a precursor of these cortical hormones. Pregnanediol is a metabolite of progesterone.*

Choriocarcinoma of the ovary: *This tumour produces progesterone.*

▼ Decreased Levels

Preeclampsia,

Eclampsia,

Threatened abortion,

Placental failure,

Fetal death: *These obstetric emergencies are associated with decreased placental viability. Progesterone is made by the placenta during pregnancy. Pregnanediol is a metabolite of progesterone, which is decreased when placental viability is threatened.*

Ovarian neoplasm: *Ovarian epithelial cancers can destroy functional ovarian tissue. Progesterone levels may decrease.*

Amenorrhea,

Ovarian hypofunction: *Without ovulation, a corpus luteum does not develop. Progesterone is not secreted, and progesterone and pregnanediol levels are lower than expected.*

RELATED TEST

Progesterone Assay (p. 429). This is a direct measurement of progesterone in serum.

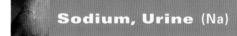

Sodium, Urine (Na)

NORMAL FINDINGS

24-hour collection: **40–250 mmol/day** (40–250 mEq/day)

Spot urine collection: **>20 mmol/L** (>20 mEq/L)

Fractional excretion: 1%–2%

Values vary, depending on the sodium content in the diet.

INDICATIONS

This test is used to evaluate fluid and electrolyte abnormalities, especially sodium. It can also be used to monitor therapy for these abnormalities.

TEST EXPLANATION

Many factors regulate sodium balance. Aldosterone causes conservation of sodium by stimulating the kidneys to reabsorb sodium, thus decreasing renal losses. Natriuretic hormone, or third factor, is stimulated by increased sodium levels. This hormone decreases renal absorption and increases renal losses of sodium. Antidiuretic hormone (ADH), which controls the reabsorption of water at the distal tubules of the kidney, affects sodium urine levels by dilution or concentration.

In the urine sodium test, sodium balance in the body is evaluated by determining the amount of sodium excreted in urine over 24 hours. Sodium is the major cation in the extracellular space. Measuring the amount of sodium in the urine is useful for evaluating patients with volume depletion, acute renal failure, adrenal disturbances, and acid-base imbalances. In the setting of acute renal failure, an increased value indicates acute tubular necrosis, whereas a low value would be typical of prerenal azotemia.

This test is also useful when the serum sodium concentration is low. For example, in patients with hyponatremia caused by inadequate sodium intake, urine sodium levels are low. However, in patients with hyponatremia caused by chronic renal failure, urine sodium concentrations are high.

Urine sodium excretions are helpful when the urine output is low (<500 mL/24 hr). However, a more accurate test to determine the cause of reduced urine output is the *fractional excretion of sodium* (FE_{Na}). FE_{Na} is the fraction of sodium actually excreted in relation to the amount filtered by the kidney. FE_{Na} is a calculation based on the concentrations of sodium (Na) and creatinine (Cr) in the blood and the urine as follows:

$$FE_{Na} = \left\{ \frac{U_{Na} \times P_{Cr}}{P_{Na} \times U_{Cr}} \right\} \times 100$$

FE_{Na} is greater than 1% and usually greater than 3% with acute tubular necrosis and severe obstruction of the urinary drainage of both kidneys. It is generally less than 1% in patients with acute glomerulonephritis, hepatorenal syndrome, and states of prerenal azotemia (such as heart failure and dehydration). FE_{Na} can also be less than 1% with acute partial urinary tract obstruction.

INTERFERING FACTORS

- Dietary salt intake may increase sodium levels.
- Drugs that may cause *increases* in urine sodium levels include antibiotics, caffeine, cough medicines, diuretics, and laxatives.
- Drugs that may cause *decreases* in urine levels of sodium include steroids.

PROCEDURE AND PATIENT CARE

Before

- Explain the procedure to the patient.
- Inform the patient that no fasting is required.

Urine Studies

11

During

- Begin the 24-hour urine collection. Discard the initial specimen, and collect all urine voided by the patient during the next 24 hours.
- ✗ Show the patient where to store the urine specimen.
- Keep the collection on ice or refrigerated during the entire 24 hours.
- On the urine container and laboratory slip, note the starting time.
- ✗ Instruct the patient to post the times of the urine collection in a prominent location to prevent the patient from accidentally discarding a specimen.
- ✗ Instruct the patient to void before defecating so that the urine is not contaminated by feces.
- ✗ Instruct the patient not to put toilet paper in the urine container.
- ✗ Encourage the patient to drink fluids during the 24 hours unless drinking is contraindicated for medical reasons.
- ✗ Instruct the patient to collect the last specimen as close as possible to the end of the 24 hours. This specimen should be added to the urine container.
- A spot urine specimen can be obtained and sent to the laboratory if information about urine sodium is needed sooner than 24 hours. In this situation, ask the patient to void in a nonsterile container, and transport the entire volume to the laboratory. The more urine available, the more accurately the spot urine specimen will reflect the 24-hour urine results.
- If FE_{Na} is ordered, venous blood is collected in a gold-top tube for serum creatinine and sodium measurement.

After

- Transport the urine specimen promptly to the laboratory.

TEST RESULTS AND CLINICAL SIGNIFICANCE

▲ Increased Levels

Dehydration: *Free water is maximally reabsorbed by the kidneys, and urine sodium is more concentrated.*

Adrenocortical insufficiency: *Aldosterone and corticosteroids stimulate sodium reabsorption in the distal renal tubules. With inadequate levels of these hormones, sodium is not reabsorbed, and large amounts are spilled into the urine.*

Diuretic therapy: *Most diuretics work by diminishing sodium reabsorption and increasing sodium loss in the kidneys.*

Syndrome of inappropriate antidiuretic hormone secretion: *ADH stimulates free water reabsorption in the kidney. With inappropriately high secretion of ADH, free water in the urine is diminished and sodium is more concentrated.*

Diabetic ketoacidosis: *The osmotic diuresis resulting from hyperglycemia tends to diminish sodium reabsorption in the kidneys. Furthermore, sodium combines with some ketotic products to further increase sodium losses into the urine.*

Chronic renal failure: *Renal reabsorption of sodium and many other products is diminished in a diseased, nonfunctioning kidney. Urine sodium levels increase.*

▼ Decreased Levels

Heart failure: *Renal blood flow is diminished with reduced cardiac output. The renin-angiotensin system is activated (see p. 48), and aldosterone production is stimulated. Aldosterone stimulates renal reabsorption of sodium, and urine levels diminish.*

Malabsorption,

Diarrhea: *Intestinal absorption of sodium is reduced. The physiologic response is to reduce sodium excretion in the urine.*

Cushing's disease: *Corticosteroids have an aldosterone-like effect on the kidney, which tends to stimulate renal reabsorption of sodium, and urine levels diminish.*

Aldosteronism: *Aldosterone stimulates renal reabsorption of sodium, and urine levels diminish.*

Inadequate sodium intake: *Intestinal absorption of sodium is very efficient. Therefore, it is rare for a nutritional deficiency to occur as sodium insufficiency severe enough to significantly diminish renal excretion. However, with sodium deficit or ongoing sodium losses treated with inadequate sodium replacement, serum sodium levels significantly diminish, and the kidneys are maximally stimulated to reabsorb sodium. Urine sodium levels diminish.*

RELATED TESTS

Sodium, Blood (p. 479). This is a direct measurement of sodium levels in serum.

Aldosterone (p. 48). More than any other hormone, aldosterone has a significant effect on blood sodium levels.

Antidiuretic Hormone (p. 83). By affecting free body water excretion, ADH alters sodium levels through dilution or concentration.

Substance Abuse Testing (Urine Drug Testing, Drug Screening, Drug Testing)

NORMAL FINDINGS

Negative

INDICATIONS

Substance abuse testing is used to identify metabolites of illegal drugs used by the person being tested.

TEST EXPLANATION

Drug testing is used mostly by employers and by law enforcement agencies. Employers use drug testing primarily to promote and protect the safety, health, and well-being of their employees. Because many industrial fatalities are attributable to substance abuse, drug-testing programs are common in the workplace. Furthermore, drug abuse is responsible for decreased productivity and increased absenteeism. Industrial testing is used at certain times: before employment, before promotion, during the annual physical examination, after an accident, or when there is reasonable suspicion. Testing at other times includes random testing or testing for follow-up surveillance of treatment.

Most commonly, a drug screen is performed. This is usually an inexpensive method of detecting small amounts of any number of metabolites of commonly used drugs. If the screen result is positive, a more accurate and quantitative test is performed on the same specimen. Drug screens are available for a variety of substances. The most common are amphetamines, barbiturates, benzodiazepines, cocaine, methamphetamine, opiates (morphine, heroin, propoxyphene, and oxycodone), cannabinoids (marijuana, whose active ingredient is tetrahydrocannabinol [THC]), and phencyclidine (PCP). Alcohol testing is used most commonly by law enforcement officers (see p. 244). Not only is drug testing helpful in identifying users, but it also acts as a deterrent to abuse. Athletes are tested for anabolic hormones that may unfairly improve their performance. Health and life insurance companies routinely test for illicit drug use.

Substance abuse testing, up until recently, consisted exclusively of urine testing. Urine is easily obtained and plentiful, and it contains a large amount of drugs and metabolites. More importantly, urine can identify drug usage for several days after the last usage. THC can be identified in the urine for several weeks in chronic users. Blood testing reflects drug usage only within the previous few hours. Saliva, breath, hair, and sweat are becoming increasingly important and accurate samples for specific drug testing. These testing methods are very expensive, however. Hair samples reveal the presence of drugs used during the previous 3 months. In addition, hair and nail samples may be used to detect or document exposure to arsenic and mercury. Nevertheless, urine testing remains the mainstay for drug testing.

♣ The Canadian Model for Providing a Safe Workplace is one best-practice policy with the purpose of ensuring a safe workplace for all workers by reducing the risks associated with the inappropriate use of alcohol and drugs. It outlines alcohol and drug testing procedures and provides guidelines for urine drug concentration limits (Table 11-1).

Toxicology screening tests for drug overdose (see Table 2-20, p. 227) and poisoning (e.g., lead and carbon monoxide poisoning; see Table 11-2 are best performed on blood. Results indicate current drug levels, which are used to determine or alter therapy. Toxicology studies are used to determine whether drug ingestion was a cause of or factor in the death of a person. They are also used to assess patients when poisoning contributes to an illness.

Urine screening is usually performed with the use of *enzyme multiplied immunoassay* (EMIT) or by *radioimmunoassay*. However, the most definitive tests entail the use of gas chromatography and mass spectrometry. If EMIT values exceed the cutoff level for any of the illicit drugs, a more definitive test is performed. Several test kits are becoming increasingly available for "in-house" drug screening. These kits can provide results in a few minutes. Results of more definitive urine or hair testing require approximately 2 to 4 days.

TABLE 11-1	Urine Drug Concentration Limits	
Drug or Classes of Drugs	**Screening Concentration Equal to or in Excess of ng/mL**	**Confirmation Concentration Equal to or in Excess of ng/mL**
Marijuana metabolite	50	15
Cocaine metabolite	150	100
Opiates	2 000	—
• Codeine	—	2 000
• Morphine	—	2 000
6-Acetylmorphine	10	10
Phencyclidine	25	25
Amphetamines	500	—
• Amphetamine	—	250
• Methamphetamine	—	250
MDMA1	500	—
• MDMA[1]	—	250
• MDA[2]	—	250
• MDEA[3]	—	250

[1] Methylenedioxymethamphetamine
[2] Methylenedioxyamphetamine
[3] Methylenedioxyethylamphetamine

TABLE 11-2   Blood Toxicology Screening

Drug	Type	Therapeutic Level[*]	Toxic Level[*]
Acetaminophen	Analgesic, antipyretic	100 *Mc*mol/L	>100 *Mc*mol/L
Alcohol	—	None	>64.8 mmol/L
Amobarbital	Sedative, hypnotic	4–22 *Mc*mol/L	>22 *Mc*mol/L
Carboxyhemoglobin (COHb [carbon monoxide poisoning])	Gas	None	>30% COHb (beginning of coma)
Glutethimide	Sedative	9–28 *Mc*mol/L	>28 *Mc*mol/L
Lead	—	None	>1.0 mmol/L
Lithium	Manic episodes of bipolar disorder	0.8–1.2 mmol/L	>2 mmol/L
Phenobarbital	Anticonvulsant	1.1–2.2 mmol/L	>170 *Mc*mol/L
Phenytoin	Anticonvulsant	40–80 *Mc*mol/L	>80 *Mc*mol/L
Salicylate	Antipyretic, anti-inflammatory, analgesic	60–170 *Mc*mol/L	>2.2 mmol/L

[*] Varies according to institution performing the test. Expressed in SI Units.

Because a positive result can have a profound effect on a person's life, job, and accountability, many drug abusers attempt to alter the urine specimen. Therefore, the urine sample is tested for odour, colour, temperature, creatinine, pH, and specific gravity to ensure that it is a proper specimen. If the specimen does not meet these assessment standards, it is rejected, and a second specimen is requested.

INTERFERING FACTORS

- Poppy seeds can cause false-positive findings of opiate use.
- Second-hand marijuana smoke can cause false-positive results.
- Ibuprofen can cause a *false-positive* finding of THC use.
- Cold remedies can cause *false-positive* findings of amphetamine use.
- Antibiotics (e.g., amoxicillin) can cause *false-positive* findings of heroin or cocaine use, or both.
- The aggressive use of diuretics can *decrease* drug levels in the urine.

PROCEDURE AND PATIENT CARE

Before
- Explain the procedure to the patient according to standard guidelines.
- Obtain a list of all medicines that the patient is taking that may alter or confound screening results including prescription, over-the-counter, and illicit drugs.

During
- Ensure that the patient provides his or her own urine. Usually, the collection of the sample is supervised by a trained health care provider, to ensure that the patient does not alter the urine specimen.
- For hair testing, cut 50 strands of hair from the scalp.

Urine Studies

11

After

- Follow the chain of custody for the specimen as provided by standard guidelines of the institution.
- Place the specimen in the required container for delivery.
- Check the temperature of urine specimens within 3 minutes after voiding. Temperature should be between 36°C and 37°C (97°F and 99°F).
- The specimen may be sent to a laboratory certified by the National Institute of Drug Abuse or accredited by the Canadian Association for Laboratory Accreditation.
- At the laboratory, the specimen is usually divided for more definitive testing if the result is above the cutoff value.

TEST RESULTS AND CLINICAL SIGNIFICANCE

Positive: *Results above the cutoff level indicate that the person tested may have used illicit drugs in the recent past. More definitive testing is then performed to confirm and quantify the presence of illicit drugs (e.g., blood sample for toxicology testing).*

RELATED TEST

Ethanol (p. 244). This is a direct measurement of alcohol level in the blood. It is another common form of drug testing used in industry and by law enforcement agencies.

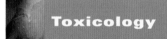

Toxicology

NORMAL FINDINGS

Table 11-2 lists the characteristics of blood toxicology.

INDICATIONS

Toxicology testing is used to evaluate for drug abuse, overdose, or poisoning.

TEST EXPLANATION

Detection of the most commonly abused nonprescription mood-altering drugs is discussed. These drugs are most commonly used in suicide attempts and chemical poisonings.

Testing for drug overdose and poisoning is best performed on blood. Results indicate immediate drug levels, which can indicate or alter therapy. Screening for use or abuse of nonprescription drugs is usually performed on urine. Urine specimens are easily obtained without any invasive procedure. Often the specimen is obtained several hours or days after the drug administration. In this case, blood levels are low but urine levels are high. Furthermore, drug metabolic products remain in the urine for longer periods, so that drug use in the previous few hours or days can be detected. The disadvantages of urine drug tests are that they cannot indicate with any degree of accuracy when the drug was used and whether the drug had any effect on the person's actions at any time. Also, the urine can be altered easily by changing the concentration (by drinking a large volume of water or adding water to the specimen), changing the pH, or adding foreign substances. Urine temperature, specific gravity, and creatinine concentration are often determined in urine specimens to ensure the specimen has not been altered. It is important to define the appropriate chain of transfer of the specimen from the moment it is obtained to the time of testing to prevent tampering.

Because of the effect on a person's life (socially, financially, and legally), positive results must be substantiated by another equally accurate test method. A popular protocol is to screen with thin-layer or gas chromatography to separate out the constituents in the specimen, followed by mass spectrometry to identify those constituents.

Toxicology studies are used to determine whether drug ingestion was a cause of or factor in a death. They are also used to assess patients when drug abuse or poisoning is contributing to an illness. Drug abuse is important to recognize in the workplace because of safety issues and in prisons because of disciplinary and safety concerns.

Commonly Abused Drugs

Marijuana (Cannabis). Marijuana is usually detected by identifying one of its metabolites (tetrahydrocannabinol) in the urine. In most laboratories, carboxy-tetrahydrocannabinol is detected, and 100 ng/mL is a cutoff value. Lower levels from passive inhalation of marijuana smoke may be detected but are not prosecutable in court. These metabolites can be present in the urine 1 hour after inhalation and for 1 to 3 days afterward.

Cocaine (Including Crack). Benzoylecgonine is a metabolite of cocaine. It is easily detectable in urine 1 to 4 hours after cocaine use and for 2 or 3 days. To indicate the timing of cocaine use, serum levels of cocaine must be determined.

Phencyclidine. Phencyclidine (PCP) or one of its metabolites is detectable in urine approximately 6 to 18 hours after use and for as long as 3 days.

Amphetamines (Especially Methamphetamine). Amphetamines are identifiable in urine approximately 3 hours after use and for approximately 1 or 2 days thereafter. Detection of amphetamines does not automatically imply abuse, because many over-the-counter cold medicines and weight loss medicines contain amphetamine analogues.

Morphine and Other Narcotic Alkaloids. Heroin, morphine, and codeine can be identified in the urine as glucuronide conjugated forms 2 hours after use and for 2 to 3 days. As with amphetamines, detection of codeine does not automatically imply abuse, because many over-the-counter pain relievers and cough-suppressive medicines contain codeine.

Barbiturates. Barbiturates can be detected in the blood, urine, or gastric contents by direct immunoassay. Detection of barbiturates does not automatically imply abuse, because barbiturates can be prescribed for therapeutic purposes.

Common Toxins

Lead. Lead diminishes the activity of delta-aminolevulinic acid (ALA) dehydrase, which converts ALA to porphobilinogen in the synthesis of heme for hemoglobin within erythroid cells. As a result, ALA accumulates in the blood and urine.

Other Heavy Metals. Heavy metals such as mercury, arsenic, bismuth, and antimony can be identified in the urine.

INTERFERING FACTORS

- The presence of detergents, bicarbonates, salt tablets, or blood in the urine can all result in inaccurate results of urine drug testing.

PROCEDURE AND PATIENT CARE

Before

- Explain the procedure to the patient or the patient's significant others.
- If the specimen is obtained for medicolegal testing, ensure that the patient or family member has signed a consent form.
- Obtain as much information as possible about the drug type, amount, and ingestion time.
- Carefully assess the patient for respiratory distress, a common adverse reaction to drug overdose.

During

- Collect blood or urine specimens as indicated. Urine specimens are collected in the presence of a trained health care provider.
- Collect gastric contents for analysis if this is indicated.
- Note that hair and nail samples may be used to detect or document exposure to arsenic and mercury.
- Identify the sample immediately and mark the patient's name on the specimen.

After

- Apply pressure or a pressure dressing to the venipuncture site.
- Assess the venipuncture site for bleeding.
- Reassess the patient for respiratory distress, a common adverse reaction to drug overdose.
- Refer the patient for appropriate drug and psychiatric counselling.
- Follow the predetermined chain of transfer of the specimen to the laboratory for testing. Each person involved in handling the specimen must document his or her place in its handling.
- Remind the patient that all positive screening results must be confirmed.

TEST RESULTS AND CLINICAL SIGNIFICANCE

Abuse or use of nonprescription drugs: *Urine is most often used in testing for these substances.*

Heavy-metal and lead poisoning: *Blood, urine, cerebrospinal fluid, and tissue specimens may all be used to identify these poisons.*

Suicide attempts: *Determination of toxic levels of drugs is much more accurately determined with blood tests, although urine may also be used.*

RELATED TESTS

Ethanol (p. 244). This is a direct measurement of alcohol level in the blood.

Carboxyhemoglobin (p. 157). This test is used to detect carbon monoxide poisoning.

Delta-Aminolevulinic Acid (p. 955). This test is used to identify lead poisoning.

Drug Monitoring (p. 227). These tests are used to help identify toxic levels of therapeutic drugs such as aspirin and acetaminophen, which are commonly involved in suicide attempts.

Substance Abuse Testing (p. 983). This test is used to detect illegal drug use.

Uric Acid, Urine

NORMAL FINDINGS

1.48–4.43 mmol/day (250–750 mg/24 hr)

INDICATIONS

Uric acid levels can be measured in both blood and urine. Urine levels of uric acid are helpful in evaluating uric acid metabolism in gout and for assessing hyperuricosuria in renal calculus formation. This test also helps to identify individuals at risk for stone formation.

TEST EXPLANATION

Uric acid is a nitrogenous compound that is the final breakdown product of purine (a DNA building block) catabolism (see p. 537 for blood uric acid level.) Seventy-five percent of uric acid is excreted by the kidneys, and 25% via the intestinal tract. Elevated uric acid levels (hyperuricemia) may be indicative of gout, a form of arthritis caused by deposition of uric acid crystals in periarticular tissue. An elevated uric acid level in the urine is called *uricosuria*. Uric acid can become supersaturated in the urine and crystallize to form kidney stones, which can block the renal system.

Uric acid is produced primarily in the liver. Urinary excretion of uric acid depends on uric acid levels in the blood, along with glomerular filtration and tubular secretion of uric acid into the urine. Elevated uric acid levels can cause nephrolithiasis and ureterolithiasis. Uric acid is not as well saturated in acidic urine. As the urine pH rises, more uric acid can exist without crystallization and stone formation. Therefore, urine known to have a high uric acid level can be alkalinized by ingestion of a strong base to prevent stone formation.

INTERFERING FACTORS

- Recent use of radiographic contrast agents may increase uric acid levels in the urine.
- Drugs that may *interfere* with test results include alcohol, anti-inflammatory preparations, salicylates, thiazide diuretics, vitamin C, and warfarin.

✔ Clinical Priorities

- This test is helpful in evaluating uric acid metabolism and gout.
- In individuals with high uric acid levels, the urine should be kept alkaline to prevent precipitation of kidney stones.

PROCEDURE AND PATIENT CARE

Before

 Explain the procedure to the patient.

Inform the patient that no special diet is usually required for the test.

During

- Begin the 24-hour urine collection. Discard the initial specimen, and collect all urine voided by the patient during the next 24 hours. A preservative may be used.
- Show the patient where to store the urine container.
- Keep the collection on ice or refrigerated during the entire 24 hours. (Note that some laboratories do not require that the specimen be kept cool.)
- On the urine container and laboratory slip, note the starting time.
- Instruct the patient to post the times of the urine collection in a prominent location to prevent the patient from accidentally discarding a specimen.
- Instruct the patient to void before defecating so that the urine is not contaminated by feces.
- Instruct the patient not to put toilet paper in the urine container.
- Encourage the patient to drink fluids during the 24 hours unless drinking is contraindicated for medical reasons.
- Instruct the patient to collect the last specimen as close as possible to the end of the 24 hours. This specimen should be added to the urine container.

After

- Transport the urine specimen to the laboratory promptly.

TEST RESULTS AND CLINICAL SIGNIFICANCE

▲ Increased Levels (Uricosuria)

Gout: *Uric acid levels are high in blood. When glomerular filtration is normal, levels are high in urine.*
Metastatic cancer,
Multiple myeloma,
Leukemias,
Cancer chemotherapy: *Rapid cell destruction is associated with rapidly growing cancers (with high cell turnover), and especially after chemotherapy for those rapidly growing tumours. This destruction causes the cells to lyse and spill their nucleic acids into the bloodstream. In the liver, these free nucleic acids are converted to uric acid. Blood and urine levels of uric acid increase.*
High-purine diet: *With increased uric acid production caused by a diet with high amounts of purines, uric acid levels in the urine are increased.*
Uricosuric drugs (e.g., ascorbic acid, calcitonin, citrate, dicumarol, estrogens, steroids, iodinated dyes, glyceryl guaiacolate, phenolsulphonphthalein, probenecid, salicylates, and outdated tetracycline): *These drugs increase uric acid excretion into the urine.*
Lead toxicity: *Heavy-metal poisoning is associated with increased uric acid tubular secretion.*

▼ Decreased Levels

Kidney disease: *With decreased glomerular filtration rate and decreased tubular secretion of uric acid, urine levels fall.*
Eclampsia: *The pathophysiologic mechanism underlying this observation is not well known.*
Chronic alcohol ingestion: *Chronic acidosis caused by excessive alcohol ingestion decreases renal tubular secretion of uric acid into the urine.*
Acidosis (ketotic [diabetic or starvation], lactic): *Renal tubular secretion of uric acid into the urine is decreased. Keto acids, as occur in diabetic or alcoholic ketoacidosis, may compete with uric acid for tubular excretion, which is another cause of decreased uric acid excretion.*

RELATED TEST

Uric Acid, Blood (p. 537). This test is used to diagnose gout.

Urinalysis (UA)

NORMAL FINDINGS

Appearance: clear
Colour: amber yellow
Odour: aromatic
pH: 4.6–8.0 (average, 6.0)
Protein (qualitative):
    0–8 mg/dL
    At rest: **<50–80 mg/24 hr** (0.05–0.08 g/day)
    During exercise: **<250 mg/24 hr** (<0.25 g/day)
Specific gravity
    Adult: 1.005–1.030 (usually, 1.010–1.025)
    Older adult: Values decrease with age
    Newborn: 1.001–1.020
Leukocyte esterase: negative
Nitrites: none
Ketones: none
Bilirubin: none
Urobilinogen: **0.5–4.0 mg/24 hr** (0.5–4.0 Ehrlich units/24 hr)
Crystals: none
Casts: none
Glucose (see urine glucose, p. 957)
    Fresh specimen: none
    24-hour specimen: **0.3–1.7 mmol/24 hr** (50–300 mg/24 hr)
White blood cells (WBCs): 0–4/low-power field
WBC casts: none
Red blood cells (RBCs): 0–3/high-power field
RBC casts: none

INDICATIONS

Urinalysis (UA) is part of routine diagnostic and screening evaluations. It can reveal a significant amount of preliminary information about the kidneys and other metabolic processes. Urinalysis is routinely performed in patients admitted to the hospital, pregnant women, and presurgical patients. It is performed for diagnostic purposes in patients with abdominal or back pain, dysuria, hematuria, or urinary frequency. It is part of routine monitoring in patients with chronic renal disease and some metabolic diseases. It is the most frequently ordered urine test.

TEST EXPLANATION

Total UA involves multiple routine tests on a urine specimen. This specimen is not necessarily a clean-catch specimen. However, if urinary tract infection (UTI) is suspected, often a midstream, clean-catch specimen is obtained. This specimen is then divided into two portions; one is sent for UA, and the other is kept in the laboratory refrigerator for culture (see p. 1007) if results of UA indicate infection. The UA report routinely includes remarks regarding the colour, appearance,

Urine Studies

11

and odour; the pH; and the presence of proteins, glucose, ketones, blood, and leukocyte esterase. In addition, the urine is examined microscopically for RBCs, WBCs, casts, crystals, and bacteria. Because this is a spot urine test, volume is not measured. Volume of urine may be important in many clinical situations; in those cases, a full 24-hour specimen is required.

Laboratory Examination

Appearance and Colour. Urine appearance and colour are noted as part of routine UA. A normal urine specimen should be clear. Cloudy urine may reflect the presence of pus (necrotic WBCs), RBCs, or bacteria; however, normal urine also may be cloudy because of ingestion of certain foods (e.g., large amounts of fat, urates, phosphates). Urine ranges from pale yellow to amber because of the pigment urochrome (product of bilirubin metabolism). The colour indicates the concentration of the urine and varies with specific gravity. Dilute urine is straw-coloured, and concentrated urine is deep amber.

An abnormal colour of urine may result from a pathologic condition or the ingestion of certain foods or medicines. For example, bleeding from the kidney colours the urine dark red, whereas bleeding from the lower urinary tract colours the urine bright red. Dark yellow urine may indicate the presence of urobilinogen or bilirubin. *Pseudomonas* infection may colour the urine green. Eating beets may colour the urine red, and rhubarb can colour the urine brown. Many frequently used drugs also may affect urine colour (Table 11-3).

TABLE 11-3	Frequently Used Drugs That May Affect Urine Colour	
Generic and (Brand) Names	**Drug Class**	**Urine Colour**
Cascara sagrada	Stimulant laxative	Alkaline urine: red; acid urine: yellow-brown
Chloroquine	Antimalarial	Rusty yellow or brown
Chlorzoxazone (Acetazone Forte)	Skeletal muscle relaxant	Orange or purple-red
Docusate calcium (Calax)	Laxative	Pink, red, red-brown
Doxorubicin Hydrochloride (Adriamycin)	Antineoplastic	Red-orange
Iron preparations (Ferrous fumerate, Iron dextran)	Hematinic	Turns dark brown or black on standing
Levodopa-Carbidopa (Sinemet)	Antiparkinsonian agent	Turns dark brown on standing
Metronidazole (Flagyl)	Anti-infective	Darkening, reddish-brown
Nitrofurantoin (Macrodantin, Macro BID)	Antibacterial	Brown-yellow
Phenazopyridine Hydrochloride (Pyridium)	Urinary tract analgesic	Orange to red
Phenothiazines (e.g., prochlorperazine [Nu-Prochlor])	Antipsychotic, neuroleptic, antiemetic	Red-brown
Phenytoin sodium (Dilantin)	Anticonvulsant	Pink, red, red-brown
Riboflavin (vitamin B2)	Vitamin	Intense yellow
Rifampin (Rifadin, Rofact)	Antibiotic	Red-orange
Triamterene Hydrochlorothiazide (Riva-Zide)	Diuretic	Pale blue fluorescent

Odour. Determination of urine odour is part of routine UA. The odour of fresh, normal urine is caused by the presence of volatile acids. Urine of patients with diabetic ketoacidosis has the strong, sweet smell of acetone. In patients with a UTI, the urine may have a foul odour. Urine with a fecal odour may indicate the presence of an enterovesical fistula.

pH. Analysis of the pH of a freshly voided urine specimen indicates the acid-base balance. The urine reflects the work of the kidneys to maintain normal pH homeostasis. Just as the lungs (respiratory component) help compensate for acid-base imbalance, so do the kidneys (metabolic component). The kidneys assist in acid-base balance by reabsorbing sodium and excreting hydrogen.

An alkaline pH is observed in a patient with alkalemia. Bacteria, UTI, or a diet with high amounts of citrus fruits or vegetables may also cause elevations in urine pH. Alkalinity of the urine is common after eating. Certain medications (e.g., streptomycin, neomycin) are effective in treating UTIs when the urine is alkaline. It is more common for the urine to be acidic. However, urine is also acidic in patients with acidemia, which can result from metabolic or respiratory acidosis, starvation, dehydration, or a diet with high amounts of meat products or cranberries.

The urine pH is useful in identifying crystals in the urine and determining the patient's predisposition to form a given type of stone. Acidity of the urine is associated with xanthine, cystine, uric acid, and calcium oxalate stones. To treat or prevent these urinary calculi, urine should be kept alkaline. Alkalinity of the urine is associated with calcium carbonate, calcium phosphate, and magnesium phosphate stones. To treat or prevent these urinary calculi, urine should be kept acidic.

Protein. Protein is a sensitive indicator of kidney function. Normally, protein is not present in the urine because the spaces in the normal glomerular filtrate membrane are too small to allow its passage. If the glomerular membrane is injured, as in glomerulonephritis, the spaces become much larger, and protein (usually albumin, because it is a smaller molecule than the globulins) seeps into the filtrate and then into the urine. If this seepage persists at a significant rate, hypoproteinemia can develop as a result of severe protein loss through the kidneys. In hypoproteinemia, the normal capillary oncotic pressure that holds fluid within the vasculature is decreased, and severe interstitial edema develops. The combination of proteinuria and edema is known as *nephrotic syndrome.*

Proteinuria (most commonly albuminuria) is probably the most important indicator of renal disease. The urine of all pregnant women is routinely checked for proteinuria, which can be an indicator of pre-eclampsia. Urinary protein is used to screen for nephrotic syndrome and for complications of diabetes mellitus, glomerulonephritis, amyloidosis, and multiple myeloma (see test for Bence-Jones protein, p. 943).

If significant protein is noted at UA, a 24-hour urine specimen should be collected so that the quantity of protein can be measured. This test can be repeated as a method of monitoring renal disease and its treatment. Usually, protein loss of more than 3000 mg in 24 hours leads to the signs and symptoms of nephrotic syndrome. If proteinuria is identified, a random urine sample can be analyzed for protein quantification. This estimate of 24-hour protein excretion is usually performed with a urine creatinine measurement, because hydration status and other factors may influence urine concentration. The normal *protein/creatinine ratio* is less than 0.15.

Glucose. See the test for blood glucose (p. 269).

Specific Gravity. Specific gravity is a measure of the concentration of particles (including wastes and electrolytes) in the urine. High specific gravity indicates concentrated urine; low specific gravity indicates dilute urine. Specific gravity is the weight of the urine in comparison with that

Urine Studies

11

of distilled water (which has a specific gravity of 1.000). Particles in the urine give it weight, or specific gravity.

Specific gravity is used to evaluate the concentrating and excretory power of the kidneys. Renal disease tends to diminish concentrating capability. As a result, chronic renal diseases are associated with low specific gravity of the urine. Specific gravity must be interpreted with regard to the presence or absence of glycosuria and proteinuria. Specific gravity is also a measurement of hydration status. With overhydration, the urine is more dilute and thus has lower specific gravity, whereas with dehydration, specific gravity can be expected to be abnormally high. Nephrotoxic diabetes insipidus is associated with very little variation in specific gravity of the urine because the kidneys cannot respond to variables such as hydration and solute load.

Measurement of urine specific gravity is easier and more convenient than measurement of osmolality (see p. 972). Specific gravity is correlated approximately with osmolality. Knowledge of specific gravity is needed to interpret the results of most parts of the UA. Specific gravity is usually evaluated with a refractometer (which measures the amount of light that can pass through a drop of urine) or a dipstick.

Leukocyte Esterase. Leukocyte esterase is a screening test used to detect leukocytes (WBCs) in the urine. Positive results indicate UTI. Some patients have no symptoms of UTI (e.g., pain or burning on urination). For this examination, chemical testing is performed with a leukocyte esterase dipstick; a shade of purple is considered a positive result. Some laboratories have established screening protocols in which a microscopic examination (see the later "Microscopic Examination of Urine Sediment" section) is performed only if results of a leukocyte esterase test are positive. Leukocyte esterase is nearly 90% accurate in revealing WBCs in urine.

Nitrites. Like the leukocyte esterase screen, the nitrite test is a screening test for identification of UTIs. Some patients have no symptoms of UTI (e.g., pain or burning on urination). This test is based on the principle that many bacteria produce reductase, an enzyme that can reduce urinary nitrates to nitrites. Chemical testing is done with a dipstick containing a reagent that reacts with nitrites to produce a pink colour, which indirectly suggests the presence of bacteria. A positive test result indicates the need for a urine culture. Nitrite screening enhances the sensitivity of the leukocyte esterase test to detect UTIs.

Ketones. Normally, no ketones are present in the urine; however, a patient with poorly controlled diabetes and hyperglycemia, or a patient on a restricted diet, may have massive fatty acid catabolism. The purpose of this catabolism is to provide an energy source when glucose cannot be transferred into the cell because of insulin insufficiency. Ketones (beta-hydroxybutyric acid, acetoacetic acid, and acetone) are the end products of this fatty acid breakdown. As with glucose, ketones spill into the urine when blood levels are elevated in patients with diabetes. Ketonuria is usually associated with poorly controlled diabetes. This test for ketonuria is also important in evaluating ketoacidosis associated with alcoholism, fasting, starvation, high-protein diets, and isopropanol ingestion. Ketonuria may occur with acute febrile illnesses, especially in infants and children.

Bilirubin and Urobilinogen. *Bilirubin* is a major constituent of bile. If bilirubin excretion is inhibited, conjugated (direct) hyperbilirubinemia results (see p. 135). Obstruction of the bile duct by a gallstone is the classic example of obstructed bilirubin excretion that causes conjugated hyperbilirubinemia. Unlike the unconjugated form, conjugated bilirubin is water soluble and can be excreted into the urine. Therefore, bilirubin in urine suggests the presence of disease affecting bilirubin metabolism after conjugation or defects in excretion (e.g., gallstones). Determination of bilirubin concentration is included in routine UA. This test is no longer very useful as a monitor of liver disease or as an indicator of severity of liver disease; serum bilirubin is more appropriate for those purposes. For screening, however, elevations in urine bilirubin concentration can indicate previously unsuspected liver injury caused by disease, gallstones, or drug toxicity. Bilirubin in the urine colours the urine dark yellow or orange.

Bilirubin is excreted via the bile ducts into the bowel. In the bowel, some of the bilirubin is transformed into *urobilinogen* by the action of bacteria in the bowel. Most of the urobilinogen is excreted from the liver back into the bowel, but some is excreted by the kidneys. If bilirubin levels are high because of overproduction, which may result from increased RBC lysis (hemolysis), urobilinogen levels are elevated. If bilirubin is high because of defects in bilirubin metabolism or obstruction of excretion, urobilinogen levels are not elevated, because excretion of bilirubin to the bowel is needed for formation of urobilinogen. Urine screening for urobilinogen is rarely performed because it is easier to determine the cause of elevations in bilirubin levels by fractionating the bilirubin into its direct and indirect components.

Microscopic Examination of Urine Sediment. Microscopic examination of the sediment from a centrifuged urine specimen provides substantial information about the urinary system. Because many different methods can be used to prepare the sediment for microscopic review, normal values may vary significantly among laboratories. Reference ranges are provided in this section to recognize marked abnormalities.

Crystals. Crystals found in the urinary sediment on microscopic examination indicate that renal stone formation is imminent, if not already present. By themselves, crystals cause no symptoms until they form stones. Even then, stones produce symptoms only when they obstruct the urinary tract. Uric acid crystals occur in patients with high serum uric acid levels (e.g., gout). Phosphate and calcium oxalate crystals (Figure 11-2) are present in the urine of patients with parathyroid abnormalities or malabsorption states. The type of crystal found varies with the disease and the pH of the urine (see previous discussion on urinary pH). Small amounts of crystalline material and even casts (see following discussion) can be observed when the specific gravity of the urine is high.

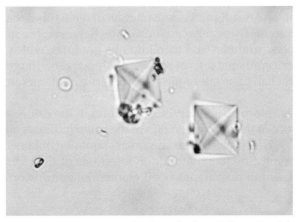

Figure 11-2 Microscopic examination of urine sediment: calcium oxalate crystals. This is the most common crystal structure seen in urine sediment. Note the classic cross-shaped internal configuration.

Casts. Casts are rectangular clumps of materials or cells that form in the renal distal and collecting tubules, where the material is maximally concentrated. These clumps of material and cells are shaped like tubules; hence the term *cast*. For casts to form, the pH must be acidic and the urine concentrated. Casts are usually associated with some degree of proteinuria and stasis within the renal tubules. There are two kinds of casts: hyaline and cellular. Casts are best seen on low power of the light microscope. Some casts are nearly clear (hyaline), and the condenser lamp must be dimmed in order to see them well.

Hyaline Casts. Hyaline casts are conglomerations of protein and are indicative of proteinuria. A few hyaline casts are normally present, especially after strenuous exercise.

Cellular Casts. Cellular casts are conglomerations of degenerated cells. Various types are described as follows.

Granular casts. Granular casts result from the disintegration of cellular material into granular particles within a WBC or epithelial cell cast. Granular casts are found after exercise and in various renal diseases. Their basic component is the same as that of the cellular material.

Fatty casts. In some diseases, the epithelial cells desquamate into the renal tubule. As the cell degenerates, fatty deposits within the cell coalesce and become incorporated with protein into casts. If casts are not formed, these fatty droplets coalesce to bigger droplets called *free oval fat bodies.* These are associated with nephrotic syndrome or nephrosis. Free oval fat bodies may also be associated with fatty emboli, which occur in patients with bone fractures.

Waxy casts. Waxy casts may also be cellular casts, hyaline casts, or present in renal failure. Waxy casts probably represent further degeneration of granular casts. They occur when urine flow through the renal tubule is diminished, in which case granular casts have time to degenerate. Waxy casts are associated with chronic renal diseases and chronic renal failure. They also occur in diabetic nephropathy, malignant hypertension, and glomerulonephritis.

Epithelial cells and casts (renal tubular casts). Epithelial cells can enter the urine at any point during the process of urinary excretion. These cells can be shed from the bladder as a result of tumour, infection, or polyps. They can result from cellular contamination of the urine by vaginal or urethral secretions. They can also result from desquamation of renal tubule cells into the lumen of the tubules and collecting system. These cells can form epithelial casts. The material in these cells can disintegrate first into coarse granules and then into fine granules, which become granular casts. The presence of occasional epithelial cells in urine is not remarkable; large numbers, however, are abnormal. Tubular (epithelial) casts are suggestive primarily of glomerulonephritis.

White blood cells and casts. Normally, few WBCs are found in the urine sediment on microscopic examination. The presence of five or more WBCs in the urine indicates a UTI involving the bladder or kidneys, or both. A clean-catch urine specimen should be obtained for further evaluation (culture). WBC casts are most frequently found in infections of the kidney (e.g., acute pyelonephritis) and are also present in poststreptococcal glomerulonephritis or inflammatory nephritis (e.g., lupus nephritis).

Red blood cells and casts. Any disruption in the blood-urine barrier—whether at the glomerular, tubular, or bladder level—causes RBCs to enter the urine. Hematuria can be microscopic or gross. Bladder, ureteral, and urethral diseases are the most common causes of RBCs in the urine. Pathologic conditions (e.g., tumours, trauma, stones, infection) that involve the mucous membrane in the collecting system can also cause hematuria. Hematuria is detected easily with routine UA. RBC casts suggest glomerulonephritis (which may be present in patients with acute bacterial endocarditis, renal infarct, Goodpasture's syndrome, vasculitis, sickle cell disease, or malignant hypertension), interstitial nephritis, acute tubular necrosis, pyelonephritis, renal trauma, or renal tumour.

INTERFERING FACTORS

Appearance and Colour
- Sperm remaining in the urethra after recent or retrograde ejaculation can cause the urine to appear cloudy.
- Urine that has been refrigerated for longer than 1 hour can become cloudy.
- Certain foods affect urine colour. Eating carrots may colour urine dark yellow; beets may colour urine red; rhubarb may colour urine reddish or brownish.
- Urine darkens with prolonged standing because of oxidation of bilirubin metabolites.
- Many drugs, given the right environment, can *alter* the colour of urine (see Table 11-3).

Odour
- Several foods (e.g., asparagus) produce characteristic urine odours.
- When urine stands for a long time and begins to decompose, it has an ammonia-like smell.

pH
- Urine pH becomes alkaline on standing because of the action of urea-splitting bacteria, which produce ammonia.
- The urine pH of an uncovered specimen becomes alkaline because carbon dioxide vaporizes from the urine.
- Dietary factors affect urine pH. Ingestion of large quantities of citrus fruits, dairy products, and vegetables turns the urine alkaline, whereas a diet with high amounts of meat and certain foods (e.g., cranberries) turns urine acidic.
- Drugs that *increase* urine pH include acetazolamide, bicarbonate antacids, and carbonic anhydrase inhibitors.
- Drugs that *decrease* urine pH include ammonium chloride, chlorothiazide, and mandelic acid.

Protein
- Transient proteinuria may be associated with severe emotional stress, excessive exercise, and cold baths.
- Radiopaque contrast media administered within 3 days before UA testing may cause false-positive results for proteinuria when turbidity is used as a measure of protein in the urine.
- Urine contaminated with prostate or vaginal secretions commonly causes findings of proteinuria.
- Diets high in protein can cause proteinuria.
- Highly concentrated urine may have a higher concentration of protein than does more dilute urine.
- Hemoglobin may cause a positive result with the dipstick method.
- Bence-Jones protein may not appear with the dipstick method.
- Drugs that may cause *increases* in protein levels include acetazolamide, aminoglycosides, amphotericin B, cephalosporins, colistin, lithium, methicillin, nafcillin, nephrotoxic drugs (e.g., arsenicals, gold salts), oxacillin, penicillamine, penicillin G, phenazopyridine, polymyxin B, salicylates, sulphonamides, tolbutamide, and vancomycin.

Specific Gravity

- Recent use of radiographic dyes increases urinary specific gravity.
- Cold causes specific gravity to be artificially high.
- Drugs that may cause *increases* in specific gravity include dextran, mannitol, and sucrose.

Leukocyte Esterase

- False-positive results may occur in specimens contaminated by vaginal secretions (e.g., heavy menstrual discharge, *Trichomonas* infection, parasites) that contain WBCs.
- False-negative results may occur in specimens containing high levels of protein or ascorbic acid.

Ketones

- Special diets (carbohydrate-free, high-protein, high-fat) may cause ketonuria.
- Drugs that may cause *false-positive* results include bromosulphophthalein, isoniazid, isopropanol, levodopa, paraldehyde, phenazopyridine, and phenolsulphonphthalein.

Bilirubin and Urobilinogen

- Bilirubin is not stable in urine, especially when exposed to light.
- Urobilinogen levels can be affected by pH. Alkaline urine indicates higher levels; acidic urine may show lower levels.
- Phenazopyridine colours the urine orange. This may produce the false impression that the patient has jaundice.
- Cholestatic drugs may *reduce* urobilinogen levels.
- Antibiotics reduce intestinal flora, which in turn *reduces* urobilinogen levels.

Crystals

- Radiographic contrast media may cause precipitation of urinary crystals.

WBCs

- Vaginal discharge may contaminate the urine specimen and factitiously cause WBCs to appear in the urine.

RBCs

- Strenuous physical exercise may cause RBC casts.
- Traumatic urethral catheterization may cause RBCs to appear in the urine.
- Overaggressive anticoagulant therapy or bleeding disorders tend to cause RBCs to appear in the urine without concomitant disease.

Clinical Priorities

- A common cause of RBCs in the urine of women is contamination because of menses. Before a more thorough evaluation is begun, determine whether the patient was menstruating when the urine specimen was obtained.
- Leukocyte esterase and nitrate tests are screening tests used to detect UTIs. Positive test results indicate the need for urine culture.
- If a UTI is suspected, a midstream, clean-catch specimen is needed.
- If a 24-hour urine collection is needed, it should be refrigerated during the collection period. A preservative may also be necessary.

PROCEDURE AND PATIENT CARE

Before

✍ Explain the procedure to the patient.

During

- Collect a fresh urine specimen in a urine container.
- If the urine specimen contains vaginal discharge or bleeding, a clean-catch or midstream specimen is needed. This requires meticulous cleaning of the urinary meatus with an iodine preparation to reduce contamination of the specimen by external organisms. The cleansing agent must then be completely removed so as not to contaminate the specimen. The midstream collection is obtained as follows:
  1. Instruct the patient to begin to urinate into a bedpan, urinal, or toilet and then stop urinating. This washes urine out of the distal part of the urethra.
  2. Correctly position a sterile urine container and have the patient void 80 to 120 mL of urine.
  3. Cap the container.
  4. Allow the patient to finish voiding.
- Testing for ketones can be performed immediately after urine collection with a dipstick.
- For testing urine specific gravity, a first-voided specimen is best.
- Specific gravity can be measured with a refractometer. Light passes through the specimen, and the refractive index (difference between the velocity of light passing through air and the specimen) is determined.
- An easier method of measuring specific gravity is the dipstick method. A dipstick is placed in the specimen, and the resulting colour is compared with a colour chart.
- To test for protein, a first-voided specimen is best. On occasion, however, a 24-hour urine collection is preferred to ensure that the protein in the urine is measured accurately.
- In most laboratories, the dipstick method is used to detect protein in the urine.
- Nitrite, leukocyte esterase, pH, and ketones are measured with the dipstick method, and the results are determined by comparison with a colour chart.
- To obtain urine sediment, a small volume (10 mL) of urine is subjected to centrifugation, and the supernatant is discarded. The remaining urine is a concentrated sediment that can be microscopically examined.

After

- Transport the urine specimen to the laboratory promptly.
- If the specimen cannot be processed immediately, refrigerate it.
- If a 24-hour urine collection is requested, the specimen should be refrigerated or preserved with formalin during the entire 24 hours.
- Casts break up as urine is allowed to sit. Urine examinations for casts should be performed with fresh specimens.

TEST RESULTS AND CLINICAL SIGNIFICANCE

Appearance and Colour

Infection: *Infection may cause turbidity and a foul smell of the urine.* Pseudomonas *infection can cause a green tint in urine.*

Gross hematuria: *RBCs in the urine cause the urine to be red. This is always a pathologic sign unless the blood is found to be from a source other than the urinary tract. Tumours, trauma, stones, and infection anywhere in the urinary tract can cause RBCs in the urine. Glomerulonephritis, interstitial nephritis, acute necrosis, and pyelonephritis are also associated with hematuria.*

Drug therapy (see Table 11-3, p. 992).
Overhydration,
Diabetes insipidus,
Diuretic therapy,
Glycosuria: *In these states, the urine is nearly colourless.*
Fever,
Excessive sweating,
Dehydration,
Jaundice: *In these states, the urine is dark yellow or orange.*
Hemoglobinuria,
Myoglobinuria,
Porphyria: *In these illnesses, the urine is wine-coloured or even dark brown.*

Odour

Ketonuria: *The presence of ketones, in association with poor glucose tolerance, causes a fruity smell.*
Urinary tract infection: *Most infections cause urine to smell foul.*
Enterovesical fistula: *This condition causes urine to smell like stool.*
Maple sugar urine: *This congenital defect in protein metabolism causes the urine to smell like burnt sugar.*
Phenylketonuria: *This disease causes the urine to smell musty.*

pH
▲ Increased Levels
Alkalemia: *The renal component of pH homeostasis causes the excretion of excess base in an effort to correct acid-base imbalance.*
Urinary tract infections: *Urea-splitting bacteria cause the urine to be alkaline as urea is converted to ammonia.*
Gastric suction,
Vomiting,
Renal tubular acidosis: *These are all associated with reduced excretion of hydrogen ion. Urine pH is increased.*

▼ Decreased Levels
Acidemia: *To maintain homeostasis, the kidneys attempt to excrete hydrogen ions, causing the urine pH to be lowered.*
Diabetes mellitus,
Starvation: *Ketone acids in association with starvation or poor glucose metabolism cause urine to be acidotic.*
Respiratory acidosis: *Hydrogen ions are excreted and the urine becomes acidotic.*

Protein
▲ Increased Levels
Nephrotic syndrome,
Glomerulonephritis,
Malignant hypertension,
Diabetic glomerulosclerosis,
Polycystic kidney disease,
Systemic lupus erythematosus,
Goodpasture's syndrome,
Heavy-metal poisoning,
Bacterial pyelonephritis,

Nephrotoxic drug therapy: *Renal disease involving the glomeruli is associated with proteinuria.*

Trauma: *Protein can spill into the urine as a result of traumatic destruction of the blood-urine barrier.*

Macroglobulinemia: *When globulin levels within the blood are increased, albumin is excreted in an attempt to maintain oncotic homeostasis.*

Multiple myelomas: *Classically, multiple myelomas produce large amounts of proteins (e.g., Bence-Jones protein) in the urine.*

Pre-eclampsia,

Heart failure: *The pathophysiologic mechanisms underlying these observations are many. In brief, albumin leaks from the glomeruli, which are temporarily damaged by these illnesses.*

Orthostatic proteinuria: *As many as 20% of normal male patients have small amounts of protein in the urine when specimens are obtained from patients in the upright position. The pathophysiologic mechanism is not known with certainty. It may be associated with passive congestion of the kidneys in the upright position. To diagnose this phenomenon, the patient should provide a urine specimen before arising and another after the patient has been up for 2 hours. The first sample has no protein; the second does.*

Severe muscle exertion: *Prolonged muscular exertion can be associated with small amounts of protein in the urine.*

Renal vein thrombosis: *Congestion of the kidneys is associated with proteinuria.*

Bladder tumour: *Tumours of the bladder secrete protein into the lumen of the bladder.*

Urethritis or prostatitis: *Inflammation in the periurethral glands or urethra can cause proteinuria.*

Amyloidosis: *Often associated with proteinuria, this condition may be so severe as to cause nephrotic syndrome. Usually, amyloidosis of the kidney is caused by other severe, ongoing disease.*

Specific Gravity

▲ Increased Levels

Dehydration: *The kidneys reabsorb all available free water; thus excreted urine is concentrated.*

Pituitary tumour or trauma: *The syndrome of inappropriate antidiuretic hormone results in excessive water reabsorption and concentrated urine.*

Decreased renal blood flow (as in heart failure, renal artery stenosis, or hypotension): *Urine is concentrated through the renin-angiotensin system and secretion of antidiuretic hormone.*

Glycosuria and proteinuria: *These particles of glucose and protein increase specific gravity.*

Water restriction,

Fever,

Excessive sweating,

Vomiting,

Diarrhea: *These five clinical conditions are associated with diminished blood volume. They cause concentration of urine, mediated through the renin-angiotensin system and secretion of antidiuretic hormone.*

▼ Decreased Levels

Overhydration: *Excess water is excreted, causing dilution of urine with low specific gravity.*

Diabetes insipidus: *Inadequate secretion of antidiuretic hormone causes decreased water reabsorption. Excess water is excreted, causing dilution of urine with low specific gravity.*

Renal failure: *In chronic renal failure the kidney loses its ability to concentrate urine through water reabsorption. Excess water is excreted, causing dilution of urine with low specific gravity.*

Diuresis: *Diuretics tend to cause dilution of urine and voluminous flow.*

Leukocyte Esterase

Possible UTI: *Detection of leukocyte esterase indicates the presence of WBCs in the urine (pyuria), which is indicative of urinary tract infection.*

Urine Studies

11

Nitrites

Possible UTI: *Reductase produced by bacteria reduces nitrates to nitrites. The presence of nitrites indicates bacterial infection somewhere in the urinary tract.*

Ketones

Poorly controlled diabetes mellitus,

Starvation,

Alcoholism,

Weight-reduction diets,

Prolonged vomiting,

Anorexia,

Fasting,

High-protein diets,

Glycogen storage diseases: *Impaired glucose metabolism causes catabolism of fat for production of energy. Ketones (beta-hydroxybutyric acid, acetoacetic acid, and acetone) are formed and spill into the urine.*

Febrile illnesses in infants and children,

Hyperthyroidism,

Severe stress or illness: *Hypermetabolic states cause excessive utilization of glucose. Fats are then broken down. Ketones form and spill into the urine.*

Excessive aspirin ingestion: *Aspirin toxicity is associated with reduced glucose production. Ketones form and spill into the urine.*

Anaesthesia: *The pathophysiologic mechanism underlying this observation is probably multifaceted. Drug effect, starvation, and severe illness can all affect ketone formation.*

Bilirubin

Gallstones,

Extrahepatic duct obstruction (e.g., tumour, inflammation, gallstone, scarring, or surgical trauma),

Extensive liver metastasis: *Direct physical obstruction of flow of bile from the biliary tree causes elevations in serum levels of conjugated (direct) bilirubin, which leads to elevations in urine levels of bilirubin.*

Cholestasis because of drugs: *Some drugs affect bilirubin metabolism and excretion after glucuronide conjugation. Elevations in serum levels of conjugated (direct) bilirubin lead to elevations in urine levels of bilirubin.*

Dubin-Johnson syndrome,

Rotor syndrome: *These congenital defects in bilirubin metabolism occur after glucuronide conjugation. This causes elevations in serum levels of conjugated (direct) bilirubin, which leads to elevations in urine levels of bilirubin.*

Urobilinogen

▲ Increased Levels

Hemolytic anemia,

Pernicious anemia,

Hemolysis because of drugs: *Hemolysis results in increased RBC destruction. This causes more heme to be catabolized into bilirubin. Increased bilirubin is excreted into the bowel. More urobilinogen is made in the bowel, reabsorbed from the gut, and excreted by the kidneys into the urine.*

Hematoma,

Excessive ecchymosis: *RBCs in these areas break down, causing large amounts of heme to be catabolized into bilirubin. Increased bilirubin is excreted into the bowel. More urobilinogen is produced in the bowel, reabsorbed from the gut, and excreted by the kidneys into the urine.*

▼ **Decreased Levels**

Biliary obstruction,

Cholestasis: *No bilirubin reaches the bowel for conversion to urobilinogen. Therefore, urine levels of urobilinogen are reduced.*

Crystals

Renal stone formation: *Stones form with crystals as a nidus for production. Crystals in small quantities are not pathologic. Crystals do provide some insight into metabolic diseases (e.g., gout, hyperparathyroidism) and other congenital defects of protein metabolism.*

Urinary tract infection: *Infection, particularly with* Proteus *organisms, is associated with crystal formation, especially if infection is chronic.*

Granular Casts and Waxy Casts

Acute tubular necrosis,

Urinary tract infection,

Glomerulonephritis,

Pyelonephritis,

Nephrosclerosis,

Chronic lead poisoning,

Exercise,

Stress,

Renal transplant rejection: *The presence of coarse and fine granular casts indicates further degeneration of cellular casts. They appear when urine flow through the collecting system is diminished, which allows time for further degeneration. As a result, nearly any renal disease or toxic effect can be associated with granular cast formation. Waxy casts represent further deterioration of granular casts over time.*

Fatty Casts

Nephrotic syndrome,

Diabetic nephropathy (Kimmelstiel-Wilson syndrome),

Glomerulonephritis associated with streptococcal infection,

Chronic renal disease (glomerulonephritis),

Mercury poisoning: *The appearance of fatty casts is classically associated with nephrotic syndrome. Any disease or poison that affects the tubular cells causes them to degenerate and desquamate into the lumen. The fatty deposits within those cells coalesce to mix with protein and to make fatty casts or free oval fat bodies.*

Fat embolism: *Approximately 50% of fat embolisms are associated with urinary fat.*

Epithelial Casts

Glomerulonephritis,

Eclampsia,

Heavy-metal poisoning: *Diseases that affect the renal tubule cells and diminish urine flow are associated with epithelial cast formation.*

Epithelial Cells

Acute renal allograft rejection,

Acute tubular necrosis,

Acute glomerulonephritis resulting from streptococcal infection: *Acute tubule cell injuries cause those cells to be destroyed and desquamate into the lumen of the tubule and to be excreted in the urine.*

Hyaline Casts

Orthostatic proteinuria,

Fever,

Strenuous exercise,

Stress: *These clinical states are often associated with short-term proteinuria and decreased urine flow through the renal collecting system. Proteinaceous (or hyaline) casts develop.*

Glomerulonephritis,

Pyelonephritis,

Heart failure,

Chronic renal failure: *These diseases are associated with chronic proteinuria and hyaline cast formation.*

Red Blood Cells and Casts

▲ Increased Red Blood Cell Levels

Primary renal diseases (e.g., glomerulonephritis, interstitial nephritis, acute tubular necrosis, pyelonephritis): *These diseases are associated with the deterioration of the blood-urine barrier.*

Renal tumour: *Renal neoplasms are friable and hypervascular. The presence of RBCs in urine is common with cancers of the kidney.*

Renal trauma: *Lacerations, contusions, and hematomas ultimately lead to blood in the urine.*

Renal stones,

Cystitis,

Prostatitis,

Tumours of the ureters and bladder,

Traumatic bladder catheterization,

Bladder trauma: *Any mucosal injury or disease can cause bleeding directly into the urine. Hematuria is usually visible to the naked eye.*

▲ Increased Red Blood Cell Cast Levels

Glomerulonephritis,

Subacute bacterial endocarditis,

Renal infarction,

Goodpasture's syndrome,

Vasculitis,

Sickling,

Malignant hypertension,

Systemic lupus erythematosus: *Bleeding from the kidneys, when associated with reduced urine flow through the kidneys, can be associated with the presence of RBC casts. The presence of RBC casts rules out the lower urinary tract as a source of bleeding.*

White Blood Cells and Casts

▲ Increased White Blood Cell Levels

Bacterial infection in the urinary tract: *The presence of WBCs in response to bacterial infections anywhere in the urinary tract can cause leukorrhea. It may be difficult to differentiate cystitis from urethritis, but it can be accomplished with the two-specimen technique. Ask the patient to void approximately 20 mL of urine into one container and the rest into another container. A higher number of WBCs in the first container indicates urethritis; a higher number in the second container indicates cystitis.*

▲ **Increased White Blood Cell Cast Levels**

Acute pyelonephritis,

Glomerulonephritis,

Lupus nephritis: *Infectious or inflammatory diseases affecting the kidney can be associated with WBC cast formation. The presence of casts rules out the lower urinary tract as a source of the infection or inflammation.*

RELATED TESTS

Glucose, Urine (p. 957). This test is included in routine UA. It warrants separate discussion, however, because of its importance.

Urine Culture and Sensitivity (p. 1007). If UA results indicate the possibility of infection, a culture and sensitivity test should be performed.

Urinary Stone Analysis (Renal Calculus Analysis)

NORMAL FINDINGS

Normally there are no stones present in urine. All stones are pathological.

INDICATIONS

Urinary stone analysis is performed to identify the chemicals that make up the kidney stone, in order to treat any underlying disease that may have caused the stone formation. This information is also used to determine the most effective methods to reduce the chance that another stone will form.

TEST EXPLANATION

Approximately 10% of all Canadians develop kidney stones; however, kidney stones occur more commonly in men than in women. Approximately 70% to 80% of all stones are composed of calcium oxalate and calcium phosphate; 10% are composed of struvite (magnesium ammonium phosphate produced during infection with bacteria that possess the enzyme urease); 9% are composed of uric acid (UA); and the remaining 1% are composed of cystine or ammonium acid urate or are diagnosed as drug-related stones. Stones ultimately arise because of a supersaturated phase of these substances from liquid to solid state.

A kidney stone can be as small as a grain of sand or as big as 2.5 cm (1 inch) or larger in diameter. Sometimes a stone can leave the kidney and move down a ureter into the bladder. From the bladder, the stone passes through the urethra and out of the body in urine. Stone passage produces renal colic that usually begins as a mild discomfort and progresses to a plateau of extreme severity over 30 to 60 minutes. If the stone obstructs the ureteropelvic junction, pain localizes to the flank; as the stone moves down the ureter, pain moves downward and

11

Urine Studies

anterior. Colic is independent of body position or motion and is described as a pressure or burning sensation.

Stones less than 5 mm in diameter have a high chance of passage; those of 5 to 7 mm have a modest chance (50%) of passage, and those greater than 7 mm almost always necessitate urologic intervention. Ideally, stone analysis is performed by infrared spectroscopy or radiographic diffraction. Renal stone burden is best gauged with computed tomography (see p. 1059) taken with 5-mm cuts, without infusion of contrast agents. The radiographic appearance and density of stones as measured by computed tomography is a guide to their composition. Approximately 90% of kidney stones can be seen on an abdominal radiograph of the kidney, ureter, and bladder (KUB; see p. 1084).

Analysis is done on a kidney stone to determine its chemical makeup. The test, done on a stone that has been passed in the urine or removed from the urinary tract during surgery, shows the type of stone, which can guide treatment and give information that may prevent more stones from forming. People who have had a kidney stone have a risk for having another one. Therefore prevention measures are important.

Diagnosing a kidney stone includes an initial evaluation based on family history, associated medical conditions, medications, and diet; biochemical blood studies; urinalysis; X-rays; and analysis of the stone itself, if obtained. It also typically includes 24-hour urine collection to analyze volume, pH, calcium, magnesium, phosphate, oxalate, urate, creatinine, sodium, citrate, and cystine. If the stone is caused by a urinary tract infection (struvite or carbonate apatite), treatment of the infection will eliminate recurrence. Treating noninfectious stones will invariably involve some form of dietary manipulation, in particular increasing water intake.

Urinary stones can be partially prevented by altering the composition of the urine. In a simplified format, the following type of stones is often treated as follows:
- Hyperuricuria, predominantly uric acid stones, and cystine stones: Alkalinize urine to increase uric acid solubility with potassium alkali two or three times daily.
- Hypercalciuria and predominantly hydroxyapatite stones: Acidify urine to increase calcium solubility. However, treatment also depends on urine pH and urine phosphate, sulphate, oxalate, and citrate concentrations. Thiazide diuretics reduce urinary calcium and increase urinary volume.
- Hyperoxaluria and calcium oxalate stones: Increase daily fluid intake and consider reduction of daily calcium.
- Magnesium, ammonium, and phosphate stones (struvite): Investigate and treat urinary tract infection.

INTERFERING FACTORS
- Tape used to attach a stone to paper may affect the ability to accurately identify the composition of the stone.

PROCEDURE AND PATIENT CARE
Before
- Explain the procedure to the patient.
- Ensure pain relief if the patient is having ureteral colic.
- Document a history of any previous urinary stones.
- Explain that there are no dietary restrictions for this test.
- Provide and explain the use of a strainer into which the patient is to urinate.

During
X Instruct the patient to urinate into the strainer provided.
X Instruct the patient to transfer any particulate matter to a container for laboratory analysis.

After
• Transport the specimen to the laboratory promptly.

TEST RESULTS AND CLINICAL SIGNIFICANCE

Urinary stone: *The composition of the stone provides information to direct further diagnosis and treatment.*

RELATED TESTS

Computed Tomography, Abdomen (p. 1059). Computed tomographic scan of the ureters and kidneys (also called *computed tomographic urography*) is the most common way to find kidney stones.

Abdominal Ultrasonography (p. 896). This is a quick method that may be used to find kidney stones.

Intravenous Pyelography (p. 1080). Intravenous pyelography can help monitor the excretion of dye through the urologic tract. An obstruction could indicate a urinary stone.

Urine Culture and Sensitivity (Urine C&S)

NORMAL FINDINGS

Negative: <10 000 colony-forming units (CFU)/mL (may indicate contamination of the specimen)
Positive: >100 000 CFU/mL, which indicates the presence of a urinary tract infection

INDICATIONS

This test is used to diagnose urinary tract infection (UTI) in patients with dysuria, frequency, or urgency. It is also indicated when patients have fever of unknown origin or when urinalysis (UA) results suggest infection.

TEST EXPLANATION

Urine culture and sensitivity tests are performed to determine the presence of pathogenic bacteria in patients with suspected UTIs. Most often, UTIs are limited to the bladder, although the kidneys, ureters, bladder, or urethra can be the locus of infection. All cultures should be performed before antibiotic therapy is initiated because the antibiotic may interrupt the growth of the organism in the laboratory. Most organisms require approximately 24 hours to grow in the laboratory, and preliminary findings can be reported at that time. Usually, 48 to 72 hours are required for growth and identification of an organism. Cultures may be repeated after appropriate antibiotic therapy to assess for complete resolution of the infection, especially UTI.

To save money in some institutions, a urine sample is collected and divided. Half is sent for UA, and the other half is kept in the laboratory refrigerator and evaluated only if results of UA indicate a possible infection (e.g., increased number of WBCs, bacteria, high pH, leukocyte esterase).

Urine Studies

11

An important part of any routine culture is assessment of the sensitivity of any bacteria that are growing in the urine to various antibiotics. The physician can then prescribe the safest, least expensive, and most effective antibiotic therapy for the specific bacteria.

INTERFERING FACTORS

- Contamination of the urine with stool, vaginal secretions, hands, or clothing causes false-positive results.
- Drugs that may affect test results include other antibiotics.

PROCEDURE AND PATIENT CARE

Before

- Explain to the patient the procedure for collecting a clean-catch (midstream) urine specimen.
- Withhold antibiotics as per the physician's order until after the urine specimen has been collected.
- Provide the patient with the necessary supplies for the collection.

During

- Note that a *clean-catch* or *midstream urine collection* is required for culture and sensitivity testing. This requires meticulous cleansing of the urinary meatus with a cleansing agent to reduce contamination of the specimen by external organisms. In uncircumcised male patients, the foreskin must be retracted. The cleansing agent must be completely removed so that it does not contaminate the urine specimen. The midstream collection is obtained as follows:
  1. Instruct the patient to cleanse the perineum from front to back with a cleansing towelette.
  2. Instruct the patient to begin to urinate into a bedpan, urinal, or toilet, and then pass the specimen container into the urine stream and collect 30 to 60 mL of urine. This allows the urine to be washed from the distal portion of the urethra and a clean specimen to be obtained.
  3. Instruct the patient to remove the specimen container before the flow of urine stops.
  4. The patient finishes voiding into the bedpan, urinal, or toilet.
  5. Cleanse the urine from the exterior of the container.
  6. Cap the container, and label the specimen.
- Note that urinary catheterization may be needed for patients who are unable to void. This procedure is not usually performed, however, because of the risk of introducing organisms into the bladder and because of patient discomfort.
- For inpatients with an *indwelling urinary catheter,* obtain a specimen by attaching a syringe at a built-in sampling port. Aspirate the urine, and place it in a sterile urine container. Usually the catheter tubing distal to the sampling port needs to be clamped for 15 to 30 minutes before aspiration of urine to allow urine to fill the tubing. After the specimen is withdrawn, remove the clamp.
- For infants and young children, collect specimens in a disposable pouch called a *U bag.* This bag has adhesive backing around the opening to attach to the child's pubic skin. Clean the child's urinary meatus before applying the bag.
- Note that *suprapubic aspiration* of urine is a safe method of obtaining urine in neonates and infants. The abdomen is prepared with an antiseptic and a local anaesthetic, and a 25-gauge needle is inserted into the suprapubic area 2.5 cm (1 inch) above the symphysis pubis. Urine is aspirated into the syringe and then transferred to a sterile urine container.

- Note that in patients with a urinary diversion (e.g., ileal conduit), catheterization should be performed through the stoma. Urine should not be collected from the ostomy pouch.
- Urine for culture and sensitivity testing should not be taken from a bedpan or brought from home, because it will be contaminated.

After

- Transport the specimen to the laboratory immediately (within 30 minutes). If this is not possible, the specimen may be refrigerated for up to 2 hours. Urine for cytomegalovirus culture, however, is rendered useless by refrigeration.
- Notify the physician of any positive results so that appropriate antibiotic therapy can be initiated.

TEST RESULTS AND CLINICAL SIGNIFICANCE

Urinary tract infection: *Urine is a good culture medium for bacteria. In case of urinary stasis, obstruction, or incomplete emptying, bacteria infect the urine. UTIs can occur as a result of ascending infections from the urethra, especially in female patients.*

RELATED TEST

Urinalysis (p. 991). This test is often performed before culture and sensitivity testing. The presence of white blood cells, leukocyte esterase, nitrites, or bacteria indicates a urinary tract infection.

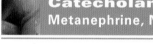

Vanillylmandelic Acid and Catecholamines (VMA; Epinephrine, Norepinephrine, Metanephrine, Normetanephrine, Dopamine)

NORMAL FINDINGS
Vanillylmandelic Acid

Adult: <35 *Mc*mol/24 hr (<6.8 mg/24 hr)
10–16 years: **12–26** *Mc*mol/24 hr (2.3–5.2 mg/24 hr)
6–10 years: **10–16** *Mc*mol/24 hr (2.0–3.2 mg/24 hr)
3–6 years: **5–13** *Mc*mol/24 hr (1.0–2.6 mg/24 hr)
Newborn: <5 *Mc*mol/24 hr (<1.0 mg/24 hr)

Catecholamines
Free Catecholamines
<590 nmol/day (<100 *Mc*g/24 hr)

Epinephrine
Adult: <109 nmol/day (<20 *Mc*g/24 hr)
Child:
   1–4 years: **0–33** nmol/24 hr (0–6 *Mc*g/24 hr)
   4–10 years: **0–55** nmol/24 hr (0–10 *Mc*g/24 hr)
   10–15 years: **2.7–110** nmol/24 hr (0.5–2.0 *Mc*g/24 hr)

11 Urine Studies

Norepinephrine
Adult: <590 nmol/day (<100 *Mcg*/24 hr)
Child:
    1–4 years: **1–170 nmol/24 hr** (0–29 *Mcg*/24 hr)
    4–10 years: **47–470 nmol/24 hr** (8–65 *Mcg*/24 hr)
    10–15 years: **89–470 nmol/24 hr** (15–80 *Mcg*/24 hr)

Dopamine
Age 4 years to adulthood: **384–2 364 nmol/day** (65–400 *Mcg*/24 hr)
≤4 years: **236–1 535 nmol/24 hr** (40–260 *Mcg*/24 hr)

Metanephrine
375–1 506 nmol/day (74–297 *Mcg*/24 hr)

Normetanephrine
89–473 nmol/day (15–80 *Mcg*/24 hr)
    Laboratories report values in various units. Check with your laboratory for correct units and values.

INDICATIONS

This 24-hour urine test for vanillylmandelic acid—also known as 3-methoxy-4-hydroxymandelic acid (VMA)—and for catecholamines is performed primarily to diagnose hypertension secondary to pheochromocytoma. It is also used to detect the presence of neuroblastomas and other rare adrenal tumours.

TEST EXPLANATION

A pheochromocytoma is a tumour of the chromaffin cells within the adrenal medulla that frequently secretes abnormally high levels of epinephrine and norepinephrine. These hormones cause episodic or persistent severe hypertension by producing peripheral arterial vasoconstriction. Dopamine is the precursor of epinephrine and norepinephrine. Metanephrine and normetanephrine are catabolic products of epinephrine and norepinephrine, respectively. VMA is the product of catabolism of both metanephrine and normetanephrine. In patients with pheochromocytoma, one or all of these substances are present in excessive quantities in a 24-hour urine collection. These hormones may be measured singularly in the urine, but the collective metabolic end product, VMA, is more easily detected because VMA concentration is much higher than any one catecholamine component.

    A 24-hour urine test is preferable to a blood test because catecholamine secretion from the tumour may be episodic and potentially could be missed at any one time. The urine provides the laboratory with a specimen that reflects catecholamine production over an entire day. It is best to perform testing when symptoms (hypertension) of the potential adrenal tumour are significant. At that time, catecholamine production is greatest and can be identified more definitely.

    In the past, these urinary tests were performed by spectrophotometric assays. Now, high-performance liquid chromatography (HPLC)–tandem mass spectrometry has improved the accuracy of this testing. Nevertheless, urine testing is cumbersome and time consuming. With HPLC, measurement of plasma-free metanephrine (see p. 372) has nearly replaced urine testing for pheochromocytoma.

INTERFERING FACTORS

- Levels of VMA may be increased by certain foods (e.g., tea, coffee, cocoa, vanilla, chocolate, cider vinegar, soda, licorice, bananas, and citrus fruit).
- Vigorous exercise, stress, and starvation may increase VMA levels.
- Levels of VMA may be artificially decreased by uremia, alkaline urine, and radiographic iodine contrast agents.
- Drugs that may cause *increases* in VMA levels include caffeine, epinephrine, levodopa, lithium, and nitroglycerin. Patients receiving L-dopa should stop taking it for 24 hours before the specimen is obtained.
- Drugs that may cause *decreases* in VMA levels include disulphiram (Antabuse), guanethidine, imipramine, monoamine oxidase inhibitors, and phenothiazines.
- Drugs that may cause *increases* in catecholamine levels include ethyl alcohol, aminophylline, caffeine, chloral hydrate, clonidine (prolonged therapy), contrast media (containing iodine), disulphiram, epinephrine, erythromycin, insulin, methenamine, methyldopa, nicotinic acid (large doses), nitroglycerin, quinidine, riboflavin, and tetracyclines.
- Drugs that may cause *decreases* in catecholamine levels include guanethidine, and salicylates (e.g., aspirin).

Clinical Priorities

- This test is used primarily to evaluate the hypertensive patient for pheochromocytoma.
- A VMA-restricted diet is essential for 2 to 3 days before and throughout the 24-hour urine collection period.
- This 24-hour urine collection requires a preservative and should be placed on ice or refrigerated during the entire 24 hours.

PROCEDURE AND PATIENT CARE

Before

- Explain the dietary restrictions and the 24-hour urine collection procedure to the patient.
- For 2 or 3 days before and throughout the 24-hour collection for VMA, place the patient on a VMA-restricted diet. Instruct the patient to avoid coffee, tea, bananas, chocolate, cocoa, licorice, citrus fruit, all foods and fluids containing vanilla, cider vinegar, soda, and aspirin. Obtain specific restrictions from the laboratory.
- Restrict the patient's use of antihypertensive medications, and sometimes all medications, during this period and possibly longer.

During

- Collect the 24-hour urine specimen. Use a preservative.
- Begin the 24-hour urine collection. Discard the initial specimen, and collect all urine voided by the patient during the next 24 hours.
- Keep the collection refrigerated or on ice during the entire 24 hours.
- Instruct the patient to post the times of the urine collection in a prominent location to prevent the patient from accidentally discarding a specimen.

Urine Studies

11

ⓧ Instruct the patient to void before defecating so that the urine is not contaminated by feces.

ⓧ Instruct the patient not to put toilet paper in the urine container.

ⓧ Encourage the patient to drink fluids during the 24 hours, unless drinking is contraindicated for medical reasons.

ⓧ Instruct the patient to collect the last specimen as close as possible to the end of the 24 hours. This specimen should be added to the urine container.

- On the laboratory slip or urine container, note the time that the last specimen was collected.
- Identify and minimize factors contributing to patient stress and anxiety. Excessive physical exercise and emotion may alter catecholamine test results by causing increased secretion of epinephrine and norepinephrine.

After

- Transmit the specimen to the laboratory as soon as the test is completed.
- Allow the patient to have foods and drugs that were restricted in preparation for the test.

TEST RESULTS AND CLINICAL SIGNIFICANCE

▲ Increased Levels

Pheochromocytomas,
Neuroblastomas,
Ganglioneuromas,
Ganglioblastomas: *These tumours can produce catecholamines. VMA levels are elevated.*
Severe stress,
Strenuous exercise,
Acute anxiety: *Catecholamine levels are elevated during physical (serious illness) or emotional stress or after heavy exercise. VMA levels are also elevated.*

RELATED TEST

Pheochromocytoma Suppression and Provocative Testing (p. 401). This is used to identify pheochromocytoma when catecholamine levels are not definitely diagnostic.

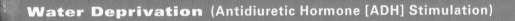

Water Deprivation (Antidiuretic Hormone [ADH] Stimulation)

NORMAL FINDINGS

In neurogenic diabetes insipidus: >9% increase in urine osmolality
In nephrogenic diabetes insipidus: <9% increase in urine osmolality
In psychogenic polydipsia: <9% increase in urine osmolality

INDICATIONS

This test is used to aid in the differential diagnosis of polyuria. Polyuria can occur as a result of neurogenic diabetes insipidus, nephrogenic diabetes insipidus, or psychogenic polydipsia.

TEST EXPLANATION

In this test, the patient is deprived of fluids. Patients who have diabetes insipidus become dehydrated quickly, as indicated by a rise in urine and serum osmolality. Patients with primary psychogenic polydipsia take a longer time to dehydrate. Next, antidiuretic hormone (ADH) is administered. Patients with neurogenic diabetes insipidus have no endogenous ADH, but their urine can become concentrated and the urine osmolality raised if ADH is provided exogenously. In patients with nephrogenic diabetes insipidus, the kidneys are insensitive to ADH, and the patients evince little or no increase in urine osmolality. Patients who have psychogenic polydipsia evince less than a 9% increase in urine osmolality.

POTENTIAL COMPLICATIONS

- Severe dehydration may occur in patients with neurogenic diabetes insipidus. If their urine output is high, they should be monitored closely during the period of dehydration.

INTERFERING FACTORS

- Diuretics can confuse the results and increase the danger of fluid restriction.

PROCEDURE AND PATIENT CARE

Before

✗ Explain the procedure to the patient.
✗ Explain the recommended fluid restriction.
   1. Patients with a urine output of less than 4000 mL/24 hr undergo fluid restriction after midnight before the test.
   2. Patients with a urine output of more than 4000 mL/24 hr begin fluid restriction at the time the test starts, because they may get dangerously dehydrated if water is restricted after midnight.
- The test usually starts at 6 AM and stops at noon.

During

- Obtain and record the patient's body weight hourly for the duration of the procedure.
- Obtain urine osmolality hourly from 6 AM to noon or until three consecutive hourly determinations show a urine osmolality increase of less than **30 mmol/kg H_2O** (30 mOsm/kg).
- At that point, measure serum osmolality. It must be greater than **288 mmol/kg H_2O** (288 mOsm/kg) for the patient to be considered adequately dehydrated and water deprived.
- If the body weight drops more than 2 kg, discontinue the test and rehydrate the patient.
- Administer the prescribed dose of vasopressin (or desmopressin, an analogue of ADH) subcutaneously.
- Measure urine osmolality 30 to 60 minutes after the injection.

After

- Rehydrate the patient with oral fluids.
- Record vital signs while the patient is in both the recumbent and erect positions to ensure that no orthostasis results from inadequate rehydration.
- Observe the venipuncture sites for bleeding.

TEST RESULTS AND CLINICAL SIGNIFICANCE

Rise in Urine Osmolality of More Than 9%

Neurogenic (or central) diabetes insipidus caused by central nervous system trauma, tumour, or infection.

Surgical ablation of pituitary gland: *ADH is not produced in affected patients, but the kidneys can respond to exogenously administered ADH by concentrating the urine.*

Little or No Increase in Urine Osmolality During Deprivation Portion of Test or After Injection

Nephrogenic diabetes insipidus caused by primary renal diseases: *Patients with nephrogenic diabetes insipidus because of chronic kidney diseases evince little or no rise in urine osmolality during the dehydration phase of the test, because the kidneys have lost their concentrating abilities. Furthermore, the kidneys are insensitive to the urine-concentrating effect of ADH.*

Hypokalemia: *Affected patients have the same lack of response as do patients with nephrogenic diabetes insipidus.*

Psychogenic polydipsia: *Affected patients frequently take longer than usual to dehydrate to the point of achieving serum osmolality of 288, and the urine osmolality rises less than 9% after vasopressin injection.*

RELATED TESTS

Antidiuretic Hormone (p. 83). This is a serum assay for direct measurement of antidiuretic hormone. This test is used in the differential diagnosis of neurogenic diabetes insipidus, nephrogenic diabetes insipidus, or psychogenic polydipsia.

Osmolality, Blood (p. 391). This test is a measurement of solute load in the serum.

Osmolality, Urine (p. 972). This test is a measurement of solute load in the urine.

Sodium, Blood (p. 479). This is a direct measurement of sodium level in the serum.

Sodium, Urine (p. 980). This is a direct measurement of sodium level in the urine.

CHAPTER 12

X-Ray Studies

NOTE: *Throughout this chapter, SI units are presented in* **boldface colour***, followed by conventional units in parentheses.*

OVERVIEW

TESTS

OVERVIEW
REASONS FOR PERFORMING X-RAY STUDIES

Because X-rays can penetrate human tissue, X-ray studies provide a valuable picture of body structures. These studies can be as simple as routine chest X-ray or as complex as dye-enhanced cardiac catheterization. There has been increasing concern because radiation exposure causes damage to the cells of the body and increases a patient's risk for developing cancer; thus, patients may want to know whether the proposed benefit of X-ray outweighs the risk involved. This can be discussed in detail with the patient's physician, but the benefits of X-ray studies generally outweigh the risks; however, risk does increase with increasing numbers of X-rays performed.

X-ray studies are used in a wide variety of clinical conditions, such as the following:

1. To evaluate dye excretion in the urinary system (e.g., with intravenous pyelography, antegrade pyelography, or retrograde pyelography).
2. To evaluate arterial occlusive disease (e.g., with arteriography of the kidney, adrenal glands, or cerebrum).
3. To evaluate the gastrointestinal (GI) tract with barium contrast medium (e.g., with barium enema study, upper GI series).
4. To evaluate bone disorders such as fractures, infections, and arthritis (with long bone X-ray).
5. To evaluate the tracheobronchial tree (with bronchography).
6. To visualize the heart chambers, arteries, and great vessels (with cardiac catheterization).
7. To evaluate the pulmonary and cardiac systems (with chest X-ray).
8. To guide needles for biopsy of tumour and aspiration of fluid.
9. To evaluate abdominal organs (with computed tomography [CT] of the abdomen).
10. To determine patency of the fallopian tubes (with hysterosalpingography).
11. To evaluate abdominal pain or trauma (with kidneys, ureter, and bladder [KUB] X-ray or with obstruction series).
12. To detect breast cancer (with mammography).

PRINCIPLES OF RADIOLOGY

X-ray images are radiographs of body structures and look like negatives of photographs. Radiography is based on the ability of X-rays to penetrate tissues and organs differently according to tissue density. X-rays are generated by a machine that passes a high-voltage electrical current through a tungsten filter in a vacuum tube (X-ray tube). As the X-ray passes through body tissues, images are formed on photographic film or a digital imaging plate. Images are produced in varying degrees of dark and light, depending on the amount of X-rays that penetrate the tissues. The greater the amount of energy absorbed, the fewer are the X-rays that reach the film or plate, and the whiter the image appears. For example, bones appear white (radiopaque) because the X-rays cannot penetrate bone to reach the film. When a bone is fractured, the break is visible as a black (radiolucent) line. Because patients with osteoporosis have less calcium in their bones, their bones appear grey and porous on X-rays. X-rays can easily penetrate air; therefore, areas filled with air or gas (e.g., lungs, bowel) appear black or very dark on X-rays. Muscles, blood, organs, and other tissues in the body appear as various shades of grey because they are denser than air but not as dense as bone.

By orienting the X-ray machine at different angles in relation to the body or a body part, different views (projections) can be obtained. The two basic views are anteroposterior, in which the X-rays pass through the front of the body (anterior) to the back (posterior), and lateral, in which the X-rays pass through the body from the side. For posteroanterior views, the X-rays pass through the back of the body to the front. Oblique views are obtained when the X-rays pass through the body at different angles according to how the patient is positioned.

Some of the many types of X-ray procedures are described as follows.

PLAIN RADIOGRAPHY

Plain radiography is performed without contrast material or other augmentation techniques. This procedure is used for routine examination of areas such as the chest, skull, abdomen, and bones.

FLUOROSCOPY

In this radiologic procedure, X-rays pass through the body to a fluorescent viewing screen that is coated with calcium tungstate. The radiologist can not only view the body organs but also observe their motion. For example, after a patient swallows barium, its flow through the upper GI tract can be followed, and after administration of a barium enema, the flow of barium through the colon can be observed. Fluoroscopy is used in angiography procedures to guide the catheter to its desired position (e.g., through the heart during cardiac catheterization). Single (spot) X-rays can be obtained for a permanent record of findings. Videotapes of fluoroscopic procedures (cineradiography) can provide a record of movement for study at a later time. Video recordings can be viewed in slow motion to aid in determining abnormal function. The major disadvantage of fluoroscopy is that it exposes the patient to more radiation than do standard X-ray procedures.

TOMOGRAPHY

In CT, computers recreate a three-dimensional, cross-sectional view of body structures after obtaining X-ray information from the entire circumference of the body. To produce a computed tomographic scan, X-rays pass through the body organs at many angles throughout 360 degrees. The variation in density of each tissue allows for variable penetration of the X-rays. Each degree of density is given a numeric value called a *density coefficient,* which is digitally computed into a shade of grey. An image is then displayed on the computer monitor as thousands of dots in various shades of grey. The image can be enhanced by repeating the computed tomographic procedure after intravenous administration of iodine-containing contrast dye. The images can be recorded. See Figures 12-12 and 12-13, p. 1063.

CONTRAST STUDIES

In some areas of the body, a contrast agent is necessary to provide better visualization of organs being studied. Contrast material can be administered orally, rectally, intravenously, percutaneously, by inhalation, or through urinary catheterization. For angiography, contrast agent is injected into a blood vessel.

The most commonly used contrast media are barium sulphate for GI studies (Box 12-1), organic iodine for vascular and renal studies, and iodized oils for myelography. These substances are radiopaque (i.e., they block the passage of X-rays) and thus provide excellent contrast enhancement of body structures. Air can also be used as a contrast medium, although it is much less commonly used now than in the past.

In addition to radiation risks associated with all radiology procedures, contrast studies pose additional potential complications. For example, iodinated dyes may cause a severe allergic reaction and nephrotoxicity (Box 12-2). Barium sulphate may cause constipation and bowel impaction.

X-Ray Studies

12

BOX 12-1 | **Clinical Responsibilities Associated With Use of Barium Sulphate**

- Barium may interfere with subsequent X-ray studies (e.g., IVP, CT). Tests necessitating the use of barium should be performed after other X-ray studies.
- Cathartics are usually required before barium tests, to prevent the possibility of false-positive findings because of food in the bowel.
- Cathartics should always be administered after barium tests, to diminish the possibility of barium or fecal impaction.
- The patient should observe the colour of stool to ensure that all barium (white) has been eliminated from the intestinal tract.
- Barium should not be administered in patients with acute colitis, especially ulcerative colitis, because it can precipitate development of toxic megacolon.
- Barium should not be administered if GI perforation is suspected. Extravasation of barium from the GI tract may be associated with multiple and recurrent abdominal abscesses.

CT, Computed tomography; *GI,* gastrointestinal; *IVP,* intravenous pyelography.

BOX 12-2 | **Nephrotoxic Effects of Contrast Medium**

Definition: Impairment in renal function, manifested by increase in serum creatinine level by more than 25% or **>44 Mcmol/L** (>0.5 mg/dL) that occurs within 48 hours after the intravascular administration of a contrast medium; in the absence of an alternative cause, contrast medium is considered the trigger

Risk Factors
- Pre-existing renal impairment (e.g., renal failure)
- Elevated serum creatinine level, particularly secondary to diabetic nephropathy
- Dehydration
- Heart failure
- Age older than 70 years
- Concurrent administration of nephrotoxic drugs (e.g., NSAIDs)

Clinical Priorities
- Ensure that the patient is well hydrated. Depending on the clinical situation, administer at least 100 mL oral or intravenous normal saline per hour, starting 4 hours before administration of contrast medium and continuing to 24 hours afterwards. Increase the volume in warm weather.
- Use low-osmolar or iso-osmolar nonionic contrast media.
- Stop administration of nephrotoxic drugs for at least 24 hours.
- If possible, use alternative imaging techniques that do not necessitate use of an iodinated contrast media.
- Do not do any of the following:
  - Administer high-osmolar contrast media
  - Administer large doses of contrast media
  - Administer mannitol and diuretics, particularly loop diuretics
  - Perform multiple studies with contrast media within hours of each other

---

NSAIDs, Nonsteroidal anti-inflammatory drugs.

DIGITAL SUBTRACTION ANGIOGRAPHY

Digital subtraction angiography is a type of computerized fluoroscopy in which venous or arterial catheterization is performed to visualize the arteries, especially the carotid and cerebral arteries. Small differences in X-ray absorption between an artery and the surrounding tissues can, through this procedure, be converted to digital information and stored. This procedure is especially useful when bone blocks the visualization of the blood vessel being studied. Digital subtraction angiography is valuable for preoperative and postoperative evaluation of patients undergoing vascular and tumour surgery.

An image "mask" is made of the area of clinical interest and stored in a computer program. After intravenous injection of contrast material, subsequent images are made. The computer program then "subtracts" the preinjection mask image from the postinjection image. This removes the appearance of all tissue images (e.g., bone) that are not needed and leaves an arterial image of high contrast. Venous injection of the dye, rather than arterial injection, averts the complications and risks associated with conventional arteriography. However, arterial injection of contrast material is more often used.

RISKS OF RADIATION EXPOSURE

All X-ray procedures carry the risk of exposure to radiation. Exposure to ionizing radiation from a single test does not pose a substantial risk; however, a number of tests can result in cumulative exposure that could present a substantial risk to the patient. Both patients and health care providers can be at risk for radiation exposure. Health care providers who are exposed at work usually wear a dosimeter or radiation badge to monitor the accumulated exposure to radiation over a period of time, usually 3 months. ♣ The Canadian Nuclear Safety Commission has set a limit of 50 mSV per year and 100 mSV over 5 years for workers exposed to X-ray radiation. For pregnant workers, the limit is much lower: 4 mSv for the entire duration of the pregnancy. Radiation exposure limits vary across provinces, but maximums limits are set by the Canada Labour Code. Pregnant workers should have their dosimeter badge monitored every 2 weeks instead of the usual 3 months. Reducing exposure for health care providers can also be achieved by wearing a lead apron and by increasing their distance away from where the X-ray is being taken.

There are three possible types of damage to the body from radiologic procedures:
1. *Somatic effects* ultimately occur in patients exposed to the harmful agent. These may include short-term effects, such as blood cell problems, or long-term effects, such as cancer.
2. *Genetic effects* include damage to future generations as a result of exposure of parental germ cells to a harmful agent. Depending on the type of damage to the germ cell, genetic effects can range from mild to severe (e.g., mental retardation).
3. *Fetal effects* occur as a result of exposure to a harmful agent during the embryonal or fetal stage of development. This type of damage is highly dependent on timing of the exposure with regard to gestational age. Damage can range from mild birth defects to childhood malignancies. The fetus is at greatest risk during early pregnancy, when organs are developing. Radiation exposure during later pregnancy, after development is complete and only growth is occurring, is far less risky to the fetus.

Because of the risks of radiation exposure, X-ray studies should not be performed more often than necessary. For this reason, patients should be adequately prepared for each test in order to reduce the need for repeated studies. Patients should be shielded from unnecessary exposure with lead aprons and gloves. During or within 10 to 12 days after normal menses, women can safely undergo diagnostic X-ray studies. Otherwise, no women of childbearing age should undergo X-ray examination unless a pregnancy test is performed and the results are negative. These restrictions exist to avoid exposure and subsequent injury to a fetus when a woman is unknowingly pregnant.

CONTRAINDICATIONS

Pregnancy is a contraindication to X-ray studies. However, sometimes the benefits of diagnostic X-ray examination outweigh the risks. In pregnant patients, every attempt should be made to minimize exposure of the fetus to X-rays (e.g., with the use of a lead apron). The contraindications listed as follows are related to the predisposing risk factors for general acute adverse reactions to specific types of X-ray studies. Specific details relative to each type of X-ray procedure are discussed later in this chapter.

1. Iodinated dye (e.g., cardiac catheterization with intravenous pyelography)
   - Allergy to shellfish or with history of adverse reactions or allergic reactions to iodinated dye; skin testing for iodine allergy is often performed before procedure
   - History of asthma, allergies, and heart disease
   - Hematologic conditions such as sickle cell disease
   - Ages younger than 1 year and older than 65 years
   - Ingestion of certain medications, such as beta blockers, nonsteroidal anti-inflammatory drugs (NSAIDs), and interleukin-2
   - Renal disorders, because iodinated contrast is nephrotoxic
   - Dehydration, because affected patients are especially susceptible to dye-induced renal failure
   - Pheochromocytoma, because a hypertensive crisis may be precipitated by the use of iodine
2. Arterial or venous puncture (e.g., cardiac catheterization, angiography)
   - Bleeding disorder, because the arterial or venous puncture site may not stop bleeding
3. Barium (e.g., upper GI series, barium enema study)
   - Suspected perforation of the colon or upper GI tract; in this situation, meglumine diatrizoate (Gastrografin), a water-soluble contrast medium, should be used instead

POTENTIAL COMPLICATIONS

- Adverse reactions or allergic reactions to iodinated dye can include flushing, itching, urticaria, and even severe life-threatening anaphylaxis (evidenced by respiratory distress, decreased blood pressure, or shock; Table 12-1). In the unusual event of anaphylaxis, diphenhydramine (Benadryl), steroids, and epinephrine are included in resuscitative efforts. Oxygen and endotracheal equipment should be on hand for immediate use. Adverse reactions may also be delayed for up to 1 week after the procedure. Delayed reactions are usually skin reactions, including maculopapular rash, erythema, urticaria, and angioedema.
- Catheter-induced complications include embolic stroke (cerebral vascular accident, myocardial infarction).
- Complications associated with the catheter insertion include arterial thrombosis, embolism, or pseudoaneurysm.
- Infection can occur at the catheter insertion site.
- Contrast-induced nephrotoxicity or an acute decrease in the renal function, manifested by an increase in baseline serum creatinine level of at least **44 $Mcmol/L$** (0.5 mg/dL), occurs within 48 hours of injection of the contrast. Acute renal failure is especially a concern for patients older than 65 years who have chronic dehydration or pre-existing mild renal failure.
- Lactic acidosis, possibly leading to renal failure and death: This is an uncommon but serious problem for patients who do not discontinue metformin (Glucophage) after an injection of contrast material. Biguanides (metformin-containing medications) must be discontinued before or at the time of the contrast injection. They are withheld for 48 hours after the injection. Metformin is restarted once normal renal function is established.

TABLE 12-1	Signs and Symptoms of Adverse Reactions to Iodinated Contrast Media, and Treatment		
Characteristic	**Mild Reaction**	**Moderate Reaction**	**Severe or Life-Threatening Reaction**
Incidence	15%	1%–2%	0.2%
Signs and symptoms	Nausea, vomiting, mild urticaria, mild pallor, pain in injected extremity	Facial, tongue, or laryngeal edema; bronchospasm; chest pain; chills and fever; severe vomiting; extensive urticaria; dyspnea; rigors (extreme shivering)	Laryngeal and pulmonary edema, hypotension, myocardial depression, cardiac arrhythmias, seizure, ventilatory failure, circulatory collapse, unconsciousness
Treatment	Retain IV access Observe until patient is fully recovered Administer antinausea medications, antihistamines, oxygen if necessary	Oxygen by mask (6–10 L/min) Administer antihistamines, possibly steroids, IV fluids, observation, bronchodilators, adrenaline if broncospasm is progressive	Call resuscitation team Ensure patency of patient's airway Elevate patient's legs Administer oxygen by mask (6–10 L/min), antihistamines, steroids, IV fluids (normal saline or Ringer lactate), bronchodilators, antiseizure medications Perform intubation and ventilation as necessary

IV, Intravenous.

INTERFERING FACTORS

Factors that can obscure X-ray visualization include the following:
- Presence of metallic objects (e.g., hemostasis clips, jewellery)
- Barium retained from previous studies
- Large amounts of fecal material or gas in the bowel
- Improper positioning
- Excessive movement

PROCEDURE AND PATIENT CARE

Specific procedures are described; however, check agency policies for each test.

Before

✍ Explain the procedure to the patient. Cooperation is necessary, because the patient must lie still during the procedure. If the patient has mobility problems or cognitive challenges, positioning and instructions may need to be modified to ensure that the X-ray is of good quality.

- If the patient is taking metformin, discuss with the health care team the need to hold the metformin prior to and/or after the test.
- Obtain the patient's informed consent for the procedure if it is required by the institution.
- Assess the patient for allergy to iodinated dye. If an allergy to iodinated contrast is suspected, inform the radiologist. The radiologist can prescribe a preparation of diphenhydramine and steroid, to be administered before testing. Hypoallergenic nonionic contrast material is usually administered for the test.
- Assess the patient for any evidence of dehydration or renal disease. Usually, blood urea nitrogen and creatinine levels are measured before administration of iodine-containing intravenous contrast material. Hydration may be required before the administration of iodine.
- Assess the patient for diabetes and to determine if the patient has recently taken metformin.
- Instruct the patient to remove all jewellery from the area to be imaged.
- Inform the patient of any fasting requirements.
- Depending on the type of test, the patient may be given nothing orally for 2 to 8 hours before testing.
- Mark the site of the patient's peripheral pulses with a pen before arterial catheterization, to enable assessment of the peripheral pulses after the procedure.
- Ensure that the appropriate coagulation studies have been performed and that the results are normal.
- For cerebral angiography, perform a baseline neurologic assessment for comparison with subsequent assessments.
- Administer sedatives if they are indicated.
- Assist the patient with bowel preparation if it is indicated. For example, a barium contrast study necessitates bowel preparation and, possibly, cleansing enemas.

During

- Instruct the patient to remain motionless throughout the testing. The patient may be asked to hold the breath while an image is being taken.

After

- If an iodine contrast dye has been used, instruct the patient to drink fluids to promote dye excretion.
- If the physician has ordered the metformin to be held, explain the reason to the patient and reinforce the need for glucose monitoring.
- If barium contrast was used, laxatives may be indicated to prevent constipation and bowel obstruction.
- Monitor the patient's vital signs. Changes may be noted because of medications used during the tests or from complications such as bleeding.
- Evaluate the patient for delayed reaction to dyes (e.g., dyspnea, rash, tachycardia, urticaria). Reactions may occur within 2 to 6 hours after the test. Treat with antihistamines or steroids.

REPORTING OF RESULTS

Radiographs are carefully reviewed and the findings reported by the radiologist. Results may be discussed with the patient at the time of testing or within a few days.

Adrenal Venography

NORMAL FINDINGS
Normal adrenal veins and normal results of an adrenal vein hormone assay

INDICATIONS
With adrenal venography, adrenal disease can be localized in preparation of proposed surgical extirpation.

TEST EXPLANATION
Adrenal venography is performed to obtain blood samples from the adrenal veins and to detect adrenal disease. Once the veins are identified, a catheter can be placed in them and blood selectively obtained from each adrenal vein.

In patients with Cushing's syndrome, the blood is analyzed for plasma cortisol. If the plasma cortisol level in the blood obtained from one side is much higher than that in the other, a unilateral adrenal tumour is causing the Cushing's syndrome. If plasma cortisol levels are bilaterally elevated, it can be concluded that the Cushing's syndrome is caused by bilateral adrenal hyperplasia.

In patients with a pheochromocytoma, adrenal venous blood is analyzed for catecholamines. If the catecholamine level on one side is much higher than that on the other, a unilateral pheochromocytoma exists on the side with the elevated levels. If the blood catecholamine levels on both sides are equally elevated, bilateral adrenal pheochromocytoma is probably present. If the adrenal venous blood levels are not elevated on either side in a patient with elevated peripheral blood catecholamine levels, the pheochromocytoma exists outside the adrenal gland (i.e., extra-adrenal pheochromocytoma).

The venous blood also can be evaluated for aldosterone, androgens, and other substances. This procedure is usually performed in approximately 1 hour by an angiographer (radiologist). The only discomfort is the groin puncture necessary for venous access.

CONTRAINDICATIONS
- Predisposing risk factors for acute adverse reactions to contrast media
- Allergy to shellfish
- Bleeding disorders, because bleeding at the venous puncture site (usually in the groin) may be difficult to stop

POTENTIAL COMPLICATIONS
- See potential complications associated with iodinated dye on p. 1021.
- Adrenal hemorrhage or necrosis caused by the pressure of dye injection, which may cause Addison's disease (adrenal insufficiency)
- Cellulitis
- Thrombophlebitis
- Bacteremia

X-Ray Studies

12

PROCEDURE AND PATIENT CARE

Before

 Explain the procedure to the patient.

- Obtain the patient's written informed consent for the procedure.
- See assessment for allergy to iodinated dye on p. 1021.
- Administer a beta-adrenergic blocker and phenoxybenzamine, an alpha-adrenergic blocker, in patients with suspected pheochromocytoma, to prevent a potentially fatal catecholamine-induced hypertensive episode.

During

- Place the patient in the supine position on the X-ray table.
- Note the following procedural steps:
  1. The patient's groin is prepared and draped in a sterile manner.
  2. After the venipuncture site is locally anaesthetized, the femoral vein is catheterized.
  3. The catheter is passed into the adrenal vein.
  4. Dye is injected to visualize the adrenal veins and to ensure that the catheter is in the adrenal vein.
  5. Blood is obtained and sent to the chemistry laboratory for assays.

After

- Evaluate the patient's vital signs frequently for signs of bleeding or hemorrhage.
- Assess the patient with a suspected pheochromocytoma for signs and symptoms of a hypertensive episode. If such an episode occurs, notify the physician immediately to obtain an order for appropriate alpha- and beta-adrenergic blocking agents.
- Assess the groin site for redness, pain, swelling, and bleeding during each vital sign check.
- Apply cold compresses to the puncture site if needed to reduce discomfort or swelling.

Home Care Responsibilities

- Monitor the puncture site for signs of bleeding (e.g., increased pulse, decreased blood pressure).
- Carefully monitor the blood pressure for a hypertensive episode.
- Assess the groin for redness, swelling, pain, or bleeding.

TEST RESULTS AND CLINICAL SIGNIFICANCE

Unilateral adrenal tumour: *Disease is limited to one side, which indicates a tumour.*

Bilateral adrenal hyperplasia: *Disease exists on both sides.*

Unilateral pheochromocytoma,

Bilateral pheochromocytoma,

Extra-adrenal pheochromocytoma: *If the catecholamine level is elevated on one side and not on the other, unilateral pheochromocytoma is present. If the level is elevated on both sides, bilateral pheochromocytomas are present. If catecholamine levels are not elevated on either side and yet catecholamine levels are elevated in the peripheral blood, the site of the pheochromocytoma is outside the adrenal glands. This is important preoperative information for the endocrine surgeon.*

RELATED TESTS

Vanillylmandelic Acid and Catecholamines (p. 1009). This test is used to identify pheochromocytoma in patients with aggressive hypertension.

Metanephrine, Plasma Free (p. 372). This is a measurement of plasma-free metanephrine. This test is more accurate than that for urinary catecholamines.

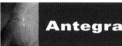

Antegrade Pyelography

NORMAL FINDINGS

Normal outline, size, and position of the renal pelvic collections system, ureters, and bladder

INDICATIONS

This procedure provides visualization of the renal pelvis for accurate placement of nephrostomy tubes.

TEST EXPLANATION

This study is used to identify the upper collecting system in an obstructed kidney to be used as a map for accurate percutaneous placement of a nephrostomy tube. This study is performed on patients who have an obstruction of the ureter and hydronephrosis. With this procedure, the renal pelvis is identified with computed tomographic imaging or ultrasonography. A needle is placed into the pelvis. Radiopaque dye is then injected, and the entire upper renal collecting system is demonstrated by obtaining X-rays in rapid succession. Proper positioning for the nephrostomy is then decided on the basis of these images.

POTENTIAL COMPLICATIONS

- Hemorrhage at the needle puncture site, because the kidney is highly vascular
- Allergic reaction to iodinated dye, which rarely occurs because the dye is not administered intravenously

PROCEDURE AND PATIENT CARE

Before

- Explain the procedure to the patient. Allow time for the patient to verbalize concerns, and allay the patient's fears.
- Obtain the patient's informed consent for the procedure.
- Assess for adverse reaction to contrast media, and inform the physician of findings.
- Check for allergy to shellfish, and inform the physician of findings.
- Check coagulation studies because of the vascularity of the kidney.

During

- The patient is placed in the prone position.
- The renal pelvis is localized by means of ultrasonography or X-ray.
- After administration of a local anaesthetic, a thin-walled needle is advanced into the lumen of the renal pelvis.
- Contrast material is injected, and X-rays in posteroanterior, oblique, and anteroposterior views are obtained.
- The nephrostomy tube is placed over guide wires, and its position is confirmed with another X-ray.

After

- The nephrostomy tube is dressed and secured by sterile technique and attached to a collection bag.
- Because the kidney is highly vascular, check vital signs as ordered to detect any evidence of bleeding.
- Note that antibiotic drugs are often recommended to avoid infection, which may be caused by instrumentation at a level above the ureteral obstruction.
- Evaluate the patient for signs of allergic reaction to dye (e.g., dyspnea, rash, tachycardia, urticaria). Reactions usually occur within 2 to 6 hours after the test. Treat with antihistamines or steroids.

TEST RESULTS AND CLINICAL SIGNIFICANCE

Ureteral stone,

Ureteral obstruction from tumour or adhesions,

Ureteropelvic or ureterovesical obstruction from a stone, tumour, or scarring,

Congenital or acquired hydronephrosis: *These conditions are evident from complete obstruction of contrast medium in the ureter, which may necessitate temporary or permanent nephrostomy placement.*

RELATED TESTS

Retrograde Pyelography (p. 1102). To visualize the ureters, they are filled with contrast medium from below (during cystoscopy, p. 626).

   Intravenous Pyelography (p. 1080). To visualize the ureters, contrast medium is injected intravenously and becomes concentrated in the kidney. This test also allows visualization of the kidneys.

Arteriography (Angiography; Renal, Mesenteric, Adrenal, Cerebral, and Lower Extremity Arteriography)

NORMAL FINDINGS

Normal arterial vasculature

INDICATIONS

Arteriography is used to evaluate arterial occlusive disease of the adrenal glands, kidneys, mesentery, brain, and lower extremity and is helpful in evaluation of suspected neoplasms arising from these structures. Arteriography provides the vascular surgeon with an accurate picture of the vascular anatomy of these structures. This is especially important in arterio-occlusive disease involving the arteries to these structures.

TEST EXPLANATION

With the injection of radiopaque contrast material into arteries, blood vessels can be visualized to determine arterial anatomy, vascular disease, or neoplasms. With a catheter usually placed through the femoral or brachial artery and into the desired artery, radiopaque contrast material is rapidly injected while X-rays are obtained. Blood-flow dynamics, abnormal blood vessels, vascular anomalies, normal and abnormal vascular anatomy, and tumour can be seen. An iodinated contrast agent is usually used to visualize the arteries. Carbon dioxide gas as a contrast material is an alternative to iodinated contrast material. When injected into a blood vessel, carbon dioxide bubbles displace blood, enabling vascular imaging. Because of the lack of nephrotoxicity, adverse reactions, and allergic reactions, carbon dioxide may be an attractive alternative for diagnostic angiography and vascular interventions in both the arterial and venous circulation.

Digital subtraction angiography allows bone structures to be obliterated from the X-ray picture. This technique is a sophisticated type of computerized process that, when used with angiography, enables better visualization of the arteries, especially the carotid and cerebral arteries, by eliminating bone structures from the image. It is especially useful when adjacent bone inhibits visualization of the blood vessel to be evaluated. For digital subtraction angiography, an image (mask) is made of the area of clinical interest and stored in the computer program. After intraarterial injection of contrast material, subsequent images are made. The computer program then "subtracts" the preinjection mask image from the postinjection image. In this way, all the undesired features (e.g., bone) are removed, and the arterial image is one of high contrast and quality.

While nearly all major blood vessels can be visualized through the technique of arteriography, the kidneys, adrenal glands, brain, and abdominal aorta (with lower extremities) are most commonly visualized. Coronary arteriography is described in the section on cardiac catheterization (p. 1047).

Renal angiography enables evaluation of blood flow dynamics, demonstration of abnormal blood vessels, and differentiation of a vascular renal cyst from hypervascular renal cancers (Figure 12-1). Arteriosclerotic narrowing (stenosis) of the renal artery is best demonstrated with this study. The angiographic location of the stenotic area is helpful information for the vascular surgeon considering repair. Complete transection of the renal artery by blunt or penetrating trauma can also be seen on the renal angiogram as total vascular obstruction. Highly vascular renal cancers can produce a "blush" of contrast material on angiography.

The adrenal gland and its arterial system can also be visualized by *adrenal arteriography*. Both benign and malignant tumour of the adrenal gland, as well as bilateral adrenal hyperplasia, can be detected easily with this technique.

Cerebral angiography provides X-ray visualization of the cerebral vascular system with the injection of radiopaque dye into the carotid or vertebral arteries (Figure 12-2). With this procedure,

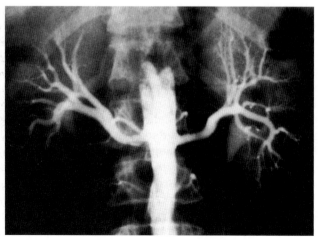

Figure 12-1 Renal arteriogram.

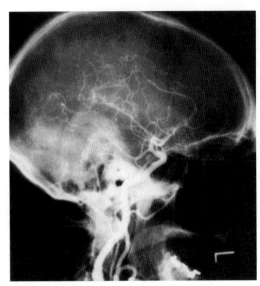

Figure 12-2 Carotid angiogram.

abnormalities of the cerebral circulation (e.g., aneurysms, occlusions, stenosis, arteriovenous malformations) can be identified. A vascular tumour is seen as a mass containing small, abnormal blood vessels. A nonvascular tumour, abscess, or hematoma appears as a mass that distorts the normal vascular contour.

Lower-extremity arteriography enables accurate identification and location of occlusions within the abdominal aorta and the arteries of the lower extremities. After the catheter is placed in the aorta or, more selectively, into the femoral artery, radiopaque dye is injected. Radiographs are obtained in timed sequence to allow X-ray visualization of the arterial system of the lower extremities. The flow of dye appears totally or almost totally blocked in arteriosclerotic vascular occlusive disease. Emboli appear as total occlusions of the artery. Arterial traumas such as lacerations or intimal tears (laceration of the arterial inner lining) likewise appear as total or near-total obstruction of the flow of dye. Aneurysmal dilation of the aorta or its branches also can be seen. Unusual arterial disorders (e.g., thromboangiitis obliterans [Buerger's disease], fibromuscular dysplasia) demonstrate classic arterial "beading," which is pathognomonic.

Lower extremity arteriography is usually performed electively in patients with symptoms and signs of peripheral vascular disease. Emergency arteriography, however, is needed when the blood flow to an extremity has ceased suddenly. Immediate surgical therapy is needed and is most effective when the surgeon knows the cause and location of the sudden occlusion. This knowledge can be obtained only with arteriography.

Arterial vascular balloon dilation and stent placement can be performed if a short-segment arterial stenosis is identified. In these instances, the wire is placed through the angiocatheter into the area of narrowing. A balloon catheter is inserted over the wire. The dilating balloon is inflated, the arteriosclerotic plaque is gently and persistently dilated, and a stent can then be placed.

With angiography, there is always a concern that the arterial puncture site may not seal, which would lead to a pseudoaneurysm. Vascular closure products have been used to seal femoral artery punctures quickly after catheterization procedures. This allows for the patient's early ambulation and hospital discharge. The injection of these materials on the vascular entrance site creates a mechanical seal by sandwiching the arteriotomy between a bioabsorbable anchor and a collagen sponge, which dissolve within 60 to 90 days.

This procedure is usually performed in approximately 1 to 2 hours by a radiologist. During the dye injection, remind the patient that an intense, burning flush may be felt throughout the body, but it lasts only a few seconds. The only discomforts are in the area of the groin puncture necessary for arterial access and from lying on a hard X-ray table for a long time.

Age-Related Concerns

- Adults older than 75 years who have chronic dehydration or mildly decreased renal function are at high risk for contrast material–induced nephrotoxicity.
- The postprocedure urinary output in older patients needs to be carefully monitored.

CONTRAINDICATIONS

- Allergy to shellfish
- History of adverse reactions or allergic reactions to iodinated dye
- Inability of patients to cooperate, or tendency to become agitated
- Pregnancy, unless the benefits of the procedure outweigh the risks of radiation exposure to the fetus
- Renal disorders, because iodinated contrast medium is nephrotoxic
- Propensity for bleeding, because the arterial puncture site may not stop bleeding
- Unstable cardiac disorders
- Dehydration, because affected patients are especially susceptible to dye-induced renal failure

POTENTIAL COMPLICATIONS

- Potential complications are associated with iodinated dye (see Table 12-1, p. 1021).
- Hemorrhage can occur at the arterial puncture site used for arterial access.
- Arterial embolism or stroke can result from dislodgement of arteriosclerotic plaque.
- Soft tissue infection can develop around the puncture site.
- Renal failure can occur, especially in older patients with chronic dehydration or mild renal failure (see Box 12-2, p. 1018).
- Dissection of the intimal lining of the artery can occur, which causes complete or partial arterial occlusion.
- Pseudoaneurysm can develop as a result of failure of the puncture site to seal.
- Hypertensive crisis: With adrenal angiography, fatal hypertensive crisis may occur in patients with pheochromocytoma. Propranolol (Inderal), a beta-adrenergic blocker, and phenoxybenzamine (Dibenzyline), an alpha-adrenergic blocker, are given for several days before the study to avert precipitation of a malignant hypertensive episode.
- In adrenal angiography, hemorrhage of the adrenal gland may lead to adrenal insufficiency.

Clinical Priorities

- Assess the patient for allergies and predisposing risk factors for general acute adverse reactions to contrast media (see Table 12-1, p. 1021).
- Perform a baseline assessment of the patient's peripheral pulses before arterial catheterization.
- Ensure that results of coagulation studies (prothrombin time, partial thromboplastin time, bleeding time) are normal before the test, because of the risk of bleeding.
- After the test, the patient is kept on bed rest for approximately 8 hours to allow complete sealing of the arterial puncture.

X-Ray Studies

12

PROCEDURE AND PATIENT CARE

Before

- ✗ Explain the procedure to the patient. Allow the patient to verbalize concerns, and allay any fears.
- Obtain the patient's written informed consent for this procedure.
- ✗ Inform the patient that a warm flush may be felt when the dye is injected.
- See assessment for allergy to iodinated dye on p. 1021.
- Determine whether the patient has been taking anticoagulants.
- The patient is kept on NPO status (nothing by mouth) for 2 to 8 hours before testing.
- Mark the site of the patient's peripheral pulses with a pen before arterial catheterization, to enable assessment of the peripheral pulses after the procedure.
- If the patient has signs of arterial occlusion, such as no peripheral pulses before the arteriography, document that fact so that it will not be suspected that arterial occlusion has resulted from the procedure at the postangiographic assessment.
- Administer preprocedural medications as ordered.
- If a pheochromocytoma is suspected, administer medications as ordered, to prevent a potentially fatal hypertensive episode.
- Ensure that the appropriate coagulation studies have been performed and that the results are normal.
- For cerebral angiography, perform a baseline neurologic assessment for comparison with subsequent assessment, potentially to diagnose stroke that may be precipitated by the study.
- ✗ Instruct the patient to remove all valuables and dental prostheses.
- ✗ Instruct the patient to void before the study, because iodinated dye can act as an osmotic diuretic.
- ✗ Inform the patient that bladder distension may cause some discomfort during the study.

During

- Note the following procedural steps:
  1. The patient may be sedated before being taken to the angiography room, which is usually within the radiology department.
  2. The patient is placed in the supine position on the X-ray table (Figure 12-3).
  3. If the femoral artery is to be used, the groin is shaved, prepared, and draped in a sterile manner.
  4. The femoral artery is cannulated, and a wire is threaded up through the artery and into or near the opening of the artery to be examined (Figure 12-4).
  5. A catheter is placed over that wire. Both the wire and catheter are visualized fluoroscopically. Because the catheter and wire have curled tips, both can be manipulated directly into the artery to be studied. The wire is removed.
  6. Iodinated contrast material is injected through the catheter with an automated injector at a preset, controlled rate, over several seconds.
  7. Serial X-rays are obtained in timed sequence to show the arterial injection, and subsequent X-rays are taken to show the venous phase of the injection.
- During adrenal angiography, monitor blood pressure for evidence of malignant hypertensive storm.

After

- X-ray studies are completed, the catheter is removed, and a pressure dressing is applied to the puncture site.
- Monitor the patient's vital signs for indications of hemorrhage every 15 minutes for the first hour and then hourly until signs are stable or as per agency protocol and policies.

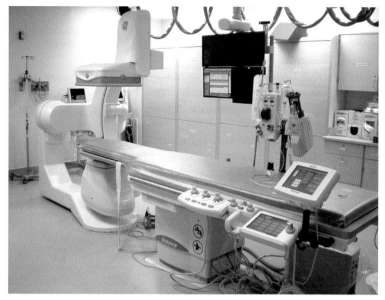

Figure 12-3 Angiography room.

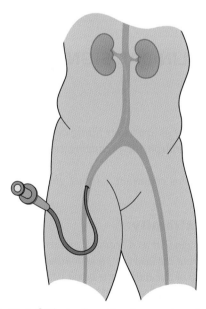

Figure 12-4 Catheter insertion for renal angiography.

- Assess the peripheral arterial pulse in the extremity used for vascular access, and compare that pulse with the preprocedural baseline values.
- If cerebral arteriography was performed, perform a neurologic assessment for any signs of catheter-induced embolic stroke syndrome.
- Observe the arterial puncture site frequently for signs of bleeding or hematoma.

- Maintain pressure at the puncture site with a 1- to 2-pound (454- to 907-g) sand bag or intravenous bag.
- Keep the patient on bed rest for approximately 8 hours after the procedure to allow complete sealing of the arterial puncture site.
- Assess the patient's extremities for signs of loss of blood supply (e.g., loss of pulses, numbness, pallor, tingling, pain, loss of sensory or motor function).
- Note and compare the colour and temperature of the involved extremity with that of the uninvolved extremity.
- Administer mild analgesics for discomfort at the arterial puncture site.
- If the patient has severe, continuous pain, notify the physician.
- Encourage the patient to drink fluids to promote dye excretion and to prevent dehydration caused by the diuretic action of the dye.
- Evaluate the patient for delayed allergic reaction to the dye (e.g., dyspnea, rash, tachycardia, urticaria). Reactions usually occur within 2 to 6 hours after the test. Treat with antihistamines or steroids.

Home Care Responsibilities

- Monitor the arterial puncture site for bleeding and hematoma.
- Monitor the vital signs for evidence of bleeding (increased pulse and decreased blood pressure).
- Instruct the patient to report any signs of numbness, tingling, pain, or loss of function in the involved extremity.
- Encourage the patient to drink fluids to prevent dehydration and to promote dye excretion.

TEST RESULTS AND CLINICAL SIGNIFICANCE

Adrenal Angiography

Pheochromocytoma,
Adrenal adenoma,
Adrenal carcinoma: *These are evident as avascular filling defects within the gland. Pheochromocytomas are epinephrine-producing or norepinephrine-producing tumours that can precipitate a hypertensive crisis during angiography.*
Bilateral adrenal hyperplasia: *In this condition, adrenal glands are usually larger and more vascular than normal.*

Arteriography of Lower Extremity

Arteriosclerotic occlusion: *This is evident as a segment of narrowing in an otherwise normal vessel.*
Embolus occlusion: *An embolus from the heart or an abdominal aortic aneurysm may obstruct an artery. Complete interruption in the flow of dye within the blood vessel is seen on arteriograms.*
Primary arterial diseases (e.g., fibromuscular dysplasia, Buerger's disease): *Arteriograms often demonstrate findings that are classic for the particular disease.*
Aneurysm: *This is a saccular dilation of a blood vessel. It can rupture or expel emboli.*
Aberrant arterial anatomy: *Variations in arterial anatomy are well known and usually well delineated by arteriography.*
Tumour neovascularity: *With vascular tumours, classical findings often include arteriovenous shunting, which causes blood to pool in these areas.*
Neoplastic arterial compression: *Nonvascular tumours compress or distort the normal vasculature.*

Brain Arteriography

Vascular aneurysm,

Vascular occlusion or stenosis,

Vascular arteriovenous malformations,

Cerebral vascular thrombosis: *Arteriographic findings are similar to those described for the lower extremities.*

Tumour,

Abscess,

Hematoma: *These abnormalities distort the normal arterial anatomy.*

Kidney Arteriography

Anatomic aberrant blood vessels: *Anatomic abnormalities involving the kidneys are common.*

Renal cyst: *This is an avascular mass in a kidney.*

Renal solid tumour: *Most renal cell carcinomas are very vascular.*

Atherosclerotic narrowing of the renal arteries: *Stenosis or total occlusion of the renal arteries causes decreases in blood flow to the kidneys. Vasopressin is stimulated through the renin-angiotensin system (p. 83). Hypertension results.*

 Barium Enema (BE, Lower GI Series)

NORMAL FINDINGS

Normal filling, contour, and patency of the colon

Normal filling of the appendix and terminal ileum

INDICATIONS

Barium contrast study of the lower gastrointestinal tract enables visualization of the colon, distal small bowel, and occasionally the appendix. It is indicated in patients with the following conditions:

- Abdominal pain (but contraindicated in patients with acute abdominal pain)
- Obvious or occult blood in the stools
- Inflammatory bowel disease
- Suspected cancer (bowel or abdominal)
- Abnormal results of an obstruction series of X-rays (see p. 1095) that indicate volvulus or colon obstruction

TEST EXPLANATION

The barium enema (BE) study consists of a series of X-rays in which the colon is visualized. It is used to demonstrate the presence and location of suspected neoplasms, polyps, tumour, diverticular disease, and inflammatory bowel disease. Anatomic abnormalities (e.g., malrotation) also can be detected. Therapeutically, the BE study may be used to reduce nonstrangulated ileocolic intussusception in children. Bleeding from diverticula can cease after a BE study.

The BE study is occasionally used to assess filling of the appendix. When clinical findings suggest possible appendicitis, failure of the appendix to fill with barium may support the diagnosis. Although the colon is the main organ evaluated with a BE study, reflux of barium into the terminal ileum also

X-Ray Studies

12

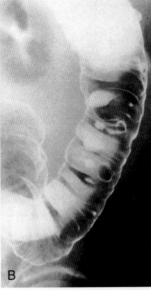
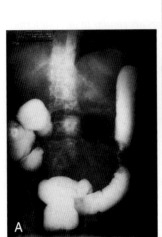

Figure 12-5 Barium enema studies. **A,** Single-contrast view illustrates obstructing circumferential carcinoma of the sigmoid colon. **B,** Double-contrast view shows multiple colonic diverticula. Diverticula on dependent surfaces are filled with barium; diverticula on nondependent surfaces appear as ring shadows.

allows adequate visualization of the distal portion of the small intestine. Diseases that affect the terminal ileum, especially Crohn's disease (regional enteritis), can be identified. Inflammatory bowel disease and fistulas involving the colon can be demonstrated with the BE study.

In many patients undergoing BE studies, air is insufflated into the colon after instillation of barium. This provides visual contrast between air and the barium. With air contrast, the colonic mucosa can be much more accurately visualized. This procedure is called an *air contrast–BE* or *double-contrast BE study,* and it is used especially when small polyps are suspected. The accuracy of the BE study to detect small colonic tumour is approximately 60%, whereas the accuracy of the air contrast–BE study to detect small colonic tumour exceeds 85% (Figure 12-5).

This test is usually performed in approximately 45 minutes in the radiology department by a radiologist. Abdominal bloating and rectal pressure occur during instillation of barium.

CONTRAINDICATIONS

- Suspected perforation of the colon: In this situation, diatrizoate (Gastrografin), a water-soluble contrast medium, is administered. No bowel preparation is performed.
- Inability of patients to cooperate: This test requires the patient to hold the barium in the rectum and colon, which is especially difficult for older adult patients.
- Megacolon: Barium may worsen this condition.

POTENTIAL COMPLICATIONS

- Colonic perforation, especially when the colon is weakened by inflammation, tumour, or infection
- Bowel impaction

INTERFERING FACTORS

- Barium in the abdomen from previous barium contrast tests may interfere with visualization of portions of the colon.
- Significant residual stool in the colon precludes adequate visualization of the entire bowel wall. Stool may be confused with polyps.
- Spasm of the colon can mimic the X-ray signs of a cancer. The use of intravenous glucagon minimizes spasm.

 Age-Related Concerns

- Typical preparation in a child may include the following:
  Age ≤2 years:
    Clear liquid diet for 24 hours before the test
    NPO status (nothing by mouth) for 4 hours before testing
    Pediatric Fleet enema the night before testing, repeated 3 hours before testing
  Age >2 years:
    Low-residue diet for 2 days before testing
    Clear liquid diet (excluding milk) for 24 hours before testing
    NPO status for 3 hours before testing
    Castor oil the day before testing:
      Age 2–4 years: 1 oz (30 mL)
      Age 5–9 years: 1.5 oz (44 mL)
      Age 10–16 years: 2 oz (59 mL)
  Saline solution enemas the night before testing only if good results were not obtained with castor oil
  Pediatric Fleet enemas until bowel movements are clear, 3 hours before testing
- Be aware of dehydration and electrolyte abnormalities. Instruct the parent to hydrate the child well with electrolyte-containing fluids after the BE study.
- The colon in the young child cannot tolerate the volume and pressure of instillation of barium that the adult colon can. Both should be reduced.
- A child cannot retain the barium long enough for complete filling of the colon. Thus, a rectal tube with a balloon on the end is used. The small balloon is inflated minimally, and the buttocks are taped tightly to prevent premature defecation of the barium.

 Age-Related Concerns: Older Adults

- Bowel preparation may be difficult for adults older than 75 years. Many older patients live alone and cannot administer an enema. Their social support system should be evaluated before the day of the BE study.
- Older adults become dehydrated easily. Hypovolemia and orthostasis can lead to falling. Furthermore, electrolyte abnormalities may develop, which can alter cardiac rhythm. Bowel preparation may have to be decreased or prolonged over several days to avert these complications. Hydration with electrolyte-containing fluids is vital.
- Older adults have reduced muscle tone and often cannot retain barium long enough for adequate visualization of the colon. A rectal tube with a balloon at the end is inserted into the rectum, and the balloon is inflated to diminish premature defecation of barium.
- Elimination of residual barium is especially important in chronically constipated older adult patients. Instruct older patients to use a mild cathartic after testing and to continue the cathartic daily until the stool is no longer white.

X-Ray Studies

12

PROCEDURE AND PATIENT CARE

Before

✗ Explain the procedure to the patient. Encourage the patient to verbalize questions and fears.

✗ Assist the patient with bowel preparation, which varies among institutions. In older patients, this preparation can be exhaustive and can cause severe dehydration. Bowel preparation usually includes diet restriction, hydration, orally ingested cathartic, and cleansing enemas.

• In most adults, typical preparation the day before examination includes the following:
  1. Give the patient clear liquids (no dairy products) for lunch and supper.
  2. Have the patient drink one glass of water or clear fluid every hour for 8 to 10 hours.
  3. 2:00 PM: Administer 240 mL of magnesium citrate or X-Prep (extract of senna fruit).
  4. 7:00 PM: Administer three 5-mg bisacodyl (Dulcolax) tablets.
  5. Keep the patient on NPO status after midnight.

• In most adults, typical preparation the day of examination includes the following:
  1. Keep the patient on NPO status.
  2. 6:00 AM: Administer a bisacodyl suppository or a cleansing enema, or both.

• Determine whether the bowel is adequately cleansed. When the fecal return is clear, preparation is adequate. If fecal return contains large, solid fecal waste or is not entirely clear, this indicates that fecal material is still being evacuated, and preparation is inadequate. Notify the radiologist, who may want to extend the bowel preparation.

• In patients with suspected bowel obstruction, no oral cathartic should be administered. If catharsis is ineffective and enemas are not evacuated, colon obstruction may be present, and the physician should be notified immediately.

✗ Suggest that the patient take reading material to the X-ray department to occupy the time while expelling the barium.

During

• Note the following procedural steps:
  1. A two- or three-way Foley-type catheter (catheter with a balloon) is inserted gently but deeply into the colon.
  2. The balloon may be slowly inflated under direct fluoroscopic control while the patient is asked to report any discomfort.
  3. The patient is asked to roll to the lateral, supine, and prone positions.
  4. Barium is dripped into the rectum through the Foley-type catheter with the help of gravity.
  5. Barium flow is monitored fluoroscopically.
  6. The colon is thoroughly examined as the barium progresses through the large colon and into the terminal ileum.
  7. The barium is drained out.
  8. If an air contrast–BE study has been ordered, air is insufflated into the large bowel.
  9. The patient is asked to expel the barium, and a postevacuation X-ray is obtained.
  10. The standard procedure for administering barium through a colostomy is to instill the contrast medium through an irrigation cone placed in the stoma. When the X-ray series is completed, the barium is allowed to be expelled from the stoma. A gentle stream of clean water for irrigation is helpful in expelling residual barium. Box 12-3 outlines special care of the patient with a colostomy.

BOX 12-3   **Special Care for the Patient With a Colostomy Undergoing a Barium Enema**

- Bowel preparation is the same, except enemas are not administered.
- The patient may be asked to irrigate the colostomy with saline solution approximately 4 hours before the test.
- If a loop colostomy is present (usually in the right upper quadrant of the abdomen), ask the physician which area of the colon is to be studied. If only the distal colon is to be evaluated, oral cathartics will not contribute to the cleansing process. Irrigation and enemas alone are used. If the proximal colon is to be studied, cathartics and proximal irrigation are used.
- Because barium cannot be retained, a balloon catheter is used.
- Elimination of barium is important. Cathartics and irrigation should be administered until the stool is no longer white.

After

- Ensure that the patient excretes as much barium as possible.
- The images should be checked by the radiologist before the patient is allowed to leave the department, because poorly exposed or blurry images should be retaken if necessary while the patient is still in the radiology department.
- Suggest the use of soothing ointments on the anal area to minimize anorectal pain that may result from the aggressive test preparation.
- Encourage ingestion of fluids containing electrolytes to avoid dehydration or electrolyte abnormalities caused by the cathartic agents.
- Encourage the patient to rest after the procedure. The cleansing regimen and BE procedure may be exhausting.

 Home Care Responsibilities

- Inform the patient that initially stools will be white. Mild cathartics should be given until the stool is no longer white. When all of the barium has been expelled, the stool will return to normal colour.
- Note that laxatives may be ordered to facilitate evacuation of the barium.

TEST RESULTS AND CLINICAL SIGNIFICANCE

Malignant tumour: *This is evident as a filling defect in the barium column with the appearance of an apple core.*

Polyps: *These are evident as round filling defects in the barium column. Stool can create the same appearance. Persistence in location throughout the study suggests polyps.*

Diverticula: *These are evident as outpouchings of the colon.* Diverticulosis *refers only to the presence of diverticula.* Diverticulitis *is an infectious inflammation surrounding the diverticula and is evident as narrowing of the barium column.*

Inflammatory bowel disease (e.g., ulcerative colitis, Crohn's disease): *This is evident as narrowing of the barium column as a result of inflammation surrounding the colon. A cobblestone-like pattern is typical of ulcerative colitis. Areas devoid of barium are typical of Crohn's disease. The rectum is usually involved in Crohn's disease and spared in ulcerative colitis. Fistulas may be evident in Crohn's disease.*

Colonic stenosis secondary to ischemia, infection, or previous surgery: *This is evident as narrowing of the barium column that does not resemble an apple core.*

Perforated colon: *Leakage of contrast material is seen with perforation. The most common cause of perforation is cancer or diverticulitis. If perforation is suspected, a water-soluble iodine-containing contrast agent should be used because it can be absorbed by the body. Barium cannot be absorbed and can cause persistence of infection.*

Colonic fistula: *This is evident from leakage of contrast agent from the colon to another organ (e.g., urinary bladder) or area of the bowel.*

Appendicitis: *Although a diagnosis of appendicitis cannot be made with certainty, it can be supported by lack of barium filling during a BE study. Of normal appendixes, however, 30% to 60% do not demonstrate filling.*

Extrinsic compression of the colon from extracolonic tumour (e.g., ovarian) or abscess: *This is evident as a convex, rounded distortion of the barium column.*

Malrotation of the gut: *In this congenital abnormality, the cecum—normally in the right lower quadrant of the abdomen—is in the left upper quadrant.*

Colon volvulus: *The cecum or sigmoid portion of the colon can turn on its mesentery and cut off flow of barium to that area of bowel. Sometimes, instillation of barium is therapeutic and can reduce the volvulus.*

Intussusception: *When the proximal portion of the bowel is invaginated into the distal portion (intussusception), the flow of barium stops at the tip of the intussusceptum. Sometimes, instillation of barium is therapeutic and can reduce the intussusception. In children, intussusception is usually caused by enlarged lymph nodes in the ileal colic area. In adults, a polypoid tumour usually is the leading cause of intussusception.*

Hernia: *Large groin hernias (usually sliding hernias) or ventral hernias can contain the colon, which is seen outside the abdomen in the hernia sac.*

RELATED TESTS

Colonoscopy (p. 619). This test provides direct visualization of the colon mucosa. It is more accurate than the BE study and enables endoscopic surgery (e.g., biopsy, polypectomy).

Small Bowel Follow-Through (p. 1109). This procedure provides visualization of the small intestine.

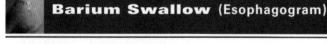

Barium Swallow (Esophagogram)

NORMAL FINDINGS

Normal size, contour, filling, patency, and position of the esophagus

INDICATIONS

The barium swallow study provides visualization of the lumen of the esophagus. It is indicated in patients with the following symptoms:

- Dysphagia
- Noncardiac chest pain
- Painful swallowing
- Swallowing abnormalities (see Swallowing Examination, p. 1113)
- Gastroesophageal reflux

TEST EXPLANATION

This barium contrast study is a more thorough examination of the esophagus than that provided by most upper gastrointestinal imaging series (p. 1117). As in most barium contrast studies, defects in normal filling and narrowing of the barium column indicate tumour, strictures, or extrinsic compression from extraesophageal masses or an abnormally enlarged heart and great vessels. Varices also appear as serpiginous linear-filling defects. Anatomic abnormalities such as hiatal hernia, Schatzki rings, and diverticula (Zenker or epiphrenic) can be seen as well.

In patients with esophageal reflux, the radiologist may identify reflux of the barium from the stomach into the esophagus. Muscular abnormalities such as achalasia and diffuse esophageal spasm can be easily detected. If perforation or rupture of the esophagus is suspected, it is best to use a water-soluble contrast medium rather than barium. Anatomic abnormalities such as sliding or paraesophageal hiatal hernias can also be detected.

This procedure is usually performed in approximately 15 to 20 minutes in the radiology department by a radiologist. No discomfort is associated with this test.

CONTRAINDICATIONS

- Evidence of bowel obstruction or severe constipation, because barium may create a stonelike impaction
- Perforated viscus, because if barium were to leak, the degree and duration of infection would be much worse; when perforation is suspected, diatrizoate (Gastrografin), a water-soluble iodine-containing contrast medium, is usually used.
- Unstable vital signs
- Inability of patients to cooperate during the test

POTENTIAL COMPLICATIONS

- Barium-induced fecal impaction

INTERFERING FACTORS

- Food in the esophagus, which prevents adequate visualization

Clinical Priorities

- This study provides a more thorough examination of the esophagus than is provided by most upper gastrointestinal X-ray studies.
- Barium is not used if perforation or rupture of the esophagus is suspected. In these cases, a water-soluble contrast agent is used.
- After the test, the use of cathartics is recommended to aid in evacuating the barium.

PROCEDURE AND PATIENT CARE

Before

 Explain the procedure to the patient.

Instruct the patient to remain on NPO status (nothing by mouth) for at least 8 hours before the test. Usually the patient is kept on NPO status after midnight on the day of the test.

- Assess the patient's ability to swallow. If the patient tends to aspirate, inform the radiologist.

During

- Note the following procedural steps:
  1. The fasting patient is asked to swallow the contrast medium. Usually this is barium sulphate in milkshake-like form; however, if a perforated viscus is suspected, diatrizoate (Gastrografin) is used.
  2. As the patient drinks the contrast agent through a straw, the X-ray table is tilted to the near-erect position.
  3. The patient is asked to roll into various positions so that the entire esophagus can be adequately visualized.
  4. With fluoroscopy or videofluoroscopy, the radiologist observes the flow of contrast medium through the entire esophagus.

After

 Inform the patient of the need to evacuate all the barium. Cathartics are recommended. Initially, stool is white, but it returns to normal colour with complete evacuation of the barium.

Home Care Responsibilities

- Inform the patient that initially stools will be white. Mild cathartics should be given until the stool is no longer white. When all of the barium has been expelled, the stool will return to normal colour.
- Inform the patient that laxatives may be ordered by the physician to facilitate evacuation of barium.

TEST RESULTS AND CLINICAL SIGNIFICANCE

Total or partial esophageal obstruction: *Usually this is caused by a cancer. However, achalasia or stricture can be so severe that it causes obstruction. Affected patients complain of dysphagia.*

Cancer: *This is most evident as narrowing in the esophagus or diminished gastroesophageal function.*

Peptic or corrosive (e.g., lye) esophagitis or ulceration: *Either of these conditions can cause bleeding, perforation, scarring, and stricture.*

Scarred strictures: *These are usually a sequela of untreated peptic or corrosive esophagitis.*

Lower esophageal rings: *These may be congenital or acquired as a result of long-term reflux.*

Varices: *Submucosal venous varices can result from prolonged portal hypertension.*

Chalasia or achalasia: *Chalasia occurs in infants who have no lower esophageal sphincter function. Affected children have gastroesophageal reflux. Achalasia is usually acquired but may be congenital. Affected patients cannot relax the lower esophageal sphincter, and esophageal obstruction (dysphagia) develops.*

Esophageal motility disorders (e.g., presbyesophagus, scleroderma, diffuse esophageal spasm): *Older patients may have asynchronous motility, which prevents swallowed food from progressing through the esophagus.*

Diverticula: *These can develop in the upper esophagus (Zenker diverticula) and be caused by spasm of the cricopharyngeus muscle (upper esophageal sphincter), or they can develop in the lower esophagus (epiphrenic diverticula) and result from paraesophageal infection.*

Extrinsic compression from extraesophageal tumour, cardiomegaly, or aortic aneurysm: *Such compression distorts the normal esophageal anatomy.*

RELATED TEST

Esophagogastroduodenoscopy (p. 636). This test enables direct visualization of the esophageal lumen.

Bone Densitometry (Bone Mineral Content [Bmc], Bone Absorptiometry, Bone Mineral Density [BMD])

NORMAL FINDINGS

Female ≥50 years: <1 standard deviation (SD) below normal (>−1.0)
Female <50 years: <2.5 SDs below normal (>2.5)
Male (all ages): <2.5 SDs below normal (>−2.5)

 Critical Values

Female ≥50 years
    Osteopenia: 1.0–2.5 SDs below normal (−1.0 to−2.5)
    Osteoporosis: ≥2.5 SDs below normal (≤−2.5)
Female <50 years
    Reduced density: ≥2.5 SDs below normal (≤2.5)
Male (all ages)
    Reduced density: ≥2.5 SDs below normal (≤−2.5)

INDICATIONS

Bone densitometry is a clinically proven and accurate method of measuring bone mineral density (BMD). It is typically applied to the central skeleton (the lumbar spine or the proximal femur) or to the whole skeleton. It can also help determine bone mineral content, which helps with the diagnosis of osteoporosis. In addition, it is used to monitor patients who are undergoing treatment for osteoporosis. Indications include the following:

- Patients of any age with suspected insufficiency (fragility) fractures
- Early premenopausal oophorectomy or estrogen-deficiency syndromes (e.g., amenorrhea)
- Plain X-rays that indicate osteopenia
- Endocrinopathies known to be associated with osteopenia (e.g., hyperparathyroidism, prolactinoma, Cushing's syndrome, male hypogonadism, hyperthyroidism)
- Unexplained or multiple fractures
- Anorexia
- Multiple myeloma
- Prolonged immobility
- Gastrointestinal malabsorption (proteins and calcium)
- Chronic renal diseases (secondary and tertiary hyperparathyroidism)
- Treatment-related osteopenia (e.g., long-term heparin, breast cancer antihormone therapy, or steroid therapy)
- Monitoring of response to treatment of osteoporosis (e.g., selective estrogen receptor modulators, bisphosphonates, calcitonins)
- Onset of menopause, to make a better informed decision regarding the risks and benefits of hormone-replacement therapy (Box 12-4)

BOX 12-4	Patients Recommended for Bone Mineral Density Testing

- Patients of any age with suspected insufficiency (fragility) fractures
- Women with estrogen deficiency (perimenopausal, postmenopausal, or after oopherectomy)
- Patients presenting with any of the following risk factors:
  1. A family history of fractures or osteoporosis
  2. Low body mass
  3. Personal history of anorexia or bulimia
  4. History of amenorrhea (>1 year before 42 years of age)
  5. Current gastrointestinal malabsorption disorder
  6. Smoking history (>1 pack/day for 5 years)
  7. Loss of height, thoracic kyphosis
- Metabolic and other disorders that could alter bone mineral density (e.g., Cushing's syndrome, chronic renal failure, primary hyperparathyroidism, hyperthyroidism, organ transplantation, or vitamin D deficiency)
- Long-term therapy with corticosteroids (glucocorticosteroids), thyroid replacement, or other medications that affect bone mineral density
- Monitoring to assess the efficacy of osteoporosis therapy

TEST EXPLANATION

Osteoporosis and osteopenia, or decreased bone mass, develop most commonly in postmenopausal women. Bones become weak and fracture easily. Diseases associated with osteoporosis include renal failure, hyperparathyroidism, and gastrointestinal malabsorption syndrome; prolonged steroid therapy and prolonged immobility are predisposing factors. The consequences of osteoporosis are generally vertebral crush fractures and hip fractures. Nationally, these fractures cost billions of health care dollars for medical treatment and long-term custodial care. More important, approximately 20% of patients older than 45 years who have hip or vertebral fracture die within 1 year as a consequence of the injury.

Methods to identify the early stages of osteoporosis are available. The earlier osteoporosis is recognized, the more effective the treatment is and the milder the clinical course is. If the diagnosis of osteoporosis is delayed until fractures occur or plain X-rays demonstrate "thin" bones, treatment is less likely to be successful.

Patients with osteoporosis should receive aggressive medical therapy, which can be expensive and is not without risks. Therefore, the diagnosis of osteoporosis must be based on accurate data: that is, bone mineral mass (best measured by BMD). Bone densitometry was developed to provide accurate and precise measurement of bone strength on the basis of bone density. Several groups of bones are routinely evaluated because they accurately represent the entire skeleton. The lumbar spine is the best representative of cancellous bone. The radius is the most easily studied cortical bone. The proximal hip (neck of the femur) is the best representative of cancellous and cortical mixed bone. Specific bone sites can be evaluated if they are symptomatic.

There are several methods of measuring BMD. The most commonly used method of determining BMD is *dual-energy densitometry* (absorptiometry). In this method, a dual-photon source is used to measure the density of the bone. With *dual-energy X-ray absorptiometry* (DEXA), two different X-ray beams produce dual photons in the X-ray spectrum. Because DEXA entails the use of two photons, more energy is produced so that bones (spine and hip [femoral neck]) surrounded by more soft tissue can be more easily penetrated. The radius can also be measured with either of these dual-energy techniques.

Several other methods of measuring BMD are available. In *quantitative computed tomography,* computed tomographic technology is used to measure central bones, especially the spine. In *single*

X-ray absorptiometry, a single X-ray beam is used to measure the density of a peripheral bone (finger, wrist, or heel). *Ultrasound absorption* (quantitative ultrasonography) can be used to measure peripheral bones (heel [calcaneus], patella, or midtibia).

Usually, bone density is reported in terms of standard deviation from mean values. *T* scores are studied to compare the patient's results with those of a group of young, healthy adults. *Z* scores are calculated to compare the patient's results with those of a group of age-matched controls. *T* scores are probably more accurate in predictive value of risk for fracture. The World Health Organization has defined *osteopenia* as bone density value of more than 1 standard deviation (SD) below peak bone mass levels in young women and *osteoporosis* as a value of more than 2.5 SDs below that same measurement scale. Most clinicians believe therapeutic intervention should be begun in patients with osteopenia to prevent progression to osteoporosis.

The data are interpreted and reported by a radiologist or a physician trained in nuclear medicine. Bone density studies take approximately 30 to 45 minutes to perform and are free of any discomfort. Only minimal radiation is used (the total dose of radiation exposure is less than for a chest X-ray study).

INTERFERING FACTORS

- Barium may artificially increase the density of the lumbar spine. Bone density measurements should not be performed within approximately 10 days after barium studies.
- Posterior vertebral calcific arthritic sclerosis can artificially increase bone density of the spine.
- Calcified abdominal aortic aneurysm can factitiously increase bone density of the spine.
- Internal fixation devices of the hip or radius factitiously increase bone density of those bones.
- Overlying metal jewellery or other objects can factitiously increase bone density.
- Previous fractures or severe arthritic changes of the bone to be studied can artificially increase its bone density.
- Metallic clips placed in the plane of the vertebra in patients who have had previous abdominal surgery can artificially increase bone density.
- Previous bone scans can factitiously decrease bone density because the photons generated from the bone as a result of the previously administered radionuclide are detected by the scintillator counter.

Clinical Priorities

- Bone densitometry was developed to provide accurate and precise measurement of bone strength based on bone density.
- According to the World Health Organization, osteopenia is present if the bone density value is more than 1 SD below peak bone mass levels in young women, and osteoporosis is present if the value is more than 2.5 SDs below the same level.
- This test should not be performed within 10 days after barium studies because barium may artificially increase the bone density of the lumbar spine.

PROCEDURE AND PATIENT CARE

Before

- The densitometer is usually calibrated by the radiologist or nuclear medicine technician before the patient's arrival.
 Inform the patient that no fasting or sedation is required.
 Explain the procedure to the patient.

✗ Ask the patient to remove all metallic objects (e.g., belt buckles, zippers, coins, keys, jewellery) that might be in the scanning path. The patient may stay dressed.

During

- The patient lies supine on an imaging table (Figure 12-6) with the legs supported on a padded box to flatten the pelvis and lumbar spine; however, a padded box must not interfere with proper positioning and must never appear in the scan field.
- Under the table, a photon generator is slowly passed under the lumbar spine.
- Above the table, a scintillation (gamma or X-ray) detector camera is passed over the patient parallel to the generator. Images of the lumbar and hip bones are projected on a computer monitor.
- Next, the foot is applied to a brace that internally rotates the nondominant hip, and the procedure is repeated over the hip. A similar procedure is performed to evaluate the radius. When the radius is examined, the nondominant arm is preferred unless there is a history of fracture in that bone.
- Note that there are numerous types of bone densitometry machines. Peripheral units that quickly scan the finger, heel, or forearm are often used to detect risk for osteoporosis. Abnormal results are followed up with the more comprehensive table procedure just described.

After

- On the computer screen, the image is of a small window of the lumbar spine, femoral neck, or distal radius. The computer calculates the number of photons not absorbed by the bone, or bone mineral content. BMD is computed as follows:

$$BMD = \left\{ \frac{\text{Bone mineral content } (g/cm^2)}{\text{Surface area of the bone } (Sv)} \right\}$$

- Findings are compared with data from healthy 25- to 35-year-old women, and the SD above or below the curve is determined. This is the T score. Positive T scores indicate that the bone is

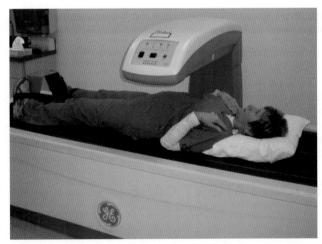

Figure 12-6 Patient undergoing bone densitometry. Note that it is not required that the patient undress. Jewellery, however, must be removed.

stronger than normal; negative *T* scores indicate that the bone is weaker than normal. *Z* scores are calculated in the same way, but the comparisons are with those in normal patients matched for age, sex, race, height, and weight.

TEST RESULTS AND CLINICAL SIGNIFICANCE

Osteopenia (low bone mass),

Osteoporosis: *Osteopenia precedes osteoporosis. The most common cause of osteoporosis is lack of sexual hormones (estrogen in female patients, testosterone in male patients). Osteopenia may result from primary ovarian failure secondary to menopause or oophorectomy or from pituitary disease. In male patients, osteopenia usually occurs in childhood in association with congenital hormone deficiencies.*

Hyperparathyroidism: *Excess parathyroid hormone mobilizes calcium from the bone, causing demineralization and bone weakening.*

Chronic renal insufficiency: *Excess phosphates that accumulate as a result of reduced glomerular filtration decrease the calcium level in the blood. Parathyroid hormone is stimulated to increase calcium levels. Excess parathyroid hormone mobilizes calcium from the bone, causing demineralization and weakening of the bones (secondary hyperparathyroidism). If after persistent parathyroid stimulation the parathyroid glands become autonomous and secrete elevated amounts of parathyroid hormone despite normal calcium levels, tertiary hyperparathyroidism develops. The bone changes are the same as described previously.*

Gastrointestinal malabsorption: *Calcium and protein cannot be absorbed. The bones are depleted of their minerals, and bone density is reduced.*

Cushing's syndrome,

Chronic steroid therapy: *Glucocorticosteroids inhibit bone mineralization and decrease bone density.*

Chronic heparin therapy: *Heparin binds calcium and other minerals. These minerals are therefore not available for bone growth. Furthermore, these minerals are mobilized from their bone stores. Bone density diminishes.*

Chronic immobility: *The pathophysiologic mechanism underlying bone demineralization in the immobilized patient is not clearly understood.*

RELATED TESTS

Bone (Long) Radiography (see following test). Plain X-rays can identify advanced bone demineralization and indicate severe osteoporosis.

Bone Turnover Markers (p. 947). N-telopeptide, bone-specific alkaline phosphatase, pyridinium, and osteocalcin are biochemical markers of bone turnover and are measured to monitor treatment for osteoporosis.

Bone (Long) Radiography

NORMAL FINDINGS

No evidence of fracture, tumour, infection, or congenital abnormalities

INDICATIONS

This X-ray study is performed to evaluate any bone for fracture, infection, arthritis, tendinitis, or bone spurs. Bone age can be determined in children to evaluate growth and development. Primary and metastatic tumour can be identified.

12   X-Ray Studies

TEST EXPLANATION

Radiographs of the long bones are usually obtained when the patient has complaints about a pertinent body area. Fractures or tumour are readily detected on X-ray studies. Severe or chronic infection involving a bone (osteomyelitis) may be detected. X-ray studies of the long bones also can detect joint destruction and bone spurring as a result of persistent arthritis. Growth patterns can be followed by serial X-ray studies of long bones, usually the wrists and hands. Healing of a fracture can be documented and monitored. Radiographs of the joints reveal the presence of joint effusions and soft tissue swelling. Calcifications in the soft tissue indicate chronic inflammatory changes of the nearby bursae or tendons. Soft tissue swelling can also be seen on these similar X-rays. Because the cartilage and tendons are not visualized directly, cartilage fractures and sprains and ligamentous injuries cannot be seen.

At least two images obtained at a 90-degree angle are required so that the bone region being studied can be visualized from two different angles (usually anteroposterior and lateral). In some bone studies (e.g., skull, spine, hip), oblique views are necessary to visualize all the parts that need to be seen.

INTERFERING FACTORS

- Jewellery or clothing can obstruct X-ray visualization of part of the bone to be evaluated.
- Previous barium studies can diminish full X-ray visualization of some of the bones surrounding the abdomen (e.g., spine, pelvis).

Clinical Priorities

- This test can determine bone age to evaluate growth and development. Usually the bones of the wrists and hands are used for this determination.
- When obtaining X-rays, shield the patient's testes or ovaries and, if the patient is pregnant, abdomen to prevent radiation exposure.

PROCEDURE AND PATIENT CARE

Before

- Explain the procedure to the patient.
- Carefully handle any injured parts of the patient's body.
- Instruct the patient to keep the extremity still while the X-ray is being obtained. This can sometimes be difficult, especially when the patient has severe pain in association with a recent injury.
- Shield the patient's testes or ovaries and, if the patient is pregnant, abdomen to prevent exposure from scattered radiation.
- Inform the patient that no fasting or sedation is required.

During

- In the radiology department, the patient is asked to place the involved extremity in several positions. An X-ray of each position is obtained.
- Note that this test is routinely performed within several minutes by a radiologic technologist.
- Inform the patient that no discomfort is associated with this test except perhaps from moving an injured extremity.

After

- Administer an analgesic for relief of pain, if it is indicated.

TEST RESULTS AND CLINICAL SIGNIFICANCE

Fractures,

Congenital bone disorders (e.g., achondroplasia, dysplasia, dysostosis): *Multiple disorders associated with bone, absence of a bone, or growth and development of bone or bone groups are detected.*

Tumour (osteogenic sarcoma, Paget's disease, myeloma, metastases): *These can be evident from osteoblastic destruction (radiolucent defects in bone) or osteoclastic reaction (radiopaque areas of bone) to the tumour.*

Infection or osteomyelitis: *These are evident from soft tissue swelling around the bone infection. Further signs may include periosteal reaction and bony destruction of the affected bone.*

Osteoporosis or osteopenia: *Bone demineralization and thinning indicate osteoporosis. Patients are at increased risk for traumatic and atraumatic fractures.*

Joint destruction (arthritis): *Degenerative and rheumatoid arthritic degenerative changes appear as narrowing of the joint space because of cartilaginous destruction. Bone spurs and other changes can be noted.*

Bone spurs: *Exophytic growths of bone at pressure points (heels and feet) can cause significant pain.*

Abnormal growth pattern: *Bone development can be evaluated with X-rays of the wrists, arms, pelvis, and skull. Comparison of findings with those normal for chronologic age provides insight and perspective into possible abnormalities in growth and development.*

Joint effusion: *Swelling and some increased radiodensity of the joint indicate effusion. This may be the result of bleeding, trauma, inflammation, or infection.*

Foreign bodies: *Radiographs of the extremities can demonstrate the presence of foreign bodies (usually in the hands and feet).*

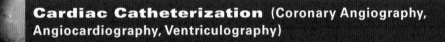

Cardiac Catheterization (Coronary Angiography, Angiocardiography, Ventriculography)

NORMAL FINDINGS

Normal heart-muscle motion, normal and patent coronary arteries, normal great vessels, and normal intracardiac pressure and volume

INDICATIONS

Cardiac catheterization is used to visualize the heart chambers, arteries, and great vessels. It is used most often to evaluate chest pain. The study is used to locate the region of coronary occlusion in patients with positive stress test results and to determine the effects of valvular heart disease. Right-sided heart catheterization is the most accurate method for determining cardiac output. It also helps with measuring right-sided heart pressures and can be used to identify pulmonary emboli (see Pulmonary Angiography, p. 1100).

TEST EXPLANATION

Cardiac catheterization enables examination of the heart, great blood vessels (aorta, inferior vena cava, pulmonary artery, and pulmonary vein), and coronary arteries. For cardiac catheterization, a catheter is passed into the heart through a peripheral vein (for right-sided heart catheterization) or artery (for left-sided heart catheterization). Through the catheter, pressures are recorded and X-ray dyes are injected. With the assistance of computer calculations, cardiac output and other

X-Ray Studies

12

measures of cardiac function can be determined. Cardiac catheterization is indicated for the following reasons:

1. To identify, locate, and quantify the severity of atherosclerotic, occlusive coronary artery disease
2. To evaluate the severity of acquired and congenital cardiac valvular or septal defects
3. To determine the presence and degree of congenital cardiac abnormalities, such as transposition of the great vessels, patent ductus arteriosus, and anomalous venous return to the heart
4. To evaluate the success of previous cardiac surgery or balloon angioplasty
5. To evaluate cardiac muscle function
6. To identify and quantify ventricular aneurysms
7. To identify and locate acquired disease of the great vessels, such as atherosclerotic occlusion or aneurysms within the aortic arch
8. To evaluate and treat patients with acute myocardial infarction
9. To insert a catheter to monitor right-sided heart pressures, such as pulmonary artery and pulmonary wedge pressures, and to measure cardiac output. Cardiac output can be measured only during right-sided heart catheterization. (Table 12-2 lists pressures and volumes used in cardiac monitoring.)
10. To dilate stenotic coronary arteries (angioplasty), to place coronary artery stents, or to perform laser atherectomy

TABLE 12-2   Pressures and Volumes Measured in Cardiac Monitoring

Parameter	Description	Normal Value
Pressures		
Routine blood pressure	Routine brachial artery pressure	90–140/60–90 mm Hg
Systolic left ventricular pressure	Peak pressure in the left ventricle during systole	90–140 mm Hg
End-diastolic left ventricular pressure	Pressure in the left ventricle at the end of diastole	4–12 mm Hg
Central venous pressure	Pressure in the superior vena cava	2–14 cm H_2O
Pulmonary capillary wedge pressure (PCWP)	Pressure in the pulmonary capillaries, an indirect measurement of left atrial pressure and left ventricular end-diastolic pressure	Left atrial: 6–15 mm Hg
Pulmonary artery pressure	Pressure in the pulmonary artery	15–28/5–16 mm Hg
Aortic artery pressure	Pressure in the aortic artery	Same as for routine blood pressure
Volumes		
End-diastolic volume (EDV)	Amount of blood present in the left ventricle at the end of diastole	50–90 mL/m²
End-systolic volume (ESV)	Amount of blood present in the left ventricle at the end of systole	25 mL/m²
Stroke volume (SV)	Amount of blood ejected from the heart in one contraction (SV = EDV − ESV)	45 ± 12 mL/m²
Ejection fraction (EF)	Proportion (fraction) of EDV ejected from the left ventricle during systole (EF = SV/EDV)	0.67 ± 0.07
Cardiac output (CO)	Amount of blood ejected by the heart in 1 min	3–6 L/min
Cardiac index (CI)	Amount of blood ejected by the heart in 1 min per square metre of body surface area (CI = CO/body surface area)	2.8–4.2 L/min/m² in a patient with 1.5 m² of body surface area

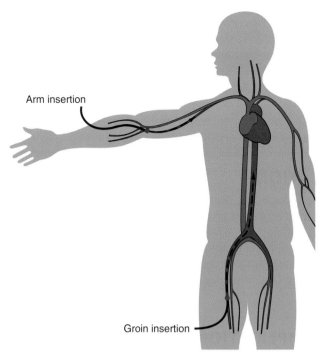

Arm insertion

Groin insertion

Figure 12-7 Two common insertion sites for left-sided cardiac catheterization: brachial and femoral artery insertion.

Cardiac catheterization is performed under sterile conditions. In right-sided heart catheterization, usually the jugular, subclavian, brachial, or femoral vein is used for vascular access. In left-sided heart catheterization, usually the right femoral artery is cannulated, or alternatively, the brachial or radial artery (Figure 12-7). As the catheter is placed into the great vessels of the heart chamber, pressures are monitored and recorded. Blood samples for analysis of oxygen content are also obtained. The catheter is advanced with appropriate guidance into the desired position. After pressures are measured, the heart chambers, valves, and coronary arteries are visualized angiographically with the injection of X-ray dye.

Percutaneous transluminal coronary angioplasty and implantation of *intracoronary stents* are therapeutic procedures that can be performed during coronary angiography in medical centres where open heart surgery is available. During this procedure, a specially designed balloon catheter is introduced into the coronary arteries and placed across the stenotic area of the coronary artery. This area can then be dilated by controlled inflation of the balloon, and a stent is subsequently placed. Coronary arteriography is then repeated to document the effects of the forceful dilation of the stenotic area. Coronary arterial stents can be placed at the site of previous stenosis after angioplasty, and they maintain patency for longer periods of time.

Atherectomy of coronary arterial plaques can be performed to more permanently open some of the hard, atheromatous plaques. Certain occlusive lesions with characteristics unfavourable for balloon angioplasty appear to be ideally suited for atherectomy. Rotational atherectomy is most commonly performed. A tiny rotating knife inside a catheter is moved to the arterial obstruction. A balloon is inflated to position the knife precisely on the fatty deposit. Then the knife shaves the fatty deposit off the wall of the artery. The shavings are collected in the catheter and removed.

Cardiac catheterization is usually performed in approximately 1 hour by a cardiologist. During the dye injection, the patient may experience a severely hot flush, which may be uncomfortable but lasts only 10 to 15 seconds. Some patients have a tendency to cough as the catheter is placed in the pulmonary artery. Provide emotional support to the patient as the X-rays are obtained, because the possibly loud noises may frighten the patient.

Age-Related Concerns

- Adults older than 75 years who have chronic dehydration or mild renal failure are at high risk for dye-induced renal failure.
- Urinary output must be carefully monitored after the procedure. Fluid intake needs to be encouraged, because dehydration may be induced by the diuretic action of the dye.

CONTRAINDICATIONS

- Inability of patients to cooperate during the test
- Patients' refusal of intervention if an amenable lesion were found
- Iodinated dye allergy in patients who have not received preventive medication for allergy
- Pregnancy, unless the benefits of the procedure outweigh the risk of radiation exposure to the fetus
- Renal disorders, because iodinated contrast material is nephrotoxic
- Propensity for bleeding (e.g., anticoagulant use), because the arterial or venous puncture site may not seal

POTENTIAL COMPLICATIONS

- Cardiac arrhythmias (dysrhythmias)
- Perforation of the myocardium
- Renal failure (see Box 12-2, p. 1018)
- Catheter-induced embolic cerebrovascular accident (stroke) or myocardial infarction
- Complications associated with the catheter insertion site, such as arterial thrombosis, embolism, or pseudoaneurysm
- Potential complications of iodinated dye (p. 1021)
- Infection at the catheter insertion site
- Pneumothorax after subclavian vein catheterization of the right side of the heart
- Hypoglycemia or acidosis, which may occur in patients who are taking metformin (Glucophage) and receive iodinated dye.

Clinical Priorities

- Assess the patient for adverse reactions or allergic reactions to iodinated dye.
- Perform a baseline assessment of the patient's peripheral pulses before catheterization.
- After the test, keep the patient on bed rest for 4 to 8 hours to allow complete sealing of the arterial puncture.
- Assess the puncture site for bleeding, hematoma, and absence of pulse.

PROCEDURE AND PATIENT CARE

Before

- Explain the procedure to the patient.
- Obtain the patient's written informed consent for the procedure.
- Allay the patient's fears and anxieties about the test. Although this test creates tremendous fear in a patient, it is performed often, and complications are rare.

⚡ Instruct the patient to abstain from oral intake for at least 4 to 8 hours before the test.
- Prepare the catheter insertion site by shaving and scrubbing the skin.
- Perform assessment for allergy to iodinated dye (p. 1021).
- Mark the patient's peripheral pulses with a pen before catheterization. This will facilitate post-catheterization assessment of the pulses in the affected and unaffected extremities.
- Provide appropriate precatheterization sedation as ordered by the physician.

⚡ Instruct the patient to void before going to the catheterization laboratory.
- Remove all valuables and dental prostheses from the patient's body before transporting the patient to the catheterization laboratory.
- Obtain intravenous access for delivery of fluids and cardiac drugs if necessary.

During

- Take the patient to the cardiac catheterization laboratory (Figure 12-8).
- Note the following procedural steps:
  1. The chosen catheter insertion site is prepared and draped in a sterile manner.
  2. The desired vessel is punctured with a needle.
  3. A wire is placed through the needle, and a sheath is placed on the wire and into the vessel.
  4. The angiographic catheter is threaded through the sheath over a guide wire to place the catheter appropriately.
  5. Once the catheter is in the desired location, the appropriate cardiac pressures and volumes are measured.
  6. Cardiac ventriculography is performed with controlled injection of contrast material.
  7. Each coronary artery is catheterized. Cardiac angiography is then carried out with controlled injection of contrast material.
  8. During the injection, X-rays are rapidly obtained.
  9. The patient's vital signs must be monitored constantly during the procedure.
  10. If angioplasty is performed, the following procedural steps are carried out:
      a. The cardiologist appropriately places the catheter and balloon at the stenotic area.
      b. As the electrocardiographic tracing is observed, the balloon is inflated, and the stenotic areas are forcefully dilated.

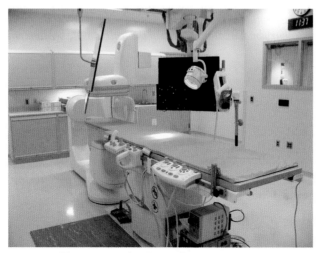

Figure 12-8 Cardiac catheterization lab.

    c. If signs of myocardial ischemia develop, the balloon is immediately deflated.

    d. The balloon is usually inflated for only 10 seconds.

11. After all required information is obtained, the catheter is removed.

12. A chemical vascular closure device designed to seal the arterial puncture site is often placed.

After

- Monitor the patient's vital signs.
- Apply pressure to the site of vascular access.
- Keep the patient on bed rest for 4 to 8 hours to allow complete sealing of the arterial puncture.
- Keep the affected extremity extended and immobilized with sandbags to decrease bleeding.
- Assess the puncture site for signs of bleeding, hematoma, or absence of pulse.
- Assess the patient's pulses in both legs. Compare these values with preprocedural baseline values.
- Encourage the patient to drink fluids to promote dye excretion and to maintain adequate hydration. Dehydration may be caused by the diuretic action of the dye. Monitor urinary output.
- Evaluate the patient for delayed allergic reaction to the dye (e.g., dyspnea, rash, tachycardia, urticaria). Reactions usually occur within the first 2 to 6 hours after the test. Treat with antihistamines or steroids.
- Inform the patient that the angiograms will be reviewed by the cardiologist and that the results will be available in 1 or 2 days.

Home Care Responsibilities

- Instruct the patient in positioning the extremity to decrease bleeding.
- Instruct the patient to check for signs of bleeding (decreased blood pressure and increased pulse).
- Instruct the patient to assess the puncture site for bleeding and hematoma.
- Instruct the patient to report any signs of numbness, tingling, pain, or loss of function in the involved extremity.

TEST RESULTS AND CLINICAL SIGNIFICANCE

Coronary artery occlusive disease: *Stenosis in one or more of the coronary arteries (or branches) can be easily identified and located for revascularization with angioplasty or coronary artery bypass grafting.*

Anatomic variation of the cardiac chambers and great vessels: *Ventricular and atrial septal defects, patent ductus arteriosus, and transposition of the great vessels are among many abnormalities that can be identified.*

Ventricular aneurysm: *Aneurysmal dilation of part of the wall muscle because of infarction and weakness is evident at ventriculography.*

Ventricular mural thrombi,

Intracardiac tumour,

Altered blood flow dynamics,

Cardiomyopathy,

Ventricular wall motion deficits,

Acquired or congenital septal defects and valvular abnormalities: *Ventricular abnormalities are most evident during the ventriculography portion of the study. Some of these abnormalities also cause hemodynamic effects, which are recognized from pressure readings performed during cardiac catheterization.*

Aortic root arteriosclerotic or aneurysmal disease,

Coronary aneurysm,

Coronary fistula,

Anomalies in pulmonary venous return,

Pulmonary emboli: *Anomalies and diseases of the great vessels are evident in the pattern of dye outflow after ventriculography.*

Pulmonary hypertension: *This condition is recognized from pressure readings performed during cardiac catheterization.*

Reduced cardiac output: *Cardiac output is most accurately assessed by right-sided heart catheterization. The right side is catheterized if cardiac output readings are required or if valvular diseases of the right side are suspected.*

Arterial oxygen desaturation: *Arterial oxygen saturation may be decreased when mixing of venous and arterial blood occurs. This may be seen with septal defects, transposition of the great vessels, or congenital shunting.*

RELATED TESTS

Cardiac Nuclear Scanning (p. 817). This test can provide similar information concerning ventricular wall function and motion. Ejection fraction (a measure of cardiac output) and blood flow dynamics can also be determined. With newer radioisotopes, sites of coronary artery occlusion can be seen.

Computed Tomography, Heart (p. 1072). This test is now being applied to the heart and coronary vessels. It holds much promise as a noninvasive substitute for cardiac catheterization.

Chest Radiography (Chest X-Ray [CXR])

NORMAL FINDINGS

Normal lungs and surrounding structures

INDICATIONS

This is the most commonly obtained X-ray study because it can indicate much information about the heart, lungs, bony thorax, mediastinum, and great vessels.

TEST EXPLANATION

Chest X-ray is important in the complete evaluation of the pulmonary and cardiac systems. This procedure is often part of the general admission screening workup in adult patients. Much information can be provided by the chest X-ray study. Repeated studies enable identification and monitoring of the following conditions:

1. Tumours of the lung (primary and metastatic), heart (myxoma), chest wall (soft tissue sarcomas), and bony thorax (osteogenic sarcoma)
2. Inflammations of the lung (pneumonia), pleura (pleuritis), and pericardium (pericarditis)
3. Fluid accumulations in the pleura (pleural effusion), pericardium (pericardial effusion), and lung (pulmonary edema)
4. Air accumulations in the lung (chronic obstructive pulmonary disease) and pleura (pneumothorax)
5. Fractures of the bones of the thorax or vertebrae
6. Diaphragmatic hernia
7. Heart size, which may vary, depending on cardiac function
8. Calcification, which may indicate large-vessel deterioration or old lung granulomas
9. Location of centrally placed intravenous access devices

Most chest X-rays are obtained at a distance of 6 feet (1.8 m), with the patient standing. The sitting or supine position also can be used, but X-rays obtained with the patient supine do not demonstrate fluid levels or pneumothorax. For a *posteroanterior* view (projection), the X-rays pass through the body from the back (posterior) to the front (anterior) (Figure 12-9, *A, B*). For an *anteroposterior* view, the X-rays pass through the body from front to back. For a *lateral* view, the X-rays enter from the side (Figure 12-10, *A, B*). For *oblique* views, X-rays pass through the body at various angles. *Lordotic* views, obtained with the patient recumbent, provide visualization of

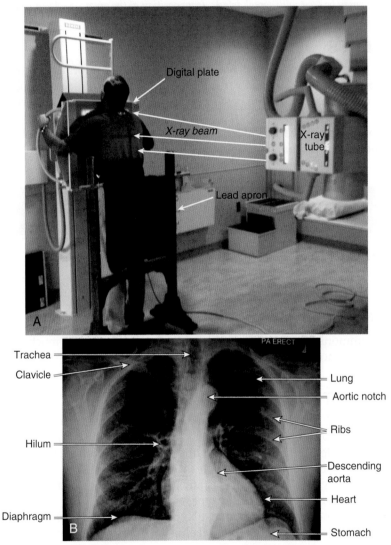

Figure 12-9 A, Routine PA view chest X-ray. Note direction of the X-ray beam from the X-ray cathode tube through the patient and to the X-ray digital receptor plate. Also note lead apron for protection from "scatter x-ray." **B,** PA chest X-ray. The diaphragm separates the abdominal contents (including the stomach) from the chest. The heart is situated in the middle of the chest, more toward the left side. The air-filled lungs are represented as dark spaces on either side of the chest. The trachea is seen as a dark shadow in the neck and upper chest. The peak of the descending aorta is the notch. The descending aorta runs vertically in front of the vertebra. The ribs, clavicle, and other bony structures can also be seen as a part of the thoracic cage.

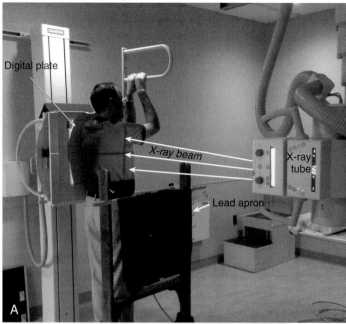

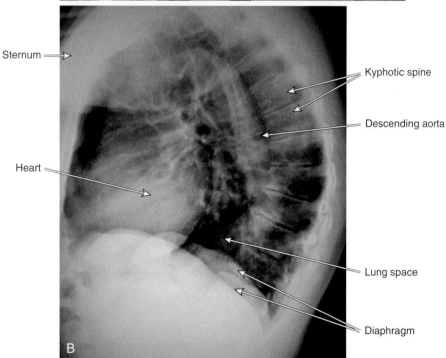

Figure 12-10 **A,** Routine lateral view chest X-ray. Note direction of the X-ray beam from the X-ray cathode tube through the patient and to the X-ray digital receptor plate. Also note lead apron for protection from "scatter x-ray." **B,** Lateral chest X-ray. The heart is situated in anterior chest under the sternum. The air-filled lungs are represented as dark spaces. The descending aorta runs vertically in front of the vertebra. The vertebral bodies are noticed in the posterior chest and are curved due to kyphosis.

X-Ray Studies

12

TABLE 12-3	Position of Patient for Identifying Suspected Problems on X-Rays
Suspected Problem	**Position Required**
Pneumothorax	Erect
Effusion	Lateral decubitus
Widened mediastinum	Erect
Cardiac enlargement	Erect
Fractured rib	Oblique
Tuberculosis	Lordotic

the apices (rounded upper portions) of the lungs and are usually used to detect tuberculosis. *Decubitus* views, obtained with the patient in the recumbent lateral position, demonstrate and localize fluid, which becomes dependent in the pleural space (pleural effusion). Table 12-3 lists the positions required for detection of various problems.

Chest X-ray studies are most accurate when performed in the radiology department. A portable X-ray machine may be brought to the patient's bedside and is often used in critically ill patients who cannot leave the nursing unit.

CONTRAINDICATIONS

• Pregnancy, unless the benefits of the procedure outweigh the risk of radiation exposure to the fetus

INTERFERING FACTORS

• Conditions (e.g., severe pain or shortness of breath because of COPD) that prevent the patient from taking and holding a deep breath
• Scarring from previous lung surgery (makes interpretation of X-rays difficult)
• Obesity (more X-rays are needed to penetrate the body in order to provide a readable X-ray)

Age-Related Concerns

• Normal aging results in changes to the ribs and vertebra; for example, the ribs become less mobile, which contributes to a decrease in lung expansion.
• Normal aging results in a decrease in the compliance of the chest wall and thus a decrease in the ability to expand the chest wall.

Clinical Priorities

• Chest x-ray studies are most accurate when performed in the radiology department but can be performed at the patient's bedside if the patient cannot leave the nursing unit.
• Patient positioning during the test depends on the suspected condition (see Table 12-3).
• To prevent radiation-induced abnormalities, a lead shield is used to cover the testicles in men, the ovaries in women, and a pregnant woman's abdomen.

Cultural Considerations

Lung tidal volume (the volume of air inspired and expired in one normal respiratory cycle) is largest in White people, followed by Black people, Asians, Native Americans, and Indigenous people. Chest X-ray results may reflect these normal cultural variations in lung tidal volumes. The chest X-ray of a White patient may show normally larger lungs on inspiration; in comparison, the chest X-ray of an Indigenous patient may show normally smaller lungs on inspiration.

PROCEDURE AND PATIENT CARE

Before

- Explain the procedure to the patient.
- Inform the patient that no fasting is required.
- Instruct the patient to remove clothing to the waist and to put on an X-ray gown.
- Instruct the patient to remove all metal objects (e.g., necklaces, pins) from his or her body so that they do not block visualization of part of the chest.
- Inform the patient that he or she will be asked to take a deep breath and hold it while the X-rays are obtained.
- Ensure that the testicles in men, the ovaries in women, and a pregnant woman's abdomen are covered with a lead shield to prevent radiation-induced abnormalities.
- Inform the patient that no discomfort is associated with chest X-ray.

During

- After the patient is correctly positioned, instruct him or her to take a deep breath and hold it until the image is taken.
- Note that X-rays are obtained by a radiologic technologist in several minutes.

After

- No special care is required after chest X-ray.

TEST RESULTS AND CLINICAL SIGNIFICANCE

Lung

Lung tumour (primary or metastatic): *This is evident as a soft tissue mass in the lung field.*

Pneumonia: *Increased opacity (lightness) in the lung field indicates pneumonia or atelectatic lung tissue.*

Pulmonary edema: *Increased opacity of the lung is indicative of pulmonary edema, most commonly from heart failure.*

Pleural effusion: *Fluid in the chest wall is evident from increased opacity outside the lung fields, particularly in the costophrenic margins. A lateral decubitus view shows layering out of free pleural fluid. Entrapped fluid, however, does not appear layered out.*

Chronic obstructive pulmonary disease: *Increased lung space is a classical finding.*

Pneumothorax: *The presence of air outside the lung space (pneumothorax) is always abnormal. If pneumothorax is large enough, chest tube insertion is necessary to release the trapped air and re-expand the lung.*

Atelectasis: *Collapse of pulmonary alveoli is evident from white patches or lines in the lung fields.*

Tuberculosis: *Tuberculosis, which is present usually in the upper lobes, is generally associated with calcification.*

Lung abscess: *Lung abscess is evident as a lung mass with a hollow (radiolucent) centre. Sometimes, fungus can grow inside an abscess.*

Congenital lung diseases (hypoplasia): *Congenital aplasia or hypoplasia of the lung tissue is evident from reduced amounts of lung tissue on the affected side.*

Pleuritis: *Thickening of the pleura indicates pleuritis, which has a viral, bacterial, neoplastic, or other cause.*

Foreign body in the chest, bronchus, or esophagus: *Swallowed, aspirated, or penetrating (bullets) foreign bodies can be easily seen.*

Heart

Cardiac enlargement: *The heart is larger than 50% to 60% of the horizontal width of the chest, as a result of heart failure or cardiomyopathy.*

Pericarditis,

Pericardial effusion: *These conditions are evident from an enlarged heart shadow.*

Chest Wall

Soft tissue sarcoma,

Osteogenic sarcoma: *These primary tumours of the bony thorax and chest wall soft tissue are evident as masses arising from those areas.*

Fracture of ribs or thoracic spine: *Best seen on lateral or oblique X-rays, fractures may be displaced or well aligned. They are usually associated with other chest trauma.*

Thoracic scoliosis: *Alterations in thoracic spinal alignment are obvious on chest X-rays.*

Metastatic tumour to bony thorax: *Osteolytic (dark) or osteoblastic (white) nodules can be seen in the bony thorax. Tumours of the breast, prostate, kidney, and lung are among the cancers that most commonly metastasize to the bones in this region.*

Diaphragm

Diaphragmatic or hiatal hernia: *This condition is evident from increased opacity in the posteroinferior mediastinum.*

Mediastinum

Aortic calcinosis: *This is evident from white lines indicating the walls of the calcified aorta.*

Enlarged lymph nodes: *Central masses in the mediastinum indicate enlargement of lymph nodes, usually of neoplastic origin.*

Dilated aorta: *This may indicate aneurysm.*

Thymoma,

Lymphoma,

Substernal thyroid: *These abnormalities are often evident as large soft tissue masses in the anterosuperior mediastinum.*

Widened mediastinum: *Cardiac enlargement, aneurysm, lymph node enlargement, or hematoma may be the cause.*

RELATED TEST

Computed Tomography, Chest (p. 1068). This test allows more detailed information concerning pathologic conditions of the chest and its structures.

Computed Tomography, Abdomen (Cat Scan, Abdomen; CT Scan, Abdomen; Helical/Spiral CT Scan, Abdomen; CT Angiography; CT Colonoscopy; Virtual Colonoscopy)

NORMAL FINDINGS

No evidence of abnormality

INDICATIONS

Computed tomography (CT) is used in evaluating abdominal organs. CT can be used to guide needles during biopsy of tumours and aspiration of fluid and in staging known neoplasms. When serially and repeatedly performed, CT is also used to monitor abdominal disease.

TEST EXPLANATION

CT of the abdomen is a noninvasive but accurate X-ray procedure used to diagnose pathologic conditions (e.g., tumour, cysts, abscesses, inflammation, perforation of the bowel, intra-abdominal bleeding, intestinal or ureteral obstruction, vascular aneurysms, and calculi) in the abdominal and retroperitoneal organs. The computed tomographic image results from the passing of X-rays through the abdominal organs at many angles. The variation in density among the tissues causes variation in the penetration of the X-rays. Each density is given a numeric value (*density coefficient*), and all these values are digitally computed into shades of grey. The resulting image is then displayed on a computer monitor (Figure 12-11). To enhance the image, the computed

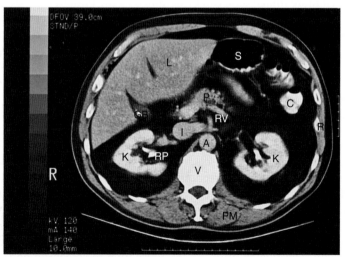

Figure 12-11 Computed tomographic scan of the abdomen. Normally, many abdominal structures can be seen on a computed tomographic scan. A, Aorta; C, the splenic flexure of the colon (contrast filled); GB, gallbladder (containing a gallstone-radiolucent area); I, inferior vena cava; K, kidney; L, liver; *P*, pancreas; PM, paraspinal muscles of the back; small R (on right side of scan), bony ribs of the lower chest; RP, pelvis of the right renal collecting system; RV, left renal vein; S, air/contrast filled stomach; V, vertebra.

tomographic scanning is repeated after intravenous administration of iodine-containing contrast material. These images can be recorded digitally.

Tumour, abscesses, trauma, cysts, and anatomic abnormalities in the liver can be seen, as can tumour, pseudocysts, inflammation, calcification, bleeding, and trauma in the pancreas. The kidneys and urinary outflow tract are well visualized.

Renal tumour and cysts, ureteral obstruction, calculi, and congenital renal and ureteral abnormalities are easily seen with the use of intravenous contrast material. Extravasation of urine secondary to trauma or obstruction can also be easily demonstrated. Adrenal tumour and hyperplasia are best diagnosed with CT. Some radiology literature indicates that the density coefficients shown on the scan may be suggestive of histologic features of the tumour.

Large tumour and perforations of the bowel can be identified with CT, especially when oral contrast material is ingested (see also the description of virtual colonoscopy). The spleen can be well visualized with CT for hematoma, laceration, fracture, tumour infiltration, and splenic vein thrombosis. The retroperitoneal lymph nodes can be evaluated. These are usually present, but all nodes with a diameter greater than 2 cm are considered abnormal. The abdominal aorta and its major branches can be evaluated for aneurysmal dilation and intramural thrombi, and the pelvic structures (including the uterus, ovaries, fallopian tubes, prostate gland, and rectum) and musculature can be evaluated for tumour, abscesses, infection, or hypertrophy. Ascites and hemoperitoneum can easily be demonstrated on a computed tomographic scan.

Dynamic CT scanning can be performed during arterial injection of dye to the organ being studied. Dynamic scanning can indicate blood flow and degree of vascularity of an organ or part of an organ in the abdomen.

Helical CT (also called *spiral* or *volume-averaging CT*) represents a marked improvement over standard computed tomographic scanning. In helical CT, data are obtained continuously as the patient is passed through the gantry. With the development in multidetector computed tomography (MDCT), much more image data can be obtained as the patient is passed through the gantry. With the use of multiple collimators (and multiple banks of detectors), large data images can be obtained in a very short period of time. The entire abdomen can be scanned in less than 30 seconds, during which most patients can hold their breath. The thicknesses of the areas imaged ("slices") are very thin (1 to 5 mm). With thin slices and rapid accession, breathing and motion distortions are minimized, and images are produced faster and are more accurate. In this computed tomographic study, 200 to 500 individual images can be obtained.

Volume imaging with three-dimensional (3D) real-time display of the volume of data allows the interpreter to visualize and analyze the data in three dimensions. With these advances in software, data can provide very accurate two-dimensional and 3D images of the intra-abdominal organs and especially the mesenteric vessels in a few seconds. This allows radiologists to see these structures from multiple views and directions.

In *3D volumetric imaging*, a 3D perspective can be added to the abdominal organs or tumour that are imaged. This provides data for virtual colonoscopy and virtual angiography. In *virtual colonoscopy,* a computed tomographic scanner and computer virtual reality software are used to look inside the body without needing to insert a colonoscope (as in conventional colonoscopy; see p. 619). Virtual colonoscopy is an appropriate alternative to screening endoscopic colonoscopy. No sedation is required, and minimal discomfort is experienced. Patients need a cleansing bowel preparation before the test. This procedure takes place in the radiology department. It begins with the insertion of a small flexible rubber tube in the rectum. Air is inserted through this tube to inflate the colon for better visualization. The air acts as a contrast medium. The test is completed in 10 to 20 minutes. Because no sedation is required, patients are free to leave the CT suite without the need for observation and recovery. Patients can resume normal activities after the procedure and can eat, work, and drive without a delay. In contrast to endoscopic colonoscopy, however, polypectomy and biopsy cannot be performed with virtual testing. If abnormalities are found with virtual colonoscopy, conventional colonoscopy is needed.

An increasingly used combination of *fusion CT/positron emission tomography (PET;* see p. 849) is now being used to provide both anatomic and physiologic information that can be fused into one image. This allows the image to locate pathologic processes and indicate whether they are benign or malignant. As directed by the principles described previously for colonoscopy, fusion CT/PET not only can provide an accurate image of the entire colon but also can indicate whether any abnormality seen is malignant.

Helical *computed tomographic arteriography* or *virtual angiography* is performed through the use of multichannel helical CT. After intravenous injection of contrast medium, CT can demonstrate the arteries in any given organ. This technology enables the creation of 3D images of the aorta and other abdominal vessels, which are particularly helpful in identifying renal artery stenosis and the hepatic vasculature for cancer-related resections. Renal computed tomographic arteriography can be used to demonstrate and evaluate each functional phase of urinary excretion. Computed tomographic angiography is becoming a viable alternative to magnetic resonance imaging (MRI) angiography to assess abdominal aneurysm, iliac vascular occlusion, arteriovenous malformations, or vascular tumour.

Computed tomographic nephrotomography is the computerized production of a 3D image of the kidneys, renal pelvis, and ureters. This is particularly helpful in identifying ureteral stone and small tumours of the kidney or collecting system.

With the increasing use and development of 3D volumetric imaging, the uses of CT have expanded to assist pathologists, coroners, and medical examiners to investigate a cadaver for clues as to the cause of death (*virtual autopsy*). These uses include CT or MRI for whole-body postmortem imaging. With these techniques, image-directed biopsies can be performed to obtain tissue for the pathologists to review. Postmortem angiography can be performed to more accurately indicate occlusive disease that may have contributed to death.

CT is usually performed in less than 10 minutes by a radiologist. If dye is used, the procedure time may be doubled because the abdomen is scanned both before and after administration of the dye. The only discomforts associated with this study are lying still on a hard table and the peripheral venipuncture. Mild nausea is common when contrast dye is used; thus, an emesis basin should be readily available. Some patients may experience a salty taste, flushing, and warmth during the dye injection.

CT can be used to aspirate fluid from the abdomen or an abdominal organ for cultures and other studies; to guide biopsy needles into areas of abdominal tumour to obtain tissue for study; and to guide catheter placement for drainage of intra-abdominal abscesses.

CT is an important part of staging and monitoring of many tumours before and after therapy. Treatment of tumours of the colon, rectum, hepatic system, breast, lungs, prostate gland, ovaries, uterus, kidneys, lymph glands, and adrenal gland commonly fails, and recurrence can be detected early with CT.

CONTRAINDICATIONS

- Allergy to shellfish
- History of adverse reactions or allergic reactions to iodinated dye
- Claustrophobia
- Pregnancy, unless the benefits of the procedure outweigh the risks of radiation exposure to the fetus
- Unstable vital signs
- Profound obesity, because the table used for CT may have weight restrictions

POTENTIAL COMPLICATIONS

- For potential complications of allergy to iodinated dye, see p. 1021.
- Acute renal failure can result from dye infusion. Adequate hydration before the procedure may reduce the likelihood of this complication (see Box 12-2, p. 1018).
- Hypoglycemia or acidosis may occur in patients who are taking metformin (Glucophage) and receive iodinated dye.

INTERFERING FACTORS

- Presence of metallic objects (e.g., hemostasis clips)
- Retained barium from previous studies
- Large amounts of fecal material or gas in the bowel
- Motion: Patients must lie still and hold their breath for several seconds as instructed; otherwise, the image can be distorted.

✓ Clinical Priorities

- Assess the patient for adverse reactions or allergic reactions to iodinated dye.
- Mild nausea is common when the contrast dye is injected. For this reason, patients are usually kept on NPO status (nothing by mouth) for 4 hours before the test.
- Most patients who are mildly claustrophobic can tolerate this study after appropriate medication with antianxiety drugs.
- Adequate hydration before the test may decrease the possibility of acute renal failure from dye infusion.
- CT can be used to guide needles into abdominal tumour for biopsy or to guide catheters into intra-abdominal abscesses for drainage.

PROCEDURE AND PATIENT CARE

Before

 Explain the procedure to the patient. Cooperation is necessary because the patient must lie still during the procedure.
- Obtain the patient's informed consent for the procedure if it is required by the institution.
- For assessment of allergy to iodinated dye, see p. 1021.

 Show the patient a picture of the CT machinery if the patient has claustrophobia. Most patients who are mildly claustrophobic can tolerate this study after appropriate medication with anti-anxiety drugs.
- Keep the patient on NPO status (nothing by mouth) for at least 4 hours before testing. However, in emergency circumstances, that requirement is not appropriate. Usually, oral contrast material is used to distinguish the gastrointestinal tract from the other abdominal organs. This is usually provided as a water-soluble contrast material that the patient drinks several hours before testing. The same contrast material can be administered rectally for improved visualization of the rectum and perirectal structures.

During

- Note the following procedural steps:
  1. The patient is taken to the radiology department and placed on the CT table (Figure 12-12).
  2. The patient then is placed in an encircling body scanner (gantry). The X-ray tube travels around the gantry, and images (scans) of the various levels of the abdomen and pelvis are

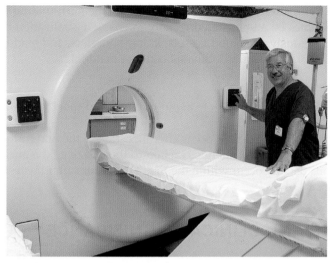

Figure 12-12 Equipment for computed tomography.

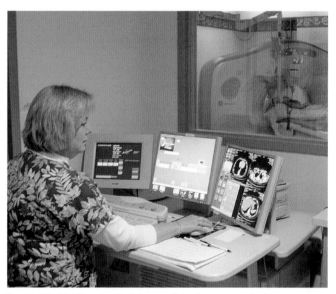

Figure 12-13 X-ray technician performing computed tomography.

obtained. Any motion will cause blurring and streaking of the final scan; therefore, the patient is asked to remain motionless during X-ray exposure. This problem is eliminated with the use of faster scanning: Data acquisition is so rapid that the entire study can be performed in less than 30 seconds. Motion and breath holding are not a problem. Television monitoring equipment allows immediate display of the computed tomographic image, which is then recorded digitally. In a separate room, the technicians manipulate the CT table and determine the level of the abdomen to be scanned (Figure 12-13). Through audio communication, the patient is instructed to hold his or her breath during X-ray exposure.
3. Better results are obtained with oral or intravenous administration of iodinated contrast dye. The gastrointestinal organs can be accurately differentiated from other abdominal organs,

and the vessels and ureters are highlighted against the surrounding structures. Contrast agent can sometimes be administered rectally to enable visualization of the pelvic organs. As described previously, the blood vessels, kidneys, ureters, and bladder are better visualized with the use of intravenous iodinated contrast material.

After

- Encourage the patient to drink fluids to avoid dye-induced renal failure and to promote dye excretion.
- Inform the patient that diarrhea may occur after ingestion of the oral contrast agent.
- Evaluate the patient for delayed allergic reaction to the dye (e.g., dyspnea, rash, tachycardia, urticaria). Reactions usually occur within the first 2 to 6 hours after the test. Treat with antihistamines or steroids.

TEST RESULTS AND CLINICAL SIGNIFICANCE

Liver

Tumour, abscess, dilation of the common bile duct: *These are evident as radiolucent (dark) filling defects in the liver parenchyma.*

Pancreas

Tumour, pseudocyst, inflammation, bleeding: *These are evident as solid or cystic masses of the pancreas.*

Spleen

Hematoma, fracture, laceration, tumour, venous thrombosis: *CT of the spleen is the most accurate method of indicating splenic trauma. Tumour, hematomas, and cysts are well demonstrated.*

Gallbladder/Biliary System

Gallstones, tumour, dilation of the common bile duct: *Gallstones are sometimes difficult to see. However, an inflammatory response around the gallbladder is evident. Dilation of the common bile duct is usually evident in the liver parenchyma.*

Kidneys

Tumour, cyst, ureteral obstruction, calculi, congenital abnormalities: *Hydronephrosis is easily evident on a computed tomographic scan. Likewise, tumour and cysts can be seen. The density of the renal mass can be computed. If the mass is the same density as water, it can safely be assumed the mass represents a cyst. CT is not as adequate as intravenous pyelography in identifying ureteral calculi or ureteral anatomic abnormalities.*

Adrenal Gland

Adenoma, cancer, pheochromocytoma, hemorrhage, myelolipoma, hyperplasia: *CT is the most accurate method of evaluating the adrenal glands. It is used not only to diagnose tumour but also to monitor neoplastic diseases that affect the adrenal glands.*

Gastrointestinal Tract

Perforation, tumour, inflammatory bowel disease, diverticulitis, appendicitis: *Although findings on CT are nonspecific as to the cause of an inflammatory mass, CT is sensitive in identification of such a mass. The location and surrounding structures aid in diagnosis of the underlying pathologic process.*

Uterus, Fallopian Tubes, Ovaries

Tumour, abscess, infection, hydrosalpinx, cyst, fibroid: *CT is accurate in evaluation of the pelvis for neoplasms of the ovaries, uterus, or cervix. Likewise, infections and abscess can be identified and drained with computed tomographic guidance.*

Prostate

Hypertrophy, tumour: *An enlarged prostate is easily seen on CT. However, benign and malignant disease cannot be differentiated.*

Retroperitoneum

Tumour, lymphadenopathy: *Sarcomas, lymphomas, and inflammation may be evident as masses of increased density in the retroperitoneum.*

Abdominal aneurysm: *The presence of an aortic aneurysm can be determined by CT. Repeated scanning can be performed to determine whether the aneurysm is expanding. A leak or rupture in the aneurysm can also be identified.*

Peritoneum

Ascites, hemoperitoneum,

Abscess: *Free and localized fluid can be seen on CT, especially if gastrointestinal contrast agent has been used. Sometimes loops of bowel can look like abscess.*

RELATED TEST

Magnetic Resonance Imaging (p. 1148). This test is less accurate than CT for identification of abdominal disease. However, it may visualize certain abdominal areas (e.g., liver and pelvis) better.

Computed Tomography, Brain (CT Scan, Brain; Computerized Axial Transverse Tomography [Catt]; Helical/Spiral CT Scan, Brain)

NORMAL FINDINGS

No evidence of disease

INDICATIONS

The first use of computed tomographic scanning was in the evaluation of the brain. The brain is well imaged with computed tomography (CT). This test is indicated when disease of the central nervous system is suspected. Specifically, CT is useful in the diagnosis of brain tumour, infarction, bleeding, and hematomas. Information about the ventricular system can also be obtained with CT. Multiple sclerosis and other degenerative abnormalities can be identified.

TEST EXPLANATION

CT of the brain consists of a computerized analysis of multiple tomographic X-ray images taken of the brain tissue at successive layers, providing a three-dimensional (3D) view of the cranial contents. The computed tomographic image provides a view from the top down. The variation in

X-Ray Studies

12

density of each tissue allows for variable penetration of the X-ray beam. An attached computer calculates the amount of X-ray penetration of each tissue, and all these values are digitally computed into shades of grey. The resulting image is then displayed digitally on a computer monitor as a photograph. The final result is a series of anatomic pictures of coronal and sagittal sections of the brain.

CT is used in the differential diagnosis of intracranial neoplasms, cerebral infarction, ventricular displacement or enlargement, cortical atrophy, cerebral aneurysms, intracranial hemorrhage and hematoma, and arteriovenous malformation. Magnetic resonance imaging (MRI; see p. 1148) is now the method of brain imaging most commonly used. However, for initial trauma evaluation and for the location and extent of subarachnoid bleeding, CT is still preferable.

Visualization of a neoplasm, previous infarction, or any pathologic process that destroys the blood-brain barrier may be enhanced by intravenous injection of an iodinated contrast dye.

Helical CT (also called *spiral* or *volume-averaging CT*) represents a marked improvement over standard CT. In helical CT, images are obtained continuously as the patient is passed through the gantry. In this way, images are produced faster and are more accurate. Because the spiral CT can image the selected area in less than 30 seconds, the entire study can be performed while patients hold their breath. Therefore, misrepresentations caused by breathing and motion are eliminated. Images are improved and scan time is reduced. This is particularly helpful in scanning uncooperative adults or children. Through volume averaging, 3D images can be created. Furthermore, when contrast material is used, the entire region can be imaged in just a few seconds after the contrast injection, thereby further improving contrast imaging.

Spiral CT is very helpful in creation of 3D images to determine accurate localization of brain tumours. Computed tomographic arteriography is performed immediately after arterial contrast injection. This technology enables the creation of 3D images of the carotid artery and its branches, which are also extremely helpful in the evaluation of cerebral vascular disease (e.g., hemorrhagic stroke).

CONTRAINDICATIONS

- History of previous adverse reactions or allergic reactions to iodinated dye
- Allergy to shellfish
- Claustrophobia
- Pregnancy, unless the benefits of the procedure outweigh the risks of radiation exposure to the fetus
- Unstable vital signs
- Profound obesity because the table used for CT may have weight restrictions

POTENTIAL COMPLICATIONS

- For potential complications of iodinated dye, see p. 1021.
- Acute renal failure can result from dye infusion. Adequate hydration before the procedure may reduce the likelihood of this complication (see Box 12-2, p. 1018).
- Hypoglycemia or acidosis may occur in patients who are taking metformin (Glucophage) and receive an iodinated dye.

PROCEDURE AND PATIENT CARE

Before

- Explain the procedure to the patient. Cooperation is necessary because the patient must lie still during the procedure.
- Obtain the patient's informed consent for the procedure if it is required by the institution.

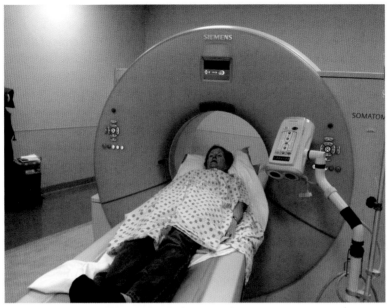

Figure 12-14 CT scan of the brain.

- Keep the patient on NPO status (nothing by mouth) for 4 hours before the study, if oral contrast medium is to be used.
- Instruct the patient to remove wigs, hairpins, clips, and partial dentures because they hamper visualization of the brain.
- For assessment of allergy to iodinated dye, see p. 1021.
- Inform the patient that he or she may hear a clicking noise as the scanner moves around the head.

During
- Note the following procedural steps:
  1. The patient lies supine on an examining table with the head resting on a platform (Figure 12-14).
  2. The scanner passes an X-ray beam through the brain from multiple angles.

After
- Encourage the patient to drink fluids to promote dye excretion and to prevent diuresis caused by the dye.
- Evaluate the patient for delayed allergic reaction to the dye (e.g., dyspnea, rash, tachycardia, urticaria). Reactions usually occur within the first 2 to 6 hours after the test. Treat with antihistamines or steroids.

TEST RESULTS AND CLINICAL SIGNIFICANCE

Intracranial neoplasm (benign or malignant): *These tumours usually are evident as soft tissue masses of increased radiolucency (darkness). Adjacent structures are distorted by the tumour's presence. Some benign tumours have calcification within.*

Cerebral infarction: *An infarction can be seen as an area of the brain that takes up no contrast material. Reduced cerebral blood flow is also noted with xenon scanning.*

X-Ray Studies

12

Ventricular displacement,

Ventricular enlargement,

Hydrocephalus: *The fluid-filled ventricles are obvious on CT as the lightest areas of the brain. Enlargement may indicate hydrocephalus, with or without increased intracranial pressure. Distortion of the ventricles may be caused by tumour or hemorrhage.*

Cortical atrophy: *Brain tissue lucency may change, and the cortical tissue appears thinner.*

Cerebral aneurysm,

Arteriovenous malformation: *Aneurysms and arteriovenous malformations are seen when intravenous contrast agent is used.*

Intracranial hemorrhage,

Hematoma,

Abscess: *These space-occupying lesions are difficult to differentiate. Serial computed tomographic scans may be helpful. In time, hemorrhage becomes more diffuse. Hematoma liquefies and becomes less radiolucent and may even calcify later. Abscess is often surrounded by edema and slowly enlarges. Epidural and subdural hematomas are evident from isodense areas of swelling that distort the nearby brain tissue.*

Multiple sclerosis: *Classic computed tomographic findings with contrast agent can indicate multiple sclerosis with a moderate degree of accuracy. White matter atrophy, periventricular plaques, and spontaneous hypolucent areas in the periventricular area are usually present.*

Brain death: *In xenon scanning, zero cerebral blood flow indicates brain death.*

RELATED TEST

Magnetic Resonance Imaging, Brain (p. 1148). MRI provides an image of the brain that is superior to CT. In most institutions, MRI has replaced CT in imaging of the central nervous system.

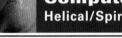

Computed Tomography, Chest (Chest CT Scan; Helical/Spiral CT Scan, Chest)

NORMAL FINDINGS

No evidence of disease

INDICATIONS

This test is used to more thoroughly evaluate suspected disease in the chest. Questionable or vague abnormalities on the routine chest X-ray can be more thoroughly evaluated with computed tomography (CT) of the chest.

TEST EXPLANATION

CT of the chest is a noninvasive but accurate X-ray procedure for diagnosing and evaluating pathologic conditions such as tumour, nodules, hematomas, parenchymal coin lesions, cysts, abscesses, pleural effusion, and enlarged lymph nodes affecting the lungs and mediastinum. Tumour and cysts of the pleura and fractures of the ribs can also be seen. When intravenous contrast material is administered, vascular structures can be identified, and aortic or other vascular abnormality can be diagnosed. With oral contrast material, the esophagus and upper gastrointestinal structures can be evaluated for tumour and other conditions. CT provides a cross-sectional view of the chest and is especially useful in detecting small differences in tissue density, thus demonstrating lesions that cannot be seen with conventional X-ray and tomography. The mediastinal structures can be visualized in a manner that cannot be equalled with conventional X-rays and tomographic scans.

The X-ray image results from the use of a body scanner (X-ray tube in a circular gantry) to deliver X-rays through the patient's chest at many different angles. The variation in density of each tissue allows for variable penetration of the X-rays. Each density is given a numeric value (*density coefficient*), and all these values are digitally computed into shades of grey. The resulting image is then displayed digitally on a computer monitor as a photograph of the anatomic area sectioned by the X-rays.

Helical CT (also called *spiral* or *volume-averaging CT*) represents a marked improvement over standard CT. In helical CT, images are obtained continuously as the patient is passed through the gantry. With the development of multidetector computed tomography (MDCT), much more image data can be obtained. With the use of multiple collimators (and multiple banks of detectors), large data images can be obtained in a very short period of time. The entire chest can be scanned in less than 30 seconds, during which most patients can hold their breath. The thicknesses of the areas imaged ("slices") are very thin (1 to 5 mm). With thin slices and rapid accession, breathing and motion distortions are minimized, and images are produced more quickly and are more accurate. This is particularly helpful in scanning uncooperative adults and children. In this computed tomographic study, 200 to 500 individual images can be obtained.

Volume imaging with three-dimensional (3D) real-time display of the volume of data allows the radiologist to visualize and analyze the data in three dimensions. With these advances in software, two-dimensional and 3D reconstructions of data can provide very accurate images of the heart (see p. 1072), lungs, chest wall, pleura, esophagus, great vessels, and soft tissue in a few seconds, allowing the radiologist to see these structures from multiple views and directions. With this new technology, *virtual bronchoscopy* and *virtual esophagoscopy* will increasingly be used in place of their invasive counterparts.

Spiral CT is considered the preferred study to identify pulmonary emboli (*computed tomographic pulmonary arteriography*). It can be performed easily and rapidly. CT of the heart (see p. 1072) can identify tiny calcifications in the coronary arteries. This finding is indicative of increased risk for an ischemic event. Pulmonary nodules are particularly well evaluated with this rapid form of CT because breathing misrepresentations are eliminated.

With the use of 3D volumetric imaging, a 3D perspective can now be added to the organs or tumours that are imaged. This provides data for *virtual angiography.*

This procedure is performed in less than 10 minutes by a radiologist. If dye is administered, the procedure time may be doubled because CT is performed before and after administration of the contrast dye. The only discomforts associated with this study are from lying still on a hard table and from the peripheral venipuncture. Mild nausea is common when contrast dye is used, and an emesis basin should be readily available. Some patients may experience a salty taste, flushing, and warmth during the dye injection.

CONTRAINDICATIONS

- History of adverse reactions or allergic reactions to iodinated dye
- Allergy to shellfish
- Claustrophobia
- Pregnancy, unless the benefits of the procedure outweigh the risks of radiation exposure to the fetus
- Unstable vital signs
- Profound obesity because the table used for CT may have weight restrictions

POTENTIAL COMPLICATIONS

- For potential complications for adverse reactions or allergic reactions to iodinated dye, see p. 1021.
- Acute renal failure can result from dye infusion. Adequate hydration before the procedure may reduce the likelihood of this complication (see Box 12-2, p. 1018).
- Hypoglycemia or acidosis may occur in patients who are taking metformin (Glucophage) and receive iodinated dye.

Clinical Priorities

- Assess the patient for adverse reactions or allergic reactions to iodinated dye.
- Mild nausea is common when the contrast dye is injected. For this reason, patients are usually kept on NPO status (nothing by mouth) for 4 hours before the test.
- Most patients who are mildly claustrophobic can tolerate this study after appropriate medication with antianxiety drugs.
- Adequate hydration before the 4-hour NPO period may decrease the possibility of acute renal failure from dye infusion.

PROCEDURE AND PATIENT CARE

Before

- Explain the procedure to the patient. Cooperation is necessary because the patient must lie still during the procedure.
- Obtain the patient's informed consent for the procedure if it is required by the institution.
- For assessment of allergy to iodinated dye, see p. 1021.
- Show the patient a picture of the CT machinery and encourage him or her to verbalize concerns about claustrophobia. Most patients who are mildly claustrophobic can tolerate this study after appropriate premedication with antianxiety drugs.
- Keep the patient on NPO status (nothing by mouth) for 4 hours before the test in the event that contrast dye is administered.

During

- Note the following procedural steps:
  1. The patient is taken to the radiology department and asked to remain motionless in a supine position.
  2. An encircling X-ray camera (body scanner) takes pictures at varying intervals and levels over the chest area. Monitor equipment allows immediate display, and the image is recorded on X-ray.
  3. Very often, intravenous dye is administered to enhance the chest image, and the X-ray studies are repeated.

After

- Encourage patients who received dye injection to drink fluids to promote dye excretion and to prevent diuresis caused by the dye.
- Evaluate the patient for delayed allergic reaction to the dye (e.g., dyspnea, rash, tachycardia, urticaria). Reactions usually occur within the first 2 to 6 hours after the test. Treat with antihistamines or steroids.

TEST RESULTS AND CLINICAL SIGNIFICANCE

Lung

Lung tumour (primary or metastatic): *This is evident as soft tissue masses in the lung fields.*

Pneumonia: *Increased lucency in the lung field indicates pneumonia or atelectatic lung.*

Pleural effusion: *Fluid in the chest wall is evident from increased lucency outside the lung fields, particularly in the costophrenic margins.*

Chronic obstructive pulmonary disease: *Increased lung space is classic for chronic obstructive pulmonary disease.*

Atelectasis: *Collapse of pulmonary alveoli is evident from white patches or lines in the lung fields.*

Tuberculosis: *Often evident in the upper lobes, chronic tuberculosis and other granulomatous diseases are usually associated with calcification.*

Lung abscess: *Lung abscess is evident as a lung mass with a hollow (radiolucent) centre. Sometimes fungus grows inside the abscess.*

Pleuritis: *Thickening of the pleura indicates pleuritis, which has a viral, bacterial, neoplastic, or other cause.*

Heart

Pericarditis,

Pericardial effusion: *These are evident as thickening of the pericardium, with or without fluid around the heart.*

Chest Wall

Soft tissue sarcoma,

Osteogenic sarcoma: *These primary tumours of the bony thorax and chest wall soft tissue are evident as masses arising from those areas of the chest.*

Fracture (ribs or thoracic spine): *This is usually associated with other chest trauma.*

Metastatic tumour to bony thorax: *Osteolytic (dark) or osteoblastic (white) nodules can be seen in the bony thorax. Breast, prostate, kidneys, and lungs are among the cancers that most commonly metastasize to the bones in this region.*

Diaphragm

Diaphragmatic or hiatal hernia: *This is evident from increased lucency in the posteroinferior mediastinum.*

Mediastinum

Aortic calcinosis: *This has the appearance of white lines indicating the walls of the calcified aorta.*

Enlarged lymph nodes: *Centrally occurring masses in the mediastinum indicate enlarged lymph nodes, usually of a neoplastic origin.*

Dilated aorta: *This is indicative of aneurysm. Dissection, if present, is obvious on computed tomographic scans of the chest.*

Thymoma,

Lymphoma,

Substernal thyroid: *These are often evident as large soft tissue masses in the anterosuperior mediastinum.*

Metastatic tumour to mediastinum: *Esophageal and upper stomach cancers may metastasize to the mediastinal lymph nodes.*

Perforation of esophagus (spontaneous [Boerhaave syndrome] or iatrogenic [after esophageal dilation]): *Meglumine diatrizoate (Gastrografin) that was previously ingested is visible free in the mediastinum.*

12 X-Ray Studies

RELATED TEST

Chest Radiography (p. 1053). This is a routine part of every thorough evaluation of the cardiopulmonary system. Although not as accurate as CT, it provides a tremendous amount of information easily.

Computed Tomography, Heart (Coronary CT Angiography, Coronary Calcium Score)

NORMAL FINDINGS

No evidence of coronary stenosis; calcium score average for age and gender

INDICATIONS

The exact role of computed tomography (CT) of the heart has not been clearly delineated. However, it holds great promise in providing information about the patency of the coronary vessels in patients who have chest pain.

TEST EXPLANATION

With the developments in multidetector computed tomography (MDCT), much data can be obtained about the heart and coronary vessels. This test is now increasingly being used to help stratify patients according to risks of future cardiac events, to instigate preventive medicinal interventions (such as statin drugs), to monitor progression of coronary vascular disease and effects of statin drugs, to evaluate chest pain, and to indicate the need for stress testing or coronary angiography.

MDCT produces fast and accurate images of the heart. With the use of multiple collimators (and multiple banks of detectors: usually 4 to 64), large data images can be obtained in a very short period of time. The entire heart can be scanned in 10 seconds, during which most patients can hold their breath. The thicknesses of the areas imaged ("slices") are very thin (1 to 5 mm). With thin slices and rapid accession, breathing and motion distortions are minimized, and images are produced more quickly and are more accurate.

With advances in software technology, two- and three-dimensional reconstructions of data can provide very accurate images of the heart and coronary vessels in a few seconds, allowing radiologists to see these structures from multiple directions. Furthermore, with shorter scanning times, when contrast material is injected intravenously, the highlighting effect can be greater, and less contrast volume is needed. The newest scanners for MDCT allow routine cardiac gating, in which the scanning is synchronized with each heartbeat, thereby eliminating further motion distortion.

MDCT is now considered the preferred study for the myocardium, cardiac chambers, cardiac valves, coronary arteries, and the great vessels, and for detection of pulmonary emboli.

Calcified atheromatous plaques can be seen and quantified (calcium score) with the use of MDCT. The assessment of coronary artery calcification has received considerable attention with regard to its potential role in the early detection of subclinical atherosclerosis and in the diagnostic workup of coronary artery disease. Coronary calcium is a surrogate marker for coronary atherosclerotic plaque. In the coronary arteries, calcifications occur almost exclusively in the context of atherosclerotic changes. Within a coronary vessel or larger segment of the vessel, the amount of coronary calcium is correlated moderately closely with the extent of atherosclerotic plaque burden.

TABLE 12-4   Categories of Agatston Lesion Scores

Agatston Lesion Score	Hounsfield Units	Risk
0	<10	Minimal
	11–100	Mild
	101–129	Mild to moderate
1	130–199	Moderate
2	200–299	Moderate
3	300–399	Moderate
4	≥400	High

Not every serious atherosclerotic coronary plaque is calcified; however, in most patients with acute coronary syndromes, coronary calcium can be detected, and the amount of calcium in these patients is substantially greater than in matched control subjects without coronary artery disease.

The *Agatston lesion score*, or the coronary calcification score, has most frequently been used to quantify the amount of coronary artery calcium on computed tomography (CT). The distribution of calcification scores in populations of individuals without known heart disease has been studied extensively. These data demonstrate that the amount of calcification increases with age. Men develop calcifications approximately 10 to 15 years earlier than women. Furthermore, in the majority of symptom-free men older than 55 years and symptom-free women older than 65 years, calcification can be detected. These data have been used to create tables that compare the amount of calcium in an individual with that in a group of people of similar age and gender (percentiles). These scores have prognostic value for determining the risk for future coronary events. A lesion score is determined on the basis of the maximal amount of coronary artery calcium as observed on CT.

Categorization of absolute Agatston scores is shown in Table 12-4.

It is well established that among individuals with Agatston scores higher than 400, the occurrence of coronary procedures (bypass, stent placement, angioplasty) is increased, as is the number of events (myocardial infarction and cardiac death) within 2 to 5 years after the test. Individuals with very high Agatston scores (>1000) have a 20% chance of suffering a myocardial infarction or cardiac death within a year. In adult patients older than 75 years, many of whom have calcification, an Agatston score above 400 is associated with a higher risk of death.

The Agatston score can vary greatly among patients with small amounts of calcium, but the variation is less pronounced for higher calcium scores (~20%). Excessively high calcium scores can inhibit the visualization of the coronary arteries. Therefore, when calcium scores are excessively high, radiopaque dye is not injected, and coronary CT cannot be carried out.

MDCT can directly and accurately visualize the coronary artery lumen after intravenous injection of a contrast agent (*coronary computed tomographic angiography*). Regular and low heart rates are a prerequisite for reliable visualization of the coronary arteries. Hence, most centres have proposed the administration of a short-acting beta blocker or a calcium-channel blocker before scanning if the heart rate exceeds 60 to 70 beats/minute. The use of sublingual nitroglycerin is also recommended in order to achieve coronary vasodilatation and maximize image quality.

CONTRAINDICATIONS

- Pregnancy
- Allergy to shellfish
- History of adverse reactions or allergic reactions to iodinated dye

X-Ray Studies

12

- Profound obesity because the table used for CT may have weight restrictions
- Unstable vital signs

POTENTIAL COMPLICATIONS

- Acute renal failure can result from dye infusion. Adequate hydration before the procedure may reduce the likelihood of this complication.
- Hypoglycemia or acidosis can occur in patients who are taking metformin (Glucophage) and receive iodinated dye.

PROCEDURE AND PATIENT CARE

Before

- Explain the procedure to the patient. The patient's cooperation is necessary because he or she must lie still during the procedure.
- Obtain the patient's informed consent for the procedure if it is required by the institution.
- Assess the patient for adverse reactions or allergic reactions to iodinated dye or shellfish.
- Assess the patient's vital signs. If the heart rate exceeds protocol levels, administer a rapid-acting beta blocker or angiotensin-converting enzyme inhibitor per protocol orders.
- Show the patient a picture of the CT machinery, and encourage the patient to verbalize concerns regarding claustrophobia. Most patients who are mildly claustrophobic can tolerate this study after appropriate premedication with antianxiety drugs.
- Keep the patient on NPO status (nothing by mouth) for 4 hours before the test.
- Inform the patient that nitroglycerine will be administered to dilate the coronary arteries and that a headache from the nitroglycerin is not uncommon.

During

- Note the following procedure for the cardiac computed tomographic scan:
  1. The patient is taken to the radiology department and asked to remain motionless in a supine position because any motion will cause blurring and streaking of the final picture.
  2. Electrocardiographic leads are applied to synchronize the electrocardiographic signal to the image data (gating).
  3. An encircling X-ray camera (body scanner) takes pictures at varying intervals and levels over the heart while the patient holds his or her breath (for ~10 seconds).
  4. Nonenhanced scanning is performed first for calcium scoring.
  5. If the calcium scoring is below threshold levels of the protocol, intravenous dye is rapidly administered through a large-bore intravenous catheter, and scanning is repeated.
  6. A fast-acting nitrate (usually nitroglycerin) is administered to maximize coronary dilatation.
- Note that a radiologist or cardiologist performs this procedure in approximately 20 minutes.
- Inform the patient that the discomforts associated with this study include lying still on a hard table and peripheral venipuncture.
- Nausea is a common sensation when contrast dye is used. An emesis basin should be readily available.
- Some patients may experience a salty taste, flushing, and warmth during the dye injection.

After

- Encourage patients to drink fluids to promote dye excretion and to prevent diuresis caused by the dye.
- See p. 1021 for appropriate interventions concerning the care of patients with adverse reactions or allergic reactions to iodinated dye.

TEST RESULTS AND CLINICAL SIGNIFICANCE

Coronary vascular disease,

Coronary vascular congenital anomalies: *The coronary vessels can be visualized completely, and any obstruction or anatomic variation is obvious.*

Ventricular aneurysm,

Aortic aneurysm or dissection,

Pulmonary emboli,

Cardiac tumour: *These anatomic abnormalities are visually obvious even before they become symptomatic.*

Myocardial scarring,

Cardiac valvular disease: *Such functional abnormalities are obvious because the normal heart muscle/ valvular motion demonstrates anatomic alterations during a cardiac cycle.*

RELATED TESTS

Cardiac Catheterization (p. 1047). This test is used to visualize the heart chambers, arteries, and great vessels. It is used most often to evaluate chest pain and to locate the region of coronary occlusion in patients with coronary occlusive disease.

Cardiac Nuclear Scanning (p. 817). This test is used to detect myocardial ischemia, infarction, cardiac wall dysfunction, and decreased ejection fraction. It is commonly used as the imaging method portion of cardiac stress testing to detect ischemia.

Cystography (Cystourethrography, Voiding, Cystography, Voiding Cystourethrography)

NORMAL FINDINGS

Normal bladder structure and function

INDICATIONS

Cystography enables X-ray visualization of the bladder. It is useful in patients with hematuria, recurrent urinary tract infections, and suspected bladder trauma.

TEST EXPLANATION

Filling the bladder with contrast material provides visualization of the bladder for X-ray study. Either fluoroscopic images or X-rays demonstrate bladder filling and collapse after emptying. Filling defects or shadows in the bladder indicate primary bladder tumour. Extrinsic compression or distortion of the bladder is seen with pelvic tumour (e.g., rectal, cervical) or hematoma (secondary to pelvic bone fractures). Extravasation of the dye is seen with traumatic rupture, perforation, and fistula of the bladder. Vesicoureteral reflux (abnormal backflow of urine from bladder to ureters), which can cause persistent or recurrent pyelonephritis, also may be demonstrated during cystography. Although the bladder is visualized during intravenous pyelography (p. 1080), primary pathologic bladder conditions are best studied by means of cystography.

A radiologist performs the study in approximately 15 to 30 minutes. This test is moderately uncomfortable if bladder catheterization is required.

12   **X-Ray Studies**

CONTRAINDICATIONS

- Urethral or bladder infection or injury, because Gram-negative sepsis can occur as a result of catheterization; existing bladder injury may be worsened by instillation of dye into the bladder

POTENTIAL COMPLICATIONS

- Urinary tract infection may result from catheter placement or instillation of contaminated contrast material.
- Adverse reactions or allergic reactions to iodinated dye are rare because the dye is not administered intravenously.

Clinical Priorities

- Assess the patient for adverse reactions or allergic reactions to iodinated dye.
- After the test, assess the patient for urinary tract infection, which may result from catheter placement or instillation of contaminated contrast material.
- Encourage the patient to drink fluids to promote dye excretion and to prevent accumulation of bacteria.

PROCEDURE AND PATIENT CARE

Before
- Explain the procedure to the patient.
- Obtain the patient's informed consent for the procedure if it is required by the institution.
- Give the patient clear liquids for breakfast on the morning of the test.
- Assure the patient that he or she will be draped to prevent unnecessary exposure.
- Insert a Foley catheter if ordered.

During
- Note the following procedural steps:
  1. The patient is taken to the radiology department and placed in the supine or lithotomy position.
  2. Unless a catheter is already present, one is placed.
  3. Approximately 300 mL (much less for children) of air or radiopaque dye is injected through the catheter into the bladder, and the catheter is clamped.
  4. X-rays are taken.
  5. If the patient is able to void, the catheter is removed and the patient is asked to urinate while films are taken of the bladder and urethra (voiding cystourethrography; Figure 12-15).
- Ensure that in male patients, a lead shield is placed over the testes to prevent irradiation of the gonads.
- The ovaries in female patients cannot be shielded without blocking bladder visualization. Ensure that female patients are not pregnant.

After
- Assess the patient for signs of urinary tract infection.
- Encourage the patient to drink fluids to promote dye excretion and to prevent accumulation of bacteria.

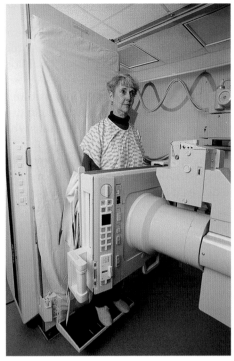

Figure 12-15 Patient positioned for voiding cystourethrography.

TEST RESULTS AND CLINICAL SIGNIFICANCE

Bladder tumour: *Primary cancers of the bladder are evident as filling defects (radiolucent shadow) in the bladder.*

Pelvic tumour or hematoma: *Any mass that distorts the pelvic anatomy is seen as external compression of the dye-filled bladder.*

Bladder trauma: *Laceration or perforation of the bladder is evident by the finding of dye outside the bladder. This is usually best demonstrated on the postvoid film.*

Vesicoureteral reflux: *Reflux of urine or dye from the bladder into the ureter is obvious with distension of the bladder with dye.*

Hysterosalpingography (Uterotubography, Uterosalpingography, Hysterogram)

NORMAL FINDINGS

Patent fallopian tubes
No defects in uterine cavity

INDICATIONS

This test is part of a workup for infertility. The result can indicate patency or obstruction of the fallopian tubes.

X-Ray Studies

12

TEST EXPLANATION

In hysterosalpingography, the uterine cavity and fallopian tubes are visualized radiographically after the injection of contrast material through the cervix. Uterine tumour, intrauterine adhesions, and developmental anomalies can be seen. Obstruction of the fallopian tubes caused by internal scarring, tumour, infection, or kinking also can be detected. A possible therapeutic effect of this test is that passage of dye through the tubes may clear mucus plugs, straighten kinked tubes, or break up adhesions. This test also may be used to document adequacy of surgical tubal ligation. Its main purpose is in the evaluation of infertility to determine whether there is any obstruction of the fallopian tubes.

This procedure is performed in approximately 15 to 30 minutes by a physician. The patient may feel occasional, transient menstrual-type cramping and may have shoulder pain caused by subphrenic irritation from the dye as it leaks into the peritoneal cavity.

CONTRAINDICATIONS

- Infections of the vagina, cervix, or fallopian tubes, because of risk of extending the infection
- Uterine bleeding, because contrast material may enter the open blood vessels; furthermore, clots may be pushed out of the uterus and into the fallopian tubes, causing obstruction
- Pregnancy, because contrast material may induce abortion

POTENTIAL COMPLICATIONS

- Infection of the endometrium (endometritis)
- Infection of the fallopian tubes (salpingitis)
- Uterine perforation
- Allergic reaction to iodinated dye or shellfish (rare because the dye is not administered intravenously)

INTERFERING FACTORS

- Fecal material or gas in the bowel may obscure visualization.
- Tubal spasm or excessive traction may cause the appearance of a stricture in a normal fallopian tube.
- Excessive traction may displace adhesions, thereby making tubes appear normal.

 Clinical Priorities

- Assess the patient for allergic reactions to iodinated dye.
- This test is not performed if pregnancy is suspected, because the contrast material might induce abortion.
- After the test, evaluate the patient for signs and symptoms of infection (e.g., fever, increased pulse rate, pain).

PROCEDURE AND PATIENT CARE

Before

- Explain the procedure to the patient. Ask the patient when she had her most recent menstrual period. If pregnancy is suspected, the test is not performed.
- Obtain the patient's informed consent for the procedure if it is required by the institution.
- Assess the patient for allergy to iodinated dye or shellfish.
- Instruct the patient to take laxatives the night before the test, if they are ordered.
- Administer enemas or suppositories on the morning of the test, if they are ordered.
- Administer sedatives (e.g., midazolam [Versed]) or antispasmodics, if they are ordered, before the test.
- Inform the patient that no food or fluid restrictions are required.
- Inform the patient that cramping and dizziness may occur after the study.

During

- Note the following procedural steps:
  1. A plain X-ray of the abdomen is often obtained before the test to ensure that preparation adequately eliminated gastrointestinal gas and feces.
  2. After voiding, the patient is placed on the fluoroscopy table in the lithotomy position.
  3. A speculum is inserted into the vagina, and the cervix is visualized and cleansed.
  4. Contrast material is injected during fluoroscopy, and X-rays are obtained.
  5. More dye is injected so that the entire upper genital tract (uterus and fallopian tubes) can be filled.
  6. This test can be considered satisfactorily performed only if the uterus and the tubes are distended to their maximal capacity or fluid flows through the fallopian tubes.

After

- Inform the patient that a vaginal discharge (sometimes bloody) may be present for 1 or 2 days after the test. A perineal sanitary pad should be worn.
- Evaluate the patient for delayed allergic reaction to the dye (e.g., dyspnea, rash, tachycardia, urticaria). Reactions usually occur within the first 2 to 6 hours after the test. Treat symptoms with antihistamines or steroids.
- Evaluate the patient for signs and symptoms of infection (e.g., fever, increased pulse rate, pain). Instruct the patient to call her physician and report these symptoms if they occur.

TEST RESULTS AND CLINICAL SIGNIFICANCE

Uterine tumour (e.g., leiomyoma, cancer) or polyps: *Filling defects in the uterus may indicate tumour.*

Developmental anomaly of the uterus (e.g., uterus bicornis): *The anatomy of the uterus can be well visualized and evaluated.*

Intrauterine adhesions: *Usually resulting from previous infection, these adhesions within the uterus can cause infertility.*

Uterine fistula: *Usually of traumatic origin (iatrogenic [e.g., during dilation and curettage]), a fistula is evident from extravasation of dye from the uterus.*

Obstruction, kinking, or twisting of the fallopian tubes secondary to adhesions: *This is indicated by stenosis or complete obstruction. Fertility is unlikely unless tubal patency is re-established.*

Extrauterine pregnancy: *Early tubal pregnancy can be demonstrated with this study, but there are better and easier ways to determine tubal pregnancy (e.g., CT of the pelvis [p. 1059]).*

Tumour of the fallopian tubes: *Tumours are evident as tubal filling defects.*

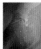

Intravenous Pyelography (IVP, Excretory Urography [Eug], Intravenous Urography [Iug, Ivu])

NORMAL FINDINGS

Normal size, shape, and position of the kidneys, renal pelvis, ureters, and bladder
Normal kidney excretory function, as evidenced by the length of time for contrast material to pass through the kidneys

INDICATIONS

Intravenous pyelography (IVP) is the radiologic test most commonly used to evaluate the urinary system because it provides much information about the kidneys, ureters, bladder, and prostate. It is indicated in patients with any of the following conditions:

- Pain compatible with the presence of urinary stones
- Blood in the urine
- Proposed pelvic surgery, to locate the ureters
- Trauma to the urinary system
- Urinary outlet obstruction
- Suspected kidney tumour

Age-Related Concerns

- In pediatric patients, fluid restrictions should be modified on the basis of age and clinical symptoms.
- Older adults are particularly vulnerable to compromised renal function. Fluid restrictions are modified for older adult patients and for patients with chronic dehydration (e.g., from chronic diarrhea).
- Because of the combination of fasting and catharsis necessary for test preparation, older adults and debilitated patients are at high risk for weakness and injury. These patients should ambulate only with assistance.

TEST EXPLANATION

IVP is a radiologic study in which radiopaque contrast material is used to visualize the kidneys, renal pelvis, ureters, and bladder. The dye is injected intravenously, filtered in the kidney by the glomeruli, and passes through the renal tubules. Images obtained at set intervals over the next 30 minutes show passage of the dye through the kidneys and ureters and into the bladder.

If a pathologic condition is suspected within the kidneys, X-rays are taken sooner in the study to best visualize the kidneys. This is sometimes referred to as the "renal phase" of IVP. If disease in the collecting system is suspected, films are taken later to better visualize the calyces, ureters, and bladder. This is sometimes called the "collecting phase" of IVP.

If the artery leading to one of the kidneys is blocked, the dye cannot enter that part of the renal system, and the artery is not visualized. If the artery is partially blocked, visualization of the contrast material takes longer than expected.

With primary glomerular disease (e.g., glomerulonephritis), the glomerular filtrate is reduced, which causes a reduction in the quantity of dye filtered. Therefore, more time is required for enough dye to enter the kidney to enable renal opacification. As a result, kidney visualization is delayed. This helps the examiner estimate renal function.

TABLE 12-5	Tests for Visualization of the Urinary System
Portion of the Urinary System	**Test**
Kidney	Computed tomography, magnetic resonance imaging
Renal pelvis and ureters	Intravenous pyelography or retrograde pyelography
Bladder	Cystography or cystoscopy
Urethra	Urethrography or cystoscopy

Defects in dye filling of the kidney can indicate renal tumour or cysts. Often, intrinsic and extrinsic tumours, stones, and scarring can partially or completely obstruct the flow of dye through the collecting system (pelvis, ureters, bladder). If the obstruction has been of sufficient duration, the collecting system proximal to the obstruction is dilated (hydronephrosis). Retroperitoneal and pelvic tumour, aneurysms, and enlarged lymph nodes also can produce extrinsic compression and distortions of the opacified collecting system.

IVP is used to assess the effect of trauma on the urinary system. Renal hematomas distort the renal contour. Renal artery laceration is suggested by nonopacification of one kidney. Laceration of the kidneys, pelvis, ureters, or bladder often causes urine leaks, which are identified from dye extravasation from the urinary system.

IVP is used to assess for congenital absence or malposition of the kidneys. Horseshoe kidneys (connection of the two kidneys), double ureters, and pelvic kidneys are typical congenital abnormalities.

To a large degree, computed tomography of the abdomen (p. 1059) has replaced the use of IVP. Table 12-5 lists diagnostic tests used to evaluate the urinary system.

CONTRAINDICATIONS

- History of previous adverse reactions or allergic reactions to iodinated dye
- Allergy to shellfish; premedication with prednisone and diphenhydramine (Benadryl) may be ordered
- Severe dehydration, which can cause renal shutdown and failure; geriatric patients are particularly vulnerable
- Renal insufficiency, as evidenced by a blood urea nitrogen value greater than 40 mg/dL, because the iodinated nephrotoxic dye can worsen kidney function
- Multiple myeloma, because the iodinated nephrotoxic dye can worsen renal function
- Pregnancy, unless the benefits of the procedure outweigh the risks of radiation exposure to the fetus

POTENTIAL COMPLICATIONS

- For potential complications of iodinated dye, see p. 1021.
- Infiltration of contrast dye can occur. This is avoided by ensuring patency of the intravenous line. In the event of infiltration, a local injection of hyaluronidase may be given to hasten absorption of iodine and resolution of the reaction.
- Renal failure can be caused by the dye. This most often occurs in older patients who already have chronic dehydration (see Box 12-2, p. 1018).
- Hypoglycemia or acidosis may occur in patients who are taking metformin (Glucophage) and receive iodinated dye.

INTERFERING FACTORS

- Fecal material, gas, or barium in the bowel may obscure visualization of the renal system.
- Abnormal renal function studies may prevent adequate visualization of the urinary tract.
- Retained barium from previous studies may obscure visualization. If studies with barium (e.g., BE study) are to be performed, they should be scheduled after IVP.

Clinical Priorities

- Assess the patient for adverse reactions or allergic reactions to iodinated dye.
- Evaluate for adequacy of renal function (blood urea nitrogen/creatinine) before IVP.
- Barium studies, if ordered, should be scheduled after IVP.

PROCEDURE AND PATIENT CARE

Before

- Explain the procedure to the patient. Inform the patient that several X-rays will be obtained over 30 minutes.
- Obtain the patient's informed consent for the procedure if it is required by the institution.
- For assessment of allergy to iodinated dye, see p. 1021.
- Give the patient a laxative (e.g., castor oil) or a cathartic, as ordered, the evening before the test.
- Inform the patient of the required food and fluid restrictions. Some institutions prefer abstinence from solid foods for 8 hours before testing; some allow a clear-liquid breakfast on the test day. For pediatric, older, and debilitated patients, fasting times are ordered on an individual basis.
- Ensure adequate hydration (intravenous or oral) before and after the test, to prevent dye-induced renal failure.
- In patients receiving high rates of intravenous fluids, infusion rates may be decreased for several hours before the study to increase the concentration of the dye within the urinary system.
- Assess blood urea nitrogen and creatinine levels. Abnormal renal function could deteriorate as a result of the dye injection.
- Give the patient an enema or suppository on the morning of the study, if it is ordered.
- If any barium studies are ordered, schedule them after completion of IVP.

During

- Note the following procedural steps:
  1. The patient is taken to the radiology department and placed in the supine position.
  2. An X-ray image of the abdomen (kidney, ureter, and bladder [KUB]; see next test) is taken to ensure that no residual stool obscures visualization of the renal system. This also helps screen for calculi in the renal collecting system.
  3. A peripheral intravenous line is started (if not in place), and a contrast dye (e.g., Hypaque, Renografin) is infused.
  4. Radiographs are obtained at specific times (usually at 1, 5, 10, 15, 20, and 30 minutes, and sometimes longer after dye administration) to follow the course of the dye from the cortex of the kidney to the bladder.
  5. Computed tomography may be performed to identify a mass.
  6. The patient is taken to the bathroom and asked to void.
  7. A postvoiding film is obtained to visualize the empty bladder.

- On occasion, it is necessary to partially occlude the ureters temporarily to obtain a better film of the collecting system in the upper part of the ureters. This is done by compressing the abdomen with an inflatable rubber tube wrapped tightly around the abdomen slightly below the umbilicus.
- The test is performed in approximately 45 minutes by a radiologist.
- Inform the patient that the dye injection often causes transient flushing of the face, a feeling of warmth, a salty taste in the mouth, or even transient nausea. Initial intravenous needle placement and lying on a hard X-ray table are the only other discomforts associated with IVP.

Home Care Responsibilities

- After the test, patients must drink a lot of fluids to re-establish their normal state of hydration.
- Instruct the patient to report decreased urine output, which may be an indication of impending renal failure.

After

- Maintain adequate oral or intravenous hydration for several hours after IVP to counteract fluid depletion caused by the test preparation procedures.
- Assess urinary output. Decreased output may be an indication of renal failure.
- Evaluate older and debilitated patients for weakness, because of the combination of fasting and catharsis necessary for test preparation. Instruct these patients to ambulate only with assistance.
- Evaluate the patient for delayed allergic reaction to dye (e.g., dyspnea, rash, tachycardia, urticaria). Reactions usually occur within the first 2 to 6 hours after the test. Treat with antihistamines or steroids.

TEST RESULTS AND CLINICAL SIGNIFICANCE

Pyelonephritis or glomerulonephritis: *Primary renal disease is evident usually as reduced opacification of the kidney with dye. This is because it takes a long time for enough dye to be filtered to the renal system to opacify the kidney.*

Kidney tumour (benign or malignant),

Renal hematoma, laceration,

Cyst or polycystic disease of the kidney: *These are usually evident as a radiolucent (dark) filling defect in the kidney parenchyma. Ultrasonography of the kidney (p. 896) helps diagnose cysts.*

Congenital abnormality of the urologic tract: *Congenital anomalies may include absence of a kidney or altered shape, size, or location of a kidney. The collecting system can be duplicated, with more than one ureter per kidney. The bladder can be divided by a congenital septum into two small bladders.*

Renal or ureteral calculi: *Calculi (stones) are evident as radiolucent filling defects that can obstruct the ureters.*

Trauma to the kidneys, ureters, or bladder: *Injury may be evident from leakage of dye from the injured organ. Hematomas appear as filling defects or radiolucent shadows.*

Tumour of the collecting system: *This can partially or completely obstruct the collecting system.*

Hydronephrosis: *This condition results from prolonged obstruction of the collecting system distal to the hydronephrotic area.*

Extrinsic compression of the collecting system (e.g., caused by tumour, aneurysm): *Nonurologic tumours or other masses can distort or obstruct the ureters or bladder.*

Bladder tumour: *This is seen as a radiolucent (dark shadow) filling defect in the bladder.*

Prostate enlargement: *This is evident as an extrinsic protrusion into the base of the bladder and inadequate emptying of the bladder because of outlet obstruction.*

RELATED TESTS

Computed Tomography, Abdomen (p. 1059). This test allows better visualization of the kidneys. The ureters are better studied with IVP.

Cystography (p. 1075). Study of the bladder after placement of radiopaque dye directly into the bladder. In this study, the dye is more concentrated, and more information concerning the bladder can be obtained.

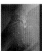 **Kidney, Ureter, and Bladder Radiography** (KUB, Flat Plate of the Abdomen, Plain Film of the Abdomen, Scout Film)

NORMAL FINDINGS

No evidence of calculi
Normal gastrointestinal gas pattern

INDICATIONS

This screening X-ray study is used to rapidly evaluate the abdomen in patients with abdominal pain or trauma. It can demonstrate pathologic conditions of the urinary or gastrointestinal system.

TEST EXPLANATION

The kidney, ureter, and bladder (KUB) X-ray is an unenhanced image of the abdomen. It is often referred to as a *plain image* or *scout image.* The KUB view is similar to the supine view on an obstruction series (see p. 1095), and the study can be performed to demonstrate the size, shape, location, and any malformations of the kidneys and bladder. The KUB study can also be used to identify calculi in these organs and in the ureters. This is often one of the first studies performed to diagnose other intra-abdominal diseases, such as intestinal obstruction, soft tissue masses, and a ruptured viscus (Figure 12-16). The KUB study is useful in detecting abnormal accumulations of gas within the gastrointestinal tract and identifying ascites. No contrast medium is used for this study.

CONTRAINDICATIONS

- Pregnancy

INTERFERING FACTORS

- Barium retained from previous studies can obscure visualization.

 Clinical Priorities

- This test is also called a *plain image* or *scout image* of the abdomen.
- This test involves no contrast dye.
- This is often one of the first tests used in the evaluation of abdominal problems.
- This test should be scheduled before any barium studies.

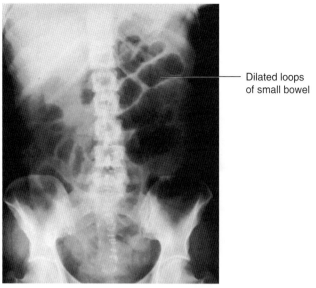

Dilated loops
of small bowel

Figure 12-16 Kidney, ureter, and bladder (KUB) X-ray of abdomen depicts multiple, somewhat dilated loops of small bowel, which is consistent with postoperative ileus.

PROCEDURE AND PATIENT CARE

Before

- Explain the procedure to the patient.
- Inform the patient that no fasting or sedation is required.
- Schedule this study before any barium studies.
- In male patients, the testicles should be shielded with a lead apron to prevent their exposure to radiation.
- In female patients, the ovaries cannot be shielded because of their proximity to the kidneys, ureters, and bladder. Ensure that the patient is not pregnant.
- Inform the patient that no discomfort is associated with this study.

During

- In the radiology department, the patient is placed in the supine position. Radiographs of the patient's abdomen are obtained (Figure 12-17).
- Note that the KUB study is performed in a few minutes by a radiologic technologist, and the results are interpreted by a radiologist.

After

- Inform the patient that results are available in approximately 1 hour.
- If intravenous pyelography or gastrointestinal studies are indicated, schedule them after completion of the KUB study.

TEST RESULTS AND CLINICAL SIGNIFICANCE

Calculi: *A calcified stone in the area of the KUB images where the ureters would be is indicative of ureteral calculi. Nearly 80% of ureteral stones can be seen on KUB images.*

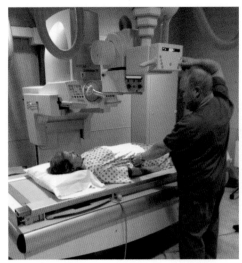

Figure 12-17 Patient positioned for a kidney, ureter, and bladder (KUB) X-ray.

Abnormal accumulation of bowel gas: *Abnormal accumulation of bowel gas can indicate intestinal obstruction or paralytic ileus.*

Ascites: *The classic "ground glass" appearance of the entire abdomen on the KUB images indicates peritoneal effusion.*

Soft tissue masses: *Large soft tissue masses can be seen surprisingly well on this plain X-ray without use of any contrast material.*

Ruptured viscus: *Free air (i.e., air outside the bowel but inside the abdomen) is indicative of a perforated viscus.*

Congenital anomalies (e.g., location, size, and number of kidneys): *Because the kidneys can be well visualized with KUB imaging, anomalies are fairly easily detected.*

Organomegaly or bladder distension: *An enlarged liver or spleen is seen as a large soft tissue mass in the right or left upper quadrant, respectively. A large soft tissue mass in the midline or pelvis is usually a distended bladder.*

RELATED TEST

Obstruction Series (p. 1095). This study includes a KUB image as part of the series of plain X-rays obtained to evaluate abdominal pain.

 Mammography (Mammogram)

NORMAL FINDINGS
Negative or benign findings

INDICATIONS
Mammography enables detection of breast cancers, benign tumour, and cysts before they are even palpable. Mammography can be performed for screening or diagnostic purposes.

Screening Mammography Recommendations

♣ **Canadian Breast Cancer Foundation and Canadian Cancer Society Screening Guidelines**.
- Women 40 years of age and older should discuss the benefits and risks of early screening with their physician or nurse practitioner.
- Women between 50 and 69 years of age should undergo mammography every 2 years.
- Women older than 70 years should discuss a screening program with their physician or nurse practitioner.
- Women whose risk for breast cancer is higher than average should talk with their health care providers about whether and how often to undergo mammography before the age of 40 years. Risk factors that increase the risk for developing breast cancer include the following:
  - Being female
  - Personal history of breast cancer
  - Family history: A woman's chance of developing breast cancer increases if her mother, sister, or daughter has a history of breast cancer (especially if it was diagnosed before the patient was 50 years of age).
  - History of carcinoma in situ
  - Certain breast changes on biopsy: A diagnosis of atypical hyperplasia (a noncancerous condition in which cells have abnormal features and are increased in number) or lobular carcinoma in situ (abnormal cells found in the lobules of the breast) increases a woman's risk of breast cancer. Women who have had two or more breast biopsies for other benign conditions also have an increased chance of developing breast cancer. This risk is increased as a result of the condition that led to the biopsies, not because of the biopsies themselves.
  - Genetic alterations (changes): Specific alterations in the *BRCA1* and *BRCA2* genes (see p. 1139).
  - Radiation therapy ("X-ray therapy"): Women who received radiation therapy to the chest (including the breasts) before 30 years of age are at an increased risk of developing breast cancer throughout their lives. This includes women treated for Hodgkin's lymphoma.
  - Reproductive history of early menstruation, late menopause, and late pregnancy or no pregnancies
  - Hormone replacement therapy or oral contraceptive ("the pill")
  - Diethystilbestrol
  - Benign breast conditions such as a typical hyperplasia
  - Dense breast
  - Obesity

When to Stop Screening

As long as a woman is in reasonably good health and would be a candidate for treatment, she should continue to be screened with mammography. However, if an individual has an estimated life expectancy of less than 3 to 5 years, severe functional limitations, or multiple or severe comorbid conditions that are likely to limit life expectancy, it may be appropriate to consider cessation of screening. Chronologic age alone should not be the reason for the cessation of regular screening.

Diagnostic Mammography

- Women older than 35 years should undergo diagnostic mammography if they have breast symptoms such as a palpable nodule or lump, breast skin thickening or indentation, nipple discharge or retraction, erosive sore of the nipple, or breast pain.

TEST EXPLANATION

Mammography is an X-ray examination of the breast. Through careful interpretation of these X-rays, the radiologist can identify cancers (Figure 12-18). In many cases, breast cancers can be detected before they become palpable. It is believed that early detection of breast cancer may improve the rate of patient survival. Radiographic signs of breast cancer include fine, stippled, clustered calcifications (white specks on the breast X-rays); a poorly defined, spiculated mass; asymmetric density; and skin thickening.

Although mammography is not a substitute for breast biopsy, results are reliable and accurate when interpreted by a skilled radiologist. The rate of detection of breast cancer with mammography is higher than 85%. This means that fewer than 15% of breast cancers are missed at mammography. Cancers that are missed are those in areas of the breast that are not well imaged by the X-ray (e.g., the high axillary tail of the breast), those in women with very dense breast tissue, or those that are too small to identify. Nearly 70% of breast cancers are not palpable and are detected only with mammography. Mammography also can detect other diseases of the breast, such as acute suppurative mastitis, abscess, fibrocystic changes, cysts, benign tumour (e.g., fibroadenoma), and intraglandular lymph nodes.

A woman receives minimal radiation exposure during mammography (~0.5 rad per view). Female patients younger than 25 years are most susceptible to the neoplastic effects of ionizing radiation; therefore, mammography is rarely recommended in young women. Most mammographic studies include two views of each breast (in the cranial-to-caudal dimension and in the medial-to-lateral dimension). It is important to inform the woman that follow-up testing is not uncommon. If the radiologist sees something that should be more thoroughly evaluated with magnified views, deeper views, or ultrasonography, the patient may be called back for further testing.

Digital mammography is a method of breast imaging in which images are captured digitally and viewed on a computer monitor, which enables the radiologist to manipulate the contrast and brightness of the images so as to miss fewer cancers. Portions of the breast image can be magnified. Results of mammography can only suggest a diagnosis of breast cancer. The diagnosis must be confirmed with microscopic histologic review of a biopsy specimen.

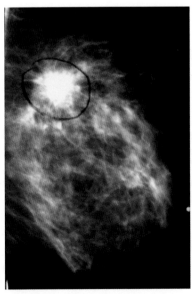

Figure 12-18 Oblique mammogram demonstrating a cancer, encircled in *red.*

Mammography is performed in approximately 10 minutes by a certified radiologic technologist. The X-rays are interpreted by an accredited radiologist. Moderate discomfort is associated with mammography. This is caused by the pressure required to compress the breast tissue while the X-rays are obtained. In patients with tender breasts, this may be especially painful. ♣ The Canadian Association of Radiologists supports the recommendations of the American College of Radiology for the standardization of mammography reporting as follows:

- Category 1: Negative
- Category 2: Benign findings noted
- Category 3: Probably benign findings; short-term follow-up is suggested
- Category 4: Suspect findings; further evaluation is indicated
- Category 5: Cancer is highly suspected
- Category 6: Known breast cancer
- Category 0: Abnormality noted for which more imaging is recommended

Mammography can also be used to locate a mammographically identified (i.e., not palpable) lesion for biopsy. The most common method is *preoperative mammographic localization* of the abnormality, followed by open biopsy. For this procedure, the patient is taken to the mammography room after having received preoperative preparation and instruction. A grid printed on transparent adhesive material is attached to the breast containing the abnormality. Craniocaudal and direct lateral views are obtained. With the grid still in place, the radiologist numbs the skin and places a needle into the abnormal area. A wire is then disengaged through the needle into the breast. Repeated mammograms are obtained. The patient is then taken to the operating room. After induction of appropriate anaesthesia, an incision is made along the wire to the abnormal tissue, which is then removed for biopsy.

Nonoperative *stereotactic biopsy* with a biopsy device is the least invasive manner of obtaining tissue from a nonpalpable mammographic abnormality. For this procedure, the patient is placed prone on a special table. Through a hole in the table, the breast is placed in a mammography machine under the table (Figure 12-19). The mammography machine is connected to a computer that

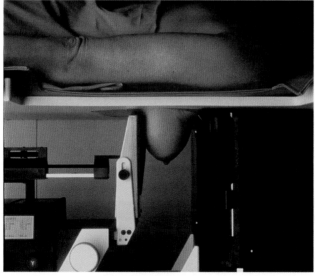

Figure 12-19 Stereotactic breast biopsy. The patient is positioned on the table with the breast pendulous through aperture. The breast is compressed with the target lesion centred in the biopsy window.

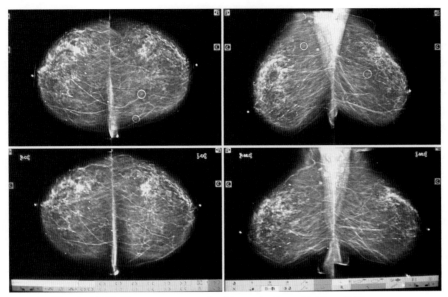

Figure 12-20 The mammography image is placed in the digitizer, and coordinates of the breast lesion are determined and displayed. These coordinates guide the needle to the precise location of the lesion, and the aspirate is drawn for biopsy.

can identify the exact location of the mammographic abnormality (Figure 12-20). The machine positions the biopsy device in alignment with the lesion. When the biopsy equipment is centred over the lesion, the needle is inserted into the lesion, and specimens are obtained for biopsy. No surgery or sutures are required. Only minimal pain is experienced, because a breast in compression has little skin pain sensation.

CONTRAINDICATIONS

- Pregnancy, unless the benefits of the procedure outweigh the risks of radiation exposure to the fetus
- Age younger than 25 years

INTERFERING FACTORS

- Talcum powder and antiperspirants give the impression of calcifications within the breast.
- Jewellery worn around the neck can preclude total visualization of the breast.
- Breast augmentation implants can inhibit total visualization of the breast. The implants are displaced, however, and the native breast tissue is imaged.
- Previous breast surgery can distort mammographic findings.

 Clinical Priorities

- The combination of mammography and close physical examination provides the best approach for detecting breast cancer at its earlier stage.
- During mammography, radiation exposure is minimal.
- Some discomfort may be experienced during breast compression. Compression is necessary for visualization of the breast.

PROCEDURE AND PATIENT CARE

Before

𝒳 Explain the procedure to the patient.

𝒳 Inform the patient that some discomfort may be experienced during breast compression. Compression allows better visualization of the breast tissue. Assure the patient that the breast will not be harmed by compression. Premenstrual women with very sensitive breasts can choose to schedule mammography 1 to 2 weeks after their menses to reduce any discomfort caused by compression required for the mammogram.

𝒳 Inform the patient that no fasting is required.

𝒳 Explain to the patient that the radiation dose used during the test is minimal.

𝒳 Instruct the patient to disrobe above the waist and put on an X-ray gown.

𝒳 Instruct the patient to report the location of any symptom or lump she may have noted.

• Markers are placed on any skin bump that may be interpreted to an abnormality on the X-ray image.

During

• Note the following procedural steps:
  1. The patient is taken to the radiology department and stands in front of a mammography machine.
  2. One breast is placed on the X-ray plate.
  3. The X-ray cone is brought down on top of the breast to compress it slowly between the broadened cone and the X-ray plate (Figure 12-21).
  4. The X-ray is exposed for a craniocaudal view.
  5. The X-ray plate is turned approximately 45 degrees medially and placed on the inner aspect of the breast.
  6. The broadened cone is brought in medially and again slowly compresses the breast. A mediolateral view is obtained.
  7. On occasion, direct lateral (90-degree) or magnified spot views are obtained to more clearly visualize an area of concern. Elongated or small cones are applied to the X-ray tube to enhance visualization of a specific area of the breast.

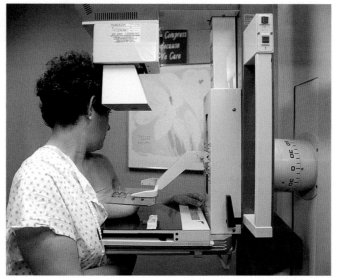

Figure 12-21 Craniocaudal positioning for mammography.

After

- Take the opportunity to instruct the patient in breast self-examination.
- If additional views are required, provide emotional support to the patient in her concerns. It is always frightening if further views are required. These additional views usually include spot magnified views, which allow the radiologist to better visualize an area of the breast.

TEST RESULTS AND CLINICAL SIGNIFICANCE

Breast cancer: *This can be evident as a radiodense (white) stellate or spiculated mass, a cluster of calcifications, or vague asymmetric radiodensity. When cancer invades the skin, the skin appears thickened. Also, the nipple can appear inverted if a subareolar cancer exists.*

Benign tumour (e.g., fibroadenoma): *Benign tumours are usually well-rounded masses with discrete borders. Sometimes fibroadenomas can degenerate, and calcifications can develop within. Colloid or medullary cancers can appear similarly well rounded.*

Breast cyst: *Cysts appear as well-rounded masses with discrete borders. Ultrasonography of the breast demonstrates the cysts to be fluid filled.*

Fibrocystic disease: *This is the most common breast finding. Nearly every woman has some degree of fibrocystic disease. On mammograms, this is seen as a vague asymmetric radiodensity (white). It can also be evident as calcifications.*

Breast abscess,

Suppurative mastitis: *The mammographic findings of infection are increased thickness of the skin, with increased radiodensity of the breast tissue.*

RELATED TESTS

Breast Ultrasonography (p. 901). An important adjunct to mammography, ultrasonography can differentiate between cystic and solid lesions.

Magnetic Resonance Imaging (p. 1148). Although MRI is a more accurate test for breast cancer, the high rate of false-positive results renders it too expensive for screening.

Myelography (Myelogram)

NORMAL FINDINGS

Normal spinal canal

INDICATIONS

Myelography provides X-ray visualization of the subarachnoid space of the spinal canal. The spinal cord, nerve roots, and surrounding meninges can be seen. This test is indicated in patients with severe back pain or localized neurologic signs that suggest that the canal is the location of disease (e.g., herniated lumbar disc).

TEST EXPLANATION

When radiopaque dye or air is placed into the subarachnoid space of the spinal canal, the contents of the canal can be fluoroscopically outlined. Spinal cord tumour, meningeal tumour, metastatic spinal tumour, herniated intervertebral discs, and arthritic bone spurs can be readily detected with this study. These lesions appear as spinal canal narrowing or as varying degrees of obstruction to the flow of the dye column within the canal. The entire canal (from lumbar to cervical areas) can be examined. Because this test is usually performed with lumbar puncture (see p. 676), it entails all the potential complications of that procedure.

Various types of contrast material can be used for myelography. Iophendylate (Pantopaque) is used as the *oil-based* medium. A *water-soluble* contrast material, metrizamide (Amipaque), is also used for myelography. This dye is absorbed by the blood and excreted by the kidneys. Another water-soluble contrast agent, iohexol (Omnipaque), is associated with a significantly lower risk of toxicity to the central nervous system than is metrizamide and is now more routinely used.

After the procedure, the patient's head and thorax should be elevated 30 to 50 degrees for approximately 6 to 8 hours to reduce upward dispersion of the dye and to prevent contact of the water-soluble agent with the cerebral meninges, which could precipitate a seizure. Bed rest for up to 6 hours may be ordered.

Magnetic resonance imaging of the spine (see p. 1148) has replaced most use of myelography.

Clinical Priorities

- Myelography can be performed with different types of contrast materials. Iophendylate (Pantopaque) is an oil-based medium; metrizamide (Amipaque) and iohexol (Omnipaque) are water-soluble contrast media. Air can also be used as the contrast medium in myelography.
- To avoid herniation of the brain, this test is contraindicated in patients with increased intracranial pressure.

CONTRAINDICATIONS

- Multiple sclerosis, because exacerbation may be precipitated by myelography
- Increased intracranial pressure, because lumbar puncture may cause herniation of the brain
- Infection near the lumbar puncture site, because this may precipitate bacterial meningitis
- Allergy to shellfish
- Adverse reactions or allergic reactions to iodinated dye

POTENTIAL COMPLICATIONS

- Headache
- Meningitis
- Herniation of the brain
- Seizures
- Hypoglycemia or acidosis in patients who are taking metformin (Glucophage) and receive iodinated dye
- Complications of iodinated dye (see p. 1021).

PROCEDURE AND PATIENT CARE

Before

 Explain the procedure to the patient.
- Obtain the patient's written, informed consent for this procedure.
- For assessment of allergy to iodinated dye, see p. 1021.

📋 Explain to the patient that he or she must lie very still during the procedure.

• Food and fluid restrictions vary according to the type of dye used. Check with the radiology department for specific restrictions.

📋 Inform the patient that he or she will be tilted into an upside-down position on the table so that the dye can properly fill the spinal canal and provide adequate visualization of the desired area.

During

• Note the following procedural steps:
    1. Lumbar puncture (see p. 676) or cisternal puncture is performed.
    2. A 15-mL sample of cerebrospinal fluid is withdrawn, and 15 mL or more of radiopaque dye is injected into the spinal canal.
    3. The patient is placed prone on the tilt table, with the head tilted down.
    4. Representative X-ray images are obtained.
    5. After myelography is performed, the needle is removed, and a dressing is applied.

After

• Note that nursing interventions after the procedure depend on the type of contrast agent used.
• After myelography, safe positioning of the patient's head is determined by the type of dye used in the procedure.
• See the section on lumbar puncture (p. 676) for appropriate postprocedure care.

Home Care Responsibilities

• Encourage the patient to drink fluids to promote dye excretion and to replace cerebrospinal fluid.
• Advise the patient to report any signs of meningeal irritation (e.g., fever, stiff neck, occipital headache, photophobia).

TEST RESULTS AND CLINICAL SIGNIFICANCE

Spinal cord tumour (e.g., astrocytoma, neurofibroma, meningioma): *These are evident as radiolucent filling defects in the column of radiopaque dye in the canal.*

Metastatic spinal tumour: *Extrinsic spinal tumours (usually metastatic) are evident as extrinsic radiolucent filling defects in the column of radiopaque dye in the canal.*

Cervical ankylosing spondylosis,

Arthritic lumbar stenosis from arthritic bone spurs: *These bone changes can compress the spinal canal and are evident as distortion of the spinal cord or nerve roots.*

Herniated intravertebral disc: *A herniated disc acts as external compression on the spinal cord or the nerve root. The most common areas of disc herniation are L4-L5 and L5-S1.*

Avulsion of nerve roots: *Traumatic avulsion of the nerve root can cause profound neurologic changes.*

Cysts: *Cysts of the spinal cord or meninges surrounding the cord are evident as extrinsic radiolucent filling defects in the column of radiopaque dye in the canal.*

RELATED TEST

Magnetic Resonance Imaging (p. 1148). This test is more accurate than myelography for viewing the spinal cord and its surrounding structures.

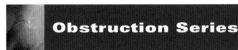

NORMAL FINDINGS

No evidence of bowel obstruction
No abnormal calcifications
No free air

INDICATIONS

This X-ray series is used for the evaluation of abdominal pain or suspected obstruction of the intestinal tract.

TEST EXPLANATION

The obstruction series is a group of X-ray images of the abdomen in patients with suspected bowel obstruction, paralytic ileus, perforated viscus, abdominal abscess, kidney stones, appendicitis, or foreign body ingestion. The series usually consists of at least two X-ray studies. The first is an *erect abdominal film,* in which both diaphragms should be visualized. The film is examined for evidence of free air under either diaphragm, which is pathognomonic for perforated viscus. This view is also used to detect air-fluid levels within the intestine; the presence of an air-fluid level is characteristic of bowel obstruction or paralytic ileus. On occasion, patients are too ill to stand erect. In this case, an X-ray can be taken with the patient in the left lateral decubitus position. If free air is present, it is visible between the liver and the right side of the abdominal wall. Air-fluid levels also can be detected.

The second view in the obstruction series is usually a *supine abdominal* X-ray study, similar to the kidney, ureter, and bladder study (p. 1084). An abdominal abscess may be seen as a cluster of tiny bubbles within a localized area. A calcification within the ureter could indicate a ureteral kidney stone. A small calcification in the right lower quadrant in a patient with pain in this quadrant may be an appendicolith. Gas distension of the bowel is characteristic of bowel obstruction or paralytic ileus.

The obstruction series can also be used to monitor the clinical course of gastrointestinal (GI) disease. For example, repeated obstruction series in patients with partial small bowel obstruction or paralytic ileus can indicate clinical worsening or improvement.

Frequently, a *cross-table lateral* view of the abdomen is included in an obstruction series to detect abdominal aorta calcification, which often occurs in older adults. The calcification represents the anterior wall of the aorta. If an aortic aneurysm is present, the calcification appears to protrude from the spine.

The *supine abdominal* view can be used as a scout image before GI or abdominal X-ray studies with contrast material (e.g., BE, p. 1033) or intravenous pyelography (IVP) (p. 1080) is performed, to ensure that nothing is obstructing adequate visualization of what needs to be studied.

The obstruction series is performed in minutes in the radiology department by a radiologic technologist; however, it can be performed at the patient's bedside with a portable X-ray machine. A radiologist interprets the images. No discomfort is associated with the study.

CONTRAINDICATIONS

- Pregnancy, unless the benefits of the procedure outweigh the risks of radiation exposure to the fetus

X-Ray Studies

12

INTERFERING FACTORS

- Previous GI barium contrast study: Although barium within the GI tract can preclude identification of other important calcifications (e.g., kidney stones), it can be helpful in outlining the GI anatomy.

PROCEDURE AND PATIENT CARE

Before

- ⟩⟨ Explain the procedure to the patient.
- Ensure that all radiopaque clothing has been removed.
- ⟩⟨ Remind the patient that no contrast agent will be used.

During

- Although the procedure varies among facilities, a supine abdominal X-ray, an erect abdominal X-ray, and perhaps a lower erect chest X-ray are usually obtained. A cross-table lateral X-ray is often also included.

After

- No special care is needed.

TEST RESULTS AND CLINICAL SIGNIFICANCE

Abdominal aortic calcification or abdominal aortic aneurysm: *Abdominal aortic aneurysm is evident by calcification in the anterior wall of the aorta, displaced significantly anterior from the vertebrae.*

Calculi: *A calcified stone in the area where the ureters would be is indicative of ureteral calculi. This finding requires further supportive evidence by means of intravenous pyelography (p. 1080). Appendicolithiasis (stone in the appendix) is suspected when a patient with right lower quadrant abdominal pain is seen to have a stone in that quadrant.*

Abdominal accumulation of bowel gas: *Abnormal accumulations of bowel gas can indicate intestinal obstruction or paralytic ileus.*

Ascites: *The classical ground-glass appearance of the entire abdomen on the supine abdominal film indicates peritoneal effusion.*

Soft tissue masses: *Large soft tissue masses or abscesses can be seen surprisingly well on this plain X-ray without contrast material enhancement.*

Ruptured viscus: *Free air (i.e., air outside the bowel but inside the abdomen) is indicative of a perforated viscus.*

Congenital anomalies in the location, size, and number of kidneys: *Because the kidneys are well seen, abnormalities of these organs are easily detected.*

Organomegaly or bladder distension: *An enlarged liver or spleen is seen as a large soft tissue mass in the right or left upper quadrant, respectively. A large soft tissue mass in the midline or pelvis is usually a distended bladder.*

Foreign body: *A bullet or other solid object is obvious on X-rays. A surgical sponge or instrument left during surgery is also visible.*

RELATED TEST

Kidney, Ureter, and Bladder Radiography (p. 1084). This is only one component of the obstruction series and therefore does not contribute as much information as does an entire obstruction series.

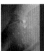

Percutaneous Transhepatic Cholangiography
(Ptc, PTHC)

NORMAL FINDINGS

Normal gallbladder and biliary ducts

INDICATIONS

This procedure allows visualization of the common bile ducts and sometimes the pancreatic duct. Patients with jaundice can be evaluated for tumour, gallstones, and other diseases.

TEST EXPLANATION

By passing a needle through the liver and into an intrahepatic bile duct, iodinated dye can be injected directly into the biliary system. The intrahepatic and extrahepatic biliary ducts, and occasionally the gallbladder, can be visualized and studied for partial or total obstruction from gallstones, benign strictures, malignant tumour, congenital cysts, and anatomic variations. This is especially helpful in patients with jaundice. If the jaundice is a result of extrahepatic obstruction, a catheter can be left in the common bile duct and used for external drainage of bile. Furthermore, a stent can be placed across a stricture to decompress the biliary system internally.

Percutaneous transhepatic cholangiography (PTHC) and endoscopic retrograde cholangiopancreatography (ERCP; p. 632) are the only methods for visualizing the biliary tree in patients with jaundice. ERCP is used more frequently because of its lower complication rate. PTHC, however, is the only way to visualize the biliary tree after most gastric surgery. On occasion (if the pancreatic duct and the common bile duct are from a common channel), part or all of the pancreatic duct can be filled with dye from the same injection. Table 12-6 lists diagnostic tests to visualize the pancreatobiliary system, along with their advantages and disadvantages.

A radiologist performs PTHC in approximately 1 hour, during which time the patient must lie still. Abdominal pain may be felt for several hours after the test. The patient also may have right-sided shoulder-top pain because of diaphragmatic irritation of leaking bile or blood.

TABLE 12-6	Diagnostic Tests to Visualize the Pancreatobiliary System	
Test	**Advantages**	**Disadvantages**
Intravenous cholangiography	Easy to perform	Poor visualization of ducts
Oral cholecystography	Easy to perform	Visualization of only the gallbladder
ERCP	Good visualization of the pancreas and common bile ducts; able to decompress the biliary system	Difficult to perform; complications possible
PTHC	Good visualization of the ducts; can be used to decompress the biliary system	Difficult to perform; complications possible
Nuclear radioscintigraphy	Easy to perform	Poor visualization of the biliary system; not specific as to disease

ERCP, Endoscopic retrograde cholangiopancreatography; *PTHC,* percutaneous transhepatic cholangiography.

X-Ray Studies

12

CONTRAINDICATIONS

- History of adverse reactions or allergic reactions to iodinated dye
- Allergy to shellfish
- Evidence of mild cholangitis, because dye injections increase biliary pressure and cause bacteremia, which may lead to septicemia and shock
- Inability of patients to cooperate and remain still
- Prolonged clotting times

POTENTIAL COMPLICATIONS

- For potential complications of iodinated dye, see p. 1021.
- Peritonitis can be caused by bile extravasation from the liver after the needle has been removed.
- Bleeding can be caused by inadvertent puncture of a large hepatic blood vessel.
- Sepsis and cholangitis can result from injection of the dye into an already infected and obstructed common bile duct. The pressure of injection pushes the bacteria into the bloodstream, causing bacteremia.

INTERFERING FACTORS

- The presence of barium from a previous upper gastrointestinal X-ray series or barium contrast study may preclude visualization of the biliary tree.

Clinical Priorities

- Assess the patient for adverse reactions or allergic reactions to iodinated dye.
- Verify that results of coagulation studies are within the normal range before this test, because bleeding is a potential complication.
- Abdominal pain after the test may be an indication of bleeding or bile extravasation.

PROCEDURE AND PATIENT CARE

Before

- Explain the procedure to the patient.
- Obtain the patient's informed consent for the procedure.
- For assessment of adverse reactions or allergic reactions to iodinated dye, see p. 1021.
- Type and crossmatch the patient's blood. Bleeding may occur, and the patient may require a transfusion or surgery.
- Verify that results of coagulation studies are within the normal range.
- Keep the patient on NPO status (nothing by mouth) after midnight on the day of the test. A laxative may be ordered.
- Premedicate the patient as indicated, usually with atropine and meperidine.

During

- Note the following procedural steps:
  1. The patient is placed supine on an X-ray table in the radiology department.
  2. The abdominal wall or lower chest wall (over the liver) is anaesthetized with lidocaine (Xylocaine).

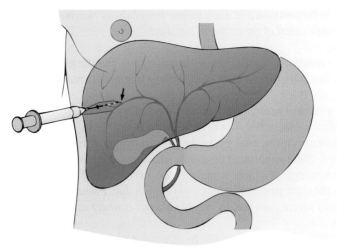

Figure 12-22 Percutaneous transhepatic cholangiography (PTHC).

3. With the use of fluoroscopic monitoring, the needle is advanced through the skin and into the liver (Figure 12-22).
4. When bile flows freely out from the liver through the needle, X-ray dye is injected.
5. X-ray images are obtained immediately.
6. If an obstruction is found, a catheter or stent is placed over a guide wire and left temporarily in the biliary tract to establish drainage and decompression of the biliary tract.

After

- Keep the patient on bed rest for several hours.
- Observe the patient for hemorrhage or bile leakage. A small amount of bleeding is normal.
- Keep the patient on NPO status (nothing by mouth) for a few hours after the test in case of the development of intra-abdominal bleeding or bile extravasation that necessitates surgery.
- Repeatedly assess the patient's vital signs for evidence of hemorrhage.
- Assess the patient for signs of bacteremia or sepsis.
- If a catheter is left in the biliary tract, establish a sterile, closed drainage system.
- Withhold high doses of pain medications that may blunt the abdominal signs associated with hemorrhage or bile extravasation.

 Home Care Responsibilities

- Instruct the patient to observe the needle insertion site for bleeding and bile leakage.
- Instruct the patient to notify the physician if fever and chills develop, inasmuch as these may indicate bacteremia or sepsis.
- Instruct the patient to report signs of bleeding (increased pulse and decreased blood pressure).

TEST RESULTS AND CLINICAL SIGNIFICANCE

Tumour, strictures, or gallstones of the hepatic or common bile duct: *These diseases cause partial or complete obstruction of the biliary tree. Tumours usually cause long strictures. Benign strictures are more likely to cause narrowing of short segments. Gallstones usually are evident as rounded radiolucent (dark) filling defects in the common bile duct. When they obstruct the common bile duct, the obstruction is visible as a soft convex cutoff of the common bile duct.*

Sclerosing cholangitis,

Biliary sclerosis: *These conditions result from inflammatory or fibrotic changes around the common bile ducts; this leads to a long stricture in most of the biliary tree and its radicals.*

Cysts of the common bile duct: *These congenital outpouchings of the common bile duct may vary in size from tiny and barely noticeable to large and voluminous. The pressure surrounding these cysts can obstruct the normal portion of the common bile duct in the closed space of the right upper quadrant of the abdomen.*

Tumour, strictures, inflammation, true cysts, or pseudocysts of the pancreatic duct: *If the pancreatic duct is visualized, these abnormalities can be identified. Pancreatic tumours are evident as long strictures. Postinflammatory strictures usually cause narrowing of short segments. Neoplastic cysts may be connected to the main pancreatic duct and fill with dye. Pseudocysts, caused by pancreatic duct disruption that follows severe pancreatitis, nearly always connect with the main pancreatic duct and therefore fill with dye.*

Anatomic biliary or pancreatic duct variations: *Duplications, aberrant entry of the pancreatobiliary ducts into the intestines and other anomalies can be identified.*

RELATED TEST

Endoscopic Retrograde Cholangiopancreatography (p. 632). This is the preferred method of visualizing the pancreatobiliary tree in the patient with jaundice.

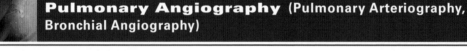

Pulmonary Angiography (Pulmonary Arteriography, Bronchial Angiography)

NORMAL FINDINGS

Normal pulmonary vasculature

INDICATIONS

Pulmonary angiography is used for patients with suspected pulmonary embolism when the lung scan yields inconclusive results. This study remains the "gold standard" for the diagnosis of pulmonary embolus; however, pulmonary angiography is generally not necessary when the perfusion scan is normal (p. 838).

TEST EXPLANATION

With injection of iodinated dye (the X-ray contrast material) into the pulmonary arteries, pulmonary angiography permits visualization of the pulmonary vasculature. Angiography is used to detect pulmonary embolism and a variety of congenital and acquired lesions of the pulmonary vessels. Box 12-5 gives an overview of the diagnosis of pulmonary embolism.

Bronchial angiography is performed in some facilities to identify sites of bleeding in the lungs. Catheters are placed transarterially into the orifice of the bronchial arteries. Radiopaque material is injected, and the arteries are visualized. If a bleeding site is identified, a sclerosing agent can be injected to prevent further bleeding.

This test is performed in approximately 1 hour by a physician. During injection of dye, the patient may feel a burning sensation at the injection site and a warm flush throughout the body.

BOX 12-5	Diagnosis of Pulmonary Embolism

Symptoms
- Shortness of breath
- Feeling of extreme anxiety
- Pleuritic chest pain

Signs
- Hypoxemia
- Tachycardia
- Pleural rub cardiac gallop
- Concomitant phlebitis

Diagnostic Tests
- Electrocardiography: right-sided heart strain
- Chest X-rays: may be normal
- Pulmonary infarct may be evident from radiodensity in affected parenchyma
- Arterial blood gases: hypoxemia, hypocapnia
- Lung scan: blood perfusion defect
- Computed tomographic angiography: clot in pulmonary artery

CONTRAINDICATIONS

- History of adverse reactions or allergies to iodinated dye
- Allergy to shellfish
- Pregnancy, unless the benefits of the procedure outweigh the risks of radiation exposure to the fetus
- Bleeding disorders

POTENTIAL COMPLICATIONS

- For potential adverse reactions or allergic reactions to iodinated dye, see p. 1021.
- Cardiac arrhythmia (dysrhythmia) in the form of premature ventricular contractions may occur during right-sided heart catheterization and may lead to ventricular tachycardia and ventricular fibrillation.
- Hypoglycemia or acidosis may occur in patients who are taking metformin (Glucophage) and receive iodinated dye.

PROCEDURE AND PATIENT CARE

Before

- Explain the procedure to the patient.
- Obtain the patient's written informed consent for the procedure.
- Inform the patient that a warm flush will be felt when the dye is injected.
- For assessment of adverse reactions or allergic reactions to iodinated dye, see p. 1021.
- Determine whether the patient has ventricular arrhythmias (dysrhythmias).
- Keep the patient on NPO status (nothing by mouth) after midnight on the day of the test.
- Administer preprocedural medications as ordered. Atropine may be administered to decrease secretions. Meperidine may be administered for sedation and relaxation.

During

- A catheter is placed into the femoral vein and passed into the inferior vena cava.
- With fluoroscopic visualization, the catheter is advanced into the main pulmonary artery, where the dye is injected.

12 **X-Ray Studies**

- X-ray images of the chest are obtained immediately in timed sequence. This allows all vessels visualized by the injection to be photographed. If filling defects are seen in the contrast-filled vessels, pulmonary emboli are present.
- If *bronchial angiography* is performed, cannulation is through the femoral artery instead of the vein.

After

- Observe the catheter insertion site for inflammation, hemorrhage, and hematoma.
- Assess the patient's vital signs for evidence of bleeding (decreased blood pressure, increased pulse).
- Apply a cold compress to the venopuncture site if necessary to reduce swelling or discomfort.

TEST RESULTS AND CLINICAL SIGNIFICANCE

Pulmonary embolism: *This is evident if one or more venous tributaries contain a clot. There may be an abrupt cutoff of the vessels as a result of complete obstruction secondary to the embolic clot.*

Congenital and acquired lesions of the pulmonary vessels (e.g., pulmonary hypertension): *Congenital anomalies in pulmonary arterial anatomy are not rare. This technique is also used for right-sided heart cardiac catheterization (p. 1047). Bronchial arterial evaluation is usually performed for pulmonary symptoms (e.g., hemoptysis).*

Tumour: *Bronchial tumour may bleed, and bronchial angiography may indicate the location.*

RELATED TESTS

Lung Scan (p. 838). When results are clearly positive, this is a very accurate method of indicating the presence of a pulmonary embolism. A negative scan is also accurate in indicating the absence of an embolism. However, all too commonly, nuclear scanning yields unclear results. Pulmonary angiography is helpful in these situations.

Pulmonary Angiography (p. 1100). This, in combination with computed tomography, is the study most commonly performed to identify pulmonary embolism.

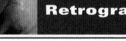

Retrograde Pyelography

NORMAL FINDINGS

Normal outline and size of the ureters and bladder
No evidence of ureteral obstruction

INDICATIONS

Retrograde pyelography provides X-ray visualization of the ureter distal to an obstruction. It is performed in patients with known obstruction of unknown cause.

TEST EXPLANATION

Retrograde pyelography enables X-ray visualization of the urinary tract through ureteral catheterization and injection of contrast material. The ureters are catheterized during cystoscopy.

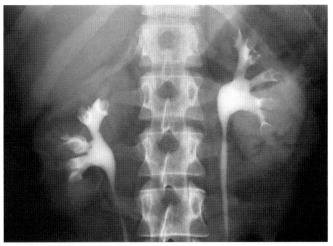

Figure 12-23 Retrograde pyelogram, obtained with patient in lithotomy position.

Radiopaque material is injected into the ureters, and X-ray images are obtained (Figure 12-23). This test can be performed even if the patient is allergic to intravenous contrast dye, because none of the dye injected into the ureters is absorbed, although allergic reactions can occur in rare cases.

Retrograde pyelography aids in X-ray examination of the ureters when visualization with intravenous pyelography (p. 1080) is inadequate or contraindicated. When a ureter is obstructed, intravenous pyelography enables visualization of only the ureter proximal to the obstruction, if anything. To visualize the distal portion of the ureter, retrograde pyelography is necessary. Also, in patients with unilateral renal disease, the involved kidney and collecting system are not visualized because renal function is poor. As a result, no dye is filtered into the collecting system by the nonfunctioning kidney. To rule out ureteral obstruction as a cause of unilateral kidney disease, retrograde pyelography must be performed. Tumour, benign strictures, tortuosity of ureters, stones, scarring, and extrinsic compression may cause ureteral obstruction. Retrograde pyelography provides complete visualization of the ureters.

Retrograde pyelography is performed in approximately 1 hour by a urologist in a cystoscopy room or an operating room. The study is uncomfortable. If awake, the patient feels pressure and an urge to void. If general anaesthesia is used, no postoperative pain is noted.

POTENTIAL COMPLICATIONS

- Urinary tract infection may result because of the invasive nature of this procedure.
- Sepsis may result because of seeding of the bloodstream with bacteria from infected urine.
- The bladder or ureter can be perforated.
- Hematuria can result from urologic instrumentation.
- Ureteral urine flow can be obstructed temporarily. Manipulation of the ureters may cause edema, which can result in temporary, partial obstruction of urine flow.
- Allergic reaction to iodinated dye can occur, but this is rare because the dye is not administered intravenously.

INTERFERING FACTORS

- Retained barium from previous X-ray studies can obscure visualization.

PROCEDURE AND PATIENT CARE

Before

- Explain the procedure to the patient.
- Obtain the patient's informed consent for the study.
- Check the patient for allergy to iodinated dye.
- If enemas are ordered for clearing the bowel, assist the patient as needed, and record the results.
- If the procedure will be performed with a local anaesthetic, allow the patient to have a liquid breakfast.
- If the procedure will be performed with the patient under general anaesthesia, follow routine general anaesthesia precautions. Keep the patient on NPO status (nothing by mouth) after midnight on the day of the test.
- Fluids may be given intravenously.
- Administer preprocedural medications as ordered 1 hour before the study. Sedatives decrease spasm of the bladder sphincter, thus decreasing patient discomfort.

During

- Note the following procedural steps:
  1. The ureteral catheters are passed into the ureters by means of cystoscopy (see Figure 4-7, p. 626).
  2. Radiopaque contrast material (Hypaque or Renografin) is injected into the ureteral catheters, and X-rays are obtained.
  3. The entire ureter and pelvis are demonstrated.
  4. As the catheters are withdrawn, more dye is injected, and more X-rays are taken to visualize the complete outline of the ureters.
  5. A delayed film is often obtained to assess the emptying capabilities of the ureter. This is usually done in approximately 5 minutes after the last injection.
  6. If obstruction is noted, a stent may be left in the ureter so that the ureter can drain.

After

- Check and record the patient's vital signs as ordered. Watch for decreased blood pressure and increased pulse as indications of bleeding.
- Observe the patient for signs and symptoms of sepsis (e.g., elevated temperature, flushing, chills, decreased blood pressure, increased pulse).
- Assess the patient's ability to void over a period of at least 24 hours. Urinary retention may be secondary to edema caused by instrumentation.
- Note the colour of the urine; a pink tinge is typically present. Report bright red blood or clots to the physician.
- Encourage the patient to drink large amounts of fluids. Dilute urine decreases dysuria. Fluids also maintain a constant flow of urine to prevent stasis and accumulation of bacteria in the bladder.
- Monitor the patient for bladder spasm. Often, belladonna-opium suppositories are given to relieve bladder spasm.
- Administer analgesics as needed.

Home Care Responsibilities

- Instruct the patient to watch for indications of bleeding (e.g., decreased blood pressure, increased pulse) and sepsis (e.g., temperature, flush, chills).
- Monitor urine output over the first 24 hours to detect urinary retention.
- Encourage the patient to drink large amounts of fluids to prevent stasis and accumulation of bacteria in the bladder.

TEST RESULTS AND CLINICAL SIGNIFICANCE

Tumour or strictures: *Primary tumours of the ureter, but most often extrinsic contiguous tumours, involve the ureters and cause partial or complete obstruction. Radiation fibrosis or primary retroperitoneal fibrosis can also cause strictures of varying degree.*

Stones: *Stones, the most common cause of ureteral obstruction, are evident on retrograde pyelography and can be removed during cystoscopy.*

Congenital anomaly: *Congenital duplications, ureteral cysts, bands, or ureteral kinking are evident with this study.*

RELATED TEST

Kidney, Ureter, and Bladder Radiography (p. 1084). This is an X-ray study of the kidneys, ureter, and bladder with the use of an intravenous contrast agent. Visualization of obstructed ureters is limited.

Sialography

NORMAL FINDINGS

No evidence of disease in the salivary ducts and related structures

INDICATIONS

This test is used to identify calculi in the salivary ducts.

TEST EXPLANATION

Sialography is an X-ray procedure used to examine the salivary ducts (parotid, submaxillary, submandibular, sublingual) and related glandular structures after injection of a contrast medium into the desired duct. The procedure is used to detect calculi, strictures, tumours, or inflammatory disease in patients with pain, tenderness, or swelling in these areas. Computed tomography of the salivary ducts is more reliable for detection of salivary parenchymal tumour or inflammation. Sialography is effective for detecting ductule calculi or strictures.

A radiologist performs this procedure in the radiology department in less than 30 minutes. The patient may feel slight pressure as the contrast medium is injected into the ducts.

CONTRAINDICATIONS

- Mouth infections (e.g., yeast infection), because the infection may be spread to the salivary glands

12

X-Ray Studies

POTENTIAL COMPLICATIONS

- Allergic reaction to iodinated dye is rare because the dye is not administered intravenously.

PROCEDURE AND PATIENT CARE

Before

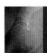 Explain the procedure to the patient. The thought of dye injection in the mouth is frightening to many patients. Provide emotional support.
- Obtain the patient's informed consent for the procedure if it is required by the institution.
 Instruct the patient to remove jewellery, hairpins, and dentures, which could obscure X-ray visualization.
 Instruct the patient to rinse the mouth with an antiseptic solution to reduce the possibility of introducing bacteria into the ductal structures.

During

- Note the following procedural steps:
  1. X-ray studies are taken before the dye injection to ensure that radiopaque stones are not present, which could prevent the contrast material from entering the ducts.
  2. The patient is placed supine on an X-ray table.
  3. The contrast medium is injected directly into the desired orifice through a cannula or special tiny catheter.
  4. Radiographs are obtained with the patient in various positions.
  5. The patient is given a sour substance (e.g., lemon juice) orally to stimulate salivary excretion of the dye.
  6. Another set of X-ray studies is obtained to evaluate ductal drainage.

After

- Encourage the patient to drink fluids to promote dye excretion.

TEST RESULTS AND CLINICAL SIGNIFICANCE

Calculi,
Strictures: *These cause obstruction of the duct draining the salivary gland.*
Tumour: *Most tumours of the salivary glands are benign and are located in the parotid gland. These tumours are demonstrated as radiolucent filling defects or distortion of the glandular ductules within the gland.*
Inflammatory disease: *Sialitis (especially parotitis) can result from viral illnesses (e.g., mumps) or bacterial infections.*

Skull Radiography

NORMAL FINDINGS

Normal skull and surrounding structures

INDICATIONS

This X-ray study is used to evaluate the skull and paranasal sinuses for trauma or disease.

TEST EXPLANATION

An X-ray of the skull provides visualization of the bones making up the skull, the nasal sinuses, and any central nervous system calcification. This study is indicated when a pathologic condition is suspected in any of these structures.

Skull fractures are easily seen as abnormal radiolucent lines in an otherwise radiopaque skull bone (Figure 12-24). Metastatic tumour of the skull can easily be seen as radiolucent spots on an otherwise normal image. Opacification of the nasal sinuses may indicate sinusitis, hemorrhage, or tumour.

Located in the middle of the brain, the pineal gland is thought to regulate biorhythms in mammals. This gland may become calcified after puberty. When calcified, the pineal gland is a useful marker and allows the midline of the brain to be easily identified on skull X-rays. Conditions such as unilateral hematoma or tumour cause a shift of the midline structures (and the calcified pineal gland) to the side opposite the site of the pathologic condition. Simple skull X-rays therefore allow easy detection of these unilateral, space-occupying lesions.

The sella turcica is the bony structure surrounding and protecting the pituitary gland. Tumours of the pituitary gland may cause an increase in size or erosion of the sella turcica. These changes can be detected on skull X-rays.

Most head trauma (or instances where skull injury is suspected) is evaluated with computed tomography of the brain. However, skull X-ray is still the best method of determining skull bone suture lines for the evaluation of children with abnormal head shape or size.

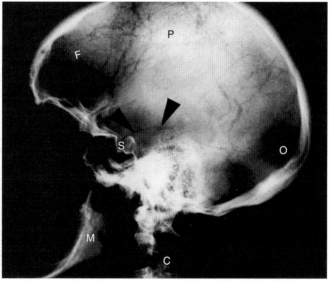

Figure 12-24 Skull X-ray, lateral view. *Arrowheads* indicate fracture line in temporal bone. *C,* Cervical vertebra; *F,* frontal bone; *M,* mandible; *O,* occipital bone; *P,* parietal bone; *S,* sella turcica.

PROCEDURE AND PATIENT CARE

Before

- Explain the procedure to the patient.
- Instruct the patient to remove all objects above the neck, because metal objects and dentures will prevent X-ray visualization of the structures they cover.
- Avoid hyperextension and manipulation of the head if surgical injuries are suspected.
- Inform the patient that no sedation or fasting is required.

During

- The patient is taken to the radiology department and placed on an X-ray table. Axial (sub-mentovertical), half-axial (Towne), posteroanterior, and lateral views of the skull are usually obtained (Figure 12-25).
- A radiologic technologist obtains the skull films in a few minutes.
- Inform the patient that the test is painless.

After

- If a glass eye is present, note this on the X-ray examination request, because it can present a confusing shadow on the X-ray.

TEST RESULTS AND CLINICAL SIGNIFICANCE

Skull fracture: *This is seen as a radiolucent line in the skull. The normal bone sutures (where the bones have grown together during normal growth and development) can look like fractures to the untrained eye.*

Metastatic tumour: *Breast cancer, Paget's disease, myeloma, and many other tumours can metastasize to the skull. Metastatic tumours can be osteolytic (radiolucent) or osteoblastic (radiopaque).*

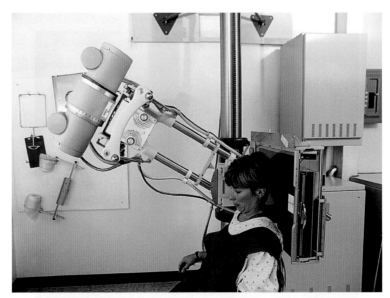

Figure 12-25 Patient positioned for a skull X-ray study (Towne view: anteroposterior projection with posterior view). A lead apron is placed on the patient to prevent unnecessary exposure to radiation.

Sinusitis: *Swelling and mucus in the sinuses are evident from increased density on the X-ray. Air-fluid levels may also be evident.*

Hemorrhage,

Tumour,

Hematoma: *When unilateral, these abnormalities cause shift of midline structures (including shift of the calcified pineal gland) to the opposite side.*

Congenital anomaly: *Many anomalies in the normal growth and development of the skull are obvious.*

RELATED TEST

Computed Tomography, Brain (p. 1065). This test can be used to evaluate the skull. Its main purpose is to evaluate the brain.

Small Bowel Follow-Through (SBF, Small Bowel Enema)

NORMAL FINDINGS

Normal positioning, motility, and patency of the small intestine

INDICATIONS

This contrast-enhanced X-ray study of the small intestine is most often used to identify and determine the cause of small bowel obstruction. It is also used to identify tumours, strictures, inflammation, and other congenital or acquired diseases of the small intestine.

TEST EXPLANATION

The small bowel follow-through (SBF) study is performed to identify abnormalities in the small bowel. Usually, the patient is asked to drink barium; in patients who cannot drink, barium can be injected through a nasogastric tube. X-rays are then obtained at timed intervals (usually 30 minutes to 1 hour) to follow the progression of the barium through the small bowel. Barium transit time may be significantly delayed as a result of both benign and malignant forms of partial obstruction or diminished intestinal motility (ileus). On the other hand, the flow of barium is faster in patients who have hypermotility of the small bowel (e.g., malabsorption syndromes). Failure of the progression through the small bowel can be observed in patients with complete mechanical small bowel obstruction. Furthermore, SBF series are helpful in identifying and defining the anatomy of small bowel fistulas (abnormal connections between the small bowel and other abdominal organs or skin). Strictures related to Crohn's disease or radiation are also evident with SBF.

A more accurate X-ray evaluation of the small intestine is enabled by the *small bowel enema* study. Barium is injected into a tube previously placed in the small bowel. This small bowel enema provides better visualization of the entire small bowel because the barium is not diluted by gastric and duodenal juices, as when the patient drinks barium. This test is especially useful in the evaluation of partial small bowel obstruction of unknown cause. Tumours, ulcers, and small bowel fistulas are more easily identified and defined with the enema.

Table 12-7 lists X-ray studies used to visualize the gastrointestinal tract. This procedure is performed in approximately 30 minutes by a radiologist in the radiology department. Inform the patient that this test is not uncomfortable.

TABLE 12-7	X-Ray Visualization of the Gastrointestinal Tract
Study	**Portion of Gastrointestinal Tract Evaluated**
Barium swallow	Esophagus
Upper gastrointestinal series	Lower esophagus, stomach, and upper duodenum
Small bowel series	Duodenum, jejunum, and ileum
Barium enema	Rectum, colon, and distal ileum

CONTRAINDICATIONS

- Complete small bowel obstruction, because the introduction of barium into an obstructed bowel may create a stonelike impaction; however, this is extremely rare
- Suspected perforated viscus, because barium may cause persistent and recurrent infections if it leaks out of the bowel; meglumine diatrizoate (Gastrografin), a water-soluble contrast medium, can be used if perforation is suspected, but it becomes diluted rapidly, minimizing the accuracy of the SBF study with this contrast medium
- Unstable vital signs because the procedure may further affect the patients' blood pressure or heart rate and rhythm; if the procedure is performed on an unstable patient, vital signs should be closely monitored during the entire time required for this study

POTENTIAL COMPLICATIONS

- Barium-induced small bowel obstruction

INTERFERING FACTORS

- Barium in the intestinal tract from a previous barium X-ray study may obstruct adequate visualization of the area of small bowel to be evaluated.
- Food or fluid within the gastrointestinal tract may give the false appearance of a filling defect because of a tumour or other mass.
- Morphine can significantly delay small bowel motility.

✓ Clinical Priorities

- More accurate evaluation of the small intestines is provided by the *small bowel enema* study, in which barium is injected through a tube placed in the small bowel.
- Barium should not be used in patients with suspected perforated viscus. In such patients, meglumine diatrizoate (Gastrografin), a water-soluble medium, is used.
- Cathartics are recommended after this test to aid in removal of the barium. Stools will return to normal colour after complete evacuation of the barium.

PROCEDURE AND PATIENT CARE

Before

- Explain the procedure to the patient.
- Instruct the patient not to eat anything for at least 8 hours before the test. In most cases, keep the patient on NPO status (nothing by mouth) after midnight on the day of the test.

- Inform the patient that the SBF series may take several hours. Suggest that the patient bring reading material or recreational items (e.g., an iPod, playing cards) to occupy the time.
- Accompany the patient to the X-ray department if vital signs are not stable.
- Arrange for transportation of the hospitalized patient back to the nursing unit between serial films.

During

- Note the following procedural steps:
  1. Barium sulphate is mixed with fluid as a milkshake, which the patient drinks through a straw.
  2. Usually, an upper gastrointestinal series is performed concomitantly with the SBF study (see p. 1117).
  3. Barium flow is followed through the upper gastrointestinal tract by means of fluoroscopy.
  4. At frequent intervals (15 to 60 minutes), repeated X-rays are obtained to monitor the flow of barium through the small intestine until barium is seen flowing into the right colon. This usually takes 60 to 120 minutes, but in patients with delayed progression of the barium, the test may take as long as 24 hours to complete.
- Small bowel enema study:
  1. In this procedure, a long, weighted tube is usually placed transorally; however, a tube also can be placed into the upper small bowel endoscopically.
  2. After the tube is in place, a thickened barium mixture is injected through the tube, and X-rays are serially obtained as described for SBF.

After

- Inform the patient of the need to evacuate all the barium. Cathartics (e.g., magnesium citrate) are recommended. Initially, stools are white but should return to normal colour with complete evacuation.

TEST RESULTS AND CLINICAL SIGNIFICANCE

Small bowel tumour: *This may be evident from partial or complete small bowel obstruction. Usually, however, tumours appear as filling defects in the column of barium in the small bowel.*

Small bowel obstruction: *Adhesions are the most common cause of small bowel obstruction, followed by extrinsic tumour, hernia, and stricture from inflammatory bowel disease in adults. Hernias, intussusception, malrotation, bowel atresia, and volvulus are most common in children. Small bowel obstruction can be partial or complete. When obstruction is complete, the barium column does not progress past the area of obstruction. When obstruction is partial, the barium does pass the area of obstruction, but abnormally slowly.*

Inflammatory small bowel disease (e.g., Crohn's disease): *Inflammatory bowel disease usually is apparent as a stricture causing partial small bowel obstruction.*

Malabsorption syndromes (e.g., Whipple's disease, celiac disease): *These are usually evident from rapid transit of contrast material through the small bowel.*

Congenital or acquired anatomic anomaly (e.g., malrotation): *Malrotation usually causes the ligament of Treitz (junction of the duodenum and jejunum) to be in the right lower quadrant instead of its normal location in the left upper quadrant. Short bowel syndrome related to surgical small bowel bypass or resection is evident from rapid transit of barium through the small bowel.*

Congenital abnormalities (e.g., small bowel atresia, duplication, Meckel diverticulum): *Bowel atresia or duplication can be noted as bowel obstruction in children. Meckel diverticulum is evident as an outpouching of the ileum. It may not be apparent until adulthood and may never cause symptoms.*

Small bowel intussusception: *An upper segment of bowel becomes invaginated (swallowed up) into a lower segment. This usually causes bowel obstruction and is most common in children.*

Small bowel perforation: *This condition is evident from leakage of contrast material out of the intestine.*

Radiation enteritis: *This becomes evident years after radiation therapy. It is demonstrated as a stricture of one or more segments of the small bowel.*

RELATED TEST

Barium Enema (p. 1033). This test is a contrast material–enhanced X-ray study of the colon. The distal portion of the small bowel is often visualized.

 Spinal Radiography (Cervical, Thoracic, Lumbar, Sacral, or Coccygeal X-Ray Studies)

NORMAL FINDINGS

Normal spinal vertebrae

INDICATIONS

Spinal X-ray is used to evaluate back or neck pain.

TEST EXPLANATION

Spinal X-ray studies may be performed to evaluate any area of the spine. They usually include anteroposterior, lateral, and oblique views of these structures. These X-rays are often obtained to assess back or neck pain, degenerative arthritic changes, traumatic fractures, tumour metastasis, spondylosis (degenerative disease of the spinal structures), and spondylolisthesis (slipping of one vertebral disc over another). Cervical spine X-ray studies are routinely performed in cases of multiple traumas to ensure absence of fracture before either the patient is moved or the neck is manipulated. However, computed tomographic scanning of the cervical vertebrae is increasingly becoming the standard of practice to ensure that there is no cervical fracture. Spinal X-rays are helpful in evaluating for spinal alignment abnormalities (e.g., kyphosis, scoliosis). Magnetic resonance imaging is another very accurate method of evaluating the spine.

CONTRAINDICATIONS

- Pregnancy, unless the benefits of the procedure outweigh the risks of radiation exposure to the fetus

PROCEDURE AND PATIENT CARE

Before

- Explain the procedure to the patient.
- If the patient can move, instruct him or her to remove any metal objects covering the area to be visualized. If the patient cannot move, ensure any metal objects are removed.
- Immobilize the patient if a spinal fracture is suspected. Apply a neck brace if a cervical spine fracture is suspected.
- Inform the patient that no fasting or sedation is required; however, if a fracture is suspected, the patient may be kept on NPO status (nothing by mouth).

During

- Note that the patient is placed on an X-ray table. Anterior, posterior, lateral, and oblique X-rays of the desired area of the spinal cord are obtained. The same views can be obtained with the patient in the standing position.
- A radiologic technologist obtains spinal X-rays in a few minutes.
- Inform the patient that no discomfort is associated with this study.

After

- Patient positioning and activity depend on test results.

TEST RESULTS AND CLINICAL SIGNIFICANCE

Degenerative arthritis changes: *Bone destruction or bone spurs are seen in patients with degenerative arthritic changes of the spinal joints.*

Metastatic tumour invasion,

Traumatic or pathologic fracture: *Of all spinal injuries, those of the cervical and lumbar portions of the spine are most frequent. Any portion, however, can be affected by metastatic neoplasm (e.g., myeloma, Paget's disease, breast or lung cancer). Bone metastasis can lead to fracture without a traumatic event.*

Scoliosis,

Spondylosis,

Spondylolisthesis: *These are anatomic alterations of spinal alignment.*

Suspected spinal osteomyelitis: *This test is helpful in detecting the infection.*

RELATED TESTS

Computed Tomography, Abdomen (p. 1059), and Computed Tomography, Chest (p. 1068). These studies demonstrate spinal anatomy and pathologic conditions better than spinal X-ray studies do. Alignment, however, is best evaluated with plain X-ray studies.

Swallowing Examination (Videofluoroscopic Swallowing Examination)

NORMAL FINDINGS

Normal swallowing function and complete clearing of X-ray material through the upper digestive tract

INDICATIONS

This test is performed to identify the cause of inability to swallow.

TEST EXPLANATION

Problems in swallowing may result from local structural diseases (e.g., tumour, upper esophageal diverticula, inflammation, extrinsic compression of the upper gastrointestinal tract) or from surgery to the oropharyngeal tract. Motility disorders of the upper gastrointestinal tract (e.g., Zenker diverticulum) and neurologic disorders (e.g., stroke syndrome, Parkinson's disease, neuropathies)

X-Ray Studies

12

also may cause difficulty in swallowing. Videofluoroscopy of the swallowing function allows the speech pathologist to delineate more clearly the exact pathologic condition in the swallowing mechanism; thus, the speech pathologist can determine the most appropriate treatment and teach the patient proper swallowing technique.

For this test, the patient swallows barium or a barium-containing meal. Videofluoroscopy is used to visualize and document the act of swallowing. Structural abnormalities and functional impairment can be identified easily with the slow-framed progression and reversal that are possible with videofluoroscopy. This test is similar to the barium swallow study (p. 1038), but finer details of swallowing can be evaluated with videofluoroscopy.

CONTRAINDICATIONS

- Aspiration of saliva; in these cases, nonswallowing methods of alimentation are required

PROCEDURE AND PATIENT CARE

Before

✗ Explain the procedure to the patient.
✗ Explain to the patient that no preparation is required.

During

- In the radiology department, the patient is asked to consume a barium-containing meal. The consistency of the meal—liquid, semisoft (e.g., applesauce), or solid (e.g., a tea biscuit)—will be determined by the speech therapist and radiologist, to simulate foods to which the patient is to be initially reintroduced. While the patient swallows, videofluoroscopy is recorded in both the lateral and the anterior positions.
- The video recording is repeatedly examined forward and backward by the radiologist and by the speech pathologist.

After

- No catharsis is required.

TEST RESULTS AND CLINICAL SIGNIFICANCE

Upper gastrointestinal tract disease,
Neuromuscular disorder,
Achalasia,
Upper gastrointestinal motility disorder (e.g., stroke syndrome, Parkinson's disease, peripheral neuropathy),
Diffuse esophageal spasms,
Zenker diverticulum: *These disorders can be associated with swallowing dysfunction at various levels in the swallowing mechanism.*

RELATED TEST

Barium Swallow (p. 1038). This test is similar to videofluoroscopy except that multiple still X-rays are obtained, and the entire swallowing mechanism cannot be fully evaluated.

T-Tube and Operative Cholangiography

NORMAL FINDINGS

Normal common bile duct with no dilation or filling defects
Good runoff of dye through the ampulla of Vater into the duodenum

INDICATIONS

Cholangiography provides visualization of the common bile ducts during and after surgery. It is most commonly used to identify stones in the common bile duct.

TEST EXPLANATION

In *operative cholangiography,* the common bile duct is directly injected with radiopaque material through the cystic duct. This is usually performed during cholecystectomy. Stones appear as radiolucent shadows. Gallstones, tumours, or strictures cause partial or total obstruction of the flow of dye into the duodenum. Visualization of the biliary duct structures enables the surgeon to see the surgical anatomy of the biliary tree. This reduces the possibility of inadvertent injury to the common bile duct during cholecystectomy. If stones in the common bile duct are demonstrated during operative cholangiography, the ducts are explored. Some surgeons perform operative cholangiography in all patients who undergo cholecystectomy. Other surgeons use specific indications for operative cholangiography, including the following:
- Jaundice
- Abnormal liver enzyme levels
- Dilation of the common bile duct
- Evidence of pancreatitis
- Evidence of small stones in the cystic duct during cholecystectomy

T-tube cholangiography is performed postoperatively after T-tube placement during an exploration of the common bile duct. Its main purpose is to detect retained stones in the common bile duct and to demonstrate good flow of contrast dye into the duodenum. This test is usually performed 5 to 10 days after surgery, with use of a T-shaped rubber tube placed in the common bile duct at surgery. If no stones are evident and there is good runoff of bile into the duodenum, the T-tube can be removed. If there are residual stones, the tube tract can be used to extract the stones.

POTENTIAL COMPLICATIONS

- Sepsis caused by increased ductal pressure with dye infusion

INTERFERING FACTORS

- Barium in the abdomen from a previous upper gastrointestinal series or BE study precludes visualization of the common bile duct.

PROCEDURE AND PATIENT CARE

Before

- Explain the procedure to the patient.
- Obtain the patient's informed consent for the main biliary procedure.

⚐ Inform the patient that no fasting or sedation is required for T-tube cholangiography. However, routine preoperative NPO status (nothing by mouth) is necessary for operative cholangiography.

⚐ Inform the patient that no discomfort is associated with these studies.

During

Operative Cholangiography

- Note the following procedural steps:
  1. The cystic duct is catheterized during cholecystectomy.
  2. Alternatively, a needle or catheter is placed in the common bile duct.
  3. The dye is injected directly into the common bile duct.
  4. Radiographs are obtained while the patient is on the operating table and are immediately reviewed by the surgeon.

T-Tube Cholangiography

- Note the following procedural steps:
  1. The patient is taken to the radiology department.
  2. A sterile dye solution is injected into the T-tube previously placed by the surgeon.
  3. X-ray images are obtained of the right upper quadrant of the abdomen with the patient placed in various positions.
- A radiologist or surgeon performs these procedures in approximately 10 minutes.

After

- Observe for signs of sepsis.
- If a T-tube has been surgically placed, establish a sterile, closed drainage system.

TEST RESULTS AND CLINICAL SIGNIFICANCE

Stones in the common bile duct: *These appear as radiolucent rounded filling defects in the column of dye within the common bile duct.*

Anatomic variations: *Many types of congenital anatomic variations in the common bile duct exist and are demonstrated at cholangiography.*

Cysts in the common bile duct: *Although rare, these cysts appear as small to large outpouchings of the common bile ducts.*

Stricture or tumour obstructing the common bile duct: *Tumour of the common bile duct (cholangiocarcinoma) or extrinsic tumour (e.g., pancreas, colon) can partially or completely obstruct the common bile duct. Benign inflammatory or posttraumatic strictures also can cause varying degrees of obstruction.*

Surgical trauma to the common bile duct: *Ligation or laceration of the common bile duct is obvious at the time of surgery with the use of cholangiography.*

RELATED TESTS

Endoscopic Retrograde Cholangiopancreatography (p. 632). This is an endoscopic procedure in which the common bile and pancreatic ducts are visualized radiographically.

Percutaneous Transhepatic Cholangiography (p. 1097). This procedure provides visualization of the common bile ducts by percutaneous access to the biliary tree through the liver.

Upper Gastrointestinal Tract Radiography (Upper GI Series, Ugi)

NORMAL FINDINGS

Normal size, contour, patency, filling, positioning, and transit of barium through the lower esophagus, stomach, and upper duodenum

INDICATIONS

This contrast-enhanced X-ray study provides visualization of the mucosa of the esophageal, gastric, and duodenum lumens. It is indicated in patients with upper abdominal pain, dyspepsia, dysphagia, early satiety, or suspected gastroduodenal obstruction.

TEST EXPLANATION

The upper gastrointestinal (GI) study consists of a series of X-rays of the lower esophagus, stomach, and duodenum; barium sulphate is usually the contrast medium. When leakage of X-ray contrast medium through a perforation of the GI tract is a concern, however, meglumine diatrizoate (Gastrografin), a water-soluble contrast medium, is used. This test can be performed in conjunction with a barium swallow study (p. 1038) or small bowel series (p. 1109), which can precede or succeed the upper GI study, respectively.

The purpose of the upper GI study is to detect ulcerations, tumour, inflammation, or anatomic malposition (e.g., hiatal hernia) of upper GI organs and obstruction in the upper GI tract. The patient drinks a beverage containing barium. As the contrast agent descends, the lower esophagus is examined for position, patency, and filling defects (e.g., tumour, scarring, varices). As the barium enters the stomach, the gastric wall is examined for benign or malignant ulcerations, filling defects (most often in cancer), and anatomic abnormalities (e.g., hiatal hernia). The patient is placed in a flat or head-down position, and the gastroesophageal area is examined for evidence of gastroesophageal reflux of barium.

As the contrast agent leaves the stomach, patency of the pyloric channel and the duodenum is evaluated. Benign peptic ulceration is the most common pathologic condition affecting these areas. Extrinsic compression caused by tumours, cysts, or enlarged diseased organs (e.g., the liver) near the stomach also can be identified on the basis of anatomic distortion of the outline of the upper GI tract.

A radiologist performs this procedure in approximately 30 minutes. The patient may be uncomfortable lying on the hard X-ray table and may occasionally experience a sensation of bloating or nausea during the test.

CONTRAINDICATIONS

- Complete bowel obstruction
- Suspected upper GI perforation; water-soluble Gastrografin should be used instead of barium
- Unstable vital signs; affected patients should be supervised during the time required for this test
- Inability of patients to cooperate, because of the necessity of frequent position changes

X-Ray Studies

12

POTENTIAL COMPLICATIONS

- Aspiration of barium
- Constipation or partial bowel obstruction caused by inspissated barium in the small bowel or colon

INTERFERING FACTORS

- Previously administered barium may block visualization of the upper GI tract.
- Poor patient performance will obscure the results.
- Incapacitated patients cannot assume the multiple positions required for the study.
- Food and fluid in the stomach give the false impression of filling defects in the stomach, which precludes adequate evaluation of the gastric mucosa.
- Patients with obtundation cannot safely drink the barium.

Clinical Priorities

- When perforation in the GI tract is a concern, meglumine diatrizoate (Gastrografin) is used instead of barium. This may cause diarrhea after the procedure.
- For an air-contrast upper GI study, the patient swallows a carbonated powder that creates carbon dioxide in the stomach and aids in visualization of the gastric mucosa.
- After the procedure, a cathartic is necessary to prevent impaction from the barium.

PROCEDURE AND PATIENT CARE

Before

 Explain the procedure to the patient. Allow the patient to verbalize concerns. Provide emotional support.

 Instruct the patient to abstain from eating for at least 8 hours before the test. In most cases, keep the patient on NPO status (nothing by mouth) after midnight on the day of the test.

 Assure the patient that the test will not cause any discomfort except for lying on the hard X-ray table and occasional sensation of bloating or nausea.

During

- Note the following procedural steps:
  1. The patient is asked to drink approximately 500 mL of barium sulphate. This is a chalky substance usually suspended in milkshake form and drunk through a straw (Figure 12-26). The drink is usually flavoured to increase palatability.
  2. After drinking the barium, the patient is moved through several position changes (e.g., prone, supine, lateral) to promote filling of the entire upper GI tract.
  3. Films are taken at the discretion of the radiologist as the flow of barium is observed fluoroscopically.
  4. The flow of barium is monitored through the lower esophagus, stomach, and duodenum.
  5. Several X-ray images are obtained throughout the course of the test.
  6. For an *air-contrast upper GI study,* the patient is asked to rapidly swallow carbonated powder. This creates carbon dioxide in the stomach, providing air contrast to the barium within the stomach and increasing visualization of the gastric mucosa.

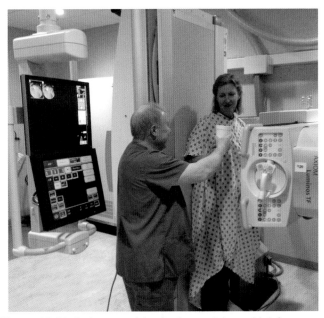

Figure 12-26 Patient receiving barium sulphate drink for upper gastrointestinal X-ray series.

After

- Inform the patient that if meglumine diatrizoate (Gastrografin) was used, significant diarrhea may develop. This contrast agent is an osmotic cathartic.
- Instruct the patient to use a cathartic (e.g., milk of magnesia) if barium sulphate was used as the contrast medium. Water absorption may cause the barium to harden and create a fecal impaction if catharsis is not carried out.
- Instruct the patient to note the stools to ensure that all of the barium has been removed. The stools should return to normal colour after the barium is completely expelled, which may take as long as a day and a half.

TEST RESULTS AND CLINICAL SIGNIFICANCE

Esophageal cancer: *Most esophageal cancers occur in the lower esophagus. They appear as a stricture or complete obstruction of the barium column.*

Esophageal varices: *Serpiginous filling defects indicate esophageal varices.*

Hiatal hernia: *There are two types of hiatal hernias. With a sliding hiatal hernia, the esophagogastric junction and upper stomach are in the chest. With the rolling type, the esophagogastric junction is normal, but the fundus of the stomach rolls up into the chest. This latter type can become incarcerated and perforate. Surgical repair is required when this condition is identified.*

Diverticula: *These can be present in the upper esophagus (Zenker) and caused by spasm of the cricopharyngeus muscle (upper esophageal sphincter), or they can be present in the lower esophagus (epiphrenic) and caused by paraesophageal infection.*

Gastric cancer: *Cancers can be evident as large polypoid filling defects within the stomach or as ulcerative masses in the wall of the stomach.*

Gastric inflammatory disease (e.g., Ménétrier disease): *Thickened rugae or gastric folds are characteristic of chronic inflammatory changes of the stomach.*

X-Ray Studies

12

Benign gastric tumour (e.g., leiomyoma): *Tumours can be small polypoid masses in the stomach or giant tumours that distort the entire upper abdomen.*

Extrinsic compression by pancreatic pseudocyst, cysts, pancreatic tumour, or hepatomegaly: *Masses in the upper abdomen can distort the stomach. Because the stomach is a large sack, it is unusual for that structure to be obstructed by extrinsic compression.*

Perforation of the esophagus, stomach, or duodenum: *Perforation is obvious when contrast material is evident outside the esophagus, stomach, or duodenum.*

Congenital abnormalities (e.g., duodenal web, pancreatic rest, malrotation syndrome): *These are congenital abnormalities that commonly cause duodenal obstruction in infants.*

Gastric ulcer (benign or malignant): *Malignancy can be ulcerative. Benign ulcers (stress or peptic) can also develop.*

Duodenal ulcer: *Most duodenal ulcers are peptic ulcers. They are most commonly seen in the bulb (the first portion) of the duodenum.*

Duodenal cancer: *This is very rare and usually is seen as a filling defect in the column of barium within the duodenum.*

Duodenal diverticulum: *These outpouchings are not uncommon, but they rarely cause symptoms.*

RELATED TEST

Esophagogastroduodenoscopy (p. 636). This endoscopic procedure provides better visualization of the upper GI organs. Furthermore, biopsy can be performed with this procedure.

 Venography, Lower Extremities (Phlebography, Venogram)

NORMAL FINDINGS

No evidence of venous thrombosis or obstruction

INDICATIONS

This contrast-enhanced X-ray study of the venous system of the lower or upper extremity is used to identify obstruction or thrombosis of the venous system in patients with a swollen arm or leg.

TEST EXPLANATION

Venography is an X-ray study designed to identify and locate thrombi in the venous system (most commonly in the extremities). Iodinated dye is injected into the venous system of the affected extremity. Radiographs are then obtained at timed intervals to visualize the venous system. Obstruction to the flow of dye or a filling defect within the dye-filled vein indicates thrombosis. Positive study results accurately confirm the diagnosis of venous thrombosis; however, negative results—although not as accurate—make the diagnosis of venous thrombosis unlikely. Often both extremities are studied, even when only one leg is suspected to contain deep-vein thrombosis. The normal extremity is used for comparison with the involved extremity. Venography is more accurate than venous Doppler imaging (p. 930) for thrombi in veins below the knee or in the femoral veins. Venography is also performed in the upper extremities to evaluate the more proximal axillary, subclavian, and innominate veins.

A radiologist performs this study in approximately 30 to 90 minutes. Venous catheterization is only as uncomfortable as a needlestick or a small incision in the foot.

The dye may cause the patient to feel a warm flush (although not as severe as with arteriography). Inform the patient that mild degrees of nausea, vomiting, or skin itching also occasionally occur.

CONTRAINDICATIONS

- Severe edema of the legs, making venous access for dye injection impossible
- Inability of patients to cooperate
- History of adverse reactions or allergic reactions to iodinated dye
- Allergy to shellfish
- Renal failure, because iodinated dye is nephrotoxic

Age-Related Concerns

- Adults older than 75 years are particularly vulnerable to renal failure, especially if they are chronically dehydrated (e.g., chronic diarrhea).
- Dehydration after the test can be exacerbated by the diuretic action of the dye.

POTENTIAL COMPLICATIONS

- For potential complications of iodinated dye, see p. 1021.
- Renal failure can occur, especially in older persons with chronic dehydration or mild renal failure (see Box 12-2, p. 1018).
- Subcutaneous infiltration of the dye can cause cellulitis and pain.
- Venous thrombophlebitis can be caused by the dye.
- Bacteremia can be caused by a break in sterile technique.
- Venous embolism may be caused by dislodgement of a deep-vein clot, induced by the dye injection.
- Hypoglycemia or acidosis may occur in patients who are taking metformin (Glucophage) and receive iodinated dye.

Clinical Priorities

- Assess the patient for adverse reactions or allergic reactions to iodinated dye.
- During the dye injection, the patient may feel a warm flush.
- The patient must be encouraged to drink large amounts of fluids after the test to prevent dehydration caused by the diuretic action of the dye.

PROCEDURE AND PATIENT CARE

Before

- Explain the procedure to the patient.
- Obtain the patient's informed consent for this procedure, if it is required.
- For assessment of adverse reactions or allergies to iodinated dye, see p. 1021.

X-Ray Studies

12

- If necessary, provide appropriate pain medication so that the patient is able to lie still during the procedure.
- Ensure that the patient is appropriately hydrated before testing. Injection of the iodinated contrast material may cause renal failure, especially in older patients.

Home Care Responsibilities

- Instruct the patient to monitor the puncture site for redness, swelling, or bleeding.
- Note that fever and chills may indicate bacteremia.
- Encourage the patient to drink fluids to promote dye excretion and to prevent dehydration caused by the injected dye.

During

- Note the following procedural steps:
  1. The patient is taken to the radiology department and placed supine on the X-ray table.
  2. Catheterization of a superficial vein on the foot is performed. This may require a surgical cutdown.
  3. An iodinated, radiopaque dye is injected into the vein.
  4. Radiographs are obtained to follow the course of the dye up the leg.
  5. Frequently, a tourniquet is placed on the leg to prevent filling of the superficial saphenous vein. All of the dye therefore goes to the deep venous system, which contains the most clinically significant thrombosis that can embolize.

After

- Continue appropriate fluid administration to prevent dehydration caused by the diuretic action of the dye.
- Observe the puncture site for infection, cellulitis, or bleeding.
- Assess the patient's vital signs for signs of bacteremia (e.g., fever, tachycardia, chills).
- Evaluate the patient for signs of delayed allergic reaction (e.g., rash, chills, fever, irritability, dyspnea, tachycardia, and urticaria). Reactions usually occur within the first 2 to 6 hours after the test. Treat reactions with antihistamines or steroids.

TEST RESULTS AND CLINICAL SIGNIFICANCE

Obstruction of venous system by thrombosis, tumour, or inflammation: *This is evident from complete obstruction of dye flow in the main vein (usually femoral or iliac).*

Acute deep-vein thrombosis: *This is evident from serpiginous filling defects in the column of dye on the wall of the vein.*

RELATED TESTS

Vascular Ultrasound Studies (p. 930). With the use of ultrasonography, blood flow within the vein can be evaluated. Obstruction to flow is easily noted. This test is less invasive and associated with less risk than is venography, and it is equally accurate (above the knee).

Venous Plethysmography. This is a manometric study of the venous system of the extremity. It enables identification of venous occlusion.

Additional Studies

NOTE: *Throughout this chapter, SI units are presented in* boldface colour, *followed by conventional units in parentheses.*

OVERVIEW

Overview, 1123

TESTS

OVERVIEW

In the preceding chapters, a multitude of diverse diagnostic tests have been organized into groups according to the specimen analyzed and the method of testing. However, a few tests, including genetic testing, could not readily be assigned to any chapter. Therefore, this chapter was created to include these important tests. There are no commonalities associated with these tests. All are described separately and in detail. Current guidelines for genetic testing in Canada are discussed, including genetic screening for breast and colorectal cancer, as well as cultural considerations for breast cancer risk. Canadian guidelines for bioterrorism testing are also included.

Allergy Skin Testing

NORMAL FINDINGS
<3-mm wheal diameter
<10-mm flare diameter

INDICATIONS

Skin testing is the most commonly used and easiest method of identifying patients who suffer from allergies. Furthermore, it is a method by which a specific allergen can be determined.

TEST EXPLANATION

When properly performed, skin testing is considered to be the most convenient and least expensive test for detecting allergic reactions. Since the early 1900s, skin testing has been a common practice for establishing a diagnosis of allergy by re-exposure of the individual to a specific allergen. Skin testing provides useful confirmatory evidence when a diagnosis of allergy is suspected on clinical grounds. The simplicity, rapidity, low costs, sensitivity, and specificity explain the crucial position skin testing has in allergy testing.

In an allergic patient, injection of the specific allergen (the substance to which the person is allergic) triggers a reaction consisting of a wheal (swelling) and flare (redness). This reaction—which is initiated by immunoglobulin E (IgE) antibodies and is mediated primarily by histamine secreted from mast cells—usually begins approximately 5 minutes after the injection and peaks at 30 minutes. In a number of patients, a "late-phase reaction" occurs; this reaction is highlighted by antibody and cellular infiltration into the area resulting in a wheal and flare that usually develops within 1 to 2 hours.

There are three commonly accepted methods of injecting the allergen into the skin. The first method is called the *prick-puncture test* or *scratch test*. In this method, the allergen is injected into the epidermis. Life-threatening anaphylaxis reactions have not been reported with this method. The second method is called the *intradermal test*. Here the allergen is injected into the dermis (creating a skin wheal). Large local reactions and anaphylaxis have been reported with this latter method. For these two tests, the allergen placement part of the test takes about 5 to 10 minutes. The third method is called the *patch test*. This takes much longer because the patient must wear the patch for 48 hours to see if there is a delayed allergic reaction. With this method, needles are not used. Instead, an allergen is applied to a patch that is placed on the skin. It is usually done to detect whether a particular substance (e.g., latex, medications, fragrances, preservatives, hair dyes, metals, resins) is causing an allergic skin irritation, such as contact dermatitis.

Patients with dermographism (nonallergic response of redness and swelling of the skin at the site of any stimulation) develop a skin wheal with any skin irritation, even if nonallergic. In such patients, a false-positive result can occur with skin testing. To avoid false-positive results, a "negative control" substance consisting of only the diluent, without an allergen, is injected at the same time as the other skin tests are performed. In patients who are immunosuppressed because of concurrent disease or medicines, the skin reaction may be blunted even in the presence of allergy. This would represent a false-negative test result. To avoid false-negative results, a "positive control" substance consisting of a histamine analogue is also injected into the forearm at the time of skin testing. This will cause a wheal-and-flare response even in a nonallergic patient, unless the patient is immunosuppressed.

For inhalant allergens, skin test results are extremely accurate. However, they are less reliable for food allergies, latex allergies, drug sensitivity, and occupational allergies. The accuracy of skin testing varies considerably because of poor injection techniques; however, when performed correctly, skin testing represents one of the major tools in the diagnosis of allergy.

CONTRAINDICATIONS

• History of anaphylaxis

POTENTIAL COMPLICATIONS

- Anaphylaxis

INTERFERING FACTORS

- Test results may be falsely positive in patients with dermographism.
- Test results may be falsely positive if the patient has a reaction to the diluent used to preserve the extract.
- Test results may be falsely negative as a result of poor-quality allergen extracts, diseases that attenuate the immune response, or improper technique.
- Infants and older adults may have decreased skin reactivity.
- Drugs that may *decrease* the immune response of skin testing include angiotensin-converting enzyme inhibitors, beta blockers, corticosteroids, nifedipine, antihistamines, and theophylline.

PROCEDURE AND PATIENT CARE

Before

- Explain the procedure to the patient.
- Observe the following skin-testing precautions:
  1. Ensure that a physician is available immediately.
  2. Ensure that medications and equipment are available for treating anaphylaxis.
- Obtain a history to evaluate the risk of anaphylaxis.
- Identify any immunosuppressive medications the patient may be taking.
- Evaluate the patient for dermographism by rubbing the skin with a pencil eraser and looking for a wheal at the site of irritation.
- Draw up 0.05 mL of 1 : 1000 aqueous epinephrine into a syringe before testing in the event of an exaggerated allergic reaction.
- A prick-puncture test should be performed, and should yield negative results, before an intradermal test.
- In general, the allergen solution is diluted 100- to 1000-fold before injection.

During

Prick-Puncture Method

- Proceed with caution in patients with current allergic symptoms.
- Pay great attention to the technique chosen for the skin test in order to obtain accurate results.
- Avoid bleeding caused by injection.
- Avoid spreading of allergen solutions beyond the injection site during the test.
- Record the skin reaction at the proper time.
- A drop of the allergen solution is placed onto the volar surface of the forearm or back.
- A 25-gauge needle is passed through the droplet and inserted into the epidermal space at an angle with the bevel facing up.
- The skin is lifted up, and the fluid is allowed to seep in. Excess fluid is wiped off after approximately 1 minute.

Intradermal Method

- Cleanse the skin area.
- With a 25-gauge needle, the allergen solution is injected into the dermis and triggers the development of a skin wheal. In this method, the bevel of the needle faces downward. A volume of between 0.01 and 0.05 mL is injected.
- In general, the allergen solution is diluted 100- to 1000-fold before injection.

After

- Evaluate the patient for exaggerated allergic response.
- In the event of a systemic reaction, a tourniquet should be placed above the testing site and epinephrine should be administered subcutaneously.
- With a pen, encircle the area of testing and mark the allergen used.
- Evaluate the skin test result at the appropriate time. Skin test results are evaluated when the reaction is mature, after approximately 15 to 20 minutes. Both the largest and smallest diameters of the wheal are determined. The measurements (in millimetres) are averaged.
- The flare is measured in the same manner.
- The patient should be observed for 20 to 30 minutes before discharge.

Patch Method

- Clean the skin area (usually back or arm).
- Apply the patches to the skin (as many as 30 can be applied).
- Instruct the patient to wear the patches for 48 hours. Tell the patient to avoid bathing or activities that cause heavy sweating.
- Tell the patient the patches will be removed at the doctor's office. Irritated skin at a patch site may indicate an allergy.

After

- Document allergen solution, location, and patient reaction.
- Evaluate the patient for exaggerated allergic response.
- In the event of a systemic reaction, a tourniquet should be placed above the testing site and epinephrine should be administered subcutaneously.
- With a pen, encircle the area of testing and mark the allergen used.
- Read the skin test at the appropriate time.
- Skin tests are read when the reaction is mature, after about 48 hours. Both the largest and smallest diameter of the wheal is determined. The measurements (in millimetres) are averaged.
- The flare is measured in the same manner.
- Observe the patient for 20 to 30 minutes before discharge.

TEST RESULTS AND CLINICAL SIGNIFICANCE

Allergy-Related Diseases

Asthma,
Dermatitis,
Food allergy,
Drug allergy,
Occupational allergy,
Allergic rhinitis,
Angioedema: *All these diseases are immunoreactive (allergic) in their pathophysiologic processes. Specific allergens, when injected or applied to the skin, cause an allergic reaction consisting of wheal and flare.*

RELATED TEST

Allergy Blood Testing (p. 56). Allergy blood testing is an alternative to allergy skin testing in diagnosing allergy as a cause of a particular symptom complex. It is also useful in identifying the particular allergen affecting a patient. It is particularly helpful when allergy skin testing is contraindicated.

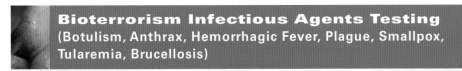

Bioterrorism Infectious Agents Testing
(Botulism, Anthrax, Hemorrhagic Fever, Plague, Smallpox, Tularemia, Brucellosis)

NORMAL FINDINGS

Negative for evidence of infectious agent

INDICATIONS

These tests are indicated if terrorism is suspected on the basis of unusual illness or when evidence of terrorism is present.

TEST EXPLANATION

Infectious agents used in bioterrorism are numerous. This discussion concerns the agents that humans are most likely to be exposed to in war or in a civilian terrorist attack. Table 13-1 summarizes specific characteristics and methods for testing of each agent. All documented cases must be reported to the Public Health Agency of Canada (PHAC).

Anthrax

Anthrax is caused by *Bacillus anthracis,* which is a spore-forming, Gram-positive rod. The organism is widely distributed in the soil, and under natural conditions, grazing animals can become infected and transfer it to people working in close contact with grazing animal products (meat, wool, or hides). It can be contracted by eating undercooked meat or inhaled from animal products (such as wool) or by inhaling the spores. Once inhaled, it is uniformly fatal without treatment.

There are three forms of anthrax disease: cutaneous, gastrointestinal, and pulmonary. Symptoms include fever, malaise, fatigue, and progression of the disease to include cutaneous lesions or pulmonary failure. Symptoms occur approximately 2 to 6 days after exposure.

Growth of the organism in sheep blood agar confirms the diagnosis. Appropriate specimens for culture are stool, blood, sputum, or the cutaneous vesicle. Treatment for this disease is early institution of antibiotics and supportive care.

Botulism Infection

The toxin produced by *Clostridia botulinum,* a spore-forming anaerobic bacterium, causes the symptoms associated with botulism. The gastrointestinal tract is the usual port of entry when the toxin itself, *C. botulinum* spores, or the actual bacterium is ingested. When ingested, the toxin produces symptoms almost immediately. If the spores or the bacterium are ingested, symptom onset may be delayed. Common sources of *C. botulinum* include undercooked meat and sauces exposed to room temperature for prolonged periods. This bacterium can be inhaled by handling the same food or by open wound contamination of soil that contains *C. botulinum.*

The toxin binds irreversibly to the presynaptic nerve terminal at the neuromuscular junction and prevents the release of acetylcholine necessary for normal muscular function. As a result, the affected person may experience bulbar palsies that cause blurring of vision, dysphagia,

TABLE 13-1 Bioterrorism Infectious Agents: Summary

Infection/Infectious Agent	Site of Entry	Sources	Specimen for Testing	Tests
Botulism/*Clostridium botulinum*	GI mucosa, skin surfaces, lungs, wound contamination	Undercooked meats, soil, dust	Blood, stool, vomitus, food	Botulinum toxin, mouse bioassay, culture for *C. botulinum*
Anthrax/*Bacillus anthracis*	Lungs, GI mucosa	Undercooked meats, inhalation of spores from animal products/skin	Sputum, blood, stool, skin vesicle, food, spores	Isolation of *B. anthracis* in a clinical specimen by immunofluorescence
Yellow fever/hantavirus, Ebola virus, multiple other viruses	Skin bite	Rodent or mosquito bites	Blood, sputum, tissue	Culture, serology to detect IgM antibodies specific for viral antigens
Plague infections/*Yersinia pestis*	Skin bite	Infected fleas	Blood, sputum, lymph node aspirate	Significant rise (≥four-fold) in serum antibody titre to *Y. pestis* F1 antigen by EIA or passive hemagglutination/inhibition titre Isolation of *Y. pestis* from body fluids
Brucellosis/*Brucella abortus, Brucella canis,* other *Brucella* species	GI mucosa, lungs, wound contamination	Infected meats and milk products	Blood, sputum, food	Isolation of *Brucella* organism from body fluids Culture of organism
Smallpox/variola virus	Lungs	Respiratory droplets, direct contact, contaminated clothing	Vesicle	Isolation of variola virus from an appropriate specimen Viral culture or viral identification with electron microscopy
Tularemia/*Francisella tularensis*	Skin, GI tract, lungs	Ingestion of contaminated plants or water	Blood, sputum, stool	Isolation of *F. tularensis* from an appropriate specimen A significant (four-fold or greater) change in serum antibody titre to *F. tularensis* antigen

EIA, Enzyme immunoassay; *GI,* gastrointestinal; *IgM,* immunoglobulin M.

dysarthria, and skeletal muscle weakness that progresses to flaccid paralysis. Symptoms begin 6 to 12 hours after ingestion of spores or bacteria from the contaminated food or approximately 1 week after wound contamination. The test used to diagnose this disease involves the identification of the toxin in the blood, stool, or vomitus of the affected individual. The food itself can also be tested. The toxin can be identified by the biologic mouse neutralization test. *C. botulinum* can also be cultured in an anaerobic environment from the stool or from contaminated food.

Treatment involves mechanical support of ventilation and nutrition. The botulinum antitoxin, which can be obtained from the U.S. Centers for Disease Control and Prevention (CDC), is the mainstay of treatment. This antitoxin presents a risk of "serum sickness" in nearly 25% of the patients who receive it.

Brucellosis

This disease is caused by various *Brucella* species: *B. abortus, B. suis, B. melitensis,* and *B. canis.* It is contracted by ingestion of contaminated milk products (especially goat's milk), through direct puncture of the skin (by butchers and farmers), or by inhalation. This multisystem disease is characterized by acute or insidious onset of fever, night sweats, undue fatigue, anorexia, weight loss, headache, and arthralgia. Hepatomegaly, splenomegaly, and spondylitis are also common. *Brucella* organisms can be cultured from a blood, sputum, or food specimen. Serologic testing is also possible. Diagnosis is confirmed by a four-fold or greater rise in *Brucella* agglutination titre between acute- and convalescent-phase serum specimens obtained 2 weeks or more apart and studied at the same laboratory. Demonstration by immunofluorescence of a *Brucella* organism in a clinical specimen is another method of diagnosis.

Hemorrhagic Fever (Yellow Fever)

This disease complex has many causative viral families, including arenavirus, bunyavirus (such as hantavirus), Filovirus (including Ebola), and flavivirus. In confirmed cases of the hantavirus pulmonary syndrome, the clinical illness is characterized by fever (oral temperature >38.3°C [101°F]) and bilateral diffuse infiltrates (may resemble acute respiratory distress syndrome [ARDS]), and the disease develops within 72 hours of hospitalization of a previously asymptomatic person. Symptoms usually develop 4 to 21 days after a mosquito or rodent bite (depending on the disease). This disease is contagious, and patients with suspect symptoms should be quarantined.

The diagnosis is determined by clinical evaluation. However, viral cultures with polymerase chain reaction, serologic tests, and immunohistochemical analysis of tissue specimens are possible. There is no specific treatment other than aggressive medical therapy and support for organ failure.

Plague

This disease is caused by the Gram-negative coccobacillus *Yersinia pestis.* In nature, it is transmitted to humans primarily by the bite of fleas or contact with other human bodily fluids. In humans, the disease takes one of four forms: bubonic (regional lymphadenitis or enlarged lymph nodes); septicemic (bloodborne); primary pneumonic (aerosol or inhalation of infectious droplets), secondary pneumonic (pneumonia resulting from hematogenous spread in bubonic or septicemic cases); or pharyngeal (pharyngitis and cervical lymphadenitis resulting from exposure to infectious droplets or ingestion of infected tissues). Pneumonic plague is, by far, the deadliest form of the disease. Symptoms may include fever, chills, headache, malaise, prostration, leukocytosis, enlarged lymph nodes, or bacterial pneumonia and respiratory failure.

The diagnosis is made from culture of the blood, sputum, or lymph node aspirate. This disease complex can be treated with antibiotics when they are started early in the course of the disease. In bioterrorism, the disease is caused by attack or spread by aerosol transmission.

Smallpox

Smallpox is a serious, contagious, and sometimes fatal infectious disease caused by the variola virus (a DNA virus). There is no specific treatment for smallpox, and the only prevention is vaccination. There are two clinical forms of smallpox. Variola major is the severe and most common form of smallpox, with a more extensive rash and higher fever. Variola minor is a less common manifestation of smallpox and a much less severe disease. A worldwide vaccination program has successfully prevented outbreaks of this disease. It is very easily spread and has the potential to cause widespread disease and death that could devastate a whole city or region.

The first symptoms of smallpox include a febrile prodrome (oral temperature >38.3°C [101°F]) and systemic symptoms (prostration, headache, back pain, abdominal pain, vomiting). This condition usually lasts 1 to 4 days and is followed by the development of a rash. The rash consists of deep, firm, well-circumscribed pustules, initially appearing as macules, evolving into papules, vesicles, and then pustules within a few days. Lesions initially appear in the oral mucosa or palate and then progress to involve the face, arms, legs, palms, and soles. As the pustules dry up and scab, the patient is no longer contagious.

Viral culture, serologic testing, immunohistochemical analysis, and electron microscopy can confirm the diagnosis. The best specimen for testing is the vesicular rash. Although there is no treatment for the disease, vaccination is available and is offered to everyone at risk for bioterrorism. In Canada, any testing related to suspected cases should be carried out only in level 4 containment facilities, and the PHAC should be contacted (1-800-545-7661) in the event of a suspected case in order to activate their emergency program.

Tularemia

This disease is caused by a Gram-negative bacterium called *Francisella tularensis*. It is contracted by drinking contaminated water or eating vegetation contaminated by infected animals or from an insect bite. It can be aerosolized and can contaminate the air or drinking water supplies. *F. tularensis* can enter through the skin by an insect bite (usually a tick or deerfly bite), and tularemia can be recognized from the presence of a lesion and swollen glands. In humans, tularemia takes three distinct forms: (1) glandular-cutaneous ulcer with regional swelling; (2) glandular-regional lymphadenopathy with no ulcer but with ocular conjunctivitis, oropharyngeal stomatitis, or tonsillitis; and (3) intestinal pain, vomiting, diarrhea, and fever. Symptoms generally appear between 2 and 10 days, but usually 3 days, after exposure.

Inhalation of the organism may produce a fever alone or fever combined with a pneumonia-like illness that is difficult to distinguish from influenza or other atypical pneumonias. Diagnosis is made from culture of the blood, sputum, or stool, and changes in serum antibody titre to *F. tularensis* antigen.

PROCEDURE AND PATIENT CARE

Before

- Maintain strict adherence to all procedures in regard to isolation or contamination of the specimen.
- Biohazard precautions are to be taken with each specimen.
- Laboratory personnel must strictly adhere to all standard/routine precautions and transmission principles.

During

- If an enema is used to obtain a botulinum stool specimen, use sterile water. Saline can negate results.
- Send enough blood for adequate testing. Usually two red-top tubes are adequate. It is best to send the blood specimens in a mixture of crushed ice and water.
- If food is sent for testing, it should be sent in its original containers.
- For anthrax or smallpox testing of a cutaneous lesion, soak one or two culture swabs with fluid from a previously unopened lesion.

After

- Identify all potential sources of contamination.
- Isolate individuals who are suspected of having a contagious disease.
- Report to the federal level (PHAC) only if cases of hantavirus pulmonary syndrome, plague, tularemia, and brucellosis are confirmed.
- Confirmed cases of the plague must also be reported to the World Health Organization, if the illness constitutes a public health emergency.
- Report to the federal level (PHAC) all confirmed, probable, and suspected cases of anthrax and smallpox.

TEST RESULTS AND CLINICAL SIGNIFICANCE

See Table 13-1.

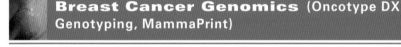

Breast Cancer Genomics (Oncotype DX Genotyping, MammaPrint)

NORMAL FINDINGS

Recurrence score <18 (on scale of 0 to 100)

INDICATIONS

In molecular genomic studies, the quantity of specific breast cancer–related genes is measured; therefore, these studies can help predict the susceptibility of cancer to chemotherapy. They also provide a powerful indicator of the likelihood of breast cancer recurrence after primary breast cancer surgery.

TEST EXPLANATION

Two genomic tests, the Onco*type* DX and the MammaPrint, are clinically validated, multigene assays that help quantitatively assess the likelihood of distant breast cancer recurrence and, in patients with newly diagnosed breast cancer, help assess the benefit from certain types of chemotherapy. In early-stage invasive breast cancer, the evaluation of the likelihood of distant recurrence is usually based on multiple pathologic factors, such as nodal status, tumour size and grade, estrogen and progesterone receptors, and *HER2* status (see p. 746). However, these factors are often inaccurate, and the recurrence risk cannot be quantified sufficiently to provide significant insight into the risks and benefits of adjuvant chemotherapy. Genomic testing is designed to provide quantitative data to assist in clinical decision making regarding the use of adjuvant systemic therapies.

In the Onco*type* DX reverse transcription polymerase chain reaction (RT-PCR) assay—performed with the use of formalin-fixed, paraffin-embedded tumour tissue—the expression of a panel of 21 genes (16 tumour-related genes and 5 reference genes) is analyzed, and the results are provided as a recurrence score (0 to 100). When this assay was developed, the gene panel was selected and the recurrence score calculation derived through extensive laboratory testing, followed by appropriate corroboration with multiple clinical studies in which the predictability of the assay was validated. In the MammaPrint, a microarray assay on fresh-frozen breast cancer tissue, the expression of 70 prognostic genes is analyzed. A 5-gene immunohistochemistry assay, the Mammostrat, entails the use of monoclonal antibody biomarkers and a diagnostic algorithm with fresh-frozen cancer tissue. Molecular genomics testing is sensitive, specific, and highly reproducible and can be used to measure the quantity of specific cancer-related genes in a wide range of body tissues.

Patients whose tumour genomics tests yield low recurrence scores have only a slight chance of recurrence and derive minimal or no benefit from chemotherapy. Patients with tumours that have high recurrence scores have a significant chance of recurrence and can experience considerable benefit from chemotherapy. At present, genomic testing is intended for patients with newly diagnosed breast cancer that is stage I or II, node negative, *HER2/neu* negative, and estrogen receptor positive. Clinical studies in populations with other cancers are currently under way.

CONTRAINDICATIONS

- Patients' refusal of adjuvant therapy, because the test is very expensive and results will not affect their treatment

PROCEDURE AND PATIENT CARE

Before

🖎 Explain the significance of the prognostic data available for the patient's tumour.
🖎 Explain the benefits of genomics in helping the physician and the patient make appropriate decisions regarding the use of adjuvant chemotherapy.
🖎 Provide the patient with emotional support throughout the postoperative period.

During

- After obtaining the specimen, the pathologist will send paraffin-embedded tissue to the centralized laboratory.
- Results will be available in approximately 2 weeks.

After

🖎 Provide education and support to patients as they evaluate their results.

TEST RESULTS AND CLINICAL SIGNIFICANCE

Breast cancer: *Patients with high recurrence scores are likely to experience early recurrence and will probably benefit from cytotoxic chemotherapy.*

RELATED TESTS

Estrogen Receptor Assay (p. 759) and Progesterone Receptor Assay (p. 781). These tests also yield prognostic indicators for breast cancer.

Breast Cancer Tumour Analysis (p. 746). *HER2/neu* is a breast cancer prognosticator and a target for monoclonal therapy.

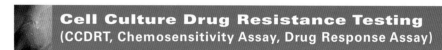

Cell Culture Drug Resistance Testing
(CCDRT, Chemosensitivity Assay, Drug Response Assay)

NORMAL FINDINGS

Cells sensitive to planned therapeutic drugs

INDICATIONS

This still-experimental test is performed to evaluate the sensitivity of a patient's cancer cells to anticancer drugs.

TEST EXPLANATION

Cell culture drug resistance testing (CCDRT) refers to testing the reaction of a patient's own cancer cells in the laboratory to drugs that may be used to treat the patient's cancer. The idea is to identify which drugs are more likely to work and which drugs are less likely to work. By avoiding the latter and choosing from among the former, the patient's probability of benefiting from the chemotherapy may be improved. There are multiple tests available for drug sensitivity testing, but all have four common steps. Cancer cells from the patient's tumour must be obtained and isolated. The cells are then isolated with various potentially therapeutic drugs. Assessment of cell survival is then performed and the results are provided. Based on those results, the clinician can recommend more appropriate chemotherapy for a particular cancer. In most cases, this testing is used for patients with refractory or recurrent epithelial tumours (usually breast or ovarian cancer).

PROCEDURE AND PATIENT CARE

Before

🖉 Explain the process to the patient. (Tumour cells are usually obtained by a surgical procedure.)

During

• Tumour cells are sent to a reference laboratory. The method of tissue preservation varies among laboratories.

After

• After the results are obtained, appropriate chemotherapy targeted to the patient's tumour cells is administered.

TEST RESULTS AND CLINICAL SIGNIFICANCE

Epithelial cancer: *This testing is still considered experimental because there is no extensive clinical experience to support its accuracy. However, a growing number of studies have shown a superior survival rate for patients treated with drugs targeting their tumour cells.*

 Chorionic Villus Sampling (CVS, Chorionic Villus Biopsy [CVB])

NORMAL FINDINGS

No genetic or biochemical disorders

INDICATIONS

Chorionic villus sampling (CVS) is performed in pregnant women whose unborn child may be at risk for a life-threatening or life-altering genetic defect. Such women include (1) those who are older than 35 years at the time of pregnancy, (2) those who have had frequent spontaneous abortions, (3) those who have had previous pregnancies with fetuses or infants with chromosomal or genetic defects (e.g., Down syndrome), and (4) those who have a genetic defect themselves (e.g., hemoglobinopathy).

TEST EXPLANATION

CVS can be performed at 8 to 12 weeks of gestation for early detection of genetic and biochemical disorders. Because CVS detects congenital defects early, first-trimester therapeutic abortions can be performed if indicated and desired.

A sample of chorionic villi from the chorion frondosum, which is the trophoblastic origin of the placenta, is obtained for analysis. These villi in the chorion frondosum appear between 8 and 12 weeks of gestation, are present throughout gestation, and are thought to reflect fetal chromosome, enzyme, and DNA content. This enables much earlier diagnosis of prenatal problems than does amniocentesis, which cannot be performed earlier than 14 to 16 weeks of gestation. Furthermore, the cells obtained with CVS are more easily cultured for karyotyping (determination of chromosomal and genetic abnormalities). Performing CVS safely requires significant experience. Although amniocentesis is the safer procedure, the cells obtained take longer to grow in culture, which delays results. At this later point, therapeutic abortion for severe genetic defects is more difficult.

POTENTIAL COMPLICATIONS

- Accidental abortion
- Infection
- Bleeding
- Amniotic fluid leakage
- Fetal limb deformities

PROCEDURE AND PATIENT CARE

Before

- Explain the procedure to the patient.
- Obtain the patient's informed consent for the procedure.

⋎ Inform the patient that no food or fluid restrictions are necessary.
⋎ Encourage the patient to drink at least 1 to 2 glasses of fluid before the test.
⋎ Instruct the patient not to urinate for several hours before the test. A full bladder enables the uterus to be an excellent reference point for pelvic ultrasonography.
• Assess the vital signs of the patient and the fetal heart rate before, during, and on completion of the test.

During

• Note the following procedural steps:
  1. The patient is placed in the lithotomy position, and a sterile speculum is placed into the previously cleansed vagina to visualize the cervix.
  2. A cannula is inserted into the cervix and uterine cavity (Figure 13-1).
  3. Under ultrasound guidance, the cannula is rotated to the site of the developing placenta.
  4. A syringe is attached, and suction is applied to obtain three or more villous samples to ensure sufficient tissue for accurate sampling.
  5. If ultrasonography indicates that the trophoblastic tissue is remote from the cervix, a transabdominal approach similar to that described for amniocentesis (p. 660) may be used.
• This procedure is performed in approximately 30 minutes by an obstetrician.
⋎ Inform the patient that discomfort associated with this test is similar to that of a Papanicolaou (Pap) smear.

After

• Some pregnant women with Rh-negative blood may receive Rho(D) immune globulin (RhoGAM) because of the risk for development of maternal antibodies to the fetal blood cells, which could threaten fetal well-being.
• Monitor vital signs, and check the woman for signs of bleeding.

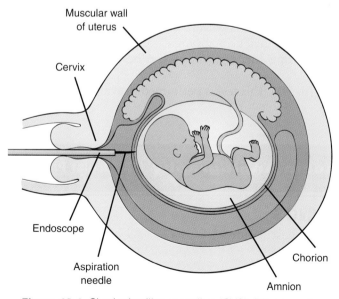

Figure 13-1 Chorionic villus sampling (CVS). Diagram of an 8-week gestation, showing endoscopic aspiration of extraplacental villi.

- Schedule an ultrasound study in 2 to 4 days to affirm continued viability of the fetus.
- Assess the vaginal area for discharge and drainage; note the colour and amount.
- Assess and educate the patient concerning signs of spontaneous abortion (e.g., cramps, bleeding) and endometrial infection (e.g., vaginal discharge, fever, crampy abdominal pain).
- Inform the patient how to obtain the results from the physician. Ensure that she understands that the results are usually not available for several weeks (although they may be available much sooner if the test is performed at a major medical centre).
- Inform the patient about genetic counselling services if they are needed.

🏠 Home Care Responsibilities

- Instruct the patient to report signs of spontaneous abortion (e.g., cramps, bleeding) immediately.
- Instruct the patient to identify and report signs of endometrial infection (e.g., vaginal discharge, fever, crampy abdominal pain).
- Instruct the patient to schedule an ultrasound study 2 to 4 days after CVS to ensure continued viability of the fetus.

TEST RESULTS AND CLINICAL SIGNIFICANCE

Chromosomal, genetic, and biochemical disorders: *Many chromosomal and genetic defects are identified by karyotyping and genetic mapping. Genetic counselling is a vital part of this sort of testing. If therapeutic abortion is an option, the patient's religious, moral, and ethical views about this decision need to be considered.*

RELATED TESTS

Pelvic Ultrasonography (p. 917). This test is used to localize trophoblastic tissue.

Amniocentesis (p. 660). This test is performed to evaluate fetal well-being and enables tissue sampling for karyotyping and genetic mapping.

Fetoscopy (p. 640). During this test, tissue can be obtained for karyotyping and genetic mapping.

Fetal Nonstress Test (p. 597). This test is performed to evaluate the viability of the fetus before, during, and after CVS.

Fluorescein Angiography (FA, Ocular Photography)

NORMAL FINDINGS

Normal retinal/choroidal vasculature

INDICATIONS

This test is performed to diagnose disease affecting the posterior structures of the eye, including the retina, choroid, and optic nerve. It is also used to monitor progression and treatment of eye disease.

TEST EXPLANATION

With the use of fluorescein angiography, the patency and integrity of the retinal circulation can be determined. It involves injection of sodium fluorescein into the systemic circulation, followed by timed-interval photographs performed with a fundus camera. The timed images are then reviewed for specific patterns indicative of disease states. The test is often repeated at intervals to monitor treatment or disease progression.

Fluorescein is a triphenylmethane dye. When the fluorescein molecules absorb light toward the end of the blue spectrum (465 to 490 nm), the molecules transform from a basal state to an excited state. In doing so, they emit light of a different wavelength (450 to 465 nm: the yellow-green portion of the light spectrum). This light emission is then recorded by a specialized camera in which very little light outside the blue spectrum is allowed to enter. The camera also has a filter that limits recording of light other than the yellow-to-green range. With digital technology, colour images can be obtained at specified times after dye injections. Before this procedure, baseline images are obtained. A 6-second bolus of approximately 5 mL of sodium fluorescein is injected into a vein in the upper extremity. Images are obtained 10 seconds later, then approximately once every second for approximately 20 seconds, and then less often. A delayed image is obtained at 5 and 10 minutes. Some physicians prefer to see a 15-minute image as well. Normal circulatory filling times are approximate:

    0 seconds: injection of fluorescein

    9.5 seconds: entrance of fluorescein into the posterior ciliary arteries

    10 seconds: choroidal flush (or pre-arterial phase)

    10 to 12 seconds: retinal arterial stage

    13 seconds: capillary transition stage

    14 to 15 seconds: early venous stage (or lamellar stage, arterial-venous stage)

    16 to 17 seconds: venous stage

    18 to 20 seconds: late venous stage

    5 minutes: late staining

Fluorescein enters the ocular circulation from the internal carotid artery via the ophthalmic artery. The ophthalmic artery supplies the choroid via the short posterior ciliary arteries and the retina via the central retinal artery. However, the route to the choroid is typically less circuitous than the route to the retina. This accounts for the short delay between the "choroidal flush" and retinal filling. Pathologic changes are characterized by either hyperfluorescence or hypofluorescence. Of the common groups of ophthalmologic diseases, diabetic retinopathy, vein occlusions, retinal artery occlusions, edema of the optic disc, and tumours can be detected with fluorescein angiography.

Fluorescein angiography is often performed to monitor the course of a disease such as diabetes, a disease that can cause the blood vessels of the retina to leak blood or fluid. Age-related macular degeneration is another disease that can cause the blood vessels of the retina to leak blood or fluid. Both diseases can be treated with a laser to help prevent loss of vision, and treatment results can be monitored with fluorescein angiography.

The test is performed and interpreted by an ophthalmologist, usually in the office setting. Results are available in less than 30 minutes.

POTENTIAL COMPLICATIONS

- Allergic reactions to fluorescein dye are rare. If they occur, they may cause a skin rash and itching. Severe allergic reactions (anaphylaxis), which are extremely rare, can be life-threatening.

PROCEDURE AND PATIENT CARE

Before

- Explain the procedure to the patient.
- Obtain the patient's informed consent for the procedure.
- Emphasize that the patient must remain still during the few seconds after fluorescein injection.
- Document any history of cataracts, prior retinal surgery, or other disease that may inhibit photography.
- Instruct the patient to remove any ocular lenses.
- Inform the patient that there are no dietary restrictions.
- Pupil dilatation can improve access to the posterior eye. Administer appropriate mydriatic medications if they are ordered. Note, however, that these medications are contraindicated for patients with glaucoma because they may increase ocular pressures to levels that may damage the eye.

During

- The patient is positioned in the fundus camera with the chin on the bar.
- The patient is told to select a spot in the far distance and stare at that spot fixedly during the examination.
- Intravenous access is obtained.
- Fluorescein dye is injected with the assistance of an autoinjector.
- Images are obtained by the ophthalmologist at timed intervals.
- This test is performed and interpreted by an ophthalmologist, usually in the office setting. Results are available in less than 30 minutes.

After

- Remove the intravenous access device, and apply pressure to the venipuncture site.
- Document the procedure and the patient's response.
- Inform the patient that fluorescein dye is excreted by the kidneys and to expect very yellow urine for the next 24 hours.

TEST RESULTS AND CLINICAL SIGNIFICANCE

▲ Increased Levels

Tumour,
Detached retina,
Trauma,
Inflammation,
Retinitis pigmentosa,
Papilledema: *Hyperfluorescence is caused by neovascularity that occurs with neoplasm or inflammation. It is also seen with destruction of vascular integrity associated with these ocular diseases.*
Diabetic retinopathy: *Capillary microaneurysms in the retina are often the earliest signs of diabetic retinopathy.*

▼ Decreased Levels

Diabetes,
Vascular disease,
Radiation to the eye,
Hemorrhage,

Edema,

Prior photocoagulation therapy: *These diseases cause hypofluorescence because the arterial flow is interrupted by these diseases.*

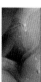

Genetic Testing (Breast Cancer [BRCA] and Ovarian Cancer, Colon Cancer, Cardiovascular Disease, Tay-Sachs Disease, Cystic Fibrosis, Melanoma, Hemochromatosis, Thyroid Cancer, Paternity [Parentage Analysis], and Forensic Genetic Testing)

NORMAL FINDINGS

No genetic mutation

INDICATIONS

Genetic testing is used to identify a predisposition to disease, establish the presence of a disease, establish or refute paternity, or provide forensic evidence used in criminal investigations.

TEST EXPLANATION

As research progresses and the Human Genome Project provides more information, precise and accurate methods of identification of normal and mutated genes are becoming more common. The use of gene amplification methods has contributed to the explosion of genetic information in regard to disease propensity. These exquisitely sensitive laboratory methods are revolutionizing the practices of medicine and law. Tests for defective genes known to be associated with certain diseases are now commonly used in screening populations of individuals who have certain phenotypes and family histories compatible with the presence of a genetic mutation. Genetic testing is done in addition to documenting a family history (pedigree). Whereas a family history is not always reliable, accurate, or available, genetic testing is very accurate in its determination of risks. Preventive medicine or surgery can be provided to eliminate disease development. Reproductive counselling and pregnancy prevention can preclude the conception of children who are likely to suffer the consequence of disease. Paternity and forensic genetic testing can accurately determine responsibility, guilt, and innocence.

The ethics and disadvantages of genetic testing are currently being discussed. Patients may face financial discrimination with regard to health or life insurance or employment if the test results are positive. In Canada, the *Personal Health Information Act (PHIA)* protects individuals from improper disclosure of personal health information without their consent; therefore, if any genetic information is to be released to a patient's employer or insurance company, the patient's consent must first be obtained. This testing may be expensive and may not be covered by insurance. The information obtained by testing may cause great emotional turmoil in affected individuals or their family. The information obtained by medical genetic testing should be shared only with the patient. If the patient chooses to allow other people access to the information, the patient must direct that release of information.

Voluntary genetic testing should always be associated with aggressive counselling and support. Because of the potential changes in life for other family members, each person receiving the genetic information must be counselled separately.

Genetic Testing for Breast Cancer and Ovarian Cancer

Inherited mutations in *BRCA* (*breast cancer*) genes increase a person's susceptibility for the development of breast cancer. *BRCA1* and *BRCA2* genes function to repair cell damage and keep breast cells growing normally. The *BRCA1* gene exists on chromosome 17; the *BRCA2* gene is on chromosome 13. These genes encode tumour suppressor proteins. Inherited mutations in *BRCA1* and *BRCA2* genes are passed from generation to generation and cause the genes to malfunction and thereby increase the person's risk for developing cancer.

Of women in the general population, approximately 12% develop breast cancer sometime during their lives; in comparison, of women who have an inherited mutation in *BRCA1* or *BRCA2*, approximately 60% develop breast cancer. Women who have an inherited mutation in those genes are approximately five times more likely to develop breast cancer than are those who do not have the mutated gene. Ovarian cancer occurs in approximately 1.4% of women in the general population, whereas it occurs in 15% to 40% of women who have the inherited mutant gene (CA-125 tumour marker). These percentages are estimates and may change as new data become available; however, it is clear that women with the mutant genes are more likely to develop breast and ovarian cancer than are women in the general population. Currently, there are no standard criteria for recommending or referring a woman for *BRCA* mutation testing. However, if a person has a family history of breast or ovarian cancer, genetic counselling may be indicated to provide more information about potential risks. Screening should be discussed with the physician to determine an individual screening plan tailored to the patient's unique situation. In addition to the recommended screening guidelines for women at average risk, a screening plan for women at high risk for breast and ovarian cancer include the recommendations outlined in Boxes 13-1 and 13-2.

These mutations have an autosomal dominant inheritance pattern; that is, women who inherit just one genetic defect can develop the phenotypic cancers. Men with *BRCA* genetic mutations (most commonly *BRCA2*) are at an increased risk for the development of breast, prostate, and colon cancer. In addition, they can pass the mutation on to their daughters. Because *BRCA* is an autosomal dominant gene, 50% of their children are at risk. Table 13-2 lists the risk factors for having an abnormal breast cancer gene.

BOX 13-1   Screening for Women at High Risk for Breast Cancer

- Monthly breast self-examination
- Annual clinical breast examination by a physician or nurse practitioner
- Annual mammography starting at the age of 30 years or younger (earlier or more often as needed)
- Annual breast magnetic resonance imaging (more often as needed; p. 1148)

BOX 13-2   Screening for Women at High Risk for Ovarian Cancer

- Transvaginal ultrasonography every 6 to 12 months
- Blood test for the CA-125 tumour marker every 6 to 12 months
- Both tests starting at the age of 25 years or 10 years before the youngest age at which ovarian cancer was diagnosed in the family (more often as needed; p. 917)

TABLE 13-2 Patients at High Risk for Abnormal Breast Cancer Gene

Patient History	Family History
Cancer diagnosed at <35 years of age	Positive or negative family history for breast cancer Blood relatives (grandmothers, mothers, sisters, aunts) on either mother's or father's side of the family who had breast cancer diagnosed at <50 years of age
Two primary breast cancers diagnosed at ~50 years of age	Blood relatives (grandmothers, mothers, sisters, aunts) on either mother's or father's side of the family who had breast cancer diagnosed at <50 years of age Women with diagnoses of both ovarian cancer and breast cancer
Cancer diagnosed at any age	Women with diagnoses of both ovarian cancer and breast cancer A family history of male breast cancer Other gland-related cancers such as pancreatic, colon, and thyroid cancer Personal history of ovarian cancer Ashkenazi Jewish (Eastern European) heritage First- or second-degree relative with *BRCA* mutation
Male breast cancer at any age	One relative with breast cancer or ovarian cancer Ashkenazi Jewish (Eastern European) heritage First- or second-degree relative with *BRCA* mutation

The value of testing a select group of women who may be at high risk for *BRCA* genetic mutations is in yielding the following information:

1. Identification of women who are at high risk for developing breast or ovarian cancer
2. Consideration of interventions for women whose test results are positive for *BRCA* mutations (e.g., prophylactic mastectomy, prophylactic oophorectomy, or chemoprevention with tamoxifen)
3. Adoption of aggressive screening surveillance testing:
   - Breast: physical examination, mammography (see p. 1086), and semiannual breast magnetic resonance imaging
   - Ovary: pelvic ultrasonography (see p. 917)
   - Semiannual CA-125 (see p. 148)
4. Estimation of potential for passing the mutated *BRCA* gene to offspring

The method of testing includes obtaining a blood sample from a patient who has breast or ovarian cancer. Through reverse-transcriptase polymerase chain reaction (RT-PCR) amplification, the DNA is sequenced and amplified for quantitation. If results are positive, blood samples of other family members are specifically tested for only that particular genetic mutation. Therefore, testing is expensive for the first person examined because the search is for any number of potential genetic mutations. However, for the other family members, testing is much less expensive because the search has been narrowed to only a single genetic mutation.

Cultural Considerations

- The frequency of finding a mutation in the *BRCA* genes is five times greater in the Ashkenazi Jewish populations than in the general population. It is not known whether this increased frequency is responsible for the increased risk of breast cancer in Jewish populations in comparison with non-Jewish populations.
- Other ethnic and geographic populations around the world also have higher frequencies of mutations, including the Norwegian, Dutch, and Icelandic peoples.

Genetic Testing for Colon Cancer

Two common types of colon cancer are associated with a strong familial link. The first type is familial adenomatous polyposis (FAP). Affected patients present with hundreds of polyps in their colon, of which one or two degenerate into cancer. The second type is hereditary non-polyposis colorectal cancer (HNPCC). HNPCC is also known as the Lynch syndrome. Patients with HNPCC are more difficult to recognize because they do not have polyps; colon cancers develop on a de novo basis.

FAP is caused by a genetic mutation at the 5q21-22 (*APC*) locus on chromosome 5. Like *BRCA* genes, these genes are responsible for the synthesis of tumour suppressor proteins. HNPCC is associated with mutations of *MLH1*, *MLH2*, and *MLH6* genes. These genes are also on chromosome 5 and are important for genome stability (prevention of chromosomal breakage and exchange). HNPCC is associated with several other cancers (Table 13-3), especially endometrial cancer.

These genetic defects are autosomal dominant; thus, an individual with just one defective gene can develop any of the phenotypic cancers. Furthermore, children of the affected parent have a 50% chance of inheriting the genetic mutation with its inherent cancer risks. Characteristics of FAP or HNPCC include the following:

1. Early-onset colorectal cancer (usually at <50 years of age)
2. Polyps in large numbers (FAP only)
3. Cancer in the proximal colon
4. Cancers that tend to be more aggressive
5. Cancers that are found at a later stage
6. Presence often in association with other cancers (endometrial, gastric, renal, ovarian, skin)

		GENERAL CANADIAN POPULATION (%)	
TABLE 13-3	**Risk for Hereditary Nonpolyposis Colorectal Cancer–Related Cancers**		
Cancer Type	**Hereditary Nonpolyposis Colorectal Cancer (%)**	**Male**	**Female**
Colorectal	80	7.5	6.4
Endometrial (body of the uterus)	60	—	2.5
Ovarian	12	—	1.5
Gastric	13	1.4	0.8

After a family meeting, genetic testing should be considered if the following criteria for HNPCC are present:

1. Three or more relatives (of whom at least one is a first-degree relative) with verified colorectal cancer
2. At least two generations of the family affected by colorectal cancer
3. One or more relatives in whom colorectal cancer was diagnosed before the age of 50 years
4. Three or more relatives with histologically verified HNPCC-associated cancer (colorectal cancer; cancer of the endometrium, small bowel, ureter, or renal pelvis), one of whom is a first-degree relative of the patient

The value of testing a family who may be at high risk for a genetic mutation is in yielding the following information:

1. Identification of individuals who are at high risk for developing colorectal or other cancers
2. Consideration of interventions for patients whose test results are positive for *APC* or *MLH* mutations (e.g., prophylactic proctocolectomy with or without hysterectomy, or chemoprevention with nonsteroidal anti-inflammatory drugs [NSAIDs], which have been shown to reduce the incidence of colon polyps and cancers)
3. Adoption of aggressive screening surveillance testing:
   • Colon: colonoscopy (p. 619)
   • Uterus: pelvic ultrasonography (see p. 617) and endometrial biopsy
4. Estimation of potential for passing the mutated *APC* or *MLH* gene to offspring

The laboratory methods of genetic testing are similar to those described for *BRCA* testing discussed previously.

Genetic Testing for Cardiovascular Disease

Because 50% of all patients with cardiovascular disease do not have the traditional risk factors (cholesterol, obesity, diabetes, and high blood pressure), these factors alone must not be relied upon in the identification of patients at high risk for cardiac disease. Although a family history is helpful in identifying families at risk for cardiovascular disease, genetic testing is more accurate and—if results are confirmatory—more predictive among individuals in such a family. The angiotensinogen (*AGT*) gene, which is on chromosome 1, demonstrates the strongest and most consistent associations with cardiovascular disease. This gene is autosomal recessive; thus, when a patient has just one *AGT* mutation, the risk for cardiovascular disease is moderately elevated, but when an individual has two *AGT* genetic mutations, the risk for cardiovascular disease is nearly triple that of the general population. Affected patients have early-age onset of hypertension, myocardial infarction, and hypertrophic cardiomyopathy. With genetic testing of individuals in families in which cardiovascular disease is rampant, early therapeutic interventions (e.g., aggressive lipid-lowering agents and aggressive use of antihypertensives) may prevent disease.

Genetic Testing for Tay-Sachs Disease

Tay-Sachs disease is characterized by the onset of severe mental and developmental retardation in the first few months of life. Affected children become totally debilitated by 2 to 5 years of age and die by 5 to 8 years. Another form of the same disease is chronic GM_2 gangliosidosis, also known as "late-onset Tay-Sachs disease." The basic defect in affected children is a mutation in the hexosaminidase gene, which is on chromosome 15. This gene is responsible for the synthesis of hexosaminidase (p. 308), an enzyme that normally breaks down a fatty substance called GM_2 gangliosides. When this enzyme is not present in sufficient quantities, gangliosides build up in the nervous system and cause the debilitating characteristics of this disease. Ashkenazi (Eastern

European) Jews are affected most often. This gene is an autosomal recessive gene. Carriers have one defective gene; in affected individuals, both genes are defective. A "carrier couple" has a 25% chance of having a child affected with the disease.

At present, there is no treatment for the disease. It is important to identify carriers so that reproductive counselling can be provided. Hexosaminidase protein testing (p. 308) has been extremely effective for identification of carriers and affected individuals. However, sometimes the results of hexosaminidase protein tests are inconclusive or uncertain. Furthermore, genetic testing is used to diagnose chronic GM_2 gangliosidosis. Both the test for the protein and that for the gene mutation are performed on a blood sample or on chorionic villus samples obtained during amniocentesis (p. 660). Genetic testing is performed by means of amino acid sequencing and comparison.

Genetic Testing for Cystic Fibrosis

Cystic fibrosis is caused by a mutation in the cystic fibrosis transmembrane conductance regulator (*CFTR*) gene. This gene encodes the synthesis of a protein that serves as a channel through which chloride enters and leaves cells. A mutation in this gene alters the cell's capability to regulate the chloride (and therefore sodium) transport. As a result, the lungs and digestive tract of patients with cystic fibrosis fill with thick mucus. As bacteria invade their mucus-filled lungs, affected patients experience frequent lung infection. As mucus blocks the pancreas, digestion becomes inefficient.

There are hundreds of potential mutations that are fatally deleterious to the *CFTR* gene. The most common mutation, which accounts for 70% of cases of cystic fibrosis, is known as the *delta AF508 mutation*. Currently, more than 30 genetic mutations are recognized to cause cystic fibrosis, and these, together with the delta AF508 mutation, account for 90% of the cases.

The *CFTR* gene is an autosomal recessive gene located on chromosome 7. A carrier has one mutated gene. The individual affected by cystic fibrosis has both defective genes. Genetic testing is now used to identify carriers of cystic fibrosis, to identify neonates with the disease, and to detect fetal disease during pregnancy. The sweat chloride test (p. 702) is a more easily performed and a less expensive means of diagnosing the disease in affected children. Therefore, the use of genetic testing for cystic fibrosis is often limited to patients with a family history of cystic fibrosis, partners of patients with cystic fibrosis, and expectant couples with a family history of cystic fibrosis. The main purpose of genetic testing for cystic fibrosis is to identify carriers who could conceive a child with cystic fibrosis.

It is important to recognize that not all patients who have the genetic mutation for cystic fibrosis will develop the disease. Furthermore, because only a few mutations that may cause cystic fibrosis can be detected, a negative test result does not necessarily eliminate the possibility of being affected by the diseases.

Genetic testing can be performed on blood samples or on samples taken during chorionic villus sampling (p. 1134) or during amniocentesis (p. 660). Polymerase chain reaction is used to amplify the locus for the *CFTR* gene. Amplification products are then hybridized to probes for the 36 most common *CFTR*-related mutations, through the use of a line probe assay. Several laboratory methods are used to separate out the sequences for study.

Genetic Testing for Melanoma

Progress in the genetics of cutaneous melanoma has led to the identification of two melanoma susceptibility genes: the tumour suppressor gene *CDKN2A*, which encodes the *p16* protein on chromosome 9p21, and the *CDK4* gene, on chromosome 12q13. The *p16* genetic mutation is by far the most common form of hereditary melanoma. Characteristics of familial melanoma include frequent multiple primary melanomas, early age at onset of first melanoma, and frequently the presence of atypical or dysplastic nevi (moles). Family members with the following characteristics may consider testing for *p16* genetic mutations in *CDKN2A*:

- Multiple diagnoses of primary melanoma
- Two or more family members with melanoma
- Melanoma and pancreatic cancer
- Melanoma and a personal/family history of multiple atypical nevi
- Relatives of a patient with a confirmed *p16* mutation

Approximately 20% to 40% of families with three or more affected first-degree relatives show inheritance of mutations in the *CDKN2A* gene. Fifteen percent of patients with multiple melanoma have a *CDKN2A* mutation. The average age at diagnosis is 35 years for those with a mutation in *CDKN2A* versus 57 years in the general population. Carriers of the *CDKN2A* gene mutation also have an increased risk for pancreatic cancer.

Once a *CDKN2A* mutation is identified, education of all family members about the need for sun protection is essential. Commencing at 10 years of age, family members should have a baseline skin examination with characterization of moles. It is recommended that an appropriately trained health care provider carry out skin examinations every 6 to 12 months. A monthly self-examination or examination by parent, partner, or family member should also be performed. Individuals should be taught about routine self-examination in the hope that this will prompt earlier diagnosis and removal of melanomas. The significance of change in shape and size of pigmented lesions should be understood, and the rules regarding asymmetry, border, colour, and diameter ("ABCD" rules) are often helpful in this regard.

Genetic Testing for Hemochromatosis

The diagnosis of hemochromatosis is traditionally established with serum iron studies. When hereditary hemochromatosis is suspected, mutation analysis of the hemochromatosis-associated *HFE* genes (*C282Y* and *H63D*) is done. Hereditary hemochromatosis, an iron overload disorder considered to be the most common inherited disease in White people, affects 1 per 500 individuals. Increased intestinal iron absorption and intracellular iron accumulation lead to progressive damage of the liver, heart, pancreas, joints, reproductive organs, and endocrine glands. Without therapy, men may develop symptoms between 40 and 60 years of age and women after menopause.

A large, but as yet undefined, fraction of people with homozygosity for this disease do not develop clinical symptoms (i.e., penetrance is low). Patients with symptoms and early biochemical signs of iron overload consistent with hereditary hemochromatosis should be tested. Relatives of individuals with hereditary hemochromatosis should also be studied. *HFE* genotyping could improve disease outcomes of the disease. If an *HFE* mutation is detected, serum iron markers are monitored at more frequent intervals, and phlebotomy therapy is initiated earlier. Early initiation of phlebotomy therapy reduces the frequency or severity of hemochromatosis-related symptoms and organ damage.

Genetic Testing for Thyroid Cancer

The rearranged during transfection (*RET*) proto-oncogene, located on chromosome subband 10q11.2, encodes a receptor tyrosine kinase expressed in tissues and tumours derived from neural crest cells. Genetic testing for *RET* germline mutation has 100% sensitivity and specificity for identifying individuals at risk for developing inherited medullary thyroid cancer: multiple endocrine neoplasia (MEN) type 2A, MEN type 2B, or familial medullary thyroid carcinoma (FMTC).

Use of the genetic assay allows earlier and more definitive identification and clinical management of individuals with a familial risk for medullary thyroid cancer. Medullary thyroid carcinoma is surgically curable if detected before it has spread to regional lymph nodes. However, lymph node involvement at diagnosis may be found in up to 75% of patients for whom a thyroid nodule is the first sign of disease. Thus, the emphasis is on early detection and intervention in families that are affected by the familial cancer syndromes of MEN types 2A and 2B and familial medullary thyroid carcinoma, which account for 25% of cases of medullary thyroid cancer.

After genetic counselling, most family members who receive positive test results undergo surgery to remove the thyroid gland. First-degree relatives of patients with medullary thyroid carcinoma that appears to be sporadic in origin also undergo testing to verify that the patient's tumour is not caused by an inheritable form of this disease. *RET* testing is considered the standard of care in families with MEN type 2A and 2B because clinical decisions are based on the results of such gene testing.

Genetic Testing for Paternity/Maternity (Parentage Analysis)

This test is used to determine whether two individuals have a biologic child-parent relationship. A paternity test determines whether a man is the biologic father of a child, and a maternity test determines whether a woman is the biologic mother of a child. Currently DNA testing is the most advanced and accurate method of determining parentage. The DNA of an individual is almost exactly the same in every cell, and when the DNA of two parents merges in sexual reproduction, the result is a unique combination of genetic DNA that can be linked back to the biologic parents. Through a comparison of the DNA sequences between individuals, it can be determined whether the DNA of one of the individuals was derived from the other.

In a DNA parentage test, the probability of parentage is 0% when the alleged parent is not biologically related and 99.9% when the alleged parent is biologically related. In rare cases, individuals have at least two distinct sets of genes (mosaicism); in that case, a false-positive or false-negative finding may result. The test specimen can be obtained with a buccal swab from the inside of the cheek; other specimens include blood, semen, nail clippings, and hair. Results are usually available in 1 to 3 weeks.

Forensic Genetic Testing

Forensic DNA testing is used with increasing frequency in today's courtrooms because of its accuracy. In a courtroom, the reliability of the evidence can protect an individual and society as a whole. Furthermore, it can quickly establish guilt or innocence beyond a reasonable doubt, unless the patient has mosaicism. Like paternity testing, forensic DNA testing is based on the fact that each individual is genetically different (except for monozygotic twins). Through the use of pyrimidine mirror repeat (PMR) chemical probes, or through restriction length polymorphism methods, the DNA content of a person can be determined from nearly any body part. Furthermore, because DNA does not change or deteriorate even after death, testing can be performed on any body part, on a cadaver, or on a live person. Specimens considered adequate for DNA testing include blood, teeth, semen, saliva, bone, nails, skin scrapings, and hair. Forensic testing is also used for body identification.

In Canada, the *DNA Identification Act* has authorized the Solicitor General of Canada to establish a national DNA data bank maintained by the Commissioner of the Royal Canadian Mounted Police. The DNA bank consists of two indexes: a crime scene index containing DNA profiles from bodily substances found at crime scenes, and a convicted offenders index, which contains DNA profiles taken from convicted offenders. Both indexes have contributed to the conviction of guilty persons and, in some cases, the exoneration of accused persons who are innocent.

CONTRAINDICATIONS

- Emotional inability to deal with the results: the wishes of family members who do not want to know the results should be respected

PROCEDURE AND PATIENT CARE

Before

✗ Explain the procedure to the patient.

✗ Inform the patient that no fasting is required.

✗ It is recommended that all patients who undergo testing receive genetic counselling.

✗ Indicate to the patient the time it will take to have the results back.

✗ Ensure that the patient is well aware of the high costs of genetic testing and that it may not be covered by all medical insurance plans.

During

• Obtain the specimen in a manner provided by the specialized testing laboratory.

Blood: This specimen is collected in a lavender-top tube. Umbilical cord blood can be used for newborns.

Buccal swab: A cotton swab is placed between the lower cheek and gums. It is twisted and then placed on a special paper or in a special container. Usually two to four swabs are requested.

Amniotic fluid: At least 20 mL of fluid is preferred.

Chorionic villus sampling: As prescribed by the testing laboratory, 10 mg of cleaned villi are obtained.

Product of conception: Approximately 10 mg of placental tissue is preserved in a sterile medium.

Other body parts: As much tissue as is available is sent for testing.

After

• If a blood specimen is obtained, apply pressure or a pressure dressing to the venipuncture site.

• Document the procedure and the patient's response.

✗ Ensure that the patient has an appointment scheduled for obtaining the results. Waiting for results is very upsetting for a patient and family. They should have a definite appointment made at a time that the results will be assuredly available.

✗ If results are abnormal, genetic and emotional counselling should be arranged.

TEST RESULTS AND CLINICAL SIGNIFICANCE

Genetic carrier state: *In this state, the person carries one autosomal genetic recessive gene mutation. Such persons rarely have any abnormal phenotype (disease characteristics). However, if two carriers conceive a child, the child has a 25% chance of having the disease.*

Affected state: *In this state, the individual has the phenotype demonstrating the genetic defect. This can occur if the person has either one autosomal dominant gene or two autosomal recessive genes. Affected people may not live long enough to have children of their own.*

RELATED TESTS

Sweat Electrolytes (p. 702). This is the definitive test for diagnosing cystic fibrosis.

Hexosaminidase (p. 308). This is the definitive test for diagnosing Tay-Sachs disease.

Mammography (p. 1086). This is the test most commonly used to screen for breast cancer.

CA-125 Tumour Marker (p. 148). This test is commonly performed to screen patients at high risk for ovarian cancer.

Magnetic Resonance Imaging (MRI, Nuclear
Magnetic Resonance Imaging [NMRI])

NORMAL FINDINGS
No evidence of disease

INDICATIONS
The indications for magnetic resonance imaging (MRI) change constantly as new uses for this technique are developed. The most important indications for MRI include evaluation of the central nervous system (CNS), namely, the neck and back; bones and joints; and the breasts.

TEST EXPLANATION
MRI is a noninvasive diagnostic technique that provides valuable information about the body's anatomy. MRI is based on how hydrogen atoms behave in a magnetic field when disturbed by radiofrequency signals. The most advantageous feature of MRI is that it does not require exposure to ionizing radiation. MRI has several advantages over computed tomography (CT), including the following:
1. MRI provides better visual contrast between normal and pathologic tissue.
2. Obscuring bone artifacts that occur with CT do not occur with MRI.
3. Because rapidly flowing blood appears dark, many blood vessels appear as dark lumens. In MRI, this provides a natural contrast between other tissues and the blood vessels.
4. Because spatial information depends only on how the magnetic fields are varied in space, it is possible to image the transverse, sagittal, and coronal planes directly with MRI.

Although the full usefulness of MRI is yet to be determined, it is currently used in evaluation of a number of areas:
1. Head and surrounding structures
2. Spinal cord and surrounding structures
3. Face and surrounding structures
4. Neck
5. Mediastinum
6. Heart and great vessels
7. Liver
8. Kidney
9. Prostate gland
10. Bone and joints
11. Breasts
12. Extremities and soft tissues

The most common uses today are visualization of the CNS, bony spine, joints, extremities, and breasts (Figures 13-2 and 13-3). MRI is not useful for evaluation of the abdomen because contrast agent is needed for adequate visualization of abdominal organs.

An important advantage of MRI is that serial studies can be performed without risk. This is useful in assessing the response of cancer to radiotherapy and chemotherapy. A major disadvantage is that fewer patients meet eligibility requirements in comparison with CT. For example, MRI of patients who require cardiac monitoring or who have metal implants, pacemakers, or cerebral aneurysm clips will result in image degradation and possible danger to the patient.

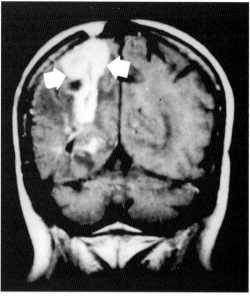

Figure 13-2 Magnetic resonance image of the skull. *Arrowheads* indicate a brain tumour, accentuated by Magnevist dye.

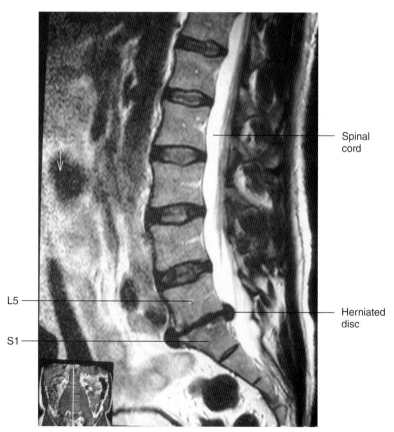

Figure 13-3 Magnetic resonance image of the spine. A herniated disc, visible between lumbar vertebra 5 and sacral vertebra 1, is compressing the spinal cord.

The uses and identifications for MRI continue to expand as new technologies emerge. For example, *magnetic resonance angiography* (MRA) is a noninvasive procedure for viewing possible blockages in arteries. MRA involves the use of radio waves and magnetic fields to visualize blood flow through the arteries. MRA has been useful in evaluation of the cervical carotid artery and large-calibre intracranial arterial and venous structures. Cardiac abnormalities, aortic aneurysm, and anatomic variants can be identified. This procedure has also proved useful in the noninvasive detection of intracranial aneurysms and vascular malformations, particularly in renal artery stenosis.

In the "time of flight" technique of *MRI of the blood vessels,* incoming blood is visualized as a bright signal; at the same time, the signal of surrounding tissue is suppressed. In the "phase contrast" method, the moving tissue (blood) is visualized, and the signal of the stationary tissue (surrounding soft tissue) is suppressed. Either method is extremely reliable, except where blood flow is turbulent (e.g., the area immediately distal to vascular stenosis). Intravenous contrast material is used to enhance the vascular differences (see the "Potential Complications" section).

The use of *MRI of the breast* has expanded markedly since 2000. When the examiner is experienced, this procedure is more sensitive than mammography or ultrasonography of the breast. MRI of the breast is often used for patients with a newly diagnosed breast cancer in order to demonstrate the extent of the tumour for preoperative planning by the surgeon. Also, MRI can detect synchronously occurring breast cancers when the second cancer in the breast is not obvious. Furthermore, lesions that previously were difficult to visualize (e.g., those close to the chest wall) are easily visualized with this technique. MRI is fast becoming the most reliable technique for breast imaging.

Magnetic resonance spectroscopy (MRS) is a noninvasive procedure that generates high-resolution clinical images according to the distribution of chemicals in the body. For example, this technique has been used to investigate myocardial metabolism without exposing the patient to ionizing radiation. MRS has also been used to assess chemical abnormalities in the brain that are associated with human immunodeficiency virus (HIV) infection without the need for a brain biopsy. MRS has been used in a wide variety of disorders, including stroke, head injury, coma, Alzheimer's disease, multiple sclerosis, tumours, and heart disease.

Because of significant improvement in *MRI of the heart* and great vessels, this noninvasive diagnostic procedure is part of mainstream of clinical cardiology practice. Cardiac MRI is already considered the procedure of choice for evaluating pericardial disease, intracardiac masses, and pericardiac masses; for imaging the right ventricle and pulmonary vessels; and for assessing many forms of congenital heart disease, especially after corrective surgery. The use of MRI is increasing in the assessment of heart function, myocardial viability, flow quantification, and coronary artery imaging. For MRI of the heart, the imaging is gated to the heartbeat by use of electrocardiographic monitoring. Often, images are obtained while patients hold their breath. These manoeuvres diminish image distortion associated with movement. The ventricle size, shape, and blood volumes can be evaluated. Cardiac valvular abnormalities, cardiac septal defects, and suspected intracardiac or pericardiac masses or thrombi can be identified. Pericardial disease (such as pericarditis or effusion) is easily identified. Ventricular muscle changes caused by ischemia or infarction can be discerned. In addition, advanced MRI techniques enable direct evaluation of the coronary vessels.

This procedure is performed in approximately 30 to 90 minutes by a qualified radiologic technologist. An injection may be used for administration of gadopentetate dimeglumine (Magnevist), used as contrast agent in MRI of intracranial, spinal, breast, or vascular lesions/anatomy. The only physical discomfort associated with MRI may be from lying still on a hard surface and possible tingling in teeth containing metal fillings. Patients' major objection to MRI testing is claustrophobia in association with being placed in the long, tubelike MRI unit. This problem is decreased if an open magnetic resonance scanner is used.

The scanning technology for MRI has undergone many advances since 2005, and a new generation of scanners has been developed, including MRI machines with short-bore magnets, open MRI machines, and stand-up MRI machines. The short-bore magnets (shorter tunnels) combine the accuracy of the traditional tunnel scanner and the comfort of open MRI, and yet they are less constrictive than the traditional MRI scanners. In open MRI, the patient lies on a table, and a large disc hovers over him or her; however, a lower-field magnet is used, and this technique therefore may not be as accurate as traditional MRI. Stand-up MRI is a more recent development that allows scanning in various positions while the patient is standing, which also thus reduces discomfort for the patient. Each of these advances in MRI technology is contributing to increased patient comfort and improved accuracy.

POTENTIAL COMPLICATIONS

- The development of nephrogenic systemic fibrosis or nephrogenic fibrosing dermopathy has been linked to gadolinium-based contrast agents: gadopentetate dimeglumine [Magnevist], gadobenate dimeglumine [MultiHance], gadodiamide [Omniscan], gadoversetamide [OptiMARK], and gadoteridol [ProHance]). There are no formal recommendations regarding cautionary action. However, it seems prudent to measure creatinine level (p. 205), blood urea nitrogen level (p. 534), or estimated glomerular filtration rate (p. 209), or a combination of these, for all patients older than 70 years and for patients known to have chronic renal insufficiency.

CONTRAINDICATIONS

- Extreme obesity because the table may have a weight restriction
- Confusion or agitation, because affected patients cannot remain still
- Unstable vital signs or need for continuous use of life-support equipment, because monitoring equipment cannot be used in the scanner room as it will be affected by the magnet (magnet-adaptive equipment is becoming available)
- Metal implants, such as pacemakers, infusion pumps, aneurysm clips, inner ear implants, and metal fragments in one or both eyes, because the magnet may move the object in the body, with possible injury to the patient
- Metal objects such as jewellery in body piercings, other jewellery, or braces; these objects should be removed before testing

INTERFERING FACTORS

- Movement of the patient during MRI causes significant distortion of images.

 Clinical Priorities

- The patient must remain motionless for long intervals during MRI because movement can distort the images.
- Many patients experience a sense of claustrophobia during this test. Sedation may be necessary. This problem is decreased with an open MRI machine.
- This test cannot be performed in patients with any implanted metal objects (e.g., pacemakers). The magnet may move the object within the body and cause injury to the patient.

PROCEDURE AND PATIENT CARE
Before

- ⟨✗⟩ Explain the procedure to the patient. Inform the patient that there is no exposure to radiation.
- • Obtain the patient's informed consent for the procedure if it is required by the institution.
- ⟨✗⟩ Inform the patient that he or she can drive without assistance after the procedure.
- ⟨✗⟩ Inform the patient that he or she may read or talk to a family member in the imaging room during the procedure, because no radiation is used.
- • Assess the patient for any contraindications to testing (e.g., aneurysm clips).
- ⟨✗⟩ If possible, show the patient a picture of the imaging machine (Figure 13-4), and encourage the patient to verbalize anxieties. Some patients may experience claustrophobia. Antianxiety

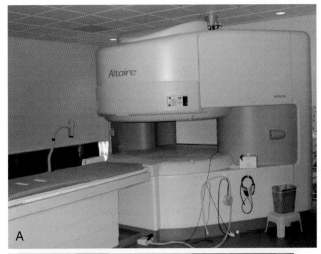

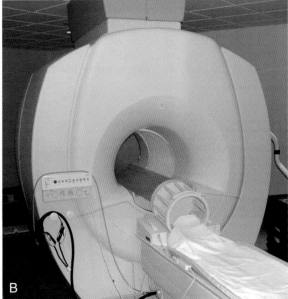

Figure 13-4 Machinery for magnetic resonance imaging (MRI). **A,** Open MRI machine. **B,** Closed MRI machine. Note that the tunnel is short and the edges are flared to minimize claustrophobia.

medications may be helpful for those with mild claustrophobia. An open MRI system can be used for these patients if one is available.

- Instruct the patient to remove all metal objects (e.g., dental bridges, jewellery, hair clips, belts, credit cards), because they will create artifacts on the scan. The magnetic field can damage watches and credit cards. Also, movement of metal objects within the magnetic field can be detrimental to anyone within the field.
- If the patient is wearing a nicotine patch (or any other patch with a metallic foil backing), instruct him or her to remove it. These patches can become intensely hot during the MRI and cause burns.
- Inform the patient that he or she will be required to remain motionless during this study. Any movement can distort the scan. Young children often are sedated for this procedure. For head and neck MRI, the patient's head may be placed in a cradle that prevents significant motion.
- Inform the patient that during the procedure he or she may hear a thumping sound. Earplugs are available if the patient wishes to use them.
- Remind the patient that a microphone inside the MRI tube allows the patient to communicate with personnel (Figure 13-5).
- Inform the patient that no fluid or food restrictions are necessary before MRI.
- For comfort, instruct the patient to empty his or her bladder before the test.

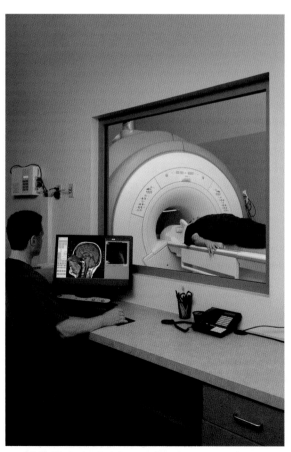

Figure 13-5 X-ray technician performing magnetic resonance imaging.

During

- Note the following procedural steps:
  1. The patient lies on a platform that slides into a tube containing the cylinder-shaped tubular magnet.
  2. The patient is instructed to lie very still during the procedure.
  3. During the procedure, the patient can talk to and hear the staff through a microphone or earphones in the imaging machine. Prism glasses can be worn so that the patient can see outside the scanner.
  4. Gadolinium meglumine (Magnevist) is a paramagnetic contrast agent that can cross the blood-brain barrier. It is especially useful for distinguishing edema from tumours. If this is to be administered, approximately 10 to 15 mL is injected in the vein. Imaging can begin shortly after the injection. No dietary restrictions are necessary before this agent is injected.

After

- No special postprocedural care is needed.
- Instruct the patient to report any nausea, vomiting, or headache to the physician, inasmuch as this may be an adverse effect of the injection.

TEST RESULTS AND CLINICAL SIGNIFICANCE

Brain

Cerebral tumour: *Natural contrast can be accentuated by varying the MRI coil. Brain tumours can be specifically diagnosed. On T1-weighted images (which depict differences in the T1, or relaxation times, of various tissues in the body), tumours are radiolucent (dark), whereas on T2-weighted images, fatty tissues are depicted as dark and fluid is depicted as radiopaque (white). For example, cerebrospinal fluid and edema appear lighter, and are thus easier to detect, on T2-weighted images. MRI is particularly useful in evaluating the pituitary gland.*

Aneurysm: *This condition is evident as compression of normal brain tissue by a small, radiopaque, enlarged vascular abnormality. Bleeding or edema may be present with aneurysmal leak.*

Arteriovenous malformation: *MRA is useful in this problem. Large arteriovenous malformations can be visible on regular MRI as large radiolucent masses in the brain tissue.*

Hemorrhage,

Atrophy of the brain,

Subdural hematoma,

Abscess: *MRI can demonstrate intracranial hemorrhage, abscess, or atrophy.*

Degenerating diseases (e.g., multiple sclerosis, hypoxic encephalopathy, encephalomyelitis): *Specific characteristics of these diseases can be detected with MRI.*

Hydrocephalus: *This condition is evident as tremendous enlargement of the ventricular system of the brain.*

Other

Herniated lumbar and cervical discs: *MRI is very sensitive for detection of these abnormalities.*

Tumour (primary or metastatic): *MRI is especially useful for detection of liver, lung, breast, and soft-tissue lesions.*

Joint disorders: *MRI is especially useful for evaluation of knee injuries.*

Destructive lesion of bone: *With multiple-weighted images, tumours, osteomyelitis, and other destructive diseases of bone, especially the spine, can be well demonstrated.*

Vascular disease: *Occlusive disease can be identified in the vessels of brain, chest, abdomen, and extremities.*

RELATED TEST

Computed Tomography, Brain (p. 1065). This test is especially useful for detecting bony abnormalities. MRI, however, provides better visualization of the CNS.

Oximetry (Pulse Oximetry, Ear Oximetry, Oxygen Saturation)

NORMAL FINDINGS

≥95%

Critical Values

≤75%

INDICATIONS

Oximetry is used to monitor arterial oxygen saturation (Sao_2) levels in patients at risk for hypoxemia. Such patients include those who are undergoing surgery, cardiac stress testing, mechanical ventilation, heavy sedation, or lung function testing and those who have multiple trauma. Oximetry is also used as an indicator of partial pressure of oxygen (Po_2) in patients who may experience hypoventilation, sleep apnea, or dyspnea. This test is commonly used to titrate oxygen levels in hospitalized patients.

TEST EXPLANATION

Oximetry is a noninvasive method of monitoring Sao_2 (i.e., ratio of oxygenated hemoglobin to total hemoglobin). Sao_2 is expressed as a percentage; for example, if Sao_2 is 95%, then 95% of the total hemoglobin available for attachment to oxygen has oxygen attached to them. Sao_2 is an accurate approximation of oxygen saturation obtained from arterial blood gas study (see p. 121). By correlating Sao_2 with the patient's physiologic status, a close estimate of Po_2 can be obtained.

Oximetry is typically used to monitor oxygenation status during the perioperative period and in patients receiving heavy sedation or mechanical ventilation. This test is also frequently used in clinical situations such as pulmonary rehabilitation programs, stress testing, and sleep monitoring. Oximetry can be used to monitor response to drug therapy (e.g., theophylline). Pulse oximetry is constantly monitored during the perioperative period, and the results are one of the discharge criteria used in the postanaesthesia unit.

Fetal Sao_2 monitoring is very useful in the monitoring of fetal well-being during delivery. When the fetal heart rate becomes significantly abnormal, Caesarean section is often performed because of concern for fetal well-being. However, fetal Sao_2 can be measured accurately, and if it is normal, Caesarean section can be avoided. The technology is based on the same principle as adult pulse oximetry except that the machine is far more sensitive to accurately read saturations of less than 70%. After membranes are ruptured, and if the fetus is in vertex position with good cervical dilatation, a specialized probe can be placed on the temple or cheek of the fetus for fetal Sao_2 monitoring. Expertise is required for appropriate placement of the sensor. The Sao_2 is displayed on a monitor screen as a percentage. The normal Sao_2 for a fetus, who is receiving oxygenated blood from the placenta, is usually between 30% and 70%. When fetal Sao_2 is less than 30% for several minutes, there is marked and progressive deterioration in fetal well-being as hypoxia and acidemia progress.

Oxygen levels can also be measured in various body tissues. For example, monitors that continuously measure tissue Po_2 are attached to a small catheter placed in the brain, heart, or peripheral muscle. Testing and monitoring of oxygen levels in brain tissue are the most common uses of this technology. Oximetry is also used to monitor the condition of the brain after severe head trauma, inasmuch as it is a measure of cerebral blood flow and pulmonary oxygenation. It is more accurate than intracranial pressure in indicating brain injury.

INTERFERING FACTORS

- Extreme vasoconstriction diminishes blood flow to the peripheral vessels, which decreases the accuracy of oximetry.
- Extreme alteration in temperature may diminish the accuracy of oximetry.
- Oximetry cannot differentiate carboxyhemoglobin saturation from Sao_2. Therefore, in cases of suspected smoke or carbon monoxide inhalation, oximetry should not be used to monitor oxygenation because the levels will be artificially elevated.
- Digital motion can alter accurate readings.
- Severe anemia affects the accuracy of comparison of oximetry and Po_2 levels.
- Fingernail polish will interrupt digital readings. The earlobe can be used as an alternative to a finger.
- Results can be affected if the patient has recently smoked a cigarette.

Clinical Priorities

- Oximetry is typically used to monitor oxygen status during the perioperative period and in patients undergoing conscious sedation. It is invaluable for titrating oxygen levels.
- Oximetry cannot differentiate carboxyhemoglobin from Sao_2. Sao_2 could be artificially elevated in patients with smoke or carbon monoxide inhalation.
- Oximetry can overestimate ABG-determined Sao_2 by as much as 2.75% in patients with severe sepsis and septic shock. ABGs are recommended when Sao_2 needs to be determined with a high degree of accuracy.
- The oximetry probe cannot be used on fingertips with nail polish. In such cases, the earlobe can be used.

PROCEDURE AND PATIENT CARE

Before
 Explain the procedure to the patient.
Inform the patient that no discomfort is associated with this study.
Inform the patient that no fasting is required.

During
- Rub the patient's fingertip or, if the ear will be used, rub the earlobe or pinna (upper portion of the ear) to increase blood flow.
- Clip the monitoring probe or sensor to the finger or ear. A beam of light passes through the tissue, and the sensor measures the amount of light the tissue absorbs (Figure 13-6).
- This study is usually performed in a few seconds by a respiratory therapist or a nurse at the patient's bedside.

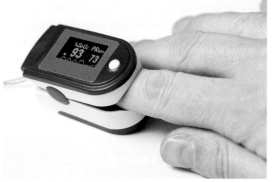

Figure 13-6 Pulse oximeter. The pulse oximeter passes a beam of light from a light-emitting diode through the vascular bed of the finger to a photodetector. The amount of light absorbed by the oxygen-saturated hemoglobin is measured by the sensor to determine the oxygen saturation level. This pulse oximeter shows an oxygen saturation of 93% and a pulse rate of 73 beats per minute.

After

- No special care is needed after oximetry.

TEST RESULTS AND CLINICAL SIGNIFICANCE

▲ Increased Levels

Increased fraction of inspired oxygen (Fio_2),

Hyperventilation: *Alveolar oxygen levels are increased by breathing more rapidly or increasing the oxygen in inspired air, Po_2 and oxygen levels can be expected to increase.*

▼ Decreased Levels

Hypoventilation,

Inadequate oxygen in inspired air (suffocation): *When ventilation is reduced enough to affect Po_2, oximetry values diminish.*

Atelectasis, mucus plug, bronchospasm, pneumothorax, pulmonary edema, acute respiratory distress syndrome, restrictive lung disease: *Nonaerated portions of the lung are still perfused with unoxygenated blood. This blood returns to the heart with little or no oxygen. The oxygen content is diluted, and oximetry values diminish.*

Atrial or ventricular cardiac septal defects: *Unoxygenated blood gains access to oxygenated blood by direct shunting. By dilution, the oxygen content of the mixed blood returning to the heart is lowered, as is that of arterial blood.*

Severe hypoventilation states (e.g., oversedation, neurologic somnolence): *Without air exchange, Po_2 levels decrease.*

Pulmonary emboli,

Chronic obstructive pulmonary disease: *These patients may experience chronic hypoxemia; therefore, oxygen therapy must be used with care in the acute setting.*

RELATED TESTS

Arterial Blood Gases (p. 121). These measurements include values for Sao_2 (the percentage of hemoglobin saturated with oxygen); Po_2 (a measure of the tension, or pressure [P], of oxygen dissolved in the plasma, which determines the force of oxygen in diffusing across the alveolocapillary membrane); and oxygen content (a calculated number that represents the amount of oxygen in the blood).

Pulmonary Function Tests (PFTs)

NORMAL FINDINGS

Vary according to patient age, sex, height, and weight

INDICATIONS

The primary reasons for performing pulmonary function studies include the following:

1. *Preoperative evaluation of the lungs and pulmonary reserve:* When planned thoracic surgery will result in loss of functional pulmonary tissue, as in lobectomy (removal of part of a lung) or pneumonectomy (removal of an entire lung), the risk of pulmonary failure is significant if the preoperative pulmonary function is already severely compromised by other diseases, such as chronic obstructive pulmonary disease (COPD).
2. *Evaluation of response to bronchodilator therapy:* In some patients with a spastic component to COPD, long-term use of bronchodilators may be useful. Pulmonary function studies performed before and after the use of bronchodilators will identify such patients.
3. *Differentiation between restrictive and obstructive forms of chronic pulmonary disease:* Pulmonary fibrosis, tumours, and chest wall trauma can result in restrictive defects that occur when ventilation is disturbed by limitation of chest expansion. Inspiration is primarily affected. Emphysema, bronchitis, and asthma can result in obstructive defects that occur when ventilation is disturbed by increased airway resistance. Expiration is primarily affected.
4. *Determination of the diffusing capacity of the lungs (D_L):* Rates are based on the difference in concentration of gases in inspired and expired air.
5. *Performance of inhalation tests in patients with inhalation allergies.*

TEST EXPLANATION

Pulmonary function tests are performed to detect abnormalities in respiratory function and to determine the extent of pulmonary abnormality. Pulmonary function tests routinely include spirometry, measurement of airflow rates, and calculation of lung volumes and capacities. Gas diffusion and inhalation tests (bronchial provocation) are also performed when requested but not routinely. Exercise pulmonary stress testing can also be performed to provide data concerning pulmonary reserve. During this staged test, the patient performs an aerobic function such as stationary biking or walking on a treadmill.

Spirometry is performed first. A spirometer is a machine that can measure air volumes. When a time element is added to the tracing, airflow rates can be determined. On the basis of age, height, weight, race, and sex, normal values for volumes and flow rates can be predicted. Values greater than 80% of predicted values are considered normal. Spirometry provides information about obstruction or restriction of airflow. Spirometry supports the diagnosis of COPD and chronic restrictive pulmonary disease.

Measurement of airflow rates provides information about airway obstruction. This portion of the study adds a time element to spirometry. When flow is plotted on the Y axis and volume is plotted on the X axis, flow/volume curves (isoflow loops) can be drawn when the patient is asked to maximally inhale, then forcefully exhale while being timed. The shape of the curve can be interpreted to identify and quantify airway obstruction. If airflow rates are significantly diminished (<60% of normal) or if further information is requested by the physician, the test can be repeated after bronchodilators are administered by nebulizer. If the airflow rates improve by 20%, use of bronchodilators may be recommended for the patient. Patients with emphysema or restrictive lung disease usually do not show improvement with bronchodilator therapy. Patients with an asthmatic component to COPD do benefit from bronchodilators.

Measurement of lung capacity (combination of two or more measurements of lung volume) can be performed with the use of nitrogen or helium washout techniques. This provides further information about air trapping within the lung.

Gas exchange studies are measurements of the D_L: that is, the amount of gas exchanged across the alveolar-capillary membrane per minute. In most laboratories, carbon monoxide is used to measure D_L because carbon monoxide has a great affinity for hemoglobin and only a small concentration is needed. Because of this affinity of hemoglobin for carbon monoxide, the only limiting factor to the transfer of the gas is its rate of diffusion across the alveolar-capillary membrane (which is what is measured). Gas exchange is abnormal in heart failure, pneumonia, and other diseases that fill the alveoli with fluid or exudate. Any disease that causes deposition of material in the interstitium of the lung (e.g., acute respiratory distress syndrome, collagen-vascular disease, Goodpasture's syndrome, pulmonary fibrosis) causes a decrease in gas exchange.

Routine Measurements

Pulmonary function tests routinely include the following measurements:

Forced Vital Capacity (FVC). FVC is the amount of air that can be forcefully expelled from a maximally inflated lung position. Values are lower than expected in obstructive and restrictive pulmonary diseases.

Forced Expiratory Volume in 1 Second (FEV_1). FEV_1 is the volume of air expelled during the first second of FVC. In obstructive pulmonary disease, airways are narrowed and resistance to flow is high. Therefore, less air can be expelled in 1 second, and FEV_1 is lower than the predicted value. In restrictive lung disease, FEV_1 is decreased because the amount of air originally inhaled is low, not because of airway resistance; therefore, the FEV_1/FVC ratio should be measured. In restrictive lung disease, a normal ratio is 80%, and in obstructive lung disease, the ratio is considerably lower. The FEV_1 value reliably improves with bronchodilator therapy if a spastic component to obstructive pulmonary disease is present.

Maximal Midexpiratory Flow (MMEF). MMEF (also known as *forced midexpiratory flow*) is the maximal rate of airflow through the pulmonary tree during forced expiration. This test is independent of the patient's effort or cooperation. MMEF volumes are lower than expected in obstructive pulmonary diseases and are normal in restrictive pulmonary diseases.

Maximal Volume Ventilation (MVV). Maximal volume ventilation (formerly known as *maximal breathing capacity*) is the maximal volume of air that a patient can breathe in and out during 1 minute. It is less than the expected value in both restrictive and obstructive pulmonary disease.

Other Measurement

A comprehensive pulmonary function study also may include evaluation of the following lung volumes and lung capacities (Figure 13-7):

Tidal Volume. Tidal volume is the volume of air inspired and expired with each normal respiration.

Inspiratory Reserve Volume (IRV). IRV is the maximal volume of air that can be inspired after the end of normal inspiration. It represents forced inspiration over and beyond tidal volume.

Expiratory Reserve Volume (ERV). ERV is the maximal volume of air that can be exhaled after normal expiration.

Residual Volume (RV). RV is the volume of air remaining in the lungs after forced expiration.

Inspiratory Capacity (IC). IC is the maximal amount of air that can be inspired after normal expiration:

$$IC = \text{Tidal volume} + IRV$$

Functional Residual Capacity (FRC). FRC is the amount of air left in the lungs after normal expiration:

$$FRC = ERV + RV$$

Vital Capacity (VC). VC is the maximal amount of air that can be expired after maximal inspiration:

$$VC = \text{Tidal volume} + IRV + ERV$$

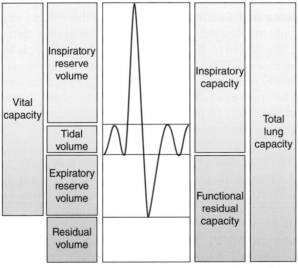

Figure 13-7 Relationship of lung volumes and capacities.

Total Lung Capacity (TLC). TLC is the volume to which the lungs can be expanded with greatest inspiratory effort:

$$TLC = Tidal\ volume + IRV + ERV + RV$$

Minute Volume. Minute volume (also known as *minute ventilation*) is the volume of air inhaled and exhaled per minute.

Dead Space. Dead space is the inhaled air that does not participate in alveolar gas exchange. It includes air within the trachea.

Forced Expiratory Flow (FEF). FEF is the portion of the airflow curve most affected by airway obstruction:

$FEF_{200-1200}$: Rate of expired air between 200 mL and 1 200 mL during FVC.

FEF_{25-75}: Rate of expired air between 25% and 75% of flow during FVC.

Peak Inspiratory Flow Rate (PIFR). PIFR is the flow rate of inspired air during maximum inspiration. An abnormal value indicates disease of the large airways (trachea and bronchi).

Peak Expiratory Flow Rate (PEFR). PEFR is the maximum airflow rate during forced expiration.

Spirometry

Spirometry is the standard method for measuring most relative lung volumes; however, it is incapable of providing information about absolute volumes of air in the lung. Thus, a different approach is necessary to measure RV, FRC, and TLC. Two of the most common methods of obtaining information about these volumes are body plethysmography and gas dilution tests.

In *body plethysmography,* the patient sits inside an airtight box and inhales or exhales to a particular volume (usually FRC), and then a shutter drops across the breathing tube. The subject makes respiratory efforts against the closed shutter. Changes in total lung volumes can be easily measured instead of calculated. From those values, assuming pressures in the box are stable, airway resistance and lung compliance can be measured. Body plethysmography is particularly appropriate for patients who have airspaces within the lung that do not communicate with the bronchial tree.

Gas dilution or *gas exchange studies* are measurements of D_L (i.e., the amount of gas exchanged across the alveolar-capillary membrane per minute). Some gases, such as helium, have densities lower than air. These gases are not affected by turbulent airflow. As a result, the use of helium provides an extremely accurate method of measuring even the most minimal airway resistance existing in small airways. This is used to test *volume of isoflow,* which is helpful in identifying early obstructive changes.

CONTRAINDICATIONS

- Pain, because of the patient's inability to cooperate with deep inspiration and expiration
- Inability to cooperate because of age or mental incapability

POTENTIAL COMPLICATIONS

- Light-headedness during the test, because of relative hyperventilation
- Fainting during FVC manoeuvre, because of Valsalva effect

- Asthmatic episode, precipitated by inhalation studies; bronchodilators may be necessary for immediate treatment

 Clinical Priorities

- Patient cooperation is essential for pulmonary function tests. These tests cannot be performed in patients with pain (e.g., from surgery, fractured ribs) or any problem that precludes cooperation (e.g., mental instability).
- Because inhalation studies can precipitate an asthmatic episode, bronchodilators must be available for immediate treatment.

PROCEDURE AND PATIENT CARE

Before

- Explain the test to the patient.
- Inform the patient that cooperation is necessary for accurate results.
- Instruct the patient not to use any bronchodilators or to smoke for 6 hours before this test (if this is requested by physician).
- Withhold the use of small-dose metered inhalers and aerosol therapy 6 hours before this study.
- Measure and record the patient's height and weight before this study to determine predicted values.
- On the laboratory slip, list any medications that the patient is taking.

During

Spirometry and Airflow Rates

- Note the following procedural steps:
  1. The unsedated patient is taken to the pulmonary function laboratory.
  2. The patient breathes through a sterile mouthpiece into a spirometer, which measures and records the desired values.
  3. The patient is asked to inhale as deeply as possible and then forcibly exhale as much air as possible. This is repeated several (usually two to three) times. The two best values are used for calculations. This test may be repeated with bronchodilators if values are deficient.
  4. The spirometer computes FVC, FEV_1, FEV_1/FVC, PIFR, PEFR, and MMEF.
  5. The patient is asked to breathe in and out as deeply and frequently as possible for 15 seconds. The total volume breathed is recorded and multiplied by 4 to obtain the maximal volume ventilation.
  6. The patient is asked to breathe in and out normally into the spirometer and then exhale forcibly from the end–tidal volume expiration point, to measure ERV.
  7. The patient is asked to breathe in and out normally into the spirometer and then inhale forcibly from the end–tidal volume expiration point, to measure IC.
  8. The patient is asked to breathe in and out maximally (but not forced), to measure VC and calculated TLC.

Gas Exchange: Diffusing Capacity of Lung

- Note the following procedural steps:
  1. The D_L for any gas can be measured as part of pulmonary function studies.
  2. The diffusing capacity of carbon monoxide ($D_L co$) is usually measured by having the patient inhale a carbon monoxide mixture.

3. $D_L$co is calculated by analysis of the amount of carbon monoxide exhaled compared with the amount inhaled.

Inhalation Tests (Bronchial Provocation Studies)
- Note the following procedural steps:
    1. These tests may be performed during pulmonary function studies to establish a cause-and-effect relationship in some patients with inhalant allergies.
    2. The methacholine chloride (Provocholine) challenge test is typically used to detect the presence of hyperactive airway disease. This test is not indicated in patients known to have asthma.
    3. Care is taken during this challenge test to reverse any severe bronchospasm with prompt administration of an inhalant bronchodilator (e.g., isoproterenol).

After

- On occasion, patients with severe respiratory problems are exhausted after pulmonary function tests and need rest.

TEST RESULTS AND CLINICAL SIGNIFICANCE

Pulmonary fibrosis,

Interstitial lung diseases: *Interstitial lung diseases are highlighted by perialveolar inflammation followed by fibrosis. Asbestosis, acute respiratory distress syndrome, radiation fibrosis, collagen-vascular diseases, Goodpasture's disease, amyloidosis, sarcoidosis, and end-stage hypersensitivity pneumonitis are some of the more common etiologic factors. Usually the FEV_1/FVC ratio is normal. Lung volumes and capacities are reduced. Hypoxemia is common. D_L is markedly reduced.*

Tumour: *Cancers of the peripheral small bronchi may not cause any changes in pulmonary function studies. Tumours of the trachea (rare) and of the large bronchi (common) cause a reduction in PIFR.*

Chest wall trauma: *Fractured ribs or recent surgery inhibits a patient's ability to cooperate fully with pulmonary function testing requirements. As a result, most lung volumes and capacities are reduced.*

Emphysema,

Chronic bronchitis,

Asthma: *Patients with COPD can be expected to have reduced airflow rates (FEV_1, FEF_{25-75}, $FEF_{200-1200}$) and abnormal airflow curves (loops). RV and ERV are increased. VC is reduced. In patients with asthma, this is reversible to a large degree with the use of bronchodilators.*

Inhalant pneumonitis (e.g., farmer's lung, miner's lung): *These patients have reduced lung volumes, impaired D_L, and exercise-induced hypoxemia. There is little airflow rate abnormality.*

Postpneumonectomy status: *As expected, lung volumes and capacities are reduced. With no pre-existing obstructive disease, no changes in airflow rates would be expected.*

Bronchiectasis: *Patients with chronic and recurrent bronchiole infection pockets have reduced airflow rates (FEV_1, FEF_{25-75}, $FEF_{200-1200}$) and abnormal airflow curves (loops), which may be reversible. They also may have some reaction to methacholine challenge.*

Airway infection: *Patients with acute bronchitis may experience transient airflow obstruction, as determined by reduced airflow rates (FEV_1, FEF_{25-75}, $FEF_{200-1200}$) and abnormal airflow curves (loops), which return to normal when the infection has resolved.*

Pneumonia: *Affected patients may have reduced lung volumes and capacities. Without other concurrent lung disease, there is no airflow obstruction. D_L is impaired.*

Neuromuscular disease: *Patients with impaired muscle strength because of neuromuscular diseases (e.g., multiple sclerosis, myasthenia gravis) have reduced lung volumes and capacities.*

Hypersensitivity bronchospasm: *Affected patients have reversible airway obstruction (FEV$_1$, FEF$_{25-75}$, FEF$_{200-1200}$) and abnormal airflow curves (loops) when induced by methacholine challenge. Airflow rates are reduced. Lung volumes may also be affected.*

RELATED TESTS

Arterial Blood Gases (p. 121). Measurements of arterial blood oxygen and carbon dioxide pressure and content are useful in determining pulmonary function and calculating lung volumes and capacities.

Chest Radiography (p. 1053). Pulmonary function can, to a small degree, be assessed with X-ray studies of the chest. Hyperexpansion of the lungs is evidence of chronic obstructive airway disease. Pulmonary fibrosis, pneumonia, and bronchiectasis may also be evident.

Sleep Studies (Polysomnography [PSG], Multiple Sleep Latency Test [MSLT], Multiple Wake Test [MWT])

NORMAL FINDINGS

Respiratory disturbance index: fewer than five episodes of apnea per hour
Normal progress through sleep stages
No interruption in nasal or oral airflow
End tidal CO_2: 30–45 mm Hg
Oximetry: >90%; no oxygen desaturation of >5%
Minimal snoring sounds
Electrocardiography: no disturbances in rate or rhythm
No evidence of restlessness
No apnea
Multiple sleep latency test: onset of sleep >9 minutes

INDICATIONS

Sleep studies are indicated in a person who snores excessively; experiences narcolepsy, excessive daytime sleeping, or insomnia; or has motor spasms while sleeping. They are also indicated in patients with documented cardiac rhythm disturbances that occur only during sleep.

TEST EXPLANATION

There are a number of types of sleep disorders. Most, however, are associated with impaired nighttime sleep and excessive daytime drowsiness. Sleep disorders can be caused by alterations in sleep times (e.g., night-shift workers), medications (stimulants), or psychiatric problems (e.g., depression, mania). In general, sleep disorders can be categorized as follows:
- *Dyssomnia:* Includes insomnia, sleep apnea, narcolepsy, and restless leg syndrome
- *Parasomnia:* Includes sleepwalking, sleep-talking, sleep terrors, and disorders of rapid eye movement (REM)

Sleep studies can identify the cause of the sleep disorders and indicate appropriate treatment. Sleep studies include polysomnography and testing for wakefulness and sleepiness. Full polysomnography would include the following assessments:
- *Electroencephalography (EEG):* Limited to two or more channels (see p. 574)

- *Electronystagmography:* Used to document eye movements (see p. 584)
- *Electromyography:* Used to demonstrate muscle movement, usually of the chin and legs (see p. 579)
- *Electrocardiography (ECG):* Used to document cardiac activity (see p. 568)
- *Chest impedance testing:* Used to monitor chest wall movement and respirations
- *Airflow monitors:* Used to measure amount of airflow in and out of the mouth and nose
- *CO_2 monitor:* Used to measure expiratory carbon dioxide levels
- *Pulse oximetry:* Used to monitor tissue oxygen levels (see p. 1155)
- *Sound sensors:* Used to document snoring sounds
- *Audio/video recordings:* Used to document restless motions and fitfulness
- *Esophageal pH probe:* Used only if gastroesophageal reflux is considered to be a cause of paroxysmal nocturnal dyspnea and coughing (see p. 717)

On occasions when sleep apnea alone is suspected, four-channel polysomnography is performed. This more simplified test includes ECG, chest impedance testing, airflow monitoring, and oximetry. Video or audio recordings, or both, are also obtained. A *sleep-screening study* is often performed to determine whether full sleep studies are indicated. This is performed by means of pulse oximetry during sleep. If no hypoxia occurs, the presence of significant sleep apnea would be highly unlikely, and full studies are not indicated.

Sleep apnea can be obstructive or central. Obstructive apnea is by far more common and is caused by muscle relaxation of the posterior pharyngeal muscles. Breathing stops for 10 to 40 seconds. Central sleep apnea is highlighted by simple cessation of breathing rather than obstructed airway. Primary cardiac events that lead to significant and transient reduction in cardiac output can also cause apnea. Apnea from either cause is associated with an increase in heart rate, a decrease in oxygen levels, changes in brain waves, and an increase in expiratory carbon dioxide. Obstructive apnea is also associated with progressively diminished airflow.

Narcolepsy is a frequent and irresistible need for sleep during daytime hours. Sleepiness can occur even during conversation or driving.

The restless legs syndrome is associated with an acute sensation of discomfort during periods of inactivity. It is difficult for affected patients to fall asleep and to stay asleep. Video monitoring identifies periodic limb movement: jerking of the legs in association with electroencephalographic evidence of sleep interruption.

Parasomnias include sleepwalking and sleep-talking. Sleep terrors, associated with sudden awakening with screaming or fighting to escape a terrifying dream that the patient cannot recall, is another example of this sleep disorder.

Another sleep disorder is REM disorder. During REM sleep, a person normally experiences varying degrees of muscle paralysis. However, patients with REM disorders do not. They may act out their dreams in a way that varies from calling out to violent behaviour. Such patients can vividly recall their dreams.

Insomnia is an inability to sleep. Although it is the most common form of sleep disorder, it is usually acute and short-lived. However, when it is persistent, a sleep study is indicated. The pretest questionnaire often pinpoints stress or restless legs syndrome.

During a sleep study, electrodes for ECG, EEG, electronystagmography, and electromyography are applied. The chest impedance belt monitors are also placed. Under video/audio monitoring, the patient is placed in a comfortable room and sleeps. During sleep, information is synchronously gathered. The various stages of sleep architecture are determined with EEG, and the physiologic changes during each stage are documented. With the use of the EEG, five stages of sleep can be identified (Table 13-4). The sleep study is repeated after the patient has been using continuous positive-airway pressure (CPAP) or a dental fixture for therapy. When the patient is receiving therapy, no sleep apnea should be noted. If the sleep apnea is significant on the first

TABLE 13-4	Stages of Sleep by Electroencephalographic Changes		
Stage	**Timing**	**Changes on EEG**	**Time Normally Spent per Stage**
I	Onset of sleep	Low voltage theta/alpha waves	3%–9%
II	Light sleep	Sleep spindles and K complexes	47%–67%
III	Deeper sleep	Delta waves	3%–21%
IV	Deep sleep/dream sleep	High-amplitude, slow delta waves	20%–29%
REM	Dreaming	Low-voltage, frequent non-alpha waves	20%–29%

EEG, Electroencephalography; *REM*, rapid eye movement.

night of study, a "split study" can be performed in which the sleep is interrupted after 4 hours and a CPAP machine is provided for the next 4 hours. During that time, appropriate CPAP settings are calibrated to reduce apneic episodes and, at the same time, minimize uncomfortable side effects.

Testing for obstructive sleep apnea is performed in a specially constructed sleep laboratory. This is a well-insulated room in which external sounds are blocked and room temperature is easily controlled. The study is performed by a certified sleep technologist and interpreted by a physician trained in sleep disorders. The study is usually completed in one night, although occasionally two nights are required. A second day is often necessary to administer the *multiple sleep latency test* or the *multiple wake test*. The multiple sleep latency test is a measure of the patient's ability to sleep during a series of structured naps. The multiple wake test is a measure of the patient's ability to stay awake during a period of what should be wakefulness.

These tests are used to diagnose narcolepsy that follows a night of inadequate sleep. These tests can also be used to determine the success of therapy for sleep disorders.

INTERFERING FACTORS
- Psychologic insomnia associated with the laboratory environment in comparison with the home
- Environmental noises, temperature changes, or other sensations
- Times for sleep testing that are different from usual times, which may affect sleep patterns and should be avoided

PROCEDURE AND PATIENT CARE
Before
- Note the following procedural steps:
- Explain the procedure to the patient.
- Instruct the patient to avoid caffeine products for several days before testing because they may delay onset of sleep.

- Sedatives are prohibited because they alter usual sleep patterns.
- Reassure the patient that monitoring equipment will not interrupt the sleeping pattern.
- Allow the patient to express concerns about video recording and other forms of monitoring.
- Several sleep rating questionnaires are completed by both the patient and his or her sleeping partner.
- Age, weight, and medical history are recorded.

During

- Electrodes for ECG, EEG, electronystagmography, and electromyography are applied. Excessive hair may need to be shaved.
- Airflow, oximetry, and impedance monitors are applied.
- Once the patient is comfortable, he or she is allowed to sleep.
- The lights are turned off, and monitoring begins before the patient is asleep.
- For polysomnography, the patient is asked to sleep per the patient's usual habits.

Multiple Sleep Latency Testing

- This test is typically performed in the morning.
- The patient is asked to nap approximately every 2 hours throughout the testing period.
- The nap is terminated after 20 minutes.
- Between naps, the patient must stay awake.

Multiple Wake Testing

- The patient is asked to stay awake and not nap during the day.
- Monitoring is similar to that described for polysomnography except for impedance, sound, and airflow monitors.

After

- On completion of the sleep cycle, the monitors and electrodes are removed.
- Test results take several days to collate and interpret.

TEST RESULTS AND CLINICAL SIGNIFICANCE

Obstructive sleep apnea: *Apneic episodes last for 10 seconds or more. Affected patients experience synchronous periods of oxygen desaturation, sleep disturbances on EEG, increase in cardiac rate, and decreased airflow.*

Central sleep apnea: *The stimulus to breathe is absent during the apneic episode. Otherwise, the findings are nearly the same as for obstructive sleep apnea. Snoring and chest impedance extremes are absent. Cardiac arrhythmia may be observed.*

Insomnia: *Affected patients demonstrate a delay in falling asleep. They may also show evidence of restless legs syndrome.*

Narcolepsy: *Affected patients demonstrate changes on EEG that are compatible with sleep rather than with napping. In the multiple sleep latency test, in which they repeatedly nap, the time they take to fall asleep is less than 5 minutes.*

Restless legs syndrome: *Affected patients experience excessive extremity motion before and after sleep.*

Parasomnia: *Affected patients may demonstrate sleepwalking or sleep-talking.*

REM disorder: *Affected patients may sleep restlessly and move about as if fighting or escaping terror.*

Tuberculin Skin Testing (TST, Tuberculin Test, Mantoux Test)

NORMAL FINDINGS

Negative (reaction <5 mm)

INDICATIONS

Tuberculin testing is performed in the following situations:
1. When a person is suspected of having active tuberculosis (e.g., patients with suspicious chest radiographic findings, productive cough with negative routine cultures, hemoptysis, or weight loss of undetermined cause)
2. When a person is at increased risk for progression to active tuberculosis
3. When a person is at increased risk for latent tuberculosis infection (LTBI; e.g., health care workers, recent immigrants, or intravenous drug abusers)
4. When a person is at low risk for LTBI but testing is required for other reasons (e.g., entrance to college)

TEST EXPLANATION

Purified protein derivative (PPD) of the tubercle bacillus is injected intradermally. If the patient is infected with or has been exposed to tuberculosis (whether active or dormant), lymphocytes recognize the PPD antigen and cause a local inflammatory reaction (Boxes 13-3 and 13-4). Although this test is used to detect tuberculosis infection, results do not indicate whether the infection is active or dormant. If test results are negative but the physician strongly suspects tuberculosis, testing with "second-strength" PPD can be performed. If these test results are negative, the

---

BOX 13-3	Criteria for Positive PPD Test Results* in Patients With No Previous PPD Results

≥5 mm (High Risk)
- Human immunodeficiency virus (HIV) infection
- Close recent contact with a person with active tuberculosis
- Patients with chest radiographic findings consistent with old, healed tuberculosis granulomatous infection

≥10 mm (Moderate Risk)
- Individuals from areas identified by the WHO as high-risk regions (e.g., Southeast Asia, sub-Saharan Africa, other areas of Africa, and Eastern Mediterranean regions)
- Intravenous drug abusers
- Economically poor individuals in the Canada and the United States
- Residents of nursing homes
- Medical conditions associated with high risk for tuberculosis (e.g., malnutrition, postgastrectomy, steroid use, cancer, diabetes)
- Worker in a long-term care facility

≥15 mm
- Individuals who do not fulfill the preceding criteria

---

* Diameter of induration 48 to 72 hours after purified protein derivative (PPD) injection.
WHO, World Health Organization.

Criteria for Positive PPD Conversion in Patients With Previously Documented Negative PPD Reaction

Age <35 years: Increase in PPD-induced induration of ≥10 mm within 2 years of most recent PPD test
Age >35 years: Increase in PPD-induced induration of ≥15 mm within 2 years of most recent PPD test

PPD, Purified protein derivative.

patient has not been exposed to tuberculosis (see p. 798 for tuberculosis culture). Results of PPD skin testing usually become positive 6 weeks after infection. Once positive, the reaction usually persists for life.

False-positive test results may occur in patients who have been vaccinated against tuberculosis or have been exposed to serial tuberculin skin tests. Successive tuberculosis testing may boost the immunologic response in patients who have previously been vaccinated, so that they appear (inaccurately) to be tuberculin converters. Tuberculin conversion is said to occur if a patient who has previously had a negative tuberculin skin test result develops a positive tuberculin skin test result at a later date. Box 13-5 lists situations in which test results may revert to negative or fail to become positive.

The PPD test also can be used as part of a series of skin tests performed to assess the immune system. If the immune system is nonfunctioning because of poor nutrition or chronic illness (e.g., neoplasia, infection, acquired immune deficiency syndrome [AIDS]), PPD test results are negative despite active or dormant tuberculosis infection. Other pathogens used in skin tests to test immune function include *Candida* organisms, mumps virus, and *Trichophyton* organisms, to which most persons in Canada and the United States have been exposed. It has been well established that any surgery is associated with greater mortality in patients with negative skin test results than in patients who react to these common pathogen skin tests. Box 13-6 lists skin tests for other diseases.

Conditions in Which PPD Test Results May Be Unexpectedly Negative*

- Fully cured tuberculosis
- Malnutrition
- Immunocompromised (e.g., from AIDS, cancer therapy, advanced cancers such as leukemia and lymphoma)
- Overwhelming infection (e.g., bacterial, viral, or miliary tuberculosis)
- Steroid therapy
- Sarcoidosis

* No reaction is demonstrated despite patient exposure, or a patient with previously positive results demonstrates negative results.
AIDS, Acquired immune deficiency syndrome; *PPD*, purified protein derivative.

Skin Tests for Other Diseases

- Schick test: Demonstrates previous exposure to diphtheria
- Dick test: Demonstrates antibody development to group A streptococci (scarlet fever)
- Allergy skin testing: Demonstrates reactions to moulds, dust, pollen, and other allergens (see p. 1123)

An alternative to skin testing is the *QuantiFERON-TB gold test,* which is a blood test used as an aid in diagnosing *Mycobacterium tuberculosis* infection (see p. 450).

Laboratory testing for tuberculosis is usually performed as part of routine prenatal evaluation in pregnant women. This may be the mother's first contact with the health care system in several years.

PPD testing is associated with no complications, except in patients known to have active tuberculosis or who have been vaccinated against tuberculosis. In these patients, local reaction may be so severe as to cause complete skin slough, which would necessitate surgical care. PPD testing will not cause active tuberculosis because the test solution contains no live organisms.

CONTRAINDICATIONS

- Active tuberculosis
- Immunization against PPD with *bacille Calmette-Guérin,* because immunized patients will demonstrate a positive reaction to PPD vaccine even if they have never had tuberculosis infection

INTERFERING FACTORS

- Subcutaneous injection of PPD may result in a negative reaction. The injection must be intradermal for induration to occur.
- Immunocompromised patients do not react to PPD despite exposure to tuberculosis.
- Improper storage of PPD can result in false-negative reactions.
- Improper dosage of PPD can result in false-negative reactions.

Clinical Priorities

- Positive PPD test results indicate previous exposure, not necessarily active infection. Active infection should be ruled out with appropriate cultures and other diagnostic tests.
- PPD testing should not be performed in patients with active tuberculosis or patients who have received bacille Calmette-Guérin vaccine, because local skin reaction may cause complete skin slough, which would necessitate surgery.
- If the immune system is nonfunctioning because of poor nutrition or chronic illness, PPD test results may be negative even if the patient has active or dormant tuberculosis infection.

Cultural Considerations

- In Canada, the incidence of tuberculosis is considerably higher among Indigenous populations than in the general population (27.5 vs. 5.0 per 100 000 population, respectively).
- Tuberculosis rates among Indigenous populations remain 8 to 10 times higher than rates among Canadians overall and 20 to 30 times higher than rates among Canadian-born, non-Indigenous populations.
- There is a disproportionate burden of tuberculosis among Canada's Indigenous populations.
- The First Nations and Inuit Health Branch of Health Canada is currently involved in renewing the Indigenous component of the Canadian Tuberculosis Strategy.

PROCEDURE AND PATIENT CARE

Before

- Explain the procedure to the patient.
- Assure the patient that tuberculosis will not develop from this test.
- Assess the patient for previous history of tuberculosis. Report a positive history to the physician.
- Evaluate the patient's history for previous PPD results and bacille Calmette-Guérin immunization.

During

- Prepare the volar (inner) forearm with alcohol, and allow it to dry.
- Intradermally inject PPD (Figure 13-8). A skin wheal (nearly 1 cm) should develop.
- Circle the area with indelible ink.
- Record the time when the PPD was injected.

After

- Read the results in 48 to 72 hours.
- Examine the test site for induration (hardening), and encircle the area of induration. Measure the area of induration (not redness) in millimetres (Figure 13-9).
- If the test results are positive, ensure that the physician is notified and that the patient is given appropriate treatment.
- If the test results are positive, check the patient's arm 4 to 5 days after the test to be certain that a severe skin reaction has not occurred.

TEST RESULTS AND CLINICAL SIGNIFICANCE

Positive Results

Tuberculosis infection,

Nontuberculous *Mycobacteria* infection: *Positive results indicate previous exposure, not necessarily active infection. Active infection should be ruled out with appropriate cultures and other diagnostic tests.*

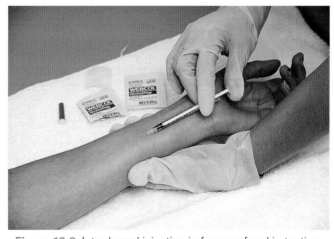

Figure 13-8 Intradermal injection in forearm for skin testing.

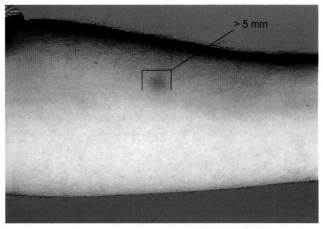

> 5 mm

Figure 13-9 Positive reading for TB.

Negative Results

Possible immunoincompetence in chronically ill patients: *Immunocompromised patients and patients who have not been exposed to tuberculosis do not react to PPD. In other patients, positive results can revert to negative (see Box 13-5). Immunocompromised patients do not respond to other common pathogens.*

RELATED TESTS

Acid-Fast Bacilli Smear (p. 735). This smear (usually with sputum specimens) is used to support the diagnosis of tuberculosis. By itself, it cannot confirm a diagnosis of tuberculosis. This smear test is also used to monitor treatment for tuberculosis.

Tuberculosis Culture (p. 798). This is the only method for confirming a diagnosis of tuberculosis. When the infecting organism is grown from culture of a specimen, the diagnosis of tuberculosis can be made, and treatment based on drug sensitivities can be started.

Chest Radiography (p. 1053). Because tuberculosis is usually an infection in the lungs as a result of inhalation of airborne infectious material, the chest X-ray study often demonstrates the results (Ghon complex) of acute granulomatous infection.

QuantiFERON-TB Gold (p. 450). This blood test can identify active and latent tuberculosis infection.

Urea Breath Test (UBT, *Helicobacter Pylori* Breath Test)

FINDINGS

<50 disintegrations per minute (if carbon-14 [^{14}C] is used)
<3% (if carbon-13 [^{13}C] is used)

INDICATIONS

This test is used to detect *Helicobacter pylori* infections. It is indicated in patients who have recurrent or chronic gastric or duodenal ulceration or inflammation. When the *H. pylori* infection is successfully treated, the ulcer or inflammation usually heals.

TEST EXPLANATION

H. pylori is a bacterium that can be found in the mucus overlying the gastric mucosa (cells that line the stomach) and in the mucosa itself. It is a risk factor for gastric and duodenal ulcers, chronic gastritis, or even ulcerative esophagitis. This Gram-negative bacillus is also a class I gastric carcinogen. Gastric colonization by this organism has been reported in approximately 90% to 95% of patients with a duodenal ulcer; in 60% to 70% of patients with a gastric ulcer; and in approximately 20% to 25% of patients with gastric cancer. There are several serologic and microscopic methods of detecting *H. pylori* (see *Helicobacter pylori* Antibodies Test, p. 292).

The urea breath test is the noninvasive test of choice for diagnosis of *H. pylori* infection. It is based on the capability of *H. pylori* to metabolize urea to carbon dioxide because of the organism's capability to produce large amount of urease. In the breath test, ^{13}C-labelled urea is administered orally. The urea is then absorbed through the gastric mucosa. If *H. pylori* is present, the urea is converted to $^{13}CO_2$. The $^{13}CO_2$ is then taken up by the capillaries in the stomach wall and delivered to the lungs, and it is exhaled. The exhaled $^{13}CO_2$ can be measured by gas chromatography or a mass spectrometer.

This test has been simplified to the point that two breath samples collected before and 30 minutes after the ingestion of urea in a liquid form suffice to provide reliable diagnostic information. Labelling urea with ^{13}C is becoming increasingly popular because it is a nonradioactive isotope of ^{14}C and is innocuous. It can be safely used in children and in women of childbearing age.

INTERFERING FACTORS

- Dietary constituents with a natural abundance of ^{13}C, such as maize, cane, and corn flour, can increase $^{13}CO_2$ levels.
- Bismuth (Pepto-Bismol) and sucralfate (Carafate) suppress mucosal uptake of the urea and interfere with test results.
- Proton pump inhibitors—such as omeprazole (Prilosec), esomeprazole (Nexium), lansoprazole (Prevacid), or pantoprazole (Protonix)—also inhibit urea absorption.

PROCEDURE AND PATIENT CARE

Before

- Note the following procedural steps:
- Explain the procedure to the patient.
- Instruct the patient to remain on NPO status (nothing by mouth) for 6 hours before testing.
- If radioactive carbon (rare) is being used, ensure that female patients are not pregnant.
- When providing the isotopic urea to the patient, instruct the patient in proper administration (per local laboratory procedure).

During

- Several minutes after the patient has swallowed the carbon dose, provide the patient with ~59 mL (2 oz) of water.
- Breath samples are collected in any one of a number of gas collection devices, depending on how and when the sample will be analyzed.

After

☒ Instruct the patient to resume medications and normal diet.

☒ If radioactive carbon was used, instruct the patient to drink plenty of fluids to facilitate excretion of the radioisotope.

TEST RESULTS AND CLINICAL SIGNIFICANCE

H. pylori infection

RELATED TESTS

Helicobacter pylori Antibodies (p. 292). This is the main serologic method of detecting *H. pylori* infection.

Esophagogastroduodenoscopy (p. 636). This endoscopic procedure is used to directly obtain a biopsy sample of the gastric mucosa for definitive identification of *H. pylori*.

Alphabetical List of Tests

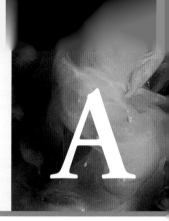

Appendix A

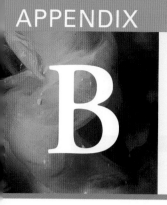

B | List of Tests by Body System

Tests in this list are grouped by the following body systems: cancer, cardiovascular, endocrine, gastrointestinal, hematologic, hepatobiliary, immunologic, miscellaneous, nervous system, pulmonary, reproductive system, skeletal system, and urologic system.

Cancer Studies

Acid phosphatase, 30
Antibody tumour imaging, 808
Bence-Jones protein, 943
Beta$_2$-microglobulin, 133
Bladder cancer markers, 946
Bone scan, 810
Breast cancer genomics, 1131
Breast cancer tumour analysis, 746
Breast ductal lavage, 673
CA 15-3 and CA 27-29 tumour markers, 146
CA 19-9 tumour marker, 145
CA-125 tumour marker, 148
Carcinoembryonic antigen (CEA), 159
Colon cancer tumour analysis, 754
Ductoscopy, 630
Estrogen receptor (ER) assay, 759
Gallium scan, 827
Mammography, 1086
Microglobulin, 967
Neuron-specific enolase, 382
Octreotide scan, 844
Papanicolaou smear, 774
Progesterone receptor assay, 781
Prostate-specific antigen, 434
Salivary gland nuclear imaging, 860
Sentinel lymph node biopsy, 866
Septin 9 DNA methylation assay, 473
Serotonin and chromogranin A, 474
Sputum cytology, 793
Squamous cell carcinoma antigen, 485
Thyroglobulin, 497

Cardiovascular Studies

Aldosterone, 48
Angiotensin, 71
Antimyocardial antibody, 95
Anti–streptolysin O titre, 109
Apolipoproteins, 116
Arteriography (renal, adrenal, cerebral, lower extremity), 1026
Aspartate aminotransferase, 130
Cardiac catheterization, 1047
Cardiac nuclear scanning, 817
Cardiac stress testing, 563
Cholesterol, 169
Computed tomography, heart, 1072
Creatine kinase, 201
2,3-Diphosphoglycerate, 224
Echocardiography, 906
Electrocardiography, 568
Electrophysiologic study, 587
Galectin-3, 258
Holter monitoring, 599
Homocysteine, 318
Intravascular ultrasonography, 914
Ischemia-modified albumin, 338
Lactate dehydrogenase, 339
Lactic acid, 343
Lipoprotein, 355
Myoglobin, 378
Natriuretic peptides, 379
Pericardiocentesis, 690
Plethysmography, arterial, 722
Tilt-table testing, 725
Transesophageal echocardiography, 927

Hepatobiliary Studies

Immunologic Studies

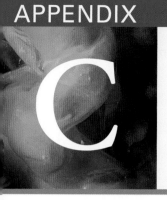

Common Testing Profiles

Note: These lists of tests may be modified or expanded depending on the clinical setting, agency protocols, and patient condition.

Acute Hepatitis

Hepatitis A IgM, 304
Hepatitis B core IgM, 304
Hepatitis B surface antigen, 304
Hepatitis C antibody, 304

Arthritis

Antinuclear antibody, 98
C-reactive protein, 199
Erythrocyte sedimentation rate, 236
Rheumatoid factor, 467
Uric acid, blood, 537

Basic Metabolic Function

Anion gap, 74
BUN, 534
Calcium, blood, 152
Carbon dioxide content, 155
Chloride, blood, 167
Creatinine, blood, 205
Creatinine clearance, 208
Glucose, blood, 269
Potassium, blood, 420
Sodium, blood, 479

Bone/Joint Profile

Alkaline phosphatase, 53
Calcium, blood, 152
Phosphate, phosphorus, 403
Uric acid, blood, 537

Cardiac Injury

Creatine kinase, 201
Myoglobin, 378
Troponins, 531

Coagulation Screening

INR, 446
Partial thromboplastin time, 396
Platelet count, 416
Prothrombin time, 446

Coma

Ammonia, 65
Anion gap, 74
Arterial blood gases, 121
Calcium, blood, 152
Lactic acid, 343
Osmolality, blood, 391
Toxicology, 986
See also "Basic Metabolic Function," this page

Complete Blood Count (CBC)

HCT, 295
HGB, 299
PLT, 416
RBC, 452
WBC, 549

Comprehensive Metabolic Function

Albumin, 440
Alkaline phosphatase, 53
ALT (SGPT), 45
Anion gap, 74
AST (SGOT), 130
ALP, 53,
Bilirubin, total, 135
Calcium, blood, 152
Carbon dioxide content, 155
Chloride, blood, 167
Creatinine, blood, 205

Glucose, blood, 269
Potassium, blood, 420
Protein, total, 440
Sodium, blood, 479
Urea nitrogen, blood (BUN), 534

Diabetes Mellitus Management

Anion gap, 74
Glucose blood, 269
Glycosylated hemoglobin (HcA$_{1c}$), 281
See also "Basic Metabolic Function," 1186, and
 "Lipids," this page

Electrolytes

Carbon dioxide content, 155
Chloride, blood, 167
Potassium, blood, 420
Sodium, blood, 479

Hemolysis

Bilirubin, 135
CBC and differential count, 187
Haptoglobin, 289
Hemoglobin, 299
Lactate dehydrogenase, 339
Reticulocyte count, 465

Hepatic Function

Albumin, 440
Alkaline phosphatase, 53
Aspartate aminotransferase, 130
Bilirubin, direct, 135
Bilirubin, indirect, 135
Bilirubin, total, 135
Globulin, 440
Protein, total, 440

Human Immunodeficiency Virus Detection

HIV serology, 310

Human Immunodeficiency Virus Monitoring

AIDS T lymphocyte cell
 markers, 161
CD4/ CD8 ratio, 161
CBC and differential count, 187
HbA$_{1c}$, 281
HIV viral load, 314
HLA-B27, 316
Hepatitis B core IgM, 304
Hepatitis B surface antigen, 304

Hepatitis C antibody, 304
Urinalysis, 991
Pregnancy test, 426

Hypertension

Cortisol, urine, 953
Metanephrine, plasma free, 372
Renin assay, plasma, 460
Urinalysis, 991
See also "Basic Metabolic Function," 1186, and
 "Thyroid Screening," 1188

Iron Deficiency Anemia

CBC and differential count, 187
Erythrocyte sedimentation rate, 236
Ferritin, 248
Iron level, total iron binding capacity, 334
Red blood cell indices, 456
Reticulocyte count, 465
Thyroid-stimulating hormone, 500
Urinalysis, 991
Stool for occult blood, 885
Vitamin B$_{12}$, 541

Lipids

Apolipoprotein, 116
Cholesterol, 169
Lipoprotein, 355
Triglycerides, 523

Obstetrics

Blood typing, 140
CBC and differential count, 187
Coombs test indirect, 191
Hepatitis B surface antigen, 304
Rubella antibody, 470
Syphilis detection, 487

Pancreatic

Amylase, blood, 67
Calcium, blood, 152
Glucose, blood, 269
Lipase, 353
Triglycerides, 523

Parathyroid

Alkaline phosphatase, 53
Calcium, blood, 152
Creatinine, blood, 205
Magnesium, 367
Parathyroid hormone, 393
Phosphate, phosphorus, 403

Appendix C

Prenatal Testing

Blood typing, 140
CBC and differential count, 187
Creatinine, blood, 205
Cytomegalovirus, 216
Glucose, blood, 269
Herpes simplex, 760
Papanicolaou smear, 774
Rubella antibody, 470
Syphilis detection, 487
Thyroxine, free, 511
Toxoplasmosis antibody titre, 519
Urea nitrogen, blood, 534
Uric acid, blood, 537
Urinalysis, 991
Urine culture and sensitivity, 1007

Renal Function

Albumin, 440
Anion gap, 74
BUN, 534
Calcium, blood, 152
Carbon dioxide content, 155
Chloride, blood, 167

Creatinine, blood, 205
Creatinine clearance, 208
Phosphate, phosphorus, 403
Potassium, blood, 420
Sodium, blood, 479

Thyroid Screening

Calcitonin, 150
Thyroglobulin, 497
Thyroid-stimulating hormone (TSH), 500
Thyroxine, free, 511
Thyroxin index, free, 514
Thyroxin total, 516

TORCH Antibody Testing

Cytomegalovirus, 216
Herpes simplex, 760
Rubella antibody, 470
Toxoplasmosis antibody titre, 519

Toxicology Screening (Urine)

Substance abuse testing, 983
Toxicology, 986

Common Abbreviations and Acronyms

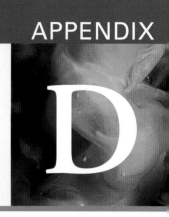

AAT	Alpha$_1$-antitrypsin
Ab	Antibody
ABEP	Auditory brainstem evoked potential
ABG	Arterial blood gas
ABI	Ankle/brachial index
ACE	Angiotensin-converting enzyme
AChR Ab	Acetylcholine receptor antibody
ACT	Activated clotting time
ACTH	Adrenocorticotropic hormone
ADH	Antidiuretic hormone
AFB	Acid-fast bacilli
AFP	Alpha-fetoprotein
A/G ratio	Albumin/globulin ratio
AIDS	Acquired immune deficiency syndrome
AIT	Agglutination inhibition test
ALA	Aminolevulinic acid
ALP	Alkaline phosphatase
ALT	Alanine aminotransferase
ANA	Antinuclear antibody
ANC	Absolute neutrophil count
ANCA	Anti–neutrophil cytoplasmic antibody
ANP	Atrial natriuretic peptide
APCA	Anti–parietal cell antibody
APTT	Activated partial thromboplastin time
ASMA	Anti–smooth muscle antibody
ASO	Anti–streptolysin O titre

AST	Aspartate aminotransferase
BAP	Bone alkaline phosphatase
β_2M	Beta$_2$-microglobulin
BE	Barium enema
BMC	Bone mineral count
BMD	Bone mineral density
BNP	Brain natriuretic peptide
BPP	Biophysical profile
BRCA	Breast cancer
BTA	Bladder tumour antigen
BUN	Blood urea nitrogen
Ca	Calcium
CBC	Complete blood cell count
CEA	Carcinoembryonic antigen
CHF	Coronary heart failure
CK	Creatine kinase
Cl	Chloride
CLO	*Campylobacter*-like organism
CMG	Cystometrography
CMV	Cytomegalovirus
CNP	C-type natriuretic peptide
CNS	Central nervous system
CO	Carbon monoxide
CO$_2$	Carbon dioxide
COHb	Carboxyhemoglobin test
COPD	Chronic obstructive pulmonary disease
CP, CPK	Creatine phosphokinase
CrCl	Creatinine clearance
CRP	C-reactive protein
C&S	Culture and sensitivity

CSF	Cerebrospinal fluid	ESR	Erythrocyte sedimentation rate
CST	Contraction stress test	EST	Exercise stress test
CT	Computed tomography	EUG	Excretory urography
cTnI	Cardiac troponin I	FA	Fluorescein angiography
cTnT	Cardiac troponin T	FBS	Fasting blood sugar (glucose)
CVB	Chorionic villus biopsy	FDP	Fibrin degradation product
CVS	Chorionic villus sampling	Fe	Iron
CXR	Chest radiograph	fFN	Fetal fibronectin
D&C	Dilation and curettage	FIT	Fecal immunochemical test
DEXA	Dual-energy X-ray absorptiometry	FOBT	Fecal occult blood test
DHEA	Dehydroepiandrosterone	%FPSA	Percent free prostate-specific antigen
DIC	Disseminated intravascular coagulation	FSH	Follicle-stimulating hormone
DM	Diabetes mellitus	FSPs	Fibrin split products
DNA	Deoxyribonucleic acid	FTA-ABS	Fluorescent treponemal antibody absorption test
DPA	Dual-photon absorptiometry	FTI	Free thyroxine index
DSA	Digital subtraction angiography	FUT	Fibrinogen uptake test
DSMA	Disodium monomethane arsenate (renal scanning)	FVL	Factor V–Leiden
DST	Dexamethasone suppression test	G6PD	Glucose-6-phosphate dehydrogenase
EBV	Epstein-Barr virus	GAD ab	Glutamic acid decarboxylase antibody
ECG	Electrocardiography	GB series	Gallbladder series
Echo	Echocardiography	GER	Gastroesophageal reflux
EEG	Electroencephalography	GER scan	Gastroesophageal reflux scan
EFS	Esophageal function study	GGTP	Gamma-glutamyl transpeptidase
EGD	Esophagogastroduo-denoscopy	GH	Growth hormone
EIA	Enzyme immunoassay	GHb	Glycosylated hemoglobin
ELISA	Enzyme-linked immunosorbent assay	GI	Gastrointestinal
EMA	Endomysial antibody	GTT	Glucose tolerance test
EMG	Electromyography	HAA	Hepatitis-associated antigen
ENG	Electroneurography	HAI	Hemagglutination inhibition
EP	Evoked potential	HAV	Hepatitis A virus
EPO	Erythropoietin	Hb	Hemoglobin
EPS	Electrophysiologic study	HBcAb	Hepatitis B core antibody
ER	Estrogen receptor	HBcAg	Hepatitis B core antigen
ERCP	Endoscopic retrograde cholangiopancreatography	HBV	Hepatitis B virus
		HCG	Human chorionic gonadotropin

HCO_3	Bicarbonate		LFTs	Liver function tests
HCS	Human chorionic somatomammotropin		LH	Luteinizing hormone
			LP	Lumbar puncture
Hct	Hematocrit		L/S ratio	Lecithin/sphingomyelin ratio
Hcy	Homocysteine		MCH	Mean corpuscular hemoglobin
HDL	High-density lipoprotein			
5-HIAA	5-Hydroxyindoleacetic acid		MCHC	Mean corpuscular hemoglobin concentration
HIDA	Hepatic iminodiacetic acid			
HIV	Human immunodeficiency virus		MCTD	Mixed connective tissue disease
HLA	Human leukocyte antigen		MCV	Mean corpuscular volume
HPL	Human placental lactogen		M/E ratio	Myeloid/erythroid ratio
HPV	Human papillomavirus		Mg	Magnesium
HSV-2	Herpes simplex virus, type 2		MI	Myocardial infarction
HTLV	Human T-cell lymphotrophic virus		MPG	Mean plasma glucose (level)
			MPV	Mean platelet volume
IAA	Insulin autoantibody		MRA	Magnetic resonance angiography
ICA	Islet cell antibody			
IFE	Immunofluorescence electrophoresis		MRI	Magnetic resonance imaging
			MRSA	Methicillin-resistant *Staphylococcus aureus*
Ig	Immunoglobulin			
IGF	Insulin-like growth factor		MUGA	Multigated acquisition (cardiac scanning)
INR	International normalization ratio			
			Na	Sodium
ITT	Insulin tolerance test		NMR	Nuclear magnetic resonance
IVC	Intravenous cholangiography			
IV-GTT	Intravenous glucose tolerance test		NMP22	Nuclear matrix protein 22
			NPO	Nothing by mouth
IVP	Intravenous pyelography		NST	Nonstress test
IVU	Intravenous urography		NTx	*N*-Telopeptide
IVUS	Intravenous ultrasonography		OB	Occult blood
K	Potassium		OCT	Oxytocin challenge test
17-KS	17-Ketosteroid		OGTT	Oral glucose tolerance test
KUB	Kidney, ureter, and bladder (radiography)		17-OCHS	17-Hydroxycorticosteroids
			O&P	Ova and parasites (stool test)
LAP	Leucine aminopeptidase		OPG	Oculoplethysmography
LATS	Long-acting thyroid stimulator		P	Phosphorus
			PAB	Prealbumin
LDH	Lactate dehydrogenase		PAI-1	Plasminogen activator inhibitor-1
LDL	Low-density lipoprotein			
LE	Lupus erythematosus		PAP	Prostatic acid phosphatase
LES	Lower esophageal sphincter		Pb	Lead

P_{CO_2}	Partial pressure of carbon dioxide	sBPP	Amyloid beta protein precursor
PET	Positron emission tomography	SER	Somatosensory evoked responses
PFTs	Pulmonary function tests		
pH	Hydrogen ion concentration	SGOT	Serum glutamic oxaloacetic transaminase
PKU	Phenylketonuria		
PMN	Polymorphonuclear	SIADH	Syndrome of inappropriate antidiuretic hormone
PNH	Paroxysmal nocturnal hemoglobinuria		
		SLE	Systemic lupus erythematosus
P_{O_2}	Partial pressure of oxygen		
PO_4	Phosphate	SPECT	Single-photon emission computed tomography
PPBS	Postprandial blood sugar		
PPD	Purified protein derivative	SSRI	Selective serotonin reuptake inhibitor
PPG	Postprandial glucose		
PR	Progesterone receptor	STS	Serologic test for syphilis
PRA	Plasma renin assay	T_3	Triiodothyronine
PSA	Prostate-specific antigen	T_4	Thyroxine
PSG	Polysomnography	TBG	Thyroxine-binding globulin
PT	Prothrombin time	TBII	Thyroid binding inhibitory immunoglobulin
PTC	Percutaneous transhepatic cholangiography		
		TBPA	Thyroxine-binding prealbumin
PTH	Parathormone, parathyroid hormone		
		TDM	Therapeutic drug monitoring
PTT	Partial thromboplastin time	TEE	Transesophageal echocardiography
PYD	Pyridium		
RAIU	Radioactive iodine uptake	TGs	Triglycerides
RAST	Radioallergosorbent test	TIBC	Total iron-binding capacity
RBC	Red blood cell	TPI	Treponema pallidum immobilization
RDW	Red blood cell distribution width		
		TRAP	Tartrate-resistant acid phosphatase
RF	Rheumatoid factor		
RIA	Radioimmunoassay	TRF	Thyrotropin-releasing factor
RPR	Rapid plasma reagin test	TRH	Thyrotropin-releasing hormone
RRA	Radioreceptor assay		
SACE	Serum angiotensin-converting enzyme	T&S	Type and screen
		TSH	Thyroid-stimulating hormone
SAECK	Sexual Assault Evidence Collection Kit		
		TSI	Thyroid-stimulating immunoglobulin
SARS	Severe acute respiratory syndrome		
		TTE	Transthoracic echocardiography
SBF	Small bowel follow-through	UA	Urinalysis

UGI	Upper gastrointestinal	VER	Visual-evoked response
UPP	Urethral pressure profile	VLDL	Very-low-density lipoprotein
US	Ultrasonography	VMA	Vanillylmandelic acid
UTI	Urinary tract infection	VPS	Ventilation/perfusion scanning
VDRL	Venereal Disease Research Laboratory (test)	WBC	White blood cell
		WNL	Within normal limits

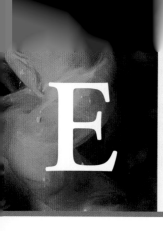

E | List of Common Blood Tests and Values

Adult Normal Range	Blood Test	Adult Normal Range	Blood Test
35–55 g/L	Albumin	< 3.4 mmol/L	Low density lipoproteins (LDL)
3-22 µmol/L	Bilirubin, total	$3.5–12.0 \times 10^9$/L	White blood cells (WBCs)
2.10–2.50 mmol/L	Calcium (Ca), total	0.65–1.05 mmol/L	Magnesium (Mg)
98–106 mmol/L	Chloride (Cl)	76–100 fL	Mean corpuscular volume (MCV)
<5.2 mmol/L	Cholesterol	1.0–1.5 mmol/L	Phosphate, Phosphorus
F: 44–97 µmol/L M: 53–106 µmol/L	Creatinine	$150–400 \times 10^9$/L	Platelet count
M: 20–215 IU/L F: 20–160 IU/L	Creatinine kinase (CPK)	3.5–5.1 mmol/L	Potassium (K)
M: $4.7–6.2 \times 10^{12}$/L F: $4.2–5.4 \times 10^{12}$/L	Red blood cell count (RBC)	0–4 µg/L	Prostate-specific antigen (PSA)
3.9–6.1 mmol/L	Glucose (fasting)	7–49 IU/L	Serum glutamic oxaloacetic transaminase (SGOT)
Nondiabetic: 4%–5.9%	Glycosylated hemoglobin (HcA$_{1c}$)	M: 13–31 µmol/L F: 5–29 µmol/L	Iron, total
M: 0.42–0.54 F: 0.37–0.47	Hematocrit (Hct)	135–145 mmol/L	Sodium (Na)
M: 140–180 g/L F: 120–160 g/L	Hemoglobin (Hb)	M: 0.45–1.71 mmol/L F: 0.40–1.52 mmol/L	Triglycerides (TGs)
> 0.91 mmol/L	High density lipoprotein (HDL)	T: <0.1 *Mcg*/L I: <0.35 *Mcg*/L	Troponins
0.9–1.1	International normalization ratio (INR)	2.9–8.2 mmol/L	Blood urea nitrogen (BUN)
45–90 IU/L	Lactate dehydrogenase (LDH)	M: 240–501 µmol/L F: 160–430 µmol/L	Uric acid

Abdul-Ghani, M., Norton, L., & Defronzo, R. (2011). Role of sodium-glucose cotransporter 2 (SGLT 2) inhibitors in the treatment of type 2 diabetes. *Endocrine Reviews, 32*, 1–17.

Alberta Nursing Association. (2010). Routine practices to reduce the risk of infectious disease. *Alberta Nurse, 66*(6), 7–8. http://www.nurses.ab.ca/Carna/index.aspx?WebStructureID=3733. Accessed May 16, 2012.

Algun, E., Topal, C., Ozturk, M., Ramazan-Sekeroglu, M., & Durmus, A. (2004). Urinary beta-2 microglobulin in renal dysfunction associated with hypothyroidism. *Journal of Clinical Practice, 58*(3), 240–243.

Baas, S., Endert, E., Fliers, E., Prummel, M., & Wiersinga, W. (2003). Establishment of reference values for endocrine test III: Primary aldosteronism. *Netherlands Journal of Medicine, 61*(2), 37–43.

Bain, L. J., Barker, W., Loewenstein, C. A., & Duara, R. (2008). Towards an earlier diagnosis of Alzheimer disease (Proceedings of the 5th MCI Symposium, 2007). *Alzheimer Disease & Associated Disorders, 22*, 99–110.

Baldea, L., Martineau, L., Benhaddou-Andaloussi, A., Arnason, J., Levy, E., & Haddad, P. (2010). Inhibition of intestinal glucose absorption by anti-diabetic medicinal plants derived from the James Bay Cree traditional pharmacopeia. *Journal of Ethnopharmacology, 132*, 473–482.

Ball, E. M., Simon, R. D., Jr., Tall, A. A., Banks, M. B., Nino-Murcia, G., & Dement, W. C. (1997). Diagnosis and treatment of sleep apnea within the community: The Walla Walla project. *Archives of Internal Medicine, 157*(4), 419–424.

Barton, S., Anderson, N., & Thammasen, H. (2005). The diabetes experiences of Aboriginal people living in a rural Canadian community. *Australian Journal of Rural Health, 13*, 242–246.

Berentsen, S. (2011). How I manage cold agglutinin disease. *British Journal of Haematology, 153*, 309–317.

Bisschop, P., Corssmit, E. P., Baas, S. J., Serlie, M. J., Endert, E., Wiersinga, W. M., et al. (2009). Evaluation of endocrine tests. C: Glucagon and clonidine test in phaeochromocytoma. *Netherlands Journal of Medicine, 67*(1), 91–95.

Borai, A., Livingston, C., Zarif, H., & Ferns, G. (2009). Serum insulin-like growth factor binding protein-1: An improvement over other simple indices of insulin sensitivity in the assessment of subjects with normal glucose tolerance. *Annals of Clinical Biochemistry, 46*, 109–113.

Borschmann, M., & Berkowitz, R. (2006). One-off streptococcal serologic testing in young children with recurrent tonsillitis. *Annals of Otology, Rhinology and Laryngology, 115*(5), 357–360.

Bowden, J. (2011). Vitamin D revisited. *Better Nutrition*, 28–30. March http://www.betternutrition.com/vitamin-d-revisited/columns/healthysolutions/1028. Accessed May 16, 2012.

British Columbia Ministry of Health Advisory Committee. (2012). *Rheumatoid arthritis: Diagnosis and management*. British Columbia Ministry of Health Advisory Committee. http://www.bcguidelines.ca/guideline_ra.html.

Burgers, A., Kokshoorn, N. E., Pereira, A. M., Roelfsema, F., Smit, J. W., Biermasz, N. R., et al. (2011). Low incidence of adrenal insufficiency after transsphenoidal surgery in patient with acromegaly: A long term follow-up study. *Journal of Clinical Endocrinology Metabolism, 96*(7), E1163–E1170.

Cakir, M., Sari, R., Tosun, O., Saka, O., & Karayalcin, U. (2006). Reproducibility of fasting and OGTT-derived insulin resistance indices in normoglycemic women. *Canadian Journal of Diabetes, 30*(1), 46–51.

Canadian Association of Radiologists, Gastrointestinal Expert Advisory Panel. (1994). *Standards for performance of adult barium enema examinations*. http://www.car.ca/uploads/standards%20guidelines/barium_enema.pdf.

Canadian Cancer Society's Steering Committee on Cancer Statistics. (2011). *Canadian Cancer Statistics 2011: Featuring colorectal cancer* (p. 2011). Toronto, ON: Canadian Cancer Society.

Canadian Centre for Occupational Health and Safety. Routine precautions. http://www.ccohs.ca/oshanswers/prevention/universa.html. Accessed May 7, 2011.

Canadian Diabetes Association. (2008). Canadian Diabetes Association 2008 clinical practice guidelines for the prevention and management of diabetes in Canada. *Canadian Journal of Diabetes, 32*(Suppl. 1).

Canadian Heart and Stroke Foundation. (2011). *Living with cholesterol: Cholesterol and healthy living.* http:// www.heartandstroke.com/site/c.ikIQLcMWJtE/b.3751077/k.FCF7/Heart_disease__Living_with_ Cholesterol.htm. Retrieved May 16, 2012.

Cappellini, M. D., & Fiorelli, G. (2008). Glucose-6-phosphate dehydrogenase deficiency. *Lancet, 371*(9606), 64–74.

Catalona, W. J., Partin, A. W., Slawin, K. M., Brawer, M. K., Flanigan, R. C., Patel, A., et al. (1998). Use of the percentage of free prostate-specific antigen to enhance differentiation of prostate cancer from benign prostatic disease. *Journal of the American Medical Association, 279*(19), 1542–1547.

Catto, A. J., Carter, A. M., Stickland, M., Bamford, J. M., Davies, J. A., & Grant, P. J. (1997). Plasminogen activator inhibitor-1 (PAI-1) 4G/5G promoter polymorphism and levels in subjects with cerebrovascular disease. *Thrombosis & Haemostasis, 77*(4), 730–740.

Centers for Disease Control and Prevention. (2014). *CDC tightened guidance for U.S. healthcare workers on personal protective equipment for ebola.* http://www.cdc.gov/media/releases/2014/fs1020-ebola-personal-protective-equipment.html.

Chatterton, R., Parker, N., Habe-Evans, M., Brky, M., Scholtens, D., & Khan, S. (2010). Breast ductal lavage for assessment of breast cancer biomarkers. *Hormonal Cancer, 1*(4), 197–204.

Cheung, C., & Shuter, J. (2010). *Pneumocystis jirovecii* prophylaxis discontinuation based upon total lymphocyte count in HIV-infected adults treated with antiretroviral therapy. *International Journal of STD and AIDS, 21,* 406–409.

Clinical and Labroatory Standards Institute. (2010). *Procedures for the Collection of Diagnostic Blood Specimens by Venipuncture; Approved Standard* (6th ed.).

College & Association of Registered Nurses of Alberta. (2010). Routine practices to reduce the risk of infectious diseases. *Alberta RN, 66*(6), 7–8.

Collinson, P. O. (1999). The need for point of care testing: An evidence-based appraisal. *Scandinavian Journal of Clinical & Laboratory Investigation: Supplement (UCR), 230,* 67–73.

Construction Owners Association of Alberta. (2014). *Canadian Model for Providing a Safe Workplace.* Author.

Cooper, T., Noonan, E., von Eckardstein, S., Auger, J., Baker, H. W., Behre, H. M., et al. (2009). World Health Organization reference values for human semen characteristics. *Human Reproduction Update, 16*(3), 231–245.

Danchin, M., Carlin, J., Devensish, W., Nola, T., & Carapetis, J. (2005). New normal ranges of antistreptolysin O antideoxyribonuclease B titres for Australian children. *Journal of Paediatric Child Health, 41,* 583–586.

Danesh, J., Wheeler, J. G., Hirschfield, G. M., Eda, S., Eiriksdottir, G., Rumley, A., et al. (2004). C-reactive protein and other circulation markers of inflammation in the prediction of coronary heart disease. *New England Journal of Medicine, 350*(14), 1387–1397.

Daniel, M., & Cargo, M. (2003). Association between smoking, insulin resistance and β-cell function in a North-western First Nation. *Diabetic Medicine, 21,* 188–193.

Decavele, A., Schouwers, S., & Devreese, K. (2011). Evaluation of three commercial ELISA kits for anticardiolipin and anti–beta$_2$–glycoprotein I antibodies in the laboratory diagnosis of antiphospholipid syndrome. *International Journal of Laboratory Hematology, 33,* 37–108.

Deeks, S., Gange, S., Kitahata, M., Saag, M., Justice, A., Hogg, R., et al. (2009). Trends in multidrug treatment failure and subsequent mortality among antiretroviral therapy–experienced patients with HIV infection in North America. *Clinical Infectious Diseases, 49*(10), 1582–1590.

DeLuca, H. F. (2004). Overview of general physiologic features and functions of vitamin D. *American Journal of Clinical Nutrition, 80*(Suppl. 6), 1689S–1696S.

Derhaschnig, U., Kittler, H., Woisetschläger, C., Bur, A., Herkner, H., & Hirschl, M. (2002). Microalbumin measurement alone or calculation of the albumin/creatinine ratio for the screening of hypertension patients. *Nephrology, Dialysis, Transplantation, 17,* 81–85.

El-Khateeb, E., Zuel-Fakkar, N., Eid, S., & Abdul-Wahab, S. (2011). Prolactin level is significantly elevated in lesional skin of patients with psoriasis. *International Journal of Dermatology, 50,* 693–696.

Ernst, D. J., Ballance, L. O., Calam, R. R., McCall, R., Smith, S. S., Szamosi, D. I., et al. (2007). *Procedures for the collection of diagnostic blood specimens by venipuncture; approved standard—6th edition (Clinical and Laboratory Standards Institute document H3-A6, Vol. 27, No. 6).* http://www.clsi.org/source/orders/free/ h3-a6.pdf. Retrieved May 29, 2012.

Etzioni, R., Ankerst, D. P., Weiss, N. S., Inoue, L. Y., & Thompson, I. M. (2007). Is prostate-specific antigen velocity useful in early detection of prostate cancer? A critical appraisal of the evidence. *Journal of the National Cancer Institute, 99*, 1510–1515.

Ezenwaka, C. (2003). Prospective study of offspring of Caribbean patient with type-2 diabetes: Results of 1 year follow-up. *Canadian Journal of Diabetes, 27*(3), 248–255.

Ferri, F. (2010). *A Practical Guide to Clinical Laboratory Medicine and Diagnostic Imaging* (2nd ed.). Philadelphia: Elsevier.

Fitzgerald, D., Patel, A., Body, S., & Garvin, S. (2009). The relationship between heparin levels and activated clotting time in the adult cardiac surgery population. *Perfusion, 24*, 93–96.

Flanagan, M., Love, S., & Hwang, S. (2010). Status of intraductal therapy for ductal carcinoma in situ. *Current Breast Cancer Rep, 2*, 75–82.

Francis, R. (2006). Calcium, vitamin D and involutional osteoporosis. *Current Opinion in Clinical Nutrition and Metabolic Care, 9*, 13–17.

Gangaram, R., Naicker, M., & Moodley, J. (2009). Comparison of pregnancy outcomes in women with hypertensive disorders of pregnancy using 24-hour urinary protein and urinary microalbumin. *International Journal of Gynecology and Obstetrics, 107*, 19–22.

Genest, J., McPherson, R., Frohlich, J., Anderson, T., Campbell, N., Carpentier, A., et al. (2009). 2009 Canadian Cardiovascular Society/Canadian guidelines for the diagnosis and treatment of dyslipidemia and prevention of cardiovascular disease in the adult—2009 recommendations. *Canadian Journal of Cardiology, 25*(10), 567–579.

Gersel-Penderson, A., Winther-Bach, F., Nissen, M., & Bach, F. (1985). Creatine kinase and β-2-microglobulin as markers of CNS metastases in patient with small cell lung cancer. *Journal of Clinical Oncology, 3*(10), 1364–1372.

Giannitsis, E., & Katus, H. A. (1999). Strategies for clinical assessment of patients with suspected acute coronary syndromes. *Scandinavian Journal of Clinical & Laboratory Investigation: Supplement (UCR), 230*, 36–42.

Grant, W., & Holick, M. (2005). Benefits requirements of vitamin D for optimal health: A review. *Alternative Medicine Review, 10*(2), 94–111.

Gray, W., Bayer-Pietsch, E., Chieco, P., Cochand, Priollet B., Desai, M., Drijkoningen, M., et al. (2007). The future of cytopathology in Europe. Will the wider use of HPV testing have an impact on the provision of cervical screening? [Review]. *Cytopathology, 18*, 278–282.

Grenache, D., Wilson, A., Gross, G., & Gronowski, A. (2010). Clinical laboratory trends in fetal lung maturity testing. *Clinica Chimica Acta, 411*, 1746–1749.

Grundy, S. M., Cleeman, J. I., Merz, C. N., Brewer, H. B., Jr., Clark, L. T., Hunninghake, D. B., et al. (2004). Implications of recent clinical trials for the National Cholesterol Education Program Adult Treatment Panel III guidelines. *Circulation, 110*(2), 227–239.

Hancock, R. D. (1993). Venipuncture vs. arterial catheter activated partial thromboplastin times in heparinized patients. *Dimensions in Critical Care Nursing, 12*(5), 238–245.

Hanley, W. (2005). Newborn screening in Canada—Are we out of step? *Paediatric Child Health, 10*(4), 203–207.

Harris, C. S., Lambert, J., Saleem, A., Coonishish, J., Martineau, L. C., Cuerrier, A., et al. (2008). Antidiabetic activity of extracts from needle, bark, and cone of *Picea glauca*: Organ-specific protection from glucose toxicity and glucose deprivation. *Pharmaceutical Biology, 46*(1), 126–134.

Harris, L., Fritsche, H., Mennel, R., Norton, L., Ravdin, P., Taube, S., et al. (2007). American Society of Clinical Oncology 2007 update of recommendations for the use of tumor markers in breast cancer. *Journal of Clinical Oncology, 25*(33), 5287–5312.

Harrison, M., Lin, H., Blakely, D., & Tanaka, H. (2011). Preliminary assessment of an automatic screening device for peripheral arterial disease using ankle-brachial and toe-brachial indices. *Blood Pressure Monitoring, 16*(3), 138–141.

Hasbun, R., Abrahams, J., Jekel, J., & Quagliarello, V. J. (2001). Computed tomography of the head before lumbar puncture in adults with suspected meningitis. *New England Journal of Medicine, 345*(24), 1727–1733.

Hemminki, K., & Chen, B. (2004). Familial association of colorectal adenocarcinoma with cancers at other sites. *European Journal of Cancer, 40*, 2480–2487.

Hirsch, R., Dent, C., Pfriem, H., Allen, J., Beekman, R. H., 3rd., Ma, Q., et al. (2007). NGAL is an early predictive biomarker of contrast-induced nephropathy in children. *Pediatric Nephrology, 22*(12), 2089–2095.

Ho, G. Y., Bierman, R., Beardsley, L., Chang, C. J., & Burk, R. D. (1998). Natural history of cervicovaginal papillomavirus infection in young women. *New England Journal of Medicine, 338*(7), 423–428.

Holdsworth, S., Boyce, N., Thomson, N., & Atkins, R. (1984). The clinical spectrum of acute glomerulonephritis and lung hemorrhage (Goodpasture's Syndrome). *Quarterly Journal of Medicine, 55*(216), 75–86.

Holick, M. F. (2007). Vitamin D deficiency. *New England Journal of Medicine, 357*, 266–281.

Hrnciarikova, D., Hyspler, R., Vyroubal, P., Klemera, P., Hronek, M., & Zadak, Z. (2009). Serum lipids and neopterin in urine as new biomarkers of malnutrition and inflammation in the elderly. *Nutrition, 25*, 303–308.

Iglesias, P., Castor, J. C., & Díez, J. J. (2011). Clinical significance of anaemia associated with prolactin-secreting pituitary tumours in men. *International Journal of Clinical Practice, 65*(6), 669–673.

Iqbal, S., Mendoza, K., Curran, M., & Lindau, S. (2007). *Salivary cotinine measurement in wave I of the National Social Life, Health & Aging Project (NSHAP)*. Chicago Core on Biomarkers in Population-Based Aging Research. http://biomarkers.uchicago.edu/pdfs/TR-Cotinine.pdf. Accessed May 16, 2012.

Iwadate, Y., Hayama, M., Adachi, A., Matsutani, T., Nagai, Y., Hiwasa, T., et al. (2008). High serum level of plasminogen activator inhibitor-1 predicts histological grade of intracerebral gliomas. *Anticancer Research, 28*, 415–418.

Jarvis, M., Primatesta, P., Erens, B., Feyebend, C., & Bryant, A. (2003). Measuring nicotine intake in populations surveys: Comparability of saliva cotinine and plasma cotinine estimates. *Nicotine and Tobacco Research, 5*, 349–355.

Kang, D., Kim, H., Oh, S., Hoon, J., Kim, H., & Min, K. (2010). Short term effect and safety of antidiuretic hormone in patients with nocturia. *International Neurological Journal, 14*, 227–231.

Knight, E. L., Fish, L. C., Kiely, D. K., Marcantonio, E. R., Davis, K. M., & Minaker, K. L. (1999). Atrial natriuretic peptide and the development of congestive heart failure in the oldest old: A seven-year prospective study. *Journal of the American Geriatric Society, 47*, 407–411.

Kohler, H. P., & Grant, P. J. (2000). Plasminogen-activator inhibitor type I and coronary disease. *New England Journal of Medicine, 342*(24), 1792–1801.

Kostka, T., Para, J., & Kostka, B. (2009). Cardiovascular disease risk factors, physical activity and plasma plasminogen in a random sample of community-dwelling elderly. *Archives of Geriatrics, 48*, 300–305.

Lanoy, E. (2009). Prognosis of patients treated with cART from 36 months after initiation, according to current and previous CD4 cell count and plasma HIV-1 RNA measurements. *AIDS, 23*, 2199–2208.

Lee, B., Al-Waili, N., Butler, G., & Salom, K. (2011). Assessment of heparin anticoagulation by Sonoclot Analyzer in arterial reconstruction surgery. *Technology in Health Care, 19*(2), 109–114.

Leenen, F., Durmais, J., Turton, P., Stratychuj, L., Nemeth, K., Lurn-Kwong, M., et al. (2008). Results of the Ontario survey on the prevalence and control of hypertension. *Canadian Medical Association Journal, 178*(11), 1441–1449.

Lensing, A. W., Doris, C. I., McGrath, F. P., Cogo, A., Sabine, M. J., Ginsberg, J., et al. (1997). A comparison of compression ultrasound with color Doppler ultrasound for diagnosis of symptomless postoperative deep vein thrombosis. *Archives of Internal Medicine, 157*(7), 765–768.

Leslie, W., Derksend, S., Prior, H., Metge, C., & O'Neil, J. (2006). The interaction of ethnicity and chronic disease as risk factors for osteoporotic fractures: A comparison in Canadian Aboriginals and non-Aboriginals. *Osteoporosis International, 17*, 1358–1368.

Leslie, W., Weiler, H., Lix, L., & Nyomba, G. (2008). Body composition and bone density in Canadian white and aboriginal women: The First Nations Bone Health Study. *Bone, 42*, 990–995.

Levin, B., Lieberman, D. A., McFarland, B., Smith, R. A., Brooks, D., Andrews, K. S., et al. (2008). Screening and surveillance for the early detection of colorectal cancer and adenomatous polyps, 2008: A joint guideline from the American Cancer Society, the US Multi-Society Task Force on Colorectal Cancer, and the American College of Radiology. *CA: A Cancer Journal for Clinicians, 58*(3), 130–160.

Lewis, S. (2011). *Medical surgical nursing* (8th ed.). St. Louis: C. V. Mosby.

Ley, S., Hegele, R. A., Connelly, P. W., Harris, S. B., Mamakeesick, M., Cao, H., et al. (2010). Assessing the association of the *HNF1A* G319S variant with C-reactive protein in Aboriginal Canadians: A population-based epidemiological study. *Cardiovascular Diabetology, 9,* 39.

Ley, S., Hegele, R. A., Harris, S. B., Mamakeesick, M., Cao, H., Connelly, P. W., et al. (2011). *HNF1A* G319S variant, active cigarette smoking and incident type 2 diabetes in Aboriginal Canadians: A population-based epidemiological study. *BMC Medical Genetics, 12*(1), 1–7.

Liu, J., Hanley, A., Young, T., Harris, S., & Zinman, B. (2006). Characteristics and prevalence of metabolic syndrome among three ethnic groups in Canada. *International Journal of Obesity, 30,* 669–676.

Longstaff, C., Rigsby, P., & Whitton, C. (2010). Calibration of the WHO 1st international standard and SSC/ISTH secondary coagulation standard for tissue plasminogen activator antigen in plasma. *Journal of Thrombosis and Haemostasis, 8,* 1855–1857.

Lorenz, M. W., Markus, H. S., Bots, M. L., Rosvall, M., & Sitzer, M. (2007). Prediction of clinical cardiovascular events with carotid intima-media thickness: A systematic review and meta-analysis. *Circulation, 115*(4), 459–467.

Mahendrappa, K. (2010). Upper limit of normal antistreptolysin-O titer in healthy school children. *Indian Pediatrics, 47,* 929.

Manuel, A., MacDonald, S., Alani, S., Moralejo, D., & Dubrowski, A. (2014). Ebola virus hemorrhagic fever: A simulation-based clinical education experience designed for senior undergraduate nursing students. *Cureus, 6*(11), e228. https://doi.org/10.7759/cureus.228.

Marrett, L., Prithwish, D., Airia, P., & Dryer, D. (2008). Cancer in Canada 2008. *Canadian Medical Association Journal, 179*(11), 1163–1170.

Martineau, L., Adeyiwola, D., Valler, D., Afshar, A., Arnason, J., & Hadda, P. (2010). Enhancement of muscle cell glucose uptake by medicinal plant species of Canada's native populations is mediated by a common metformin-like mechanism. *Journal of Ethnopharmacology, 127,* 396–406.

Masood, S., & Bui, M. (2002). Prognostic and predictive value of *HER2/neu* oncogene in breast cancer. *Microscopy Research and Technique, 59,* 102–108.

Matheson, A., Wilcox, M., Flanagan, J., & Walsh, B. (2010). Urinary biomarkers involved in type 2 diabetes: A review. *Diabetes Metabolism Research and Reviews, 26,* 150–171.

Matrat, A., Veysseyre-Balter, C., Trolliet, P., Villar, E., Dijoud, F., Bienvenu, J., et al. (2011). Simultaneous detection of anti-C2q and anti–double stranded DNA autoantibodies in lupus nephritis: Predictive value for renal flares. *Lupus, 20,* 28–34.

Mayrand, M. H., Duarte-Franco, E., Rodrigues, I., Walter, S. D., Hanley, J., Ferenczy, A., et al. (2007). Human papillomavirus DNA versus Papanicolaou screening tests for cervical cancer. *New England Journal of Medicine, 357*(16), 1579–1588.

McHenry, C., Hunter, S., McCormick, M., Russell, C., Smye, M., & Atkinson, A. (2011). Evaluation of the clonidine suppression test in the diagnosis of phaeochromocytoma. *Journal of Human Hypertension, 25*(7), 451–456.

McPherson, R., Frohlich, J., Fodor, G., & Genest, J. (2006). Canadian Cardiovascular Society position statement—Recommendations for the diagnosis and treatment of dyslipidemia and prevention of cardiovascular disease. *Canadian Journal of Cardiology, 22*(11), 913–927.

Mercuri, M., Sheth, T., & Natarajan, M. K. (2011). Radiation exposure from medical imaging: A silent harm? *Canadian Medical Association Journal, 183*(4), 413–414.

Miller, E. (2007). Nutrition and osteoporosis: Focus on vitamin D. *Journal of Musculoskeletal Medicine, 24*(6, Suppl), S14–S15.

Motyckova, G., & Marali, M. (2011). Laboratory testing for cryoglobulins. *American Journal of Hematology, 86,* 500–502.

Mujoomda, M., Moulton, K., & Nkansah, K. (2010). *Positron emission tomography (PET) in oncology; A systematic review of clinical effectiveness and indications for use.* Ottawa, ON: Canadian Agency for Drugs and Technologies in Health–Health Technology Inquiry Service.

Mullins, M. D., Becker, D. M., Hagspiel, K. D., & Philbrick, J. T. (2000). The role of spiral volumetric computed tomography in the diagnosis of pulmonary embolism. *Archives of Internal Medicine, 160*(3), 293–298.

Murphy, M. J., & Berding, C. B. (1999). Use of measurements of myoglobin and cardiac troponins in the diagnosis of acute myocardial infarction. *Critical Care Nursing, 19*(1), 58–66.

Mussolino, M. E., Looker, A. C., Madans, J. H., Edelstein, D., Walker, R. E., Lydick, E., et al. (1997). Phalangeal bone density and hip fracture risk. *Archives of Internal Medicine, 157*(4), 433–438.

Namasivayan, S., Kalra, M., Torres, W., & Small, W. (2006). Adverse reactions to intravenous iodinated contrast media: A primer for radiologists. *Emergency Radiology, 12,* 210–215.

National Cancer Institute. (2011). *BRCA1 and BRCA2: Cancer risk and genetic testing.* http://www.cancer .gov.cancertopics/factsheet/Risk/BRCA.

National Cholesterol Education Program, National Institutes of Health, & National Heart, Lung, and Blood Institute. (2001). *Third report of the National Cholesterol Education Program (NCEP) Expert Panel on Detection, Evaluation and Treatment of High Blood Cholesterol in Adults (Adult Treatment Panel III).* NIH Publication No. 01-3670. http://www.nhlbi.nih.gov/guidelines/cholesterol/atp3xsum.pdf. Accessed May 16, 2012.

Newman, D., Pugia, M., Lott, J., Wallace, J., & Hiar, A. (2000). Urinary protein and albumin excretion corrected by creatinine and specific gravity. *Clinical Chimica Acta, 294,* 139–155.

Ng, S. B., & Khoury, J. D. (2009). Epstein-Barr virus in lymphoproliferative processes: An update for the diagnostic pathologist. *Advances in Anatomic Pathology, 16*(1), 40–55.

Nordberg, A. (2008). Amyloid plaque imaging in vivo: Current achievement and future prospects. *European Journal of Nuclear Medicine & Molecular Imaging, 35*(Suppl. 1), S46–S50.

Nouh, M., Mohamed, M. M., El-Shinawi, M., Shaalan, M. A., Cavallo-Medved, D., Khaled, H. M., et al. (2011). Cathepsin B: A potential prognostic marker for inflammatory breast cancer. *Journal of Translational Medicine, 9*(1), 1–8.

Nozaki, N., & Pestronk, A. (2009). High aldolase with normal creatine kinase in serum predicts a myopathy with perimysial pathology. *Journal of Neurosurgical Psychiatry, 80,* 904–909.

O'Brien, J. T. (2007). Role of imaging techniques in the diagnosis of dementia. *British Journal of Radiology, 80*(Special No. 2), S71–S77.

O'Brien, J. T., Paling, S., Barber, R., Williams, E. D., Ballard, C., McKeith, I. G., et al. (2001). Progressive brain atrophy on serial MRI in dementia with Lewy bodies, AD, and vascular dementia. *Neurology, 56,* 828–834.

Odeniyi, I., Fasanmade, O., Ajala, M., & Ohwovoriole, A. (2010). Comparison of low dose and standard dose adrenocorticotropin stimulation tests in healthy Nigerians. *African Journal of Medical Science, 39*(2), 113–118.

Olaison, L., Hogevik, H., & Alestig, K. (1997). Fever, C-reactive protein, and other acute-phase reactants during treatment of infective endocarditis. *Archives of Internal Medicine, 157*(8), 885–892.

Ontario Association of Medical Laboratories. (2009). *Guidelines for reporting laboratory test results.* http://oaml.com/wp-content/uploads/2016/05/OAML-Guidelines-for-Reporting-Revised-Sept-2-09-FINAL.pdf. Retrieved July 4, 2017.

Ontario Ministry of Health & Long Term Care/Provincial Infectious Diseases Advisory Committee. (2010). *Routine practices and additional precautions in all health care settings.* Toronto, ON: Author. http://www .oahpp.ca/resources/documents/pidac/Routine%20Practices%20and%20Additional%20Precautions.pdf.

O'Shaughnessy, J. A. (2002). Recent advances in the treatment of metastatic breast cancer. *Clinical Oncology Updates, 5*(2), 1–20.

Ozturk, L., Mansour, B., Pelin, Z., Celikoglu, F., & Gokhan, N. (2002). Adaptation to nocturnal intermittent hypoxia in sleep-disordered breathing: 2,3 Diphosphoglycerate levels: A preliminary study. *Sleep and Hypnosis, 4*(4), 143–148.

Pagana, K. D., & Pagana, T. J. (2009). *Mosby's diagnostic and laboratory test references* (9th ed.). St. Louis: Mosby.

Panel on Antiretroviral Guidelines for Adults and Adolescents. (2012). *Guidelines for the use of antiretroviral agents in HIV-1-infected adults and adolescents.* Washington, D.C.: U.S. Department of Health and Human Services. http://www.aidsinfo.nih.gov/ContentFiles/AdultandAdolescentGL.pdf.

Periard, M. (2003). Adverse effects and complications related to the use of barium sulphate contrast media for radiological examinations of the gastrointestinal tract. *Canadian Journal of Medical Radiation Technology, 34*(3), 3–9.

Parente, D. B., Gasparetto, E. L., da Cruz, L. C., Jr., Domingues, R. C., Baptista, A. C., Carvalho, A. C., et al. (2008). Potential role of diffusion tensor MRI in the differential diagnosis of mild cognitive impairment and Alzheimer's disease. *American Journal of Roentgenology, 190,* 1369–1374.

Pearson, T. A., Mensah, G. A., Alexander, R. W., Anderson, J. L., Cannon, R. O., 3rd., Criqui, M., et al. (2003). Markers of inflammation and cardiovascular disease: Application to clinical and public health practice: A statement for healthcare professionals from the Centers for Disease Control and Prevention and the American Heart Association. *Circulation*, *107*, 499–511.

Peuralinna, T., Tanskanen, M., Mäkelä, M., Polvikoski, T., Paetau, A., Kalimo, H., et al. (2011). APOE and AβPP gene variation in cortical and cerebrovascular amyloid-β pathology and Alzheimer's disease: A population-based analysis. *Journal of Alzheimer's Disease*, *26*(2), 377–385.

Pickhardt, P. J., Choi, J. R., Hwang, I., Butler, J. A., Puckett, M. L., Hildebrandt, H. A., et al. (2005). Computed tomographic virtual colonoscopy to screen for colorectal neoplasia in asymptomatic adults. *New England Journal of Medicine*, *349*(23), 2191–2200.

Plebani, M., & Zaninotto, M. (1999). Cardiac marker: Present and future. *International Journal of Clinical & Laboratory Research*, *29*(2), 56–63.

Polascik, T. J., Oesterling, J. E., & Partin, A. W. (1999). Prostate-specific antigen: A decade of discovery— What we have learned and where we are going. *Journal of Urology*, *162*, 293–306.

Pollex, R., Hanley, A., Zinman, B., Harris, S., Khan, H., & Hegele, R. (2006). Metabolic syndrome in Aboriginal Canadians: Prevalence and genetic associations. *Atherosclerosis*, *184*, 121–129.

Potter, P., Perry, A., Stockert, P., & Hall, A. (2016). *Fundamentals of nursing* (8th ed.). St. Louis: C. V. Mosby.

Potter, S. R., Reckwitz, T., & Partin, A. W. (1999). The use of percent free PSA for early detection of prostate cancer. *Journal of Andrology*, *20*(4), 449–453.

Public Health Care Agency of Canada. (2014). Interim guidance-ebola virus disease: Infection prevention and control measures of borders, healthcare settings and self-monitoring at home. *Canada Communicable Disease Report*, *40*, 15. www.phac-aspc.gc.ca/id-mi/vhf-fvh/ebola-ipc-pci-eng.php.

Public Health Agency of Canada. (2006). Management and treatment of specific infections: Human immunodeficiency virus infections. In *Canadian Guidelines on Sexually Transmitted Infections*. http:// www.phac-aspc.gc.ca/std-mts/sti-its/.

Public Health Agency of Canada. (2007a). *Canadian nosocomial infection surveillance program*. Ottawa, ON: Author. http://www.phac-aspc.gc.ca/nois-sinp/survprog-eng.php.

Public Health Agency of Canada. (2007b). *Infection prevention and control best practices for long term care, home and community care including health offices and ambulatory clinics*. http://www.phac-aspc.gc.ca/amr-ram/ ipcbp-pepci/pdf/amr-ram-eng.pdf.

Public Health Agency of Canada. (2008a). *Canadian guidelines of sexually transmitted infections*. Public Health Agency of Canada. http://www.phac-aspc.gc.ca/std-mts/sti-its/guide-lignesdir-eng.php.

Public Health Agency of Canada. (2008b). The rising challenge of Lyme borreliosis in Canada. *Canada Communicable Disease Report*, *34*(1). http://www.phac-aspc.gc.ca/publicat/ccdr-rmtc/08vol34/dr-rm3401a-eng.php.

Public Health Agency of Canada. (2011). *Bioterrorism and emergency preparedness*. http://www.phac-aspc .gc.ca/ep-mu/bioem-eng.php.

Raff, G., Abidov, A., Achenbach, S., Berman, D. S., Boxt, L. M., Budoff, M. J., et al. (2009). SCCT guidelines for the interpretation and reporting of coronary computer tomographic angiography. *Journal of Cardiovascular Computer Tomography*, *3*(2), 122–136.

Randox Laboratories. (2011). *Anti–streptolysin-O 2 (ASO 2) latex-enhanced immunoturbidimetric assay*. http://www.randox.com/brochures/PDF%20Brochure/LT082.pdf.

Rao, J. K., Weinberger, M., Oddone, E. Z., Allen, N. B., Landsman, P., & Feussner, J. R. (1995). The role of antineutrophil cytoplasmic antibody (c-ANCA) testing in the diagnosis of Wegener granulomatosis. *Annals of Internal Medicine*, *123*(2), 925–932.

Ravikovich, E., Messersmith, T., McCormick, G., & McCormick, K. (2002). Effect of oral fluid intake on urinary albumin excretion in diabetes mellitus. *Journal of Diabetes and Its Complications*, *16*, 310–312.

Riaz, S., Alam, S. S., Srai, S. K., Skinner, V., Riaz, A., & Akhtar, M. W. (2010). Proteomic identification of human urinary biomarkers in diabetes mellitus type 2. *Diabetes Technology and Therapeutics*, *12*(12), 979–988.

Rice, M. S., & MacDonald, D. C. (1999). Appropriate roles of cardiac troponins in evaluating patients with chest pain. *Journal of the American Board of Family Practice*, *12*(3), 214–218.

Ridker, P. M. (1999). Evaluating novel cardiovascular risk factors: Can we better predict heart attacks? *Annals of Internal Medicine*, *130*(11), 933–937.

Ridker, P. M., Buring, J. E., Cook, N. R., & Rifai, N. (2003). C-reactive protein, the metabolic syndrome, and risk of incident cardiovascular events: An 8-year follow-up of 14,719 initially healthy American women. *Circulation, 107*, 391–397.

Righini, M., Legal, G., Perrier, A., & Bournameaux, H. (2005). The challenge of diagnosing pulmonary embolism in elderly patients: Influence of age on community used diagnostic tests and strategies. *Journal of the American Geriatric Society, 53*, 1039–1045.

Rohlfing, C. L., Little, R. R., Wiedmeyer, H. M., England, J. D., Madsen, R., Harris, M. I., et al. (2000). Use of GHb (HbA1c) in screening for undiagnosed diabetes in the U.S. population. *Diabetes Care, 23*(2), 187–191.

Ronchi, C. L., Ferrante, E., Rizzo, E., Giavoli, C., Verrua, E., Bergamaschi, S., et al. (2008). Long-term basal and dynamic evaluation of hypothalamic-pituitary-adrenal (HAP) axis in acromegalic patients. *Clinical Endocrinology, 69*(4), 608–612.

Ronco, G., Giorgi-Rossi, P., Carozzi, F., Dalla Palma, P., Del Mistro, A., De Marco, L., et al. (2006). Human papillomavirus testing and liquid-based cytology in primary screening of women younger than 35 years: Results at recruitment for a randomised controlled trial. *Lancet Oncology, 7*(7), 547–555.

Rosen, C. J., & Tenenhouse, A. (1998). Biochemical markers of bone turnover. *Postgraduate Medicine, 104*(4), 101–114.

Ross, R. (1999). Atherosclerosis—An inflammatory disease. *New England Journal of Medicine, 340*, 115–126.

Rothmann, S. A. (2007). *Semen analysis: The test techs love to hate.* http://www.mlo-online.com/articles/0407/0407cover_story.pdf.

Rowley, K., Daniel, M., & O'Dea, K. (2005). Screening for diabetes in indigenous populations using glycated haemoglobin: Sensitivity, specificity, post-test likelihood and risk of disease. *Diabetic Medicine, 22*, 833–839.

Rypins, E., & Kipper, S. L. (2000). Scintigraphic determination of equivocal appendicitis. *American Surgeon, 66*(9), 891–895.

Saraux, A., Berthelot, J., Devauchelle, V., Bendaoud, B., Chalès, G., Le Henaff, C., et al. (2003). Value of antibodies to citrulline-containing peptides for diagnosing early rheumatoid arthritis. *Journal of Rheumatology, 30*(12), 2535–2539.

Savarino, V., Vigneri, S., & Celle, G. (1999). The 13C urea breath test in the diagnosis of *Helicobacter pylori* infection. *Gut, 45*(Suppl. 1), I18–I22.

Scott, J. D., Fernando, K., Banerjee, S. N., Durden, L. A., Byrne, S. K., Banerjee, M., et al. (2001). Birds disperse ixodid (Acari: Ixodidae) and *Borrelia burgdorferi*–infected ticks in Canada. *Journal of Medical Entomology, 38*(4), 493–500.

Seeley, W. W., & Miller, B. L. (2012). Dementia. In D. L. Longo, A. S. Fauci, D. L. Kasper, S. L. Hauser, J. L. Jameson, & J. Loscalzo (Eds.), *Harrison's principles of internal medicine* (18th ed.). http://www.accessmedicine.com/content.aspx?aID=9146233. Retrieved May 29, 2012.

Sethi, S., Kaushik, K., Mohandas, K., Sengupta, C., Singh, S., & Sharma, M. (2003). Anti–streptolysin O titers in normal healthy children of 5–15 years. *Indian Pediatrics, 40*(11), 1068–1071.

Shariat, S. F., Casella, R., Khoddami, S. M., Hernandez, G., Sulser, T., Gasser, T. C., et al. (2004). Urine detection of survivin is a sensitive marker for the noninvasive diagnosis of bladder cancer. *Journal of Urology, 171*(2, Part 1), 626–630.

Siegel, J. D., Rhinehart, E., Jackson, M., Chiarello, L., & the Healthcare Infection Control Practices Advisory Committee. (2007). *Guideline for isolation precautions: Preventing transmission of infectious agents in healthcare settings.* http://www.cdc.gov/niosh/docket/archive/pdfs/NIOSH-219/0219-010107-siegel.pdf. Accessed May 16, 2012.

Silfen, M., Manibo, A., McMahon, D., Levine, L., Murphy, A., & Oberfield, S. (2001). Comparison of simple measures of insulin sensitivity on young girls with premature menarche: The fasting glucose to insulin ratio may be a simple and useful measure. *Journal of Clinical Endocrinology and Metabolism, 86*(2), 2863–2868.

Siminoski, K., O'Keeffe, M., Lévesque, J., Hanley, D., & Brown, J. (2011). Canadian Association of Radiologists technical standards for bone mineral densitometry reporting. *Canadian Association of Radiologists Journal, 62*(3), 166–175.

Singh, H., Bernstein, C., Samadder, J., & Ahmed, R. (2011). Screening rates for colorectal cancer in Canada: A cross-sectional study. *CMAJ, Open, 3*(2).

Skoll, A., Louis, P., Amiri, N., Delisle, M., & Lalji, S. (2006). The evaluation of the fetal fibronectin test for prediction of preterm delivery in symptomatic patients. *Journal of Obstetrics and Gynecology Canada, 28*(3), 206–213.

Solomon, P. R., & Murphy, C. A. (2008). Early diagnosis and treatment of Alzheimer's disease. *Expert Review of Neurotherapeutics, 8*, 769–780.

Steer, A., Vidmar, S., Ritika, R., Kado, J., Batzloff, M., Jenney, A. W., et al. (2009). Normal ranges of streptococcal antibody titers are similar whether streptococci are endemic to the setting or not. *Clinical Vaccine Immunology, 16*(2), 172–175.

Stevens, L. A., Coresh, J., Schmid, C. H., Feldman, H. I., Froissart, M., Kusek, J., et al. (2008a). Estimating GFR using serum cystatin C alone and in combination with serum creatinine: A pooled analysis of 3418 individuals with CKD. *American Journal of Kidney Disease, 51*(3), 395–406.

Stevens, T., Conwell, D. L., Zuccaro, G., Jr., Van Lente, F., Lopez, R., Purich, E., et al. (2008b). A prospective crossover study comparing secretin-stimulated endoscopic and Dreiling tube pancreatic function testing in patients evaluated for chronic pancreatitis. *Gastrointestinal Endoscopy, 67*(3), 458–466.

Stief, T. (2008). Antithrombin III determination in nearly-undiluted plasma. *Laboratory Medicine, 39*(1), 46–48.

Stoeck, K., & Zerr, I. (2011). Cellular immune activation markers neopterin and beta 2-microglobulin are not elevated in the cerebrospinal fluid of patients with Creutzfeldt-Jakob disease. *Journal of Neuroimmunology, 233*, 228–232.

Stolzenber-Solomon, R. Z., Vieth, R., Azad, A., Pietinen, P., Taylor, P. R., Virtamo, J., et al. (2006). A prospective nested case-control study of vitamin D status and pancreatic cancer risk in male smokers. *Cancer Research, 66*(20), 10213–10219.

Stratton, J., Chandler, W. L., Schwartz, R. S., Cerqueira, M. D., Levy, W. C., Kahn, S. E., et al. (1991). Effects of physical conditioning on fibrolytic variables and fibrinogen on young and old health adults. *Circulation, 83*, 1692–1697.

Smolyar, D., Tirado-Bernardini, R., Landman, R., Lesser, M., Young, I., & Poretsky, L. (2003). Comparison of 1-µg and 250-µg corticotropin stimulation tests for the evaluation of adrenal function in patient with acquired immunodeficiency syndrome. *Metabolism, 52*(5), 647–651.

Soldin, S., Brugnara, C., & Wong, E. (2005). *Pediatric reference intervals* (5th ed.). Washington, D.C.: American Association for Clinical Chemistry Press.

Soule, S., Van Zyl Smit, C., Parolis, G., Attenborough, S., Peter, D., Kinvig, S., et al. (2000). The low dose ACTH stimulation test is less sensitive than the overnight metyrapone test for the diagnosis of secondary hypoadrenalism. *Clinical Endocrinology, 53*(2), 221–227.

Sousa-Junior, E., Alencar, A., & da Silva, B. (2009). Analysis of Ki-67 and Bcl-2 protein expression in normal colorectal mucosa of women with breast cancer. *European Journal of Cancer, 45*, 3081–3086.

Sullivan, J. M. (2011). Caring for older adults after surgery. *Nursing, 41*(4), 48–51.

Sutinen, J. (1998). Etiology of central nervous system infections in the Philippines and the role of serum C-reactive protein in excluding acute bacterial meningitis. *International Journal of Infectious Diseases, 3*(2), 88–93.

Tal, S., Gurevich, A., Guller, V., Gurevich, I., Berger, D., & Levi, S. (2002). Risk factors for recurrence of *Clostridium difficile*–associated diarrhea in the elderly. *Scandinavian Journal of Infectious Diseases, 34*, 594–597.

Thaler, L., & Blevins, L. (1998). The low dose adrenocorticotropin stimulation test in the evaluation of patients with suspected central adrenal insufficiency. *Journal of Clinical Endocrinology and Metabolism, 83*(8), 2726–2729.

Thorwarth, W., & Lentle, B. (2002). Standard for performance of adult dual- or single-energy X-ray absorptiometry (DXA/pDXA/SXA). In *Canadian Association of Radiologists*. http://old.car.ca/Files/bone_densito_1999.pdf.

Trimbath, J., & Giardiello, M. (2002). Review article: Genetic testing and counselling for hereditary colorectal cancer. *Alimentary Pharmacology and Therapeutics, 16*, 1843–1857.

van Meurs, J. B., Dhonukshe-Rutten, R. A., Pluijm, S. M., van der Klift, M., de Jonge, R., Lindemans, J., et al. (2004). Homocysteine levels and the risk of osteoporotic fracture. *New England Journal of Medicine, 350*(20), 2033–2041.

Ventolini, G., Neiger, R., Hood, D., & Belcastro, M. (2006). Changes in the threshold of fetal lung maturity and neonatal outcome of infants delivered electively before 39 weeks gestation: Implications and cost-effectiveness. *Journal of Perinatology, 26*(5), 264–267.

Verburg, F., Kirchgässner, C., Hebestreit, H., Steigerwald, U., Lentjes, E. G., Ergezinger, K., et al. (2011). Reference ranges for analytes of thyroid function in children. *Hormone and Metabolism Research, 43*(3), 422–426.

Vogester, M., & Jacob, K. (2001). B-type natriuretic peptide (BNP): Validation of an immediate response assay. *Clinical Laboratory, 47*, 29–33.

Wang, J., Godbold, J., & Sampson, H. (2008). Correlation of serum allergy (IgE) tests performed by different assay systems. *Journal of Allergy and Clinical Immunology, 21*(5), 1219–1224.

Warner, E., Foulkes, W., Goodwin, P., Meschino, W., Blondal, J., Paterson, C., et al. (1999). Prevalence and penetrance of *BRCA1* and *BRCA2* gene mutations in unselected Ashkenazi Jewish women with breast cancer. *Journal of the National Cancer Institute, 91*(14), 1241–1247.

Wilson, B., Cowan, H., Lord, J., Zuege, D., & Zygun, D. (2010). The accuracy of pulse oximetry in emergency department patients with severe sepsis and septic shock: A retrospective cohort study. *BMC Emergency Medicine, 10*(9). http://www.biomedcentral.com/1471-227X/10/9.

Winn-McMillan, T., & Karon, B. (2005). Comparison of the TDx-FLM II and lecithin to sphingomyelin ratio assays in predicting fetal lung maturity. *American Journal of Obstetrics and Gynecology, 193*(3), 778–782.

World Health Organization. (2010). *International statistical classification of diseases and related health problems, 10th revision.* http://apps.who.int/classifications/icd10/browse/2010/en. Retrieved July 4.

Wu, A., Lewandrowski, K., Gronowski, A., Grenache, D., Sokoll, L., & Magnani, B. (2010). Antiquated tests within the clinical pathology laboratory. *American Journal of Managed Care, 16*(9), e220–e227.

Yap, M., Vinod, S. K., Shon, I. A., Fowler, A., Lin, M., Gabriel, G., et al. (2010). The registration of diagnostic versus planning fluorodeoxyglucose positron emission tomography/computer tomography in radiotherapy planning for non–small cell lung cancer. *Clinical Oncology, 22*(7), 554–560.

Yeh, E. T., & Willerson, J. T. (2003). Coming of age of C-reactive protein. *Circulation, 107*, 370–372.

Zanocchi, B., Poli, M., & Molaschi, L. (2005). The ankle-brachial index is not related to mortality in elderly subjects living in nursing homes. *Angiology, 56*(6), 693–697.

Zorzi, A., Wabi, G., MacNab, A., & Panagiotopoulos, C. (2009). Prevalence of impaired glucose tolerance and the components of metabolic syndrome in Canadian Tsimshian Nation youth. *Canadian Journal of Rural Medicine, 14*(2), 61–67.

Chapter 2

2-1, 2-2: Courtesy John Crowell, Memorial University of Newfoundland; 2-3: Courtesy Sandra A. Pike-MacDonald; 2-5, 2-7: Wilson, S. F., & Thompson, J. M. (1990). *Respiratory disorders*. St. Louis: Mosby; 2-10: © Ed Reschke; 2-11: Mahon, C., Smith, L. A., & Burns, C. (1998). *An introduction to clinical laboratory science*. Philadelphia: Saunders; 2-12: The Canadian Journal of Cardiology and the Canadian Cardiovascular Society; 2-16: Lewis, S. M., Heitkemper, M. M., Dirksen, S. R., O'Brien, P. G., & Bucher, L. (2008). *Medical-surgical nursing: Assessment and management of clinical problems* (7th ed.). St. Louis: Mosby; 2-18: Patton, K. T., & Thibodeau, G. A. (2016). *Anatomy and physiology* (9th ed.). St. Louis: Mosby; 2-20, 2-25: Belcher, A. E. (1993). *Blood disorders*. St. Louis: Mosby.

Chapter 3

3-1: Courtesy Cardiac Science; 3-2, 3-4: Beare, P. G., & Myers, J. L. (Eds.). (1998). *Adult health nursing* (3rd ed.). St. Louis: Mosby; 3-5: Copyright © yacobchuk/iStock/Thinkstock.com; 3-6: Chipps, E., Clanin, N., & Campbell, V. (1992). *Neurologic disorders*. St. Louis: Mosby; 3-7: From Gates, P. (2010). *Clinical neurology: A primer*. Chatswood, Australia: Churchill Livingstone; 3-8: Sigler, B. A., & Schuring, L. T. (1994). *Ear, nose, and throat disorders*. St. Louis: Mosby; 3-9: Copyright Dorling Kindersley: Gary Ombler; 3-10: Perkin, G. D. (2011). *Atlas of clinical neurology* (3rd ed.). Philadelphia: Saunders; 3-11: Copyright © anamejia18/iStock/thinkstock.com; 3-12: Copyright © anasimin/iStock/thinkstock.com.

Chapter 4

4-1: Doughty, D., & Jackson, D. B. (1993). *Gastrointestinal disorders*. St. Louis: Mosby; 4-2: Gregory, B. (1994). *Orthopaedic surgery*. St. Louis: Mosby; 4-6: Modified from Hacker, N. F., & Moore, J. G. (1998). *Essentials of obstetrics and gynecology* (3rd ed.). Philadelphia: Saunders; 4-12: Black, J. M., & Hawks, J. H. (2009). *Medical-surgical nursing: Clinical management for positive outcomes* (8th ed.). St. Louis: Saunders.

Chapter 5

5-3, 5-5: Beare, P. G., & Myers, J. L. (Eds.). (1998). *Adult health nursing* (3rd ed.). St. Louis: Mosby; 5-4: Wilson, S. F., & Thompson, J. M. (1990). *Respiratory disorders*. St. Louis: Mosby.

Chapter 7

7-2, 7-3: Redrawn from Black, J. M., Hawks, J. H., & Keene, A. M. (2001). *Medical-surgical nursing: Clinical management for positive outcomes* (6th ed.). Philadelphia: Saunders; 7-4: Lewis, S. M., Heitkemper, M. M., Dirksen, S. R., Bucher, L., & Camera, I. M. (2011). *Medical-surgical nursing: Assessment and management of clinical problems* (8th ed.). St. Louis: Mosby; 7-9, 7-11, 7-12: Grimes, D. E. (1991). *Infectious diseases*. St. Louis: Mosby; 7-10: Mahon, C., Smith, L.A., & Burns, C. (1998). *An introduction to clinical laboratory science*. Philadelphia: Saunders.

Chapter 8

8-3, 8-4: Chipps, E., Clanin, N., & Campbell, V. (1992). *Neurologic disorders*. St. Louis: Mosby; 8-5, 8-6: Canobbio, M. M. (1990). *Cardiovascular disorders*. St. Louis: Mosby.

Chapter 9

9-1: Potter, P. A., et al. (2017). *Fundamentals of nursing* (9th ed.). St. Louis: Elsevier.

Chapter 10

10-1, 10-2, 10-13: Canobbio, M. M. (1990). *Cardiovascular disorders.* St. Louis: Mosby; 10-3: Rumack, C. M. (2011). *Diagnostic ultrasound* (4th ed.). Philadelphia: Mosby. 10-4: Wakefield, R. J., & D'Agostino, M. A. (2010). *Essential applications of musculoskeletal ultrasound in rheumatology.* Philadelphia: Saunders. 10-6: Brundage, D. J. (1992). *Renal disorders.* St. Louis: Mosby; 10-10, 10-14: Image courtesy Philips Medical. All rights reserved. 10-15: Phillips, N. (2017). *Berry & Kohn's operating room technique* (13th ed.). St. Louis: Mosby.

Chapter 11

11-1: Proctor, D. (2017). *Kinn's the medical assistant: An applied learning approach* (13th ed.). St. Louis: Elsevier. 11-2: Brunzel, N. A. (2018). *Fundamentals of urine and body fluid analysis* (4th ed.). St. Louis: Elsevier.

Chapter 12

12-1, 12-22: Brundage, D. J. (1992). *Renal disorders.* St. Louis: Mosby; 12-2, 12-25: Chipps, E., Clanin, N., & Campbell, V. (1992). *Neurologic disorders.* St. Louis: Mosby; 12-5, 12-16: Doughty, D., & Jackson, D. B. (1993). *Gastrointestinal disorders.* St. Louis: Mosby; 12-8: Image used with permission, Flagstaff Medical Center, Northen Arizona Healthcare. All rights reserved; 12-15: Gray, M. (1992). *Genitourinary disorders.* St. Louis: Mosby; 12-19, 12-20: Edge, V., & Miller, M. (1994). *Women's health care.* St. Louis: Mosby; 12-21: Belcher, A. E. (1992). *Cancer nursing.* St. Louis: Mosby.

Chapter 13

13-2: Pagana, K. D., & Pagana, T. J. (1994). *Diagnostic testing and nursing implications: A case study approach* (4th ed.). St. Louis: Mosby; courtesy Holy Spirit Magnetic Imaging Center, Mechanicsburg, PA; 13-5: Copyright © jgroup/iStock/thinkstock.com; 13-6, Copyright © juanrvelasco/iStock/thinkstock.com; 13-8: Wilson, S. F., & Thompson, J. M. (1990). *Respiratory disorders.* St. Louis: Mosby. 13-9: Helbert, M. (2017). *Immunology for medical students* (3rd ed.). Philadelphia: Elsevier.

Index

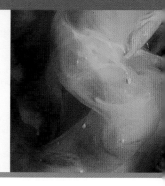

Note: Page numbers followed by *f* indicate figures, *t* indicate tables, and *b* indicate boxes.